# DESK ENCYCLOPEDIA OF ANIMAL AND BACTERIAL VIROLOGY

# DESK ENCYCLOPEDIA OF ANIMAL AND BACTERIAL VIROLOGY

**EDITOR-IN-CHIEF**

Dr BRIAN W J MAHY

ELSEVIER

AMSTERDAM • BOSTON • HEIDELBERG • LONDON • NEW YORK • OXFORD
PARIS • SAN DIEGO • SAN FRANCISCO • SINGAPORE • SYDNEY • TOKYO
Academic Press is an imprint of Elsevier

ACADEMIC
PRESS

Academic Press is an imprint of Elsevier
Linacre House, Jordan Hill, Oxford, OX2 8DP, UK
525 B Street, Suite 1900, San Diego, CA 92101-4495, USA

**British Library Cataloguing in Publication Data**
A catalogue record for this book is available from the British Library

**Library of Congress Cataloguing in Publication Data**
A catalogue record for this book is available from the Library of Congress

ISBN: 978-0-12-375144-7

For information on all Elsevier publications
visit our website at books.elsevier.com

Printed and bound by CPI Group (UK) Ltd, Croydon, CR0 4YY

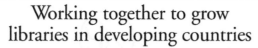

# EDITOR-IN-CHIEF

**Brian W J Mahy MA PhD ScD DSc**
*Senior Scientific Advisor,*
*Division of Emerging Infections and Surveillance Services,*
*Centers for Disease Control and Prevention,*
*Atlanta GA, USA*

# ASSOCIATE EDITORS

**Dennis H Bamford, Ph.D.**
Department of Biological and Environmental Sciences
and Institute of Biotechnology, Biocenter 2,
P.O. Box 56 (Viikinkaari 5),
00014 University of Helsinki,
Finland

**Charles Calisher, B.S., M.S., Ph.D.**
Arthropod-borne and Infectious Diseases Laboratory
Department of Microbiology, Immunology and Pathology
College of Veterinary Medicine and Biomedical Sciences
Colorado State University
Fort Collins
CO 80523
USA

**Andrew J Davison, M.A., Ph.D.**
MRC Virology Unit
Institute of Virology
University of Glasgow
Church Street
Glasgow G11 5JR
UK

**Claude Fauquet**
ILTAB/Donald Danforth Plant Science Center
975 North Warson Road
St. Louis, MO 63132

**Said Ghabrial, B.S., M.S., Ph.D.**
Plant Pathology Department
University of Kentucky
201F Plant Science Building
1405 Veterans Drive
Lexington
KY 4050546-0312
USA

**Eric Hunter, B.Sc., Ph.D.**
Department of Pathology and Laboratory Medicine, and
Emory Vaccine Center
Emory University
954 Gatewood Road NE
Atlanta Georgia 30329
USA

**Robert A Lamb, Ph.D., Sc.D.**
Department of Biochemistry,
Molecular Biology and Cell Biology
Howard Hughes Medical Institute
Northwestern University
2205 Tech Dr.
Evanston
IL 60208-3500
USA

**Olivier Le Gall**
IPV, UMR GDPP, IBVM,
INRA Bordeaux-Aquitaine, BP 81,
F-33883 Villenave d'Ornon Cedex
FRANCE

**Vincent Racaniello, Ph.D.**
Department of Microbiology
Columbia University
New York, NY 10032
USA

**David A Theilmann, Ph.D., B.Sc., M.Sc**
Pacific Agri-Food Research Centre
Agriculture and Agri-Food Canada
Box 5000, 4200 Highway 97
Summerland
BC V0H 1Z0
Canada

**H Josef Vetten, Ph.D.**
Julius Kuehn Institute, Federal Research Centre for
Cultivated Plants (JKI)
Messeweg 11-12
38104 Braunschweig
Germany

**Peter J Walker, B.Sc., Ph.D.**
CSIRO Livestock Industries
Australian Animal Health Laboratory (AAHL)
Private Bag 24
Geelong
VIC 3220
Australia

# ASSOCIATE EDITORS

# PREFACE

The *Desk Encyclopedia of Animal and Bacterial Virology* is the third of a series of four volumes that reproduce many of the chapters in the third edition of the *Encyclopedia of Virology*, edited by Brian W J Mahy and Marc H V van Regenmortel, published by Academic Press/Elsevier 2008. It contains 79 chapters that relate to animal and bacterial virology. The first section includes 34 chapters that describe general features of farm and other animals of agricultural importance. Section 2 contains 20 chapters describing other animal viruses, and Section 3 has four chapters on avian viruses. In section 4, 10 chapters are devoted to viruses affecting aquatic species such as fish and crustaceans. The volume concludes with Section 5, which contains 11 chapters, and deals with viruses that infect bacteria (bacteriophages).

In bringing all these topics under one cover, it is hoped that the book will provide a convenient reference source and an up-to-date introduction to recent advances in animal and bacterial virology. Along with the first volume of the series, on *General Virology*, this book provides excellent material for a teaching course in virology for students of veterinary science.

Brian W J Mahy

# CONTRIBUTORS

**S Adhya**
National Institutes of Health, Bethesda, MD, USA

**D J Alcendor**
Johns Hopkins School of Medicine, Baltimore, MD, USA

**C Apetrei**
Tulane National Primate Research Center, Covington, LA, USA

**A G Bader**
The Scripps Research Institute, La Jolla, CA, USA

**J K H Bamford**
University of Jyväskylä, Jyväskylä, Finland

**J W Barrett**
The University of Western Ontario, London, ON, Canada

**T Barrett**
Institute for Animal Health, Pirbright, UK

**M N Becker**
University of Florida, Gainesville, FL, USA

**K L Beemon**
Johns Hopkins University, Baltimore, MD, USA

**H U Bernard**
University of California, Irvine, Irvine, CA, USA

**P D Bieniasz**
Aaron Diamond AIDS Research Center, The Rockefeller University, New York, NY, USA

**B A Blacklaws**
University of Cambridge, Cambridge, UK

**J-R Bonami**
CNRS, Montpellier, France

**H Bourhy**
Institut Pasteur, Paris,France

**P R Bowser**
Cornell University, Ithaca, NY, USA

**D B Boyle**
CSIRO Livestock Industries, Geelong, VIC,Australia

**M A Brinton**
Georgia State University, Atlanta, GA, USA

**F J Burt**
University of the Free State, Bloemfontein, South Africa

**S J Butcher**
University of Helsinki, Helsinki, Finland

**G Carlile**
CSIRO Livestock Industries, Geelong, VIC, Australia

**J W Casey**
Cornell University, Ithaca, NY, USA

**R N Casey**
Cornell University, Ithaca, NY, USA

**D Chapman**
Institute for Animal Health, Pirbright, UK

**M Chen**
University of Arizona, Tucson, AZ, USA

**J E Cherwa**
University of Arizona, Tucson, AZ, USA

**V G Chinchar**
University of Mississippi Medical Center, Jackson, MS, USA

**M G Ciufolini**
Istituto Superiore di Sanità, Rome, Italy

**J K Craigo**
University of Pittsburgh School of Medicine, Pittsburgh, PA, USA

**M St J Crane**
CSIRO Livestock Industries, Geelong, VIC, Australia

**B H Dannevig**
National Veterinary Institute, Oslo, Norway

**A J Davison**
MRC Virology Unit, Glasgow, UK

**R C Desrosiers**
New England Primate Research Center, Southborough, MA, USA

**L K Dixon**
Institute for Animal Health, Pirbright, UK

**R L Duda**
University of Pittsburgh, Pittsburgh, PA, USA

**J P Dudley**
The University of Texas at Austin, Austin, TX, USA

**B M Dutia**
University of Edinburgh, Edinburgh, UK

**M L Dyall-Smith**
The University of Melbourne, Parkville, VIC, Australia

**A Ensser**
Virologisches Institut, Universitätsklinikum, Erlangen, Germany

**B A Fane**
University of Arizona, Tucson, AZ, USA

**F Fenner**
Australian National University, Canberra, ACT, Australia

**I Greiser-Wilke**
School of Veterinary Medicine, Hanover, Germany

**A J Gubala**
CSIRO Livestock Industries, Geelong, VIC, Australia

**D Haig**
Nottingham University, Nottingham, UK

**T Hatziioannou**
Aaron Diamond AIDS Research Center, The Rockefeller University, New York, NY, USA

**G S Hayward**
Johns Hopkins School of Medicine, Baltimore, MD, USA

**R W Hendrix**
University of Pittsburgh, Pittsburgh, PA, USA

**M de las Heras**
University of Glasgow Veterinary School, Glasgow, UK

**S Hertzler**
University of Illinois at Chicago, Chicago, IL, USA

**J Hilliard**
Georgia State University, Atlanta, GA, USA

**D M Hinton**
National Institutes of Health, Bethesda, MD, USA

**L E Hughes**
University of St. Andrews, St. Andrews, UK

**A D Hyatt**
Australian Animal Health Laboratory, Geelong, VIC, Australia

**A R Jilbert**
Institute of Medical and Veterinary Science, Adelaide, SA, Australia

**W E Johnson**
New England Primate Research Center, Southborough, MA, USA

**P D Kirkland**
Elizabeth Macarthur Agricultural Institute, Menangle, NSW, Australia

**R P Kitching**
Canadian Food Inspection Agency, Winnipeg, MB, Canada

**N Knowles**
Institute for Animal Health, Pirbright, UK

**G Kurath**
Western Fisheries Research Center, Seattle, WA, USA

**M E Laird**
New England Primate Research Center, Southborough, MA, USA

**J C Leong**
University of Hawaii at Manoa, Honolulu, HI, USA

**J-H Leu**
National Taiwan University, Taipei, Republic of China

**M L Linial**
Fred Hutchinson Cancer Research Center, Seattle, WA, USA

**H L Lipton**
University of Illinois at Chicago, Chicago, IL, USA

**C-F Lo**
National Taiwan University, Taipei, Republic of China

**A Mankertz**
Robert Koch-Institut, Berlin, Germany

**M Marthas**
University of California, Davis, Davis, CA, USA

**P A Marx**
Tulane University, Covington, LA, USA

**W S Mason**
Fox Chase Cancer Center, Philadelphia, PA, USA

**A A McBride**
National Institutes of Health, Bethesda, MD, USA

**G McFadden**
The University of Western Ontario, London, ON, Canada

**G McFadden**
University of Florida, Gainesville, FL, USA

**P S Mellor**
Institute for Animal Health, Woking, UK

**A A Mercer**
University of Otago, Dunedin, New Zealand

**P P C Mertens**
Institute for Animal Health, Woking, UK

**T C Mettenleiter**
Friedrich-Loeffler-Institut, Greifswald-Insel Riems, Germany

**C J Miller**
University of California, Davis, Davis, CA, USA

**S Mjaaland**
Norwegian School of Veterinary Science, Oslo, Norway

**V Moennig**
School of Veterinary Medicine, Hanover, Germany

**R C Montelaro**
University of Pittsburgh School of Medicine, Pittsburgh, PA, USA

**R W Moyer**
University of Florida, Gainesville, FL, USA

**A Müllbacher**
Australian National University, Canberra, ACT, Australia

**A A Nash**
University of Edinburgh, Edinburgh, UK

**J C Neil**
University of Glasgow, Glasgow, UK

**L Nicoletti**
Istituto Superiore di Sanità, Rome, Italy

**D J O'Callaghan**
Louisiana State University Health Sciences Center, Shreveport, LA, USA

**N Osterrieder**
Cornell University, Ithaca, NY, USA

**S A Overman**
University of Missouri – Kansas City, Kansas City, MO, USA

**M Palmarini**
University of Glasgow Veterinary School, Glasgow, UK

**I Pandrea**
Tulane National Primate Research Center, Covington, LA, USA

**T A Paul**
Cornell University, Ithaca, NY, USA

**A E Peaston**
The Jackson Laboratory, Bar Harbor, ME, USA

**K Porter**
The University of Melbourne, Parkville, VIC, Australia

**S L Quackenbush**
Colorado State University, Fort Collins, CO, USA

**A J Redwood**
The University of Western Australia, Crawley, WA, Australia

**M Regner**
Australian National University, Canberra, ACT, Australia

**W K Reisen**
University of California, Davis, CA, USA

**T Renault**
IFREMER, La Tremblade, France

**J F Ridpath**
USDA, Ames, IA, USA

**E Rimstad**
Norwegian School of Veterinary Science, Oslo, Norway

**J Rovnak**
Colorado State University, Fort Collins, CO, USA

**D J Rowlands**
University of Leeds, Leeds, UK

**P Roy**
London School of Hygiene and Tropical Medicine, London, UK

**B E Russ**
The University of Melbourne, Parkville, VIC, Australia

**M D Ryan**
University of St. Andrews, St. Andrews, UK

**M Salas**
Universidad Autónoma, Madrid, Spain

**S K Samal**
University of Maryland, College Park, MD, USA

**B Schaffhausen**
Tufts University School of Medicine, Boston, MA, USA

**J M Sharp**
Veterinary Laboratories Agency, Penicuik, UK

**G R Shellam**
The University of Western Australia, Crawley, WA, Australia

**G Silvestri**
University of Pennsylvania, Philadelphia, PA, USA

**N Sittidilokratna**
Centex Shrimp and Center for Genetic Engineering and Biotechnology, Bangkok, Thailand

**M A Skinner**
Imperial College London, London, UK

**L M Smith**
The University of Western Australia, Crawley, WA, Australia

**E J Snijder**
Leiden University Medical Center, Leiden, The Netherlands

**T E Spencer**
Texas A&M University, College Station, TX, USA

**K M Stedman**
Portland State University, Portland, OR, USA

**P G Stockley**
University of Leeds, Leeds, UK

**M J Studdert**
The University of Melbourne, Parkville, VIC, Australia

**R Swanepoel**
National Institute for Communicable Diseases, Sandringham, South Africa

**G J Thomas Jr.**
University of Missouri – Kansas City, Kansas City, MO, USA

**A N Thorburn**
The University of Melbourne, Parkville, VIC, Australia

**S Trapp**
Cornell University, Ithaca, NY, USA

**J-M Tsai**
National Taiwan University, Taipei, Republic of China

**R Tuma**
University of Helsinki, Helsinki, Finland

**A Uchiyama**
Cornell University, Ithaca, NY, USA

**M de Vega**
Universidad Autónoma, Madrid, Spain

**P K Vogt**
The Scripps Research Institute, La Jolla, CA, USA

**P J Walker**
CSIRO Australian Animal Health Laboratory, Geelong, VIC, Australia

**P J Walker**
CSIRO Livestock Industries, Geelong, VIC, Australia

**R P Weir**
Berrimah Research Farm, Darwin, NT, Australia

**R A Weisberg**
National Institutes of Health, Bethesda, MD, USA

**S P J Whelan**
Harvard Medical School, Boston, MA, USA

**R G Will**
Western General Hospital, Edinburgh, UK

**J Winton**
Western Fisheries Research Center, Seattle, WA, USA

**J K Yamamoto**
University of Florida, Gainesville, FL, USA

# CONTENTS

## SECTION II: OTHER ANIMAL VIRUSES

## SECTION III: AVIAN VIRUSES

# ANIMAL VIRUSES OF AGRICULTURAL IMPORTANCE

# African Horse Sickness Viruses

**P S Mellor and P P C Mertens,** Institute for Animal Health, Woking, UK

## Glossary

**Ascites** Abnormal collection of fluid in the abdominal cavity.

**Cecum** The first part of the large intestine.

**Choroid plexus** A highly vascular membrane and part of the roof of the brain that produces cerebrospinal fluid.

**Culicoides** Genus of blood-feeding dipterous insects also known as biting midges.

**Cyanosis** Bluish discoloration of the skin or mucus membranes caused by lack of oxygen in the blood.

**Ecchymotic** Diffuse type of hemorrhage larger than a petechia.

**Fascial** A band of fibrous tissue that covers the muscles and other organs.

**Hydropericardium** Excessive collection of serous fluid in the pericardial sac.

**Hydrothorax** Excessive collection of serous fluid in the thoracic cavity.

**Petechiae** Pinpoint to pinhead-sized red spots under the skin that are the result of small bleeds.

**Purpura hemorrhagica** Hemorrhages in skin, mucous membranes and other tissues. First shows red then darkening into purple, then brownish-yellow.

**Supraorbital fossae** Holes in the skull situated above the eye socket.

**TCID$_{50}$** 50% tissue culture infective dose.

## Introduction

African horse sickness virus (AHSV) causes a noncontagious, infectious, insect-borne disease of equids (African horse sickness – AHS) that was first recognized in Africa in the sixteenth century. The effects of the disease, particularly in susceptible populations of horses, can be devastating with mortality rates often in excess of 90%. Although AHS is normally restricted to Africa (and possibly north Yemen), the disease has a much wider significance as a result of the ability of AHSV to spread, without apparent warning, beyond the borders of that continent. For these reasons the virus has been allocated OIE 'serious notifiable disease' status (i.e., communicable diseases which have the potential for very rapid spread, irrespective of national borders, which are of serious socioeconomic or public health consequence and which are of major importance in the international trade of livestock or livestock products).

## Taxonomy, Properties of the Virion and Genome

*African horsesickness virus* is a species of the genus *Orbivirus* within the family *Reoviridae*. The virus is nonenveloped, approximately 90 nm in diameter and has an icosahedral capsid that is made up of three distinct concentric protein layers (**Figure 1**), and which is very similar to the structure of bluetongue virus (the prototype orbivirus). Nine distinct serotypes of AHSV have been identified by the specificity of interactions between the more variable viral proteins that make up the outermost layer of the virus capsid (VP2 and VP5), and neutralizing antibodies that are normally generated during infection of a mammalian host. The outer capsid layer surrounds the AHSV core particle (~70 nm diameter), which has a surface layer composed of 260 trimers of VP7 attached to the virus subcore. These VP7 trimers form a closed icosahedral lattice, which is made up of five- and six-membered rings that are visible by electron microscopy, giving rise to the genus *Orbivirus* (from the Latin '*orbis*' meaning ring or cycle – **Figure 2**). The VP7 trimers synthesized in infected cells sometimes form into large hexagonal crystals, composed entirely of six-membered rings, which can be observed by both electron and light microscopy. The VP7 lattice on the core surface helps to stabilize the thinner and more fragile subcore layer, which is composed of 120 copies of VP3 arranged as 12 dish-shaped decamers that interact, edge to edge, to form the complete innermost capsid layer. This subcore shell also contains the three minor viral proteins (VP1, VP4, and VP6) that form approximately 10 transcriptase complexes, associated with the 10 linear segments of dsRNA that make up the virus genome.

The five viral proteins present in the AHSV core particle and two of the nonstructural proteins (NS1 and NS2) that are also synthesized within the cytoplasm of infected cells are relatively more conserved than the outer capsid proteins. NS1 forms long tubules within the infected cell cytoplasm that are characteristic of orbivirus infections. NS2 is a major component of the granular matrices (viral inclusion bodies or VIBs) that represent the major site of viral RNA synthesis and particle assembly during the replication of AHSV and other orbiviruses (**Figure 3**). These more conserved AHSV proteins contain serogroup-specific epitopes, which cross-react between different AHSV serotypes and can therefore be used as a basis for serological assays to distinguish AHSV from the members of other *Orbivirus* species (e.g., *Equine encephalosis virus* (EEV)).

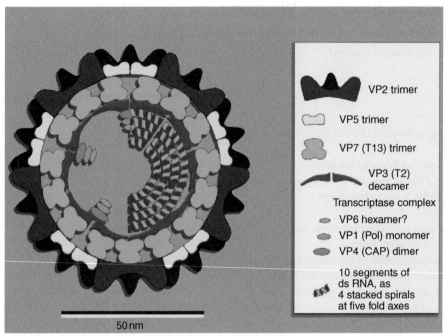

**Figure 1** Diagram of the African horse sickness virus particle structure, constructed using data from biochemical analyses, electron microscopy, cryo-electron microscopy, and X-ray crystallography. Courtesy of P.P.C. Mertens and S. Archibald – reproduced from Mertens PPC, Maan S, Samuel A, and Attoui H (2005) Orbivirus, Reoviridae. In: Fauquet CM, Mayo MA, Maniloff J, Desselberger U, and Ball LA (eds.) *Virus Taxonomy: Eighth Report of the International Committee on Taxonomy of Viruses*, pp. 466–483. San Diego, CA: Elsevier Academic Press, with permission from Elsevier.

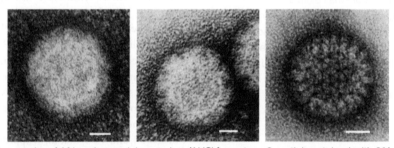

**Figure 2** Electron micrographs of African horse sickness virus (AHSV) serotype 9 particles stained with 2% aqueous uranyl acetate (left) virus particles, showing the relatively featureless surface structure; (center) infectious subviral particles (ISVP), containing chymotrypsin cleaved outer capsid protein VP2 and showing some discontinuities in the outer capsid layer; (right) core particles, from which the entire outer capsid has been removed to reveal the structure of the VP7(T13) core-surface layer and showing the ring-shaped capsomeres (line represents 20 nm). Reproduced from Mertens PPC, Maan S, Samuel A, and Attoui H (2005) Orbivirus, Reoviridae. In: Fauquet CM, Mayo MA, Maniloff J, Desselberger U, and Ball LA (eds.) *Virus Taxonomy: Eighth Report of the International Committee on Taxonomy of Viruses*, pp. 466–483. San Diego, CA: Elsevier Academic Press, with permission from Elsevier.

AHSV genome segment 10 encodes two small but largely similar proteins, NS3 and NS3a, that are translated from two in-frame start codons near the upstream end of the genome segment (see **Figure 4**). These proteins, which (by analogy with bluetongue virus) are thought to be involved in the release of virus particles from infected cells, are also highly variable in their amino acid sequence, forming into three distinct major clades. The biological significance of sequence variation in NS3/3a is uncertain, although it is clearly independent of virus serotype.

AHSV serotypes 1–8 are typically found only in restricted areas of sub-Saharan Africa while serotype 9 is more widespread and has been responsible for virtually all epizootics of AHS outside Africa. The only exception is the 1987–90 Spanish–Portuguese outbreak that was due to AHSV serotype 4.

AHSV is relatively heat resistant; it is stable at 4 and −70 °C but is labile between −20 and −30 °C. It is partially resistant to lipid solvents. At pH levels below 6.0 the virus loses its outer capsid proteins, reducing its infectivity for mammalian cell systems, although the

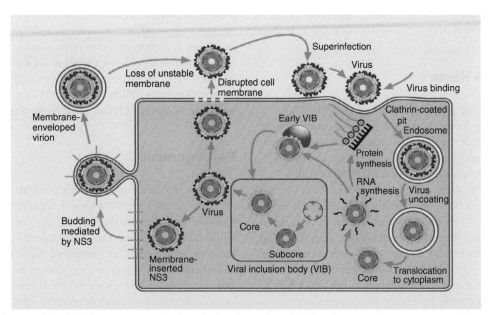

**Figure 3**   Diagram of the AHSV replication cycle, based primarily on that of BTV and other members of the family *Reoviridae*. Virus adsorption involves components of the outer capsid, although cell entry may also involve VP7(T13). VP2 (possibly also VP5) is involved in cell attachment. VP5 may be involved in penetration of the cell membrane (release from endosomes into the cytoplasm) and the expressed protein can induce cell fusion. The outer capsid layer is lost during the early stages of replication, which activates the core-associated transcriptase complexes. These synthesize mRNA copies of the 10 genome segments, which are then translated into the viral proteins. These mRNAs are also thought to combine with newly synthesized viral proteins, during the formation and maturation of progeny virus particles. The viral inclusion bodies (VIBs) are considered to be the sites of viral morphogenesis and viral RNA synthesis. Negative RNA strands are synthesized on the mRNA templates, within nascent progeny particles, reforming the dsRNA genome segments. The smallest particles containing RNA that are observed within VIBs are thought to represent progeny subcore particles. The outer core protein (VP7(T13)) is added within the VIB and the outer CP at the periphery of the VIB. Reproduced from Mertens PPC, Maan S, Samuel A, and Attoui H (2005) Orbivirus, Reoviridae. In: Fauquet CM, Mayo MA, Maniloff J, Desselberger U, and Ball LA (eds.) *Virus Taxonomy: Eighth Report of the International Committee on Taxonomy of Viruses*, pp. 466–483. San Diego, CA: Elsevier Academic Press, with permission from Elsevier.

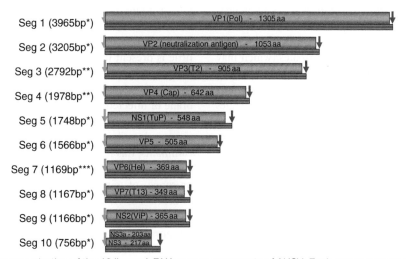

**Figure 4**   The genome organization of the 10 linear dsRNA genome segments of AHSV. Each genome segment encodes a single viral protein, with the exception of genome segment 10 which has two in-frame and functional initiation codons near the upstream end of the segment. *Data derived from AHSV-9. **Data derived from AHSV-4. ***Data derived from AHSV-6 (see: www.iah.bbsrc.ac. uk/dsRNA_virus_proteins/AHSV.htm). Like other members of the family *Reoviridae,* each AHSV genome segment contains conserved terminal sequences immediately adjacent to the upstream and downstream termini (+ve strand (green arrow) 5′-GUU$^A$/$_U$A$^A$/$_U$.........AC$^A$/$_U$UAC-3′ (red arrow)) (www.iah.bbsrc.ac.uk/dsRNA_virus_proteins/CPV-RNA-Termin.htm).

core particle retains a lower level of infectivity until it is disrupted at ~pH 3.0.

## Vertebrate Hosts

Equids are by far the most important vertebrate hosts of AHSV and the horse is the species most susceptible to disease, with mules and European donkeys somewhat less so. African donkeys are fairly resistant to clinical AHS, while zebra are usually only affected subclinically.

Occasionally, dogs or wild carnivores may become infected with AHSV by ingesting virus-contaminated equid meat and can die from the disease. Some reports also suggest that they can be infected by insect bite but most authorities believe that they play little or no part in the epidemiology of AHS and are merely dead-end hosts.

AHS is not a zoonosis. Although at least four human cases of severe disease have been documented, these were all infections acquired in an AHSV vaccine plant under conditions unlikely to be duplicated elsewhere.

## Clinical Signs

AHSV can cause four forms of disease in equids and these are discussed in ascending order of severity.

Horse sickness fever is the mildest form of disease involving only a rise in temperature and possibly, edema of the supraorbital fossae; there is no mortality. It occurs following the infection of horses with less virulent strains of virus, or when some degree of immunity exists. It is usually the only form of disease exhibited by the African donkey and zebra.

The cardiac or subacute form of disease has an incubation period of about 7–14 days and then the first clinical sign is fever. This is followed by edema, first of the supraorbital fossae and surrounding ocular tissues (which may also exhibit hemorrhage), then extending to other areas of the head, neck, and chest. Petechial hemorrhages may appear in the conjunctivae and ecchymotic hemorrhages on the ventral surface of the tongue. Colic is also a feature of the disease. The mortality rate in horses from this form of disease may be as high as 50% and death usually occurs within 4–8 days of the onset of fever.

The next most severe is the mixed form of AHS which is a combination of the cardiac and pulmonary forms with mortality rates in horses as high as 80%.

The pulmonary form is peracute and may develop so rapidly that an animal can die without prior indication of disease. Usually, there will be marked depression and fever (39–41 °C) followed by onset of respiratory distress. Coughing spasms may also occur, the head and neck tend to be extended, and severe sweating develops. There may be periods of recumbence and terminally, frothy fluid or foam may be discharged from the nostrils. Death is from congestive heart failure or asphyxia and the mortality rate in horses is frequently over 90%. During epizootics in naive populations of horses all forms of disease can occur but the mixed and pulmonary forms usually predominate, so mortality rates well in excess of 80% are likely, making AHS one of the most lethal of all horse diseases.

## Pathogenesis

On entry into the vertebrate host, initial multiplication of AHSV occurs in the regional lymph nodes. This is followed by dissemination throughout the body via the blood (primary viremia) and subsequent infection of the lungs, spleen, and other lymphoid tissues, and certain endothelial cells. Virus multiplication in these tissues and organs gives rise to secondary viremia, which is of variable duration and titer dependent upon a number of factors including host species. Under natural conditions, the incubation period to the commencement of secondary viremia is less than 9 days, although experimentally it has been shown to vary between 2 and 21 days. In horses, a virus titer of up to $10^{5.0}$ TCID$_{50}$ ml$^{-1}$ may be recorded but viremia usually lasts for only 4–8 days and has not been detected beyond 21 days. In zebra, viremia occasionally extends for as long as 40 days but peaks at a titer of only $10^{2.5}$ TCID$_{50}$ ml$^{-1}$. Viremia in donkeys is intermediate between that in horses and zebra in titer and duration, while in dogs it is considered to be very low level and transitory.

In experimentally infected horses, high concentrations of AHSV accumulate in the spleen, lungs, caecum, pharynx, choroid plexus, and most lymph nodes. Subsequently, virus is found in most organs, probably due to their blood content. In the blood, virus is associated with the cellular fraction (both red blood cells and the buffy coat) and very little is present in the plasma. This may be similar to the situation that occurs with bluetongue virus, in infected ruminants where virus is sequestered in the cell membrane of infected red blood cells and is thereby protected from the effects of humoral antibody. This leads to both virus and antibody circulating in the system together. In ruminants, this leads to extended viremia. This seems not to occur with AHSV in horses although viremia in the presence of circulating antibody has been reported in zebra. For AHSV, the onset of viremia usually corresponds with the appearance of fever and persists until it disappears.

In experimentally infected horses, exhibiting the peracute form of disease, antigen is found primarily in the cardiovascular and lymphatic systems and to a lesser extent throughout the body. In animals with horse sickness fever, antigen is concentrated in the spleen, with lesser amounts elsewhere. The main locations of antigen are endothelial cells (suggesting that they are a primary target for the virus) and large cells of the red pulp of the spleen. The presence of antigen in large mononuclear cells and surrounding lymphoid follicles suggests that these cells might also be involved in virus replication and in the transport of viral protein to the lymphoid follicles.

## Pathology

### Macrolesions

These vary in accordance with the type of disease. In the pulmonary form, the most conspicuous lesions are interlobular edema of the lungs and hydrothorax. The subpleural and interlobular tissues are infiltrated with a yellowish gelatinous exudate and the entire bronchial tree may be filled with a surfactant, stabilized froth. Ascites can occur in the abdominal and thoracic cavities and the stomach mucosa may be hyperemic and edematous.

In the cardiac form, the most prominent lesions are gelatinous exudate in the subcutaneous, subfascial and intramuscular tissues, and lymph nodes. Hydropericardium is seen and hemorrhages are found on the epicardial and/or endocardial surfaces. Petechial hemorrhages and/or cyanosis may also occur on the serosal surfaces of the cecum and colon. In these instances, a distinct demarcation can often be seen between affected and unaffected parts. This may be due to a selective involvement of endothelial cells. As in the pulmonary form, ascites may occur but edema of the lungs is usually absent.

In the mixed form of AHS, lesions common to both the pulmonary and cardiac forms of the disease occur.

### Microlesions

The histopathological changes are a result of increased permeability of the capillary walls and consequent impairment in circulation. The lungs exhibit serous infiltration of the interlobular tissues with distension of the alveoli and capillary congestion. The central veins of the liver may be distended, with interstitial tissue containing erythrocytes and blood pigments while the parenchymous cells show fatty degeneration. Cellular infiltration can be seen in the cortex of the kidneys while the spleen is heavily congested. Congestion may also be seen in the intestinal and gastric mucosae, and cloudy swelling in the myocardial and skeletal muscles.

### Epidemiology and Transmission

AHSV is widely distributed across sub-Saharan Africa. It is enzootic in a band stretching from Senegal and Gambia in the west to Ethiopia and Somalia in the east, and reaching as far south as northern parts of South Africa. The virus is probably also enzootic in northern Yemen, the only such area outside the African continent. From these zones, the virus makes seasonal extensions both northward and southward in Africa. The degree of extension is dependent mainly upon the climatic conditions and how these affect the abundance, prevalence, and seasonal incidence of the vector insects. More rarely, the virus has spread much more widely and has extended as far as Pakistan and India in the east and Spain and Portugal in the west. However, prior to the 1987–91 Spanish, Portuguese, and Moroccan outbreaks, AHSV had been unable to persist for more than 2–3 consecutive years in any area outside sub-Saharan Africa or Yemen.

AHSV is transmitted between its vertebrate hosts almost exclusively via the bites of hematophagous arthropods. Various groups have been implicated over the years, ranging from mosquitoes to ticks, but certain species of *Culicoides* biting midge are considered to be by far the most significant vectors. Biting midges act as true biological vectors and support virus replication by up to 10 000-fold. Subsequent to feeding upon a viremic equid, susceptible species of *Culicoides* become capable of transmission after an incubation period of 8–10 days at 25 °C. This period lengthens as the temperature falls, and becomes infinite below 15–18 °C. The incubation or prepatent period in the vector is the time interval necessary for ingested virus to escape from the gut lumen by entering and replicating in the mid-gut cells, and then for progeny virus particles released into the hemocoel to reach and replicate in the salivary glands. Transovarial or vertical transmission of AHSV by biting midge vectors does not occur.

*Culicoides imicola*, a widely distributed species found across Africa, southern Europe, and much of Asia, is the major vector of AHSV and has long been considered to be the only important field vector. However, a closely related species, *C. bolitinos*, has recently been identified as a second vector in Africa, and the North American *C. sonorensis* (= *variipennis*) is a highly efficient vector in the laboratory. The identification of additional vectors is likely.

In general, *Culicoides* species have a flight range of less than a few kilometers. However, in common with many other groups of flying insects, they have the capacity to be transported as 'aerial plankton' over much greater distances. In this context, a considerable body of evidence suggests that the emergence of AHSV from its enzootic zones may sometimes be due to long-range dispersal flights by infected vectors carried on the prevailing winds.

### Diagnosis

In enzootic areas, the typical clinical features of AHS (described earlier) can be used to form a presumptive diagnosis. Laboratory confirmation should then be sought. The specimens likely to be required are:

1. *Blood for virus isolation.*
2. *Tissues for virus isolation (or for antigen detection by ELISA or RT-PCR-based assays)*: Spleen is best, followed by lung, liver, heart, and lymph nodes.
3. *Serum for serological tests*: Preferably, paired samples should be taken 14–28 days apart.

Confirmation of AHS is by one or more of the following:

1. Identification of the virus in submitted samples by the group specific, antigen detection ELISA or RT-PCR–based assays. AHSV RNA can be identified by RT-PCR assays using virus-species-specific oligonucleotide primers. This identification can be confirmed by sequence analyses of the resulting cDNA products and comparison to sequences previously determined for reference strains of AHSV and other orbiviruses.
2. Isolation of infectious virus in suckling mice or embryonating hens' eggs identification first by the group-specific antigen-detection ELISA, and then by the serotype-specific, virus neutralization or RT-PCR tests.
3. Identification of AHSV-specific antibodies by the group-specific antibody detection ELISA, CF, or the serotype-specific virus neutralization tests.

## Differential Diagnosis

The clinical signs and lesions reported for AHS can be confused with those caused by the closely related EEV. Many aspects of the epidemiology of the diseases caused by these two viruses are also similar. They have a similar geographical distribution and vertebrate host range and the same vector species of *Culicoides*. As a result, both can occur simultaneously in the same locations and even in the same animal. Fortunately, rapid, sensitive, and specific ELISAs are available to enable the detection of the antigen and antibody of both the AHSV and EEV, and if used in conjunction can provide a rapid and efficient differential diagnosis.

Several other diseases may also be confused with one or other of the forms of AHS. The hemorrhages and edema reported in cases of purpura hemorrhagica and equine viral arteritis may be similar to those seen in the pulmonary form of AHS, although with AHS the edema tends to be less extensive and the hemorrhages are less numerous and widespread. The early stages of babesiosis (*Babesia equi* and *B. caballi*) can be confused with AHS, particularly when the parasites are difficult to demonstrate in blood smears.

## Treatment

Apart from supportive treatment, there is no specific therapy for AHS. Affected animals should be nursed carefully, fed well, and given rest as even the slightest exertion may result in death. During convalescence, animals should be rested for at least 4 weeks before being returned to light work.

## Control

Importation of equids from known infected areas to virus-free zones should be restricted. If importation is permitted, animals should be quarantined for 60 days in insect-proof accommodation prior to movement

Following an outbreak of AHS in a country or zone that has previously been free of the disease, attempts should be made to limit further transmission of the virus and to achieve eradication as quickly as possible. It is important that control measures are implemented as soon as a suspected diagnosis of AHS has been made and without waiting for confirmatory diagnosis. The control measures appropriate for outbreaks of AHS in enzootic and epizootic situations are described in Mellor and Hamblin.

## Further Reading

Coetzer JAW and Guthrie AJ (2004) African horsesickness. In: Coetzer JAW and Tustin RC (eds.) *Infectious Diseases of Livestock*, 2nd edn, pp. 1231–1246. Cape Town: Oxford University Press.

Hess WR (1988) African horse sickness. In: Monath TP (ed.) *The Arboviruses: Epidemiology and Ecology*, vol. 2, pp. 1–18. Boca Raton, FL: CRC Press.

Howell PG (1963) African horsesickness. In: *Emerging Diseases of Animals*, pp. 71–108. Rome: FAO Agricultural Studies.

Lagreid WW (1996) African horsesickness. In: Studdert MJ (ed.) *Virus Infections of Equines*, pp. 101–123. Amsterdam: Elsevier.

Meiswinkel Venter GJ and Nevill EM (2004) Vectors:*Culicoides* spp. In: Coetzer JAW and Tustin RC (eds.) *Infectious Diseases of Livestock*, 2nd edn, pp. 93–136. Cape Town: Oxford University Press.

Mellor PS (1993) African horse sickness: Transmission and epidemiology. *Veterinary Research* 24: 199–212.

Mellor PS (1994) Epizootiology and vectors of African horse sickness virus. *Comparative Immunology, Microbiology and Infectious Diseases* 17: 287–296.

Mellor PS, Baylis M, Hamblin C, Calisher CH, and Mertens PPC (eds.) (1998) *African Horse Sickness*. Vienna: Springer.

Mellor PS and Hamblin C (2004) African horse sickness. *Veterinary Research* 35: 445–466.

Mertens PPC and Attoui H (eds.) (2006) Phylogenetic sequence analysis and improved diagnostic assay systems for viruses of the family *Reoviridae*. http://www.iah.bbsrc.ac.uk/dsRNA_virus_proteins/ReoID/AHSV-isolates.htm (accessed July 2007).

Mertens PPC and Attoui H (eds.) (2006) The dsRNA genome segments and proteins of African horse sickness virus (AHSV).

http://www.iah.bbsrc.ac.uk/dsRNA_virus_proteins/AHSV.htm (accessed July 2007).

Mertens PPC, Attoui H, and Bamford DH (eds.) (2007) The RNAs and proteins of dsRNA viruses. http://www.iah.bbsrc.ac.uk/dsRNA_virus_proteins/orbivirus-accession-numbers.htm (accessed July 2007).

Mertens PPC, Duncan R, Attoui H, and Dermody TS (2005) Reoviridae. In: Fauquet CM, Mayo MA, Maniloff J, Desselberger U, and Ball LA (eds.) Virus Taxonomy: Eighth Report of the International Committee on Taxonomy of Viruses, pp. 447–454. San Diego, CA: Elsevier Academic Press.

Mertens PPC, Maan S, Samuel A, and Attoui H (2005) Orbivirus, Reoviridae. In: Fauquet CM, Mayo MA, Maniloff J, Desselberger U, and Ball LA (eds.) Virus Taxonomy: Eighth Report of the International Committee on Taxonomy of Viruses, pp. 466–483. San Diego, CA: Elsevier Academic Press.

Sellers RF (1980) Weather, host and vectors: Their interplay in the spread of insect-borne animal virus diseases. Journal of Hygiene Cambridge 85: 65–102.

Walton TE and Osburn BI (eds.) (1992) Bluetongue, African Horse Sickness and Related Orbiviruses. Boca Raton, FL: CRC Press.

## Relevant Website

http://www.oie.int – OIE data on AHSV outbreaks.

# African Swine Fever Virus

**L K Dixon and D Chapman,** Institute for Animal Health, Pirbright, UK

## Glossary

**Multigene family** Genes that are derived by duplication and therefore related to each other.
**Hemadsorption** Binding of red blood cells around infected cells.

## History and Geographical Distribution

African swine fever virus (ASFV) infection has been established over very long periods in areas of eastern and southern Africa, specifically in its wildlife hosts the warthog (*Phacochoerus aethiopicus*), the bushpig (*Potamochoerus porcus*), and the soft tick vector (*Ornithodoros moubata*). The virus is well adapted to these hosts, in which it causes inapparent persistent infections.

The disease caused by the virus, African swine fever (ASF), was first reported in the 1920s when domestic pigs came into contact with infected warthogs. Since then, ASF has spread to most sub-Saharan African countries. The first trans-continental spread of the virus occurred in 1957 to Portugal, via infected pig meat. Following a reintroduction of virus in 1960, ASF remained endemic in Spain and Portugal until the 1990s. During the 1970s and 1980s, ASF spread to other European countries, as well as Brazil and the Caribbean. Outside Africa, ASF is now endemic only in Sardinia, but within Africa ASF continues to cause major economic losses and has spread to countries such as Madagascar which were previously free from infections.

Analysis of the genomes of different virus isolates showed that those from wildlife sources in eastern and southern Africa are very diverse, reflecting long-term evolution in geographically separated host populations. Isolates from domestic pigs in western and central Africa, Europe, the Caribbean, and Brazil obtained over a 40 year period were all very closely related, suggesting that they were derived from a few introductions from wildlife reservoirs that have spread through pig populations. It is possible that these virus strains have been introduced into previously uninfected wildlife reservoirs in western and central Africa. Domestic pig isolates are more diverse in eastern and southern Africa. This suggests that several introductions of virus from wildlife hosts into domestic pigs have occurred in these regions.

## Transmission

In its sylvatic cycle, ASFV is maintained by a cycle of infection involving warthogs and the soft tick vector *O. moubata*. Ticks are thought to become infected by feeding on young warthogs, which develop transient viremia. Virus replicates to high titers in ticks and can be transmitted between different developmental stages, sexually between males and females, and transovarially. Warthogs can become infected by bites from infected ticks. Although virus is present in adult warthog tissues, high viremia is not detected, and direct transmission between adult warthogs may therefore be limited. For this reason the tick vector is thought to play an important role in the transmission cycle involving these hosts (**Figure 1**).

In many African countries, ASF has become established as an enzootic disease in domestic pigs and is maintained in the absence of contact with warthogs. Within pig populations, virus can spread by direct contact between

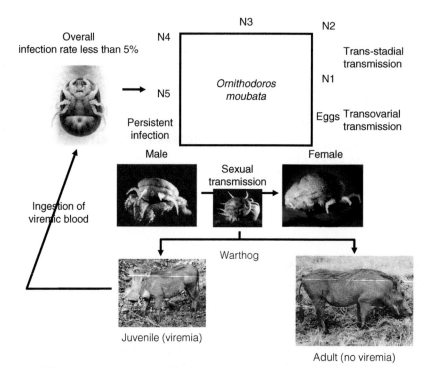

**Figure 1** Transmission of ASFV between warthogs and *O. moubata* ticks. Ticks become infected by feeding on young warthogs, which develop a transient viremia. Virus replicates in ticks and is transmitted between different nymphal stages (N1–N5), transovarially, and transexually between males and females. Ticks remain infected over long time periods and can transmit virus to the warthogs on which they feed. Direct transmission between warthogs is thought to be infrequent since viremia is low in adult warthogs. In contrast, direct transmission between infected pigs occurs readily.

pigs, which develop a high viremia, or by ingestion of infected meat or other material. However, tick vectors may also play an important role in maintaining infection in areas where they are present. The virus can replicate in other species of *Ornithodoros* including *O. erraticus*, which played a role in maintaining infection in southern Spain and Portugal. There is no vaccine available, and disease control relies on rapid diagnosis and implementation of quarantine.

## Pathogenesis

Most ASFV isolates cause an acute hemorrhagic fever with mortality approaching 100% in domestic pigs and wild swine (*Sus scrofa domesticus* and *S. s. ferus*) within 8–14 days post infection. Some moderately virulent isolates have been described that have a reduced mortality of around 30–50%. Low virulence isolates, which cause few disease signs and very low mortality, were also identified in the Iberian peninsula.

In pigs infected with virulent or moderately virulent ASFV isolates, viremia can peak at over $10^8$ hemadsorption units 50 ml$^{-1}$. However, pigs that recover generally have lower levels of viremia and reduced replication in tissues. Only sporadic low viremia is observed in pigs

infected with low virulence isolates, although moderate levels of virus replication are detected in lymphoid tissues. Persistence for long periods in recovered pigs demonstrates that the virus has effective mechanisms to evade host defense systems.

Virus replication in macrophages is observed at early times post infection, and only at later stages of disease has infection been reported in a variety of cell types, including endothelial cells, megakaryocytes, platelets, neutrophils, and hepatocytes. Thus, virus infection of macrophages is probably the primary event leading to the hemorrhagic pathology.

In common with other viral hemorrhagic fevers, ASF is characterized by damage involving induction of apoptosis in vascular endothelial cells, and this contributes to vascular permeability. This is thought to be caused by factors released from virus-infected macrophages in the early stages of disease. In the later stages of disease, the appearance of fibrin degradation products and the presence of numerous fibrin thrombi in blood indicate the development of disseminated intravascular coagulation.

Massive apoptosis of lymphocytes is observed in lymphoid tissues in pigs infected with virulent ASFV isolates. Since neither T nor B lymphocytes are infected directly by the virus, apoptosis is presumed to be caused by factors released from or on the surface of virus-infected macrophages. Observations that ASFV can act as a B-cell mitogen have suggested a model to explain lymphocyte apoptosis. This model proposes that dramatic depletion of T cells occurs by apoptosis induced by factors from infected macrophages early in infection. B cells are activated by virus infection but, because of T-cell depletion, do not receive survival signals from T cells (such as CD154 interaction), and this results in B-cell apoptosis. This dramatic depletion of T and B lymphocytes impairs the immune response to infection.

## Virus Structure

Virus particles are approximately 200 nm in diameter and have a complex multilayered structure (**Figure 2**). The nucleoprotein core contains the virus genome and enzymes and other proteins that are packaged into virus particles and used in the early stages of infection following virus entry. These include a DNA-dependent RNA polymerase, mRNA capping and polyadenylation enzymes, and other factors required for early gene transcription. The core is surrounded by a core shell and an internal envelope onto which the

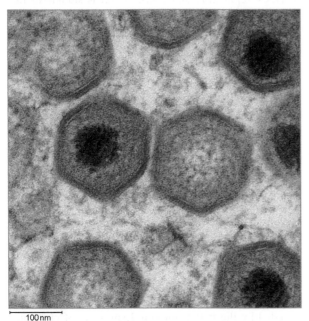

100 nm

**Figure 2** ASFV structure. An electron micrograph of mature and immature virions is shown. Mature particles contain a dense nucleoprotein core containing the DNA genome and proteins that include enzymes required for early gene transcription. This is surrounded by an internal envelope derived from the endoplasmic reticulum on which the icosahedral capsid is assembled. Immature particles differ in that the nucleoprotein core has not condensed to a dense structure and the icosahedral structure is not complete. Extracellular virus particles contain an additional envelope layer derived from the plasma membrane. Electron micrographs were kindly provided by Dr. Paul Monagahan and Pippa Hawes, Institute for Animal Health, Pirbright.

icosahedral capsid is assembled. Although earlier reports suggested that this internal membrane consists of a collapsed double membrane layer, it has also been suggested that only one membrane layer is present. Extracellular virions contain a loosely fitting external envelope which is derived by budding through the plasma membrane.

The capsid consists of a hexagonal arrangement of capsomers that appear as 13 nm long hexagonal prisms each with a central hole. The intercapsomer distance is about 8 nm, and the triangulation number has been estimated at between 189 and 217, corresponding to a capsomer number between 1892 and 2172. The number of virion proteins has been estimated at over 50 by two-dimensional gel electrophoresis. In addition to the virus-encoded enzymes, which are packaged into virions, 16 virus genes that encode virion structural proteins have been identified. Of these, two encode polyproteins (pp220 and pp60) which are processed by proteolytic cleavage by a virus-encoded SUMO-like protease into virion proteins p150, p37, p14, p34, or p35, and p15, respectively. Some of these proteins have been localized in virus particles by immunogold electron microscopy. The products of the pp220 polyprotein are localized in the core shell. Proteins p12, p24, and the CD2-like protein EP402R are present in the external region of virions. Seven of the virion proteins identified contain transmembrane domains.

## Genome Structure

The virus genome consists of a single molecule of linear, covalently close-ended double-stranded DNA that is 170–192 kbp in size. The end sequences are present in two flip-flop forms that are inverted and complementary with respect to each other. Adjacent to both termini are inverted repeats, which consist of tandem repeat arrays and vary in length between 2.1 and 2.5 kbp. The complete genome sequences of one tissue-culture adapted ASFV isolate and nine field isolates have been determined. The number of open reading frames (ORFs) encoding proteins ranges between 160 and 175 depending on the isolate, and these are closely spaced and distributed on both DNA strands. The genome is A+T rich ($\sim$61%).

## Replication

### Virus Entry

The main target cells for ASFV replication are macrophages. Those macrophages that express cell surface markers characteristic of intermediate and late stages of differentiation are permissive for infection. Virus enters cells by receptor-mediated endocytosis (**Figure 3**). Recombinant scavenger receptor CD163 has been shown to bind to virus particles and to inhibit virus infection, suggesting that it may act as a virus receptor. Antibodies against

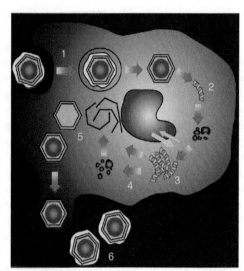

**Figure 3** ASFV replication cycle. Virus particles enter cells by receptor-mediated endocytosis (1), and early gene expression begins in the cytoplasm using enzymes and factors packaged in the nucleoprotein core (2). Replication of full-length genomes takes place in cytoplasmic perinuclear factory regions, although an early stage of replication of subgenomic fragments occurs in the nucleus (3). Following the start of DNA replication, late gene expression occurs and virus structural proteins are synthesized (4). Virion assembly takes place in the virus factories (5) and virus particles are released by budding through the plasma membrane, during which process they gain an extra membrane (6).

recombinant virus proteins p12, p72, and p54 inhibit virus binding to cells, and those against p30 inhibit virus internalization. This suggests that these proteins have a role in these processes. Virus entry requires a fusion event between the viral envelope and the limiting membrane of the endosome at low pH. Following entry, virus cores are transported to perinuclear assembly sites via the microtubule network.

## DNA Replication and mRNA Transcription

Early virus gene transcription begins in the cytoplasm immediately following virus entry, using virus-encoded RNA polymerase, mRNA capping and polyadenylation enzymes, and factors packaged in the nucleoprotein core. Proteins encoded by early genes include enzymes and factors needed for later stages of the replication cycle.

A shift in the pattern of gene transcription occurs after the onset of DNA replication in the cytoplasm. Intermediate and late gene classes have been identified, and transcription of the latter is dependent on the onset of DNA replication. The similarity in the temporal pattern of gene expression suggests that ASFV transcription follows a similar regulation cascade to that of poxviruses. In general, transcription factors required for the next phase of transcription are synthesized in the previous phase. Late genes encode virion structural proteins and enzymes, and include factors such as RNA polymerase and early transcription

factors that are packaged into virus particles for use during the next round of infection. Transcription of some early genes continues throughout the replication cycle.

Those virus promoters that have been mapped are short A+T-rich sequences that are located close upstream from the translation initiation codons. Transcription of all gene classes terminates at a sequence consisting of at least seven consecutive T-residues, which are often located within downstream coding regions. Increasing the number of T-residues causes transcription to terminate more efficiently. Virus mRNAs are capped at the 5′ end and polyadenylated at the 3′ end.

Although ASFV transcription is independent of host RNA polymerase II, productive infection requires the presence of the cell nucleus. The reasons for this are unknown, although a role in the early stages of DNA replication has been indicated by data showing replication of subgenomic length DNA fragments in the nucleus. One suggestion is that a nuclear primase may be necessary to initiate virus DNA replication.

Replication of full-length genomes occurs in the cytoplasmic factory regions via head-to-head concatamers, which are resolved to unit-length genomes and packaged into virus particles in the factories. The mechanism of DNA replication and transcription is similar to that of poxviruses, although an early phase of poxvirus DNA replication in the nucleus has not been detected.

## Assembly

Virus morphogenesis takes place in perinuclear factory regions that are adjacent to the microtubule organizing center. Virus factories resemble aggresomes since they are surrounded by a vimentin cage and increased numbers of mitochondria. Aggresomes are formed in response to cell stress and function to remove misfolded proteins, and the virus may take advantage of this cellular stress response to form its assembly sites. Progeny virus particles are assembled from precursor membranes that are thought to be derived from the endoplasmic reticulum. These membranes are incorporated as an inner envelope into virus particles and become an icosahedral structure by the progressive assembly of viral capsid protein p72. Assembly of the p72 protein into virions requires a chaperone encoded by the B602L protein. Expression of virus protein p54 (encoded by the E183L gene) is required for recruitment of envelope precursors to factory regions. This transmembrane protein is inserted into the endoplasmic reticulum when expressed in cells. It also binds to the LC8 chain of the microtubule motor dynein via a motif in its cytoplasmic domain, and this may provide a mechanism for the recruitment of membranes to virus assembly sites. The core shell is formed beneath the inner envelope by the consecutive assembly of the core shell and the DNA-containing nucleoid. Envelopment and capsid formation require calcium gradients and ATP. Expression and processing of the p220 polyprotein is required for packaging of the nucleoprotein core, and when its expression is suppressed empty virus particles accumulate in factories and can be observed budding through the plasma membrane. Both ASFV and poxviruses assemble in the reducing environment of the cell cytosol and encode proteins involved in a redox pathway that is involved in formation of disulfide bonds in some proteins in the factory. The ASFV B119L protein has been demonstrated to be a flavine adenine dinucleotide-linked sulfhydrl oxidase that is not incorporated into virus particles but is required for efficient virion maturation. The B119L protein interacts with the A151R protein, which contains a CXXC motif similar to that found in thioredoxins, and this binds to virion structural protein E248R. Possibly, all these proteins are components of a system for formation of disulfide bonds in virions.

The virus protein E120R binds to DNA and to capsid protein p72, suggesting a possible role in packaging of the genome. This protein is also required for transport from assembly sites to the plasma membrane, which occurs on microtubules using the conventional kinesin motor. Extracellular virus has an additional loose fitting external lipid envelope that is probably derived by budding through the plasma membrane.

## Virus-Encoded Proteins

Comparison of the complete genomes of ten virus isolates shows that 109 ORFs are present as single copies.

The known functions of the proteins encoded include enzymes involved in replication and transcription of the virus genome, virion structural proteins, and proteins involved in evading host defenses. Many virus encoded-proteins are not essential for replication in cells but have roles in host interactions, which are important for virus survival and transmission (**Figure 4** and **Table 1**).

## Proteins Involved in DNA Replication and Repair and mRNA Transcription and Processing

The virus encodes enzymes involved in nucleotide metabolism, such as thymidine and thymidylate kinases, ribonucleotide reductase and deoxyuridine triphosphatase. Although several of these are nonessential for replication in dividing tissue-culture cells, they are required for efficient replication in macrophages, which are nondividing and have small pools of precursor deoxynucleotide triphosphates required for incorporation into DNA. The virus encodes a DNA polymerase type B and a PCNA-like DNA clamp involved in replication of the genome. ASFV also encodes a putative DNA primase and helicase that is related to enzymes involved in binding to origins

of replication and are probably involved in initiating DNA replication. An ERCC4-like nuclease is related to the principle Holliday junction resolvase, Mus81, of eukaryotes, and the virus also encodes a lambda-type exonuclease. These enzymes may be involved in resolution of the concatamers formed during virus replication.

A DNA polymerase type X, which is the smallest known, together with an ATP-dependent-DNA ligase and AP endonuclease comprise the components of a minimalist DNA base excision repair mechanism. The requirement of the AP endonuclease for efficient replication in macrophages, but not tissue-culture cells, supports the hypothesis that this repair system is an adaptation to virus replication in the highly oxidizing environment of the macrophage cytoplasm, which is likely to cause high levels of DNA damage.

Transcription of virus genes does not require the host RNA polymerase II, indicating that the virus encodes all of the enzymes and factors required. Genes with similarity to five subunits of RNA polymerase have been identified. The gene encoding the mRNA capping enzyme contains all three domains required for this function, namely a triphosphatase, a guanyl transferase, and a methyltransferase. Since transcription takes place in the cytoplasm, no introns are present in genes and the virus does not encode enzymes involved in splicing. An FTS-J-like RNA methyltransferase is encoded, which could play a role in stabilizing rRNA in infected cells.

The virus specifies several enzymes that might be involved either in regulating the virus replication cycle or in modulating the function of host proteins or cellular compartments. These enzymes include a serine/threonine protein kinase, a ubiquitin conjugating enzyme, and a prenyl transferase. The latter two enzymes are not encoded by other viruses.

## Proteins Involved in Evading Host Defenses

A number of conserved ORFs encode proteins involved in evading host defense systems. The virus replicates in macrophages, which have important roles in activating and orchestrating the innate and adaptive immune responses. By interfering with macrophage function the virus can thus disrupt both of these types of host response. One protein, A238L, inhibits activation of the host transcription factor nuclear factor kappa B (NF-κB) and also inhibits calcineurin phosphatase activity. Calcineurin-dependent pathways, such as activation of NFAT transcription factor, are therefore inhibited. This single protein may prevent transcriptional activation of the wide spectrum of immunomodulatory genes whose expression depends on these transcription factors. So far, A238L has been shown to inhibit transcription of cyclooxygenase 2 (COX2) mRNA, thus inhibiting production of prostaglandins, which have a pro-inflammatory role. A238L has also been shown to inhibit transcription from the tumor necrosis factor (TNF)-α promoter.

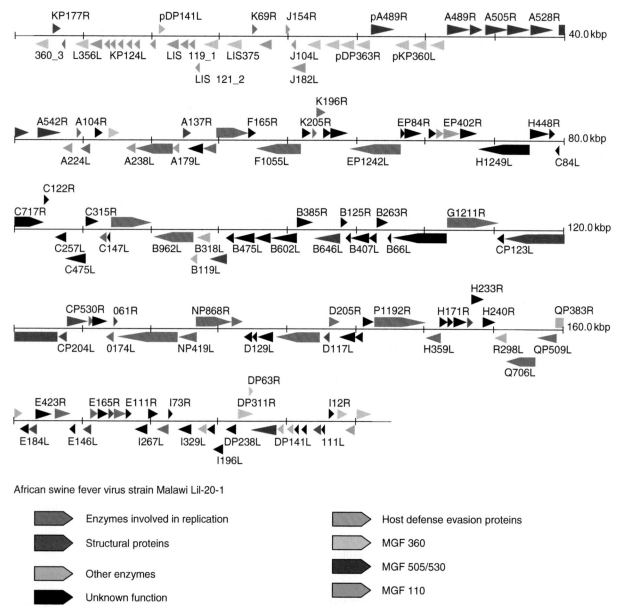

**Figure 4** Genome map of the Malawi LIL20/1 isolate. Arrows show the size and direction in which protein-coding regions are transcribed. The colors indicate protein functional class or membership of MGFs.

In addition, the virus encodes a transmembrane protein (EP402R or CD2v), which has an extracellular domain that resembles the host CD2 protein. The host CD2 protein is involved in stabilizing the interaction between T cells and antigen-presenting cells. CD2v causes binding of red blood cells to infected cells and extracellular virions, and this may help to hide virus particles and infected cells from components of the host immune system. Deletion of the CD2v gene reduces virus dissemination in infected pigs and *in vitro* abrogates the ability of ASFV to inhibit proliferation of bystander lymphocytes in response to mitogens. The cytoplasmic tail of this protein differs from that of the host protein and binds to a cellular adaptor protein (SH3P7/mabp1), which has roles in endocytosis, transport through the Golgi, and signaling pathways. This interaction may modulate functions of SH3P7/mabp1.

One protein (designated NL-S, l14L, or DP71L) is related in its C-terminal domain to a herpes simplex virus-encoded neurovirulence factor (ICP34.5) and host GADD34 proteins. These proteins act as regulatory subunits of protein phosphatase 1 (PP1). The ASFV protein is required for virus-induced activation of PP1, and its predominantly nuclear location indicates a possible function in regulating host gene transcription.

**Table 1**  Functions of ASFV genes

| | Gene name in BA71V isolate | Alternative names | Predicted protein size (kDa) |
|---|---|---|---|
| *Nucleotide metabolism, transcription, replication, and repair* | | | |
| Thymidylate kinase | A240L | | 27.8 |
| Thymidine kinase | K196R | | 22.4 |
| dUTPase* | E165R | k1R | 18.3 |
| Ribonucleotide reductase (small subunit) | F334L | | 39.8 |
| Ribonucleotide reductase (large subunit) | F778R | | 87.5 |
| DNA polymerase β | G1211R | | 139.8 |
| DNA topoisomerase type II* | P1192R | i7R | 135.5 |
| Proliferating cell nuclear antigen (PCNA) like | E301R | j15R | 35.3 |
| DNA polymerase family X* | O174L | | 20.3 |
| DNA ligase* | NP419L | g3L | 48.2 |
| Putative DNA primase | C962R | | 111.2 |
| AP endonuclease class II* | E296R | k4R | 33.5 |
| RNA polymerase subunit 2 | EP1242L | g2L | 139.9 |
| RNA polymerase subunit 6 | C147L | g6L | 16.7 |
| RNA polymerase subunit 1 | NP1450L | | 163.7 |
| RNA polymerase subunit 3 | H359L | j1L | 41.3 |
| RNA polymerase subunit 5 | D205R | i2R | 23.7 |
| Helicase superfamily II | A859L | | 27.8 |
| Helicase superfamily II similar to origin binding protein | F1055L | | 123.9 |
| Helicase superfamily II | B962L | | 109.6 |
| Helicase superfamily II | D1133L | g10L | 129.3 |
| Helicase superfamily II | Q706L | j10L | 80.4 |
| Helicase superfamily II | QP509L | | 58.1 |
| Transcription factor SII | I243L | k9L | 28.6 |
| Guanyl transferase* | NP868R | g4R | 29.9 |
| Poly A polymerase large subunit | C475L | | 54.7 |
| FTS-J-like methyl transferase domain | EP424R | | 49.3 |
| ERCC4 nuclease domain | EP364R | | 40.9 |
| Lambda-like exonuclease | D345L | | 39.4 |
| *Other enzymes* | | | |
| Prenyl transferase* | B318L | | 35.9 |
| Serine protein kinase* | R298L | j8L | 35.1 |
| Ubiquitin conjugating enzyme* | I215L | k13L | 24.7 |
| Nudix hydrolase* | D250R | g5R | 29.9 |
| *Host cell interactions* | | | |
| IAP apoptosis inhibitor* | A224L | 4CL | 26.6 |
| Bcl-2 apoptosis inhibitor* | A179L | | 21.1 |
| IkB homolog and inhibitor of calcineurin phosphatase* | A238L | 5EL | 28.2 |
| C-type lectin-like* | EP153R | | 18.0 |
| CD2-like. Causes hemadsorbtion to infected cells* | EP402R | CD2v, Mw8R | 45.3 |
| Similar to HSV ICP34.5 neurovirulence factor | DP71L | I14L, NL | 8.5 |
| Nif S-like | QP383R | j11R | 42.5 |
| *Structural proteins and proteins involved in morphogenesis* | | | |
| P22 | KP177R | P22 | 20.2 |
| Histone-like | A104R | | 11.5 |
| P11.5 | A137R | | 21.1 |
| P10 | A78R | P10 | 8.4 |
| P72 major capsid protein. Involved in virus entry | B646L | P72, P73 | 73.2 |
| P49 | B438L | P49 | 49.3 |
| Chaperone. Involved in folding of capsid | B602L | 9RL | 45.3 |
| ERV1-like. Involved in redox metabolism* | B119L | 9GL | 14.4 |
| SUMO 1-like protease. Involved in polyprotein cleavage | S273R | | 31.6 |
| P220 polyprotein precursor of p150, p37, p14, p34. Required for packaging of nucleoprotein core | CP2475L | | 281.5 |
| P32 phosphoprotein. Involved in virus entry | CP204L | P30, P32 | 23.6 |

Continued

**Table 1**    Continued

| | Gene name in BA71V isolate | Alternative names | Predicted protein size (kDa) |
|---|---|---|---|
| P60 polyprotein precursor of p35 and p15 | CP530R | | 60.5 |
| P12 attachment protein | O61R | P12 | 6.7 |
| P17 | D117L | i11L | 13.1 |
| J5R | H108R | j5R | 12.5 |
| P54 (j13L) Binds to LC8 chain of dynein, involved in virus entry | E183L | j13L, p54 | 19.9 |
| J18L | E199L | j18L | 22.0 |
| pE248R | E248R | k2R | |
| P14.5 DNA binding. Required for movement of virions to plasma membrane | E120R | k3R | 13.6 |

The functions of the virus encoded-genes are shown. Those which have been experimentally confirmed are marked with an asterisk. The designated gene names in the BA71V isolate sequence are shown and alternative names used in the literature. The predicted sizes of the encoded proteins are shown.

Three virus proteins are known to inhibit apoptosis and therefore are predicted to prolong survival of infected cells and facilitate virus replication. These include proteins which are similar to the cellular apoptosis inhibitors Bcl-2 and IAP. The Bcl-2 homolog is expressed early and thought to be essential for virus infection, whereas the IAP homolog is nonessential, is expressed late, and packaged into virus particles. The IAP homolog may play a more critical role in the tick vector.

## Multigene Families

A large proportion of the ASFV genome encodes multigene families (MGFs) consisting of related protein-coding regions that are present in multiple copies and vary in number between different isolates. MGF 360 is the largest and contains between 11 and 19 copies in different genomes; MGF 505/530 contains between 8 and 10 copies; MGF 110 between 5 and 13; MGF 300 between 3 and 4; and MGF 100 between 2 and 3. In addition, the virus genomes contain between 1 and 3 copies of one of the virus structural proteins, p22. Comparison of the genomes of high and low virulence isolates has identified a fragment encoding 6 copies of MGF 360 and 2 copies of MGF 530 which are absent from the genome of the nonpathogenic isolate. These genes were also implicated in virulence and control of interferon-alpha production by deletion from the genome of a virulent isolate. The tissue-culture adapted isolate also has a deletion from a region close to the right end of the genome encoding five ORFs. These ORFs may facilitate virus replication in macrophages since the tissue-culture adapted isolate replicates poorly in primary macrophages.

The large investment in MGFs implies that they offer a selective advantage to the virus. However, their roles are largely unknown.

## Classification and Relationship with Other Virus Families

ASFV was first classified as a member of the family *Iridoviridae* because of its large size, cytoplasmic location, and double-stranded DNA genome. However, studies of replication strategy and the genome revealed similarities with the *Poxviridae*, although the viruses differ structurally. ASFV was therefore placed as the species *African swine fever virus* into a separate virus family, the *Asfarviridae*, of which it is the sole member of the single genus, the *Asfivirus* genus. ASFV has also been considered to be part of a larger grouping of nucleo-cytoplasmic large DNA viruses (NCLDV) which, apart from the families mentioned above, includes the family *Phycodnaviridae* (large DNA viruses that infect blue-green algae) and the genus *Mimivirus* (which infect amebae). Replication of all families in the NCLDV grouping involves at least some stage in the cytoplasm, although each family has varying requirements for host nuclear functions. For example, both ASFV and poxviruses encode their own RNA polymerase which is packaged into virus particles so that transcription of early genes begins immediately following virus entry. Members of the *Iridoviridae* have a greater requirement for the nucleus since virus particles do not contain an RNA polymerase and early virus gene transcription and replication take place in the nucleus and are initiated by host enzymes. At later stages, virus DNA replication, transcription, and virus assembly take place in the cytoplasm. Less is known about the replication strategies of the *Phycodnaviridae* and *Mimivirus*, although they exhibit a greater involvement of nuclear functions in replication compared to the *Poxviridae* and *Asfarviridae*.

Analysis of the gene complements of different families in the grouping has indicated that the ancestral NCLDV may have encoded at least 40 genes involved in replication, transcription, packaging, and assembly. Each family has evolved to encode genes that represent adaptations to its particular ecological niche. Genome analysis suggests there are two major lineages, one consisting of the *Poxviridae* and *Asfarviridae* and other of the *Iridoviridae*, *Phycodnaviridae*, and *Mimivirus*.

Comparison of the NCLDV families suggests that genes have been acquired by horizontal transfer from eukaryotic and prokaryotic hosts as well as possibly from other viruses. However, there are few genes which show evidence of recent acquisition. Another feature of the NCLDV is the presence of MGFs which have evolved by processes of gene duplication and sequence divergence. The remarkable adaptation of ASFV to replicate in its tick vector suggests that its ancestor may have replicated only in arthropods and later acquired the ability to replicate also in mammalian hosts. The independence of the virus from host transcriptional machinery facilitates virus replication in both mammalian and arthropod hosts since the gene promoters do not have to be recognised by both the mammalian and arthropod host transcriptional machinery. This could have facilitated the jump from arthropod to mammalian hosts. However, ASFV also encodes proteins (such as CD2v) that are clearly derived from a higher eukaryotic host, suggesting that growth in such hosts has substantially influenced ASFV evolution. Replication in macrophages provides the virus with opportunities to manipulate the host response to infection. This advantage may offset difficulties encountered by replicating in the harsh, microbiocidal environment of the macrophage cytoplasm.

## Future Prospects

Over the last decade our knowledge of ASFV-encoded proteins involved in virus entry and assembly, as well as those with roles in evading host defenses and causing virulence, has increased dramatically. Likewise, our knowledge of host protective immune responses and of some of the virus proteins important in their induction has increased. These advances will help the development of effective vaccines to control this economically important disease. As with other large DNA viruses, the ASFV genome may be viewed as a repository of genes that have co-evolved with its hosts and serve to manipulate host defense responses. These genes will continue to provide tools for understanding host antiviral pathways and potential leads for discovery of new immunomodulatory drugs.

Investigations of the unique replication strategy and evolutionary niche of ASFV will aid our understanding of many aspects of virus host interactions and pathogenesis, as well as mechanisms of virus replication and evolution.

*See also:* Viruses Infecting Euryarchaea.

## Further Reading

Afonso CL, Piccone ME, Zaffuto KM, *et al.* (2004) African swine fever virus multigene family 360 and 530 genes affect host interferon response. *Journal of Virology* 78: 1858–1864.

Andres G, Alejo A, Salas J, and Salas ML (2002) African swine fever virus polyproteins pp220 and pp62 assemble into the core shell. *Journal of Virology* 76: 12473–12482.

Borca MV, Carrillo C, Zsak L, *et al.* (1998) Deletion of a CD2-like gene, 8-DR, from African swine fever virus affects viral infection in domestic swine. *Journal of Virology* 72: 2881–2889.

Brun A, Rivas C, Esteban M, Escribano JM, and Alonso C (1996) African swine fever virus gene A179L, a viral homologue of bcl-2, protects cells from programmed cell death. *Virology* 225: 227–230.

Carrascosa JL, Carazo JM, Carrascosa AL, Garcia N, Santisteban A, and Vinuela E (1984) General morphology and capsid fine-structure of African swine fever virus-particles. *Virology* 132: 160–172.

Cobbold C, Whittle JT, and Wileman T (1996) Involvement of the endoplasmic reticulum in the assembly and envelopment of African swine fever virus. *Journal of Virology* 70: 8382–8390.

Dixon LK, Escribano JM, Martins C, Rock DL, Salas ML, and Wilkinson PJ (2005) *Asfarviridae*. In: Fauquet CM, Mayo MA, Maniloff J, Desselberger U, and Ball LA (eds.) *Virus Taxonomy: Eighth Report of the International Committee on Taxonomy of Viruses*, pp. 135–143. San Diego, CA: Elsevier Academic Press.

Gomez-Puertas P, Rodriguez F, Oviedo JM, Brun A, Alonso C, and Escribano JM (1998) The African swine fever virus proteins p54 and p30 are involved in two distinct steps of virus attachment and both contribute to the antibody-mediated protective immune response. *Virology* 243: 461–471.

Iyer LM, Balaji S, Koonin EV, and Aravind L (2006) Evolutionary genomics of nucleo-cytoplasmic large DNA viruses. *Virus Research* 117: 156–184.

Miskin JE, Abrams CC, and Dixon LK (2000) African swine fever virus protein A238L interacts with the cellular phosphatase calcineurin via a binding domain similar to that of NFAT. *Journal of Virology* 74: 9412–9420.

Powell PP, Dixon LK, and Parkhouse RME (1996) An IκB homolog encoded by African swine fever virus provides a novel mechanism for downregulation of proinflammatory cytokine responses in host macrophages. *Journal of Virology* 70: 8527–8533.

Revilla Y, Callejo M, Rodriguez JM, *et al.* (1998) Inhibition of nuclear factor κB activation by a virus-encoded IκB-like protein. *Journal of Biological Chemistry* 273: 5405–5411.

Takamatsu H, Denyer MS, Oura C, *et al.* (1999) African swine fever virus: A B cell-mitogenic virus *in vivo* and *in vitro*. *Journal of General Virology* 80: 1453–1461.

Tulman ER and Rock DL (2001) Novel virulence and host range genes of African swine fever virus. *Current Opinion in Microbiology* 4: 456–461.

Yanez RJ, Rodriguez JM, Nogal ML, *et al.* (1995) Analysis of complete nucleotide sequence of African swine fever virus. *Virology* 208: 249–278.

# Akabane Virus

**P S Mellor,** Institute for Animal Health, Woking, UK
**P D Kirkland,** Elizabeth Macarthur Agricultural Institute, Menangle, NSW, Australia

## Glossary

**Arthrogryposis (AG)** Rigid fixation of the joints, usually in flexion but occasionally in extension.
*Culicoides* Blood-feeding dipterous insects also known as biting midges.
**Dystocia** Abnormal or difficult birth.
**Encephalomyelitis** Inflammation both of the brain and the spinal cord.
**Porencephaly** Disease of the brain with the formation of small cavities in the brain substance.
**Hydranencephaly (HE)** A condition in which the brain's cerebral hemispheres are almost or completely absent and replaced by sacs filled with cerebrospinal fluid.
**Kyphosis** Outward curvature of the spine causing a humped back.
**Nystagmus** Rapid involuntary oscillation of the eyes.
**Scoliosis** Lateral deviation of the normal vertical line of the spine.
**Torticollis** Twisting of the neck that causes the head to rotate or tilt.

## Introduction

Akabane virus was originally isolated from mosquitoes in Japan, in the summer of 1959, 'Akabane' being the name of the village where the virus was first isolated. Subsequently, it has been shown to occur widely in Africa, Australia, throughout Asia and the Middle East, its distribution being determined by the occurrence of its insect vectors which are predominantly biting midges from the genus *Culicoides*.

The virus is important in veterinary pathology because it is able to cross the placenta of cattle, sheep, and goats causing a range of congenital defects, principally arthrogryposis (AG) and hydranencephaly (HE), and abortion. The virus can be widespread without evidence of disease because it usually produces asymptomatic infections in adult animals. It is only when pregnant, serologically naive adults are infected early in pregnancy that the virus may cross the placenta to cause damage to the fetus. Evidence of the damage only becomes apparent some months later with the birth of the affected young – by which time the viruses have been eliminated from both mother and offspring and so cannot be isolated from them. This meant that for many years Akabane virus was not connected to these clinical manifestations, until careful epidemiological observations and the development of appropriate serological tests confirmed the association.

## Taxonomy, Properties of the Virion and Genome

Akabane virus is a member of the genus *Orthobunyavirus* in the family *Bunyaviridae*. Several related viruses (Aino, Cache Valley, Peaton, and Tinaroo) have been shown under experimental conditions to have the potential to cross the ruminant placenta but only Aino in Australia and Japan and Cache Valley in the USA have been recognized as pathogens in the field.

The Akabane virion is spherical in shape and is *c.* 90–100 nm in diameter. A lipid envelope with projecting glycoprotein peplomers surrounds the viral genome which consists of three separate segments of single-stranded RNA. Each segment is of a different length. The large segment encodes the viral transcriptase, the medium segment two glycoproteins, and the small segment the internal nucleoprotein. Each of the segments also encodes a nonstructural protein.

The virus is acid labile and is readily inactivated by chloroform, ether, and trypsin. It is also very heat labile and is inactivated at 56 °C in a few minutes and loses about 0.3 log of infectivity per hour at 37 °C. However, it remains viable in blood samples kept at 4 °C for several months and can be stored indefinitely at −80 °C or lower.

## Vertebrate Hosts

The virus has been isolated from cattle, sheep, and goats. Antibodies have also been detected in horses, pigs, camel, red deer, and a wide selection of African wildlife ranging from various species of antelope to hippopotamus, elephant, and giraffe.

There are no known cases of human disease caused by Akabane virus even though some of the mosquito species from which the virus has been isolated (*Aedes vexans, Culex tritaeniorhynchus,* and *Anopheles funestus*) regularly bite humans. However, the role of mosquitoes as vectors remains unclear and limited serological surveys have not found evidence of human infection. Further, the *Culicoides* species that are known vectors of the virus rarely bite humans.

## Clinical Signs

When Akabane virus infects pregnant cattle, sheep, or goats, the virus is able to replicate in and cross the ruminant placenta causing a variety of congenital abnormalities in the fetus. The range and severity of these abnormalities are dependent upon the stage of gestation at infection. In adult animals, however, infection is usually subclinical and in endemic areas most breeding age animals will have acquired an active immunity during early life sufficient to prevent the virus from reaching the developing fetus. In these situations, the virus exists as a 'silent' infection and no evidence of disease is seen. The pathogenic effects of Akabane infection are usually observed only when the vector spreads beyond the limits of its endemic areas under favorable conditions, to enter regions where many adult animals are still susceptible and therefore able to be infected during pregnancy. In such situations, an epidemic in cattle, sheep, or goats may be noticed by an increased incidence of abortions and premature births in late autumn or early winter. Calves infected close to term may be born with encephalitis, often apparent clinically as a flaccid paralysis. Some strains of Akabane virus may also cause encephalitis in newborn calves and, infrequently, in older animals. This is followed by the birth of calves, lambs, or kids with a range of congenital defects, principally AG and HE (see **Figures 1** and **2**). Young with these defects may be stillborn or delivered alive at term. AG is characterized by fixation of the joints in flexion (most frequently) or extension. The birth of some arthrogrypotic

animals is associated with dystocia, necessitating embryotomy or cesarean section to save the dam. Young born with HE may show blindness, nystagmus, deafness, dullness, slow suckling, paralysis, and lack of coordination. They may survive for several months if hand-reared but often die from misadventure. In cattle herds with animals at different stages of pregnancy, there will be a succession of defects, initially with cases of AG and later calves with HE. In sheep and goats, due to the shorter period of gestation and narrower range at which the fetus is susceptible, affected progeny born may show one or more of the defects of AG and HE concurrently.

Epidemics of AG/HE disease due to Akabane virus have been recorded in Japan, Australia, Israel, and Turkey, the most severe involving 30 000 calves in Japan and approximately 8000 calves in Australia. The incidence of affected progeny varies depending on the strain of virus. In naturally infected cattle, the incidence of AG and HE varies from 25% to 50% but in sheep that have been experimentally infected with different virus strains, the incidence of abnormal lambs can vary from 15% to 80%.

## Pathogenesis

In naturally infected cattle, there is an incubation period of a few days followed by a viremia of 3–6 days duration. This is not usually associated with clinical signs in the adult animal. From about day 12 post infection, virus-neutralizing antibodies begin to be detected in the circulation.

The sequence of events leading to fetal infection involves virus replication in the endothelial cells of the placenta, then the trophoblastic cells, and finally in the fetus itself. The ability of the virus to produce congenital damage depends upon the stage of gestation at which fetal infection occurs. Fetal Akabane virus infection is characterized by a predictable chronological sequence of

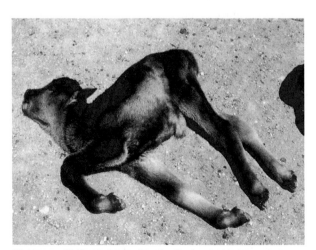

**Figure 1** Calf with AG and torticollis due to Akabane virus infection.

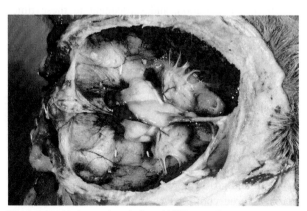

**Figure 2** Akabane virus-induced HE in a calf.

congenital defects directly referable to the fetal age at which infection has occurred. The bovine fetus is susceptible from about 90 days through to term while the ovine and caprine are most susceptible between 28 and 56 days of gestation. In sheep and goats, defects are less common than in cattle because of both the limited gestational range and the fact that small ruminants are less likely to be pregnant during the virus transmission period.

In cattle, the defects occur over a longer period and are seen in consistent sequence. The first abnormalities to appear in live neonates are nonsuppurative encephalitis and encephalomyelitis, the outcome of infection late in gestation. Arthrogrypotic neonates follow as a result of infection in the fifth and sixth months of gestation, then more severe malformations including porencephaly and HE reflecting infection in the third and fourth months. When AG is first observed, only one joint on a single limb might be affected, but in cases that are born later (infected earlier) the abnormalities are more severe with changes in several joints on all limbs. Calves affected with severe AG after infection early in the fifth month of gestation may show early changes in the brain with small cystic lesions of porencephaly. The lesions of HE then develop as a result of infection in the third and fourth months of gestation. As calves are born later in an outbreak, the lesions of HE will progress in severity, initially being seen as small focal cystic cavities but soon progressing to large fluid-filled cavities. In calves with severe lesions, the cerebral hemispheres are completely absent and only fluid-filled meninges remain but the brainstem and cerebellum remain unaffected.

The replication of Akabane virus and its tissue tropisms in the fetus are determined by fetal age, the presence of rapidly dividing cells, and the development of immunocompetence. The most severe lesions occur in fetuses infected during the early stages of organogenesis. In cattle the most severe lesions occur after infection between 70 and 90 days of gestation and in sheep and goats between 28 and 36 days. Immunocompetence develops in calves from about 90 days and in lambs from 65–70 days of gestation, and subsequent to these times virus is rapidly eliminated from the fetal tissues. As a result, virus cannot be isolated from calves and lambs delivered at term but may be isolated from a fetus that is aborted soon after infection.

## Pathology

AG and HE are the main gross lesions of Akabane disease but cervical scoliosis, torticollis, and kyphosis also occur. In sheep and goats, there may also be pulmonary hypoplasia. Arthrogrypotic calves exhibit restrictions to movements of the limb joints exclusively as a result of changes to the soft tissues. The joint surfaces are normal and the bones are unaffected. In affected limbs, the muscles are usually reduced in size and paler in color than normal. This is a result of both neurogenic muscular atrophy and also from primary infection of the muscles.

Microscopically, there is a severe loss of myelinated fibres in the lateral and ventral funiculi of the spinal cord, and of ventral horn neurons and nerve fibers in the ventral spinal nerves. However, white matter is unaffected.

In HE calves, the cerebral cortex is represented only by a thin shell of brain tissue, perhaps only the meninges, filled with fluid (**Figure 2**). The meninges may be thickened. In most cases, the brainstem is intact and the cerebellum appears normal.

During the early stages of an outbreak of Akabane disease, there may be calves which are incoordinate or unable to stand at birth. No gross pathological lesions are found in such animals but microscopically there is a mild to moderate nonsuppurative acute encephalomyelitis, most evident in the gray matter of the mid- and posterior brain.

## Epidemiology and Transmission

Most of Africa, the Middle East, southern Asia, Japan, Korea, and Australia may be regarded as being endemic for Akabane virus. Papua New Guinea and the island countries of the Pacific, however, are free from infection. The geographical distribution of this virus is controlled completely by the distribution, seasonal activity, and abundance of its insect vectors.

Akabane virus was first isolated in Japan in 1959 from mosquitoes of the species *Ae. vexans* and *Cx. tritaeniorhynchus*. Then, in 1968, it was isolated in Australia from the biting midge *Culicoides brevitarsis*. More recently, isolations have also been made from *An. funestus* in Kenya, and from *Culicoides* species such as *C. oxystoma* in Japan, *C. imicola* (**Figure 3**) and *C. milnei* in Zimbabwe, *C. imicola* in Oman, *C. brevitarsis* and *C. wadai* in Australia, and a mixed pool consisting mainly of *C. imicola* in South Africa. The virus has been shown to replicate in *C. sonorensis* (=*C. variipennis*) by up to 1000-fold, and transmission occurs after 7–10 days incubation at 25 °C. As *C. sonorensis* is widely distributed and abundant in North America, this suggests that should Akabane virus gain entry to that continent, transmission would be likely. The virus has also been shown to replicate in *C. brevitarsis* and reaches the salivary glands of infected individuals after 10 days incubation. In Australia, *C. brevitarsis* is the only biting insect whose distribution correlates closely with the distribution of Akabane antibodies in cattle. The development of antibodies also coincides with the seasons when *C. brevitarsis* is active. Furthermore, *C. brevitarsis* feeds upon sheep and horses in Australia, in which species antibodies to Akabane virus have been found.

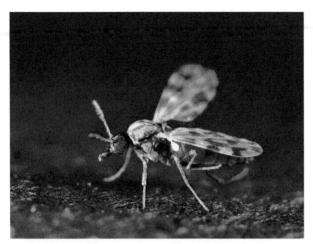

**Figure 3** *Culicoides imicola*, a vector of Akabane virus.

These findings suggest that in Australia *C. brevitarsis* is the principal vector of Akabane virus. No close correlation has yet been reported between any mosquito species and Akabane virus distribution, and as replication and transmission of the virus have not been demonstrated in any mosquito species, this suggests that *Culicoides* species are likely to be the major vectors of Akabane virus and mosquitoes are of lesser importance. Akabane virus persists in nature by alternate cycling of the virus between the midges and its mammalian hosts after biting of the mammalian host by the insects. Transovarial (vertical) transmission of Akabane virus has not demonstrated.

In Australia, the principal vector *C. brevitarsis* spreads Akabane virus throughout an endemic area that extends across the north of the country and southward along the east coast. Within this area, virus transmission occurs annually, so breeding animals are usually infected early in life before becoming pregnant and few Akabane cases occur. Under harsh climatic conditions, usually drought, the distribution of the midge may retreat northward and toward the coast, reducing the extent of infection for one or perhaps two seasons. On resumption of the usual pattern of spread, a susceptible population of pregnant females will be infected at the margins of the range of the midge, resulting in small disease outbreaks. Under the influence of very favorable conditions of higher rainfall and mild temperatures, the insect may spread further south and inland than is usual and result in virus transmission in highly susceptible livestock populations. Large outbreaks will then occur with abortions noticed in late autumn and calves with AG/HE begin to appear in midwinter and spring, from July through to September.

Outbreaks of Akabane disease in Japan also show seasonal and geographic clustering, with most cases occurring from September to March. In Israel, disease outbreaks have occurred from November to June and in western Turkey during early spring (March). The differences in timing are presumably related to the abundance of the vector insects as influenced by climate.

## Diagnosis

Sporadic cases of AG/HE due to Akabane virus often remain undiagnosed. However, when there is a cluster of cases, a teratogenic virus should be considered as a possible cause.

Because Akabane virus does not persistent in the fetus, attempts to isolate virus from affected newborn calves, lambs, and kids are uniformly unsuccessful. Nevertheless, virus may be isolated from the tissues (e.g., brain, spinal cord, skeletal muscle) of fetuses that are aborted early in pregnancy. Virus isolation is usually conducted by inoculation of a continuous cell line and the polymerase chain reaction (PCR) assay has been used to reliably detect viral RNA in fetal tissues.

Akabane infection is most frequently confirmed serologically. Serum from affected calves, lambs, and kids should be collected prior to suckling to enable detection of specific antibodies to Akabane virus. As virus-specific antibodies are produced in fetuses after they become immunocompetent, the detection of antibodies to this virus in serum and body fluids prior to suckling is considered to confirm an *in utero* infection. An examination of the abomasum for milk curd should be made to confirm that the calf has not suckled. As a further check, a serum sample from the dam should also be taken and the two samples tested in parallel for antibodies to Akabane and other common viruses. If the serum of the neonate contains a similar range of antibodies to the dam, it would suggest that suckling has taken place. If only antibodies to Akabane virus are detected in the serum of the neonate but there are antibodies to several in its dam's serum then the evidence is strong that it has been infected *in utero*.

The virus neutralization test is the most specific serological test available but enzyme-linked immunosorbent assays (ELISAs) have also been developed that are either Akabane specific or Simbu serogroup specific.

## Differential Diagnosis

Other viral teratogens may be associated with *in utero* infections and the delivery of neonates with congenital defects. Of the bunyaviruses, Aino virus has been linked with congenital AG/HE in cattle, though the lesions of the cerebrum are less symmetrical than those due to Akabane virus and the cerebellum may also be affected. In sheep in the USA (where Akabane virus is exotic), Cache Valley virus is a possible cause. Other viral agents that may cause defects include bluetongue, Rift Valley fever, Wesselsbron, border disease, and bovine viral diarrhea viruses. An important differential feature of Akabane infection in cattle is that the cerebellum is unaffected. Individual agents may be confirmed by using virus-specific serology to test precolostral serum or fluid from body cavities (e.g., pericardial or pleural fluid).

A range of noninfectious causes of congenital AG and HE in calves, lambs, and kids should also be considered and include maternal intoxication (e.g., by ingestion of toxic plants) or an inherited defect. The detection of elevated immunoglobulin G (IgG) levels in precolostral serum or fluids will differentiate between infectious and noninfectious causes of congenital defects.

## Prophylaxis and Control

There are two main approaches to the prophylaxis of Akabane virus infections: vaccination and management strategies to control or avoid vectors.

### Vaccination

Vaccination is the main method of prophylaxis and Akabane vaccines have been produced in Japan and Australia.

In Japan and Australia, inactivated vaccines have been developed that induce high antibody titers after two doses given with a 4 week interval. In trials, these vaccines prevented development of a viremia and fetal infection on challenge or after natural exposure and were safe when used in pregnant animals. As antibody titers decline fairly rapidly, annual revaccination is recommended. In Japan, a live attenuated vaccine has also been produced by serial passage of Akabane virus in cell culture. When used in cattle this vaccine induces high titers of neutralizing antibodies without pyrexia, leucopoenia, or viremia and virus was not recoverable from the organs or the fetuses of vaccinated animals. It also prevented infection of the bovine fetus on challenge with virulent Akabane virus. However, in pregnant ewes, the vaccine induced a viremia and frequently caused intrauterine infection of the fetus, so this vaccine is not recommended for use in sheep.

### Vector Control and Management Strategies

At present, vector control is considered to be impractical partly because of inadequate knowledge of vector biology over much of the global range of Akabane virus and partly because vector control can be prohibitively expensive. Further, absolute control of vectors is impossible and animals only need to be bitten by a single virus-infected vector for infection to occur. Possible control measures involve elimination or reduction in the vector-breeding sites (damp organically enriched soil or large herbivore dung) and direct insecticide attack on adult vectors. Susceptible hosts may also be protected from the bites of vectors by the use of insect repellents or by screening animal housing with insect-proof nets or mesh.

An important measure to minimize losses due to Akabane virus is to avoid the movement of susceptible pregnant animals into virus-endemic areas during the vector season. Such inadvertent movements have resulted in significant losses.

*See also:* Vector Transmission of Animal Viruses.

## Further Reading

Al-Busaidy SM, Mellor PS, and Taylor WP (1988) Prevalence of neutralising antibodies to Akabane virus in the Arabian Peninsula. *Veterinary Microbiology* 17: 11–149.

Charles JA (1994) Akabane virus. *Veterinary Clinics of North America: Food Animal Practice* 10: 525–546.

Inaba Y and Matumoto M (1990) Akabane virus. In: Dinter Z and Morein B (eds.) *Virus Infections of Ruminants*, pp. 467–480. Oxford: Elsevier.

Jagoe S, Kirkland PD, and Harper PAW (1993) An outbreak of Akabane virus induced abnormalities in calves following agistment in an endemic region. *Australian Veterinary Journal* 70: 56–58.

Jennings DM and Mellor PS (1988) *Culicoides*: Biological vectors of Akabane virus. *Veterinary Microbiology* 21: 125–131.

Kirkland PD and Barry RD (1986) The economic impact of Akabane virus and cost effectiveness of Akabane vaccine in New South Wales. In: St. George TD, Kay BH, and Blok J (eds.) *Arbovirus Research in Australia*, pp. 229–232. Brisbane: CSIRO.

Kirkland PD, Barry RD, Harper PAW, and Zelski RZ (1988) The development of Akabane virus induced congenital abnormalities in cattle. *Veterinary Record* 122: 582–586.

Matumoto M and Inaba Y (1980) Akabane disease and Akabane virus. *Kitasato Archives of Experimental Medicine* 53: 1–21.

St. George TD and Kirkland PD (2004) Diseases caused by Akabane and related Simbu-group viruses. In: Coetzer JAW and Tustin RC (eds.) *Infectious Diseases of Livestock,* 2nd edn., vol. 2, pp. 1029–1036. Cape Town: Oxford University Press.

St. George TD and Standfast HA (1989) Simbu group viruses with teratogenic potential. In: Monath TP (ed.) *The Arboviruses: Epidemiology and Ecology,* vol. 4, pp. 145–166. Boca Raton, FL: CRC Press.

Taylor WP and Mellor PS (1994) The distribution of Akabane virus in the Middle East. *Epidemiology and Infection* 113: 175–185.

# Animal Rhabdoviruses

**H Bourhy,** Institut Pasteur, Paris, France
**A J Gubala,** CSIRO Livestock Industries, Geelong, VIC, Australia
**R P Weir,** Berrimah Research Farm, Darwin, NT, Australia
**D B Boyle,** CSIRO Livestock Industries, Geelong, VIC, Australia

## Glossary

**Dipterans** Insects having usually a single pair of functional wings (anterior pair) with the posterior pair reduced to small knobbed structures and mouth parts adapted for sucking or lapping or piercing.
**Hematophagous** Feeding on blood.
**Homopterans** Insects having membranous forewings and hind wings.
**Orthopterans** Insects having leathery forewings and membranous hind wings and chewing mouthparts.

## Introduction

RNA viruses of the family *Rhabdoviridae* comprise arthropod-borne agents that infect plants, fish, and mammals, as well as a variety of non-vector-borne mammalian viruses. The *Rhabdoviridae* presently comprises six genera, and members of three of these genera – *Vesiculovirus*, *Lyssavirus*, and *Ephemerovirus* – have been obtained from a variety of animal hosts and vectors, including mammals, fish, and invertebrates. The remaining three rhabdovirus genera are more taxon-specific in their host preference. Novirhabdoviruses infect numerous species of fish, while cytorhabdoviruses and nucleorhabdoviruses are arthropod-borne and infect plants. Rhabdoviruses are the etiological agents of human diseases that cause serious public health problems. Some of them can also cause important economic loss in plants and livestock. Other than the well-characterized rhabdoviruses that are known to be important for agriculture and public health, there is also a constantly growing list of rhabdoviruses (presently 85), isolated from a variety of vertebrate and invertebrate hosts, that are partially characterized and are still awaiting definitive genus or species assignment.

## History and Classification

Commencing in the 1950s, monitoring programs have been established in tropical regions of Africa, America, Southeast Asia, and northern Australia to detect and identify arboviruses of medical or veterinary importance.

In Australia, the use of sentinel cattle herds monitoring associated with insect and vertebrate trapping has provided a means of monitoring the ecology of endemic arboviruses that infect livestock and humans, and an early warning system for incursions of exotic arboviruses and insect vectors. In most other regions, these programs have been based on the collection of viruses from terrestrial vertebrates and hematophagous arthropods. As a result, many new and uncharacterized rhabdoviruses have been isolated. The considerable range of likely vectors and hosts and the wide geographical distribution seen among these isolates highlights the diversity of animal rhabdovirus evolution and ecological adaptation.

The isolation of viruses in the early years was primarily performed in suckling mice by intracranial inoculation with clarified supernatant fluid obtained after grinding of pools of collected arthropods. The mice were then observed daily for at least 14 days and those that showed signs of illness were euthanized and the brains were removed for extraction and subsequent passage in mice to amplify the virus. In more recent times, virus isolations have been made by routine propagation through embryonated eggs or mosquito (*Aedes albopictus* C6/36 or *Aedes pseudoscutellaris* AP 61), baby hamster kidney (BHK-21), African green monkey kidney epithelial (Vero), hamster kidney (CER), or swine kidney (PS) cell lines. Monolayers are observed daily until cytopathic effect (CPE) is observed, at which point the cell culture medium is clarified at low-speed centrifugation and aliquots of virus are stored frozen at −70 °C. Generally, the presence of virus has been verified by indirect immunofluorescent assays (IFAs) and electron microscopy.

Unknown viruses have been classified as members of the *Rhabdoviridae* by electron microscopy, based on their bullet-shaped morphology – a characteristic trait of members of this family (**Figure 1**). Subsequently, the assessment of antigenic relationships between these unknown viruses and other viruses worldwide has been performed using serological tests. Immune reagents have been developed for tentative assignment of the unclassified viruses by IFA, complement fixation (CF), virus neutralization (VNT) assays, hemagglutination inhibition (HI), and more recently enzyme-linked immunosorbent assays (ELISAs). However, many of these isolates have revealed no relationship with any known rhabdovirus. Up to seven different antigenic groups have been

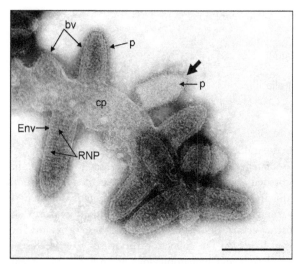

**Figure 1**  Electron micrograph of a negative-stained cell infected with Wongabel virus, representative of the nonassigned rhabdoviruses. Viruses are budding (bv) from a cell process (cp). The viruses are bullet-shaped, possess an envelope (Env), surface projections (peplomers) (p), and an internal helical ribonucleocapsid (RNP). The peplomers (p) consisting of trimers of viral glycoprotein can also be observed on the surface of the virus not penetrated by stain (short thick arrow). Scale = 200 nm. Electron micrograph courtesy 'Electron Microscopy and Iridoviruses Group', CSIRO-AAHL.

defined. Gene sequencing and phylogenetic relationships have been progressively applied to complete this initial virus taxonomy.

Other than the approved species, tentative species have been proposed in each of the four currently recognized genera of animal rhabdoviruses: 19 in the genus *Vesiculovirus*, 5 in the genus *Lyssavirus*, 3 in the genus *Ephemerovirus*, and 2 in the genus *Novirhabdovirus*. There remain six serogroups of animal rhabdoviruses (altogether comprising 20 different viruses) that have not yet been assigned to an existing genus: the Bahia Grande group, Hart Park group, Kern Canyon group, Le Dantec group, Sawgrass group, and Timbo group. A further 43 unassigned animal rhabdoviruses are listed in the *Eighth Report of the International Committee on Taxonomy of Viruses* (Eighth ICTV Report). Serological surveys conducted using sera collected from livestock, various wildlife and humans from Australia, Asia, and the Pacific region have revealed potential animal hosts and the geographical distribution for some of these viruses. However, for most of the uncharacterized rhabdoviruses information is limited. Although links between disease and the uncharacterized rhabdoviruses have not been made, recent studies have provided insights into their genetic composition and have revealed that wide genetic diversity exists among them, beckoning more intensive study of this family of viruses.

## Virion Properties

### Morphology

Rhabdovirus virions are 100–400 nm long and 50–100 nm in diameter (**Figure 1**). Viruses appear bullet-shaped. From the outer to the inner side of the virion, one can distinguish the envelope covered with viral glycoprotein spikes and, internally, the nucleocapsid with helical symmetry consisting of the nucleoprotein tightly bound to genomic RNA.

### Genome Organization and Genetics

All rhabdoviruses contain a genome consisting of a non-segmented single-stranded negative-sense RNA molecule with a size in the range of approximately 8.9–15 kbp. This RNA molecule contains at least five open reading frames (ORFs) encoding five virion proteins in the order (3'–5'): nucleoprotein (N); phosphoprotein (P); matrix protein (M); glycoprotein (G); and polymerase (L). Viruses in the genus *Ephemerovirus* contain several additional ORFs between the G and L genes, which encode a second glycoprotein ($G_{NS}$) and several other nonstructural proteins. Similarly, in the genus *Novirhabdovirus*, a sixth functional cistron between the G and L genes encodes a nonstructural protein (NV) of unknown function. The unclassified rhabdoviruses, sigma virus infecting flies (*Drosophila* spp.) and plant rhabdoviruses in the genera *Cytorhabdovirus* and *Nucleorhabdovirus* also contain an additional ORF which is located between the P and M genes. Flanders virus from mosquitoes (*Culista melanura*) has a complex arrangement of genes and pseudogenes in the same genome region. Nucleotide sequence analysis of Tupaia virus from the tree shrew (*Tipiai belangeri*) has identified an additional gene encoding a small hydrophobic protein between the M and G genes, and genome sequence analysis of Wongabel virus, an unassigned rhabdovirus isolated from biting midges (*Culicoides austropalpalis*), has revealed that it contains five additional genes that appear to be novel. The function of these other proteins (including additional glycoproteins) is not yet known. Therefore, despite preservation of a characteristic particle morphology, the *Rhabdoviridae* includes viruses that display a wide genetic diversity (**Figure 2**).

Relatively low sequence identities across the *Rhabdoviridae* prevent the construction of a family phylogeny. One approach to determining the phylogenetic relationships among the rhabdoviruses, as well as the identification of new viral species, is to utilize the conserved regions that have been identified in alignments of the N and L genes.

## Evolutionary Relationships

A molecular phylogenetic analysis of 56 rhabdoviruses, including 20 viruses which are currently unassigned or

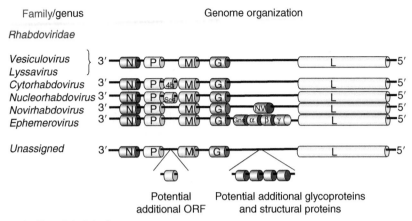

**Figure 2** Genome organization of rhabdoviruses.

**Table 1** Unassigned rhabdoviruses from Australia and Papua New Guinea

| Virus name | Isolated from | Neutralizing antibody detected | Year of isolation | Location |
|---|---|---|---|---|
| Almpiwar | *Ablepharus boutonii virgatus* (skink) | Skink, cattle, horse, sheep, kangaroo, bandicoot, various birds, human | 1966 | Mitchell River, Queensland |
| Charleville | *Phlebotomus* spp. (sand fly) *Gehyra australis* (gecko) *Lasiohelea* spp. (biting midge) | Human | 1969 | Charleville, Queensland |
| Coastal Plains | Cattle | Buffalo, cattle (Australia and Papua New Guinea) | 1981 | Beatrice Hill[a], Northern Territory |
| Humpty Doo | *C. marksi*, *Lasiohelea* spp. (biting midge) | Unknown | 1975 | Beatrice Hill, Northern Territory |
| Joinjakaka | Mixed Culicines (mosquito) | Cattle | 1966 | Sepik District, Papua New Guinea |
| Koolpinyah | Cattle (*Bos indicus* x *Bos taurus*) | Cattle | 1985 | Berrimah Farm, Northern Territory |
| Kununurra | *Ad. catasticta* (mosquito) | Unknown | 1973 | Kununurra, Western Australia |
| Ngaingan | *C. brevitarsis* (biting midge) | Wallaby, kangaroo, cattle | 1970 | Mitchell River, Queensland |
| Oak Vale | *Cx. edwardsi* (mosquito) | Ferral pigs | 1981 | Peachester, Queensland |
| Parry Creek | *Cx. annulirostris* (mosquito) | Unknown | 1973 | Kununurra, Western Australia |
| Tibrogargan | *C. brevitarsis* (biting midge) | Buffalo, cattle | 1976 | Peachester, Queensland |
| Wongabel | *C. austropalpalis* (biting midge) | Sea birds | 1979 | Wongabel, Queensland |
| CSIRO75 (Harrison Dam virus) | *Cx. annulirostris* (mosquito) | Unknown | 1975 | Beatrice Hill, Northern Territory |
| CSIRO1056 | *C. austropalpalis* (biting midge) | Unknown | 1981 | Samford, Queensland |
| DPP1163 (Holmes Jungle virus) | *Cx. annulirostris* (mosquito) | Cattle, buffalo, humans | 1987 | Darwin, Northern Territory |
| OR559 (Little Lilly Creek virus) | *Cx. annulirostris* (mosquito) | Unknown | 1974 | Kununurra, Western Australia |
| OR1023 (Ord River virus) | *Cx. annulirostris* (mosquito) | Unknown | 1976 | Kununurra, Western Australia |

[a]Beatrice Hill, NT has in the past been known as Coastal Plains.

assigned as tentative species within the *Rhabdoviridae*, has been reported by using the sequences from a region of block III of the L polymerase (**Table 1** and **Figure 3**). Block III is predicted to be essential for RNA polymerase function because it is conserved among all L proteins, and mutations in this region abolish polymerase activity. This phylogenetic analysis produced an evolutionary tree that generally, although not entirely, conforms to accepted serological

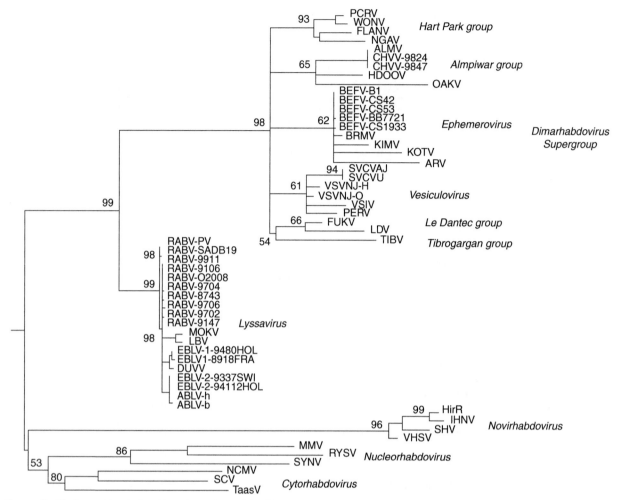

**Figure 3**  Phylogenetic relationships of members of the *Rhabdoviridae* based on a maximum likelihood analysis of a 158-amino-acid residue alignment of the L polymerase region. The established rhabdovirus genera as well as the newly proposed groups are indicated. Horizontal branches are drawn to scale and quartet puzzling frequencies are shown for key nodes (values in italics are for genera, groups, and supergroups, while all other quartet puzzling frequencies are shown in normal font). The tree is midpoint rooted for purposes of clarity only and all potential outgroup sequences were deemed too divergent to include in the analysis. Adapted from Bourhy H, Cowley JA, Larrous F, Holmes EC, and Walker PJ (2005) Phylogenetic relationships among rhabdoviruses inferred using the L polymerase gene. *Journal of General Virology* 86: 2849–2858.

groupings and taxa within the *Rhabdoviridae*. In particular, members of four genera – *Lyssavirus, Novirhabdovirus, Cytorhabdovirus,* and *Nucleorhabdovirus* – obtained from a variety of host species, including mammals, fish, arthropods, and plants, can be easily distinguished and fall into relatively well-supported clades. Although the vesiculoviruses and ephemeroviruses also fall into clear monophyletic groups, they are less well supported, and each genus contains some unclassified viruses. Furthermore, kotonkan virus, which causes clinical ephemeral fever in cattle but has previously been classified as a lyssavirus, is very clearly clustered with members of the genus *Ephemerovirus*. Lastly, there is some evidence that the two groups of plant rhabdoviruses – the cytorhabdoviruses and nucleorhabdoviruses – form a distinct clade. Taastrup virus which remains unassigned is related to cytorhabdoviruses.

Strikingly, this phylogenetic analysis has also identified four more monophyletic groups of currently unclassified rhabdoviruses, which have variable support values. First, Wongabel, Parry Creek, Flanders, and Ngaingan viruses formed a distinct cluster, with high levels of support. We refer to this as the Hart Park group, based on the serologic grouping of Flanders virus in the Hart Park serological group. Second, a tentatively named Almpiwar group containing Almpiwar, Humpty Doo, Charleville, and Oak Vale viruses was also identified. Although this grouping had a lower support, the Almpiwar and Charleville viruses possess almost indistinguishable sequences in the L gene region and each has been associated with infection in lizards. Another group, consisting of the Le Dantec and Fukuoka viruses, and herein referred to as the Le Dantec group, was also seen to form a distinct cluster. Finally, the phylogenetic position of Tibrogargan virus was ambiguous.

Common rhabdovirus sequence motifs have also been found in the central region of the N gene. Phylogenetic analysis of partial N gene sequences indicated that two viruses isolated from bats from various regions of the world, Oita virus and Mount Elgon bat virus, were grouped in a monophyletic cluster. Kolongo virus (Africa) and Sandjimba virus (Asia) also formed a distinct clade together with Tupaia virus (Asia). In this analysis, Flanders virus, sea trout virus, sigma virus, Kern Canyon virus, and Rochambeau virus remained isolated on the phylogenetic tree.

Phylogenetic analysis of both partial N and L gene sequences of Obodhiang virus and kotonkan virus has indicated that they should be classified as members of the genus *Ephemerovirus*.

## Host Range and Virus Propagation

### Transmission

Many of the rhabdoviruses replicate in and are transmitted by insect vectors. Plant-infecting rhabdoviruses are transmitted by vectors including aphids, planthoppers, and leafhoppers. Several animal rhabdoviruses (e.g., ephemeroviruses and vesiculoviruses) are known to be transmitted by hematophagous insects such as mosquitoes and biting midges. The widespread ability of rhabdoviruses to infect insects has led to the hypothesis that this virus family has evolved from an ancestral insect virus and that the host range is largely determined by the insect host. Sigma virus (SIGMAV) does not appear to have any vertebrate host but can be transmitted congenitally in flies (*Drosophila* spp.).

A number of important biological conclusions can be drawn from the rhabdovirus phylogeny based on the L gene. First, assuming a midpoint rooting of the tree, there is major split between those viruses that infect fish (novirhabdoviruses) or infect plants and employ arthropods as vectors (cytorhabdoviruses and nucleorhabdoviruses) – and those viruses that infect both mammals or lizards and dipterans (dimarhabdoviruses, sigla for dipteran-mammal-associated rhabdovirus). Such a division illuminates the biology of a number of key rhabdoviruses. For example, although vesicular stomatitis virus (VSV) is responsible for a disease of horses, cattle, and pigs, and can be transmitted directly by transcutaneous or transmucosal routes, the virus replicates in a wide range of hosts, including insects, and there is good evidence that VSV may employ insect vectors as at least one of its mechanisms of transmission. Similarly, bovine ephemeral fever virus, which is frequently found in Australasia and Africa, is also dipteran-transmitted, using vectors such as biting midges and culicine and anopheline mosquitoes. Finally, viruses assigned by the L-based phylogenetic analysis to the four

new groups (Le Dantec, Tibrogargan, Hart Park, and Almpiwar groups) have all been found to infect dipterans and in some cases also mammals (Tibrogargan, Le Dantec, and Ngaingan viruses) or lizards (Charleville virus).

Importantly, there is, as yet, no evidence for a virus making the link between plant rhabdoviruses, novirhabdoviruses of fish, or dimarhabdoviruses. Furthermore, the uncertainty over branching order at the root of the tree makes it difficult to determine whether the ancestral mode of transmission in rhabdoviruses was vector or nonvector transmission. However, the major phylogenetic division between these groups indicates that the biology of the rhabdoviruses could be strongly influenced by mode of transmission and by the host (plant, fish, or mammals) and vector species (orthopterans, homopterans, or dipterans).

## Clinical Features and Pathology

For most of the uncharacterized rhabdoviruses, links with disease have not yet been made. The only virus isolated from a natural infection in humans is Le Dantec virus. As indicated above, kotonkan virus causes clinical ephemeral fever in cattle and deer. Fukuoka virus has also been isolated from the blood of febrile calves.

## Serogroups of Nonassigned Rhabdoviruses (As Recognized in the Eighth ICTV Report)

### Hart Park Group

Phylogenetic analyses of the L gene have indicated that Flanders virus (FLANV), Ngaingan virus (NGAV), Parry Creek virus (PCV), and Wongabel virus (WONV) cluster with Hart Park virus (HPV) and are possible members of the Hart Park group. FLANV was isolated in 1961 from a pool of engorged female *Culista melanura* mosquitoes that were collected in Long Island, New York, USA. Similar viruses have been collected from different mosquito species in various parts of the United States. FLANV has also been isolated from the blood of house sparrows, red-winged blackbirds, and from the spleen of an oven bird. HPV was isolated in 1955 from a pool of female *Culex tarsalis* collected at Hart Park, California. NGAV (strain MRM14556) was isolated in 1970 from a pool of biting midges (*Culicoides brevitarsis*) that were collected at Mitchell River Aboriginal community in northern Queensland. This arbovirus has also been found to multiply in experimentally infected mosquitoes (*Aedes aegypti*). Serological surveys have indicated that NGAV infects wallabies, and possibly kangaroos and cattle, although its role in disease in these animals is unknown. IFA, CF, and VNT results place NGAV in the Tibrogargan antigenic group.

PCV (strain OR189) was isolated in 1973 from mosquitoes (*Culex annulirostris*) that were collected at Parry Creek near Kununurra, Western Australia. WONV (strain CSIRO264) was isolated in 1979 from biting midges (*Culicoides austropalpalis*) collected at Wongabel on the Atherton Tableland of northern Queensland. Morphological examination has revealed bullet-shaped particles $(80–90) \times (160–180)$ nm in dimension (**Figure 1**). This species of biting midge has been observed to have a feeding preference for birds. Although no link has been established between WONV and disease, neutralizing antibodies were detected in sea birds collected off the Great Barrier Reef. No neutralizing antibodies were detected in human sera from island residents in this region. Two other viruses, Mossuril virus (MOSV) and Kamese virus (KAMV), have been classified with the Hart Park group based on antigenic relationships only, as they were not included in any phylogenetic analysis. MOSV was first identified in 1959 in Mozambique and later in Central African Republic. It was isolated from mosquitoes (*Culex sitiens*, *Culex decens*, *Culex perfusus*, *Culex pruina*, *Culex telesilla*, *Culex Weschei*, and *Culex tigripes*) and birds (*Andropadus virens* and *Cliuspassrer maccrourus*). KAMV was first identified in Uganda in 1967 and then in Central African Republic. It has been isolated from culicine mosquitoes (*Culex annulioris*, *Aedes africanus*, *Culex decens*, *Culex perfuscus*, *Culex pruina*, and *Culex tigripes*).

## Le Dantec Group

At the L gene amino acid level, Fukuoka virus (FUKAV) and Le Dantec virus (LDV) appear to be related, although FUKAV was previously classified in the Kern Canyon group on the basis of its antigenic properties (see below). LDV was originally recovered in 1965 from a patient with a febrile illness, headaches, and spleen and liver hypertrophy in Senegal. In CF tests with other known rhabdoviruses, Le Dantec virus was found to be antigenically related to Keuraliba virus, a previously ungrouped agent isolated from rodents (*Tatera kempi*) in Senegal in 1968. FUKAV was first isolated from biting midges, *Culicoides punctalis* and *Culex tritaeniorhynchus* in 1986, and subsequently isolated from blood of calves with fever and leucopoenia.

## Bahia Grande Group

Bahia Grande (BGV) (prototype strain TB4–1054), Reed Ranch (RRV)(TB4–222), and Muir Springs (MSV) viruses (76V-23524) were first obtained from salt-marsh mosquitoes (*Culex*, *Aedes*, *Anopheles*, and *Psorophora* spp.) collected between 1972 and 1979 in west Texas, New Mexico, Louisiana, Colorado, North Dakota, and south Texas. Structural analysis of the prototype strain of BGV

from Texas has revealed five proteins. Comparative oligonucleotide fingerprint maps has shown 51–86% sharing of the large oligonucleotides between BGV (strain TB4–1054) and 11 other antigenically related isolates but not with MSV (strain 76V-23524), an antigenically distinct isolate from mosquitoes collected in Colorado. A serological survey for antibody to BGV has shown that humans, cattle, sheep, reptiles, and wild mammals from south Texas have neutralizing antibodies to this virus.

## Timbo Group

Chaco virus (CHOV) was isolated from *Ameiva ameiva ameiva* and *Kentropyx calcaratus* lizards in Brazil in 1962. Timbo virus (TIMV) was isolated from *Ameiva ameiva ameiva* lizards in Brazil. The optimal growth temperature of these viruses is approximately $30\,°C$.

## Sawgrass Group

New Minto virus (NMV) was isolated from *Haemaphysalis leporis-palustris* (Packard) ticks removed from snowshoe hares (*Lepus americanus* Erxleben) in east central Alaska in 1971. This virus is serologically (complement fixation and neutralization tests) related to Sawgrass virus. Sawgrass virus (SAWV) was isolated for the first time in Florida in 1964 from *Dermacentor variabilis* ticks removed from a raccoon, and later from *Haemophysalis leporis-palustris* ticks. Connecticut virus (CNTV) was first isolated in 1978 from a pool of nymphal *Ixodes dendatus* ticks removed from eastern cottontail rabbits (*Sylvilagus floridanus*) trapped in Connecticut, USA. Neutralizing antibodies have been detected in the eastern cottontail population in Connecticut, suggesting tick–rabbit maintenance cycle.

## Kern Canyon Group

Kern Canyon virus (KCV) was first isolated in 1956 from a pool of spleen and heart tissues from *Myotis yumanensis* bats in Kern County, California. KCV is not related to other groups or viruses classified in established genera according to the N gene phylogeny. Barur virus (BARV) was isolated from rodents (*Mus booduga*) and from ixodid ticks (*Haemaphysolis intermedia*) in 1961 in Mysore State, India and later, in 1971, from a pool of *Mansonia uniformis* mosquitoes in Kono Plain, Kenya. FUKAV was first grouped with KCV based on its antigenic properties. According to recent phylogenetic studies, it seems more related to the Le Dantec group. Nkolbisson virus (NKOV) was first isolated from *Aedes* sp., *Culex* sp., and *Eretmapodites* sp. mosquitoes in Cameroon in 1965. It was later isolated from Culicidea in the Ivory Coast, and from humans in the Republic of Central Africa.

## Other Groups as Proposed by Phylogenetic Analyses but Not Yet Recognized in the Eighth ITCV Report

### Almpiwar Group

Recent analysis of the L gene of different rhabdoviruses has suggested that Almpiwar virus (ALMV), Charleville virus (CHVV), Oak Vale virus (OVRV), and Humpty Doo virus (HDOOV) share a high genetic similarity, and they have been proposed to constitute the Almpiwar group.

ALMV (strain MRM4059) was isolated in 1966 from the skink *Ablepharus boutonii virgatus* at the low-lying plains of the Mitchell River Aboriginal community on the Gulf of Carpentaria in northern Queensland (**Figure 4**). Antibody to this virus has been detected in this species of skink. The virus optimally replicates at 30 °C in cell culture, which further supports the presumption that it is a reptilian virus. Although ALMV has never been isolated from arthropods, evidence of multiplication and passage of the virus in experimentally infected mosquitoes (*Culex fatigans*) supports the assumption that it is an arbovirus. No antigenic relationship has been found by complement fixation or neutralization test to any other known or suspected arboviruses. Although evidence indicates the presence of neutralizing antibodies to ALMV in sera from several different vertebrates, including humans, the significance of these results is considered uncertain. While ALMV and Charleville virus (CHVV) (see below) were each isolated from

lizards (of different species) captured at Mitchell River, the viruses appear to share no serological relationship.

CHVV (strain Ch9824) was initially isolated in 1969 from sandflies (*Phlebotomus* spp.) collected near Charleville in southern Queensland. The following year, CHVV was isolated from the heart, liver, and lung of a lizard (*Gehyra australis*), and from a pool of biting midges (*Lasiohelea* spp.), each collected at Mitchell River in northern Queensland. Multiplication of this virus was demonstrated in experimentally infected mosquitoes (*A. aegypti*), supporting the possibility that it may be an arbovirus. CHVV was analyzed by complement-fixation test against all known Australian arboviruses (including ALMV, see above) but no relationships were found. Limited evidence suggests the presence of neutralizing antibody to CHVV in humans (1 of 30 sera tested).

OVRV (strain CSIRO1342) was isolated on nine occasions in 1984 from mosquitoes (*Culex edwardsi*) that were collected near a sentinel cattle herd located at Peachester near Brisbane in Queensland. OVRV was also isolated once from mosquitoes (*Aedes vigilax*) in Darwin, Northern Territory in January 1984. OVRV is not neutralized by any antiserum prepared against known Australian arboviruses. However, antiserum to this virus has been shown to cross-react with Kimberley virus (genus *Ephemerovirus*) by IFA. No antibodies to OVRV were detected in cattle sera collected at the same time from the same area, but neutralizing antibodies were found in feral pigs. Although it has been suggested that OVRV may be cycling between mosquitoes and an undefined avian host, this virus did not successfully replicate in cattle egrets, unlike Kununurra virus (KNAV) which is also suspected to have an avian host.

Humpty Doo virus (strains CSIRO79 and 80) was isolated between the years 1974 and 1976 from biting midges (*Culicoides marksi* and *Lasiohelea* spp.) that were collected at Beatrice Hill, near Darwin in the Northern Territory.

### Tibrogargan Group

At the L amino acid level, Tibrogargan virus (TIBV) is likely to be a member of the proposed 'dimarhabdovirus supergroup'. However, it appears to be considerably different from the other members of this supergroup. Complement fixation tests have indicated that Coastal Plains virus (CPV) is serologically related to TIBV, but cross-neutralization tests using rabbit antisera prepared to each of these viruses indicated that they are distinct.

TIBV (prototype strain CSIRO132) was isolated from a pool of biting midges (*Culicoides brevitarsis*) that were collected during a 2-week summer period in 1976 at a farm near Peachester, near Brisbane, Queensland. Shortly after isolation, analysis of the virus by complement fixation and hemagglutination inhibition tests did not reveal any relationships with other known or suspected

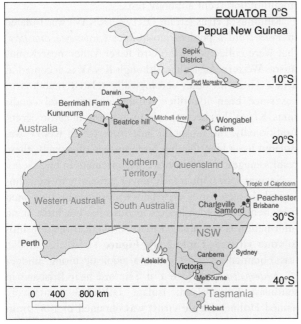

**Figure 4** Map of Australia and Papua New Guinea showing locations from which unassigned animal rhabdoviruses were isolated.

arboviruses from Australia, Papua New Guinea, or elsewhere in the world. However, further studies have indicated that TIBV and CPV are antigenically related, but distinguishable by VNT tests. Subsequent tests performed using sera collected during the mid-1970s indicated the presence of neutralizing antibodies to TIBV in cattle from New Guinea, and in a region from northern Australia spanning as far south as the central coast of New South Wales. This distribution mirrors the geographical distribution of the biting midge *C. brevitarsis*. Some sentinel cattle herds have been found to be up to 100% seropositive for neutralizing antibodies. Neutralizing antibodies were also found in water buffalo in far north Australia, but no evidence of neutralization has been found in sera from a range of other animal species including humans. Despite the high prevalence of neutralizing antibodies in the tested cattle and water buffalo, there are no records of the direct isolation of this virus from any vertebrate, and it has not been directly linked with disease.

CPV (strain DPP53) was isolated from the blood of a healthy steer (*Bos taurus*) in 1981 at Coastal Plains Research Station near Darwin in the Northern Territory. Although TIBV was isolated from biting midges, CPV was isolated directly from cattle and it is therefore not conclusively an arbovirus. However, the geographic distribution of neutralizing antibodies to CPV in cattle sera in Australia and Papua New Guinea appears to correspond to the distribution of the biting midge *C. brevitarsis*, which is the known vector of TIBV. Neutralizing antibody to CPV has also been detected in the sera of water buffalo, dogs, and one horse, but not in sera from humans, deer, pigs, or wallabies collected in the same areas.

### Mount Elgon Bat Virus Group

Nucleoprotein gene sequence analysis has indicated that Mount Elgon Bat virus (MEBV) and Oita virus (OITAV) form a distinct clade. Although they do not group by this analysis with the other vesiculoviruses, MEBV is currently classified as a tentative species of the genus *Vesiculovirus*. OITAV (296/1972) was isolated in 1972 from the blood of a wild horseshoe bat *Rhinolophus cornutus* (*Temminck*) in Japan. This virus causes lethal encephalitis in mice through the intracerebral route. MEBV was first isolated in 1964 in Kenya from bats (*Rhinolophus hildebrandtii*).

### Kolongo and Sandjimba Group

Kolongo virus (KOLV) and Sandjimba virus (SJAV) form a monophyletic clade based on analysis of the central region of the N gene. KOLV and SJAV were isolated in 1970 in Central African Republic from birds (*Euplected afra* and *Acrocephalus schoenbaeus*, respectively). Tupaia virus (TUPV) (a tentative species of the genus *Vesiculovirus* according to the Eighth ITCV Report) has been shown to join the same clade, although quite distantly.

### Other Nonassigned Rhabdoviruses

'Sigma virus' (SIGMAV) is the agent responsible for $CO_2$ sensitivity in *Drosophila melanogaster*. It is a noncontagious rhabdovirus which is transmitted through gametes.

Rochambeau virus (RBUV) was first isolated from mosquitoes (*Coquillettidia albicosta*) in French Guiana in 1973. It is classified as a tentative species of the genus *Lyssavirus* in the Eighth ICTV Report and is not related to any other dimarhadovirus, according to the phylogenetic analysis of the central region of the nucleoprotein.

Joinjakaka virus (strain MK7837) (JOIV) was isolated in 1966 from a pool of mixed mosquitoes (*Culicines*) that were aspirated from human bait at Joinjakaka, Sepik River District of Papua New Guinea. No relationship has been found between JOIV and any other known or putative arboviruses by complement fixation tests. Evidence suggests that cattle in Queensland have tested positive for antibody to JOIV by serum neutralization tests, but this study is not well documented.

Koolpinyah virus (KOOLV) was isolated from heparinized blood collected from two bulls (*Bos indicus-taurus* cross) at Berrimah Farm near Darwin in the Northern Territory in 1985 (strain DPP819) and 1986 (strain DPP883). In 1985, three additional bulls in the herd located at Berrimah developed neutralizing antibody to KOOLV, as did a sheep experimentally inoculated with blood from one of the bulls. KOOLV has been reported to be related serologically to Parry Creek virus (PCRV) and kotonkan virus (KOTV) by cross-neutralization tests, and to KOTV, PCRV, Obhodiang virus, and SJAV by indirect immunofluorescent antibody tests.

Kununurra virus (strain OR194) (KNAV) was isolated in 1973 from a pool of mosquitoes (*Aedeomyia catasticta*) that were collected in the Ord River Valley near Kununurra, Western Australia. Although KNAV is accepted as a new virus, no other serologically related rhabdovirus has since been identified. Under experimental conditions, KNAV has been shown to multiply in cattle egrets. Additionally, the mosquito host from which KNAV was isolated has a bird-feeding preference. Collectively, these results suggest that this virus may circulate in birds.

Several other apparently novel viruses with morphological characteristics of rhabdoviruses have been isolated from hematophagous insects in Australia but little or no information is available on their serological relationships to other viruses (**Table 2** and **Figure 1**). Isolate CS1056 was obtained in 1981 from a pool of biting midges (*C. austropalpalis*) collected at Samford near Brisbane in southeast Queensland. Isolate DPP1163 (tentatively named Holmes Jungle virus) was obtained in 1987 from mosquitoes (*C. annulirostris*) collected at Palm Creek near Darwin in the Northern Territory. Neutralizing antibody to this virus has been detected in cattle, buffalo, and humans, but there is no known association with

**Table 2**   Representative isolates of the genera and groups of rhabdoviruses used for the phylogenetic analysis of the L gene

| Genus | Name | UA /TS[a] | Abbreviation | Species from which it was isolated and from which neutralizing antibodies were identified | Origin[b] | Year of first isolation |
|---|---|---|---|---|---|---|
| Nucleorhabdovirus | Rice yellow stunt virus | | RYSV | Leafhopper | | |
| | Sonchus yellow net virus | | SYNV | Aphid | | |
| | Maize mosaic virus | | MMV | Leafhopper (Peregrinus maidis) | | |
| Cytorhabdovirus | Northern cereal mosaic virus | | NCMV | Leafhopper (Laodelphax striatellus) | Japan | |
| | Strawberry crinkle virus | | SCV | Aphid (Fragaria spp.) | Chile | |
| | Taastrup virus | UA | TaasV | Leafhopper (Psammottetix alienus) | Denmark | |
| Novirhabdovirus | Infectious hematopoietic necrosis virus | | IHNV | Rainbow trout (Onchorynchus mykiss)/ Invertebrate reservoirs? | | |
| | Viral hemorragic septicemia virus | | VHSV | Rainbow trout (Onchorynchus mykiss)/ Invertebrate reservoirs? | | |
| | Snakehead rhabdovirus | TS | SHV | Sneakhead fish (Ophicephalus striatus) | | |
| | Hirame rhabdovirus | UA | HirR | | | |
| Ephemerovirus | Adelaide River virus | | ARV | Bos taurus | Australia | 1981 |
| | Berrimah virus | | BRMV | Bos taurus | Australia | 1981 |
| | Kimberley virus | TS | KIMV | Bos taurus | Australia | 1980 |
| | Kotonkan virus | UA | KOTV | Culicoides species | Nigeria | 1967 |
| | Bovine ephemeral fever virus | | BEFV | Bos taurus, An. Bancrofti | Australia, China | 1968 |
| | Obodhiang virus | UA | OBOV | Mansonia uniformis | Sudan | 1963 |
| Almpiwar Group | Humpty Doo virus | UA | HDOOV | Lasiohelea species, Culicoides marski. cattle | Australia | 1975 |
| | Charleville virus | UA | CHVV | Phlebotomus species (sand fly), Lasiohelea species (biting midge) lizard (Gehyra australis), human | Australia | 1969 |
| | Almpiwar virus | UA | ALMV | Ablepharus boutonii virgatus, skink, cattle, horse, sheep, kangaroo, bandicoot, birds, human | Australia | 1966 |
| | Oak-Vale virus | UA | OVRV | Culex species, Culex edwardsi, Aedes vigilax, ferral pigs | Australia | 1981 |
| Tibrogargan Group | Tibrogargan virus | UA | TIBV | Culicoides brevitarsis, water buffaloes, cattle | Australia | 1976 |
| | Coastal Plains | UA | CPV | Cattle | Australia, Papua New Guinea | 1981 |
| Hart Park Group | Parry Creek virus | UA | PCRV | Culex annulirostris | Australia | 1972 |
| | Hart Park virus | UA | HPV | Culex tarsalis, birds | USA | 1955 |
| | Wongabel virus | UA | WONV | Culicoides austropalpalis, sea birds | Australia | 1979 |
| | Flanders virus | UA | FLANV | Culiseta melanura, Culex pipiens quinquefasciatus, Cx. salinarus, Cx. territans, Cx. restuans, Cx. tarsalis, Seiurus aurocapillus, birds | New York, USA | 1961 |

Continued

**Table 2**    Continued

| Genus | Name | UA /TS[a] | Abbreviation | Species from which it was isolated and from which neutralizing antibodies were identified | Origin[b] | Year of first isolation |
|---|---|---|---|---|---|---|
| | Ngaingan virus | UA | NGAV | *Culicoides brevitarsis*, wallaby, kangaroo, cattle | Australia | 1970 |
| | Mossuril virus | UA | MOSV | *Culex sitiens, Culex decens, Culex perfusus, Culex pruina, Culex telesilla, Culex weschei, Culex tigripes*, birds (*Andropadus virens* and *Cliuspassrer maccrourus*) | Mozambique, Central African Republic | 1959 |
| | Kamese virus | UA | KAMV | *Culex annulioris, Aedes africanus, Culex decens, Culex perfuscus, Culex pruina* and *Culex tigripes* | Uganda, Central African Republic | 1967 |
| Le Dantec and Kern Canyon Group | Le Dantec virus | UA | LDV | Human | Senegal | 1965 |
| | Fukuoka virus | UA | FUKV | *Culicoides punctatus*, calves | Japan | 1982 |
| | Keuraliba virus | UA | KEUV | Rodents (*Tatera kempi, taterillus* sp.) | Senegal | 1968 |
| *Vesiculovirus* | Perinet virus | TS | PERV | Mosquitoes: *Anopheles coustani, Culex antennatus, Culex gr pipiens, Mansonnia uniformis* Others: *Phlebotomus berentensis* | Madagascar | 1978 |
| | Vesicular stomatitis virus New Jersey | | VSNJV | *Sus scrofa* ; *Bos taurus, Culex nigripalpus, Culicoides species, Mansonia indubitans* | USA | 1949 |
| | Vesicular stomatitis virus Indiana | | VSIV | *Bos taurus* | USA | 1925 |
| | Spring viremia of carp virus | TS | SVCV | *Cyprinus carpio* | Yougoslavia | 1971 |
| *Lyssavirus* | Mokola virus | | MOKV | Cat | Zimbabwe | 1981 |
| | Lagos bat virus | | LBV | Bat (*Eidolon helvum*) | Nigeria | 1956 |
| | European Bat Lyssavirus subtype 1 | | EBLV-1 | Bat (*Eptesicus serotinus*) | | |
| | European Bat Lyssavirus subtype 2 | | EBLV-2 | Bat (*Myotis daubentonii, Myotis dasycneme*) | | |
| | Duvenhage virus | | DUVV | Human | Rep. South Africa | 1986 |
| | Australian bat lyssavirus | | ABLV | Human, bat (*Pteropus* species) | Australia | 1996 |
| | Rabies virus | | RABV | | | |

[a]UA, unassigned species and unclassified viruses; TS, tentative species.
[b]Precise location of isolates from Australia and Papua New Guinea is given on **Figure 4**.

disease. Isolate CSIRO75 (tentatively named Harrison Dam virus) was isolated in 1975 from mosquitoes (*C. annulirostris*) at Beatrice Hill, near Darwin in the Northern Territory. No information is available on the prevalence of antibodies in domestic or native animals. Isolate OR559 (tentatively named Little Lily Creek virus) was isolated from mosquitoes (*C. annulirostris*) collected at Kununurra in the Ord River region of Western Australia in 1974. Isolate OR1023 (tentatively named Ord River virus) was obtained in 1976, also from mosquitoes (*C. annulirostris*) collected at Kununurra. No other information is yet available about these viruses. Recent evidence suggests that KNAV might not be a rhabdovirus, but further studies are required to confirm this.

Two unassigned rhabdoviruses were isolated from birds during surveillance for arboviral encephalitis in the northeastern United States. Rhode Island virus strains RI-166 and RI-175 were each isolated from brain tissue of dead pigeons (*Columba livia*) collected at two localities in Rhode Island in summer 2000. Farmington virus designated CT-114 was originally isolated from an unknown wild bird captured in central Connecticut in 1969. Both viruses infect birds and mice, as well as monkey kidney cells in culture.

## Future Perspectives

The list of viruses described here is not complete and more viruses will certainly be characterized in the near future. Although there is strong phylogenetic support for the dimarhabdovirus supergroup, the precise branching order within this group cannot be resolved on the L or N gene data. Indeed, there is a clear need for further phylogenetic studies within the dimarhabdovirus supergroup, particularly with respect to the demarcation of genera, which currently is influenced more by genome structure than host/vector relationships. There is some evidence that some of these viruses contain additional genes that are not present in lyssaviruses and vesiculoviruses. Although the functions of these additional proteins are not understood, revealing the evolution of genome complexity may be an important factor in resolving the taxonomy of this supergroup.

## Further Reading

Bourhy H, Cowley JA, Larrous F, Holmes EC, and Walker PJ (2005) Phylogenetic relationships among rhabdoviruses inferred using the L polymerase gene. *Journal of General Virology* 86: 2849–2858.

Calisher CH, Karabatsos N, Zeller H, *et al.* (1989) Antigenic relationships among rhabdoviruses from vertebrates and hematophagous arthropods. *Intervirology* 30: 241–257.

Fu ZF (2005) Genetic comparison of the rhabdoviruses from animals and plants. In: Fu ZF (ed.) *Current Topics in Microbiology and Immunology, Vol. 292: The World of Rhabdoviruses*, p. 1. Berlin: Springer.

Hogenhout SA, Redinbaugh MG, and Ammar ED (2003) Plant and animal rhabdovirus host range: A bug's view. *Trends in Microbiology* 11: 264–271.

Karabatsos N (1985) *International Catalogue of Arboviruses Including Certain Other Viruses of Vertebrates*. San Antonio, TX: American Society of Tropical Medicine and Hygiene.

Kuzmin IV, Hughes GJ, and Rupprecht CE (2006) Phylogenetic relationships of seven previously unclassified viruses within the family *Rhabdoviridae* using partial nucleoprotein gene sequences. *Journal of General Virology* 87: 2323–2331.

## Relevant Websites

http://www.pasteur.fr – CRORA Report. This report involves all the data collected by Pasteur Institute and ORSTOM, since 1962, more than 6000 isolated strains of 188 arboviruses or mixed arboviruses. For each virus identified by the CRORA, all the observed hosts or vectors are given, with the number of collected strains in each country, viral properties of collected strains, and bibliographical references concerning them.

http://www.ncbi.nlm.nih.gov – ICTV database on *Rhabdoviridae*, International Committee on Taxonomy of Viruses, NCBI.

# Arteriviruses

**M A Brinton,** Georgia State University, Atlanta, GA, USA
**E J Snijder,** Leiden University Medical Center, Leiden, The Netherlands

## History

Equine arteritis virus (EAV) was first isolated in 1953 in Bucyrus, Ohio from the lung tissues of an aborted fetus during an epidemic of abortions and arteritis in pregnant mares. However, an equine disease similar to that caused by EAV was first observed in the late 1800s. At the time of its discovery, EAV was distinguished from equine (abortion) influenza virus.

Lactate dehydrogenase-elevating virus (LDV) was discovered by accident in 1960 during a study to find methods for early detection of tumors in mice. A five- to tenfold increase in lactate dehydrogenase (LDH) levels in serum 4 days after inoculation of mice with either Ehrlich carcinoma cells or cell-free extracts suggested that an infectious agent was responsible for the observed LDH elevation.

Porcine respiratory and reproductive syndrome was first observed in North America in 1987 and in Europe in 1990. This disease has also been referred to as porcine epidemic abortion and respiratory syndrome (PEARS), swine infertility and respiratory syndrome (SIRS), and mystery swine disease (MSD). The causative agent of the disease is now referred to as porcine respiratory and reproductive syndrome virus (PRRSV).

Simian hemorrhagic fever virus (SHFV) was isolated in 1964 during outbreaks of a fatal hemorrhagic fever disease in macaque colonies in the US, Russia, and Europe. A number of additional SHFV outbreaks in macaque colonies have occurred since the 1960s. The most 'famous' of these was the one in Reston, Virginia, which occurred in conjunction with an Ebola virus outbreak in the same facility.

## Taxonomy and Classification

On the basis of virion size and morphology as well as the positive polarity of the RNA genome, LDV and EAV were originally classified within the family *Togaviridae*. In 1996, following the sequence analysis of their genomes, EAV, LDV, SHFV, and PRRSV were classified as species within a new family, *Arteriviridae*, genus *Arterivirus*. EAV was designated the prototype of this family. At the same time, the family *Arteriviridae* was classified together with the family *Coronaviridae* in the order *Nidovirales*. This order also includes two additional virus groups, the toroviruses (a genus in the *Coronaviridae* family) and the family *Roniviridae*. The arterivirus genome shares similar general organizational features and conserved replicase motifs with corona-, toro-, and ronivirus genomes, but is only about half their size. In addition, arterivirus particles are smaller than those of other nidoviruses, differ from them morphologically, and are the only ones to have an isometric nucleocapsid structure.

## Geographic Distribution

Viruses with biological properties identical to those of LDV have been isolated from small groups of wild mice (*Mus musculus*) in Australia, Germany, the US, and UK. Natural infections with EAV and EAV-induced disease in horses and donkeys have been documented in North America, Europe, and Japan and anti-EAV antibodies have been detected in horse sera from Africa and South America, indicating that EAV infection is geographically widespread. Natural PRRSV infections in pigs have been reported in North America, Europe, and Asia. SHFV infection in captive patas monkeys has been documented and this virus has also been detected in the blood of wild-caught patas and African green monkey as well as baboons, suggesting that these African primates are the natural hosts for SHFV.

## Host Range and Virus Propagation

Natural infections with EAV occur only in horses and donkeys. Field isolates of EAV can be readily obtained from field samples (semen, fetal tissues, and buffy coats) using RK-13 cells. Laboratory strains of EAV have been successfully grown in primary cultures of horse macrophages and kidney cells, rabbit kidney cells, and hamster kidney cells and also in cell lines, such as BHK-21, RK-13, MA-104, and Vero.

LDV replicates efficiently in all strains of laboratory and wild *Mus musculus* and somewhat less efficiently in the Asian mouse *Mus caroli*. Numerous attempts to infect other rodents such as rats, hamsters, guinea pigs, rabbits, deer

mice (*Peromyscus maniculatus*), and dwarf hamsters (*Phodopus sungorus*) with LDV have not been successful. LDV replicates only in primary murine cell cultures that contain macrophages, such as spleen, bone marrow, embryo fibroblast, and peritoneal exudate cell cultures. Although peritoneal cultures prepared from starch-stimulated adult mice contain 95% phagocytic cells, only 6–20% of these cells support LDV replication as demonstrated by autoradiographic, *in situ* hybridization, immunofluorescence and electron microscopic techniques, suggesting that LDV infects an as yet uncharacterized subpopulation of macrophages. A much higher percentage of cells in peritoneal exudate cells obtained from infant mice are susceptible to virus infection.

Natural infections with PRRSV were thought to be restricted to pigs. However, one report suggested that chickens and mallard ducks may be susceptible to the virus. PRRSV can replicate in primary cultures of porcine alveolar macrophages and macrophages from other tissues. Some, but not all, isolates of PRRSV can be adapted to replicate in a subclone of the MA-104 cell line.

Natural infections with SHFV occur in several species of African primates, namely *Erythrocebus patas*, *Cercopithecus aethiops*, *Papio anuibus* and *Papio cynocephalus*. SHFV infection of members of the genus *Macaca* has occurred in primate facilities in a number of countries and was associated with a fatal hemorrhagic fever. Isolates of SHFV can replicate in primary cultures of rhesus aveolar lung macrophages or peripheral macrophages and some isolates can replicate efficiently in the MA-104 cell line.

Maximum arterivirus yields after infection of susceptible cell cultures are observed by 10–15 h after infection. The maximum titers obtained for LDV and PRRSV are $10^6$–$10^7$ $ID_{50}$ ml$^{-1}$ and can exceed $10^8$ PFU ml$^{-1}$ for EAV and SHFV.

## Properties of the Virion

Arterivirus particles are spherical, enveloped, and 40–60 nm in diameter (**Figures 1(a)** and **1(b)**). Unfixed virions undergo distortion and disintegration during standard negative staining procedures. The virion surface appears rather smooth. The virion capsid is icosahedral and about 25–35 nm in diameter. Buoyant densities of 1.13–1.17 g cm$^{-3}$ and sedimentation coefficients of 214S to 230S have been reported for arteriviruses. Virions can be stored indefinitely at −70 °C but are heat labile. For instance, the infectivity of LDV samples in plasma decreased by half after 4 weeks at −20 °C and by about 3.5 logs after storage for 32 days at 4 °C. Virus in media supplemented with 10% serum is stable for 24 h at room temperature, but completely inactivated by heating at 58 °C for 1 h. Virions are fairly stable between pH 6 and pH 7.5, but are rapidly inactivated by high or low pH.

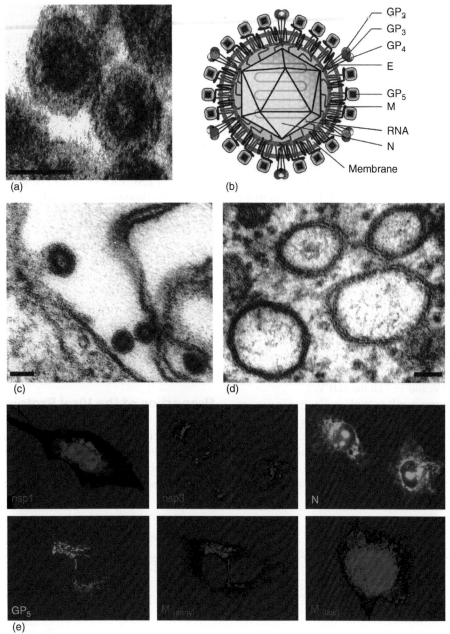

**Figure 1** (a) An electron micrograph of extracellular PRRSV particles. (b) Schematic representation of an arterivirus particle and its seven structural proteins. (c) An electron micrograph of EAV particles budding from smooth membranes in (or close to) the Golgi region of infected baby hamster kidney cells (BHK-21) cells. (d) An electron micrograph of typical double-membrane vesicles found in the cytoplasm of arterivirus-infected cells that have been implicated in replication complex formation and viral RNA synthesis. (e) Localization of selected EAV nonstructural and structural proteins in infected BHK-21 cells by immunofluorescence microscopy. In contrast to all other nsps (e.g., nsp3), the N-terminal replicase subunit nsp1 only partially localizes to the perinuclear region and is partially targeted to the nucleus. The double-labeling for nsp3 and the N protein shows that a considerable part of the latter co-localizes with the viral replication complex, whereas another fraction of the N protein is targeted to the nucleus. Early in infection, double-labeling for the major glycoprotein GP$_5$ and the M protein showed almost complete co-localization of the two proteins in the Golgi complex, in the form of the heterodimer that has been found to be critical for virus assembly. Later in infection, the M protein accumulates in the endoplasmic reticulum. Scale = 50 nm (a, c–d). (a) Reprinted from Snijder EJ and Meulenberg JM (1998) The molecular biology of arteriviruses. *Journal of General Virology* 79: 961–979. (b) Reprinted from Snijder EJ, Siddell SG, and Gorbalenya AE (2005) The order Nidovirales. In: Mahy BWJ and ter Meulen V (eds.) *Topley and Wilson's Microbiology and Microbial Infections, Vol. 1: Virology*, 10th edn., pp. 390–404. London: Hodder Arnold. (c, d) Reprinted from Snijder EJ and Meulenberg JM (1998) The molecular biology of arteriviruses. *Journal of General Virology* 79: 961–979. (e) Images courtesy of Yvonne van der Meer and Jessika Zevenhoven, Leiden University Medical Center, The Netherlands.

Virus is efficiently disrupted by low concentrations of nonionic detergent.

The locations of the seven structural proteins in an EAV virion are indicated schematically in **Figure 1(b)**. The icosahedral capsid is composed of the nucleocapsid (N) protein. The major envelope glycoproteins, $GP_5$ and M, form a disulfide-linked heterodimer. The minor glycoproteins $GP_2$, $GP_3$, and $GP_4$ form a disulfide-linked heterotrimer. $GP_2$–$GP_4$ heterodimers have also been detected in EAV virions. Although all six of these proteins were shown to be required for EAV and PRRSV infectivity, not all of the minor structural proteins have been identified so far in the other arteriviruses and the nomenclature for the SHFV structural proteins differs due to an insertion in the 3' region of the SHFV genome. Virions bud into the lumen of cytoplasmic vesicles (**Figure 1(c)**).

## Properties of the Genome

Arterivirus genomes are single-stranded RNAs of positive polarity that contain a 3' poly(A) tract of approximately 50 nucleotides in length and a type I cap at the 5' end. The genome lengths are 12.7 kb for EAV, 14.1 kb for LDV, 15.1 kb for PRRSV, and 15.7 kb for SHFV.

The large nonstructural or 'replicase' polyproteins are encoded by open reading frames (ORFs) 1a and 1b and occupy the 5' three-fourths of the genome. ORF 1b is translated only when a −1 ribosomal frameshift occurs in the short ORF 1a/ORF 1b overlap region. A 'slippery sequence' upstream of a pseudoknot directs frameshifting

and for EAV, a frameshifting efficiency of 15–20% has been reported. ORF 1a encodes three or four proteases that post-translationally cleave the pp1a and pp1ab polyproteins at multiple sites into the mature viral nonstructural proteins (**Figure 2**). The lengths of the ORF 1a regions of the different arteriviruses vary. ORF 1b encodes major conserved domains, in particular an RNA-dependent RNA polymerase, a putative zinc-binding domain, an RNA helicase, and a nidovirus uridylate-specific endoribonuclease. The multiple 3'-proximal ORFs (**Figure 2**) encode the structural proteins. There are six such ORFs in the genomes of EAV, PRRSV, and LDV, while SHFV contains nine ORFs downstream of ORF 1b. Limited sequence homology suggests that the SHFV ORFs 2a, 2b, and 3 may be duplications of ORFs 4, 5, and 6, respectively. In most cases, adjacent structural protein genes of arteriviruses are in different reading frames and overlap. Conserved transcription-regulating sequences (TRSs; **Figure 3**) are located at the 3' end of the genomic leader sequence (leader TRS) and upstream of each of the 3'-proximal ORFs (body TRSs). RNA hairpin structures are located near the 5' end of the genome (including a leader TRS-presenting hairpin) and also in the 3' NTR.

## Properties of the Viral Proteins

Arterivirus proteins that are encoded at the 5' end of the genome are translated directly from the genomic RNA as polyproteins (pp1a and pp1ab; **Figure 2**). The proteins generated from these ORFs contain all functions

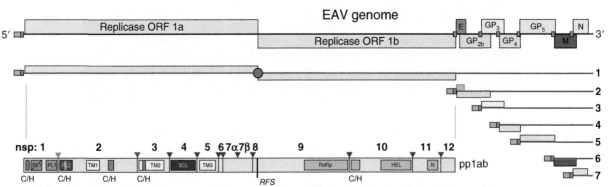

**Figure 2** Arterivirus genome organization and expression are illustrated using the family prototype EAV as an example. The genomic open reading frames are indicated and the names of the corresponding proteins are given. Below the genome, the nested set of mRNAs found in infected cells is depicted, with RNA1 being identical to the viral genome and subgenomic RNAs 2–7 being used to express the structural protein genes located in the 3'-proximal quarter of the genome. With the exception of the bicistronic mRNA2, the subgenomic mRNAs are functionally monocistronic. The EAV replicase gene organization is depicted in the polyprotein pp1ab from the replicase (pp1a is identical to the nsp1–8 region of pp1ab). Ribosomal frameshift (RFS) delineates the boundary between amino acids encoded in ORF 1a and ORF 1b and arrows represent sites in pp1ab that are cleaved by papain-like proteases (yellow and blue) or the main (3CL) protease (red). The proteolytic cleavage products (nsps) are numbered and the locations of various conserved domains are highlighted. These include domains with conserved Cys and His residues (C/H), putative transmembrane domains (TM), protease domains (PL1, PL2, and 3CL), the RNA-dependent RNA polymerase domain (RdRp), helicase (HEL), and uridylate-specific endoribonuclease (N). Adapted from Siddell SG, Ziebuhr J, and Snijder EJ (2005) Coronaviruses, toroviruses, and arteriviruses. In: Mahy BWJ and ter Meulen V (eds.) *Topley and Wilson's Microbiology and Microbial Infections, Vol. 1: Virology*, 10th edn., pp. 823–856. London: Hodder Arnold.

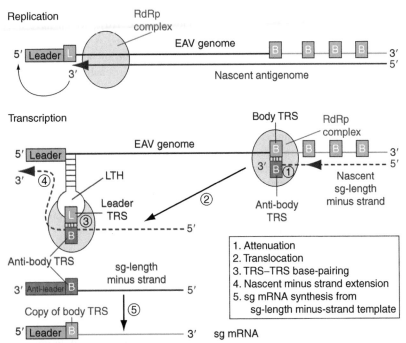

**Figure 3** Arterivirus RNA synthesis (using a hypothetical virus that produces four subgenomic (sg) mRNAs). Both replication (top panel) and transcription (bottom panel) are depicted. In the 'replication mode', the RdRp produced a full-length minus-strand RNA (antigenome) that serves as the template for synthesis of new genomic RNA. In the 'transcription mode', minus-strand RNA synthesis is thought to be discontinuous and regulated by transcription-regulating sequences (TRSs). Body TRSs (B) in the genome would act as attenuators of minus-strand RNA synthesis. Subsequently, the nascent minus strand, with an anti-body TRS at its 3′ end, would be redirected to the 5′-proximal region of the genomic template by a base-pairing interaction with the leader TRS (L) that (for EAV) has been shown to reside in a leader TRS hairpin (LTH) structure. Following the addition of the anti-leader to the nascent minus strands, the sg-length minus strands would then serve as templates for sg mRNA synthesis.

required for viral RNA synthesis. Both pp1a/pp1ab contain multiple papain-like cysteine proteases and a chymotrypsin-like (or '3C-like') serine protease (**Figure 2**). The EAV papain-like cysteine proteases each cleave at a single site. The nsp4 serine protease, or main protease, cleaves at six sites in the pp1a region and at three additional sites in the ORF 1b-encoded part of pp1ab. Due to the existence of two alternative processing cascades (minor and major pathways) a variety of processing intermediates and mature proteins are generated from the C-terminal half of pp1a. In total, 13 (EAV) or 14 (PRRSV/LDV) mature proteins are (predicted to be) generated from the arterivirus replicase polyproteins. Three hydrophobic regions in pp1a are thought to be important for membrane association of the viral replication–transcription complexes. With the exception of nsp1, which is partly found in the nucleus, the rest of the nonstructural proteins localize to endoplasmic reticulum-derived double-membrane structures (**Figure 1(d)**) in the perinuclear region (**Figure 1(e)**). The mature ORF 1b-encoded proteins (nsp9–nsp12) are thought to be the primary enzymes of the viral replication–transcription complexes that direct viral RNA synthesis.

The proteins encoded in the 3′-proximal quarter of the genome are expressed from six (nine for SHFV) overlapping subgenomic mRNAs (a 3′ co-terminal nested set; **Figure 2**). Although the subgenomic mRNAs, with the exception of the smallest one, are structurally polycistronic, in general only the 5′ terminal ORF is translated. An exception is mRNA 2, which is bicistronic encoding $GP_{2b}$ and E. The nucleocapsid (N) protein is encoded by ORF 7 (ORF 9 in SHFV). Analysis of the crystal structure of the C-terminal domain of the PRRSV N protein suggests that arteriviruses have a unique capsid-forming domain. The M protein which is encoded by ORF 6 (ORF 8 in SHFV), is a triple-membrane-spanning protein and the major nonglycosylated envelope protein. The major envelope glycoprotein is encoded by ORF 5 (ORF 7 in SHFV). $GP_{2b}$, $GP_3$, and $GP_4$ are each about 20 kDa in size and are minor envelope glycoproteins (EAV, **Figure 2**). $GP_{2b}$ and $GP_4$ ($GP_{4b}$ and $GP_6$ in SHFV) are class I integral membrane proteins. A soluble, non-virion-associated form of PRRSV $GP_3$ is released from infected cells. E is an unglycosylated small hydrophobic minor envelope protein. The PRRSV E protein has been shown to possess ion channel protein-like properties.

The nonstructural protein nsp1 and the N protein have been detected in the nucleus as well as the cytoplasm (**Figure 1(e)**). However, the biological significance of the nuclear localization of these two viral proteins is currently not known.

## Replication

Cell tropism is determined in part at the level of a receptor on the cell surface, since in some cases cells that are nonpermissive for an arterivirus have been reported to be productively infected after transfection of viral genomic RNA. Evidence for a specific saturable, but as yet unidentified receptor for LDV on a subpopulation of murine macrophages has been reported. LDV-immune complexes are also infectious and can infect macrophages via Fc receptors. Sialoadhesin (sialic acid-dependent lectin-like receptor 1), a macrophage-restricted, cell surface protein, has been shown to mediate the internalization of PRRSV by alveolar macrophages. Heparin sulphate on the cell surface and sialic acid on the virion are also thought to play a role in entry. PRRSV has been reported to enter cells via a low pH-dependent endocytic pathway. Soon after infection, both EAV and LDV particles have been observed in small vesicles that appear to be clathrin-coated. The existence of an additional level of host restriction at the endosomal membrane fusion or uncoating steps was suggested by the observation that nonsusceptible cells expressing recombinant sialoadhesin could internalize virus but rarely became productively infected.

The arterivirus replication cycle occurs in the cytoplasm of infected cells. After the incoming genomic RNA is uncoated, it is translated to produce polyproteins pp1a (1727–2502 amino acids) and pp1ab (3175–3959 amino acids) and then becomes the template for minus-strand synthesis (**Figure 3**). Either a full-length minus-strand RNA, that then serves as a template for genomic RNA synthesis, or subgenomic minus strands, that then serve as the templates for subgenomic mRNA synthesis, can be produced. The subgenomic RNAs are thought to be produced by a mechanism of discontinuous minus-strand RNA synthesis that utilizes conserved primary (TRSs) and higher-order RNA structures as signals for producing a subgenomic minus-strand template for each subgenomic mRNA. Subgenomic mRNAs are 3′-coterminal and contain a common 5′ leader sequence that is identical to the 5′ terminus of the genomic RNA. *cis*-Acting regulatory signals required for arterivirus replication have been mapped to the ~300 nt at each end of the genome. Host proteins also appear to be involved in the regulation of arterivirus RNA synthesis.

The co-localization of N with replicase complexes (**Figure 1(e)**) suggests that genome encapsidation may be coordinated with genome synthesis. New virions form via budding of preformed capsids into the lumens of smooth endoplasmic reticulum and/or Golgi complex membranes (**Figure 1(c)**). Arterivirus envelope proteins localize to intracellular membranes and recent data suggest that the formation of the GP$_5$–M heterodimer is required for budding (**Figure 1(e)**). Mature virions in the lumens of these vesicles are then transported to the exterior of the cell and released.

The formation of cytoplasmic double-membrane vesicles (**Figure 1(d)**), which have been implicated in viral RNA synthesis, is characteristic of arterivirus-infected cells. Infection of primary macrophages by EAV, SHFV, PRRSV, and probably also LDV is cytocidal. Laboratory strains of EAV, SHFV, and PRRSV cause obvious cytopathology in the continuous cell cultures that they infect, such as MA-104 cells. Infected cells become rounded by 24–36 h after infection and release from the tissue culture flask. Apoptosis has been reported in PRRSV-infected primary porcine alveolar macrophages and MA-104 cell cultures as well as in testicular germ cells in pigs. However, other studies with PRRSV showed that necrosis, not apoptosis, was the main cause of death of infected cells.

## Genetics

Evidence for virulence variants of all arteriviruses has been obtained. One strain of LDV isolated from C58 tumor-bearing mice and designated LDV-C was shown to efficiently induce neurologic disease in a few susceptible inbred mouse strains, such as AKR and C58, both of which are homozygous for the *Fv-1$^n$* allele. Subsequent studies showed that neuropathogenic and non-neuropathogenic isolates coexist in most LDV pools. The number of glycosylation sites in the ectodomain of GP$_5$ varies in different LDV strains and it has been postulated that antibodies bind less efficiently to virions with extensive glycosylation in this region. A neurovirulent strain of PRRSV has also been reported. Virulent and avirulent mutants of EAV have been identified on the basis of the severity of the diseases they cause. Attenuated vaccine strains of EAV and PRRSV and a number of temperature-sensitive mutants of EAV have been selected. SHFV isolates that produce acute asymptomatic infections and ones that cause persistent, asymptomatic infections in patas monkeys have been reported. EAV and PRRSV infectious cDNA clones have been constructed and provide a means for analyzing the virulence determinants via reverse genetics.

## Evolution

Evidence of RNA recombination has been obtained by genome sequencing for both LDV and PRRSV after co-infections with different strains of the same virus type and it is thought that RNA recombination is the mechanism responsible for the observed gene duplication in the SHFV genome. Sequence comparisons of various field isolates of either PRRSV or EAV indicate that the sequences of the M and N proteins are more conserved than those of the virion glycoproteins. The extent of the divergence of the sequences of European and North

American PRRSV isolates indicates that these two virus populations represent subspecies and also suggests that the ability to cause porcine disease arose independently in geographically separated virus populations. Phylogenetic analysis of the arteriviruses indicated that PRRSV is most closely related to LDV and that SHFV is more closely related to both of these viruses than to EAV. Although the host specificity of LDV has experimentally been shown to be restricted to mouse species, it has been postulated that PRRSV arose when wild boars became infected with LDV after they ate infected wild mice and that wild boars then introduced a divergent 'LDV' virus into domestic pigs independently in North America and Europe.

The nidoviruses represent a distinct evolutionary lineage among positive-strand RNA viruses. Although the organization of the conserved replicase motifs in the arterivirus genome is very similar to that of the other nidoviruses (coronaviruses, toroviruses, and roniviruses), the structural protein genes of these viruses are apparently unrelated (**Figure 1**). This level of divergence may be related to a high frequency of RNA recombination that appears to be a characteristic of nidovirus replicases and may be a byproduct of the mechanism of discontinuous RNA synthesis utilized by these viruses for subgenomic RNA production. The ancestral nidovirus has been postulated to have had an icosahedral capsid. If via a recombination event with another type of virus, the progenitor of the coronavirus/torovirus lineage acquired an N protein that could form a helical nucleocapsid, then packaging restrictions on genome size would have been lost, allowing genome size expansion via further recombination events and divergence from the arterivirus branch.

### Serologic Relationships and Variability

Attempts to demonstrate antigenic cross-reactivity between EAV, LDV, PRRSV, and SHFV have not been successful with one exception. Antibodies produced to a single linear LDV neutralization site located in $GP_5$ neutralized both LDV and PRRSV. Monoclonal antibodies elicited by one strain of LDV did not bind to the proteins of most other LDV isolates in Western blots, suggesting that serologic variants of LDV exist. Variation in PRRSV N epitopes has been observed between North American and European virus isolates and a high degree of heterogeneity has been observed between strains of PRRSV within the ectodomain of $GP_4$, which contains a secondary neutralization epitope.

### Transmission

There is no evidence for transmission of any of the arteriviruses via insect vectors. Horizontal transmission of both EAV and PRRSV occur via the respiratory route as well as via the venereal route by virus in the semen of persistently infected 'carrier' males. Vertical transmission of PRRSV *in utero* has been reported.

Nothing is currently known about the incidence of transmission of LDV in wild mouse populations. In the laboratory, unless the cage mates are fighting males, LDV is rarely transmitted between mice housed in the same cage, even though infected mice excrete virus in their feces, urine, milk, and saliva. However, transmission of LDV from mother to the fetus via the placenta and to pups via breast milk/saliva has been documented within the first week after infection of the mother. Since LDV in mice and SHFV in patas monkeys is produced throughout the lifetime of persistently infected animals, the transfer of fluids or tissues from an infected animal to an uninfected one results in the inadvertent transfer of infection. Historically the most frequent mode of transmission of LDV among laboratory mice and SHFV from patas monkeys to macaques has been through experimental procedures such as the use of the same needle for sequential inoculation of several animals. Currently, the most frequent sources of LDV contamination are pools of other infectious agents or tumor cell lines that have been repeatedly passaged in mice, especially those first isolated in the 1950s. Such materials should be checked for the presence of LDV. Infectious agent stocks can be 'cured' of LDV by passage in a continuous cell line or a different animal species. Tumor cell stocks can be 'cured' by *in vitro* culture for several passages. It has been suggested but not proven that SHFV can be transmitted between macaques via the respiratory route.

### Tissue Tropism

The primary target cells for all four arteriviruses are macrophages. Measurement of the amount of virus in various tissues during natural EAV infections indicated that lung macrophages and endothelial cells were the first host cells to be infected. Bronchial lymph nodes subsequently became infected and then the virus spread throughout the body via the circulatory system. In fatally infected horses, lesions are found in subcutaneous tissues, lymph nodes, and viscera. The progression of PRRSV infection in pigs is likely to be similar to that observed with EAV. However, although PRRSV is thought to be naturally transmitted by aerosols, experimental transmission by this route has been difficult to achieve. PRRSV has been reported to replicate in testicular germ cells which could result in excretion of virus into the semen. LDV replicates in an uncharacterized subpopulation of murine macrophages. Virus target cells are located in tissues as well as in the blood. Cells containing LDV-specific antigen have been identified in sections of liver and spleen by indirect immunofluorescence. In spleen, the virus-infected cells are nucleated and located in the red pulp. In liver, only Kupffer cells contained LDV-specific antigen. In C58 and AKR mice infected with a neurotropic strain of LDV, virus replication was demonstrated in ventral motor neurons by *in situ* hybridization.

## Pathogenicity and Clinical Features of Infection

Serological evidence indicates that even though EAV is widespread in the horse population, it rarely causes clinical disease. Both EAV and PRRSV can cause either persistent asymptomatic infections or induce various disease symptoms such as respiratory disease, fever, necrosis of small muscular arteries, and abortion. The severity of disease caused by EAV and PRRSV depends on the strain of virus as well as the condition and age of the animal. The most common symptoms of natural EAV infections in horses are anorexia, depression, fever, conjunctivitis, edema of the limbs and genitals, rhinitis, enteritis, colitis, and necrosis of small arteries. If clinical symptoms occur, they are most severe in young animals and pregnant mares. Infections in pregnant mares are often inapparent, but result in a high percentage (50%) of abortions. Young animals occasionally develop a fatal bronchopneumonia after infection, but natural infections are not usually life-threatening. In contrast, about 40% of pregnant mares and foals experimentally inoculated with EAV die as a result of the infection. Horses infected with virulent EAV isolates develop a high fever, lymphopenia, and severe disease symptoms. Symptoms observed in PRRSV-infected pigs include fever, anorexia, labored breathing, and lymphadenopathy. Lesions are observed in the lungs and infected pregnant sows produce weak or stillborn piglets.

Mice infected with LDV usually display no overt symptoms of disease. A distinguishing feature of LDV infections is the chronically elevated levels of seven serum enzymes, LDH (eight- to tenfold), isocitrate dehydrogenase (five- to eightfold), malate dehydrogenase (two- to threefold), phosphoglucose isomerase (two- to threefold), glutathione reductase (two- to threefold), aspartate transaminase (two- to threefold), and glutamate-oxaloacetate transaminase (two- to threefold). A decrease in the humoral and cellular immune response to non-LDV antigens is observed during the first 2 weeks following LDV infection. Thereafter, the immune response to other antigens is normal. In immunosuppressed C58 and AKR mice, neurovirulent isolates of LDV can induce a sometimes fatal poliomyelitis. In these mice, immunosuppression is required to delay antibody production until after virus has reached the central nervous system (CNS) and infected susceptible ventral motor neurons. LDV-infected neurons become the targets of an inflammatory response. In mice 6 months of age or older, paralysis of one or both hindlimbs and sometimes a forelimb is observed. In younger C58 mice, poliomyelitis is usually subclinical.

Isolates of SHFV that induce persistent, asymptomatic infections and ones that cause acute, asymptomatic infections of patas monkeys have been reported. All SHFV isolates cause fatal hemorrhagic fever in macaque monkeys. Infected macaques develop fever and mild edema followed by anorexia, dehydration, adipsia, proteinuria, cynosis, skin petechia, bloody diarrhea, nose bleeds, and occasional hemorrhages in the skin. The pathological lesions consist of capillary-venous hemorrhages in the intestine, lung, nasal mucosa, dermis, spleen, perirenal and lumbar subperitoneum, adrenal glands, liver, and periocular connective tissues. These signs and symptoms are not unique to SHFV-infected animals, since they are also observed after infection of macaques with other types of hemorrhagic fever viruses such as Ebola virus. Although the SHFV-induced lesions are widespread in infected animals, the level of tissue damage is not severe. Even so, mortality in macaques infected with SHFV approaches 100% and occurs within 1 or 2 weeks after infection.

## Pathology and Histopathology

In horses experimentally or fatally infected with EAV, the most common gross lesions are edema, congestion, and hemorrhage of subcutaneous tissues, lymph nodes, and viscera. Microscopic investigation of tissues from chronically infected horses, which had mildly swollen lymph nodes and slightly increased volumes of pleural and peritoneal fluids, revealed extensive lesions consisting of generalized endothelial damage to blood vessels of all sizes as well as severe glomerulonephritis. Both types of lesions are thought to be caused by the deposition of viral immune complexes. Extensive capillary necrosis leads to a progressive increase in vascular permeability and volume, hemoconcentration, and hypotension. During the terminal stages of the disease, lesions are also found in the adrenal cortex, and degenerative changes are observed in the bone marrow and liver. Focal myometritis is observed in infected pregnant mares and is thought to be the cause of deficiencies in the fetal and placental blood supply. The resulting anoxia is probably the cause of abortion.

Although most LDV infections are inapparent in mice, some histopathogenic changes are observed in infected animals. As described above, the serum levels of seven enzymes are chronically elevated in LDV-infected mice. Normally, an increase in serum levels of tissue enzymes is the result of tissue damage, but in LDV-infected animals little tissue damage is observed. Although there are five naturally occurring LDH isozymes in mouse plasma, only the level of isozyme LDVV is elevated in LDV-infected mice. Studies have indicated that the increase in enzyme levels is primarily the result of a decreased rate of enzyme clearance. A subpopulation of Kupffer cells involved in receptor-mediated endocytosis of LDH is severely diminished in mice by 24 h after LDV infection. It has been postulated that LDV replication in these cells causes their death and results in increased LDH serum levels. Splenomegaly, characterized by a greater than 30% increase in spleen weight, occurs in about 40% of the mice infected with LDV. The increase in spleen weight is observed by 24 h after infection and persists for up to a month. A marked necrosis of lymphocytes in thymic-dependent areas occurs during the first 4 days after LDV infection together with a transient decrease in the number of circulating T lymphocytes between 24 and 72 h after infection. A transient decrease in peritoneal macrophages is also observed between the first and tenth day of infection. Despite the lifelong presence of circulating viral immune complexes and the demonstration of some LDV antibody deposits in the kidneys of LDV-infected mice as early as 7 days after infection, these animals do not develop kidney disease. It has been suggested that nephritis does not develop in these chronically infected mice because of the inability of the majority of the LDV–antibody complexes to bind C1q. Low levels of C1q-binding activity can only be detected between days 10 and 18 after LDV infection. LDV infection can alter the outcome of concomitant autoimmune disease, probably through modulation of the host-immune responses. LDV infection can also trigger the spontaneous production of different types of autoantibodies, possibly as a result of polyclonal B-lymphocyte activation.

The CNS lesions in neurovirulent LDV-infected C58 and AKR mice are located in the gray matter of the spinal cord and, occasionally, in the brainstem and consist of focal areas of inflammatory mononuclear cell infiltrates in the ventral horn. Virus-specific protein and nucleic acid have been detected in ventral motor neurons, and maturing virions in these neurons have been observed by electron microscopy.

## Immune Response

Antibodies in sera obtained from animals infected with EAV or PRRSV recognize virion proteins N, M, $GP_5$, and $GP_2$. Neutralizing antibodies are primarily directed to $GP_5$ and the neutralization epitopes of EAV, LDV, and PRRSV have been mapped to the ectodomain of this protein. For EAV, there are four major $GP_5$ conformational neutralization sites that are interactive. Also, for EAV, interaction between $GP_5$ and M is required for neutralization. For LDV and PRRSV, the major neutralization site is located in the N-terminus of $GP_5$. A secondary neutralization site for PRRSV has been mapped to the ectodomain of $GP_4$. The neutralization epitopes of SHFV have not yet been studied.

Anti-EAV antibodies can be detected in horses 1–2 weeks after infection with virulent or avirulent strains of the virus. Complement-fixing, antiviral antibodies peak 2–3 weeks after the initiation of infection and then decline. Neutralizing antibody peaks between 2 and 4 months after infection. An increase in neutralizing antibodies usually leads to virus clearance. Often after 8 months, anti-EAV antibody can no longer be detected by complement-fixation or neutralization assays. However, in some animals the virus persists and viral immune complexes continue to circulate.

The first month of infection of pigs with PRRSV is characterized by high viremia and disease symptoms. A vigorous antiviral antibody response can be detected by ELISA beginning 7–9 days after infection but these antibodies have little neutralizing activity. Beginning at about a month after infection, neutralizing antibody can be detected and peaks between 1 and 2 months after infection. Viremia is reduced to very low levels but virus continues to be produced from infected cells in tissues for at least 5 months. Usually, the infection eventually is completely cleared, but in some cases it continues to persist.

In LDV-infected mice, which always become persistently infected, antiviral $GP_5$ and N antibody that is primarily of the IgG2a subclass is produced as early as 6–10 days after infection. The production of this antibody is dependent on functional T helper cells. Plasma from LDV-infected mice has a much higher nonspecific binding activity than plasma from uninfected mice; virus-specific binding measured by enzyme-linked immunosorbent assay (ELISA) usually cannot be detected until the plasma has been diluted at least 1:400. Some virus neutralization by this early antibody has been demonstrated but is incomplete due to the presence of virus quasispecies that are resistant to neutralization. Anti-LDV antibody that is not complexed to virus can be detected by 15 days after infection, indicating that antibody is present in excess of virus in chronically infected mice. Although the presence of anti-LDV antibodies does not prevent infection of macrophages, it does effectively neutralize neurovirulent LDV strains and so protects motor neurons from becoming infected. LDV-infected mice display a polyclonal humoral response and anti-LDV antibody apparently accounts for only a small portion of this polyclonal response. The mechanism by which LDV infection activates B cells polyclonally is currently not known, but mice immunized with inactivated virus do not develop a polyclonal response. Autoantibodies to a variety of cellular components (autoimmune antibodies) have been detected in mice chronically infected with LDV.

SHFV isolates that produce acute infections in patas monkeys induce high levels of neutralizing antibody, whereas SHFV isolates that induce persistent infections induce low titers of non-neutralizing antibody. Antibodies to virus that causes acute infection do not cross-neutralize virus that causes persistent infection. In macaques, death from an SHFV infection occurs before an effective adaptive immune response can be elicited.

LDV-infected animals develop cytotoxic T cells that can specifically recognize and lyse virus-infected macrophages. However, this cytotoxic response is not able to clear the infection. Whether anti-LDV cytotoxic T cells persist indefinitely in chronically infected mice or eventually disappear due to clonal exhaustion is disputed. A cytotoxic T-cell response as indicated by IFNγ-producing T cells can be detected in PRRSV-infected pigs starting about a month (the same time that neutralizing antibody appears) after infection and lasts at least a year.

Although the production of neutralizing antibody and cytotoxic T cells is delayed in EAV- and PRRSV-infected animals, these responses are usually effective in clearing the infection. However, in some EAV and PRRSV infections and in all LDV infections, persistent infections develop even though good levels of neutralizing antiviral antibodies and helper and cytotoxic T-cell responses are elicited. The mechanisms by which these viruses evade clearance by the adaptive immune system include extensive glycosylation of the major glycoprotein $GP_5$ that masks the major neutralization epitope of some strains of the virus, and enhanced infection of macrophages by infectious viral immune complexes via cell surface Fc receptors. Neutralization escape virus variants have been reported to arise during persistent LDV infections and may also arise during persistent infections with other arteriviruses. An immunodominant decoy epitope located just upstream of the neutralization epitope in PRRSV $GP_5$ induces a strong non-neutralizing antibody response and may be responsible for the weak/absent induction of neutralizing antibodies during the first month of infection.

## Prevention and Control

Avirulent and virulent strains of EAV and PRRSV have been isolated. A number of live attenuated vaccines and killed vaccines are commercially available for both EAV and PRRSV. The live vaccines are more efficacious in providing protection and induce a longer-lasting immunity than the killed vaccines. Although these vaccines induce immunity against disease, immunized animals are not completely protected from reinfection. Animals immunized with live vaccines can spread virus and can become persistently infected. Outbreaks of disease due to reversion of live PRRSV vaccines have been reported. To allow discrimination between natural and vaccine infections, markers have been engineered into one EAV live vaccine. Recent vaccine development efforts have focused on the utilization of recombinant virus vectors, such as Venezuelan equine encephalitis virus and pseudorabies, or DNA vectors to express $GP_5$ or both $GP_5$ and M.

The current lack of rapid diagnostic assays for the detection of LDV and SHFV in persistently infected animals means that it is still a time-consuming task to identify animals with inapparent infections. Care should be taken not to inadvertently transfer arteriviruses from a persistently infected animal to other susceptible animals. Cells and infectious agent pools obtained from animals that might be persistently infected with an arterivirus should be checked for viral contamination before they are injected into a susceptible animal.

## Future Perspectives

Arteriviruses have so far been isolated from mice (LDV), horses (EAV), pigs (LV), and monkeys (SHFV). It seems likely that other host species, including humans, harbor additional members of this virus family. However, such viruses will be difficult to find if the natural hosts develop asymptomatic infections. Little is yet known about the functional roles of the arterivirus proteins in the virus life cycle. Recent studies suggest that the arterivirus nucleocapsid and envelope proteins have unique properties. The intense current interest in dissecting the structure and function of the SARS-coronavirus replicase may provide new insights for similar analyses of the arterivirus replicase. The availability of reverse genetic systems for several of the arteriviruses will not only aid the further molecular characterization of these viruses but will also facilitate the study of viral pathogenesis and antiviral immunity as well as the development of improved vaccines.

## Further Reading

Balasuriya UB and Maclachlan NJ (2004) The immune response to equine arteritis virus: Potential lesions for other arteriviruses. *Veterinary Immunology and Immunopathology* 102: 107–129.

Coutelier J-P and Brinton MA (2006) Lactate dehydrogenase-elevating virus. In: Fox JG, Newcomer C, Smith A, Barthold S, Quimby F, and Davidson M (eds.) *The Mouse in Biomedical Research*, 2nd edn., pp. 215–234. San Diego, CA: Elsevier.

Delputte PL, Costers S, and Nauwynck HJ (2005) Analysis of porcine reproductive and respiratory syndrome virus attachment and internalization: Distinctive roles for heparan sulphate and sialoadhesin. *Journal of General Virology* 86: 1441–1445.

Godeny EK, de Vries AAF, Wang XC, Smith SL, and de Groot RJ (1998) Identification of the leader–body junctions for the viral subgenomic mRNAs and organization of the simian hemorrhagic fever virus genome: Evidence for gene duplication during arterivirus evolution. *Journal of Virology* 72: 862–867.

Gorbalenya AE, Enjuanes L, Ziebuhr J, and Snijder EJ (2006) Nidovirales: Evolving the largest RNA virus genome. *Virus Research* 117: 17–37.

Lopez OJ and Osorio FA (2004) Role of neutralizing antibodies in PRRSV protective immunity. *Veterinary Immunology and Immunopathology* 102: 155–163.

Murtaugh MP, Xiao ZG, and Zuckermann F (2002) Immunological responses of swine to porcine reproductive and respiratory syndrome virus infection. *Viral Immunology* 15: 533–547.

Pasternak AO, Spaan WJM, and Snijder EJ (2006) Nidovirus transcription: How to make sense...? *Journal of General Virology* 87: 1403–1421.

Plagemann PGW and Moennig V (1992) Lactate dehydrogenase-elevating virus, equine arteritis virus, and simian hemorrhagic fever virus: A new group of positive-strand RNA viruses. *Advances in Virus Research* 41: 99–192.

Siddell SG, Ziebuhr J, and Snijder EJ (2005) Coronaviruses, toroviruses, and arteriviruses. In: Mahy BWJ and ter Meulen V (eds.) *Topley and Wilson's Microbiology and Microbial Infections, Vol. 1: Virology*, 10th edn., London: Hodder Arnold.

Snijder EJ and Meulenberg JM (1998) The molecular biology of arteriviruses. *Journal of General Virology* 79: 961–979.

Snijder EJ, Siddell SG, and Gorbalenya AE (2005) The order Nidovirales. In: Mahy BWJ and ter Meulen V (eds.) *Topley and Wilson's Microbiology and Microbial Infections, Vol. 1: Virology*, 10th edn., London: Hodder Arnold.

Snijder EJ and Spaan WJM (2007) Arteriviruses. In: Knipe DM, Howley PM, Griffin DE, *et al.* (eds.) *Fields Virology*, 5th edn., pp. 1337–1356. Philadelphia, PA: Lippincott Williams and Wilkins.

Wieringa R, de Vries AAF, van der Meulen J, *et al.* (2004) Structural protein requirements in equine arteritis virus assembly. *Journal of Virology* 78: 13019–13027.

Ziebuhr J, Snijder EJ, and Gorbalenya AE (2000) Virus-encoded proteinases and proteolytic processing in the *Nidovirales. Journal of General Virology* 81: 853–879.

# Bluetongue Viruses

**P Roy,** London School of Hygiene and Tropical Medicine, London, UK

## Glossary

**Arthrogryposis** Persistent flexure or contracture of a joint.

**Campylognathia** A condition marked by misalignment of the jaws leading to a twisted appearance of the face.

**Hemoconcentration** An increase in the concentration of red blood cells in the circulating blood.

**Hemorrhagic** Related to bleeding.

**Hydranencephaly** Related to the abnormal buildup of cerebrospinal fluid in the ventricles of the brain.

**Hydropericardium** A noninflammatory accumulation of fluid within the linings surrounding the heart.

**Hydrothorax** An accumulation of serous fluid in the cavity of the chest.

**Hypotension** Abnormally low blood pressure.

**Mucosal edema** The presence of abnormally large amounts of fluid in the intercellular tissue spaces of the connective tissue lining the internal cavities of the body.

**Prognathia** A condition marked by abnormal protrusion of the lower jaw.

**Pulmonary edema** A state of increased interstitial fluid within the lung that leads to flooding of the lung alveoli with fluid.

**Serosal hemorrhages** Bleeding in the delicate membranes of connective tissue which line the internal cavities of the body.

**Thrombotic** Related to formation of thrombus; that is, an aggregation of blood factors, frequently causing vascular obstruction at the point of its formation.

**Triskelions** A shape consisting of three protruding branches radiating from a common center.

## History

Bluetongue disease (initially known as 'malarial catarrhal fever') was first observed in the late eighteenth century in sheep, goats, cattle, and other domestic animals, as well as in wild ruminants (e.g., white-tailed deer, elk, and pronghorn antelope) in Africa. A distinctive lesion in the mouths of the infected animals with severely affected, dark blue tongues was a characteristic symptom. That the disease was caused by a filterable agent was discovered in 1905. The first confirmed outbreak outside of Africa occurred in sheep in Cyprus in 1924 and this was followed by a major outbreak in 1943–44 with 70% mortality. The disease was recognized subsequently in the USA in 1948 and in Southern Europe in 1956 where approximately 75% of the affected animals died. The outbreaks of bluetongue disease in the Middle East, Asia, Southern Europe, and the USA in the early 1940s and 1950s led to its subsequent description as an 'emerging disease'. To date, based on serum-neutralization tests, 24 different serotypes have been isolated in tropical, semitropical, and temperate zones of the world including Africa, North and South America, Australia, Southeast Asia, the Middle East, and, more recently, Southern and Central Europe. An important factor in the distribution of bluetongue virus (BTV) worldwide is the availability of suitable vectors, usually biting midges (gnats) of the genus *Culicoides*.

## Properties of the Virion

*Bluetongue virus* is the type species of the genus *Orbivirus* within the family *Reoviridae*. Details of the structure, genetics, and molecular properties of orbiviruses have been gleaned largely from studies of BTV. BTV and other orbiviruses are nonenveloped with two concentric protein shells and a genome consisting of ten double-stranded RNA (dsRNA) segments. BTV virions (550S) are architecturally complex icosahedral structures and are composed of seven discrete proteins that are numbered VP1 to VP7 in order of their decreasing size. When viewed by electron microscopy (EM), negative-stained, 550S BTV particles exhibit a poorly defined surface structure with a 'fuzzy' appearance. Complete virions are relatively fragile and the infectivity of BTV is lost easily in mildly acidic conditions. The outer capsid of BTV consists of two major proteins (VP2 and VP5) which constitute approximately 40% of the total protein content of the virus. Both proteins are removed shortly after infection to yield a transcriptionally active core (470S) particle (see schematic, **Figure 1**) which, in contrast to virions, is fairly robust. They are composed of two major proteins (VP7 and VP3), three minor proteins (VP1, VP4, and VP6), and the dsRNA genome. The cores may be further uncoated to form subcore particles (390S) that lack VP7. The 470S cores can be derived from virions *in vitro* by physical or proteolytic treatments that remove the outer capsid and cause activation of the BTV transcriptase. Considerable information on the three-dimensional (3-D) structures of BTV particles and proteins has been generated in recent years.

## Virion Structure and Outer Capsid Proteins

In contrast to negative staining, cryoelectron microscopy (cryo-EM) of intact BTV particles shows the icosahedral morphology of the mature particle, with a diameter of 86 nm. The outer layer consists of 60 sail-shaped, spike-like structures made up of VP2 (110 kDa) trimers and of 120 globular structures made up of VP5 (59 kDa) trimers (**Figure 2**). The most external part of the outer capsid is the propeller-shaped triskelion blade of VP2, the tip of which bends upward, perpendicularly to the plane of the virus. These bent tips give the entire virion a diameter of ~88 nm

and extend from the main body of the particle by 3 nm. Interspersed between the triskelions and lying more internally are the globular VP5 trimers, each with a ~6 nm diameter. These are also entirely exposed in the virion, not covered by VP2, and both proteins make extensive contacts with the core VP7 layer underneath.

## Core Particle and Proteins

The core particles derived from purified virus by proteolytic treatment have been analyzed by cryo-EM and by X-ray crystallography. The icosahedral core has a diameter of 73 nm and a triangulation number of 13 ($T = 13$) with the surface layer made up of 260 VP7 (38 kDa) trimers. Trimers are arranged around 132 distinctive channels (three types: I, II, and III) as six-member rings, with five-member rings at the vertices of the icosahedrons (**Figure 3**). The five quasiequivalent trimers form a visible protomeric unit (P, Q, R, S, T). Each trimer consists of two distinct domains, 'upper' (an antiparallel β-sandwich) and 'lower' (mainly α-helical), which are twisted in such a way that the top domain of one monomer rests upon the lower domain of an adjacent monomer and the interaction between monomers is extensive. The lower domains are attached to an inner shell (59 nm in diameter) made up of 120 VP3 (103 kDa) molecules arranged as 60 dimers with $T = 2$ symmetry (**Figure 4**). Each molecule consists of three distinct domains: a rigid 'carapace' domain, an 'apical' domain, and a 'dimerization' domain. Five of the VP3 dimers form a decamer with fivefold axes of symmetry, and 12 decamers, each a convex disk shape, are arranged together to form the complete VP3 shell.

Much of the genomic RNA can also be detected as an electron-dense region within the central core space. The dsRNA appears to be highly ordered, and approximately 80% of the entire genome can be modeled as four distinct

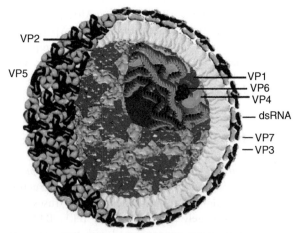

**Figure 1**  A schematic diagram of bluetongue virus (BTV) showing the positions and structural organizations of BTV components. Reproduced courtesy of professor David Ian Stuart.

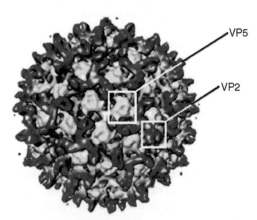

**Figure 2**  Surface representations of the 3-D cryo-EM structures (22 Å resolution) of BTV. Whole particle showing sail-shaped triskelion propellers (VP2 trimers) in red and globular domains (VP5 trimers) in yellow.

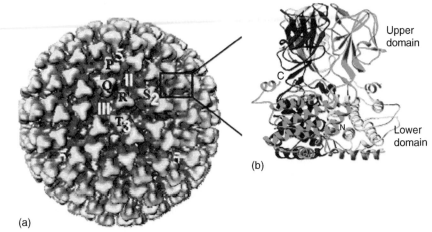

(a)

(b)

**Figure 3**  Three-dimensional structures of BTV core and VP7 protein. (a) Surface representations of the 3-D cryo-EM structures of BTV core (700 Å in diameter) viewed along the icosahedral threefold axes showing the 260 trimers of VP7 (in blue). The five quasiequivalent trimers (P, Q, R, S, and T) and the locations of channels II and III are marked. (b) The trimer image of the VP7 atomic structure solved at 2.8 Å resolution. Two domains of the molecule are indicated. The view is shown from the side. Note the flat base of the trimer lies in a horizontal plane in this view.

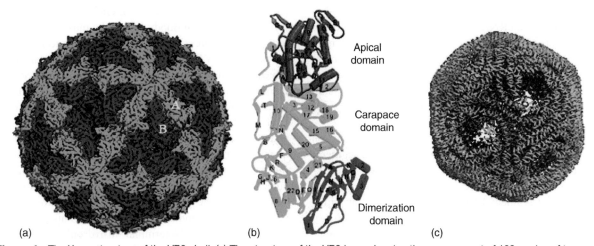

(a)                                    (b)                                    (c)

**Figure 4**  The X-ray structure of the VP3 shell. (a) The structure of the VP3 layer showing the arrangement of 120 copies of two conformationally distinct types of VP3 molecules, 'A' shown in green and 'B' shown in red. (b) Structure of VP3 molecule shown as a thin triangular plate consisting of three domains as indicated. (c) The model diagram of genomic dsRNA that has been built into the four layers of electron density in the core.  Reproduced courtesy of professor David Ian Stuart.

concentric layers that have center-to-center spacing between RNA strands of 26–30 Å.

The arrangement of three internal minor proteins within the VP3 layer is not discernible in the core structure. However, cryo-EM of core-like particles (CLPs) consisting of VP3 and VP7 together with two minor proteins, VP1 (150 kDa) and VP4 (78 kDa), though lacking the genome, and VP6 has revealed a flower-shaped complex formed by VP1 and VP4, directly beneath the icosahedral fivefold axes. The exact position of the smallest minor protein VP6 (35 kDa) remains unclear although it forms a stable hexamer *in vitro* in the presence of BTV RNA, indicating that it is closely associated with genomic RNA.

## The Virus Genome

The BTV genome comprises ten dsRNA segments in equimolar amounts which appear to be organized in an orderly fashion as four distinct layers within the core. The RNA segments, numbered 1–10 in order of migration by polyacrylamide gel electrophoresis (PAGE), were historically referred to as large, medium, and small segments (i.e., L1–L3, M4–M6, and S7–S10). Their relative order of mobility may vary according to the electrophoretic conditions used (agarose gel vs. PAGE) and the dsRNA profiles of members representing each orbivirus serogroup are generally distinctive and different from those of other members of the family *Reoviridae.*

The complete sequences of all ten dsRNA segments of a number of BTV serotypes (BTV-10 being completed as early as in 1989) are available. Each segment has six nucleotides at the 3' end and eight nucleotides at the 5' end conserved in each messenger sense RNA (mRNA) strand. For BTV-10, the genome is 19 218 bp in length with a molecular weight of $1.3 \times 10^7$ Da and the individual sizes of BTV-10 RNAs range from 3954 bp (segment 1, molecular weight $2.7 \times 10^6$ Da) to 822 bp (segment 10, molecular weight $5 \times 10^5$ Da). The 5' noncoding regions range from 8 nt (segment 4) to 34 nt in length (segment 6) while the 3' noncoding sequences are generally longer, that is, from 31 nt (segment 5) to 116 nt (segment 10) in length.

The 5' and 3' terminal sequences of the ten mRNA strands of BTV have inverted complementarity capable of forming intramolecular hydrogen bonds (i.e., end-to-end hydrogen bonding) and share some common features (e.g., a looped-out sequence proximal to the 3' termini). Apart from segment 2 and segment 5 (segment 6 in agarose gels) that code for the two outer capsid proteins (VP2 and VP5), all other eight RNA segments are highly conserved. Despite this sequence conservation, some genetic diversity exists for each RNA segment representing the various BTV serotypes as well as for various isolates within a single serotype. In addition, high-frequency segment reassortment occurs between different BTV serotypes in cell cultures, vertebrate hosts, or *Culicoides* vectors to generate new genotype combinations. Thus, both genetic drift and genetic shift contribute to BTV evolution.

Apart from segment 10, each of the AUG codons on the positive-sense mRNA strand of each of the segments initiates a single long open reading frame (see **Table 1**). There are two methionine codons in the same reading frame in the segment-10 RNA sequences, one at triplet 20–22 and the other at triplet 59–61, encoding two overlapping proteins. Thus, segment 10 codes for two nonstructural proteins, NS3 and NS3A. In addition to the seven structural proteins, two major nonstructural proteins (NS1, NS2) are also synthesized in infected cells. **Table 1**

summarizes the coding assignments of the ten genome segments of BTV-10.

## Viral Replication

The basic features of the BTV replication cycle, including the transcription process and the conservative mode of genome replication, are similar to those of reoviruses and rotaviruses. Unlike reoviruses or rotaviruses, however, BTV and other orbiviruses multiply in arthropods as well as in vertebrate hosts. Also, in view of the structural differences, it is likely that some stages of BTV replication and morphogenesis are unique.

### Attachment and Entry into Cells

BTV adsorbs rapidly to susceptible cells at both 4 and 37 °C. The cell receptor for BTV is not known although it binds to a sialoglycoprotein via the outer capsid protein VP2 in mammalian cells. VP2 is the serotype determinant and viral hemagglutinin protein, elicits serotype-specific virus-neutralizing antibody, and is the most variable protein among different serotypes. Although protease-treated particles with VP2 cleavage products attached are fully infectious, removal of VP2 results in loss of virus infectivity in mammalian cells. Core particles, however, are infectious only for invertebrate cells.

The attachment of VP2 leads to receptor-mediated endocytosis by clathrin-coated vesicles which are subsequently lost when large endocytic vesicles form. Only the early endosomes are involved in BTV entry. BTV entry into the cytoplasm requires endosomal acidic pH which allows the second outer capsid protein VP5 to permeabilize the endosomal membrane. This occurs via the function of the N-terminal 40 hydrophobic residues which act as a 'pore-forming' peptide, analogous to the fusion peptides of envelope viruses. Thus, VP2 makes an initial contact with the host cell and VP5 mediates the

**Table 1**    Coding assignments and function of the BTV-10 viral RNA segments

| Genome segment[a] | Size (kbp) | Protein | Protein size (kDa) | Location | Function |
|---|---|---|---|---|---|
| Seg. 1 (L1) | 3.954 | VP1 | 149.5 | Core | Polymerase |
| L2 | 2.926 | VP2 | 111 | Outer shell | Attachment protein |
| L3 | 2.772 | VP3 | 103 | Core | Structural |
| M4 | 2.011 | VP4 | 764 | Core | Capping enzyme |
| M5 | 1.770 | NS1 | 644 | Tubules | Trafficking? |
| M6 | 1.639 | VP5 | 591 | Outer shell | Fusion protein |
| S7 | 1.156 | VP7 | 385 | Core | Insect cell attachment |
| S8 | 1.123 | NS2 | 409 | Nonstructural | RNA selection |
| S9 | 1.046 | VP6 | 357 | Core | Helicase |
| S10 | 0.822 | NS3 | 256 | Nonstructural | Egress |

[a]Genome segment nomenclature based on order of migration by electrophoresis. In some gel systems the migration of segments 5 and 6 is frequently, but not always, reversed.

penetration of the host cell membrane by destabilizing the endosomal membrane. Core particles lacking both VP2 and VP5 proteins then enter the cytoplasm.

## Transcription

In the cytoplasm, core particles do not disassemble further but initiate the transcription of the viral genome, and newly synthesized viral mRNAs, capped but not polyadenylated, are extruded into the cytoplasm. When intact cores, isolated from virus particles, are activated *in vitro* by the presence of magnesium ions and nucleoside triphosphate (NTP) substrates, distinct conformational changes can be seen around the fivefold axes of the core, forming pores in the VP3 and VP7 layers through which mRNAs are extruded. The role of each internal minor protein in genome replication activity has been established using individual purified proteins.

The smallest minor protein VP6, which is rich in basic amino acids (Arg, Lys, and His), binds both single-stranded RNAs (ssRNAs) and dsRNAs and, in isolation, has the ability to unwind dsRNA substrates *in vitro*. The protein exhibits physical properties characteristic of other helicases, including being hexameric, and has the ability to form ring-like structures in the presence of BTV RNAs. Mutation of amino acid residues in the active site destroys the catalytic activity of the protein.

The replication of viral dsRNA occurs in two distinct steps. First, plus-strand RNAs (mRNAs) are transcribed and extruded from the core particle. Second, the plus-strand RNAs serve as templates for the synthesis of new minus-strand RNAs. The largest core protein VP1 (150 kDa), in soluble form, has the ability to both initiate and elongate minus-strand synthesis *de novo*, but the catalytic activity is lost when a GDD motif (amino acids 287–289), the polymerase signature motif, is mutated.

The third minor protein VP4 is the mRNA-capping enzyme. The purified, soluble, recombinant VP4 alone has the ability to synthesize type 1-like 'cap' structures on uncapped BTV transcripts *in vitro*, and 'cap' structures are identical to those found on authentic BTV mRNAs. Thus, VP4 possesses methyltransferase, guanylyltransferase, and RNA triphosphatase activities. The recently resolved atomic structure has shown how distinct domains of this single protein perform each of these catalytic activities consecutively.

In summary, each of the three minor proteins of the BTV core has the ability to function on its own. Together they constitute a molecular motor that can unwind RNAs, synthesize ssRNAs of both polarities, and modify the 5′ termini of the newly synthesized mRNA molecules. The transcripts are not produced in equimolar amounts from the ten segments of BTV; the smaller genome segments are generally the most frequently transcribed, although segment-6 RNA (encoding NS1) is synthesized more abundantly than segment-10 (the smallest) RNA (encoding NS3). The molar ratios of the ten different BTV mRNAs remain the same throughout the infection cycle. The ratios of mRNAs synthesized *in vivo* and *in vitro* are similar.

Much less is known about the *in vivo* RNA replication mechanisms of BTV. It is believed that, like reoviruses and rotaviruses, the packaged plus-strand RNA serves as a template for synthesis of a minus strand, and once the minus strand is synthesized, the dsRNA remains within the nascent progeny particle. As discussed, VP1 acts as the replicase enzyme but the roles of other proteins in minus-strand synthesis remain undefined.

## Protein Synthesis and Replication

In tissue culture, the first BTV-specific proteins are detectable 2 h post infection and the rate of protein synthesis increases rapidly until 12–13 h post infection, after which it slows down but continues until cell death. BTV infection of mammalian cells, in contrast to insect cells, leads to a rapid inhibition of cellular macromolecular synthesis and the induction of a robust apoptotic response triggered via multiple apoptotic pathways.

Two NS proteins, NS1 (64 kDa) and NS2 (41 kDa), are synthesized abundantly early in BTV infection and coincide with two virus-specific intracellular structures, tubules, and viral inclusion bodies (VIBs), respectively. By contrast, synthesis of NS3 and NS3A (26 and 25 kDa) varies from barely detectable to highly expressed, depending on the host cells, and may correlate with virus release.

Tubules are present in large numbers, mostly in perinuclear locations, and are made up of helically coiled NS1 dimers, on average 52.3 nm in diameter and ~1 μm long. The exact role of tubules or NS1 dimers in virus replication is not known. During BTV infection, VIBs are found in the infected cells, predominantly near the nucleus. VIBs act as the nucleation site for newly synthesized proteins that form the core structure and transcripts as well as the subsequent assembly of subviral particles. The major component of VIBs is the phosphoprotein NS2. Phosphorylation plays a key role in the formation of VIBs and may be involved in stabilizing NS2 folding. The cellular protein kinase, casein kinase II (CKII), is responsible for NS2 phosphorylation via two serine residues.

Soluble NS2 and NS2 in VIBs have a strong affinity for ssRNA. NS2 preferentially binds BTV transcripts via specific hairpin structures, an indication of its role in the recruitment and selection of BTV mRNA during virus replication and RNA packaging. Since phosphorylation of NS2 is not necessary for recruitment of core components, but important for VIB formation, phosphorylation and dephosphorylation of NS2 is plausibly a dynamic process that controls the assembly and release of core particles.

## Capsid Assembly

The assembly of BTV capsids requires a complex and highly ordered series of protein–protein interactions. The use of CLPs and virus-like particles (VLPs), together with structure-based mutagenesis, has revealed the key principles that drive the assembly process. The VP3 shell appears to play the major role in the initiation of core assembly with formation of VP3 decamers and the complex formed with VP1 and VP4. These assembly intermediates subsequently recruit the viral RNA, and possibly VP6, prior to completion of the assembly of the VP3 subcore and the addition of VP7 trimers. Initially, multiple sheets of VP7 trimers form around different nucleation sites and thus it is likely that a number of strong VP7 trimer–VP3 contacts act as multiple equivalent initiation sites and that a second set of weaker interactions then 'fill the gaps' to complete the outer core layer. The VP7 layer gives increased rigidity and stability to the core particle. Assembly of the core takes place entirely within VIBs and assembled core is released from VIBs prior to the simultaneous addition of VP2 and VP5, which most likely occurs within the vimentin component of the cytoskeleton.

## Egress from Host Cells

The majority of mature virus particles remain cell-associated in mammalian cells, causing substantial cytopathic effect. However, some particles bud through the cell membrane or move in groups through a local disruption of the plasma membrane. NS3 (229 aa) and its shorter form NS3A (216 aa) are the only BTV glycoproteins and are associated with smooth-surfaced, intracellular vesicles. NS3/NS3A proteins have long N-terminal and shorter C-terminal cytoplasmic domains connected by two transmembrane domains and a short extracellular domain. A single glycosylation site is present in the extracellular domain of BTV NS3. The NS3/NS3A proteins are synthesized at very low levels in infected mammalian cells but at very high levels in invertebrate cells where there is nonlytic virus release. The NS3 protein is localized at the site of the membrane where viruses or VLPs are released. NS3 may cause local disruption of the plasma membrane, allowing virus particles to be extruded through a membrane pore without acquiring a lipid envelope. The N-terminal residues of NS3 interact with the calpactin light chain (p11) of the cellular annexin II complex, itself involved in membrane secretory pathways. The interaction of p11 with NS3 may direct NS3 to sites of active cellular exocytosis, or NS3 could become part of an active extrusion process. NS3 is also capable of interaction with Tsg101, a cellular protein implicated in the intracellular trafficking and release of a number of enveloped viruses. Interactions of both p11 and Tsg101 with

NS3 appear to impact the nonlytic release of virions from infected cells. The significance of these interactions for BTV egress becomes more apparent in the light of the observation that the other cytoplasmic domain of the protein, situated at the C-terminal end, interacts specifically with the BTV outer capsid protein VP2. Current data suggest that NS3 makes use of host proteins and acts as an intermediate to facilitate the release of newly synthesized progeny virus across the cell membrane.

## Pathogenesis

BTV produces a spectrum of conditions from subclinical infection to severe and fatal disease, depending on virus strain and host species. Virus is transmitted to vertebrate hosts through blood-feeding insect vectors and infectious particles migrate to lymph nodes where they initially replicate and subsequently spread to spleen, thymus, and other lymph nodes. In the final phase of infection, the virus begins circulating in the bloodstream and can persist for several months. In certain vertebrate hosts (e.g., cattle), BTV can induce a prolonged viremia. BTV binds to glycophorins on the surface of bovine and ovine erythrocytes where it may remain in an infectious state as invaginations of the erythrocyte cell membrane for prolonged periods of time. This precludes contact with antibody and T cells and thus provides multiple opportunities for transmission by infection of blood-sucking midges.

The role of leukocytes in cell-associated viremia is less certain, although BTV has been recovered from bovine mononuclear cells during the early stage of infection. A characteristic feature of BTV pathogenesis is the ability of viruses to replicate in and to damage endothelial cells with tropisms for cells representing distinct anatomic sites. Infection of endothelial cells is followed by infection of vascular smooth muscle cells and pericytes. These then undergo lytic infections, resulting in virus-induced vascular injury and a cascade of pathophysiologic events characterized by capillary leakage, hemorrhage, and disseminated intravascular coagulation. Clinically, these events are manifested by mucosal edema, hemoconcentration, pulmonary edema, hydrothorax, hydropericardium, serosal hemorrhages, other hemorrhagic and thrombotic phenomena, hypotension, and shock. A curious feature of BTV infection in sheep is hemorrhage at the base of the pulmonary artery. Generally, sheep develop potentially fatal hemorrhagic disease and have extensive endothelial cell infections, whereas cattle typically develop subclinical infections and have only minimal endothelial infections. Thus, BTV and other related orbiviruses in their respective large animal hosts have pathophysiologic features resembling other viral hemorrhagic fevers.

Infection of pregnant cattle and sheep with BTV can result in maternal death, abortion and fetal death, or congenital anomalies including runting, blindness, deafness, hydranencephaly, arthrogryposis, campylognathia, and prognathia.

## Epidemiology

In many countries, the prevalence of BTV infection is high in ruminants although clinical disease is often not recorded. The epidemiology of bluetongue disease can be considered in the context of three major zones of infection: an endemic zone (generally subclinical infection), an epidemic zone (disease occurs at regular intervals), and an incursive zone (disease occurs usually only at extended intervals, but when it does occur, the epidemic is often extensive). Transmission of BTV is influenced by both the distribution and biology of insect vectors and the weather pattern, and different strains of the virus are perpetuated within distinct ecosystems and in separate geographic regions by different vector species. This has been emphasized by the application of molecular genotyping techniques which have given further insights into the epidemiology of BTV and the extent of BTV evolution. Indeed molecular epidemiology studies have demonstrated the basis of the recent European emergence of BTV and how changes in BTV epidemiology coincide with climate changes which appear to have increased both the distribution and size of vector insect populations in the region. It is also evident that bluetongue viruses have crossed from the original insect vector species (e.g., *Culicoides imicola*) and are now being transmitted by novel vectors (e.g., *C. obsoletus* and *C. pulicaris*) that are abundant across Central and Northern Europe. As a result, many of the serotypes associated with the initial outbreaks have persisted and spread across much of Southern and Central Europe.

## Immunity

Neutralizing antibodies, which play major role in protection against reinfection, appear within 8–14 days of virus infection. Although BTV infection results in the production of antibodies to all ten proteins, the outer capsid protein VP2 alone is sufficient to induce protective neutralizing antibodies. Cell-mediated immunity (CMI) also plays an important role in recovery from infection and protection against reinfection. Cytotoxic (CD8+) cells responsive *in vitro* to BTV antigens have been demonstrated in the blood of cattle and sheep during the first week of infection and observed to peak at 2 weeks post infection. Both cross-reactive and serotype-specific cytotoxic T-lymphocyte (CTL) responses occur in BTV-infected animals. The role of CMI in protection against BTV infection has been demonstrated in sheep in which possible transfer of specific CD8+ cells conferred protection on challenge with live virus. Immunity was major histocompatibility complex (MHC) restricted and thus was host specific.

## Prevention and Control

Despite the high morbidity and mortality associated with BTV infection, little attention has been given to the development of efficacious vaccines. Early vaccination attempts included the use of virus in the serum of sheep which had recovered from the disease. This mild strain of the virus, which had been serially propagated in sheep, was used as an attenuated vaccine for more than 50 years despite evidence that it was not entirely safe and the resultant immunity was not adequate.

The only vaccines currently in use are live-attenuated vaccines developed by serial passage of BTV in embryonated chicken eggs. These are administered as polyvalent vaccines consisting of a total of 15 serotypes. Sheep develop BTV antibodies by 10 days post-vaccination. The antibody response reaches a maximum at 4 weeks and may persist up to 1 year. There is a temporal relationship between the increase in neutralizing antibody titer and clearance of virus from the peripheral circulation. However, there are several problems associated with these vaccines including incomplete protection and reversion to virulence. Attenuated virus can also be transmitted by insects from vaccinated sheep to other animals. This poses risks since live virus vaccine is teratogenic in pregnant sheep and may cause fetal death and abnormalities.

To avoid the problems encountered by live virus vaccines, a number of inactivated vaccines have been developed in various countries and are used locally. Many experimental trials have also been undertaken using VP2 antigen and VLPs as candidate vaccines. VP2 administered at high dose (>100 μg per dose) alone or together with VP5 (~20 μg per dose) has been demonstrated to be protective against virulent virus challenge in sheep. VLPs (containing the four major proteins) appear to be highly protective at a lower dose (10 μg per dose) and have generated protective immunity for up to 15 months. However, despite their high protective efficacy and safety, no subunit vaccines are yet available commercially. One of the likely reasons for lack of interest in these vaccines is the lower demand of BTV vaccine in the Western countries, but this may change following the recent emergence of BTV in Europe.

## Future Perspectives

BTV has been a major focus for understanding of the molecular biology of the *Reoviridae* and has served as a model system for the other members of the genus *Orbivirus*. Significant recent advances have been made in understanding the structure–function relationships of

BTV proteins and their interactions during virus assembly. By combining structural and molecular data, it has been possible to make progress on the fundamental mechanisms used by the virus to invade, replicate in, and escape from susceptible host cells. Evidence has been obtained for the role of cellular proteins in non-enveloped virus entry and egress.

Despite these advances, some critical questions remain unanswered. In particular, host–virus interactions during virus trafficking is one area needing intense attention in the future. Exactly how each genome segment is packaged into the progeny virus is another outstanding question. One of the major drawbacks of research with BTV and other members of *Reoviridae* has been the lack of availability of a suitable system for genetic manipulation of the virus and this has limited our understanding of the replication processes. However, in a recent major development in BTV research, live virus has been rescued by transfection of BTV transcripts. There is no doubt that this will soon be extended to establish *in vitro* manipulative genetic systems and will allow molecular and structural studies of individual BTV proteins to be placed in the context of the whole virus.

## Further Reading

Boyce M and Roy P (2007) Recovery of infectious bluetongue virus from RNA. *Journal of Virology* 81: 2179–2186.

Eaton BT, Hyatt AD, and Brookes SM (1990) The replication of bluetongue virus. In: Roy P and Gorman BM (eds.) *Current Topics in Microbiology, Vol. 162: Bluetongue Viruses*, pp. 89–118. Berlin: Springer.

Huismans H and Verwoerd DW (1973) Control of transcription during the expression of the bluetongue virus genome. *Virology* 52: 81–88.

MacLachlan NJ (1994) The pathogenesis and immunology of bluetongue virus infection of ruminants. *Comparative Immunology, Microbiology, and Infectious Diseases* 17: 197–206.

Mertens PPC, Maan S, Samuel A, and Attoui H (2005) *Reoviridae* – Orbivirus. In: Fauquet CM, Mayo MA, Maniloff J, Desselberger U,, and Ball LA (eds.) *Virus Taxonomy: Eighth Report of the International Committee on Taxonomy of Viruses*, pp. 466–483. New York: Academic Press.

Noad R and Roy P (2006) Bluetongue virus assembly and morphogenesis. In: Roy P and Gorman BM (eds.) *Current Topics in Microbiology and Immunology, Vol. 309: Reoviruses: Entry, Assembly and Morphogenesis*, pp. 87–116. Berlin: Springer.

Parsonson IM (1990) Pathology and pathogenesis of bluetongue infections. In: Roy P and Gorman BM (eds.) *Current Topics in Microbiology and Immunology*, Vol. 162: *Bluetongue Viruses*, pp. 119–141. Berlin: Springer.

Roy P (2005) Bluetongue virus proteins and particles and their role in virus entry, assembly and release. In: Roy P (ed.) *Virus Structure and Assembly, Vol. 64*, pp. 69–114. New York: Academic Press.

Roy P (2006) Orbiviruses and their replication. In: Knipe DM and Howley PM (eds.) *Field's Virology*, 5th edn., pp 1975–1997. Philadelphia, PA: Lippincott–Raven Publishers.

Stott JL and Osburn BI (1990) Immune response to bluetongue virus infection. In: Roy P and Gorman BM (eds.) *Current Topics in Microbiology and Immunology, Vol. 162: Bluetongue Viruses*, pp. 163–178. Berlin: Springer.

Verwoerd DW, Huismans H, and Erasmus BJ (1979) Orbiviruses. In: Fraenkel-Contrat H and Wagener RR (eds.) *Comprehensive Virology*, vol. 14, pp. 163–178. New York: Plenum.

# Bovine and Feline Immunodeficiency Viruses

**J K Yamamoto,** University of Florida, Gainesville, FL, USA

## History

Since the isolation of human immunodeficiency virus (HIV) in 1983, the search for its counterpart in domestic and laboratory animals was initiated in a number of laboratories. Bovine immunodeficiency virus (BIV) was isolated in 1969 from a Louisiana dairy cow (called R29) during an intensive search for bovine leukemia virus (BLV). However, the viral sequencing of the frozen cell preparation from this cow was not performed until 1987, when this isolate ($BIV_{R29}$) was determined to be a lentivirus. Unlike the long history of BIV discovery, feline immunodeficiency virus (FIV) was isolated in 1986 from two laboratory cats inoculated with tissues derived from stray cats found in Petaluma, California. The stray cats were from a private cattery with high incidence of mortality and immunodeficiency-like syndrome. The isolated virus, called feline T-lymphotropic virus, resembled HIV in biochemical and morphological characteristics and was renamed FIV in 1988. Viral sequencing in 1989 confirmed this isolate (FIV-Petaluma, $FIV_{Pet}$) to be a lentivirus. BIV and FIV infections are prevalent worldwide and each has a distinctive impact on the survival of its host.

## Taxonomy and Classification

Based on nucleotide sequence analysis, both BIV and FIV belong to the genus *Lentiviruses* in the family *Retroviridae*. Phylogenetic tree analyses of Pol sequences indicate that

BIV is related to caprine arthritis encephalitis virus (CAEV), whereas FIV is related to the equine infectious anemia virus (EIAV). Both BIV and FIV are distantly related to the primate lentiviruses, HIV and SIV. Serosurvey for BIV has identified a bovine lentivirus, called Jembrana disease virus (JDV), which causes an acute disease with 17% mortality in Balinese cattle. The full nucleotide sequence of JDV demonstrates that JDV is more closely related to BIV than to other lentiviruses.

FIV has been classified into five clades or subtypes (A–E) based on *env* and *gag* sequence analyses. Both serological and sequence analyses suggest that wild cats are infected with species-specific FIV. Eighteen of 37 nondomestic feline species, including lions, pumas, ocelots, leopards, cheetah, and Pallas cats (**Figure 1(b)**), are infected with species-specific FIV. Lion FIV-Ple and puma FIV-Pco are currently classified into three subtypes (A–C) and two subtypes (A, B), respectively. Based on *pol-RT* sequence, domestic FIV (FIV-Fca) is more closely related to puma FIV-Pco and ocelot FIV-Lpa than to other nondomestic FIV. Recent serological and *pol-RT* sequence analyses demonstrated species-specific FIV infection in Hyaenidae species (spotted hyena FIV-Ccr), the closest relative to the feline family.

## Geographic Distribution

The global distribution of BIV infection was determined by serological survey. BIV infection was found in Europe; North, Central, and South America; Asia; Middle East; Australia; New Zealand; and Africa (**Figure 1(a)**). In the USA, BIV infection was more prevalent in cattle herds from Southern states than those from Northern states. Standard serological survey has difficulty distinguishing BIV infection from JDV infection due to antibody cross-reactivity in the capsid protein (CA). JDV infection was reported on the island of Bali and neighboring districts in Indonesia.

A recent survey concluded that cattle in Australia have antibodies to a lentivirus antigenically more closely related to JDV than BIV.

The worldwide prevalence of FIV infection in domestic cats was determined by serosurvey and confirmed by sequence analysis (**Figure 1(b)**). In general, FIV subtypes are distributed according to the geographic location. Subtype B FIV was the predominant global subtype with higher prevalence in USA, Canada, eastern Japan, Argentina, Italy, Germany, Austria, and Portugal. Subtype A was the next predominant subtype with prevalence in

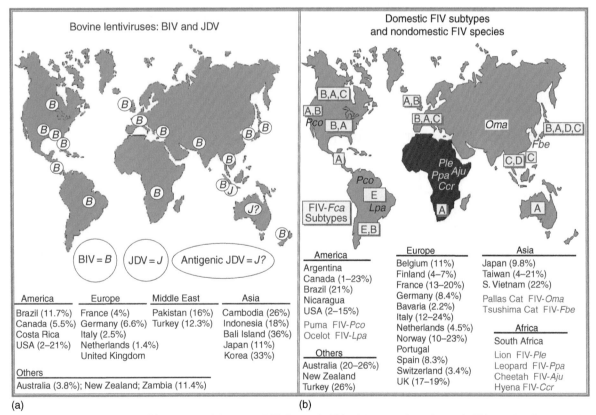

(a)                    (b)

**Figure 1** Global distribution of (a) bovine lentiviruses and (b) domestic FIV subtypes and nondomestic FIV species. Seroprevalence rates of BIV, JDV, and domestic FIV-Fca (prevalence in high risk group) are described in the parentheses next to the corresponding country. Nomenclatures of the nondomestic FIV in wild cats and hyena are shown in the prevalent country or continent.

western USA, western Canada, Argentina, Nicaragua, northern Japan, Australia, Germany, Italy, Netherlands, France, Switzerland, United Kingdom, and South Africa. Subtype C was detected predominantly in Vietnam, northern Taiwan, Japan, southern Germany, and British Columbia; subtype D in southern Japan and Vietnam; and subtype E in Brazil and Argentina.

## Virion and Genome Structure

BIV, JDV, and FIV are RNA viruses with two identical single-stranded RNA molecules of approximately 8.5, 7.7, and 9.5 kb per genome, respectively. The viral genomes, viral enzymes, and nucleoproteins (NC) involved in viral assembly are all packaged within the nucleocapsid core (**Figure 2(a)**). The mature core is shaped like a cone, typical of primate lentiviruses. Viral enzymes are protease (PR), reverse transcriptase (RT), and integrase (IN) encoded by the *pol* gene. FIV also produces a deoxyuridine triphosphatase (dUTPase or DU), which is unique to certain ungulate lentiviruses and important for replication in nondividing macrophages or resting T lymphocytes. The virus core, composed of CA, is surrounded by the matrix protein (MA), which coats the inner surface of viral envelope membrane. FIV has a myristoylated MA, similar to that of HIV and SIV. In contrast, BIV has a nonmyristoylated MA, typical of ungulate lentiviruses (EIAV, maedi-visna virus (MVV)). Myristoylation is important in targeting Gag to the inner surface of plasma membrane. The viral envelope (Env) consists of surface (SU) and transmembrane (TM) glycoproteins, projecting from the lipid bilayer derived from host plasma membrane.

BIV, JDV, and FIV have a genomic organization of *5′-LTR-gag-pol-env-LTR-3′*, like all retroviruses. The viral RNA is reverse-transcribed into double-stranded DNA in the cell cytoplasm, which are transported into the cell nucleus and then integrated into the host genome as viral provirus using viral IN. A genome-length mRNA, transcribed from the provirus, is translated into the Gag and Gag-Pol precursor polyproteins. These polyproteins are cleaved by the viral protease into MA, CA, and NC from Gag and PR, RT, DU (only FIV), and IN from Pol (**Figure 2(b)**). Similarly, the spliced *env* mRNA is translated into the Env precursor polyprotein, which is subsequently cleaved by a cellular protease into SU and TM. Like other lentiviruses, the BIV, JDV, and FIV genomes are more complex in organization than other retroviruses by containing regulatory genes that are found in the open reading frames (*orfs*) overlapping or flanking the 5′ and 3′ ends of the *env* gene. These viruses do not possess a *nef* gene or produce Nef protein. BIV *orfs* contain *tat, rev, vpy, vpw, vif,* and *tmx* genes but JDV *orfs* have no *vpy* and *vpw*. Tat is a spliced gene product that binds to viral transcripts to enhance transcribing polymerase activity. Rev is a

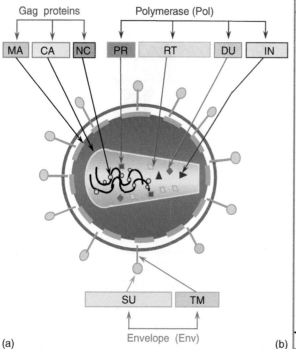

(a)

| Viral components | FIV | BIV |
|---|---|---|
| *Gag proteins* | | |
| Capsid (CA) | p24 | p26 |
| Matrix (MA) | p15 | p16 |
| Nucleoprotein (NC) | p7 | p13 |
| | | |
| *Pol proteins* | | |
| Protease (PR) | p13* | p11* |
| Reverse Transcriptase (RT) | p61* | p64 |
| Integrase (IN) | p31 | p32* |
| | | |
| *Env glycoproteins* | | |
| Surface Env (SU) | gp95–gp100 | gp100 |
| Transmembrane Env (TM) | gp39 | gp45 |
| | | |
| *Regulatory proteins* | | |
| Regulator of expression of viral protein (Rev) | p23 | p23 |
| Virus infectivity factor (Vif) | p29 | Vif** |
| Transactivator (Tat) | ?*** | p14 |
| Virus protein y (Vpy) | None | p10* |
| Virus protein w (Vpw) | None | p7* |
| Transmembrane x (Tmx) | None | p19 |

* Predicted value; ** Predicted; *** 79 aa Tat-like protein

(b)

**Figure 2** General structure of (a) BIV and FIV with (b) the size designations of structural proteins, enzymes, and regulatory proteins.

spliced gene product that is important in production and transport of viral RNA transcripts. Vpy and Vpw are speculated to have similar function as HIV-1 Vpu and Vpr. Vpu is involved in increasing virion release, while Vpr promotes the transport of the DNA pre-integration complex into the cell nuclei. Tmx has been detected in infected cells but its function remains unknown. FIV has four main *orfs* (*orf 1–4*). FIV *orf 1* appears to be analogous to the HIV-1 *vif* gene. Vif acts late in the viral life cycle and is needed for optimal production of virions. FIV *orf 2* (also called *orf A*) was speculated to be the first exon of the *tat* gene (encoding a 79 aa Tat-like protein) but recently was reported to be related to the *vpr* gene found in primate lentiviruses. FIV *orf 3* (3′ end of *orf A* or *orf 2*) and *orf 4* (*orf H*) are analogous to the exons of the *rev* gene found in HIV and SIV.

## Host Range and Virus Propagation

BIV has been isolated from dairy and beef cattle, and buffaloes. In addition, rabbits, goats, and sheep can be experimentally infected with BIV. BIV infects primary cells from bovine embryonic tissues (lung, brain, thymus, and spleen) and established cell lines of epithelial bovine trachea, canine fetal thymus, and embryonic rabbit epidermis, but does not infect human cell lines. Monocytes and macrophages are the major cell types infected by BIV. Recent studies show low-level infection in T cells and B cells from BIV$_{R29}$-infected cattle.

Domestic FIV has limited host range with productive infection found only in felid species. In contrast, nondomestic FIV sequence was recently identified in Hyaenidae species. Puma FIV-pco and lion FIV-Ple cause persistent infection in laboratory cats without clinical disease. Domestic FIV has been found in the wild cat population, Tsushima cat (*Felis bengalensis euptilura*), and may present problems for the conservation of this endangered species. FIV of domestic cats infects macrophages, endothelial cells, glial cells, B cells, CD8$^+$ T cells, and CD4$^+$ T cells. *In vitro* infection has been demonstrated in feline astrocytes, fibroblastic Crandell feline kidney cells, feline T cell lines, macaque peripheral blood mononuclear cell (PBMC), and low-level-to-defective infection in human cell lines. Experimental inoculation with domestic FIV grown in macaque PBMC resulted in FIV infection of macaques. However, there has been no evidence of zoonotic transmission and productive infection of humans with FIV.

## Genetics and Evolution

Due to the difficulty of isolating BIV from infected cattle, only a few full sequences, all from the USA (Louisiana,

Florida, and Oklahoma), are available. Genetic variability of different USA strains shows as much as 10% variation in the *pol* and considerably more at the *env*. Genetic variability was also assessed by analyzing polymerase chain reaction (PCR)-amplified short sequences of *env* and *pol*. Phylogenetic analysis of the *SU* gene showed clustering of Asian isolates distinct from USA isolates. Moreover, inter- and intra-animal *env* variations were observed in BIV$_{R29}$-infected rabbits, suggesting the potential development of quasispecies. Only one Bali JDV isolate has been fully sequenced and therefore, little is known about the genetics of JDV.

Due to the wide genetic variability between worldwide isolates, FIV is classified into five subtypes (A–E). Studies on mutation rates in FIV *env* and *gag* show positive selective pressure for *env* mutations, consistent with reports that HIV *env* has a high mutation rate compared to *gag* and *pol*. PCR analyses of FIV variants isolated within individual cats over a 3 year period indicate that sequence variation in *env* increases over time, with later isolates showing divergence of 0.5–1.5%. Hence, the divergence of the variants within individual cats appears to be twofold less than those variants from an HIV-1-positive individual. Superinfections and recombinations have been reported for FIV much like those reported for HIV-1. Phylogenetic analyses suggest domestic FIV originated from a lineage associated with the wild cat lentivirus (see the section titled 'Taxonomy and classification').

## Serologic Relationships and Variability

Sera from BIV-infected cattle reacted to CA from HIV-1, SIV, EIAV, and JDV, and vice versa. Strongest serum cross-reactivity to CA was observed between BIV- and JDV-infected cattle. Sera from BIV$_{R29}$-infected cattle contained virus-neutralizing antibodies (VNAs) to BIV$_{R29}$ throughout 5 years post infection (pi), but these VNAs did not cross-neutralize Florida BIV$_{FL112}$. The *env* sequences between BIV and JDV and among BIV, HIV-1, SIV, and EIAV are less conserved. Consequently, cross-neutralization of HIV-1, SIV, and EIAV with sera from BIV-infected cattle is not expected.

Sera from cats infected with different FIV strains reacted to prototype FIV$_{Pet}$. The cross-reactivity of the infected sera has been the basis for the commercial FIV diagnostic kit. Sera from wild cats infected with nondomestic lentivirus cross-reacted predominantly to CA p24 and lesser degree to MA p15 of domestic FIV, and vice versa. Sera from HIV-1-positive subjects cross-reacted to domestic FIV p24 and vice versa. Rabbit polyclonal antibodies to ungulate lentiviruses, MVV and CAEV, also reacted to domestic FIV at p24 and p15, demonstrating the evolutionarily conserved epitopes on p24 and p15. In general,

FIV-specific VNAs can neutralize closely related strains but not divergent strains. Preliminary studies suggest that a loose correlation exists between the genotype based on *env* sequence and the VNAs elicited by infected cats.

## Epidemiology

Global distribution of BIV infection in dairy and beef cattle has a seroprevalence of 1.4–33% (**Figure 1(a)**). Clinical signs were more frequently observed in BIV-infected dairy cattle than in BIV-infected beef cattle. This may be due to fewer stress factors in beef cattle than in dairy cattle. In some countries, BIV infection was higher in the dairy cattle than the beef cattle, because of the management practices (hand-feeding pooled colostrums/milk to dairy calves) and the longer lifespan (more risk of exposure) of the dairy cattle than the beef cattle. The global prevalence of FIV infection is 1–26% in the high-risk populations (symptomatic cats) (**Figure 1(b)**) and 0.7–16% in the healthy (minimal to no-risk) populations. FIV infection is found more frequently in cats >5 years of age than in younger cats and rarely in cats <1 year of age. Furthermore, free-roaming cats have the highest incidence of infection as compared to indoor cats. Male cats are 2–3 times more likely to be infected than female cats. Since male cats are territorially aggressive and have higher incidence of wounds and bite abscesses, the high prevalence of FIV infection in male free-roaming cats is consistent, with the major mode of FIV transmission being via biting.

## Transmission and Tissue Tropism

BIV has been detected in the spleen, liver, brain, lymph nodes, and PBMC of infected cattle. Based on PCR analysis of purified cell populations from $BIV_{R29}$-infected cattle, BIV is pantropic and infects $\alpha\beta$ T cells, $\gamma\delta$ T cells, B cells, and monocytes/macrophages. The cellular receptor for BIV is still unknown. Transmission of BIV is by exposure to contaminated blood, contaminated milk/colostrum, and possibly by sexual contact. *In utero* vertical transmission was reported. BIV was detected by PCR in embryo and occasionally in semen from infected cattle. Controversy exists about the BIV PCR detection in the semen and on the viability of BIV from the PCR-positive frozen semen and embryos, which are the sources for artificial insemination. Transmission by arthropod vector has been suggested but the evidence for this mode is lacking. Transmission by ingesting contaminated colostrum/milk was also suspected since BIV was detected in milk. Moreover, iatrogenic transmission (reused hypodermic syringe and equipment for pregnancy examination, de-horning, artificial insemination, and castration) of contaminated blood is suspected to be the main source of passing the infection to large numbers of uninfected cattle.

Although significant CD4$^+$ T-cell loss occurs during FIV infection, the feline CD4 molecule is not the receptor for FIV. The primary cellular receptor for domestic FIV was recently identified to be feline CD134, also called OX40. CD134 is a member of tumor necrosis factor receptor family that is transiently expressed on activated T cells. FIV cannot use human CD134 as receptor to infect human cells, but can use both feline and human CXCR4, a chemokine receptor, as co-receptor. It has been speculated that CXCR4 can also serve as primary cellular receptor for FIV. Based on experimental transmission studies, the major route of FIV transmission is through bites from infected cats. This transmission route is consistent with the epidemiological studies and with the fact that cats shed significant amounts of virus in saliva. FIV transmission by ingestion of virus via grooming and licking bleeding wounds of an infected cat cannot be excluded, since oral administration of infected blood can cause infection. FIV infection was demonstrated by experimental vaginal and rectal inoculation, and FIV was isolated from vaginal swab and semen of infected cats. Another route of transmission is by ingesting contaminated colostrum/milk of infected queens. Experimental studies suggest the possibility of transplacental infection and transmission during birth through a contaminated birth canal. In conflict with these experimental observations is the low incidences of FIV infection in cats <1 years of age and in kittens born to chronically infected queens, suggesting that vertical transmission of FIV may be rare in nature.

## Clinical Features and Infection

Experimental $BIV_{R29}$ infection of dairy cattle caused lymphocytosis, hypertrophic regional lymph nodes, and hypertrophic hemal lymph nodes, which was identical to the lymphoid changes observed in cow R29. Seroconversion and virus recovery also demonstrated BIV infection. Unlike cow R29, clinical disease was not observed in the experimentally infected cattle. Naturally infected dairy cows had lymphoid changes similar to the experimentally infected cattle, and a portion of the population displayed postparturition problems. These included foot problems, mastitis, diarrhea, pneumonia, neuropathy, and decreased milk production. Clinical signs in beef cattle were less frequent when compared to dairy cattle. Infected beef cattle grew normally and gained weight but displayed dullness, lumbering gait, and enlarged subcutaneous hemal lymph nodes. The low pathogenicity of BIV has been described in a number of studies. In contrast, JDV infection of Bali (*Bos javanicus*) cattle had pronounced clinical disease with mortality of 17% and was more pathogenic than BIV or JDV infection of Ongole (*Bos taurus*) and Friesian (*Bos indicus*) cattle.

The immunological hallmark of FIV infection is depletion of peripheral $CD4^+$ T cells and reduced CD4:CD8 ratios, leading to B- and T-cell dysfunctions and hypergammaglobulinemia. The clinical stages of FIV infection are similar to human AIDS in several ways. The acute stage of experimental FIV infection was characterized by immunological abnormalities followed by depression, fever, diarrhea, neutropenia, and persistent generalized lymphadenopathy. FIV was primarily detected in lymphoid tissues followed by dissemination of the virus into nonlymphoid organs. Both antibodies against FIV and virus recovery from PBMC persisted throughout infection. The FIV load in the blood was lower and $CD4^+$ T-cell decline was slower at the asymptomatic stage than acute stage. By late symptomatic stage, the animals were severely immunosuppressed and displaying wasting syndrome, neurological disorders, and persistent secondary opportunistic infections. The virus load was extremely high at this stage, and FIV was readily isolated from nonlymphoid tissues and organs, such as kidney, saliva, and central nervous system (CNS). Lymphomas with and without FIV proviral integration were reported in naturally and experimentally infected cats, including B-cell lymphoma of more unusual extranodal forms (predominantly in the neck and head). The major clinical manifestations observed in naturally infected cats were a progressively degenerative immune disorder, neurological disorders, wasting syndrome, and persistent secondary opportunistic infections. The specific signs were chronic oral diseases, chronic upper respiratory tract disease, chronic enteritis, chronic conjunctivitis, anorexia, fever of unspecified origin, and recurrent cystitis. Abnormal behavioral problems, lymphosarcoma, and myeloproliferative disease were observed in a small proportion of affected cats.

## Pathology and Histopathology

Experimental $BIV_{R29}$ infection of dairy cattle caused B-cell lymphocytosis, hypertrophic regional lymph nodes with lymphoid hyperplasia, and primary hypertrophic hemal lymph nodes with follicular lymphoid hyperplasia. The lymph nodes and hemal lymph nodes during natural infection showed hyperplasia followed by follicular exhaustion and dysfunction, and follicular hypoplasia with atrophy and central follicular depletion especially of T-dependent zones in severe cases. Infected cattle developed early atypical proliferation of lymphocytes in lymphoid tissue followed by recurrent opportunistic infections, loss of circulating monocytes, poor body condition, and weight loss. Encephalitis was diagnosed with lesions of lymphocytic infiltration into the meninges and perivascular spaces, and foci of microglia and astrocytosis. Overall, the primary lesions were in the brain, lymphoid tissue, and feet (lymphocyte infiltration of hoof tissues).

Secondary diseases included nerve paralysis, persistent mastitis, septicemia, laminitis, secondary pododermatitis (plasmacytic inflammation), gastrointestinal diseases, bronchopneumonia, and subcutaneous and intramuscular abscesses.

Major histopathological changes during acute stage of experimental FIV infection were observed in the lymphoid tissues. In the first three weeks pi, lymphoid hyperplasia was observed in the lymph nodes, tonsils, spleens, and gut-associated lymphoid tissues. A majority of the FIV-infected cells were found in the germinal centers of lymphoid follicles of these tissues. Some infected cells were observed in the paracortex and medullary cords of lymph nodes, and in periarterial lymphoid sheaths and red pulp of the spleen. Shortly after, cats developed myeloid hyperplasia in the bone marrow and cortical involution, thymitis, and follicular hyperplasia of the medulla in the thymus. Both T cells and monocytes/macrophages were infected with FIV at an early phase of the acute stage, followed by infection of B cells. By early symptomatic stage, lymph nodes displayed follicular hyperplasia, involution, and lymphoid depletion, and by late phase, destruction of nodal architecture with involution and depletion of lymphoid follicles.

The CNS disease of FIV resembles those induced by HIV, and includes perivascular mononuclear cell infiltrates, glial nodules and diffuse gliosis of gray and white matter, and neuronal loss. Similar to HIV, neurotropic FIV strains infect microglia, astrocytes, and brain microvascular endothelial cells, but do not infect neuronal cells. Both anti-FIV antibodies and FIV virions have been isolated from cerebral spinal fluid (CSF) of infected cats, in addition to the elevated IgG index detected in the CSF. Like HIV, the level of FIV infection in the CNS cannot account for the cognitive/motor function abnormalities observed in these cats, suggesting that cytokines induced during CNS infection may play a key role in FIV neuropathogenesis. Neurological abnormalities included limb paresis, delayed righting and pupillary reflexes, behavioral changes, delayed visual and auditory evoked potentials, decreased spinal and peripheral nerve conduction velocities, and sleep abnormalities (e.g., increased awake time with decreased rapid eye movement) similar to sleep disturbances described in AIDS patients.

## Immune Response

Antibodies to p26 followed by antibodies to Env developed during early $BIV_{R29}$ infection, while a transient CD4/CD8 ratio decrease developed 2–7 weeks pi. This decrease was attributed to the greater $CD8^+$ cell increase than the slight $CD4^+$ cell increase. No significant $CD4^+$ cell or CD4/CD8 ratio decreases were observed throughout 5 years pi, even though persistent infection was demonstrated by the continued presence of TM-specific antibodies and VNAs. High VNA titers resulted in faster detection of virus, indicating high viral load. The role that VNAs play during natural pathogenesis of BIV is still unclear. It has been speculated that cellular immunity such as BIV-specific cytotoxic T lymphocytes (CTLs) may control the infection from progressing into clinical disease. However, decreased proliferation responses to T-cell mitogen and depressed T-dependent antibody responses to recall antigens at 4 and 5 years pi suggest loss in functional T-cell responses. In another study, B-cell lymphocytosis but no changes in $CD4^+$ cells and $CD8^+$ cells were observed in cattle infected with slightly pathogenic $BIV_{FL112}$. Although BIV infection does not cause $CD4^+$ cell loss, signs of T-cell dysfunction appear to develop upon prolonged infection.

Both the exposure dose and the FIV strain infecting the cats determine the nature of humoral and cellular immunity generated against the virus. Some strains do not elicit high or even significant VNAs even though high antibody titers to SU and TM are produced. Upon experimental infection with a moderate dose of FIV, anti-FIV antibodies were detected as early as 3 weeks pi, followed by VNAs starting 6–9 weeks pi. A decrease in primary proliferative response to only foreign antigen (none to T-cell mitogens and recall antigen) was observed at 5 weeks pi, the earliest time point tested. Hence, selective defects in primary antigen-specific response of naive $CD4^+$ T-helper cells are the early signs of T-cell dysfunction. Meanwhile, PBMC developed CTL responses to FIV Gag and Env at 7–9 and 16 weeks pi, respectively. The time of CD4/CD8 inversion depended greatly on the FIV strain used, with a moderate dose of pathogenic strains causing CD4/CD8 inversion as early as 4–6 weeks pi. In general, the $CD4^+$ T-cell loss accounted for the CD4/CD8 ratio inversion with most strains, but $CD8^+$ T-cell increases also contributed to this inversion in a number of strains. A defect in proliferative response of memory T cells to recall antigen developed at about 19 weeks pi. Decreased T-cell mitogen responses developed upon prolonged infection when considerable CD4/CD8 ratio inversion prevailed. B-cell dysfunctions were milder and were decreased primary antibody responses to T-dependent antigens and increased serum IgG levels, indicative of virus-specific B-cell hyperactivity. In addition, functional abnormalities in macrophages, neutrophils, and natural killer cells were observed in the FIV-infected cats.

## Prevention and Control

The control of BIV infection in animal food relies on the practice of testing and preventing the spread of BIV infection by decreasing iatrogenic transmission through improved management practices. Public health concern appears to be minimal, since there is no evidence of BIV zoonosis and the virus in milk is readily inactivated by pasteurization. The importance of BIV infection to the cattle industry depends on the severity of the economic losses resulting from lower milk production and poor beef quality. Similarly, the need for developing a BIV vaccine will hinge on the perception of the cattle industry rather than the significance this virus has as an animal model for AIDS.

Experimental FIV vaccine trials, ranging from inactivated single-subtype virus vaccine to proviral DNA vaccine, were performed with minimal-to-no success against homologous (identical to vaccine strains) and heterologous strains. A commercial dual-subtype FIV vaccine, consisting of inactivated subtype A and D viruses, was released in USA in 2002. This vaccine was effective against homologous strains, heterologous subtype A strains, and subtype B strains. This vaccine induced VNAs to closely related FIV strains from subtypes A and D. The vaccine protection against subtype B viruses was achieved in the absence of VNAs to challenge viruses, suggesting the importance of vaccine-induced cellular immunity. Both the prototype and commercial dual-subtype vaccines induced strong FIV-specific $CD4^+$ T-helper and $CD8^+$ CTL responses. Since there is no evidence of FIV zoonosis, the efforts to develop FIV-specific antiretroviral drugs have been limited. Only few antiretroviral drugs for HIV-1 therapy have been tested in infected cats. These include azidothymidine (AZT), 9-(2-phosphonylmethoxyethyl) adenine, dideoxycytidine 5′-triphosphate, dideoxycytidine, lamivudine (3TC), cyclosporine A, interferon-α, and commercial HIV-1 protease inhibitors. Prophylactic 2 week therapy with a high-dose AZT/3TC combination, started either 3 days before or on the day of FIV inoculation, resulted in 100% and 67% protection of cats from infection, respectively. Although the prophylaxis with nucleoside analogs was remarkable, the therapeutic use of the aforementioned drugs, including nucleoside analogs, was somewhat disappointing. Like HIV-1 drug therapy, FIV therapy will require multiple drug combination with each drug inhibiting different stages of FIV replication cycle.

## Future

The importance of BIV infection to the cattle industry is still unclear. The current strategy is to contain BIV infection by methodical testing and imposing management practices that prevent the spread of BIV. More information about the genetic and pathogenic evolution of BIV is needed to assess whether fatal pathogenic strains can evolve from current low-pathogenic strains. Overall, the policies set by cattle industry and government agencies will influence the extinction or survival of BIV infection in cattle.

FIV infection causes an important disease in domestic pet cats. The commercial vaccine was effective against strains from global subtypes A and B, and should be able to contain the global spread of FIV. However, the inability of current FIV diagnostics (enzyme-linked immunosorbent assay (ELISA) and immunoblot assay) to distinguish vaccinated cats from FIV-infected cats has caused a dilemma in the use of this vaccine. This problem can be resolved by developing sensitive molecular diagnostics or a vaccine that does not conflict with current FIV diagnostics. Identifying the protective vaccine epitopes should assist in designing a vaccine that is devoid of diagnostic epitopes. Moreover, FIV research on vaccines will provide new insights to HIV vaccine development for humans. The recent discovery of fatal pathogenic FIV strains (10% acute mortality) demonstrates the pathogenic evolution of FIV similar to HIV-1 immunopathogenesis. Hence, FIV infection is not only important for feline medicine but serves as an important small animal model for testing novel antiretroviral drugs, immunotherapy, and vaccine approaches for HIV/AIDS.

*See also:* Equine Infectious Anemia Virus; Simian Immunodeficiency Virus: Animal Models of Disease; Simian Immunodeficiency Virus: General Features; Simian Immunodeficiency Virus: Natural Infection; Visna-Maedi Viruses.

## Further Reading

Bachmann MH, Mathiason-Dubard C, Learn GH, *et al.* (1997) Genetic diversity of feline immunodeficiency virus: Dual infection, recombination, and distinct evolutionary rates among envelope sequence clades. *Journal of Virology* 71: 4241–4253.

Burkhard MJ and Dean GA (2003) Transmission and immunopathogenesis of FIV in cats as a model for HIV. *Current HIV Research* 1: 15–29.

Evermann JE, Howard TH, Dubovi EJ, *et al.* (2000) Controversies and clarifications regarding bovine lentivirus infections. *Journal of the American Veterinary Medical Association* 217: 1318–1324.

Podell M, March PA, Buck WR, and Mathes LE (2000) The feline model of neuroAIDS: Understanding the progression towards AIDS dementia. *Journal of Psychopharmacology* 14: 205–213.

Snider TG, Hoyt PG, Jenny BF, *et al.* (1997) Natural and experimental bovine immunodeficiency virus infection in cattle. *The Veterinary Clinics of North America. Food Animal Practice* 13: 151–176.

St-Louis M-C, Cojocariu M, and Archambault D (2004) The molecular biology of bovine immunodeficiency virus: A comparison with other lentiviruses. *Animal Health Research Reviews* 5: 125–143.

Troyer JL, Pecon-Slattery J, Roelke ME, *et al.* (2005) Seroprevalence and genomic divergence of circulating strains of feline immunodeficiency virus among Felidae and Hyaenidae species. *Journal of Virology* 79: 8282–8294.

Uhl EW, Heaton-Jones TG, Pu R, and Yamamoto JK (2002) FIV vaccine development and its importance to veterinary and human medicine: A review. *Veterinary. Immunology and Immunopathology* 90: 113–132.

Wilcox GE, Chadwick BJ, and Kertayadnya G (1995) Recent advances in the understanding of Jembrana disease. *Veterinary Microbiology* 46: 249–255.

# Bovine Ephemeral Fever Virus

**P J Walker,** CSIRO Livestock Industries, Geelong, VIC, Australia

## Glossary

**Epicardium** The outer layer of heart tissue.
**Hypocalcemia** A low level of calcium in the circulating blood.
**Leucopenia** A decreased total number of white blood cells in the circulating blood.
**Pericardial fluid** Fluid within a double-walled sac that contains the heart and the roots of the great blood vessels.
**Sternal recumbency** Reclined in a position of comfort on the chest bone.
**Synovial membranes** Connective tissue membranes lining the cavities of the freely movable joints.
**Thoracic fluid** Fluid in the chest cavity.

## Introduction

Bovine ephemeral fever virus (BEFV) is an arthropod-borne rhabdovirus that causes a disabling and sometimes lethal disease of cattle (*Bos taurus, Bos indicus,* and *Bos javanicus*) and water buffaloes (*Bubalus bubalis*). Unapparent infections can also occur in cape buffalo, hartebeest, waterbuck, wildebeest, deer, and possibly goats. Bovine ephemeral fever (BEF) was first recorded in East Africa and Egypt during the late nineteenth century. However, BEF (which is also variously called three-day sickness, bovine enzootic fever, bovine influenza, and stiffsiekte) is thought to have been endemic since antiquity in much of tropical and subtropical Africa, and Asia. As the name suggests, BEF is often characterized by the rapid onset of and recovery from clinical signs that can include a bi- or multiphasic fever, ocular and nasal discharge, muscle stiffness, anorexia, rumenal stasis, lameness, and sternal recumbency. Although mortality rates rarely exceed 1–2%, a particularly severe outbreak in Taiwan in 1996 has been reported to have resulted in the death or culling of 11.3% of a population of 110 247 dairy cattle on 516 farms. Severe infections commonly occur in larger, more valuable animals. Morbidity rates may approach 100% with significant economic impacts including loss of milk production, temporary infertility in bulls, abortion, loss of condition in beef herds, and disablement of draft animals at the time of harvest. The economic consequences of BEF can be significant. An outbreak of BEF in Israel in 1999 has been estimated to have cost, on average $280 per lactating cow and $112 per nonlactating cow. In Australia, sweeping epidemics in the 1970s have been estimated to have caused industry-wide losses exceeding $200 million in today's values. Due to limitations on the importation of livestock and semen from animals with evidence of BEFV infection, the disease can also have significant impact on international trade.

## Taxonomic Classification

BEFV is classified in the order *Mononegavirales*, family *Rhabdoviridae* as the type species of the genus *Ephemerovirus*. Ephemeroviruses have morphological and genetic characteristics common to all rhabdoviruses, including an enveloped, bullet-shaped virion containing a nonsegmented, negative-sense, single-stranded (ss) RNA genome. However, unlike viruses classified in other established rhabdovirus taxa, ephemeroviruses share the unusual characteristic of two type 1 transmembrane glycoproteins (G and $G_{NS}$) that are related in amino acid sequence and appear to have arisen by gene duplication. Other recognized species in the genus include *Berrimah virus* (BRMV) and *Adelaide River virus* (ARV). These viruses have each been isolated from cattle in northern Australia and also appear to be transmitted by biting insects. Tentative species in the genus include Kimberley virus (KIMV), Malakal virus (MALV), and Puchong virus (PUCV), each of which is closely related serologically to BEFV. KIMV has been isolated from *Culex annulirostris* mosquitoes and *Culicoides brevitarsis* midges in Australia, and from healthy cattle. MALV was isolated in Sudan and PUCV in Malaysia, each from *Mansonia uniformis* mosquitoes. Potential vertebrate hosts for these viruses are yet to be identified. Although BEFV is the only ephemerovirus known to be associated with disease, Kotonkan virus (KOTV), which was originally isolated from *Culicoides* spp. in Nigeria, does cause an ephemeral fever-like illness in cattle. Recent phylogenetic studies using the N gene and segments of the L gene suggest that KOTV, as well as Obodhiang virus (OBOV) which was isolated from

*Mansonia uniformis* mosquitoes in Sudan, should also be classified as ephemeroviruses. It has also been suggested that all arthropod-borne rhabdoviruses, including the ephemeroviruses, vesiculoviruses, and a large number of other unclassified rhabdoviruses share a common ancestor and should form a larger taxonomic group for which the name 'dimarhabdovirus' (dipteran-mammalian rhabdovirus) has been proposed (**Figure 1**).

## Geographic Distribution

BEFV is known to occur in most tropical and subtropical regions of Africa, Asia, and Australia. The disease occurs throughout much of Africa and in Asian countries south of a line that includes Israel, Iraq, Iran, Syria, India, Pakistan, Bangladesh, southern and central China, and east to Taiwan, and southern Japan. It occurs throughout Southeast Asia, parts of New Guinea, and in most of northern and eastern Australia. It does not occur in New Zealand or the islands of the Pacific, or in the Americas, or Europe, where it is considered an important exotic pathogen. There is reported serological evidence of infection in southern Russia but the disease has not been described. The distribution of BEFV is determined by the geographic range of available insect vectors and is limited by international trade restrictions on live animals and semen showing evidence of infection.

## Epizootiology

Bovine ephemeral fever is a seasonal disease. It occurs principally in the summer and early autumn, and with the onset of the monsoon season in Asia. Outbreaks are usually associated with periods of high rainfall which precipitate the emergence of insect vectors in large numbers. BEFV can also spread in epizootics that follow the pattern of prevailing winds with a general southward movement in the Southern Hemisphere and northward movement above the Equator. Wind-borne movement of insect vectors is the likely mechanism of spread. Vectors include biting midges (*Culicoides* spp.) and mosquitoes, in which the virus replicates. BEFV has been isolated from *Culicoides brevitarsis*, *Culicoides coarctatus*, *Anopheles bancroftii*, a mixed pool of mosquito species in Australia, and from a mixed pool of biting midges in Africa. The virus has also been recovered from several other species of biting midge and mosquito following experimental infection. The abundance and distribution of insects from which BEFV has been isolated suggests that several major vectors may be involved in transmission. There is no evidence of direct transmission of BEFV between cattle, even when encouraged by smearing nasal or ocular discharges on mucosal surfaces.

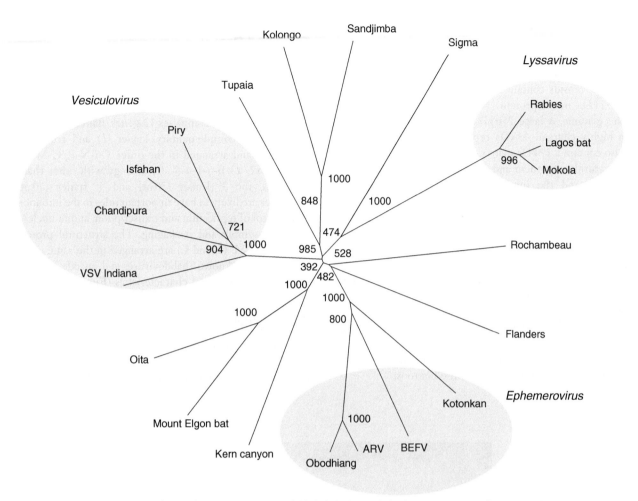

**Figure 1**   Phylogenetic tree of partial N gene sequences of 20 rhabdoviruses infecting mammals and/or insects. The tree was generated from a Clustal X alignment of the sequences by the neighbor-joining method and presented graphically using Treeview software. The viruses include representatives of three rhabdovirus genera: *Ephemerovirus* (BEFV, ARV, Obodhiang virus, and Kotonkau virus); *Vesiculovirus* (VSV Indiana, Chandipura, Isfahan, and Piry viruses); and *Lyssavirus* (rabies, Mokola, and Lagos bat viruses). Unclassified rhabdoviruses include Sandjimba, Rochambeau, Flanders, Kern Canyon, Mount Elgon bat, Oita, Tupaia and Kolongo, and sigma viruses. Confidence in branch nodes was determined by bootstrap analysis on 1000 replicates (indicated as numbers).

## Pathology and Pathogenesis

Bovine ephemeral fever is principally an inflammatory disease. The incubation period is normally 2–4 days. Viremia usually persists for 1–3 days and peaks approximately 24 h before the onset of fever. The initial sites of infection are not known but the virus has been isolated from neutrophils and reticuloendothelial cells of the lungs, spleen, and lymph nodes. There is also evidence of infection in synovial membranes, epicardium and aorta, and in cells derived from synovial, pericardial, thoracic, and abdominal fluids. There is not widespread tissue damage. The primary lesion is a vasculitis affecting the endothelium of small vessels of synovial membranes, tendon sheaths, muscles, facia, and skin. The onset of fever and other clinical signs is accompanied by marked leucopenia, relative neutrophilia, elevated plasma fibrinogen, and elevated levels of cytokines including interferon α, interleukin 1, and tissue necrosis factor. There is also a significant hypocalcemia that is thought to be responsible for sternal recumbency. The major clinical signs can be treated very effectively with anti-inflammatory drugs.

## Virion Structure and Morphogenesis

BEFV virions are enveloped, bullet-shaped particles (approximately $70 \times 180$ nm) containing a precisely coiled, helical nucleocapsid with 35 cross-striations at an interval of 4.8 nm. Virions have a prominent axial channel intruding from the base and typically are more cone-shaped than commonly observed for viruses in other genera of animal rhabdovirus (e.g., lyssaviruses and vesiculoviruses). The envelope contains a single 81 kDa class

1 transmembrane glycoprotein (G) that forms visible projections on the virion surface. The G protein mediates cell attachment and entry, is the target for virus-neutralizing antibodies, and induces protective antibodies in cattle. Nucleocapsids contain a negative-sense ssRNA genome, a 52 kDa nucleoprotein (N) which is tightly bound to the genome, a large 250 kDa replicase protein (L), and a highly charged 43 kDa replicase cofactor (P). Virions also contain a 29 kDa matrix protein (M) which is a major structural component and appears to lie between nucleocapsids and the inner surface of the lipid envelope (**Figure 2**).

Viral replication is cytoplasmic and morphogenesis occurs primarily at the plasma membrane in association with accumulations of a filamentous, granular, intracytoplasmic matrix. However, late in infection, there is a proliferation of plasma membrane, cells become highly vacuolated, and virions are observed both at the plasma membrane and within cytoplasmic vacuoles. Following budding as cone-shaped extrusions, virions accumulate in extracellular spaces. The general characteristics of viral morphogenesis appear to be similar in infected mammalian cell cultures and mouse neurons.

## BEFV Genome Organization and the Encoded Proteins

The 14 900 nt BEFV genome is the largest known for any rhabdovirus and one of the largest and most complex genomes for any nonsegmented, negative-sense RNA virus. The genome comprises 12 genes, flanked by terminal, partially complementary leader ($l$) and trailer ($t$) sequences, and arranged in the order 3′-$l$-N-P/C-M-G-$G_{NS}$-α1/α2/α3-β-γ-L-$t$-5′. By analogy with other rhabdoviruses, the 3′ leader (50 nt) and 5′ trailer (70 nt) sequences are likely to have important roles in the initiation and control of replication and transcription, and in nucleoprotein assembly and packaging. The structural protein genes (N, P, M, G, and L) are arranged in the same order as for all other known rhabdoviruses and encode proteins with similar functional characteristics (**Figure 3**).

### The N Protein

The BEFV N gene encodes the 431 amino acid nucleoprotein (N). The N protein is a highly hydrophilic, RNA-binding protein containing 14.4% basic residues

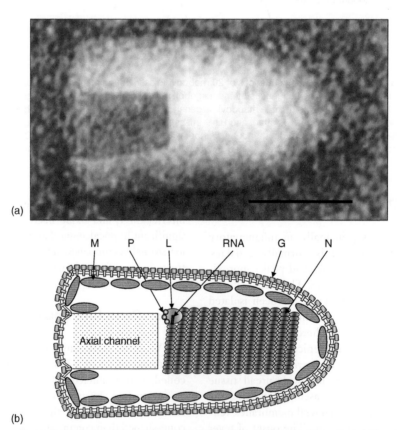

(a)

(b)

**Figure 2** (a) Negative-contrast electron micrograph of a purified BEFV virion. (b) Schematic representation of the BEFV virion. Structural proteins N, P, M, G, and L, and the negative-sense ssRNA genome are indicated. The axial channel is also depicted. The size and relative quantities of the proteins do not accurately reflect the content in virions. Scale = 50 nm (a).

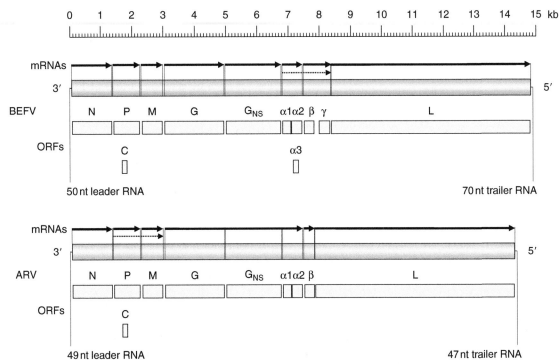

**Figure 3** Illustration of the genome organization and transcription strategy of BEFV and ARV. Solid arrows indicate the major transcriptional products. Minor transcripts are indicated by dotted arrows. The length of the ARV L protein is estimated from the alignment of available sequences with those of BEFV.

(lysine, arginine, and histidine) distributed relatively evenly throughout the molecule. Seven of these residues are highly conserved in rhabdoviruses and are involved in RNA-binding and stabilizing the interaction. The N protein also contains 14.6% acidic residues (glutamate and aspartate) that are less evenly distributed with significant clustering in a short domain near the C terminus. A similar acidic domain in the rabies N protein is a phosphorylation site involved in binding P protein to nucleocapsids. The BEFV N protein is also phosphorylated when packaged in virions and contains a similar phosphorylation site in this acidic domain.

## The P Protein

The P gene encodes the 278 amino acid, highly hydrophilic P protein. It corresponds to the polymerase-associated phosphoproteins of rabies virus (RV) and vesicular stomatitis virus (VSV) which are components of nucleocapsids and act as essential cofactors to the L protein during transcription and replication. The BEFV P protein has not been observed to be phosphorylated when extracted from virions but is phosphorylated when expressed from a recombinant baculovirus in insect cells. The BEFV P gene also contains an alternative open reading frame (ORF) encoding a 48 amino acid, highly basic 5.8 kDa polypeptide. This protein has not been detected in BEFV-infected cells and it is not known if it is expressed. However, alternative ORFs in the

P gene occur in vesiculoviruses and are a common feature of many viruses in the *Mononegavirales*. As in VSV, the BEFV C protein has two potential initiation codons, suggesting it could be expressed in two different forms.

## The M Protein

The M gene encodes the 691 amino acid, basic, hydrophilic protein that corresponds to the matrix protein (M) of rabies and VSV. The M protein is a major component of rhabdovirus virions and has been shown to have important functions in regulation of viral replication and transcription, inhibition of host cell protein synthesis and induction of apoptosis, and in budding of nucleocapsids at cytoplasmic membranes. The BEFV M protein has been shown to be phosphorylated when extracted from virions but not when expressed from a recombinant baculovirus in insect cells. This is consistent with observations that phosphorylation of the VSV M protein occurs at a late stage in viral assembly. The BEFV M protein also contains a 'late domain' sequence motif (PPSY) which, in VSV and several other RNA viruses, is essential for efficient budding from infected cells.

## The G Protein

The BEFV G gene encodes the 623-amino-acid virion transmembrane glycoprotein (G). The G protein is a class 1 membrane protein. It shares significant amino acid sequence identity with other animal rhabdovirus G proteins and contains a core of conserved cysteine residues suggesting preservation of fundamentally similar secondary structure. The G protein contains five potential N glycosylation sites, three of which appear to align with similar sites in VSV and/or rabies virus. The G protein is responsible for cell docking and entry, and is the target of virus-neutralizing antibodies for which the major binding sites have been defined (see below).

## The L Protein

The L gene encodes the 2144-amino-acid RNA-dependent RNA polymerase (L protein). The L protein is a structural component of nucleocapsids that, in cooperation with the N and P proteins, forms the ribonucleoprotein (RNP) complex that is responsible for replication and transcription of the viral genome. The BEFV L protein shares a high level of sequence similarity with other rhabdovirus L proteins and contains all of the conserved sequence motifs associated with the major functional domains; these include the polymerase catalytic site and other regions involved in replication, transcription, initiation, elongation, and termination, 3' polyadenylation, 5' capping, and cap methylation.

## The G$_{NS}$ Protein

The BEFV nonstructural protein genes are located in a 3442 nt region of the genome between the G gene and L gene. Immediately downstream of the G gene is a second gene encoding a class 1 transmembrane glycoprotein (G$_{NS}$). The 90 kDa G$_{NS}$ protein is abundant in infected cells but has not been detected in virions. It is related in structure and sequence to the BEFV virion G protein and other rhabdovirus G proteins and the evidence suggests that it has arisen by gene duplication. The G$_{NS}$ protein contains eight potential N-glycosylation sites and, as the size by sodium dodecyl sulfate-polyacrylamide gel electrophoresis (SDS-PAGE) is approximately 21 kDa in excess of the calculated molecular weight of the unmodified polypeptide, it appears to be highly glyscosylated. Sequence alignments indicate that it shares 10 of 12 cysteine residues that appear to form the core of secondary structure common to all animal rhabdoviruses. However, the G$_{NS}$ protein does not share antigenic sites with the BEFV G protein and antibody to G$_{NS}$ does not neutralize the infectivity of BEFV produced in either mammalian or insect cells. It has been shown to accumulate at the cell surface in association with amorphous structures but not with budding or mature virions. The function of the G$_{NS}$ is currently unknown.

## The Small Nonstructural Proteins

Downstream of the G$_{NS}$ gene is a complex region of the genome-encoding proteins that appear to be unique to BEFV and other ephemeroviruses. None of these proteins has yet been detected in virions or BEFV-infected cells. The α-gene coding region contains three long ORFs (α1, α2, and α3). The α1 ORF encodes an 88 amino acid, 10.6 kDa protein. It features a central transmembrane domain comprising 16 hydrophobic amino acids bounded by arginine residues, and a highly basic C-terminal domain in which 12 of 18 amino acids are lysine or arginine residues. This structure suggests α1 may function as a viroporin, a class of proteins that causes cytopathic effects by increasing membrane permeability. The BEFV α1 protein has been shown to be cytotoxic when expressed in insect cells from a recombinant baculovirus vector. The α2 ORF encodes a 116 amino acid, 13.7 kDa polypeptide. It overlaps the α3 ORF which encodes a 51 amino acid, 5.7 kDa polypeptide that contains an unusual triple repeat of isomers of the sequence KLMEE at intervals of four residues. The β-gene encodes a 107 amino acid, 12.3 kDa polypeptide. The γ-gene encodes a 114 amino acid, 13.5 kDa polypeptide. The α2, α3, β, and γ products share no sequence homology with known viral proteins (other than ARV, see below) and their functions are yet to be determined.

## BEFV Transcription

The RNP complex, comprising the RNA genome and the N, L, and P proteins, is the active replication and transcription unit of the virus. As for other rhabdoviruses, BEFV transcription from the (−) RNA genome generates 5' methylated, capped, and polyadenylated mRNAs by a progressive mechanism that initiates and terminates at short, conserved sequences flanking each gene. For each of the structural protein genes (N, P, N, G, and L), and the nonstructural glycoprotein gene (G$_{NS}$), transcription initiates at the sequence UUGUCC and terminates at the polyadenylation signal GUAC [U]$_7$. Transcription of the α-, β-, and γ-coding regions is more complex. The α-coding region is translated as an α1-α2-α3 polycistronic mRNA that initiates at UUGUCC but terminates at the variant polyadenylation signal GUUC [U]$_7$. This variant signal appears to cause incomplete termination and partial read-through of a longer tri-cistronic α-β-γ mRNA. The β gene is also immediately followed by a variant polyadenylation signal (GUAC [U]$_6$). However, the truncated (U$_6$) palindrome does not allow transcription termination, and reinitiation does not occur at a UUGUCC sequence located immediately in advance of the γ gene. As a result, the β- and γ-coding regions are transcribed as a bi-cistronic mRNA that initiates at UUGUCC upstream of the β ORF and terminates at the functional GUAC [U]$_7$

polyadenylation signal downstream of the γ ORF. This polyadenylation signal overlaps the L gene initiation sequence by 21 nt, requiring an upstream repositioning of the polymerase to commence L gene transcription. A similar arrangement for L gene transcription has been observed for several other nonsegmented (−) RNA viruses.

## ARV Genome Organization and Transcription

The genome organization and transcription strategy of ARV are similar to those of BEFV. However, there are subtle differences that reveal aspects of genome evolution and the control of gene expression in ephemeroviruses. The ARV genome includes the five structural protein genes that are common to all rhabdoviruses (N, P, M, G, and L). Each of the proteins encoded in these genes is similar in size and shares a high level of sequence identity with the corresponding BEFV proteins. Like BEFV, the ARV P gene also contains an alternative ORF that encodes a basic protein of similar size (7.4 kDa) to the BEFV C protein. The ARV 3′ leader sequence (49 nt) is similar in size to the BEFV leader RNA and shares a high level of sequence identity (21/22 nt) in the U-rich terminal domain. The ARV 5′ trailer sequence (47 nt) is shorter than the BEFV trailer RNA (70 nt), primarily due to the absence of a 26 nt direct repeat of the BEFV leader sequence that occurs in the BEFV trailer RNA. The function (if any) of this direct repeat is not known. The A-rich 5′ terminal region of the ARV trailer RNA shares only moderate sequence identity (15/21 nt) with the BEFV trailer, and is partially complementary (18/21 nt) to the U-rich ARV 3′ leader. This complementarity reflects the specificity of interaction of the polymerase with both the (−) RNA genome and (+) RNA antigenome during replication.

Like BEFV, the ARV genome encodes a second, class 1 transmembrane glycoprotein ($G_{NS}$) immediately downstream of the G gene. ARV $G_{NS}$ is also nonstructural and shares significant amino acid sequence identity with the BEFV $G_{NS}$ protein, as well as the G proteins of BEFV and other animal rhabdoviruses. ARV $G_{NS}$ has eight potential N-glycosylation sites, four of which appear to align with sites in BEFV $G_{NS}$. There is a high level of preservation of cysteine and proline residues with BEFV $G_{NS}$, suggesting a similar folded secondary structure. The ARV and BEFV $G_{NS}$ glycoproteins also appear to have preserved a core of cysteine residues conserved in rhabdovirus G proteins and is crucial for maintaining a fundamentally similar secondary structure. A proline-rich motif that, in VSV, forms a crucial 'P' helix in the membrane fusion domain, is also present in the BEFV and ARV G proteins. The 'P' helix motif is also present in BEFV $G_{NS}$ but it is absent from the ARV $G_{NS}$ protein. However, unlike the BEFV G protein, BEFV $G_{NS}$ does not induce cell fusion

when expressed in insect cells from a recombinant baculovirus vector. The biological significance of these observations will not be clear until further studies are conducted to better define the functions of ephemerovirus $G_{NS}$ proteins.

Between the $G_{NS}$ and L genes, ARV also contains a complex region encoding several proteins of uncertain function. The genes in this region are arranged in the order −$G_{NS}$-α1/α2-β-L-*t*-5′. The α1 ORF encodes a membrane-spanning, nonstructural protein with a highly basic C-terminal domain which is similar to the BEFV α1 protein and may well also function as a viroporin. The ARV α2 and β ORFs encode proteins similar in size to the corresponding BEFV proteins but, although the overall sequence similarity is relatively high, there is no significant sequence identity. A 17 kDa protein reported in purified ARV virions is similar in size to that predicted for the β protein. The α3 and γ ORFs are not present in the ARV genome.

The ARV transcription strategy is somewhat different from that of BEFV. Only the N-gene, L-gene, and β-gene are transcribed solely as monocistronic mRNAs. For the N-gene and L-gene, transcription initiates and terminates at standard UUGUCC and GUAC [U]$_7$ signals flanking each gene. Transcription of the β-gene initiates at the variant UUGUCU sequence and terminates at GUAC [U]$_7$. The P-gene and the M-gene are transcribed both as high abundance monocistronic mRNAs and a lower abundance (approximately 10%) bicistronic P/M mRNA. Each initiates at UUGUCC and the M-gene terminates at GUAC [U]$_7$. However, the P-gene terminates at the leaky variant signal GCAC [U]$_7$. The G-, $G_{NS}$-, and α-genes are transcribed primarily as a long polycistronic mRNA that initiates at UUGUCG upstream of the G-gene and terminates at GUAC [U]$_7$ following the α-gene. Corrupted termination/polyadenylation signals following the G-gene (GUAC [U]$_4$C [U]$_2$) and the $G_{NS}$-gene (GUGC [U]$_2$C [U]$_4$) appear to allow a very low level of termination and transcription initiation at UUGUCC signals immediately preceding both the $G_{NS}$- and α-genes. As for the BEFV γL junction, there is an overlap (22 nt) of the β-L gene junction in ARV, highlighting the importance of polymerase repositioning in the control of L gene expression. There is also a high level of nucleotide sequence identity between the α-β and β-γ gene junctions in BEFV, and between the ARV β-L gene junction and the BEFV γL gene junction. This suggests that the BEFV γ-gene may have evolved as a consequence of β-gene duplication. It appears, therefore, that gene duplication may have an important role in ephemerovirus evolution.

## Antigenic Variation

As defined either by cross-protection experiments in cattle, or by cross-neutralization tests in mice, or in cell cultures, BEFV exists as a single serotype globally. The relative antigenic stability of BEFV is most likely due to the occurrence of viremia and vector-borne transmission several days prior to the appearance of significant levels of virus-neutralizing antibodies. The BEFV virion G protein is the target of neutralizing antibody and four major neutralization sites have been identified and mapped to the amino acid sequence. Antigenic site G1 is a linear site that maps as two minimal B-cell epitopes at each end of the sequence spanning amino acids $Y^{487}$ to $K^{503}$ in the 'stem' domain of the G protein. This domain appears to be a unique feature of ephemeroviruses. Antigenic site G2 is conformational. It is located adjacent to two cysteine residues ($C^{172}$ and $C^{182}$) that appear to form a disulfide bridge linking a tight glycosylated loop structure in the folded G protein. Site G3 is the major conformational site comprising two partially overlapping elements (G3a and G3b). The site encompasses three different domains of the cysteine-rich 'head' structure of the folded G protein spanning $Q^{49}$ to $D^{57}$, $K^{215}$ to $E^{229}$, and $Q^{265}$. Similarly complex antigenic sites map to corresponding regions of other animal rhabdoviruses, again supporting the view that essential elements of G protein secondary structure are preserved. Site G4 is a linear site. It has not yet been mapped to the G-protein sequence but it is known to be conserved in BRMV and KIMV which are also neutralized by site G4 monoclonal antibodies. (Amino acid residues are numbered here to include the N-terminal

signal peptide that is cleaved during maturation of the G protein; **Figure 4**).

Limited natural antigenic variation has been reported between BEFV isolates. Variations in sites G3a and G3b have been identified among 70 Australian BEFV isolates collected from diverse locations between 1956 and 1992. There appears to be a temporal basis for the shift in site G3a which is present in most strains isolated after 1973. Comparison of prototype Australian and Chinese BEFV isolates has also indicated variations in site G3a. In Taiwan, variations have been reported in sites G1 and G3. The pattern of amino acid substitutions indicates that the isolates cluster into those which included the 1984 Taiwanese vaccine strain (Tn73) and those which were isolated after 1986. It is possible that incomplete protection provided by available BEF vaccines is contributing to antigenic instability in the G protein.

## Immune Response and Vaccination

Natural BEFV infection induces a strong neutralizing antibody response and apparently durable immunity. Following experimental infection, neutralizing IgG antibody appears 4–5 days after the onset of clinical signs and peaks within 1–4 weeks. Although there are some reports that cattle with high levels of neutralizing antibody can be susceptible to experimental challenge, other evidence

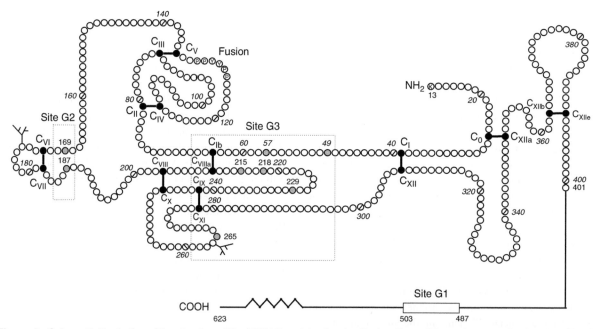

**Figure 4**  Schematic illustration of the structure of the BEFV G protein showing the locations of the major neutralization sites (G1, G2, and G3) and the predicted fusion domain including the highly conserved poly-proline helix (PPYYPP). Amino acids known to be located in the major antigenic sites are indicated as shaded circles. Disulfide bridges are assigned according to previous predictions from sequence alignments with other rhabdoviruses and from the known crystallographic structure of the low-pH form of the VSV G protein. Amino acids are numbered from the first residue of the translated protein, prior to removal of the N-terminal signal peptide.

suggests a good correlation between protection and neutralizing antibody. Colostral antibody has also been shown to protect calves against experimental challenge. High levels of cytokines circulate during the acute phase of infection but little is known of the role of innate or adaptive cell-mediated immunity in recovery from infection or protection against natural or experimental challenge.

Several forms of live-attenuated, inactivated, subunit, and recombinant BEFV vaccines have been reported and vaccines of varying format are produced for commercial use. Live-attenuated vaccines have been produced in mice and in cell cultures. In general, live vaccines are relatively effective in inducing protection but require at least two doses in adjuvant to generate durable immunity. Inactivated vaccines have been produced by treatment of BEFV with formalin or β-propiolactone, but have generally poor efficacy. Consecutive vaccinations with live-attenuated and killed preparations have also been used with some success. A purified G-protein subunit vaccine delivered in Quil A adjuvant has been shown to provide reliable protection following a two-dose treatment at an interval of 21 days. Recombinant BEFV vaccines employing the BEFV G protein delivered in vaccinia and capripox viral vectors have also been trialed.

*See also:* Animal Rhabdoviruses; Fish Rhabdoviruses; Vesicular Stomatitis Virus.

## Further Reading

Inaba Y, Kurogi H, Takahashi A, et al. (1974) Vaccination of cattle against bovine ephemeral fever with live attenuated virus followed by killed virus. *Archiv fur die Gesamte Virusforschung* 44: 121–132.

Kirkland PD (2002) Akabane and bovine ephemeral fever virus infections. *Veterinary Clinics of North America: Food Animal Practice* 18: 501–514.

Kongsuwan K, Cybinski DH, Cooper J, and Walker PJ (1998) Location of neutralizing epitopes on the G protein of bovine ephemeral fever rhabdovirus. *Journal of General Virology* 79: 2573–2578.

Kuzmin IV, Hughes GJ, and Rupprecht CE (2006) Phylogenetic relationships of seven previously unclassified viruses within the family *Rhabdoviridae* using partial nucleoprotein gene sequences. *Journal of General Virology* 87: 2323–2331.

McWilliam SM, Kongsuwan K, Cowley KA, Byrne KA, and Walker PJ (1997) Genome organization and transcription strategy in the complex G$_{NS}$-L intergenic region of bovine ephemeral fever rhabdovirus. *Journal of General Virology* 78: 1309–1317.

Nandi S and Negi BS (1999) Bovine ephemeral fever: A review. *Comparative Immunology, Microbiology, and Infectious Diseases* 22: 81–91.

St. George TD (1990) Bovine ephemeral fever virus. In: Dinter Z and Morein B (eds.) *Virus Infections of Vertebrates, Vol. 3: Virus Infections of Ruminants*, pp. 405–415. Amsterdam: Elsevier.

Theodoridis A, Giesecke WH, and Du Toit IJ (1973) Effects of ephemeral fever on milk production and reproduction of dairy cattle. *The Onderstepoort Journal of Veterinary Research* 40: 83–92.

Tomori O, Fagbami A, and Kemp G (1974) Kotonkan virus: Experimental infection of Fulani calves. *Bulletin of Epizootic Diseases of Africa* 22: 195–200.

Tordo N, Benmansour A, Calisher C, et al. (2005) *Rhabdoviridae*. In: Fauquet CM, Mayo MA, Maniloff J, Desselberger U,, and Ball LA (eds.) *Virus Taxonomy: Eighth Report of the International Committee on Taxonomy of Viruses*, pp. 623–644. San Diego, CA: Elsevier Academic Press.

Uren MF, St. George TD, and Zakrzewski H (1989) The effect of anti-inflammatory agents on the clinical expression of bovine ephemeral fever. *Veterinary Microbiology* 19: 99–111.

Venter GJ, Hamblin C, and Paweska JT (2003) Determination of the oral susceptibility of South African livestock-associated biting midges, *Culicoides* species, to bovine ephemeral fever virus. *Medical and Veterinary Entomology* 17: 133–137.

Walker PJ (2005) Bovine ephemeral fever in Australia and the World. In: Fu Z and Kaprowski H (eds.) *The World of Rhabdoviruses. Current Topics in Microbiology and Immunology*, vol. 292, pp. 57–80. Berlin: Springer.

Walker PJ, Byrne KA, Riding GA, et al. (1992) The genome of bovine ephemeral fever rhabdovirus contains two related glycoprotein genes. *Virology* 191: 49–61.

Wang YH, McWilliam SM, Cowley JA, and Walker PJ (1994) Complex genome organization in the G$_{NS}$-L intergenic region of Adelaide River rhabdovirus. *Virology* 203: 63–72.

# Bovine Herpesviruses

**M J Studdert,** The University of Melbourne, Parkville, VIC, Australia

## History

Although some of the clinical diseases caused by herpesviruses in members of the family Bovidae have been recognized for centuries, it was not until the first and probably most important alphaherpesvirus now called bovine herpesvirus 1 (BHV1) was isolated in the late 1950s from the genital disease coital exanthema (also called infectious pustular vulvovaginitis (IPV) in the female) and from the respiratory disease infectious bovine rhinotracheitis (IBR) that any of these diseases was confirmed to be caused by a herpesvirus. Historically, IPV and its male counterpart infectious pustular balanoposthitis (collectively the male and female diseases are termed coital exanthema or *blaschenausschlag*) were commonly described diseases in central Europe throughout the nineteenth century. It was common for a single bull in a village to serve all the female cattle in that village and, where distances were small, also in nearby villages, and *blaschenausschlag* was a frequently observed sequel to mating. The isolation of IBR virus in 1957 and IPV virus in 1958, and subsequent work that established that the two viruses were essentially identical, led to the designation of BHV1.

Around 1970, a distinctly different, but BHV1-related, alphaherpesvirus was recognized as a cause of encephalitis. This virus is designated BHV5 pending identification of its definitive host, which may not be European cattle.

The alphaherpesvirus BHV2 was recognized as a cause of pseudolumpy skin disease and, as an independent syndrome, mammillitis, in about 1960, although both diseases were known clinically well before this time.

An alphaherpesvirus with a natural history similar to that of BHV1 was isolated from goats in the mid-1960s. An increasing number of alphaherpesviruses, again assumed to have a natural history similar to BHV1, have been isolated from various deer and other wild ruminant species. Curiously, no alphaherpesvirus has been isolated from sheep.

A slowly growing, highly cell-associated gammaherpesvirus, uncertainly associated with a number of disease syndromes in cattle, is designated BHV4.

The disease bovine malignant catarrhal fever (MCF) has been described for at least a century and the causative gammaherpesvirus of the African form of the disease, formerly designated BHV3 (sometimes BHV4), was first isolated in 1968. However, the natural host for the best-characterized MCF gammaherpesvirus, acquired by European cattle, as originally reported in southern Africa, is the wildebeest (*Connochaetes gnu*) and this virus is now termed alcelaphine herpesvirus 1 (AlHV1). A poorly characterized gammaherpesvirus (OvHV1) associated with ovine pulmonary adenomatosis has been described and a second ovine gammaherpesvirus (OvHV2) is the cause of sheep-associated bovine MCF.

An increasing number of gammaherpesviruses have been identified in normally free-ranging ruminant species when they are farmed or held in zoological collections. Several of these viruses have caused MCF-like syndromes when transmitted to other in-contact ruminant species.

## Classification

Members of the family *Herpesviridae* (in the proposed order *Herpesvirales*) that infect certain members of the family *Bovidae* are classified in the subfamilies *Alphaherpesvirinae* or *Gammaherpesvirinae*. Some of the viruses are listed in **Table 1**, which also lists their respective genera, together with some other salient properties, where known, including nucleotide composition and genome size. All of the ruminant alphaherpesviruses are classified in the genus *Varicellovirus* with the notable exception of BHV2, which is classified in the genus *Simplexvirus* because it is most closely related to human herpes simplex virus. All of the ruminant gammaherpesviruses have been

proposed as members of the new genus *Macavirus* (*maca* is short for MCF) with the exception of BHV4, which remains in the genus *Rhadinovirus*.

## Structure

Each of the viruses listed in **Table 1** has a typical herpesvirus morphology. Virions are enveloped and about 150 nm in diameter. The double-stranded DNA genome is spooled within the capsid. There is an icosahedral nucleocapsid 100 nm in diameter composed of 162 hollow capsomers (150 hexamers and 12 pentamers). The nucleocapsid is surrounded by a layer of globular material called the tegument that is enclosed by a typical bilayer lipoprotein envelope in which are embedded glycoproteins, which generally appear as projecting spikes in negatively stained electron micrographs. There are about 12 distinct glycoproteins associated with the envelope spikes. Though the size of the DNA genome varies (**Table 1**), there is evidence that there are up to 76 open reading frames (genes) minimally coding for a corresponding number of individual proteins. About 40 of these proteins are structural (i.e., associated with the virion), while the remainder are nonstructural, being found only in infected cells. Repeat DNA sequences are found in the genomes of all bovine herpesviruses. For the alphaherpesviruses a set of two inverted repeats bracket the so-called short region of the genome, and in the case of BHV2 only a second set of inverted repeats bracket the so-called long region. The gammaherpesviruses have a set of terminal repeat structures, within each of which a variable number of tandemly repeated sequences is found.

## Replication

Virus replication occurs in the nucleus of cells, and in the case of alphaherpesviruses typically results in the production of a rapid cytopathic effect, with characteristic large intranuclear, eosinophilic inclusion bodies present in appropriately stained preparations. Some of the gammaherpesviruses can be cultivated in monolayer cell cultures, where they produce a cytopathic effect, but others have not been isolated in cell cultures. The replication cycle involves at least three classes of genes termed $\alpha$, $\beta$, and $\gamma$ or immediate early, early, and late, the synthesis of which is coordinately regulated in a cascade manner during the replication cycle.

Herpesviruses transcribe sets of micro (mi)RNAs that add complexity to understanding the replication cycle and the host–virus relationship and change views of the antiviral roles of RNA interference (RNAi), also known as gene silencing. Rather than being inhibited, many herpesviruses appear to be able to usurp or divert

**Table 1**  Herpesviruses of the family Bovidae and some other ruminant species

| Virus | Abbreviation | Disease names/synonyms | Subfamily | Genus[a] | Genome Size (kbp) | Genome G+C (mol.%) |
|---|---|---|---|---|---|---|
| Bovine herpesvirus 1 | BHV1 | Infectious bovine rhinotracheitis; infectious pustular vulvovaginitis; coital exanthema | Alphaherpesvirinae | Varicellovirus | 135 | 72 |
| Bovine herpesvirus 2 | BHV2 | Bovine mammilitis; Allerton virus; pseudolumpy skin disease | Alphaherpesvirinae | Simplexvirus | 133 | 64 |
| Bovine herpesvirus 4 | BHV4 | Movar virus | Gammaherpesvirinae | Rhadinovirus | 160[b] | 41 |
| Bovine herpesvirus 5 | BHV5 | Bovine encephalitis | Alphaherpesvirinae | Varicellovirus | 135 | 74 |
| Bovine herpesvirus 6 | BHV6 | Bovine lymphotropic HV | Gammaherpesvirinae | Macavirus | | |
| Bubaline herpesvirus 1 | BuHV1 | Buffalo HV | Alphaherpesvirinae | Varicellovirus | | |
| Elk herpesvirus 1 | ElHV1 | Elk HV related to BHV1 | | | | |
| Caprine herpesvirus 1 | CapHV1 | Goat HV1 | Alphaherpesvirinae | Varicellovirus | | |
| Caprine herpesvirus 2 | CapHV2 | Goat HV2 | Gammaherpesvirinae | Macavirus | | |
| Ovine herpesvirus 1 | OvHV1 | Sheep pulmonary adenomatosis-associated HV | | | | |
| Ovine herpesvirus 2 | OvHV2 | Cause of sheep-associated bovine malignant catarrhal fever | Gammaherpesvirinae | Macavirus | 160[b] | 52[b] |
| Cervid herpesvirus 1 | CerHV1 | Red deer HV | Alphaherpesvirinae | Varicellovirus | | |
| Cervid herpesvirus 2 | CerHV2 | Reindeer HV | Alphaherpesvirinae | Varicellovirus | | |
| Alcelaphine herpesvirus 1 | AlHV1 | Wildebeest HV, cause of malignant catarrhal fever of European cattle | Gammaherpesvirinae | Macavirus | 155–160[b] | 46[b] |
| Alcelaphine herpesvirus 2 | AlHV2 | Barbary red deer HV, cause of malignant catarrhal fever of Jackson's hartebeest | Gammaherpesvirinae | Macavirus | | |

[a]Viruses listed in proposed genus *Macavirus* are currently in genus *Rhadinovirus* or are unclassified.
[b]Sizes shown include the terminal repeats, which vary in total size around 25–30 kbp. G + C contents exclude the terminal repeats.

the host RNA silencing machinery to their advantage. Herpesvirus-encoded miRNAs can act in *cis* to ensure accurate expression of viral genomes or in *trans* to modify the expression of host RNA transcripts.

## Geographic Distribution

In general, each of the bovine alphaherpesviruses occurs worldwide, paralleling the distribution of the host species. The bovine alphaherpesviruses, with minor exceptions, have a restricted host range. None is known to infect nonbovine species; most are restricted to the primary host species.

Increasing numbers of gammaherpesviruses have been identified in normally free-ranging (exotic) ruminant species that have been farmed or held in zoological collections, and several of these viruses have caused MCF-like syndromes when transmitted to other in-contact ruminant species. At least six members of the MCF virus group of ruminant gammaherpesviruses have been identified thus far. Four of these viruses are clearly associated with clinical disease: alcelaphine herpesvirus 1 (AlHV-1) carried by wildebeest (*Connochaetes* spp.); ovine herpesvirus 2 (OvHV-2), ubiquitous in domestic sheep; caprine herpesvirus 2 (CapHV-2), endemic in domestic goats; and the virus of unknown origin that caused classic MCF in white-tailed deer (*Odocoileus virginianus*, MCFV-WTD). Gammaherpesviruses in the MCF virus group have been found in musk ox (*Ovibos moschatus*), Nubian ibex (*Capra nubiana*), and gemsbok (South African oryx, *Oryx gazella*). Gammaherpesviruses have also been found in bighorn sheep, bison, black-tailed deer, mule deer, fallow deer, elk, and addax.

## Antigenic Relationships

Bovine herpesviruses are genetically stable, with only a single antigenic type described for each species and no major changes in antigenicity over time recognized. Some intratypic (within species) differences are detectable using restriction endonuclease DNA fingerprinting, but these differences have not been correlated with major antigenic differences in the proteins coded for by the regions where variable sequences have been identified.

## Epidemiology

In general, transmission of the alphaherpesviruses requires close contact, particularly the kinds of physical contact that bring moist epithelial surfaces into apposition (e.g., coitus, or licking and nuzzling as between mother and offspring). In large, closely confined populations such as cattle feedlots or zoo collections, short-distance aerosol is an important mode of transmission.

Most of the bovine gammaherpesviruses are recognized when they are transmitted to heterologous hosts. For example, MCF in European cattle is acquired from wildebeest, sheep, or other nondomestic (exotic) ruminant species. Where exotic species are the source of infection, more often than not the transmissions occur outside of the natural geographic habitat of the transmitting host.

The gammaherpesviruses are probably transmitted primarily via nasal secretions in both the natural host and to the heterologous hosts that develop MCF. The latter transmission cycle is probably much less efficient, at least for some of the viruses, since many cases of MCF are sporadic. It is only recently that cell-free OvHV2 virions have been demonstrated in nasal secretions of sheep, which is a reflection of the highly cell-associated nature of gammaherpesviruses.

## Pathogenesis

Alphaherpesviruses typically cause localized lesions, particularly of mucosal surfaces of the respiratory and genital tracts or, less commonly, the skin. Progression is characterized by the sequential production of vesicles, pustules, and shallow ulcers that become covered by a pseudomembrane and heal after 10–14 days, usually without scar formation (**Figure 1**).

Generalized alphaherpesvirus infections may occur in very young calves or in a fetus prior to abortion. Encephalitis produced by bovine encephalitis herpesvirus (BHV5) occurs as a consequence of spread of virus from the nasal cavity to the brain, via trigeminal nerve branches.

The gammaherpesvirus BHV4 is associated with low-grade clinical infection. MCF is a uniformly fatal disease associated with mucosal erosions, ophthalmia, and encephalitis that appear to be immune mediated. Lesions are characterized by infiltration and proliferation of lymphocytes. It is still not clear which lymphocyte population is the site of latency; both B and T lymphocytes have been implicated for different gammaherpesviruses. Immune complexes of viral antigen are probably also produced and contribute to the pathology.

Latency is a hallmark of bovine herpesviruses. The genome, probably as a circularized episome, persists in ganglion cells, typically the trigeminal and sciatic in the case of alphaherpesviruses, and in white blood cells in the case of gammaherpesviruses. From these sites of latency, virus is periodically shed to give rise to recurrent disease, shedding, and transmission to in-contact animals.

BHV1 establishes latency in sensory neurons of trigeminal ganglia, and in germinal centers of pharyngeal tonsil and similar sites related to the genital tract. BHV1 reactivates

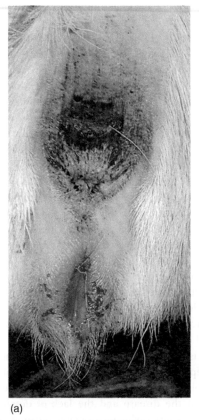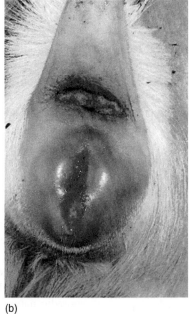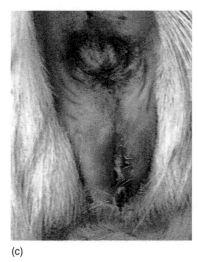

(a) (b) (c)

**Figure 1** As examples of alphaherpesvirus genital disease, three naturally occurring cases (a (early case), b, c) of acute, primary, infectious pustular vulvovaginitis in 8-month-old does caused by caprine herpesvirus 1 are shown. The extent of the individual vesicular/ pustular lesions on the vaginal mucosa is not well shown because of the swelling, and the pain associated with closer examination. Reproduced from Piper KL, Fitzgerald CJ, Ficorilli N, and Studdert MJ (2008) Isolation of caprine herpesvirus 1 from a major outbreak of infectious pustular vulvovaginitis in goats. *Australian Veterinary Journal* 86: 136–138, with permission.

periodically from latency, virus is shed, and consequently virus transmission occurs. Two RNA transcripts, the latency-related RNA and ORF-E RNA, are abundantly expressed in trigeminal ganglia of latently infected cattle, and these transcripts probably regulate the BHV1 latency–reactivation cycle.

## Clinical Diseases

The alphaherpesvirus BHV1 causes coital exanthema and IBR. Both diseases are a consequence of lesions of the mucous membrane at the two sites. The extent and severity of the lesions may vary from mild, subclinical disease to acute, complicated and severe clinical disease that is more likely to occur in the case of IBR in feedlot cattle, where the disease is complicated by secondary bacterial infections. Complicated cases of IBR extending to pneumonitis in feedlot cattle may be fatal.

BHV1 may occasionally cause enteritis in calves. Encephalitis caused by BHV1 has not been confirmed; all cases of alphaherpesvirus encephalitis in cattle have been caused by the distinctly different virus BHV5. In

groups of young calves the mortality caused by BHV5 encephalitis may approach 100%.

Mammilitis caused by BHV2 may be acute, leading to loss of skin from the teats, udder, and perineal regions following vesicle and pustule formation. Pseudolumpy skin disease caused by BHV2 appears to be a consequence of viremic spread, possibly as a cell-associated viremia with localization of the virus in the skin resulting in large golf-ball-sized subcutaneous swellings. These eventually resolve after a course of 3–4 weeks.

BHV6 was identified in bovine B-lymphoma cells and peripheral blood mononuclear cells.

The natural history of caprine herpesvirus 1 is similar to that of BHV1, with disease characterized by a variety of clinical signs including conjunctivitis and lesions of the genital tracts and sometimes the respiratory and gastrointestinal tracts. Abortion may occur.

The red deer and reindeer alphaherpesviruses probably cause clinical disease and have a similar natural history to BHV1.

Bovine MCF in European cattle is caused by alcelaphine herpesvirus 1 or 2 or ovine herpesvirus 2. The disease follows an incubation period of 3 weeks and is characterized by fever, depression, leucopenia, profuse nasal and ocular discharge, generalized lymphadenopathy, extensive mucosal erosions, central nervous system signs, and bilateral ophthalmia that begins as a keratoconjunctivitis and extends to a panophthalmitis. Death, which is invariable, occurs about 1 week after the onset of clinical signs.

Caprine herpesvirus 2 causes clinical MCF when transmitted to farmed white-tailed deer. The transmission pattern of caprine herpesvirus 2 in goats is similar to that of ovine herpesvirus 2 in sheep, with nasal secretions believed to be the major mode of transmission.

Ovine herpesvirus 2 is a noncultivable, lymphotropic gammaherpesvirus that asymptomatically infects most sheep, but causes MCF in cattle, bison, and, somewhat surprisingly, pigs and deer. A uniformly fatal enteric form of MCF caused by ovine herpesvirus 2 was identified in American bison (*Bison bison*) at a large feedlot in the American Midwest in 1998. An estimated 150 bison died. Clinical onset was acute, and most affected bison died within 1–3 days following the onset of clinical disease.

## Immune Response

Both antibody and cell-mediated immune responses are generated during herpesvirus infections. Neutralizing antibody primarily directed against envelope glycoproteins is probably important in long-term immunity. Viral antigens, some of which may be nonstructural immediate early and early proteins, are incorporated into the cell membrane and serve as targets for cytotoxic T lymphocytes. The immune response associated with infection does not prevent the establishment of latency and its role in regulating reactivation of latent virus and recurrent disease and shedding is debated. A central contradiction of herpesvirus immunity is that following natural infection immune animals are also animals that are infected for life.

## Prevention and Control

BHV1 genital disease can be controlled by eliminating carrier cattle identified either serologically or by reactivation and isolation of virus following the administration of corticosteroids such as dexamethasone. Alternatively, where it is important to do so, such as for bulls in artificial breeding centers, a two-herd system may be established. IBR is often associated with stress of transport, intercurrent disease, overcrowding and the mixing together of cattle from different sources, all of which are typically associated with feedlot operations. Awareness and minimization of these predisposing factors can reduce the severity of clinical disease. In an increasing number of countries, test and slaughter programs have achieved total eradication of BHV1 from national herds.

In many parts of the world, including North America, control of BHV1 is achieved by vaccination with conventional live attenuated or inactivated vaccines. With parts of Europe being BHV1 free, the ability to differentiate infected from vaccinated animals has become critical for trade. Live and killed glycoprotein E-deleted marker vaccines are now widely used in Europe, in combination with glycoprotein-based diagnostic tests to monitor cattle. There is debate about the cost and sustainability of eradication programs other than in limited settings such as artificial insemination centers or small countries. Conventional inactivated and attenuated vaccines are less efficacious in neonates because of interference by virus-specific, passively derived maternal antibody. Alternative vaccine types, such as those incorporating CpG oligonucleotides as adjuvant for recombinant protein vaccines or DNA vaccines, are being explored.

Vaccines are not generally available for the control of other bovine or other ruminant herpesvirus diseases.

The epidemiology of BHV2 is not well understood and a possible approach to prevention and control would be to consider removal of known infected cattle.

Since MCF is acquired from a heterologous host (wildebeest, sheep, goats, or other ruminant species), it is clearly preventable by avoiding such contacts. The often-sporadic nature of the disease and the lack of detailed knowledge of the putative sheep-associated virus make avoidance difficult. In zoological collections, bovid species known to harbor alcelaphine herpesviruses 1 and 2 or any of the other gammaherpesviruses should not be cohabited with those species known to be susceptible to MCF.

## Future

Continued progress in understanding the molecular biology of the bovine herpesviruses, including full genome sequencing such as already reported for some viruses including BHV1, BHV4, BHV5, and AlHV1, will occur. Characterization of the transcripts and proteins of the viruses will be taken forward. Progress in developing better vaccines and diagnostic reagents for BHV1 including those based on recombinant DNA technologies, including DNA vaccines, will continue. How effective these new vaccines and diagnostic tests will be in national and international eradication programs is a question of will and financial commitment. The unusual epidemiologies of BHV2 and BHV5 are matters for future inquiry. Further progress in the unusual pathogenesis of MCF and the characterization of the sheep-associated virus responsible for many cases of MCF in the Western world are a part of ongoing work. It may be anticipated that the number of new heterologous host transmission cycles of gammaherpesviruses leading to highly fatal MCF outbreaks will continue to increase, and definition of these should lead to better control measures where ruminant species cohabit. There are many members of the family *Bovidae* for which neither alphaherpesviruses nor gamma-herpesviruses have been identified, and over time it may be expected that more of these viruses will be isolated and characterized.

*See also:* Pseudorabies Virus.

## Further Reading

Jones C, Geiser V, Henderson G, *et al.* (2006) Functional analysis of bovine herpesvirus 1 (BHV-1) genes expressed during latency. *Veterinary Microbiology* 113: 199–210.

Li H, Gailbreath K, Flach EJ, *et al.* (2005) A novel subgroup of rhadinoviruses in ruminants. *Journal of General Virology* 86: 3021–3026.

Murphy FA, Gibbs EPJ, Horzinek MC, and Studdert MJ (eds.) (1999). *Herpesviridae.* In: *Veterinary Virology*, 3rd edn., ch.18, pp. 301–325. New York: Academic Press.

O'Toole D, Li H, Sourk C, Montgomery DL, and Crawford TB (2002) Malignant catarrhal fever in a bison (*Bison bison*) feedlot, 1993–2000. *Journal of Veterinary Diagnostic Investigation* 14: 183–193.

Pfeffer S, Sewer A, Lagos-Quintana M, *et al.* (2005) Identification of microRNAs of the herpesvirus family. *Nature Methods* 2: 269–276.

Piper KL, Fitzgerald CJ, Ficorilli N, and Studdert MJ (2008) Isolation of caprine herpesvirus 1 from a major outbreak of infectious pustular vulvovaginitis in goats. *Australian Veterinary Journal* 86: 136–138.

Rovnak J, Quackenbush SL, Reyes RA, Baines JD, Parrish CR, and Casey JW (1998) Detection of a novel bovine lymphotropic herpesvirus. *Journal of Virology* 72: 4237–4242.

Taus NS, Oaks JL, Gailbreath K, Traul DL, O'Toole D, and Li H (2006) Experimental aerosol infection of cattle (*Bos taurus*) with ovine herpesvirus 2 using nasal secretions from infected sheep. *Veterinary Microbiology* 116: 29–36.

Thiry J, Keuser V, Muylkens B, *et al.* (2006) Ruminant alphaherpesviruses related to bovine herpesvirus 1. *Veterinary Research* 37: 169–190.

Thonur L, Russell GC, Stewart JP, and Haig DM (2006) Differential transcription of ovine herpesvirus 2 genes in lymphocytes from reservoir and susceptible species. *Virus Genes* 32: 27–35.

van Drunen Littel-van den Hurk S (2006) Rationale and perspectives on the success of vaccination against bovine herpesvirus-1. *Veterinary Microbiology* 113: 275–282.

# Bovine Spongiform Encephalopathy

**R G Will,** Western General Hospital, Edinburgh, UK

## Introduction

Bovine spongiform encephalopathy (BSE) is a prion disease of cattle, which was first identified in 1986, and has subsequently become a source of widespread concern for policymakers and public health. To date, more than 184 000 cases have been identified in the UK and more than 5000 cases in other countries, primarily, but not exclusively, in Europe. The origin of BSE is unknown, but may have been related to scrapie contamination of cattle feed, with amplification of the epidemic through within-species recycling of infection. Legislative measures, including restrictions on the feeding of ruminant protein to ruminants, has led to a decline in annual numbers of identified cases in most countries, and there is a possibility that the introduction and implementation of appropriate control measures will lead to the eradication of BSE.

In 1996, a new form of human prion disease, variant Creutzfeldt–Jakob disease (vCJD), was identified in the UK, and epidemiological and laboratory data indicate that this disease is a zoonosis caused by infection with BSE, probably through past dietary exposure to infection. The human population in the UK and many European countries were exposed to significant titers of BSE infectivity over a period of years from about 1980, but the possibility of an extensive epidemic of vCJD has not, as yet, materialized.

There has been a relatively limited and declining annual mortality rate in the UK and, with the exception of France, only isolated cases in other, mainly European, countries. However, future outbreaks of vCJD, perhaps related to polymorphisms in the human prion protein gene (*PRNP*), cannot be excluded and concern for public health has increased with the demonstration of transmission of vCJD through blood transfusion. Accurate predictions of future numbers of cases are hampered by many uncertainties including the mean incubation period of human BSE infection and the prevalence of sub- or preclinical infection in exposed populations.

## BSE

### Clinical and Subclinical Infection

All prion diseases are degenerative conditions of the central nervous system and present with progressive and fatal neurological disorders. The clinical features of BSE include weight loss, reduced milk yield, ataxia and hyperesthesia, progressing to recumbency and death. Although there is a wide age range of affected cattle, the majority of cases are aged 4–6 years. Identification of clinically affected animals is critical to analysis of the epidemiology of BSE and for protection of public health, but depends on recognition of the clinical phenotype or active testing in abattoirs. As in other prion diseases, BSE has a protracted incubation period, in BSE a mean of about 5 years prior to the onset of clinical signs, and infectivity may be present in some tissues, particularly in the pre-terminal stages. However, the tissue distribution of infectivity in BSE is relatively restricted in comparison to other prion diseases such as sheep scrapie. Effective protection of public health depends on accurate case identification in the field or testing for the presence of disease in the abattoir to prevent clinically unrecognized cases entering the human food chain.

Passive surveillance for BSE has proved to be a relatively inefficient strategy for case identification and varies by country according to available skills and resources and the size of the cattle population. Active testing for BSE in abattoirs by examination of the obex region of the brain stem for disease-associated prion protein ($PrP^{Sc}$) has proved to be a reliable method of identifying infected animals. This has allowed more precise information on the course of the BSE epidemic, although the costs of systematic testing of cattle populations are significant.

Infectivity in prion diseases is not restricted to the central nervous system and may involve peripheral tissues, particularly in the lymphoreticular system, in which the agent replicates during the incubation period prior to neuroinvasion and clinical disease. In order to minimize human exposure to infection from preclinical or unrecognized clinical cases, many countries have introduced a ban on certain bovine tissues from entering the human food chain from apparently healthy cattle. A 'specified bovine offal' ban was introduced in the UK in 1989 and an extended list of tissues, the 'specified risk materials' in other European countries in 2000. Implementation and enforcement of these measures is essential to protect public health in countries with a significant risk of human exposure to BSE.

The original list of proscribed tissues was based on information from previous studies in sheep scrapie, but experimental pathogenesis studies have subsequently provided information on the tissue distribution of infectivity in BSE during the incubation period and in the clinical phase. Infectivity in BSE can be identified in tonsil at 10 months after challenge, in terminal ileum after 6–18 months, in the dorsal root ganglia at 32 months, with clinical onset and involvement of brain at 35 months. Many tested tissues have been negative by bioassay in mice and a restricted range of tissue by similar studies in cattle, indicating that the anatomical distribution of BSE is relatively restricted in comparison to other prion diseases such as sheep scrapie. A more extensive tissue involvement in BSE, including involvement of sciatic nerve, has been suggested by the development of more sensitive techniques for the identification of either $PrP^{Sc}$ or infectivity.

## The Origin of BSE

BSE was first identified in the UK in 1986 and epidemiological investigation indicated that the disease was a common source epidemic caused by infection in cattle feed in the form of meat and bone meal. This hypothesis has been strongly supported by the decline in the BSE epidemic in the UK about 5 years after a ban on feeding ruminant protein to cattle and the effectiveness of similar measures in other countries.

The original hypothesis was that the initial source of infection was sheep scrapie, which had been inadvertently included in cattle feed, and that sufficient levels of infection had been present to cross the 'species barrier' between sheep and cattle. Circumstantial evidence of a change in the production methods for meat and bone meal in the 1970s provided an explanation for the timing of the initial cases and the subsequent extensive epidemic was attributed to subsequent recycling of infected cattle tissues to cattle. An alternative hypothesis for the origin of BSE is that this was due to the development of spontaneous disease in a single animal, which was used in the production of meat and bone meal and recycling of infection within the cattle population resulted in an epidemic.

The true origin of BSE is unknown and will probably never be established with certainty. However, any hypothesis must be consistent with the origin of BSE in the UK rather than any other country. The UK had a large sheep population, a high incidence of scrapie, and a practice of feeding meat and bone meal to calves. If spontaneous BSE actually occurs, by analogy with sporadic CJD, the probability of a spontaneous case will be proportionate to the size of the cattle population and that in the UK was smaller than some other countries such as the USA, Australia, and New Zealand, and the latter two countries are believed to be free of scrapie and BSE.

## Epidemiology

The first cases of BSE in the UK probably occurred in the early 1980s and the subsequent epidemic peaked in 1992 and then declined as a result of the ban on feeding ruminant protein to ruminants, introduced in the UK in 1988 (**Figure 1**). At its peak, more than 30 000 clinical cases were identified annually by passive surveillance, although it is likely that there was under-ascertainment of cases, particularly in the early years of the epidemic and before the introduction of an active abattoir testing program. In addition, mathematical models suggest that at least 1 000 000 preclinically infected cattle may have entered the human food chain in the 1980s prior to the introduction of measures to minimize human exposure to BSE.

To date, more than 40 000 affected cattle born after the introduction of the ruminant feed ban have been

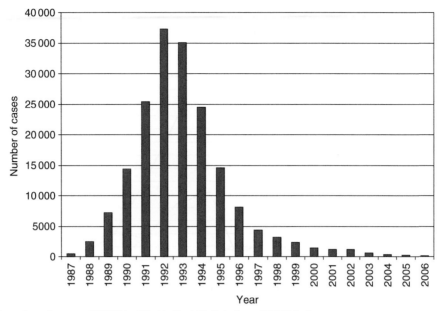

**Figure 1** Annual number of cases of BSE identified in the UK. Data from OIE Website.

identified, indicating that this measure was not fully enforced. There is no good evidence of alternative vertical or lateral routes of transmission in BSE. A likely explanation for these cases is that meat and bone meal was still being fed to other species such as pigs and poultry and that cross contamination in feed mills resulted in continuing cattle exposures. A reinforced feed ban, prohibiting the feeding of meat and bone meal to any farmed species, was introduced in 1996 and only 140 cases of BSE born after this date have been identified, possibly linked to importation of animal feed. An experimental challenge study in BSE has shown that as little as 1 mg of infected brain is sufficient to cause infection by the oral route. It is of note, however, that the BSE epidemic continues to decline and in 2006 there were only 114 cases in the UK.

Live cattle and bovine products, including cattle feed, were exported from the UK in the 1980s and early 1990s and from other European countries in later years. It is likely that the risk of cattle exposure to BSE has a widespread geographical distribution. BSE was identified in Ireland in 1989, in Portugal and Switzerland in 1990, in France in 1991, and has subsequently been identified in all original member states of the European Union (EU). A ban on feeding ruminant protein to ruminants was introduced in the EU in 1994 and an SRM ban in 2000, although some countries introduced these measures earlier. In contrast to the UK, the passive surveillance system appears to have been relatively inefficient in identifying cases of BSE in most countries (with the exception of Switzerland), and it was with the introduction of a mandatory abattoir testing program in 2000–01 that some countries first identified indigenous BSE (e.g., Denmark, Germany,

Italy, and Spain), with resulting extensive public concern. It is likely that cases of BSE may not have been identified in preceding years and the true size of BSE outbreaks in some counties, although limited in relation to the size of the UK epidemic, is unknown. In recent years, there has been a decline in the number of cases in almost all European countries (**Figure 2**), underlining the importance of introducing and enforcing measures to prevent the recycling of infection within cattle populations.

Cases of BSE have been found in small numbers in non-European countries, including Canada (9), Israel (1), Japan (31), and the USA (2, including 1 that originated in Canada). Despite the limited numbers of these cases, their identification has had important implications for trade. The possibility that risk of BSE may have been widely disseminated has resulted in a recommendation that all countries carry out a risk assessment, taking into account the possibility of importation of relevant risk materials and the possibility of recycling infection within cattle populations. Active abattoir testing for BSE can be an efficient means of identifying cases of BSE, but the precise populations to be tested, that is, normal slaughter, fallen stock, casualty animals, etc., and the numbers of required tests in specific populations are controversial. Over 10 000 000 cattle are currently tested per annum in the EU at a cost of 45 euros per test, with 561 positives in 2005.

New and atypical forms of BSE have been identified through the active testing programs, Cases of a novel form of BSE defined by a differential neuropathology and biochemical prion protein characteristics, bovine amyloidotic spongiform encephalopathy, were first recognized in Italy, and subsequently a small number of cattle

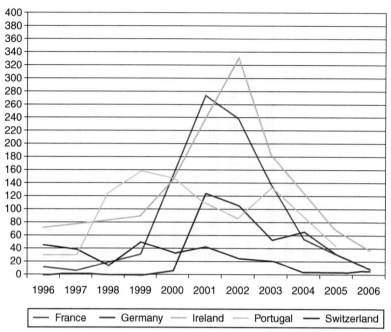

**Figure 2** Annual number of cases of BSE identified in some European countries. Data from OIE Website.

with brain prion protein characteristics different from both the Italian cases and BSE itself have been found, mainly in Europe. The total number of atypical BSE cases identified is currently 18 and the majority are in the older age groups (>10 years) and most had no clinical signs. The origin of these cases is unknown (curiously no cases have yet been identified in the UK) and the implications for human health, if any, are uncertain.

## Variant CJD

### Clinical and Subclinical Infection

vCJD presents clinically with psychiatric symptoms, including depression and withdrawal, followed after a mean of 6 months by progressive ataxia and cognitive impairment, associated with involuntary limb movements. The mean survival is 14 months. vCJD affects younger age groups than in sporadic Creutzfeldt–Jakob disease (sCJD) with a mean age at death of 29 years (range 16–74 years), and it has been proposed that this may be related to either age-related susceptibility or variation in dietary exposure by age. All tested clinical cases have been methionine homozygotes at codon 129 of the human prion protein gene (*PRNP*).

The pathogenesis of vCJD is distinct from other human prion diseases as there is evidence of significant involvement of peripheral tissues and in particular the lymphoreticular system, including lymph nodes, spleen, appendix, and tonsil, in addition to the central nervous system. Infectivity is also present in peripheral nerves and large intestine and PrP$^{Sc}$ in enteric plexus, adrenal, ileum,

and skeletal muscle. Infectivity may be present in some peripheral tissues during the incubation period and act as a source of potential secondary iatrogenic infection, for example, through blood transfusion.

The prevalence of sub- or preclinical infection has not been established with certainty in any population, but anonymized screening of appendectomy and tonsillectomy specimens in the UK has led to estimates that there may be a minimum prevalence of infection of 237 per million, translating to about 4000 individuals in the age group 10–30 years who are currently infected, taking account of the age distribution of those from whom specimens were sourced. Two out of the three positive appendix specimens were analyzed for codon 129 genotype and both were valine homozygotes, suggesting that individuals with this genetic background may be susceptible to infection with BSE.

### The Origin of vCJD

The hypothesis of a causal link between BSE and vCJD is supported by a range of evidence. The clinical and pathological phenotypes are remarkably consistent and distinct from previous experience. The characteristic neuropathological findings, including widespread deposition of florid plaques of PrP$^{Sc}$, have not been recognized previously in human prion disease, and review of archive tissues in a number of countries has failed to identify any case with the typical pathological phenotype prior to the identification of vCJD in the UK. Retrospective review of deaths certified under a range of rubrics and review of neuropathology in a limited number of these cases have failed to identify past cases of unrecognized vCJD. This evidence strongly suggests that vCJD is a new disease.

Laboratory studies have demonstrated that the infectious agent in vCJD is almost identical to the BSE agent in terms of incubation period and brain lesion distribution in experiments carried out on wild-type and transgenic mice. The biochemical characteristics of the $PrP^{Sc}$ deposited in the brain in vCJD are similar to BSE and distinct from other human prion diseases. Macaque monkeys inoculated experimentally with BSE develop florid plaques similar to those in vCJD. These studies indicate that the BSE agent is the cause of vCJD.

It has been proposed that BSE-infected humans through past dietary exposure, probably to high-titer bovine tissues and, in particular, spinal cord, dorsal root ganglia, and products containing mechanically recovered meat. Direct evidence of this hypothesis is lacking, not least because of the difficulties in investigating exposures that may have taken place years or even decades in the past. Furthermore, details of dietary history are necessarily obtained from surrogate witnesses because of the cognitive impairment that develops in vCJD. A case-control study comparing dietary exposures in cases of vCJD and age-matched population controls is consistent with increased risk through past oral intake of food products likely to have contained high levels of BSE infectivity, but the potential biases in this study compromise any firm conclusions. It is however of note that the mortality rate of vCJD is approximately double in the north when compared to the south of the UK, and this may reflect regional differences in past dietary exposures. Neither descriptive analyses nor case-control studies have provided evidence of any plausible alternative route of BSE exposure in vCJD cases, including past occupation or previous surgery.

The occurrence of a novel form of human prion disease, vCJD, in a country with a potentially new risk factor, BSE, first raised the possibility that these conditions were linked. Importantly, data from a harmonized system for surveillance of CJD in Europe indicated, in 1996, at the time vCJD was first found in the UK, that similar cases had not been identified in other countries. Improved efficiency of surveillance in the UK was therefore unlikely to explain the identification of this new disease. Subsequently, cases of vCJD have been found in other countries, but the fact that some of the cases occurred in countries with a very limited risk of exposure to indigenous BSE and had a history of residence in the UK during the time of maximal human exposure to BSE supports the concept that BSE is indeed the cause of vCJD.

## Epidemiology

Up to February 2007, 165 cases of vCJD have been identified in the UK, all but three of which are presumed to be related to past dietary exposure to BSE. The annual number of deaths from vCJD in the UK peaked in 2000 with 28 cases and has subsequently declined to 5 deaths in both 2005 and 2006 (**Figure 3**). Fears of a large epidemic have receded, but there remains the possibility of further outbreaks of cases related to BSE infection in individuals with a heterozygous or valine homozygous genotype at codon 129 of *PRNP* and it is possible that such cases may occur with an extended incubation period and perhaps with a different clinical and pathological phenotype. It is also likely, by analogy with other human prion diseases such as kuru, that there will be an extended tail to the epidemic with a low annual number of deaths for years or even decades.

Cases of vCJD have been found in a number of other countries, mainly, but not exclusively, in Europe (**Table 1**). To date, 21 cases have been identified in France with a peak in annual deaths some 5 years later than in the UK, consistent with a mathematical model which attributes the French cases to exposure to exports of BSE-infected materials from the UK rather than to indigenous BSE. Cases of vCJD are attributed by country according to the

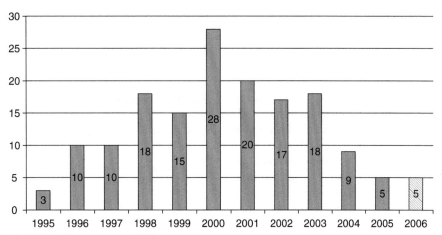

**Figure 3** Number of vCJD deaths per annum (UK).

**Table 1**    Number of vCJD cases per country (Feb. 2007)

| Country | Total number of primary cases (number alive) | Total number of secondary cases: blood transfusion (number alive) | Residence in UK >6 months during period 1980–96 |
|---|---|---|---|
| UK | 162 (6) | 3 (1) | 165 |
| France | 21 (1) | | 1 |
| Rep. of Ireland | 4 (1) | | 2 |
| Italy | 1 (0) | | 0 |
| USA | 3[a] (0) | | 2 |
| Canada | 1 (0) | | 1 |
| Saudi Arabia | 1 (1) | | 0 |
| Japan | 1[b] (0) | | 0 |
| Netherlands | 2 (0) | | 0 |
| Portugal | 1 (1) | | 0 |
| Spain | 1 (0) | | 0 |

[a]The third US patient with vCJD was born and raised in Saudi Arabia and has lived permanently in the United States since late 2005. According to the US case report, the patient was most likely infected as a child when living in Saudi Arabia.
[b]The case from Japan had resided in the UK for 24 days in the period 1980–96.

country of normal residence at the time of the onset of clinical symptoms. This does not necessarily correlate with the country in which exposure to BSE took place and it is of note that 2/3 US cases, 2/4 Irish cases, and the single Canadian case all had a history of extended residence in the UK during 1900–96 and were probably exposed to BSE in the UK rather than the country of attribution. The third US case had lived for most of his life in the country of origin, Saudi Arabia, and a further case has been identified from this country, which is not known to have BSE. One possibility is that human BSE exposure was related to exports from the UK, a matter of concern as exports from the UK and other European countries were distributed worldwide. The single case of vCJD in Japan could be related to this factor, although the individual had also spent a short period of time in the UK. It is of note that, although Italy did import bovine material from the UK and has indigenous BSE, only a single Italian case of vCJD has been identified and that was in 2001, with no new cases for 6 years. Although measures to minimize human exposure to high-titer bovine tissues were introduced in continental Europe more than 10 years after the UK, it is likely that the total number of vCJD cases in other countries will be significantly less than in the UK.

Concerns about the public health implications of BSE and vCJD have increased with the identification of transfusion transmission of vCJD. Four recipients of non-leucodepleted red cells, donated by individuals who later developed vCJD, have either developed vCJD ($n = 3$) or have become sub- or preclinically infected ($n = 1$). In the latter case, an individual who died of an intercurrent illness was found to have immunostaining for $PrP^{Sc}$ in spleen and one lymph node. The three clinical cases were methionine homozygotes and the preclinical case a heterozygote at codon 129 of $PRNP$, thus indicating that methionione homozygotes are not the only ones susceptible to secondary infection. In all four instances of

transmission of infection by blood transfusion, the donation had been given months to years prior to clinical onset in the donor, indicating that infection is present in blood during the incubation period. The three clinical cases developed symptoms between 6 and ~9 years after transfusion, and it is of note that the four infections developed out of a total cohort of 26 individuals who survived at least 5 years after transfusion, indicating that this route is an efficient mechanism of transmitting vCJD infection from person to person. Although transfusion transmission of vCJD has only been identified in the UK, individuals with vCJD who had previously donated blood have been found in France, Spain, Ireland, and Saudi Arabia.

There is no evidence, to date, of secondary transmission of vCJD through plasma-derived products, contaminated surgical instruments, or vertically from mother to child and, although risk assessments suggest that the risks by some of these routes are limited, the period of observation is currently too short to exclude the possibility of alternative routes of transmission in the future, taking account of the potentially extended incubation periods in these diseases. A range of measures have been introduced in many countries to limit the risks of secondary transmission of vCJD, including, for example, deferral of blood donors with a history of extended residence in the UK.

## Further Reading

Bradley R (1998) An overview of the BSE epidemic in the UK. *Developments in Biological Standard* 93: 65–72.

Brown P, McShane LM, Zanusso G, and Detwiler L (2007) On the question of sporadic or atypical bovine spongiform encephalopathy and Creutzfeldt–Jakob disease. *Emerging Infectious Diseases* 12(12): 1816–1821.

Collee JG and Bradley R (1997) BSE: A decade on – Part 1. *Lancet* 349: 636–641.

Collee JG and Bradley R (1997) BSE: A decade on – Part 2. *Lancet* 349: 715–721.

Cousens S, Everington D, Ward HJT, Huillard J, Will RG, and Smith PG (2003) The geographical distribution of variant Creutzfeldt–Jakob disease in the UK: What can we learn from it? *Statistical Methods in Medical Research* 12: 235–246.

Hewitt PE, Llewelyn CA, Mackenzie J, and Will RG (2006) Creutzfeldt–Jakob disease and blood transfusion: Results of the UK Transfusion Medicine Epidemiology Review study. *Vox Sanguins* 91: 221–230.

Hilton DA, Ghani AC, Conyers L, *et al.* (2004) Prevalence of lymphoreticular prion protein accumulation in UK tissue samples. *Journal of Pathology* 203: 733–739.

Kimberlin RH (1996) Speculations on the origin of BSE and the epidemiology of CJD. In: Gibbs CJ, Jr. (ed.) *Bovine Spongiform Encephalopathy: The BSE Dilemma*, pp. 155–175. New York: Springer.

Valleron A-J, Boelle P-Y, Will R, and Cesbron J-Y (2001) Estimation of epidemic size and incubation time based on age characteristics of vCJD in the United Kingdom. *Science* 294: 1726–1728.

Ward HJT, Everington D, Cousens SN, *et al.* (2006) Risk factors for variant Creutzfeldt–Jakob disease: A case-control study. *Annals of Neurology* 59: 111–120.

Wells GAH, Scott AC, Johnson CT, *et al.* (1987) A novel progressive spongiform oncephalopathy in cattle. *Veterinary Record* 121: 419–420.

Wilesmith JW, Ryan JBN, and Atkinson MJ (1991) Bovine spongiform encephalopathy: Epidemiological studies of the origin. *Veterinary Record* 128: 199–203.

Wilesmith JW, Wells GAH, Cranwell MP, and Ryan JB (1988) Bovine spongiform encephalopathy: Epidemiological studies. *Veterinary Record* 123: 638–644.

Will RG, Ironside JW, Zeidler M, *et al.* (1996) A new variant of Creutzfeldt–Jakob disease in the UK. *Lancet* 347: 921–925.

World Health Organisation, Food and Agricultural Organisation, Office International des Epizooties (2002) Technical Consultation on BSE: Public health, animal health, and trade.

## Relevant Website

http://www.oie.int – OIE website.

# Bovine Viral Diarrhea Virus

**J F Ridpath,** USDA, Ames, IA, USA

Published by Elsevier Ltd.

## Glossary

**Biotype** Designation based on expression of cytopathic effect in cultured epithelial cells.
**Cytopathic effect** Alteration in the microscopic appearance of cultured cells following virus infection.
**Genotype** Group designation determined by genetic sequence comparison.
**Hemorrhagic syndrome** Form of severe acute bovine viral diarrhea (BVD) characterized by high morbidity and mortality as high as 50%. Clinical signs include hemorrhages throughout digestive system, high fevers, and bloody diarrhea. While similar in clinical presentation to mucosal disease it differs in that it is the result of an uncomplicated acute infection, only one biotype is present (noncytopathic) and it is not 100% fatal.
**Mucosal disease (MD)** Form of BVD characterized by low morbidity and 100% mortality. Clinical signs include severe and bloody diarrhea, sores in the mouth, and rapid wasting. MD occurs in animals born persistently infected with a noncytopathic BVDV that are subsequently superinfected with a cytopathic bovine viral diarrhea virus (BVDV). While similar in clinical presentation to hemorrhagic syndrome it differs in that it only occurs in persistently infected

animals, two biotypes of virus are present, and it is 100% fatal.
**Persistent infection** Results from infection with noncytopathic virus during the first 125 days of gestation. The infected fetus develops an immune tolerance to the virus and sheds virus throughout its subsequent lifetime. Cytopathic BVDV are not able to establish persistent infections.
**Species** A fundamental category of taxonomic classification, ranking below a genus or subgenus and consisting of related organisms grouped by virtue of their common attributes and assigned a common name.

## Introduction

Bovine viral diarrhea viruses (BVDVs) present the researcher and veterinary clinician with arguably the most complicated combination of clinical presentation, pathogenesis, and basic biology of all bovine viral pathogens (**Figure 1**). There are two distinct species of BVDV (BVDV1 and BVDV2), two distinct biotypes (cytopathic and noncytopathic), two states of infection (acute and persistent), five recognized forms of clinical acute

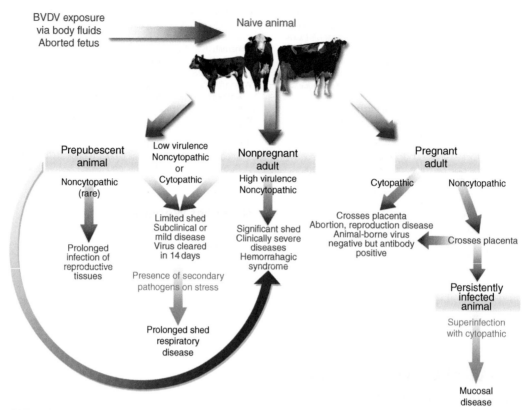

**Figure 1** BVDV infections. Clinical presentation following BVDV infection is dependent on viral strain, viral biotype, viral virulence, age of host, reproductive status of host, and presence of other pathogens. Acute uncomplicated BVDV infections are always accompanied by a loss of immune tissue and circulating lymphocytes.

presentation (acute BVDV infection, severe acute BVDV infection, hemorrhagic BVDV infection, acute BVDV infection/bovine respiratory disease (BRD), and acute BVDV infection/immunosuppression), and one clinical presentation that is the sequeale of a persistent infection with one biotype followed by an acute infection with the other biotype. While BVDV infections are most commonly associated with cattle, they also occur in a wide variety of domesticated and wild ruminants including white tail and mule deer, bison, elk, and sheep.

In the last 10 years a host of advances in BVDV research and diagnostics have led to the development of improved diagnostics and burgeoning eradication/control programs. While the economic impact of BVDV is largely due to affects of acute infections, persistently infected animals are the most frequent vector. Thus, identification and removal of persistently infected animals is key to effective control strategies.

## History

### First Reports of BVD and MD

Bovine viral diarrhea (BVD) was first reported as a 'new' disease of cattle observed in New York dairies in 1946. The

first report, by Dr. Francis Fox of Cornell University, described a 'rinderpest like' disease characterized by leukopenia, high fever, depression, diarrhea and dehydration, anorexia, salivation, nasal discharge, gastrointestinal erosions, and hemorrhages in various tissues. In the five initial herds in which it was observed, morbidity rates ranged from 33% to 88% and mortality rates ranged from 4% to 8%. In addition, fetal abortions were observed 10 days to 3 months following infection. It was shown that this disease could be transmitted experimentally. Rinderpest virus was ruled out as a causative agent because sera from convalescent animals did not neutralize rinderpest virus and cattle that had recovered from BVD were not resistant to rinderpest virus infection.

In 1953 another disease was reported in the US. Given the name mucosal disease (MD), it was characterized by severe diarrhea, fever, anorexia, depression, profuse salivation, nasal discharge and gastrointestinal hemorrhages, erosions, and ulcers. The gut-associated lesions were similar to, but more severe, than those reported for BVD. However, unlike BVD, MD could not be transmitted experimentally. In addition, while BVD outbreaks were marked by high morbidity but low mortality, MD usually only infected a small number of animals in the herd but once contracted was invariably fatal. Based on differences in lesions, transmissibility, and morbidity/mortality rates MD and BVD were initially thought to have different causative agents.

## Isolation of Virus

In 1957 Dr. James Gillespie of Cornell University isolated a noncytopathic virus as the causative agent of BVD. Three years later, in 1960, he isolated a cytopathic virus from a MD case. Cross-neutralization studies demonstrated that the viral agents associated with BVD and MD were the same and led to the realization that BVD and MD were different disease manifestations of infection with the same agent. The agent was termed bovine viral diarrhea virus (BVDV). While BVDV was identified as the causative agent, the etiology of MD, now referred in the literature as BVD-MD, remained a puzzle. In the late 1960s several research groups reported that animals succumbing to MD had persistent BVDV infections. It was also noted that persistently infected animals did not mount a serological immune response to the virus that they carried. The observations that fetal bovine serum was frequently contaminated with BVDV and that BVDV infections could be detected in newborn and one-day-old calves suggested that persistent infection might arise from *in utero* exposure.

## Release of First MLV Followed by Reports of pvMD

Because cytopathic strains could be more easily detected, quantitated, and studied in tissue culture than noncytopathic strains, the discovery of cytopathic BVDV was a boon to the study of BVDV. In 1964, the first cytopathic BVDV strain discovered (Oregon C24 V) was incorporated into a modified live multivalent vaccine. Soon it was reported that subsequent to use of this vaccine a minority of animals became sick with MD-like symptoms and died. These cases were referred to as postvaccinal MD (pvMD).

Further investigation revealed that the vaccinated animals that succumbed to pvMD responded with serum antibodies to the other components of the vaccine but did not respond to the BVDV component. This suggested that the susceptibility to pvMD might be correlated with failure of the immune system to recognize BVDV. Questions raised by pvMD lead to the elucidation of the etiology of MD.

## Unraveling the Etiology of MD

By the early 1970s the prevailing wisdom was that calves with persistent BVDV infections were uniformly unthrifty and usually died within the first few months of life. In a series of papers published in the late 1970s and early 1980s, Arlen McClurkin of the USDA's National Animal Disease Center (then known as the National Animal Disease Laboratory or NADL) reported persistent infection and immune tolerance in apparently healthy adult animals. Calves born to persistently infected (PI) cows were persistently infected at birth indicating maternal transmission. Further, McClurkin was able to generate persistently infected calves by exposing seronegative cows to noncytopathic BVDV between 42 and 125 days gestation. He followed the fate of the PI calves he generated and observed the following:

1. while many PI animals appeared weak and had congenital malformations, some appear apparently normal;
2. while that majority of PI animals died soon after birth, some lived to breeding age;
3. PI lines of cattle could be generated by breeding PI animals; and
4. PI animals spontaneously developed MD.

Using the McClurkin studies as a springboard, Joe Brownlie (Institute for Animal Health, Compton Laboratory, UK) and Steve Bolin (NADC/ARS/USDA) in separate but nearly concurrent studies experimentally reproduced MD in PI cattle. In the Brownlie study a cytopathic virus isolated from an animal that died from MD was inoculated into healthy PI herd mates. Both animals succumbed to MD. In the Bolin study, PI cattle were infected with noncytopathic and cytopathic strains of BVDV. Only those animals receiving cytopathic BVDV developed MD. Both studies concluded that cattle born persistently infected with a noncytopathic BVDV succumb to MD later in life when they are superinfected with a cytopathic BVDV. Follow-up studies revealed that the noncytopathic and cytopathic viruses isolated from individual MD cases were antigenically similar. At this point the origin of the cytopathic virus remained a mystery.

## Discovery of the Molecular Basis for Biotype

The first two BVDV strains to be sequenced were the cytopathic strains Osloss (European origin, sequence published in 1987 by L. De Moerlooze) and NADL (North American origin, sequence published in 1988 by M. Collett). Studies of proteins associated with BVDV replication in cultured cells, done during this same time period, demonstrated that cytopathic BVDV could be distinguished from noncytopathic BVDV by the production of an extra nonstructural protein (now known as NS3). This protein is a smaller version of a nonstructural now known as NS2-3 (**Figure 2**). Comparison of the sequences of the cytopathic viruses Osloss and NADL to noncytopathic viruses from the genus *Pestivirus* revealed insertions in the region of the genome coding for the NS2-3. Subsequent studies, in which the NS2-3 coding region of cytopathic and noncytopathic viral pairs isolated

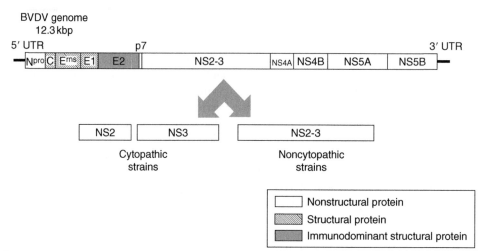

**Figure 2**  BVDV genome. The organization of the single-stranded RNA genome of BVDV is shown. The cleavage of the NS2-3 protein to NS2 and NS3 is observed with cytopathic, but not noncytopathic, isolates.

from MD cases were sequenced, revealed that nearly all cytopathic viruses had host-cell genetic sequences or duplicated BVDV genetic sequences inserted into the NS2-3 region when compared to their noncytopathic counterparts. These studies suggested that cytopathic viruses arise from noncytopathic viruses by a recombinational event.

## Segregation of BVDV into Two Genotypes

Studies done in the late 1980s and early 1990s, comparing vaccination cross-protection and monoclonal antibody binding, revealed antigenic variability among BVDV strains. While these studies indicated that there was considerable variation among BVDV strains, no standard means of grouping viruses based on these variations was generated. Meanwhile, based on hybridization analysis and sequence comparison, several groups evaluated the 5′ untranslated region (UTR) as a target for polymerase chain reaction (PCR) tests designed to detect the wide range of BVDV strains or to differentiate BVDV strains from other pestiviruses.

Concurrent to this research a highly virulent form of BVD, termed hemorrhagic syndrome, was reported in Canada and the US. While the first report of BVDV in 1946 described a severe acute disease, the most commonly reported form of acute uncomplicated BVD between the 1950s and late 1980s was a mild or subclinical infection. Acute BVDV infections came to be regarded as clinically unimportant and textbooks of the day stated that the transmission of the virus between healthy immunocompetent cattle was probably insignificant. The potential for infection with BVDV to result in clinical disease was downplayed and the research focused on the consequences of transplacental infections and the

pathogenesis of BVD-MD. However, the recognition of hemorrhagic syndrome in the late 1980s and early 1990s brought the concept of severe acute BVD once more to the forefront. Case records of cattle admitted to the Cornell College of Veterinary Medicine for the years 1977–87 revealed that 10% of clinically acute BVD infections in adult cattle were associated with thrombocytopenia. During this period an outbreak in the state of New York resulted in 50 of 100 animals in a milking herd becoming ill and 20 of them subsequently dying. Clinical signs included high temperatures, bloody diarrhea, hemorrhages, and prolonged bleeding from venipuncture sites. This disease came to be considered as a distinct form of severe acute BVD termed hemorrhagic syndrome. Severe acute BVD cases were reported with increasing frequency in North America in the early 1990s. These outbreaks were particularly devastating in the Canadian provinces of Quebec and Ontario. The disease in some ways resembled MD, but differed in that it was transmissible to normal non-PI cattle and that only one virus, from the noncytopathic biotype, was present. In 1994, in separate studies, Charles Pellerin (Institut Armand-Frappier, University of Quebec, Canada) and Julia Ridpath (NADC/ARS/USDA) performed phylogenetic analysis of BVDV strains, isolated from animals suffering from hemorrhagic syndrome and arrived at the same conclusion. The BVDV strains associated with the outbreaks of hemorrhagic syndrome belong to a genetic group (genotype) clearly distinct from the BVDV strains commonly used, at that time, in vaccine production, diagnostic tests, and research. The newly recognized group of BVDV was designated BVDV genotype II, while the group containing the strains used in vaccines, detection, and research was termed BVDV genotype I. The names of these two genotypes were later modified to BVDV1 and BVDV2 in keeping with taxonomic conventions in use with other viruses. It was further noted that viruses from the BVDV2 genotype were also isolated from PI calves born to dams that had been vaccinated with vaccines based on BVDV1 isolates. In 2005 the Eighth Report of the International Committee on Taxonomy of Viruses officially classified BVDV1 and BVDV2 as separate and distinct species within the genus *Pestivirus*.

In the late 1990s there was some speculation that BVDV2 strains represented newly emerging viruses that originated in the US as a result of use of vaccines by US producers and were then transferred to Europe. While BVDV2 strains were first recognized in 1994, retrospective characterization of strains collected from BVDV outbreaks in Ontario that occurred between 1981 and 1994 demonstrated that BVDV2 were present in North America at least since the early 1980s. However, the first isolate, retrospectively identified as BVDV2, described in the literature was isolated in Europe prior to 1979. Interestingly, this strain was isolated from a pig and was referred to as an atypical classical swine fever virus (CSFV).

### Emergence of BVDV Reduction/Eradication Programs

In the decades after the first description of BVD and the discovery of its causative agent, systematic reduction/eradication programs were not considered. This was partially due to an underestimation of the economic impact of BVDV infections and the lack of suitable diagnostics. In the mid-1990s studies began to appear showing the sizable economic impact BVDV infections have on beef and dairy industries worldwide. Initially, veterinarians and producers assumed that vaccination alone could substantially reduce the incidence of BVDV infections. However, by the late 1990s it became apparent that four decades of vaccination had not reduced the incidence of BVDV. At this time, better diagnostics, particularly for the detection of PI animals, began to be developed. Concurrently, in the Scandinavian countries, programs designed around a strict testing and removal program for PI accompanied by movement restrictions for infected herds resulted in near eradication of BVDV in those countries by 2005. The success of these efforts encouraged other European countries and US producers to implement reduction/eradication programs. The Scandinavian programs, which were conducted in countries with a relatively low incidence of both BVD and cattle densities, eschewed the use of vaccines and were based solely on the test and removal of PI cattle. In areas of the world in which cattle densities are high and BVDV is endemic, current control programs are focused on a combination of test and removal of PI's, systematic vaccination, and consistent biosecurity.

## Characteristics of BVDV

### Characteristics Common to Both BVDV1 and BVDV2

All BVDV belong to the genus *Pestivirus* within the family *Flavivirus*. The BVDV virion is an enveloped, spherical particle 40–50 nm in diameter that consists of an outer lipid envelope surrounding an inner protein shell or capsid that contains the viral genome. The capsid appears as an electron-dense inner core with a diameter of approximately 30 nm. The lipid envelope that surrounds the virion is pleomorphic which impedes purification of infectious particles by banding in sucrose gradients and identification by electron microscopy. The $M_r$ of the virion is estimated as $6.0 \times 10^7$ and the buoyant density in sucrose is 1.10–1.15 gm cm$^{-3}$.

The viral genome consists of a single strand of positive-sense RNA, that in the absence of insertions is about 12.3 kbp long and codes for a single open reading frame (ORF). The ORF is preceded and followed by relatively long UTRs on the 5′ and 3′ ends of the genome (**Figure 2**). Similar to other members of the genus *Pestivirus*, BVDV1 and BVDV2 viruses encode two unique proteins, $N^{pro}$ and $E^{rns}$. The nonstructural protein $N^{pro}$ is encoded at the very beginning of the ORF and is a proteinase, whose only known function is to cleave itself from the viral polypeptide. The $E^{rns}$ is an envelope glycoprotein that possesses an intrinsic RNase activity.

All *Pestivirus* species, including BVDV1 and BVDV2, are antigenically related. However, neutralizing antibody titers found in convalescent sera are typically several-fold higher against viruses from the same species as compared to viruses from other *Pestivirus* species. Both BVDV1 and BVDV2 viruses may exist as one of two biotypes, cytopathic and noncytopathic. The noncytopathic biotype is the predominant biotype in both BVDV species. Noncytopathic viruses from both the BVDV1 and the BVDV2 species can cross the placenta and establish persistent infections. All BVDV strains, regardless of species or biotype, are lymphotrophic and acute infection always results in destruction of immune tissues. The extent of the loss of immune tissue and the accompanying immunosuppression is dependent on viral strain.

Virions are stable within a pH range of 5.7–9.3. Infectivity is not affected by freezing but decreases at temperatures above 40 °C. Like other enveloped viruses, BVDV are inactivated by organic solvents and detergents. Other methods of inactivation include trypsin treatment (0.5 mg ml$^{-1}$, 37 °C, 60 min), ethylenimine (reduction of 5 log10 units using 10 mM at 37 °C for 2 h), electron beam irradiation (4.9 and 2.5 kGy needed to reduce virus infectivity 1 log10 unit for frozen and liquid samples, respectively), and gamma irradiation (20–30 kGy).

## Differences between BVDV1 and BVDV2

While severe disease and death loss have been reported in association with both BVDV1 and BVDV2 strains, severe acute BVD and hemorrhagic syndrome have only been reproduced experimentally with BVDV2 strains. Aside from severe acute BVDV, which is only caused by a small proportion of BVDV2 strains, it is difficult to distinguish BVDV1 infections from BVDV2 infections based on clinical signs. Further, while virulence is strain dependent, clinical presentation may also be affected by immune status, reproductive status, stress, and the presence of secondary pathogens.

BVDV1 and BVDV2 strains are antigenically distinct as demonstrated by serum neutralization using polyclonal sera and monoclonal antibody binding. The practical significance of antigenic differences is indicated by the birth of BVDV2 PI animals to dams that had been vaccinated against BVDV1 strains. While modified live BVDV1 vaccines may induce antibodies against BVDV2 strains, the titers average one log less than titers against heterologous BVDV1 strains. These observations have lead to the inclusion of both BVDV species in BVDV vaccines.

While the first studies segregating BVDV strains into two different genotypes were based on comparison of the 5′ UTR, differences between BVDV1 and BVDV2 strains are consistently found throughout the genome. Based on complete genomic sequence comparisons, the genetic sequences of BVDV1 and BVDV2 differ from each other as much as other member species of the genus *Pestivirus*, such as CSFV and border disease virus, differ from each other. The level of the genetic difference was the basis for declaring BVDV1 and BVDV2 to be two separate and distinct species.

## Molecular Biology of BVDV

### Viral Genome

The single-stranded RNA genome of BVDV codes for one long ORF (approximately 4000 codons in the absence of insertions). The ORF is bracketed by relatively large 5′ (360–390 bp) and 3′ (200–240 bp) UTRs. The 5′ terminus does not contain a cap structure and there is no poly(A) tract present at the 3′ end. Similar to the genomes of other pestiviruses, both BVDV1 and BVDV2 genomes terminate at the 3′ end with a short poly(C) tract. Sequence identity is highest between BVDV1 and BVDV2 strains in the 5′ UTR region. It is thought that conservation of 5′ UTR sequences is related to formation of tertiary structures required for internal ribosomal entry-mediated initiation of translation. While sequence conservation between BVDV1 and BVDV2 is high in the 5′ UTR, there are two short regions that are notable for

their variability. These are located between nucleotides 208–223 and nucleotides 294–323 (nucleotide position numbers based on the sequence of BVDV1-SD-1). (Although BVDV1a-NADL and BVDV2-890 are the type virses for genotypes BVDV1 and BVDV2, respectively, both genomes have inserted sequences. Insertions can cause confusion when indicating genomic location based on nucleotide number. For this reason BVDV1a-SD-1 is used as the reference for nucleotide position. It was the first noncytopathic BVDV1 sequenced and does not have an insertion. The accession number for BVDV1a-SD-1 is M96751.) Sequence variations in these regions have been exploited in PCR-based tests designed to differentiate BVDV1 strains from BVDV2 strains.

### Viral Proteins

#### Structural proteins

The large ORF is translated as a polyprotein. The order of the individual viral proteins within the polyprotein is as follows: $N^{pro}$-C-$E^{rns}$-E1-E2-p7-NS2/3-NS4A-NS4B-NS5A-NS5B (**Figure 2**). The polyprotein is processed co- and post-translationally by host and viral proteases. The proteins associated with the mature virion (structural proteins) are C, $E^{rns}$, E1, and E2. C is the virion nucleocapsid protein. $E^{rns}$, E1, and E2 are associated with the outer envelope of the BVDV virion. These three proteins are highly glycosylated and possess the antigenic determinants of the virus. It is not known whether the $E^{rns}$ and E1 possesses neutralizing epitopes that are important in disease control. The E2 protein is the immunodominant structural protein and possesses neutralizing epitopes that function in disease control. Protective antibodies induced by killed vaccines are predominantly against the E2. Monoclonal antibodies (Mab's) produced against the E2 have been used to differentiate between BVDV1 and BVDV2 strains.

#### Nonstructural proteins

The first viral protein encoded by the BVDV ORF is the nonstructural protein, $N^{pro}$. This protein, as discussed above, is unique to the genus *Pestivirus*. Its only known function is to cleave itself from the polyprotein. The next nonstructural protein, p7, follows the structural protein E2 in the polyprotein. While the role of this cell-associated protein is unknown, it is hypothesized that it is required for production of infectious virus but not for RNA replication. The p7 protein is inefficiently cleaved from the E2 during processing of the polyprotein. This leads to two intracellular forms of E2 with different C termini (E2 and E2-p7). However, neither p7 or E2-p7 are found associated with infectious virus.

Following p7 is the serine protease, NS2-3. As discussed above, in BVDV strains from the cytopathic biotype the NS2-3 is cleaved to NS2 and NS3 (**Figure 2**). Both the uncleaved NS2-3 and the cleaved NS3 act as serine proteases that cleave the remaining nonstructural proteins from the polyprotein. The function of the NS2 is unknown. It is not required for RNA replication and its cleavage from the NS2-3 does not affect serine protease activity. Purified BVDV NS3 also possesses RNA helicase and RNA-stimulated NTPase activities and all three activities (serine protease, RNA helicase, and RNA-stimulated NTPase) are essential to virus viability. While antibodies to the NS2-3 and NS3 do not neutralize infectivity, these proteins possess immunodominant epitopes. The NS2-3 and NS3 (but not the NS2), are strongly recognized by polyclonal convalescent sera and animals vaccinated with modified live vaccines have as nearly a strong antibody response to the NS2-3 and/or NS3 protein as to the E2 structural protein. In contrast, animals vaccinated with inactivated (killed) vaccines primarily react with structural proteins and not the NS2-3 or NS3. The difference in recognition of NS2-3 or NS3 may be useful in differentiating between immune responses to inactivated vaccines and immune responses to natural infection.

The NS4A and NS4B proteins are similar in size, composition, and hydrophobicity to the NS4A and NS4B proteins of other flaviviruses. NS4A acts as a cofactor for the NS2-3 and NS3 serine protease activity. NS4B and NS5A probably are replicase complex components. RNA polymerase activity has been demonstrated for the NS5B protein.

## Viral Replication

### Viral uptake

Uptake of virus appears to be a multistep process that occurs by endocytosis. In the initial step, the virus attaches to the cell surface through interaction of $E^{rns}$ envelope protein and a docking glycosaminoglycan receptor molecule. The next step is mediated by attachment of the E2 envelope protein to the low-density lipoprotein receptor (LDLR) followed by internalization via endocytosis.

### Release of genomic RNA, translation, and replication

The mechanism of release of genomic RNA into the cell cytoplasm is unknown but probably involves acidification of endocytic vesicles. Following release, the genomic RNA must act as mRNA, directing the translation of viral proteins. The translated viral proteins provide functions necessary for RNA replication, protein processing (protease cleavages), and protein trafficking, but are insufficient to perform all or perhaps even most of the

functions required. Thus, the virus relies on host cell machinery to provide many functions required for virus replication. The most important of these host-provided functions is protein synthesis. After translation to produce viral proteins, RNA replication begins with the synthesis of complementary negative strands. It has been proposed that a secondary structure motif in the 5′ UTR enables the switch of viral RNA from a template for translation to a template for replication. Using these negative strands as templates, genome-length positive strands are synthesized by a semiconservative mechanism involving replicative intermediates and replicative forms. Because viral proteins are not detected on the surface of infected cells, it is thought that virions mature in intracellular vesicles and are released by exocytosis. A substantial fraction of the infectious virus remains cell associated.

## Detection and Control

BVDV diagnostics have focused on the detection of PI animals. Virus isolation on cultured bovine cells remains the gold standard. However, due to ease and lower expense, antigen detection by either immunohistochemistry or antigen capture ELISA or nucleic acid detection by RT-PCR are gaining favor. Both killed and modified live vaccines are available for the prevention of BVD. Control by vaccination alone is compromised by the heterogeneity observed among BVDV strains, lack of complete fetal protection afforded by vaccination, and the failure to remove PI animals from cattle populations.

*See also:* Classical Swine Fever Viruses.

## Further Reading

Dubovi ED, Brownlie J, Donis R, et al. (eds.) (1996) *International Symposium on Bovine Viral Diarrhea Virus: A 50 Year Review*. Ithaca, NY: Cornell University.

Goyal SM and Ridpath JF (eds.) (2005) *Bovine Viral Diarrhea Virus: Diagnosis, Management and Control*. Ames, IA: Blackwell Publishing.

Houe H, Brownlie J,, and Steinar Valle P (eds.) (2005) *Bovine Virus Diarrhea Virus (BVDV) Control, Vol. 72: Preventive Veterinary Medicine*. Special Issue. Amsterdam: Elsevier Academic Press.

Smith RA (consulting ed.) and Brock KV (guest ed.) (2004) *Veterinary Clinics of North America Food animal practice. Vol. 20: Bovine Viral Diarrhea Virus: Persistence is the Key*. Philadelphia, PA: Saunders.

Thiel H-J, Collett MS, Gould EA, et al. (2005) Family *Flaviviridae*. In: Fauquet CM, Mayo MA, Maniloff J, Desselberget U,, and Ball LA (eds.) *Virus Taxonomy Classification and Nomenclature of Viruses*, 8th edn., pp. 981–998. Amsterdam: Elsevier Academic Press.

# Capripoxviruses

**R P Kitching,** Canadian Food Inspection Agency, Winnipeg, MB, Canada

## Glossary

**Abomasal** Pertaining to the fourth stomach of ruminants.
**Agalactia** Shortage of milk supply.
**Myiasis** Infestation with maggots.
**Hydropic** Accumulating water.

## History

Sheeppox and goatpox are malignant pox diseases of sheep and goats easily recognizable by their characteristic clinical signs, and described in the earliest texts on animal diseases. Lumpy skin disease (Neethling) of cattle (LSD), however, was first described in 1929 in Northern Rhodesia (Zambia), having apparently been absent from domestic cattle until that time. From Zambia, LSD spread south to Botswana and Zimbabwe, and by 1944 the disease appeared in South Africa, where it caused a major epizootic, affecting over 6 million cattle. In 1957, LSD was first diagnosed in Kenya, and was thought at the time to be associated with the introduction of a flock of sheep affected with sheeppox on the farm. Since then LSD has been present in most of the countries of sub-Saharan Africa, often associated with large epizootics followed by periods in which the disease is only rarely reported. In 1988, LSD caused a major outbreak in Egypt, and in 1989 it spread from Egypt to a village in Israel. This was the first time that a diagnosis of LSD outside of Africa had been supported by laboratory confirmation.

## Taxonomy and Classification

The viruses that cause sheeppox, goatpox, and LSD are all members of the genus *Capripoxvirus*, in the subfamily *Chordopoxvirinae* of the family *Poxviridae*, and have morphological, physical, and chemical properties similar to vaccinia virus. Originally, the viruses were classified according to the species from which they were isolated, but comparisons of their genomes indicate that the distinction between them is not so clear, and that recombination events occur naturally between isolates from different species. This is reflected in the ability of some strains to cause disease in both sheep and goats and in experimental results which show that all the sheep isolates examined could infect goats, and that goat isolates could infect sheep.

The epidemiological relationship between sheeppox and goatpox isolates and cattle isolates is less clear, apparent in differences in the geographical distribution of sheeppox and goatpox and LSD (see below). However, some isolates recovered from sheep and goats in Kenya have genome characteristics very similar to cattle isolates. It has been proposed that confusion can be reduced by referring to the malignant pox diseases of sheep, goats, and cattle, including Indian goat dermatitis and Kenyan sheep and goatpox, as capripox. It is envisaged that when sufficient isolates have been examined biochemically, no clear distinction will be possible between sheep, goat, and cattle isolates, but a spectrum will emerge in which some strains have clear host preferences while others will be less defined and will naturally infect the host with which they come into contact.

## Geographical and Seasonal Distribution

Capripox of sheep and goats is enzootic in Africa north of the equator, the Middle East and Turkey, Iran, Afghanistan, Pakistan, India, Nepal, and parts of the People's Republic of China, and, in 1986, Bangladesh. Sheeppox was eradicated from Britain in 1866, and from France, Spain, and Portugal in 1967, 1968, and 1969, respectively. Sporadic outbreaks still occur in Europe, for instance in Italy in 1983 and Greece and Bulgaria both in 1995 and 1996, and Greece in 1997 and 2000. In 2005, goatpox was first reported in Vietnam, following its introduction from China.

LSD is enzootic in the sub-Saharan countries of Africa and is still present in Egypt. The single outbreak in Israel was eradicated by slaughter of affected and in-contact cattle.

There is no clear seasonality to outbreaks of capripox in sheep and goats. In enzootic areas, lambs and kids are protected against infection with capripoxvirus for a variable time dependent on the immunity of the mother. However, the spread of LSD is related to the density of biting flies and consequently major enzootics have been associated with humid weather when fly activity is greatest.

## Host Range and Virus Propagation

Among domestic species, capripoxvirus is restricted to cattle, sheep, and goats. Experimentally, it is possible to infect cattle, sheep, or goats with isolates derived from any of these three species, although clinically the reaction following inoculation may be indiscernible. Viral genome analysis using restriction endonucleases has identified fragment size characteristics by which it is possible to classify strains into cattle, sheep, or goat isolates. However, the identification of strains that have intermediate characteristics between typical sheep and goat isolates does suggest the movement of strains between these species. Analysis of some Kenyan isolates derived from sheep and goats shows very close homology with cattle LSD isolates.

The involvement of the African buffalo (*Syncerus caffer*) in the maintenance of LSD has not been clearly established. Some surveys have shown the presence of capripoxvirus antibody in buffalo, while others have failed to show its presence. Buffaloes clinically affected with LSD have not been described. Experimental infection of giraffe (*Giraffe camelopardalis*), impala (*Aepyceros melampus*), and gazelle (*Gazella thomsonii*) has resulted in the development of clinical disease.

*Bos indicus* cattle are generally less susceptible to LSD and develop milder clinical disease than *Bos taurus*, of which the fine-skin Channel Island breeds are particularly susceptible. Similarly, breeds of sheep and goats indigenous to capripoxvirus enzootic areas appear less susceptible to severe clinical capripox than do imported European or Australian breeds.

Capripoxvirus will grow on the majority of primary and secondary cells and cell lines of ruminant origin. Primary lamb testes cells are considered the most sensitive system for isolation and growth of capripoxvirus. The virus produces a characteristic cytopathic effect (cpe) on these cells which can take up to 14 days for field isolates, but can be as short as 3 days for well-adapted strains.

Isolates of capripoxvirus derived from cattle have been adapted to grow on the chorioallantoic membrane of embryonated hens' eggs, although attempts to grow isolates from sheep and goats in eggs have been unsuccessful. Vaccine strains of capripoxvirus have been adapted to grow on Vero cells. Capripoxvirus will not grow in any laboratory animals.

## Genetics

Less is known concerning the specific genetics of capripoxvirus than is known about the orthopoxvirus genome. Studies on field isolates taken from cattle suggest that the virus is very stable, as *Hin*dIII restriction endonuclease digest patterns of isolates from the 1959 Kenya outbreak of LSD are identical to those obtained from 1986 LSD isolates. However, recombination has been shown to occur between cattle and goat isolates and this could be the natural method by which the virus evolves. By analogy with the orthopoxviruses, it is also likely that sequences are deleted or repeated within the genome in the normal replicative cycle.

The genomes of those capripoxvirus isolates that have been sequenced, representing isolates from cattle, sheep, and goats, have a 96% nucleotide homology along their entire length of approximately 150 kbp.

Sheep and goat isolates have 147 putative genes and LSD isolates an additional nine. However, the sheep and goat isolates have these nine in a disrupted form, suggesting that the LSD virus is the more ancient progenitor. This is clearly not consistent with the apparent first appearance of LSD in 1929. Nevertheless, the published sequences have shown a range of genes coding for host cell protein homologs, in common with many identified in the orthopoxviruses. In fact, in the central region of the genome, there is a high degree of similarity (*c.* 65%) with amino acid sequences found in other poxvirus species, in particular suipoxvirus, yatapoxvirus, and leporipoxvirus. These sequence studies and those reported from India suggest that distinction can be made between sheep and goat isolates, but limited numbers were studied; however, some isolates examined from the Middle East show less evidence of host-species-specific sequences.

## Evolution

The capripoxviruses have evolved into specific cattle, sheep, and goat lines, but, as has been described above, intermediate strains exist, particularly those with cattle and goat genome characteristics. In Kenya, there is evidence of movement of strains between all three species, but the absence of sheeppox or goatpox in LSD enzootic areas in southern Africa, and the absence of LSD outside of Africa, would suggest that host-specific strains are being maintained and presumably are continuing to evolve.

## Serologic Relationships and Variability

Polyclonal sera fail to distinguish in the virus neutralization test between any of the isolates of capripoxvirus so far examined. Sheep, goats, or cattle that have been infected with any of the isolates are totally resistant to challenge with any of the other isolates. On this basis, it has been possible to use the same vaccine strain to protect all three species. No monoclonal antibodies are as yet available against capripoxvirus, but it can be expected that differences will emerge between strains using these reagents.

Capripoxviruses share a precipitating antigen with parapoxviruses, but no cross-immunity has been shown between these two genera, or between capripoxvirus and any other poxvirus genera.

## Epizootiology

In sheeppox and goatpox enzootic areas the distribution of disease is frequently a reflection of the traditional form of husbandry. For instance, in the Yemen Arab Republic, the sheep and goat flocks kept on the grassland of the central plateau and better irrigated regions of the coastal plain move about in search of food, frequently mixing with flocks from neighboring villages at water holes, and in this situation disease is restricted to the young stock. Animals over 1 year of age have a solid immunity. The animals belonging to villages in the more mountainous regions and the arid areas of the coastal plain are isolated by terrain or semidesert from mixing with animals from other villages. It is not known what is the critical number of animals required to maintain capripoxvirus within a single population but it is over a thousand adult animals, which is the approximate village sheep and goat populations. In these villages, disease is usually only seen following the introduction of new animals, typically from market, and generally affects animals of all age groups. The disease spreads through the village, usually within 3–6 months, and then disappears in the absence of more susceptible animals. Occasionally, even within areas of high sheep and goat density, it is possible to encounter animals that have been kept totally isolated in the confines of a domestic residence, and these may remain susceptible to infection until adult.

In Sudan, large numbers of sheep and goats are trekked from the west to the large collecting yards and markets of Omdurman, outside Khartoum. Here also, it is possible to see capripox infection in adult animals. Many of the flocks originate in villages which, like in the Yemen, are isolated from their neighbors. Capripoxvirus does not persist in these villages, and as a result the animals acquire no resistance, and are fully susceptible when they first encounter disease on the long journey across Sudan. Animals being exported from countries that are free of capripoxvirus may suffer a similar fate when they arrive in a capripoxvirus enzootic area, as often seen in Australian or New Zealand sheep imported into the Middle East.

In a study of 49 outbreaks of capripox in the Yemen, only 8 were reported to affect both sheep and goats, the remaining 41 causing clinical disease in either sheep or goats. It is possible that both sheep and goats could have been involved in more than the eight outbreaks, but that the disease was inapparent in one species; whether, therefore, the species in which the disease was inapparent could transmit virus and become a vector for disease has not been determined. In Kenya, capripox is frequently encountered in both sheep and goats within the same flock, and there is the possibility that the same strain of capripoxvirus could also cause LSD in cattle.

The epidemiology of sheeppox, goatpox, and LSD is similar; the severity of outbreaks depends on the size of the susceptible population, the virulence of the strain of capripoxvirus, the breed affected (indigenous animals tending to be less susceptible to clinical disease than imported), and, with LSD, the presence of suitable insect vectors. Morbidity rates vary from 2% to 80%, and mortality rates may exceed 90%, particularly if the infection is in association with other disease or bad management.

## Transmission and Tissue Tropism

Under natural conditions, capripoxvirus is not transmitted very readily between animals, although there are circumstances when transmission appears very rapid; for example, in association with factors that damage the mucosae, such as peste des petits ruminants infection or feeding on abrasive forage. Animals are most infectious soon after the appearance of papules and during the 10-day period before the development of significant levels of protective antibody. High titers of virus are present in the papules, and those papules on the mucous membranes quickly ulcerate and release virus in nasal, oral, and lachrymal secretions, and into milk, urine, and semen. Viremia may last up to 10 days, or in fatal cases until death. Those animals that die of acute infection before the development of clinical signs and those that develop only very mild signs or single lesions rarely transmit infection, while those that develop generalized lesions produce considerable virus and are highly infectious. Aerosol infection over a few meters only, as with other poxvirus infections, is probably the usual form of transmission. Contact transmission of LSD virus under experimental conditions in the absence of insect vectors has only rarely been reported. Biting flies are significant in the mechanical transmission of LSD, and *Stomoxys calcitrans* and *Biomyia fasciata* have been implicated. There are probably a number of insects capable of mechanically transmitting LSD virus, but insects such as mosquitoes, which preferentially feed on hyperemic sites such as papules and if interrupted inoculate a new host intravenously, are considered the most likely to be involved in outbreaks characterized by large numbers of affected animals with generalized infections. Experimentally, *S. calcitrans* has also been shown to be capable of transmitting sheeppox and goatpox, and mosquitoes have transmitted LSD virus under experimental conditions.

During the recovery phase following infection, the papules on the skin become scabs. It is relatively easy to demonstrate virions in the scab, but difficult to isolate virus on tissue culture, probably because of the complexing of antibody and virus within the scab. Capripoxvirus is reported to remain viable in wool for 2 months and in contaminated premises for 6 months, and is reported to remain infectious in skin lesions of cattle for 4 months. The true epidemiological significance of the virus within the scab, and ultimately the environment, is not clear. It has been suggested that the protein material that envelops the virus within the type A intracytoplasmic inclusion bodies of infected cells protects the virus in the environment.

There is no evidence for the existence of animals persistently infected with capripoxvirus. Transplacental transmission of capripoxvirus may be possible in association with simultaneous pestivirus infection, as may occur with pestivirus-contaminated capripox vaccine.

Capripoxvirus can be isolated from the leukocytes during viremia, and has been isolated from lesions in the liver, urinary tract, testes, digestive tract, and lungs; however, the cells of the skin and skin glands and the internal and external mucous membranes appear to be the major sites of virus replication.

## Pathogenicity

There is considerable variation in the pathogenicity of strains of capripoxvirus. Little is known concerning the genes responsible in the capripoxvirus genome for virulence or host restriction; some preliminary results have been published.

## Clinical Features of Infection

The incubation period of capripox infection, from contact with virus to the onset of pyrexia, is approximately 12 days, although it frequently appears longer as transmission is often not immediate between infected and susceptible animals. Following experimental inoculation of virus, the incubation period is approximately 7 days, and this is similar to that shown experimentally using biting flies to transmit virus.

The clinical signs of malignant disease are similar in sheep, goats, and cattle. Twenty-four hours after the development of pyrexia of between 40 and 41 °C, macules (2–3 cm diameter areas of congested skin) can be seen on the white skin of sheep and goats, particularly under the tail. Macules are not seen on the thicker skin of cattle, and are frequently missed on skin of pigmented sheep and goats. After a further 24 h, the macules swell to become hard papules of between 0.5 and 2 cm diameter, although they may be larger in cattle. In the generalized form of capripox, papules cover the body, being concentrated particularly on the head and neck, axilla, groin, and perineum, and external mucous membranes of the eyes, prepuce, vulva, anus, and nose. In cattle, these papules may exude serum, and there may be considerable edema of the brisket, ventral abdomen, and limbs. The papules on the mucous membranes quickly ulcerate, and the secretions of rhinitis and conjunctivitis become

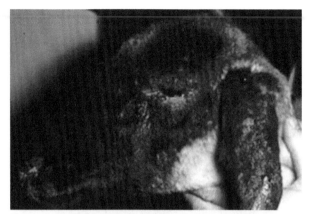

**Figure 1** Sheeppox showing rhinitis and conjunctivitis.

mucopurulent (**Figure 1**). Keratitis may be associated with the conjunctivitis.

All the superficial lymph nodes, particularly the prescapular, are enlarged. Breathing may become labored as the enlarged retropharyngeal lymph nodes put pressure on the trachea. Mastitis may result from secondary infection of the lesions on the udder.

The papules do not become vesicles and then pustules, typical of orthopoxvirus infections. Instead, they become necrotic, and if the animal survives the acute stage of the disease, change to scabs over a 5–10 day period from the first appearance of papules. The scabs can persist for up to a month in sheep and goats, whereas in cattle the necrotic papules that penetrate the thickness of the skin may remain as 'sitfasts' for up to a year.

Severe disease is accompanied by significant loss of condition, agalactia, possibly secondary abortion, and pneumonia. Eating, drinking, and walking may become painful, and death from dehydration is not uncommon. Secondary myiasis is also a major problem in tropical areas.

## Pathology and Histopathology

The lesions of capripox are not only restricted to the skin, but also may affect any of the internal organs, in particular the gastrointestinal tract from the mouth and tongue to the anus, and the respiratory tract. In generalized infections, papules are prominent in the abomasal mucosa, trachea, and lungs. Those in the lungs are approximately 2 cm in diameter, and papules may coalesce to form areas of gray consolidation (**Figure 2**).

In affected skin, there is an initial epithelial hyperplasia followed by coagulation necrosis as thrombi develop in the blood vessels supplying the papules. Histiocytes accumulate in the areas of the papules, and the chromatin of the nuclei of infected cells marginates. The cells appear stellate as their boundaries become poorly defined, and many undergo hydropic degeneration with

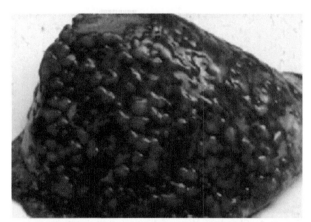

**Figure 2** Sheeppox showing severe lung lesions.

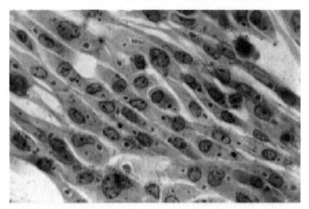

**Figure 3** Capripoxvirus growing in lamb testis cells showing many intracytoplasmic inclusion bodies. Magnification ×400.

the formation of microvesicles. Intracytoplasmic inclusion bodies are present in infected cells of the dermis and also in the columnar epithelial cells of the trachea where frequently gross lesions may not be apparent. These are initially type B inclusions at the sites of virus replication (**Figure 3**), but later in infection they are replaced by type A inclusions (see above). The maximum titer of virus is obtained from papules approximately 6 days after their first appearance.

## Immune Response

Capripoxvirus, like orthopoxvirus, is released from an infected cell within an envelope derived from modified cellular membrane. The enveloped form of the virus is more infectious than the nonenveloped form, which can be obtained experimentally by freeze–thawing infected tissue culture. By analogy with orthopoxvirus, antigens on the envelope and on the tubular elements of the virion surface may stimulate protective antibodies. Animals immune to nonenveloped virus are still fully susceptible to the enveloped form. Passively transferred antibody,

either colostral or experimentally inoculated, will protect susceptible animals against generalized infection; however, in the vaccinated or recovered animal, there is no direct correlation between serum levels of neutralizing antibody and immunity to clinical disease. Antibody may limit the spread of capripoxvirus within the body, but it is the cell-mediated immune response that eliminates infection. In sheep, major histocompatibility complex-restricted cytotoxic T-lymphocytes are required in the protective immune response to orthopoxvirus infection, and therefore probably also capripoxvirus infection.

Immune animals challenged with capripoxvirus by intradermal inoculation develop a delayed-type hypersensitivity reaction at the challenge site. This may not be apparent in animals with high levels of circulating antibody. It has been suggested that the very severe local response shown by some cattle at the site of vaccination against LSD may be a hypersensitivity reaction due to previous contact with the antigens of parapoxvirus.

There is total cross-immunity between all strains of capripoxvirus, whether derived from cattle, sheep, or goats.

## Prevention and Control

In temperate climates, capripox can be effectively controlled by slaughter of affected animals, and movement control of all susceptible animals within a 10 km radius for 6 months. In tropical climates, particularly in humid conditions when insect activity is high, movement restrictions are not sufficient and vaccination of all susceptible animals should be considered. In outbreaks of LSD, it is not considered necessary to vaccinate sheep and goats, although theoretically cattle strains of virus could infect them. Similarly, in outbreaks of capripox in sheep and goats, cattle are not normally vaccinated.

Countries in which capripoxvirus is absent can maintain freedom by preventing the importation of animals from infected areas. There is always a possibility that skins from infected animals could introduce infection into a new area, although there have been no proven examples of this. The insect transmission of capripoxvirus into Israel from Egypt over a distance of between 70 and 300 km would indicate that it is impossible for countries neighboring enzootic areas to totally secure their borders.

In enzootic areas, annual vaccination of susceptible animals with a live vaccine will control the disease. Calves, kids, and lambs up to 6 months of age may be protected by maternal antibody, but this would only occur if the mother had recently been severely affected with capripox. Although maternal antibody will inactivate the vaccine, it is advisable to vaccinate all stock over 10 days of age. No successful killed vaccines have been developed for immunization against capripoxvirus infection, other than those that give only very short-term immunity.

## Future Perspectives

Capripox of sheep and goats is present in most of Africa and Asia, whereas LSD is restricted to Africa. There is no good explanation as to why LSD has not spread into the Middle East and India, carried by the considerable trade in live cattle. Unless there is a reservoir host in Africa which is required for the maintenance of the cattle-adapted capripoxvirus, it can be anticipated that LSD will spread out of Africa, with major economic consequences.

While considerable attention has been given to vaccinia virus as a vector of other viral genes for development as a recombinant vaccine, little attention has been given to capripoxvirus as a potential vector vaccine. Although its use would be restricted to the not inconsiderable capripoxvirus enzootic area, it would have the advantage of not being infectious to humans, and be a useful vaccine in its own right.

The high degree of homology between the genomes of capripoxvirus isolates from different species and the apparent differences between their virulence and host preference would make them good candidates for studying the genetic basis of virulence and host specificity.

*See also:* Leporipoviruses and Suipoxviruses.

## Further Reading

Black DN, Hammond JM, and Kitching RP (1986) Genomic relationship between capripoxvirus. *Virus Research* 5: 277–292.

Carn VM and Kitching RP (1995) An investigation of possible routes of transmission of lumpy skin disease (Neethling). *Epidemiology and Infection* 114: 219–226.

Gershon PD, Ansell DM, and Black DN (1989) A comparison of the genome organization of capripoxvirus with that of the orthopoxviruses. *Journal of Virology* 63: 4703–4708.

Gershon PD, Kitching RP, Hammond JM, and Black DN (1989) Poxvirus genetic recombination during natural virus transmission. *Journal of General Virology* 70: 485–489.

Kitching RP, Bhat PP, and Black DN (1989) The characterization of African strains of capripoxvirus. *Epidemiology and Infection* 102: 335–343.

Kitching RP, Hammond JM, and Taylor WP (1987) A single vaccine for the control of capripox infection in sheep and goats. *Research in Veterinary Science* 42: 53–60.

Tulman ER, Afonso CL, Lu Z, Zsak L, Kutish GF, and Rock DL (2001) Genome of lumpy skin disease virus. *Journal of Virology* 75: 7122–7130.

Tulman ER, Afonso CL, Lu Z, et al. (2002) The genomes of sheeppox and goatpox viruses. *Journal of Virology* 76: 6054–6061.

# Circoviruses

**A Mankertz,** Robert Koch-Institut, Berlin, Germany

## Glossary

**Apoptosis** Programmed self-induced cell death.

**Botryoid** Grape-like appearance.

**Bursa of Fabricius** Specialized organ in birds, that is necessary for B-cell development.

**Chimera** Virus created from two or more different genetic sources.

**Koch's postulates** Four criteria that must be fulfilled in order to establish a causal relationship between an agent and a disease.

**Mono/polycistronic mRNA** mRNA is termed polycistronic when it contains the genetic information to translate more than one protein, monocistronic if only one protein is encoded.

**Phylogenetic tree** Depicts the evolutionary interrelationships among species that are believed to have a common ancestor.

**Rolling-circle replication (RCR)** Mechanism of replication which takes its name from the characteristic appearance of the replicating DNA molecules, a special feature of RCR is the uncoupling of the synthesis of the two DNA strands.

## Circovirus Taxonomy

Circoviruses contain a covalently closed circular single-stranded DNA (ssDNA) genome with sizes between 1759 and 2319 nt. The circular nature of their genomes, which are the smallest possessed by animal viruses, has led to the family being termed *Circoviridae*. Differences in organization of the viral genomes and capsid morphology led to their classification into two different genera.

*Chicken anemia virus* is the only species member of the genus *Gyrovirus*, while the genus *Circovirus* currently comprises *Porcine circovirus type 1* and *Porcine circovirus type 2*, *Psittacine beak and feather disease virus*, *Pigeon circovirus*, *Canary circovirus*, and *Goose circovirus*. Duck circovirus (DuCV), finch circovirus (FiCV), and gull circovirus (GuCV) are members of tentative species in the genus, while the circoviruses of raven (RaCV) and starling (StCV) have been discovered only recently and are therefore not yet included in the taxonomic classification.

The reported size range for the chicken anemia virus (CAV) virion is 19.1–26.5 nm, the genome is of (–) polarity, and the open reading frames (ORFs) are overlapping. Only one mRNA molecule is produced from a promoter/enhancer region; it encodes three partially overlapping ORFs. CAV shows homology to the newly identified ssDNA viruses in humans, torque teno virus (TTV) and the related torque teno mini virus (TTMV), which are members of the unassigned genus *Anellovirus*. The noncoding regions of CAV and TTV are G/C-rich and show a low level of nucleotide homology. In addition, CAV and TTV specify structural proteins that contain two amino acid motifs with putative roles in rolling-circle replication (RCR) and nonstructural proteins that exhibit protein phosphatase activity. CAV and TTV are separately classified, since their sequence homology is limited and only one mRNA is produced from CAV, while splicing has been detected in TTV and TTMV. Phylogenetic investigation of the family *Circoviridae* revealed that CAV has no close relationship to the genus *Circovirus* (**Figure 1**).

Members of the genus *Circovirus* differ in several aspects from CAV, because they display a smaller particle size (12–20.7 nm, **Figure 2**), their ambisense genomes

(**Figure 3**) are divergently transcribed, and splicing has been reported. The viruses of the genus *Circovirus* show homology in genome organization and protein sequences and function to the plant-infecting viruses of the family *Nanoviridae* and *Geminiviridae*.

## Virion Structure

The size for the CAV virion has been reported as 19.1–26.5 nm and 12–20.7 nm for circoviruses (**Figure 2**).

The virions of CAV, porcine circovirus type 1 (PCV1) and porcine circovirus type 2 (PCV2), are each comprised of one structural protein, for which sizes of 50 (CAV), 30 (PCV1), and 30 kDa (PCV2) have been estimated, respectively. Psittacine beak and feather disease virus (PBFDV) is reported to contain three proteins (26, 24, and 16 kDa). The protein composition of the other avian circoviruses is not known, but putative structural proteins have been identified by homology searches. All capsid proteins have a basic N-terminal region containing several arginine residues, which is expected to interact with the packaged DNA. Virions do not possess an envelope. Investigation of the structures of CAV, PCV1, and PCV2 revealed that all have an icosahedral $T = 1$ structure containing 60 capsid protein molecules arranged in 12 pentamer clustered units. PCV2 and BFDV show similar capsid structures with flat pentameric morphological units, whereas chicken anemia virus displayed protruding pentagonal trumpet-shaped units.

## Pathogenesis of Circoviruses

### Circoviruses and Gyroviruses Induce Diseases

Circoviruses are supposed to be host specific or to have narrow host ranges. The fecal–oral route of transmission

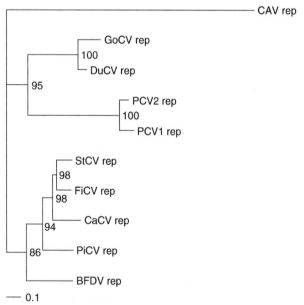

**Figure 1** Phylogenetic tree of members of the family *Circoviridae*. The amino acid sequences of the Rep proteins of the members of the genus *Circovirus* (GoCV, DuCV, BFDV, PiCV, StCV, FiCV, CaCV, PCV1, PCV2) and of the only member of the genus *Gyrovirus* (CAV) were compared. Analysis was performed using the MacVector program package by analyzing 100 data sets.

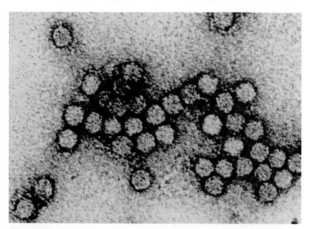

**Figure 2** Electron microscope picture of particles of PCV1. PCV1 particles in an immunoaggregation with a PCV1 hyperimmuneserum (180 000-fold magnification, negative contrasting with 1% UAc).

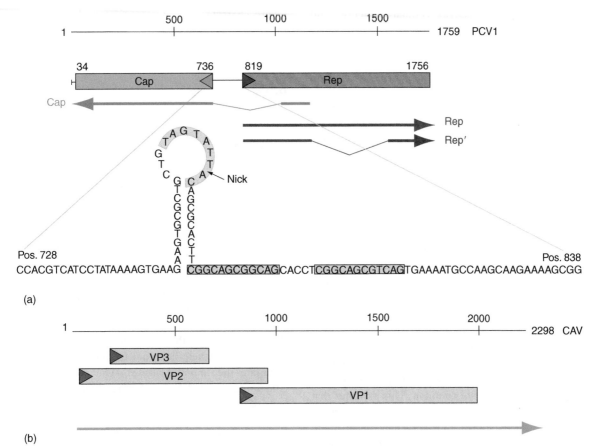

(a)

(b)

**Figure 3** Genomic organization of PCV1 member of the type species of the genus *Circovirus* and CAV member of the type species of the genus *Gyrovirus*. ORFs are shown in open boxes, the direction of transcription is indicated by triangles. Transcripts are indicated by arrows, splice processes by dotted lines. (a) PCV1, the species type of the genus *Circovirus*, is shown. The ambisense genomic organization is outlined, that is, both strands of the replicative form are coding for proteins. Therefore, the two major genes Rep and Cap are divergently transcribed. Between the start points of Rep and Cap, the origin of viral replication is located. This element is drawn to a larger scale, displaying its characteristic features, a putative hairpin, and adjacently located repeats. An arrow indicates the position where Rep and Rep' restrict the replicative intermediate to initiate the replication.(b) CAV is a member of the type species of the genus *Gyrovirus*. Its genome is of the 'negative-sense' type, that is, the viral strand does not encode genetic information, it has to be converted into a dsDNA version, from which one polycistronic mRNA is produced. Splice processes have not been observed.

is likely, but vertical transmission has been reported in some cases. With the exception of PCV1, all known circoviruses are pathogens, which cause immune suppression and damage in the lymphoreticular tissues.

CAV infections occur mainly in young chicken. The main targets of CAV replication are cells in the bone marrow (hemocytoblasts) and precursor lymphocytes in the thymus. Characteristic symptoms are aplastic anemia and hemorrhagic lesions, watery blood, pale bone marrow, lymphoid depletion, atrophy of thymus and bursa, and swollen and discolored liver. Since macrophages recovered from infected birds produce less interleukin 1 (IL-1) and the pathogenicity of co-infecting viruses such as Marek's disease virus, infectious bursal disease virus, and Newcastle disease virus are enhanced, immune suppression is thought to play a role in CAV-induced pathogenesis.

Another intensively studied circoviral disease is psittacine beak and feather disease (PBFD). PBFD is the most

common disease in cockatoos and parrots and is typically detected in young birds. Deformation of beak, claws, and feathers, lethargy, depression, weight loss, and severe anemia are the most prominent symptoms.

Young pigeon disease syndrome (YPDS) is a multifactorial disease in which PiCV is assumed to induce immunosuppression in young birds, which suffer from ill-thrift, lethargy, anorexia, and poor race performance. Depletion of splenic and bursal lymphocytes was seen and bacterial agents as *Escherichia coli* and *Klebsiella pneumoniae* were isolated more frequently from PiCV-infected birds. Inclusion bodies were present in various organs, especially the bursa of Fabricius.

In CaCV-infected neonatal canary birds, a condition known as 'black spot' has been reported. It is associated with abdominal enlargement, gall bladder congestion, failure to thrive, dullness, anorexia, lethargy, and feather disorder. Histological changes as lymphofollicular hyperplasia, lymphoid necrosis, cellular depletion, and cystic atrophy are observed in the thymus and the bursa of Fabricius. A general feature of circovirus infection is the formation of globular or botryoid, basophilic inclusion bodies in the cytoplasm, in which the virus may form paracrystalline arrays.

PCV1 and PCV2 seem to be restricted to pigs. PCV2 is the etiological agent of a new disease in swine, the so-called post-weaning multisystemic wasting syndrome (PMWS), and may be involved in several other porcine circoviral diseases (PCVDs) like porcine dermatitis and nephropathy syndrome (PDNS) or porcine respiratory disease complex. PMWS was first recognized in Canada in 1991. Since then it has been described as a major economic concern in virtually all pig-producing areas of the world. PMWS primarily occurs in pigs between 60 and 80 days old. Maternal antibodies confer titer-dependent protection against PCV2 infection – higher titers are generally protective, but low titers are not. PMWS is characterized by wasting, respiratory signs, enlargement of superficial inguinal lymph nodes, diarrhea, paleness of the skin or icterus, but the clinical signs are often variable. The most consistent feature of PMWS is a generalized depletion of lymphocytes. Secondary infections with opportunistic organisms are common. This indicates that the immune system is involved in the pathogenesis of PMWS. On affected farms, mortality may reach up to 40%, but it can be reduced, if special management plans are implemented. In the first attempts, experimental reproduction of the disease according to Koch's postulates has led to an amazing variety of results, since no symptoms were seen as well as histopathological lesions or a full-blown PMWS. The symptoms of the disease were aggravated when piglets were infected in which the immune system had been stimulated either by a prior vaccination or by a co-infection with porcine parvovirus (PPV) or porcine reproductive and respiratory syndrome virus (PRRSV). These and other findings indicate that PMWS is a multifactorial disease, in which not only factors such as the status of the immune system and genetic predisposition but also practical aspects such as nutrition and vaccination policy may influence the onset of the disease and the severity of the symptoms.

### Diagnosis of Circoviral Diseases

In general, diagnosis of circoviral diseases is based on detection of the virus by culture, polymerase chain reaction (PCR), immunohistochemistry or *in situ* hybridization, or detection of antibodies against the circovirus by serology. PBFD can also be diagnosed on the basis of feathering abnormalities. PCV2 is a ubiquitous virus and also prevalent in healthy pigs; therefore, diagnosis of PMWS must concurrently meet three criteria: (1) the presence of compatible clinical signs, (2) the presence of moderate to severe characteristic microscopic lymphoid lesions, and (3) the presence of moderate to high amount of PCV2 within these lesions.

### PCV1 and PCV2

A striking difference is seen in the pathogenicity of PCV1 and PCV2. No disease is attributed to PCV1, while PCV2 is the etiological agent of PMWS, a new emerging disease of swine. What may be the molecular basis for this distinct feature? The genomes of the two strains are highly conserved, especially the origin of replication (80% sequence homology) and the Rep gene (82%). Exchange of replication factors between PCV1 and PCV2 did not reveal differences, since the Rep protein of PCV1 (Rep/PCV1) replicated its cognate origin as well as the heterotype origin of PCV2 (and vice versa), suggesting that pathogenesis may not be linked to the replication factors. A higher degree of sequence deviation is found in the Cap genes with less than 62% homology between PCV1 and PCV2. Chimeras of PCV1 and PCV2 have been produced and tested for their potential to induce PMWS and to stimulate the immune answer. The chimera PCV2/1, containing the PCV1 capsid gene cloned into the backbone of the pathogenic PCV2 genome, was compared to a chimera PCV1/2, containing the PCV2 capsid gene in the nonpathogenic PCV1 genome. Both variants displayed similar growth characteristics *in vitro*. Gross lesions significant for PMWS were not observed, but PCV1/2 induces protective immunity to wild-type PCV2 challenge in pigs, indicating that it may be an effective vaccine candidate. ORF3 is comprised by the rep gene and may also contribute to the pathogenesis of PCV2, because its sequence differs significantly in PCV1 and PCV2 and induction of apoptosis has been reported.

### Interaction with the Immune System

PCV2 provides a valuable model for gaining insight into how ssDNA viruses interact with the host immune system and for understanding their pathogenesis. PCV2 is intriguing in its ability to persist in macrophages and dendritic cells without replication although its infectivity is retained. When natural interferon (IFN)-producing cells responded to an inducer of cytokine synthesis, their co-stimulatory function, which induces myeloid dendritic cell maturation, was clearly impaired in case of a concurrent PCV2 infection. Stimulation of the porcine immune system with IFN-$\alpha$ and IFN-$\gamma$ causes increased replication of PCV2 *in vivo*, while no changes were observed in IL-1-, IL-6-, tumor necrosis factor alpha (TNF-$\alpha$)-, or IL-10-treated cells. With the circumstantial evidence compiled over the last years, one may assume that PMWS can be considered as an acquired immunodeficiency syndrome of pigs although direct evidence for this hypothesis is still missing.

## Molecular Biology of Circoviruses

### Genome Organization of Circoviruses

The genomes of all circoviruses are composed from a circular ssDNA molecule with a size between 1759 and 2319 nt and therefore display the smallest genomes possessed by mammalian viruses. Nevertheless, members of the genera *Circovirus* and *Gyrovirus* show remarkable differences in their genome organization.

The genomes of CAV isolates are either 2298 or 2319 nt in size. Part of the noncoding region of the genome is G–C-rich and able to form putative hairpin structures. The three genes are encoded by the viral (–)strand, therefore CAV has a negative-sense genome organization. One major polycistronic mRNA (2.0 kbp) is transcribed from the circular double-stranded (ds) replication form (RF), which is produced after infection. The nontranscribed region of the genome contains transcription initiation and termination signals and a tandemly arranged array of four or five 19 nt repeats with which promoter–enhancer activity is associated. Within this sequence, estrogen response element consensus half-sites were found, resembling the arrangement that can be recognized by the nuclear receptor superfamily. Since expression from the CAV promoter was significantly increased with estrogen treatment, members of the nuclear receptor superfamily may provide a mechanism to regulate CAV activity.

The hypothesis that the circular ssDNA genome replicates using the RCR mechanism is supported by the presence of the conserved nonanucleotide motif within the CAV genome, at which RCR is initiated in other circular ssDNA replicons, but it is not located at the apex of a putative hairpin. The presence of two amino acid motifs typical for enzymes involved in RCR within VP1 also suggests that this structural protein possesses DNA replication function, while its basic N-terminus implies that this protein is involved in capsid formation, too. This would be highly unlike the genus *Circovirus*, where two distinctly encoded proteins perform the two most elementary functions of replication and packaging of the genome. Coding regions of the avian and porcine circoviruses are arranged divergently resulting in an ambisense genome organization and creating two intergenic regions, a larger one between the 5′ ends of the two major ORFs rep and cap and a shorter one between their 3′ ends. In case of PCV1 and PCV2, the non-coding regions between the ATGs of the rep and cap gene comprise the origin of viral genome replication. Similar genomic structures are found in members of the families *Geminiviridae* and *Nanoviridae*.

## Viral ORFs and Proteins

Synthesis of three virus proteins is directed from the CAV genome. VP1 (52 kDa) is encoded by ORF1 and may combine the function of a structural protein as well as the initiator of replication. VP2 (26 kDa) is a protein phosphatase encoded by ORF2. VP2 protein phosphatase activity is required for efficient replication. It may also have a role as a scaffolding protein during virion assembly. Co-expression of both VP1 and VP2 is necessary for the induction of neutralizing antibodies. VP3 is a 14 kDa virulence factor known to induce apoptosis in transformed cell lines and has been called 'apoptin'.

Two major ORFs are encoded by the genomes of PCV1 and PCV2, encoding the viral functions for replication (Rep and Rep′) and a structural protein (Cap). A similar genomic structure is seen in the avian circoviruses. Several smaller ORFs have been found by computer analyses, but with the exception of ORF3 of PCV, which seems to be involved in pathogenesis and apoptosis, their expression has not been studied yet. The largest ORF of the ambisense organized circoviruses is located on the viral plus-strand (V1). It encodes the Rep protein (312 or 314 aa). Three motifs conserved in enzymes mediating replication in the RCR mode and a dNTP-binding domain have been identified. Both Rep proteins reside in the nucleus of infected cells. Phylogenetic analyses suggest that circovirus Rep proteins may have evolved by a recombination event between the Rep protein of nanoviruses and an RNA-binding protein encoded by picorna-like viruses or a helicase of prokaryotic origin. The second largest ORF of all circoviruses is located on the complementary strand (C1) and encodes the major structural protein Cap protein (234 aa), which displays a basic N-terminus rich in arginine residues. This suggests that this region is involved in binding to viral DNA. Some avian circoviruses use alternative start codons for Cap translation. After expression in bacteria and insect cells, Cap of PCV assembled into virus-like particles when viewed by electron microscopy. Cap has been shown to reside mostly in the nucleoli, but shuttling to the cytoplasm occurs during the infectious cycle. ORF3 is encoded counterclockwisely by ORF1. It encodes a protein that is not essential for PCV replication but has been reported to induce apoptosis.

## Transcription of PCV

The promoter of the cap gene of PCV has been mapped to a fragment at 1168–1428, that is, $P_{cap}$ is located within the rep gene. $P_{cap}$ is not regulated by virus-encoded proteins. The cap transcript starts at nucleotide 1238 with an untranslated leader sequence of 119 nt (1238 to 1120) joined to exon 2 of the ORF1 transcript at nucleotide 737, immediately adjacent to the start point of translation. Processing of this RNA has presumably evolved to avoid synthesis of another protein initiated at an internal start codon in the intron. The start of the rep transcript of PCV1 has been mapped to nucleotide $767 \pm 10$. The promoter of the rep gene, $P_{rep}$, is comprised within a fragment, nucleotides 640–796. $P_{rep}$ overlaps the intergenic region and the origin of replication. $P_{rep}$ is repressed by the Rep protein by binding to hexamers H1 and H2; these elements are involved in initation of replication, too. Mapping the rep mRNA revealed synthesis of several transcripts in PCV1 and PCV2. A full-length transcript directs synthesis of the Rep protein (312 aa, 35.6 kDa). In a spliced transcript, removal of an intron (nucleotides 1176 to 1558) results in synthesis of a truncated protein, which has been termed Rep′. Rep′ is truncated to 168 aa (19.2 kDa) and, due to a frameshift, the last 49 aa are expressed in a different reading frame. Comparison of the ratio of Rep and Rep′ transcript with a real-time PCR discriminating between the two transcripts indicated a variation of the ratio of the two transcripts in correlation to time. Replication of PCV is dependent on expression of both proteins. Splicing of Rep proteins is a well-known feature in other small ssDNA viruses (e.g., *Mastrevirus*), but, in contrast to PCV, one Rep protein is sufficient for replication of these viruses.

## Replication of Circoviruses

Although the main target for viral replication still remains unknown, PCV2 was seen *in vivo* in a variety of cell types including hepatocytes, enterocytes, epithelial and endothelial cells, lymphocytes, smooth muscle cells, and fibroblasts. This broad range of cells that support PCV2 infection indicates that PCV2 does not enter the cell via a rarely expressed receptor. When binding of PCV2 to monocytic cells was investigated, it became evident that surface proteins and glycosaminoglycans heparan sulfate and chondroitin sulfate B are attachment receptors for PCV2. This result is supported by the finding that the heparan sulfate binding motif (XBBXBX; B = basic amino acid, X = neutral/hydrophobic amino acid) is present on the PCV2 capsid protein. PCV2 enters the cells predominantly via clathrin-mediated endocytosis and requires an acidic environment for infection.

Replication of PCV has been studied in detail. PCVs are supposed to replicate their genomes using a circular, ds RF intermediate, which is produced by host cell DNA polymerases during the S phase of cell division. The origin of replication of PCV has been mapped to a fragment comprising the intergenic region between the start points of the two major ORFs (**Figure 3**).

Replication of these fragments cloned into a vector was observed after co-transfection of porcine kidney cells with plasmids expressing the rep gene. By sequence alignment, analogous elements can be identified for all other circoviruses with the exception of CAV. The origin of replication is characterized by a potential stem–loop structure with a nonamer (5′-TAGTATTAC; **Figure 3**) in its apex. Mutagenesis of the nonamer resulted in inactivation of PCV replication. Adjacent to the nonamer, short repeats are located, which serve as the binding site for the rep gene products. Nonamer, stem–loop, and adjacent short repeats are conserved in all other circoviruses, in the families *Nanoviridae* and *Geminiviridae*, and, although to a lesser extent, in many replicons replicating via RCR. The conserved elements in the *cis*-acting origin of replication as well as RCR signatures in the *trans*-acting Rep protein amino acid (aa) sequence (see below) indicate an RCR-like replication mechanism for the circoviruses.

## Functional Analyses of PCV-Encoded Proteins

Truncation of the rep gene as well as site-directed mutagenesis of the four conserved motifs abrogated replication of PCV, indicating that the rep gene products are indispensable. The roles of Rep and Rep′ of PCV have been analyzed in detail.

*Binding to DNA.* Rep and Rep′ bind *in vitro* to fragments of the origin of replication containing the stem–loop structure plus the conserved nonamer and the four hexamer (H) repeats (5′-CGGCAG; H1 to H4). Proteins bind either the two inner (H1/H2) or the two outer (H3/H4) hexamers. A minimal binding site (MBS) has been identified for Rep and Rep′ protein using truncated substrates: the Rep MBS was mapped to the right leg of the stem–loop plus the two inner hexamer repeats H1/H2, while the MBS of Rep′ was composed of only the two hexamer repeats H1/H2. Gel shift assays also revealed presence of several complexes, indicating that variable amount of proteins may be bound.

*Replication.* The covalently closed, ssDNA genome of PCV replicates via a dsDNA replicative intermediate. The replication occurs by RCR whereby a single-stranded break is introduced by Rep or Rep′ leading to a free 3′-hydroxyl group serving as a primer for subsequent DNA synthesis. Replication does occur when Rep plus Rep′ protein are expressed in the cells, indicating that both proteins are essential for replication from the PCV origin. This is in contrast to other ssDNA viruses, for example, AAV2 or members of the genus *Mastrevirus*, in which spliced Rep proteins are produced, but are not essential for viral replication. Rep and Rep′ cleave the viral strand between nucleotides 7 and 8 *in vitro* within the conserved nonanucleotide located at the apex of a putative stem–loop structure. In addition, Rep and Rep′ join viral ssDNA fragments, implying that these proteins also play a role in the termination of virus DNA replication. This joining activity is strictly dependent on preceding substrate cleavage and the close proximity of origin fragments accomplished by base pairing of the stem–loop structure. This dual 'nicking/joining' activity associated with Rep and Rep′ are pivotal events underlying the RCR-based replication of porcine circoviruses in mammalian cells. Although presence of the palindrome plus a single H sequence is sufficient for PCV replication, a tandem repeat arrangement is more stable. Within the H sequence, selected nucleotides at specific positions are critical for Rep-associated protein recognition and for viral DNA replication.

*Repression of the Rep gene promoter $P_{rep}$.* When the influence of virus-encoded proteins upon $P_{rep}$ was investigated, it became apparent that $P_{rep}$ is repressed by its own gene product Rep but not by Rep′ or Cap. This finding illustrates that Rep protein initiates replication and controls its own transcription by binding to hexamers H1/H2. Interestingly, Rep′ also binds to H1/H2, but this does not result in repression of $P_{rep}$ activity. Since mutagenesis of H1/H2 decreases but does not inactivate $P_{rep}$ transcription, features other than binding of Rep may be necessary for repression of $P_{rep}$, for example, interaction of Rep protein with transcription factors. $P_{cap}$ is not regulated by Cap, Rep, and Rep′.

*Interaction.* Studies investigating the interaction of PCV-encoded proteins are bemusing, because the results were depending on the system used for expression. While two hybrid analysis in bacteria revealed interaction of Rep and Cap, this was not observed in yeast cells, suggesting that post-translational modifications of Rep and Cap may significantly modulate their function. Rep and Rep′ have been observed to interact in yeast cells and this observation was reproduced by immuno-precipitation in mammalian cells, the natural target of PCV.

*Localization.* Rep and Rep′ protein co-localize in the nucleoplasm of infected cells, but no signal was seen in the nucleoli. The localization did not change during the infection cycle. Rep and Rep′ carry three potential nuclear localization signals (NLSs) in their identical N-termini. Proteins mutated in their NLSs demonstrated that NLS1 and NLS2 mediate the nuclear import, whereas NLS3 enhances the nuclear accumulation of the replication proteins. In contrast to Rep and Rep′, the localization of the Cap protein was restricted to the nucleoli in plasmid-transfected cells. In PCV-infected cells, Cap was localized in the nucleoli in an early stage, while it was seen later on in the nucleoplasm and the cytoplasm. This signifies that Cap is shuttling between distinct cellular compartments during the infection cycle. Since Rep, Rep′, and Cap are all located in the nucleus, this points out that DNA replication and encapsidation of the circular closed ssDNA probably occur in the nucleus and not in cytoplasmic compartments. The biological function of the early localization of Cap to the nucleoli remains unclear. Nucleolar localization has been described for proteins of many DNA and RNA viruses and it has been proposed that virus proteins enter the nucleoli to support viral transcription or influence the cell cycle.

## Conclusion

Although the family *Circoviridae* comprises only a relatively small number of viruses, the increasing number of publications demonstrates rising interest. This may not only be related to the fact that circoviruses induce severe multifactorial diseases, which compromise and unbalance the immune system, but also to the fact that the apparent simplicity of the circovirus genome contrasts highly with the complex and poorly understood pathogenesis. Hopefully, this will induce many question-solving studies, enabling us to improve our understanding of these intriguing viruses in the future.

## Further Reading

Cheung AK (2004) Palindrome regeneration by template strand-switching mechanism at the origin of DNA replication of porcine circovirus via the rolling-circle melting-pot replication model. *Journal of Virology* 78: 9016–9029.

Clark EG (1997) Post-weaning wasting syndrome. *Proceedings of the American Association of Swine Practitioners* 28: 499–501.

Crowther RA, Berriman JA, Curran WL, Allan GM, and Todd D (2003) Comparison of the structures of three circoviruses: Chicken anemia virus, porcine circovirus type 2, and beak and feather disease virus. *Journal of Virology* 77: 13036–13041.

Darwich L, Segales J, and Mateu E (2004) Pathogenesis of postweaning multisystemic wasting syndrome caused by porcine circovirus 2: An immune riddle. *Archives of Virology* 149: 857–874.

Fenaux M, Opriessnig T, Halbur PG, Elvinger F, and Meng XJ (2004) A chimeric porcine circovirus (PCV) with the immunogenic capsid gene of the pathogenic PCV type 2 (PCV2) cloned into the genomic backbone of the nonpathogenic PCV1 induces protective immunity against PCV2 infection in pigs. *Journal of Virology* 78: 6297–6303.

Finsterbusch T, Steinfeldt T, Caliskan R, and Mankertz A (2005) Analysis of the subcellular localization of the proteins Rep, Rep′ and Cap of porcine circovirus type 1. *Virology* 343: 36–46.

Gibbs MJ and Weiller GF (1999) Evidence that a plant virus switched hosts to infect a vertebrate and then recombined with a vertebrate-infecting virus. *Proceedings of the National Academy of Sciences, USA* 96: 8022–8027.

Krakowka S, Ellis JA, McNeilly F, Ringler S, Rings DM, and Allan G (2001) Activation of the immune system is the pivotal event in the production of wasting disease in pigs infected with porcine circovirus-2 (PCV-2). *Veterinary Pathology* 38: 31–42.

Mankertz A, Mueller B, Steinfeldt T, Schmitt C, and Finsterbusch T (2003) New reporter gene-based replication assay reveals exchangeability of replication factors of porcine circovirus types 1 and 2. *Journal of Virology* 77: 9885–9893.

Miller MM, Jarosinski KW, and Schat KA (2005) Positive and negative regulation of chicken anemia virus transcription. *Journal of Virology* 79: 2859–2868.

Misinzo G, Delputte PL, Meerts P, Lefebvre DJ, and Nauwynck HJ (2006) Porcine circovirus 2 uses heparan sulfate and chondroitin sulfate B glycosaminoglycans as receptors for its attachment to host cells. *Journal of Virology* 80: 3487–3494.

Segales J, Allan GM, and Domingo M (2005) Porcine circovirus diseases. *Animal Health Research Reviews* 6: 119–142.

Steinfeldt T, Finsterbusch T, and Mankertz A (2006) Demonstration of nicking/joining activity at the origin of DNA replication associated with the Rep and Rep′ proteins of porcine circovirus type 1. *Journal of Virology* 80: 6225–6234.

Tischer I, Gelderblom H, Vettermann W, and Koch MA (1982) A very small porcine virus with circular single-stranded DNA. *Nature* 295: 64–66.

Todd D, Bendinelli M, Biagini P, *et al.* (2005) Circoviridae. In: Fauquet C, Mayo MA, Maniloff J, Desselberger U,, and Ball LA (eds.) *Virus Taxonomy: Eighth Report of the International Committee on Taxonomy of Viruses*, pp. 327–334. San Diego, CA: Elsevier Academic Press.

# Classical Swine Fever Virus

**V Moennig and I Greiser-Wilke,** School of Veterinary Medicine, Hanover, Germany

## Glossary

**CPE** Viruses can have a cytopathic effect on infected cells, that is, they either kill cells or change their properties.

**DI** Defective interfering particles lack part(s) of their genome and they depend on complete helper virus for replication; they interfere with the replication of the helper virus by competing for essential enzymes.

**ELISA** Enzyme-linked immunosorbent assays are widely used for virological and serological diagnosis. Samples can be processed automatically and results are read using optical methods.

**IFT** Immunofluorescense tests utilize specific antibodies conjugated with fluorescent dye. Viral antigens can be visualized after binding of conjugated antibodies.

**MLV** Modified live vaccines consist of attenuated viruses that have lost their pathogenic properties and cause an infection without significant clinical signs in the vaccine.

**PLA** Enzymes like peroxidase can be conjugated to virus-specific antibodies. Binding of these antibodies to viral antigens located in infected cells can be visualized by adding substrate to the antigen–antibody–enzyme complex.

**qPCR** Real-time PCR allows monitoring of the polymerase chain reaction in real time on a computer screen. In contrast to gel-based PCR systems qPCR yields semi-quantitative results.

**VNT** Virus neutralization tests are tissue-culture-based assays for the detection and quantification of virus neutralizing antibodies. Of all antibody detection tests they are generally considered the 'gold standard'.

## Introduction

Classical swine fever (CSF), formerly known as hog cholera, is a highly contagious viral disease of swine with high morbidity and mortality especially in young animals. Due to its economic impact it is notifiable to the Office International des Epizooties (OIE (World Organisation for Animal Health)). First outbreaks of the disease were observed in 1833 in Ohio, USA. The aetiological agent was long assumed to be a bacterium (hog cholera bacillus), until de Schweinitz and Dorset demonstrated in 1903 that the agent was filterable. CSF has been eradicated in Australia, Canada, the US, and almost all member states of the European Union (EU). Vaccination is banned in these countries. However, outbreaks of CSF still occur intermittently in several European countries in either wild boar or domestic pigs. The latter can cause large economic losses. During the last 16 years in the EU, close to 20 million pigs were euthanized and destroyed because of control measures imposed to combat CSF epizootics, causing total costs of about 5 billion euros. In many countries worldwide, CSF is still a major problem. In 2004, a total of 38 member states of the OIE reported CSF outbreaks.

## Virus Properties

### Genome Organization and Protein Expression

CSF virus (CSFV) is an enveloped virus with a diameter of $c.$ 40–60 nm. The single-stranded RNA genome has a size of 12.3 kb. It has positive polarity with one open reading frame (ORF) flanked by two nontranslated regions (NTRs). The 5′ NTR functions as an internal ribosomal entry site (IRES) for cap-independent translation initiation of the large ORF that codes for a polyprotein of about 3900 amino acids. The polyprotein is co- and post-translationally processed by viral and cellular proteases.

From 11 viral proteins, four constitute the structure of the particle, namely three envelope glycoproteins ($E^{rns}$, E1, and E2) and one core (C) protein. The remaining seven nonstructural proteins are $N^{pro}$, p7, NS2-3, NS4A, NS4B, NS5A, and NS5B. The main target for neutralizing antibodies is the viral envelope glycoprotein E2. To a lesser extent, the host's immune system produces neutralizing antibodies to $E^{rns}$. This viral envelope glycoprotein occurs as a disulfide-bonded homodimer in the virus particle, and is also secreted by CSFV-infected cells. $E^{rns}$ was shown to be a potent ribonuclease specific for uridine. $N^{pro}$ has an autoproteolytic activity that achieves cleavage from the downstream nucleocapsid protein C. *In vitro*, it had been shown that $N^{pro}$ interferes with the induction of interferon $\alpha/\beta$, and *in vivo* CSFV with a deletion in the $N^{pro}$ gene was able to infect pigs but had lost its pathogenicity.

## Replication

CSFV replicates in cell lines from different species, for example, pigs, cattle, sheep, and rabbit. For most purposes, the viruses are cultivated in porcine cells. Virus replication is restricted to the cytoplasm of the cell and normally does not result in a cytopathic effect (CPE). The first progeny virus is released from the cells at 5–6 h post infection. Virion assembly occurs on membranes of the endoplasmic reticulum, and full virions appear within cisternae. They are released via exocytosis or cell lysis.

Cytopathic isolates of CSFV occur only sporadically, and most of them are defective interfering (DI) particles. Their genomes have large internal deletions, consisting mainly of the genomic regions coding for the structural proteins. The DI particles are strictly dependent on a complementing helper virus for replication.

## Taxonomy and Classification

CSFV belongs together with viruses in the species *Bovine viral diarrhea virus 1* (BVDV-1), BVDV-2, and viruses in the species *Border disease virus* (BDV) to the genus *Pestivirus*, in the family *Flaviviridae*. Classification of CSFV strains and isolates is currently performed by genetic typing. For this purpose, three regions of the CSFV genome are used, mainly 190 nt of the E2 envelope glycoprotein gene, but also 150 nt of the 5′ NTR, and 409 nt of the NS5B polymerase gene. The phylogenetic tree shows that the CSFV isolates can be divided into three groups with three or four subgroups: 1.1, 1.2, 1.3; 2.1, 2.2, 2.3; 3.1, 3.2, 3.3, 3.4. CSFV groups and subgroups show distinct geographical distribution patterns, which is important for epidemiologists. Whereas isolates belonging to group 3 seem to occur solely in Asia, all CSF virus isolates of the last 15 years isolated in the EU belonged to one of the subgroups within group 2 (2.1, 2.2, or 2.3) and

were clearly distinct from historic CSFV of group 1, that are still being used as CSFV laboratory reference viruses. In contrast, current representatives of group 1 viruses continue to cause outbreaks in South America and Central America, and in the Caribbean. Interestingly, CSFVs of all groups have been found in various locations in Asia (**Figure 1**).

## Antigenic Relationships and Variability

All pestiviruses were originally classified according to their host origin and the disease they cause. Later, it was found that they are not restricted to their original hosts and that they are serologically related, for example, BVDV and BDV have the capacity to naturally infect many other ruminant species and pigs. The same applies for CSFV, although its extended host range has only been determined experimentally and does not seem to reflect natural conditions. Detailed studies on the antigenic relationship between CSFV and ruminant pestiviruses have been performed using monoclonal antibodies and neutralization studies.

In recent years, progress in molecular biology has allowed a more precise assessment of their relationship. Several genomic regions have been used to study genetic diversity, for example, the 5′ NTR and genes coding for proteins ($N^{pro}$, C, and E2). Phylogenetic analysis confirmed the classification of the genus *Pestivirus*, comprising CSFV, BVDV-1, BVDV-2, and BDV, and has revealed at least one additional species, a pestivirus isolated from giraffe.

There is as yet little knowledge concerning the evolution of CSFV, although some analyses have been performed, albeit using short regions of the genome only. These results are difficult to interpret as, in contrast to other RNA viruses, CSFV has little tendency to accumulate mutations. Extensive genomic analyses of isolates obtained between February 1997 and March 1998 in the Netherlands emphasized the genetic stability of CSFV even in the highly variable antigenic region of the E2 gene during a major epidemic that lasted longer than 1 year.

## Transmission and Host Range

Members of the family Suidae, in particular domestic pigs (*Sus scrofa domesticus*) and European wild boar (*Sus scrofa scrofa*), are the natural hosts of CSFV. Blood, tissues, secretions, and excretions from an infected animal contain the virus. Transmission occurs mainly by the oral–nasal route, though infection through the conjunctiva, mucous membrane, by skin abrasion, insemination, and percutaneous blood transfer (e.g., common needle, contaminated instruments) may occur. Airborne transmission is not thought to be important in the epizootiology of

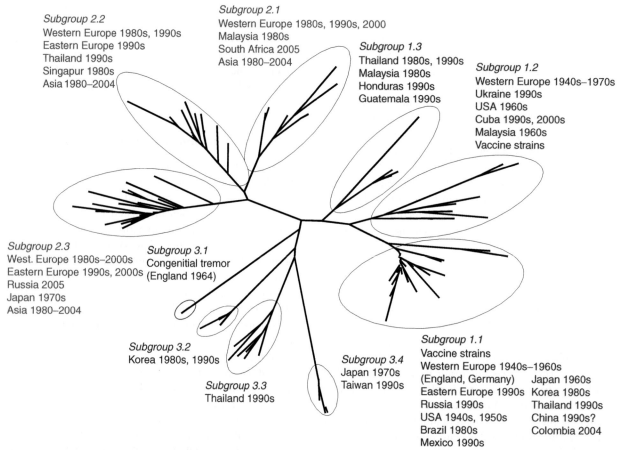

*Subgroup 2.2*
Western Europe 1980s, 1990s
Eastern Europe 1990s
Thailand 1990s
Singapur 1980s
Asia 1980–2004

*Subgroup 2.1*
Western Europe 1980s, 1990s, 2000
Malaysia 1980s
South Africa 2005
Asia 1980–2004

*Subgroup 1.3*
Thailand 1980s, 1990s
Malaysia 1980s
Honduras 1990s
Guatemala 1990s

*Subgroup 1.2*
Western Europe 1940s–1970s
Ukraine 1990s
USA 1960s
Cuba 1990s, 2000s
Malaysia 1960s
Vaccine strains

*Subgroup 2.3*
West. Europe 1980s–2000s
Eastern Europe 1990s, 2000s
Russia 2005
Japan 1970s
Asia 1980–2004

*Subgroup 3.1*
Congenitial tremor
(England 1964)

*Subgroup 3.2*
Korea 1980s, 1990s

*Subgroup 3.3*
Thailand 1990s

*Subgroup 3.4*
Japan 1970s
Taiwan 1990s

*Subgroup 1.1*
Vaccine strains
Western Europe 1940s–1960s
(England, Germany)      Japan 1960s
Eastern Europe 1990s   Korea 1980s
Russia 1990s              Thailand 1990s
USA 1940s, 1950s        China 1990s?
Brazil 1980s              Colombia 2004
Mexico 1990s

**Figure 1**   Diversity and geographical distribution of CSF virus isolates. The unrooted neighbor-joining phylogenetic tree was calculated using 190 nt of E2 sequences from 108 CSF viruses. The nomenclature of virus subgroups is as suggested by Paton DJ *et al.* Adapted from Paton DJ, McGoldrick A, Greiser-Wilke I, *et al.* (2000) Genetic typing of classical swine fever virus. *Veterinary Microbiology* 73: 137–157.

CSFV, but such transmission could occur between mechanically ventilated units within close proximity to each other.

Experimental transmission of CSFV to goats, sheep, cattle, peccaries (*Tayassu tajacu*), and rabbits was successful, while other vertebrates, for example, racoons, mice, and pigeons did not support the propagation of the virus. Of all species, the rabbit has been of major importance because it was, and in some countries still is, used for the attenuation of CSFV and for large-scale production of live vaccine virus.

## Clinical Features

The incubation period in individual animals is 3–10 days. Since transmission from animal to animal may be slow, in large holdings symptoms of CSF may only become evident several weeks after virus introduction ('herd incubation'). The severity of clinical signs mainly depends on the age of the animal and the virulence of the virus. In older breeding pigs, the course of infection is often mild or even subclinical. The virulence of a CSFV isolate is difficult to determine on a rational basis, as the same CSFV isolate can cause different forms of disease depending on age, breed, and immune status of the host animal. Basically acute, chronic, and prenatal forms of CSF can be distinguished, and there is no classical pattern of symptoms that is invariably associated with the disease.

## Acute CSF

Most piglets up to 12 weeks of age develop a severe form of acute CSF with high fatalities, whereas older breeding animals may only show mild symptoms. A constant finding in young animals is pyrexia higher than 40 °C. Initial signs are anorexia, lethargy, huddling together, conjunctivitis, respiratory symptoms, and constipation followed by diarrhea. Neurological signs are frequently seen, such as a staggering gait with weakness of hind legs, incoordination of movement, and convulsions. Hemorrhages of the skin are frequently observed on the ear, tail, abdomen, and the lower part of the limbs during the second and third week after infection until death. Virus is shed from the infected animal by all secretions and excretions. CSFV causes severe leukopenia and immunosuppression, which often leads to secondary enteric or respiratory infections. The signs of these secondary infections can mask or overlap the most typical signs of CSF and may mislead the veterinarian. With increasing age of the infected pigs (fattening and breeding animals), clinical signs are less specific and recovery is frequent. The infection is terminated by a strong, predominantly humoral immune response. First neutralizing antibodies against CSFV become detectable 2–3 weeks post infection.

## Chronic CSF

The chronic form of CSF is always fatal. It develops in a low percentage of infected animals, when pigs are not able to mount an effective immune response to overcome the virus. Initial signs are similar to those characteristic for the acute infection. Later, predominantly nonspecific signs are observed, for example, intermittent fever, chronic enteritis, and wasting. Animals usually survive for 2–4 months before they die. Until death, CSFV is constantly shed from the onset of clinical signs. Antibodies may be temporarily detected in serum samples, as the immune system begins to produce antibodies, although they are not able to eliminate the virus. Consequently, the antibodies are complexed by circulating virus and cease to be detectable. Since clinical signs of chronic CSF are rather nonspecific, a broad range of other diseases must be considered for differential diagnosis.

## Prenatal and Late Onset CSF

Although the course of infection in sows is often subclinical, CSFVs, as do other pestiviruses, cross the placenta of pregnant animals, thereby infecting fetuses during all stages of pregnancy. The outcome of transplacental infection depends primarily on the time of gestation and on viral virulence. Abortions and stillbirths, mummification, and malformations are observed after infection during early pregnancy. In breeding herds, this leads to a reduction in the fertility index of the affected pig herd. Infection of sows from about 50 to 70 days of pregnancy may lead to the birth of persistently viremic piglets, which may be clinically normal at birth and survive for several months. After birth, they usually show poor growth ('runt'), wasting, or occasionally congenital tremor. This course of infection is referred to as 'late onset CSF' and the outcome is fatal. During their lifetime, these animals constantly shed large amounts of virus and are dangerous virus reservoirs, spreading and maintaining the infection within the pig population. This feature of CSFV infection is comparable to cattle or sheep persistently infected with BVDV and BDV, respectively.

## Pathology and Histopathology

After infection, the tonsils are the location of primary virus replication. Thereafter, the agent progresses to neighboring lymphoreticular tissues. Through lymph channels the virus reaches regional lymph nodes, from where it spreads to the blood vascular system. Massive secondary virus replication takes place in spleen, bone marrow, and visceral lymph nodes. Major targets for the virus are cells of the immune system. In the peripheral blood, main target cells for the virus appear to be monocytes. In later stages of the disease, infected lymphocytes as well as granulocytes are found. Early events that are not completely understood play a significant role in the pathogenesis and manifestation of CSF. As early as 24 h post infection with virulent virus, that is, when animals are still asymptomatic and 2–4 days before virus can be detected in the peripheral blood, a progressive lymphopenia is observed resulting in severe immunosuppression. The reason for the massive cell death is not clear; however, a direct interaction with the virus can be ruled out. Viral $E^{rns}$ has been shown to induce apoptosis in lymphocytes of different species. Since this protein is secreted in large quantities from infected cells, it is conceivable that it causes massive destruction of lymphocyte populations. An additional or an alternative mechanism of cell death, respectively, might be triggered by cytokines that are activated shortly after infection, for example, tumor necrosis factor-$\alpha$ (TNF-$\alpha$), interleukin-1$\beta$ (IL-1$\beta$) and IL-1$\alpha$, as well as IL-6.

A severe thrombocytopenia develops once infected animals develop fever and virus is detectable in peripheral blood. Currently, there are two explanations for thrombocyte depletion: (1) abnormal peripheral consumption of thrombocytes may be responsible for thrombocytopenia; and (2) progressive degeneration of megakaryocytes, which is observed to begin at day 1 p.i., can result in cell death and shortage of thrombocyte production. It is not clear whether direct or indirect effects are responsible for the latter phenomenon. In analogy to the clinical picture, the severity of pathological lesions depends on time of infection, age of the animal, and virulence of the strain.

In acute cases, pathological changes visible on postmortem examination are observed most often in lymph nodes, spleen, and kidneys. Kidney parenchyma may display a yellowish brown colour. Infarctions of the spleen are considered pathognomonic; however, they are rarely observed. Lymph nodes are swollen, edematous, and hemorrhagic. Hemorrhages of the kidney may vary in size from petechial to ecchymotic. Petechiae can also be observed in the mucous membranes of other organs, for example, urinary bladder, larynx, epiglottis, and heart, and may be widespread over the serosae of the abdomen and chest. Inflammation in the respiratory, gastrointestinal, and urinary tract often are sequelae of secondary infections. Severe pneumonia sometimes is complicated by interstitial edema. Tonsils may display necrotic foci caused by micro infarcts followed by secondary infection. A nonpurulent encephalitis is often present.

In chronically infected animals, pathological changes are less pronounced, especially an absence of hemorrhages on organs and serosae. Instead, thymus atrophy, lymphocyte depletion in peripheral lymphatic organs, and hyperplasia of the renal cortex are often observed. In animals displaying chronic diarrhea, necrotic and ulcerative lesions on the ileum, the ileocaecal valve, and the rectum are found. 'Button' ulcers in the large intestine are pathognomonic, though rare. In cases of congenital infection, a proportion of piglets may show incomplete development of the cerebellum or other developmental abnormalities, such as atrophy of the thymus.

## Epizootiology

Primary outbreaks in CSF-free regions usually occur as a consequence of the feeding of swill containing infected pork. Although this practice is officially banned in almost all CSF-free and many other countries, it is still the major risk factor for the importation of the infection into CSF-free populations of domestic pigs or wild boar. The most common route for the spread of the infection among pigs is virus excretion by infected pigs via saliva, feces and urine, and oronasal virus uptake by uninfected animals. Further sources of infection are natural breeding and artificial insemination, since the virus is also excreted in sperm. Trade of live pigs, including at auction sales, has been shown to be the most frequent cause of virus spread from herd to herd. Other farming activities, for example, livestock shows, visits by feed dealers, and rendering trucks are also high-risk factors. Infected pregnant sows ('carrier sows') may give birth to persistently infected piglets that play an important role in the spread of the infection. CSF in small holdings, commonly called 'backyard holdings', is particularly difficult to control. Swill feeding, lack of animal registration and movement control, poor hygiene and lack of education of pig owners, as well as lack of awareness of private and government veterinarians facilitate the further spread and persistence of the infection in backyard pig populations.

CSF outbreaks in wild boar or feral pigs can be caused by contaminated garbage or 'spillover' from CSFV-infected domestic pigs. The outcome of these outbreaks mainly depends on the size and density of the wild boar populations affected. Outbreaks in small populations that live within natural confines, such as valleys, tend to be self-limiting. In contrast, infections leading to outbreaks in large areas and dense populations often become endemic. Most of the older animals survive the infection and become immune. Piglets become susceptible with waning maternal immunity and then can serve as reservoirs for the perpetuation of the infection. Most fatalities are registered in the young age class. CSFV in wild boar or feral pigs is a threat to any local domestic pig holding and strict measures have to be taken to avoid the spread to domestic pigs.

## Diagnosis

The majority of outbreaks of CSF are diagnosed tentatively on clinical grounds, especially in the severe acute form of disease. However, a number of diseases must be considered for differential diagnosis: acute African swine fever leads to a very similar clinical and pathological picture. Erysipelas, porcine reproductive and respiratory syndrome, cumarin poisoning, purpura hemorrhagica, postweaning multisystemic wasting syndrome, porcine dermatitis and nephropathy syndrome, *Salmonella* or *Pasteurella* infections, or any enteric or respiratory syndrome with fever not responding to antibiotic treatment may display features resembling CSF. Infections of pigs with related ruminant pestiviruses occasionally cause similar symptoms and cross-reactions in diagnostic laboratory tests. In conditions of reduced fertility, CSF, next to parvovirus infections, porcine reproductive and respiratory syndrome, leptospirosis, and Aujeszky's disease (pseudorabies), should be considered in the differential diagnosis. In any case, suspected CSF outbreaks need to be verified using laboratory diagnostic methods. Techniques for the detection of CSFV and virus-specific antibodies are well established and they are described in detail in the Manual of Standards of the OIE as well as in the Diagnostic Manual attached to Decision 2002/106/EC.

### Virus Isolation in Cell Culture

Virus isolation using susceptible porcine cell cultures is still considered the standard method for the direct diagnosis of CSFV infection. Suitable samples are whole blood, buffy coat, plasma, serum or clarified organ suspensions from tonsils, spleen, kidney, or gut lymph nodes. Since CSFV does not cause a CPE, the infection must be visualized by fixing and staining the cells. Antigen can then be detected either by direct or indirect immunofluorescence tests (IFTs), or by immunoperoxidase assays (PLAs), using conjugated virus-specific polyclonal or monoclonal antibodies. Virus isolation is time consuming, but the virus isolates can be stored and used for further analyses, for example, genotyping, and it allows the establishment of strain collections.

### Direct Antigen Detection

Antigen detection may be carried out on fixed cryosections of organs, using IFT or PLA with polyclonal or monoclonal antibodies. The tests yield results quickly and they are often used for a first laboratory investigation in a suspected case. However, due to limited sensitivity, a CSF suspicion cannot be ruled out in case of a negative result. The correct interpretation of results requires well-trained and experienced personnel.

Commercially available antigen capture enzyme-linked immunosorbent assays (ELISAs) are used for analyzing blood, buffy coat, organ suspension, plasma, or serum samples. Although the method yields quick results (4 h), its usefulness is limited due to its low sensitivity. It is only suitable for herd diagnosis and not for individual animals. In the near future, the ELISA will most probably be replaced by polymerase chain reaction after reverse transcription of the genome (reverse transcription-polymerase chain reaction, RT-PCR) using pools of samples.

### Detection of Viral Nucleic Acid by PCR

RT-PCR is becoming an increasingly important tool for the diagnosis of CSFV. Evaluation of RT-PCR can be performed either by agarose gel electrophoresis, or by real-time techniques (RT-qPCR). As laboratory equipment is becoming reliable and also more affordable, coupling of liquid handling robotics for nucleic acid isolation and RT-qPCR is becoming practicable. Another advantage of both the standard gel-based RT-PCR and the RT-qPCR is that, due to their high sensitivities, pooled samples can be tested. In particular, the use of RT-qPCR allows rapid and reliable testing of herds at the perimeter of an outbreak in order to avoid preemptive slaughter. Despite the advantages that RT-PCR methodology may have over conventional diagnostic tests, it is extremely vulnerable to false negative or false positive results. False negative results can arise when the nucleic acid is degraded, or when the reaction mixture contains inhibitors. Due to its high sensitivity, false positive results may arise from contaminations, either from sample to sample or from other sources. This implies that before diagnostic laboratories can replace any test, their RT-PCR protocols have to be validated, and regular participation in proficiency testing must prove that performance of the methods used is accurate. In addition, specification concerning sensitivity of the detection must be defined. This is important when samples are pooled. In summary, analytical performance must be equal to or better than that of the standard method, that is, isolation of CSFV in permissive cells.

### Antibody Detection

CSFV-specific antibodies in pig populations are sensitive indicators for the presence of the infection. Hence, serological tests are valuable tools for diagnosis and surveillance. CSFV infection mainly induces antibodies against viral proteins E2, $E^{rns}$, and NS3. Detectable levels of antibodies appear 2–3 weeks post infection and persist lifelong in recovered animals. The virus neutralization test (VNT) is the most sensitive and versatile assay. It is very useful for quantifying neutralizing antibodies as well as for discriminating between infections with CSFV or ruminant pestiviruses. This often becomes necessary since, irrespective of its clinical status, a pig herd or single animal seropositive for CSFV is considered as CSFV infected, unless an involvement of CSFV is ruled out. In contrast, in the case of BDV or BVDV infections in pigs, no disease control measures are taken. The choice of test viruses should take into account the local epidemiological situation. While the above-mentioned differentiation is often possible, the VNT is not able to discriminate between antibody titers due to CSFV field infection and antibody titers resulting from immunization with modified live CSFV vaccines. As it relies on cell culture technology, the test is labor intensive and time consuming, and it is not suitable for mass screening of samples. Therefore, it is mainly used for cases where an accurate quantitative and discriminatory assessment of antibody levels is required.

For routine serological investigation, ELISAs are suitable. These tests are either designed as blocking or as indirect ELISAs. They are widely used for screening of antibodies during and after outbreaks, for monitoring of CSFV infections in wild boar, and to test coverage of immunization of wild boars after vaccination. In general, ELISAs are less sensitive than VNTs. However, although ELISAs have some limitations considering specificity and/or sensitivity, they yield results quickly and they are well suited for mass screening of animals, and on a herd basis they are suitable to detect field virus infections.

## Immune Response

Live CSFV infection induces a B-cell as well as a T-cell response, while inoculation of inactivated virus elicits only a B-cell response. The cellular immune response has not been thoroughly investigated. Antibodies are produced against viral proteins NS3, E2, and $E^{rns}$. Antibodies against E2 and to a lesser extent $E^{rns}$ are protective. Neutralizing antibodies against CSFV are regarded as the most important specific defence against infection and disease. This is in accord with the immune responses to other pestivirus infections. There is some antigenic variation among CSFV isolates, but not to the extent observed with ruminant pestiviruses. Therefore, convalescent animals have a stable and long-lasting, if not lifelong, immunity against all variants of CSFV.

## Vaccination

First attempts to vaccinate against swine fever date back to the beginning of the last century, when pigs were infected with live virus and simultaneously treated with serum from immune pigs. This high-risk practice was replaced in the 1940s by the use of inactivated and modified live vaccines (MLVs). While the inactivated vaccines proved rather inefficient, MLV turned out to be highly efficacious and safe in pigs of any age, for example, the GPE⁻ and the lapinized Chinese strain (C-strain) of CSF. The latter is probably the most popular MLV against CSF. When properly used, MLVs are powerful tools for prophylactic protection of domestic pigs against CSF. In countries still struggling with endemic CSF, vaccines are being used in order to limit economical damage. The systematic use of these vaccines often was and is the first step in the eradication of CSF. In countries that have eradicated the infection, prophylactic vaccination is usually banned, mainly because animals vaccinated with conventional MLV (e.g., the C-strain) cannot be distinguished serologically from animals that have recovered from field infection and thus the CSF-free status of the country would not be regained. However, in emergency situations, vaccination may be used, followed by international trade restrictions for vaccinated animals and their products for at least 6 months. For EU member states, provisions have been made in directive 2001/89/EC for limited vaccination of domestic pigs in cases of severe outbreak emergencies.

In order to overcome the severe restrictions after vaccination, novel marker vaccines have been developed. They are based on the concept that the pattern of antibodies against CSFV from a vaccinated animal can be distinguished from that of an animal which has recovered from a field virus infection. The recently developed E2 subunit CSFV marker vaccines induce neutralizing antibodies against the E2 glycoprotein only. Consequently, CSFV antibodies which are not directed against the E2 glycoprotein are indicative of an infection with wild-type CSFV. With the availability of E2 glycoprotein-based subunit marker vaccines against CSFV, two discriminatory ELISAs were developed as companion tests that detect antibodies directed against the E$^{rns}$ glycoprotein. Positive results are indicative of the exposure to wild-type CSFV. The development of subunit marker vaccines was a major step forward. Compared to MLV, a few shortcomings have to be taken into account when using subunit marker vaccines. In comparison with conventional MLV, full immunity after subunit vaccination is slow (c. 21 days). Sometimes, a booster vaccination is needed, and it does not induce sterile immunity, for example, transplacental transmission of CSFV cannot be completely prevented. However, it was shown that the E2 subunit vaccine was able to stop virus spread among pigs that were vaccinated 10 days earlier. The discriminatory tests are suitable for herd diagnosis but they must not be used to assess the serological status of individual animals. Most likely the limitations of the first generation of marker vaccines

may be overcome by a second generation of live marker vaccines. Candidates are being developed. Viral vectors carrying the E2 gene of CSFV or chimeras using the genomes of the CSFV C-strain and BVDV are promising candidates.

## Prevention and Control

There is no specific treatment for CSF. In countries where CSF occurs endemically, infected animals are killed and destroyed and vaccination is used to prevent further spread of the virus. Countries free of CSF usually implement measures to avoid outbreaks of the disease. The most effective sanction to prevent introduction of CSFV into a free pig population is the ban of swill feeding and the control of trade. Attempts must be made to prevent the illegal importation of meat and meat products. Professional farms must comply with standard biosecurity rules. In order to eradicate the disease, a system for the registration and identification of all holdings and pigs should be in place. This greatly facilitates the traceability of animal movements. In case CSFV has been introduced, eradication programs are based principally on the destruction of infected and serologically positive animals. In order to avoid trade restrictions, vaccination is usually prohibited. Despite continued efforts to control CSF, outbreaks have occurred intermittently in several European countries. In areas with high pig densities very high numbers of pigs had to be culled in order to stop virus spread, and in these cases direct and indirect economical damage was very high. For example, in the course of the 1997 CSF epidemic in the Netherlands, approximately 12 million pigs had to be destroyed and total economic losses amounted to more than 2 billion euro. In severe outbreak situations, an emergency vaccination option is available. Thus far, emergency vaccination has never been used in Western Europe.

Epidemics of CSF in wild boar populations may be long-lasting and difficult to control. Oral vaccination campaigns using MLV sometimes accompanied by specific hunting measures have been shown to be suitable tools to shorten the duration of these epidemics.

## Perspectives

The fascinating pathogenesis of CSFV displays similarities with other hemorrhagic diseases. Further elucidation of determinants of viral virulence and virus interaction with the host animal will contribute to the understanding of hemorrhagic diseases.

Control and eradication of CSFV will remain a challenge for many years to come. In CSF-free countries with a highly developed pig industry and densely populated livestock areas, the control of CSF outbreaks will change from the presently practiced excessive culling of pigs to a more sophisticated disease control strategy using sensitive and specific diagnostic tools (e.g., RT-PCR), for the tracing of virus at the perimeters of outbreaks, combined with emergency marker vaccination, preferably with a live marker vaccine, which is yet to be developed.

In countries where CSF is endemic and where a sizable proportion of pigs are held in backyards, extensive vaccination with MLV, in combination with movement controls and epidemiological surveillance, might help to control this pestilence. Of prime importance is thorough education in order to increase knowledge and awareness of all parties involved.

## Further Reading

Anonymous (2001) Council Directive 2001/89/EC on community measures for the control of classical swine fever. *Official Journal of the European Communities* L 316/5.

Anonymous (2002) Commission Decision 2002/106/EC approving a Diagnostic Manual establishing diagnostic procedures, sampling methods and criteria for evaluation of the laboratory tests for the confirmation of classical swine fever. *Official Journal of the European Communities* L 39/71.

Armengol E, Wiesmüller K-H, Wienhold D, *et al.* (2002) Identification of T-cell epitopes in the structural and nonstructural proteins of classical swine fever virus. *Journal of General Virology* 83: 551–560.

Bouma A, de Smit AJ, de Kluijver EP, Terpstra C, and Moormann RJ (1999) Efficacy and stability of a subunit vaccine based on glycoprotein E2 of classical swine fever virus. *Veterinary Microbiology* 66: 101–114.

Meyers G and Thiel HJ (1996) Molecular characterization of pestiviruses. *Advances in Virus Research* 47: 53–118.

Moennig V, Floegel-Niesmann G, and Greiser-Wilke I (2003) Clinical signs and epidemiology of classical swine fever: A review of new knowledge. *Veterinary Journal* 165: 11–20.

Paton D and Greiser-Wilke I (2003) Classical swine fever – An update. *Research Veterinary Science* 75: 169–178.

Paton DJ, McGoldrick A, Greiser-Wilke I, *et al.* (2000) Genetic typing of classical swine fever virus. *Veterinary Microbiology* 73: 137–157.

Reimann I, Depner K, Trapp S, and Beer M (2004) An avirulent chimeric pestivirus with altered cell tropism protects pigs against lethal infection with classical swine fever virus. *Virology* 322: 143–157.

Ruggli N, Bird BH, Liu L, Bauhofer O, Tratschin D-J, and Hofmann MA (2005) N$^{pro}$ of classical swine fever virus is an antagonist of double-stranded RNA-mediated apoptosis and IFN-α/β induction. *Virology* 340: 265–276.

Stegeman A, Elbers A, de Smit H, Moser H, Smak J, and Pluimers F (2000) The 1997/1998 epidemic of classical swine fever in the Netherlands. *Veterinary Microbiology* 73: 183–196.

Thiel H-J, Plagemann PGW, and Moennig V (1996) Pestivirus. In: Fields B (ed.) *Virology*, 3rd edn., pp. 1059–1073. Philadelphia: Lippincott-Raven Publishers.

# Enteroviruses of Animals

**L E Hughes and M D Ryan,** University of St. Andrews, St. Andrews, UK

## Introduction

In the 1950s, the use of monkey kidney cell cultures for the growth of poliovirus revealed the presence of simian viruses and further study showed some of these to have properties consistent with enteroviruses. In parallel, investigations of viruses infecting domestic animals also revealed the presence of enteroviruses (and enterovirus-like particles) in pigs and cattle. Enteroviruses have since been isolated from African buffalo, water buffalo, sheep, goat, deer, and impala and many have been shown to be related to bovine enterovirus isolates.

In the past, the classification of enteroviruses was primarily based upon the physico-chemical properties of virions, growth in tissue-cultured cell lines, and by serotyping. In practice, this can be difficult with some isolates being poorly recognized by the reference antisera, or, the occurrence of (misleading) cross-reactivities between serotypes. The expansion of the sequence database together with more sensitive cloning/sequencing techniques have facilitated the elucidation of the genome structures of many picornaviruses. Such analyses have replaced other techniques in the classification of picornaviruses, and this article discusses characteristics which are important for the classification of animal enteroviruses.

## Animal Enteroviruses

### Bovine Enteroviruses

Bovine enteroviruses (BEVs) are endemic in cattle in many regions of the world with infection typically asymptomatic and apparently healthy animals acting as carriers. There has, however, been some association of BEVs with diarrhoea and abortion. Studies in Spain have shown that BEV is widespread and variants co-circulate in cattle around the country, with the virus less prevalent in cattle from extensive farms (69%) than in cattle from intensive farms (94%). Analysis of samples collected from a farm in the USA indicated that the virus was present in the spring in 2–4-month-old calves but that the infection had probably been cleared by summer.

Recently, it has been shown that infectious virus particles are present in water from animal watering tanks, pastures, and streams/rivers in regions where BEVs are endemic, demonstrating the ability of these viruses to survive in aqueous environments. Interest in these viruses has widened over recent years with proposals that they can be utilized as markers for fecal contamination of the environment. BEVs have also been proposed as surrogate viruses for evaluating FMDV contamination of farms and the evaluation of extraction/detection techniques.

### Porcine Enteroviruses

Historically, the more economically significant diseases of pigs caused by the porcine enteroviruses (PEVs) included neurological disorders (Teschen/Talfan disease), fertility disorders, dermal lesions, pneumonia, and diarrhoea. With the major reappraisal of the taxonomy of these viruses, these diseases are now associated with the teschoviruses (see below).

### Swine Vesicular Disease Virus

Swine vesicular disease virus (SVDV) causes a highly contagious disease of pigs that spreads rapidly through contact with infected pigs and a contaminated environment. The disease is variable from mild or subclinical infections to lesions on the snout and feet that are indistinguishable from those caused by FMDV. For this reason, routine surveillance of SVDV is maintained in European countries.

SVDV was first described in Italy in 1966 and since then, numerous outbreaks have occurred throughout Europe and Asia. SVDV was largely eradicated from Europe during the 1970s and 1980s, but a new strain, possibly originating in the Far East, entered Europe during 1992. This strain spread to the Netherlands, Belgium, Portugal, Spain, and Italy. In 2003–04, clinical outbreaks were only reported in Portugal (leading to the slaughter of 2168 pigs) while subclinical infections are continuously detected in southern Italy. A long-term study of pigs infected with a recent Italian isolate showed the vRNA and virus could be detected long after the initial infection, and provided good preliminary evidence that this virus can establish persistent infections.

### Simian Enteroviruses

Many simian viruses – including enteroviruses – were isolated from a range of nonhuman primate tissue-cultured cells used in biomedical research and vaccine development and from primates used for biomedical research. Twenty enterovirus serotypes were defined, with cross-reactivity in some cases. All these isolates were, however, distinct in that they did not show cross-reactivity with the (then) known human enteroviruses. Very little is known about the pathogenesis of these viruses. Simian enterovirus A (A-2 plaque virus) was isolated from a human, but caused viremia in tamarin monkeys 1–2 weeks post inoculation. Virus could not be detected in fecal samples.

### 'Animal' versus 'Human' Enteroviruses

Viruses of the genus *Enterovirus* of the family *Picornaviridae* primarily cause infections of the gastrointestinal tract, where large numbers of progeny virions are produced and shed in the feces. The virus particles are stable in a wide range of pH, temperature, and salinity conditions and may remain infective in the environment for long periods.

A number of viruses formerly thought to be enteroviruses are now known to be members of other genera. Presently, those animal viruses assigned to the enteroviruses include SVDV, BEV-1 and -2, and PEV-9 and -10.

Currently five human and three animal species comprise the genus *Enterovirus*. The separation of the genus into human and animal species is not as clear as in the past. Nucleotide sequence and serological data strongly suggest that some viruses have passed from man to domestic animals, or vice versa. For many years, SVDV was known to have a close relationship with human coxsackievirus B5 (CBV-5) and, indeed, this animal enterovirus is now classified in the species *Human enterovirus B* (HEV-B). The antigenic and molecular relationships between the two viruses suggest that CBV-5 crossed from humans to pigs – probably in the early 1950s – and has since adapted to the new host.

Another human enterovirus, type 70 (EV70; spp. *Human enterovirus D*) first appeared in humans in 1969 causing widespread outbreaks of acute hemorrhagic conjunctivitis. In a small proportion of cases (1:10 000–1:17 000), this generally benign ocular infection was accompanied by a disease with a presentation very similar to poliomyelitis. Interestingly, studies on animal sera collected prior to the human outbreaks showed the presence of anti-EV70 antibodies in cattle, sheep, swine, chickens, goats, dogs, and wild monkeys. EV70 disappeared from the human population in the 1980s, but the data suggest that this human disease was the result of a zoonosis.

Recent sequence analyses of simian enteroviruses has shown that some of these viruses are closely related to viruses within the species *Human enterovirus A*, while others are proposed as new members of *Human enterovirus B*. It is not surprising, therefore, that the present 'human' enterovirus classification scheme contains several animal viruses.

## Genome Structure and Classification

The classification of picornaviruses has been in a state of flux for a number of years. Originally classification was based on serological, pathogenic and biophysical properties, but now genome structure is paramount. In some instances, such analyses confirmed previous classifications, while in others reclassification occurred – either by simply renaming, regrouping, or, more fundamentally, by the formation of new genera.

## Entero- and Rhinovirus Genome Structures

Briefly, a viral protein (VPg), is covalently linked to the 5′ end of the genome and followed by a nontranslated region, the 5′ NTR (**Figure 1(a)**). A single, long, open reading frame (ORF) encodes a polyprotein of ~2200 aa. The N-terminal domain of the polyprotein (P1) comprises the four capsid proteins, while the replicative proteins comprise the central domain (P2) and C-terminal domain (P3) of the polyprotein. The full-length translation product predicted by the single ORF is not observed within infected cells due to rapid, intramolecular, proteolysis by the two virus-encoded proteinases, 2A$^{pro}$ and 3C$^{pro}$ (**Figure 1(a)**). The P1, P2, and P3 'primary' cleavage products subsequently undergo proteolytic processing to yield the individual virus proteins. After the stop codon, there is a short 3′ NTR and a poly(A) tail (**Figure 1(a)**).

A few, but major, differences between the genomes of enteroviruses and other genera are now of prime importance in the classification of viruses within the *Picornaviridae*. Specifically, the RNA secondary structural features of the 5′ NTR (**Figure 1(b)**), the presence/absence of an L protein at the N-terminus of the polyprotein (**Figure 1(c)**), and the nature of the 2A region of the polyprotein (**Figure 1(d)**) are now taken to be the

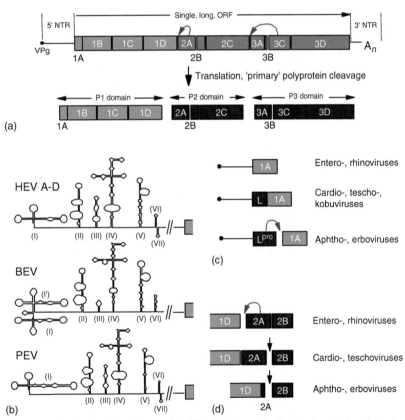

**Figure 1** Enterovirus genome organization. The oligopeptide VPg (3B) is covalently attached to the 5′ terminus of vRNA. The long 5′ nontranslated region (5′ NTR) precedes the single, long, ORF (boxed area). The polyprotein comprises three domains: the capsid proteins precursor (P1; green boxed areas) and the nonstructural replication protein domains P2 and P3 (blue boxed areas). The 3′ portion of the genome comprises a short 3′ NTR and a poly(A) tail. The 'primary' (cotranslational) cleavages of the polyprotein mediated by the 2A and 3C proteinases are shown (red curved arrows) (a). The type 1 IRES RNA secondary structural features together with the individual domain features (I–VII) are shown for *Human enteroviruses A–D* (HEV A–D), bovine enterovirus (BEV), and porcine enterovirus (PEV) (b). In the case of enteroviruses, the N-terminal portion of the polyprotein is the capsid protein 1A (VP4), whereas in cardio- and teschoviruses, for example, the polyprotein starts with an L protein. Aphtho- and erbovirus polyproteins commence with an L proteinase (L$^{pro}$) which cleaves at its own C-terminus (c). Entero- and rhinovirus 2A proteins are proteinases (2A$^{pro}$) which cleave the polyprotein to form their own N-termini, whereas the 2A proteins of other genera (cardio-, tescho-, aphtho-, and erboviruses) mediate a cotranslational ribosome 'skipping' effect (producing an apparent prolyprotein cleavage), but these 2A proteins are not proteinases (d).

discriminative features. It has been shown, however, that comparison of VP1 (1D) sequences alone is sufficient to assign isolates to enterovirus species. Note that the high-level of recombination within noncoding regions and regions encoding nonstructural proteins (see below) means care should be taken when comparing sequences from these regions for taxonomic purposes.

### The 5′ nontranslated region

The 5′ terminal ~100 nt of picornavirus vRNA folds into a cloverleaf-shaped structure (domain I; **Figure 1(b)**). A large proportion of the remainder of the 5′ NTR forms a complex secondary structure comprising multiple domains which functions as an internal ribosome entry site (IRES). This region confers a cap-independent mode of initiation of translation of the viral RNA: the $^{7me}G$ cap structure associated with eukaryotic mRNAs is replaced in picornaviruses by the oligopeptide 3B (or VPg) covalently linked to the 5′ terminus of vRNA. While the 5′ NTR has the same functions across the *Picornaviridae*, there are differences in the overall structure and this may be used to aid the classification of viruses. The entero- and rhinoviruses have a 'type 1' IRES (**Figure 1(b)**), while many of the other picornaviruses have a type 2 IRES.

### The leader protein

A leader protein (L) is present at the N-terminus of the polyprotein in the aphtho-, erbo-, cardio-, tescho-, and kobuviruses (**Figure 1(c)**). In the cardioviruses, L has been shown to interact with Ran-GTPase disrupting nucleocytoplasmic trafficking of cellular proteins. In the aphtho- and erboviruses, however, L is a papain-like proteinase ($L^{pro}$). This proteinase cleaves at its own C-terminus and is involved in shut-off of host cell protein synthesis via cleavage of eIF4G. Expression of the erbovirus L protein in cells did not, however, lead to efficient inhibition of cap-dependent translation. In the entero- and rhinoviruses, no L protein is present: the N-terminus of the polyprotein is the capsid protein, VP4 (1A).

### The 2A protein

Picornavirus 2A proteins are diverse in sequence and function (**Figure 1(d)**). The 2A proteins of entero- and rhinoviruses are very similar, and are structurally related to the small subclass of serine proteinases – although the active site nucleophile is not serine, but cysteine. They catalyze an intramolecular proteolytic cleavage at their own N-termini (*in cis*), separating the structural protein polyprotein domain (P1) from the nonstructural proteins (P2, P3; **Figure 1(a)**). Importantly, this virus-encoded proteinase also cleaves a host-cell translation factor (like $L^{pro}$), the initiation factor eIF4G, which brings about the 'shut-off' of host-cell (cap-dependent) mRNA translation.

The 2A regions of all other picornaviruses are quite different (**Figure 1(d)**). In the case of the aphtho-, cardio-, erbo-, and teschoviruses, the 2A protein is not a proteinase. This type of 2A may be identified by a C-terminal –NPG– motif. In these cases, the N-terminal residue of protein 2B is, invariably, proline. An apparent 'cleavage' of the nascent polyprotein occurs between the glycine and proline residues at the 2A/2B junction (-NPG ⇓ P-). This processing event is not, however, proteolytic but rather mediated by a translational effect termed ribosome 'skipping'.

## Genome Structure of BEV

The genome organizations of several BEV isolates have been reported. BEV 5′ NTRs range from 812 to 822 nt and are unusual in that the 5′ cloverleaf-like secondary structure is duplicated (domains I and I′; **Figure 1(b)**). Furthermore, the putative domains III and VI of the IRES region differ in size and shape from other enteroviruses. The ORF varies from 6498 nt in BEV-2 to 6525 nt in BEV-1. The 3′ NTRs of BEV are 71–75 nt and although the predicted folding pattern (two stem–loop structures – a potential pseudoknot-like element) resembles other enteroviruses, no nucleotide sequence similarity exists.

Originally classified into several serotypes, only two serotypes (BEV-1 and BEV-2) are now recognized within the species *Bovine enterovirus*. A recent study has suggested, however, that the taxonomy of these viruses be revised. Sequence comparisons provided data that the bovine enteroviruses form two major clusters characterized by structural features and levels of sequence identity. These clusters have been designated BEV-A and BEV-B and appear to correlate with the two serotypes BEV-1 and BEV-2. It is also suggested that these clusters represent species, rather than serotypes. Further subgrouping within the clusters is proposed with BEV-A comprising two geno-/serotypes and BEV-B comprising three geno-/serotypes.

## Genome Structure of PEV

Sequence analyses of what were formerly regarded as PEVs have shown that all but three now form the genus *Teschovirus*. Based upon the presence of an L protein and the nature of the 2A proteins, it is further proposed that one of these three, PEV-8 (together with some simian enteroviruses; see below) forms a new genus – *Sapelovirus*. The two remaining 'true' enteroviruses are PEVs 9 and 10. The 5′ NTR of PEV-9 is 809 nt (814 nt for PEV-10). Both 5′ NTRs are predicted to adopt a secondary structure similar to that of the human enteroviruses. However, the 5′ cloverleaf has a unique insertion that enlarges domain I (**Figure 1(b)**). Interestingly, this domain has been previously shown to bind the 3CD proteinase in poliovirus and rhinovirus 14, forming a ribonucleoprotein complex required for initiation of positive-strand RNA synthesis. The long ORFs encode a polyprotein (2168 aa – PEV9; 2171 aa – PEV10) with a very similar organization to other enteroviruses (**Figure 1(a)**). The 3′ NTRs of both viruses are similar in sequence and length (72 nt – PEV9; 71 nt – PEV10), and predicted to form two stem–loop structures.

## Genome Structure of SVDV

Complete genome sequences of the virulent J1′73 strain of SVDV and the avirulent H3′76 strain have been determined. Furthermore, partial sequences (5′ NTR, capsid protein VP1, protein 3BC) have been determined from a large number of isolates for epidemiological studies. The genome structure is very similar to that of the other enteroviruses (**Figure 1(a)**). Although only a single serotype, SVDV shows high genetic variability. The IRES is very similar to the human enterovirus type 1 IRES (**Figure 1(b)**; spp. HEV-B), although variability between isolates was observed in the 'spacer' region extending from the 3′ end of the IRES to the initiation codon. Indeed, several isolates had blocks of sequence (6–125 nt) deleted in this region.

A key determinant of virulence was mapped to a single residue within the 2A proteinase. Residue 20 of the avirulent H3′76 strain is isoleucine, the virulent J1′73 strain, arginine (this site is adjacent to His21, a component of the catalytic triad of 2A$^{pro}$). Pigs were infected with viruses rescued from an infectious copy of the virulent strain bearing mutations at this single site. Each mutant tested showed much reduced virulence correlating with the different efficiencies of the two forms of the proteinase to promote translation of the vRNA.

## Genome Structure of Simian Enteroviruses

Formerly, the 20 simian picornaviruses were provisionally classified as enteroviruses. Analysis of partial (5′ NTR, VP1, and 3D) sequences showed that the simian viruses SV2, -16, -18, -42, -44, -45, and -49 are not enteroviruses, but comprise a new genus *Sapelovirus*. The complete genome sequence of SV2 confirmed that this virus was not an enterovirus since it does not possess a type 1 IRES and is thought, like PEV-8, to possess an L protein. The sequence of the 2A protein was quite different to other picornaviruses, although the presence of the conserved motif –GxCG– (also present in PEV-8) suggests that SV2/PEV8 2A proteins may be proteinases. If these viruses do possess an L protein and a 2A proteinase, then they represent an interesting link between the enteroviruses and other genera.

Analyses of the 5′ NTR and VP1 sequences showed that A13, SV19, -26, -35, -43, -46 were members of *Human enterovirus A*, SA5 a member of *Human enterovirus B*, and SV6, N125 plus N203 were related, but apparently form a new enterovirus species most closely related to *Human enterovirus A*. The complete genome sequence of simian enterovirus A (A-2 plaque virus) showed an organization characteristic of enteroviruses (**Figure 1(a)**), but along with SV4 and SV28 forms another new enterovirus species, this time most closely related to *Human enterovirus B*.

## Virus Replication

Most of the receptors identified for picornaviruses belong to the immunoglobulin superfamily or the integrin receptor family. However, the receptors for the animal enteroviruses remain to be determined. Internalization occurs via endocytosis, and as the endosome undergoes acidification, changes in the virion structure lead to the release of the vRNA into the cytoplasm. The vRNA acts as an mRNA; the first step of replication is, therefore, translation of the single, long ORF. The autocatalytic processing by the virus-encoded proteinases 2A$^{pro}$ and 3C$^{pro}$ produces the three 'primary' processing products P1, P2, and P3 (**Figure 1(a)**) – the full-length (predicted) translation product is not observed. Subsequently further, 'secondary', proteolytic processing of these precursors occurs mediated by 3C$^{pro}$. In the case of poliovirus, it has been demonstrated that the P1 capsid protein precursor is processed not by 3C$^{pro}$, but by 3CD$^{pro}$ – also a proteinase. The function of the vRNA soon switches from that of an mRNA, to that as a template for −ve strand synthesis. The −ve-strand RNA then serves as a template for the synthesis of +ve-strand RNA. A large excess (∼80-fold) of +ve-, over −ve-, sense RNA is observed. Although the RNA-dependent RNA polymerase (3D$^{pol}$) is an enzyme, overall the replication of vRNA is not 'enzymic' as such, since protein 3B is used to prime RNA synthesis and is covalently linked to the 5′ terminus of both +ve- and −ve-sense RNA.

A characteristic feature of picornavirus replication is the disappearance of the Golgi apparatus concomitant with the appearance of virus-induced vesicles. It is upon these structures that RNA replication occurs; proteins 2C and 3A are key players in this remodeling of the endomembrane system. An increase in the intracellular level of $Ca^{2+}$ is also observed; protein 2B has been shown to function as a 'viroporin' releasing calcium ions stored in the endoplasmic reticulum.

Recombination occurs with high frequency, reported to be in the region of 10%. The polymerase complex, together with the nascent strand, may 'switch' template and complete the synthesis of the vRNA from another parent. Analyses of recombinants have shown that viable progeny arise largely from template switching within noncoding regions, or regions encoding nonstructural proteins.

The process by which vRNA is encapsidated is not clear. A feature of this process is the 'maturation' cleavage of VP0 (1AB) into VP4 and VP2 (1B) – again poorly understood. Replication is rapid with cell death and release of progeny virions occurring within ~9 h for BEV and SVDV for most cell types.

## Virion Structure and Properties

Particles have a buoyant density of $1.30–1.34\,g\,ml^{-1}$ in cesium chloride gradients, are resistant to ether, and stable throughout a wide range of pH (3–10). The ability to tolerate low pH is seen as an adaptation to survive passage through the acidic conditions of the stomach. Under the electron microscope, particles are seen as icosahedrons, 25–30 nm in diameter (**Figure 2(a)**). Capsids are nonenveloped, comprising 60 copies of each of the capsid proteins VP4, VP2, VP3 (1C), and VP1. Capsid proteins are arranged into protomers and 60 of these structural units form an icosahedron (symmetry: pseudo $T = 3$; **Figure 2(b)**).

The atomic structures of both BEV and SVDV capsids have been determined. The folding pattern of BEV polypeptides VP1–3 is similar resulting in an eight-stranded antiparallel β-sheet structure. The VP4 protein is much smaller than the other capsid proteins, and lies across the inner surface of the capsid. The N-terminus of VP4 is close to the icosahedral fivefold axes of symmetry and the C-terminus close to the threefold axes. Furthermore, in all picornaviruses, the N-terminal residue of VP4 is covalently bonded to a myristic acid group giving the capsid five symmetry-related myristoyl moieties around the inner surface of the capsid, a channel running from the inner to outer surface at this point. It has been proposed that the myristic groups attached to the VP4 proteins may insert into the host membrane aiding entry.

A radial depth-cued image of the BEV particle is shown in **Figure 2(c)**. The topologies of the BEV major capsid proteins and the overall architecture of the virion

are similar to those of related picornaviruses. Some differences were observed, however; the external loops are relatively truncated giving a comparatively 'smooth' appearance. A 'canyon' receptor binding region (running around the fivefold axes of symmetry) is observed in the structures of polio- and rhinoviruses. In BEV, this depression is partially filled by a five-residue extension of the G-H loop of VP3. The extended VP3 loop of BEV has been implicated in receptor binding, although the cell-surface receptor has not been identified. BEV is usually cultured in hamster kidney (BHK-21) cells but is known to be readily adaptable to grow in human cervical carcinoma (HeLa) cells to equivalent titer and can cause cytopathic effect in an extensive range of cell types *in vitro*. The BEV receptor is, therefore, thought to be a ubiquitous cell-surface glycoprotein. The crystal structure also revealed that the virus maintains a hydrophobic pocket within VP1, occupied by a specific 'pocket factor' which appears to be myristic acid. The pocket factor is thought to stabilize the capsid and it has been proposed that a kinetic equilibrium exists between occupied and unoccupied pocket states, with occupation inhibiting 'uncoating' of the vRNA. In purified BEV preparations, a small proportion of the precursor protein VP0 is detected and it is suggested that in a few protomers this precursor remains uncleaved. This maturation cleavage is completely absent in the genera *Parechovirus* and *Kobuvirus* – these viruses possessing only three structural proteins.

The crystal structures of two SVDV isolates, UK/27/72 and SPA/2/93, have been reported. These two structures are in agreement and are similar to those of other enteroviruses, with SVDV being most similar to coxsackievirus B3 (CBV-3). The major capsid proteins (VP1–3) possess the conserved β-sheet structure with some notable differences. VP1, making up most of the outer surface area, is often the most variable, and while the β-sheet is conserved, the connecting loops vary in length between SVDV and CBV-3. Five copies of VP1 associate to form each of the fivefold vertices, and in SVDV it has been noted that an arginine residue from each of the five VP1s

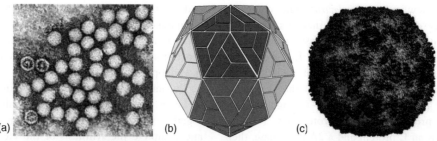

**Figure 2** The structure of enterovirus particles. (a) A negatively stained electron microscopic image of enterovirus shows unenveloped particles ~25 nm in diameter. (b) The icosahedral structure of the particle is shown. Five copies each of capsid proteins 1A–D form a pentamer, twelve of which form the complete particle. (c) A radially depth-cued image produced from the X-ray crystallographic data of the BEV particle showing surface projections (dark blue) – particularly notable at the fivefold axis of symmetry. The particle is smoother than the surface of other enteroviruses. Rasmol image courtesy of Dr. J.-Y. Sgro, University of Wisconsin, USA.

form a crown at the apex of the fivefold axes of symmetry. The hydrophobic pocket formed by VP1 is also present in SVDV and electron density clearly showed that this accommodates a fatty acid pocket factor. The hydrophobic pocket situated at the base of the canyon extends from a pore on the surface inward, until it is blocked by VP1 loops. In CBV-3, the pocket factor has been identified as palmitic acid. The dimensions of the pocket are similar in CBV-3 and SVDV, but in the case of SVDV the electron density suggests that the pocket factor is a longer molecule – similar to sphingosine.

The VP2 and VP3 proteins alternate around the threefold axes of symmetry. The VP2 of SVDV possesses a puff region composed of two sequential loops between sheets E and F, with the second loop being more exposed on the surface. This is the least conserved area between SVDV and CBV-3. Furthermore, in poliovirus, this area has been implicated in the binding of the virus to its cell-surface receptor. The C-terminus of the VP3 protein is external and forms a major surface protrusion termed the 'knob'; this structure is present in SVDV and CBV-3. VP3 is also important in the stability of the pentamer with fivefold neighboring VP3 proteins forming a β-cylinder.

VP4 is situated on the inner surface of the capsid and is the most conserved of the capsid proteins. The central region of this protein was found to be disordered with little secondary structure. VP4 begins close to the fivefold axes and snakes toward the nearest threefold axes, with the C-terminus of VP4 lying close to the N-terminus of VP2. The N-terminal glycine of VP4 is covalently attached to myristic acid and the myristoyl groups of adjacent VP4s group around the fivefold axes, under the VP3 β-cylinder. In general, the surface structure of SVDV is very similar to that of coxsackieviruses.

Rather than a continuous, circular, canyon in SVDV, there are five distinct depressions. The C-terminus of VP3, the first loop of the VP2 puff, and residues of the C-terminal VP1 loop form a ridge between these depressions. Further depressions are present on the twofold axes with the enclosing four walls composed of symmetrically related pairs of VP2 and VP3. SVDV, the six CBV serotypes (CBV-1–6), and many adenoviruses share a common receptor on human cells. The coxsackieadenovirus receptor (CAR) has two immunoglobulin-like extracellular domains, a transmembrane domain and a cytoplasmic domain. Cryoelectron microscopy has provided evidence that CAR binds into the canyon of CBV-3, mostly interacting with VP1 but with contributions from VP2 and VP3. CBV-5 (thought to have given rise to SVDV in pigs) uses CAR as a primary receptor and decay-accelerating factor (DAF;

CD55) as a co-receptor. Recent isolates of SVDV have been shown to have lost the ability to bind human DAF but have not developed the ability to bind pig DAF, suggesting that SVDV may have adapted to use another co-receptor which is tailored to the new host.

## Concluding Remarks

Understandably, in terms of research effort, for many years the animal enteroviruses have been the poor cousins of their human 'relatives'. The greatly expanded sequence database has led to a wholesale reappraisal of the taxonomy of these viruses. It is clear that within this group close relationships exist between animal and human viruses and that viruses have passed from man to animals, and vice versa. The high mutation rate in combination with high frequency of recombination means these viruses can rapidly adapt to new host species. Animal enteroviruses are, therefore, worthy of study not only for their intrinsic interest and economic impact but, through enzoonosis, they pose an ever-present threat to human health.

## Further Reading

Hughes AL (2004) Phylogeny of the *Picornaviridae* and differential evolutionary divergence of picornavirus proteins. *Infections, Genetics and Evolution* 4: 143–152.

Hyypia T, Hovi T, Knowles NJ, and Stanway G (1997) Classification of enteroviruses based on molecular and biological properties. *Journal of General Virology* 78: 1–11.

Krumbholz A, Dauber M, Henke A, *et al.* (2002) Sequencing of porcine enterovirus groups II and III reveals unique features of both virus groups. *Journal of Virology* 76: 5813–5821.

Oberste MS, Maher K, Flemister MR, *et al.* (2000) Comparison of classic and molecular approaches for the identification of untypeable enteroviruses. *Journal of Clinical Microbiology* 38: 1170–1174.

Oberste MS, Maher K, and Pallansch MA (2002) Molecular phylogeny and proposed classification of the simian picornaviruses. *Journal of Virology* 76: 1244–1251.

Oberste MS, Maher K, and Pallansch MA (2003) Genomic evidence that simian virus 2 and six other simian picornaviruses represent a new genus in *Picornaviridae*. *Virology* 314: 283–293.

Pöyry T, Kinnunen L, Hovi T, and Hyypiä T (1999) Relationships between simian and human enteroviruses. *Journal of General Virology* 80: 635–638.

Zang G, Haydon DT, Knowles NJ, and McCauley JW (1999) Molecular evolution of swine vesicular disease virus. *Journal of General Virology* 80: 639–651.

Zell R, Dauber M, Krumbholz A, *et al.* (2001) Porcine teschoviruses comprise at least eleven distinct serotypes: Molecular and evolutionary aspects. *Journal of Virology* 75: 1620–1631.

Zell R, Krumbholz A, Dauber M, Hoey E, and Wutzler P (2006) Molecular-based reclassification of the bovine enteroviruses. *Journal of General Virology* 87: 375–385.

# Equine Infectious Anemia Virus

**J K Craigo and R C Montelaro,** University of Pittsburgh School of Medicine, Pittsburgh, PA, USA

## History

Equine infectious anemia (EIA), colloquially known as swamp fever, has been documented in numerous diverse geographical areas and is currently considered a worldwide disease that occurs only in members of the family Equidae. EIA was first identified as an infectious disease of horses by veterinarians in France in 1843. In 1904, the infectious organism that caused EIA was identified as a 'filterable agent', making EIA one of the first animal diseases to be assigned a viral etiology.

Despite this early identification of the equine infectious anemia virus (EIAV), the characterization of this virus was extremely slow because of the difficulties experienced in the isolation and propagation of the virus in cell culture. Thus, the major focus on the control of EIA has been the development of regulatory policies that involve the identification and elimination of EIAV-infected horses. More recently, advances in animal vaccine strategies and the demand for animal models for AIDS vaccine development have provided renewed impetus to the development of an EIAV vaccine to prevent virus infection. EIAV also offers an important model for the role of antigenic variation in a persistent retrovirus infection.

## Classification

EIAV is classified as a member of the genus *Lentivirus* based on criteria of virion morphology, serological properties, and genomic sequence homologies. There has been no formal further subdivision of EIAV isolates into subtypes.

## Properties of the Virion

The EIAV particle has the general morphology of a lentivirus, including an oblong core enclosed in a viral envelope with surface projections (**Figure 1**). The oblong core observed in EIAV is characteristic of lentiviruses, in contrast to the icosahedral cores found in most oncoviruses. This distinctive structural feature was the initial indication that HIV-1 was related to EIAV and a member of the lentivirus rather than the oncovirus subfamily of retroviruses. The virus particles appear roughly spherical in the electron microscope (**Figure 2**), although there are various degrees of polymorphism depending on the sample preparation. The overall diameter of the virion is approximately 100 nm. The surface projections extend about 7 nm and appear to be distributed on the viral surface in a symmetrical pattern.

## Properties of the Genome

The EIAV genome consists of a dimer of single-stranded, positive-sense RNA. The genomic organization of EIAV is characteristic of a complex retrovirus, but is the simplest and smallest of characterized human and animal lentiviruses (**Figure 3**). The viral RNA contains about 8200 bp and contains three major genes (*gag, pol,* and *env*) encoding viral structural proteins and three minor genes (*tat, S2,* and *rev*) that encode nonstructural proteins that regulate various aspects of virus replication. The order of the EIAV genome is 5'-R-U5-*gag-pol-env*-U3-R-3'. The *tat* and *S2* genes are encoded as distinct alternate reading frames within the *pol–env* intergenic region, while

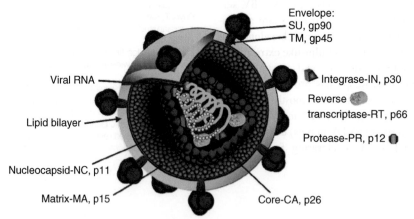

**Figure 1** Virion morphology and protein organization of EIAV.

the *rev* gene is encoded by alternate reading frames contained at the beginning of the *env* gene sequences and following the 3′ end of the *env* gene. The relatively small size of the EIAV genome compared to other lentiviruses is primarily due to the much smaller size of the *pol–env* intergenic region.

The EIAV *gag* gene encodes the four viral core proteins in the order of 5′-p15-p26-p11-p9–3′, while the *env* gene encodes the two envelope glycoproteins of the virus in the order of 5′-gp90-gp45–3′. The *pol* gene encodes a complex of enzymes with an organization of 5′-protease-reverse transcriptase-RNase H-dUTPase-integrase-3′. As with other lentiviruses, the EIAV *tat* and *rev* genes encode important regulatory proteins that either transactivate virus transcription (Tat) or control viral transcription patterns (Rev) after infection of host cells. The function of the 8 kDa protein encoded by the *S2* gene remains to be defined, although mutation studies of this gene indicate that it is not essential for *in vitro* viral replication and results in a single $\log_{10}$ reduction in viral replication in equines. The terminal LTR sequences of EIAV contain the usual complex of transcriptional regulatory domains distinctive of lentiviruses.

## Properties of the Viral Proteins

The proteins encoded by the *gag* and *env* genes of EIAV constitute the major structural proteins of the virus (cf. **Figure 1**). The gp90 protein is a highly glycosylated, hydrophilic surface (SU) protein that forms the outermost

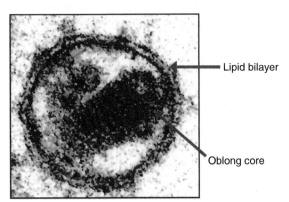

**Figure 2**  Transmission electron micrograph of an EIAV particle.

knobs of the envelope projections, while the gp45 is a sparsely glycosylated, hydrophobic transmembrane (TM) protein that forms the membrane-spanning spike of the envelope projection. There are approximately 300 copies each of the envelope glycoproteins per virion, and the surface projections are composed of trimers of gp90 and gp45. The final component of the EIAV envelope structure is the fatty acylated p15 that forms a continuous matrix (MA) immediately beneath the lipid bilayer of the virus particle. The virion core shell or capsid (CA), composed predominantly of p26 molecules, encloses a helical ribonucleoprotein complex containing the basic nucleoprotein (NP), p11, and various polymerases (RT, IN, and DU) in close association with the viral RNA genome. The location of the final core protein, p9, is not certain, but it has been proposed as a linker protein between the core shell and envelope matrix. Recent experiments have indicated that the EIAV p9 protein mediates late stages of viral budding.

The *gag*-encoded proteins of the virus are present in molar amounts that are at least tenfold greater than the envelope glycoproteins, in the range of 3000–5000 copies per virus particle. In contrast, the *pol*-encoded enzymes appear to be present in the virus at levels of about 10 molecules per virion.

## Replication Strategy

The EIAV replication cycle is characteristic of retroviruses in general and lentiviruses in particular (summarized in **Figure 4**). Viral recognition, attachment, and penetration of target cells is believed to be mediated by specific interaction of the viral envelope glycoproteins and cellular receptor proteins contained in the plasma membrane. Until recently, there were no recognized receptors for EIAV. Recently, a cellular receptor for EIAV, designated ELR1, has been identified as a member of the tumor necrosis family of receptors (TNFRs). Once inside the target cell cytoplasm, the virus reverse transcriptase copies the single-stranded RNA genome into double-stranded DNA provirus that is then transported to the nucleus of the cell. There is no evidence for translation of the incoming EIAV genome at this stage of infection. Once inside of the cell nucleus, the EIAV integrase mediates apparently random but limited incorporation of the

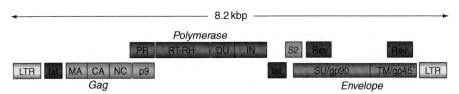

**Figure 3**  Organization of the EIAV genome indicating viral genes (italic print) and the respective proteins encoded by these genes (block print).

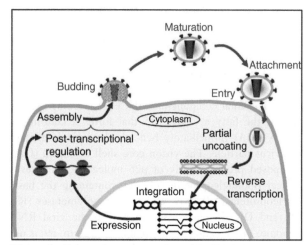

**Figure 4** Schematic representation of the EIAV life cycle.

provirus DNA into cellular chromosomes, although some extrachromosomal viral DNA is always present in productively infected cells. There is typically a total of about 10 copies of proviral DNA per infected cell. Cytopathic infections by EIAV have been correlated with higher ratios of integrated to unintegrated proviral DNA.

Transcription of the proviral DNA by cellular polymerases produces a complex pattern of viral messenger RNA species whose relative proportions may differ depending on the virus strain and target cell. In all instances, the predominant EIAV transcripts are an 8.2 kbp transcript representing the full-length genomic RNA and translated to produce the *gag* and *pol* gene products, and a 3.5 kbp mRNA that is a singly spliced transcript translated to produce the viral envelope proteins. Lentivirus-infected cells usually contain in addition to these major viral transcripts, a heterogeneous population of small multiply spliced RNA that are used to produce the various regulatory proteins. In the case of EIAV, however, infected cells reveal only minute quantities of these small, multiply spliced RNA species. The relatively low abundance of small transcripts may in part reflect the relative genetic simplicity of EIAV and the lack of extensive splicing to ensure production of all of the minor viral genes. On the other hand, it is intriguing that the 3.5 kbp transcript is in fact a tricistronic messenger that can produce by *in vitro* translation the viral Tat and Rev proteins in addition to the more abundant envelope glycoproteins. The use of a tricistronic messenger may represent a novel mechanism of maximizing genetic efficiency in EIAV replication.

The viral Gag and Env proteins are initially produced as polyproteins that are cleaved into the mature virion components by a combination of viral and cellular proteases. The only modification documented in the core proteins is a fatty acylation at the N terminus of the matrix protein, p15. The envelope proteins are modified by N linked glycosylation. Although the gp90 and gp45

polypeptides contain about 400 amino acid residues, the gp90 contains an average of 17 potential N linked glycosylation sites, while the gp45 contains only about five potential glycosylation sites. By comparison to HIV-1 gp120, it is assumed that all potential glycosylation sites are occupied by complex oligosaccharides.

The precise mechanisms of EIAV assembly have not been completely dissected, although it is assumed that it follows the general model for retrovirus assembly. It appears to be a highly concerted process that is mediated by interactions between the viral Gag polyproteins and host cofactors. Accordingly, the viral envelope glycoproteins are initially inserted into the plasma membrane to create distinct sites of virus assembly at which the Gag polyprotein is accumulated beneath the membrane lipid. Subsequently, Gag proteins recruit host cellular components that also regulate the endocytic pathway for assembly and budding. To date, early (AP-2) and late endocytic proteins (TSG101) as well as the actin cytoskeleton have been associated with EIAV virion production. The intermediate viral proteins are next cleaved into the mature virion proteins as the particle buds from the cell surface and is released to produce progeny virions.

## Epidemiology, Geographic and Seasonal Distribution

EIAV has been diagnosed in many areas of the world and is considered a worldwide disease of horses. Although localized outbreaks of disease can occur, the incidence of EIAV-infected horses is the highest in tropical and subtropical climates, presumably due to the longer warm seasons and more abundant populations of insect vectors that may transmit EIAV among horses. During the past 20 years, the EIAV infection rate reported by the USDA has dropped from about 4% to less than 0.2%. However, these testing results do not reflect the general horse population as less than 10% of the horses in the United States are tested for EIA, usually because of requirements for transportation across state lines or for participation in organized shows or races. General surveys of unregulated herds in the Southeast United States demonstrate infection rates of up to 15%. EIAV infections are especially prevalent in Central and South America, where limited surveys of Latin American countries have demonstrated infection rates in unregulated herds frequently approach 50% indicating that EIAV infection is epidemic in these areas. Although the probability of EIAV infection by insect vectors is greatest during seasons that are warm, infections can occur throughout the year via mechanical transfers of blood by hypodermic needles and other veterinary instruments. Sexual transmission of EIAV has not been demonstrated to date.

## Host-Range and Virus Propagation

EIAV appears to infect only members of the family Equidae. There is no evidence to support the concept of natural or experimental infections of humans or of other mammalian species. EIAV infection of horses results in high levels of virus replication, persistent infection, and clinical disease. EIAV infection of donkeys produces only limited virus replication, presumably a persistent infection, but no signs of clinical disease.

Field strains of EIAV can only be propagated *in vitro* in cultures of equine monocyte or macrophage cells, where virus infection typically produces a cytopathic effect within several days. Large-scale production of EIAV is limited to cell culture-adapted strains of virus that can be grown in primary cultures of equine dermal cells or fetal equine kidney cells and in a limited selection of non-equine continuous cell lines, including canine fetal thymus (Cf2th) cells and the Fea and FEF feline cell lines. The cell-adapted strains of EIAV are noncytopathic to these permissive cell lines. Field strains of EIAV retain their pathogenic properties when propagated in leukocyte cultures, but usually become avirulent when adapted to other types of cell cultures. Cell-adapted strains of EIAV that retain their virulence have been produced by back passage of avirulent cell-adapted strains in ponies or horses. There is no evidence for infection of cultured human cells by EIAV.

EIAV production in cell cultures is most easily detected by the presence of viral antigens or reverse transcriptase activity in culture media.

## Genetics

Like other retroviruses, EIAV replication is mediated by a virion reverse transcriptase (RT) that copies the viral RNA genome into proviral DNA that is found in the nucleus of infected cells randomly integrated into the cellular chromosome and as extrachromosomal molecules. There are typically only about 10 copies of EIAV DNA per infected cell. EIAV replication in horses is characterized by relatively rapid and diverse genomic mutations that produce an apparently wide variety of variant virus strains. Analyses of sequential antigenic variants of EIAV from experimentally infected horses suggest that the rate of mutation in the envelope gene of the virus is greater than $10^{-2}$ base substitutions per site per year. The fidelity of DNA synthesis by purified EIAV RT has been measured *in vitro*, and an average error rate of 1/700 bp has been estimated. This value is similar to the *in vitro* error rate calculated for human immunodeficiency virus (1/700 bp), but is significantly higher than the rate observed for oncovirus RT such as avian myeloblastosis virus (1/3000 bp). The error-prone nature of EIAV RT

produces significant biological diversity that is important in EIAV persistence and pathogenesis. As demonstrated for HIV and SIV, recombination between variant EIAV genomes in infected cells may also contribute to genetic diversification during persistent infection.

## Evolution

Phylogenetic analyses based on the nucleotide sequences of various retroviruses indicate that EIAV is most closely related to the ungulate lentiviruses (visna-maedi virus, caprine arthritis-encephalitis virus, and bovine immunodeficiency virus) and equally divergent from the human and simian immunodeficiency viruses (**Figure 5**).

Studies of EIAV evolution through analyses of sequence variation during persistent infection in experimentally infected equids have clearly identified dynamic changes in envelope sequences that alter viral antigenic properties, evidently as a result of immune selection. Variation of the envelope gene has therefore served as a distinct marker for analysis of viral population evolution. Detailed molecular characterization of envelope variation during sequential disease cycles in experimentally infected ponies revealed the presence of distinct EIAV envelope variants with each wave of viremia. Examination of inapparent stage viral populations from the plasma of ponies indicated that evolution of the viral quasispecies is continuous, even with relatively low levels of detectable virus replication in the periphery or tissues. These results suggest that even in the absence of detectable plasma virus, viral populations, most likely in tissue reservoirs, continue to replicate and evolve, seeding the plasma with new viral quasispecies.

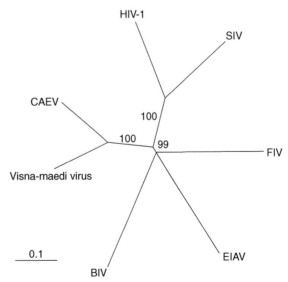

**Figure 5** Phylogenetic tree of the complete genomes of identified lentiviruses.

## Serologic Relationships and Variability

Field and laboratory isolates of EIAV display a remarkable variability in antigenic properties. The core proteins of the virus contain conserved antigenic determinants that are the basis of current serological diagnostic assays. The viral glycoproteins also contain a limited number of conserved antigenic determinants, but predominantly present an array of variable antigenic sites that can be distinguished by their reactivity with monoclonal antibodies or by neutralization with polyclonal immune serum from infected horses. The range of variation observed among EIAV isolates has precluded any classification of virus strains on the basis of serological properties.

Immune serum from EIAV-infected horses is reactive with the respective major core protein of most animal and human lentiviruses, but not with any of the major core proteins of oncoviruses. Immune serum taken from other species infected with a lentivirus generally do not reveal a cross-reactivity with EIAV or with other lentiviruses. This one-way serological reactivity suggests that horses infected with EIAV uniquely recognize a conserved lentivirus-specific, antigenic determinant.

## Transmission and Tissue Tropism

Blood from persistently infected horses is the most important source of EIAV for transmission; *in utero* transmissions of EIAV from mare to foal are evidently very rare. This blood transfer can be affected by man or blood-feeding vectors. EIAV has been shown to remain infectious on hypodermic needles for up to 96 h, emphasizing the potential for transmission via routine animal husbandry or veterinary medical practices. However, the mechanical transmission of EIAV by arthropods, especially horseflies, is generally accepted as the major natural means of transmission in the field. Transmission of EIAV by a single horsefly carrying only approximately 10 nl of virus-infected blood has been documented under experimental conditions.

The target cell during persistent EIAV infections appears to be exclusively cells of the monocyte/macrophage lineage; there is no evidence for infection of lymphocytes as observed with some other lentiviruses. The virus burden in infected horses is predominantly in tissue macrophage found in liver, kidney, and spleen with much lower levels of virus found in lymph nodes, bone marrow, or in circulating monocytes. Thus, the relatively high levels of viremia ($10^{4-6}$ $TCID_{50}$) observed during episodes of chronic EIA evidently result primarily from the production and release of virus from infected tissue macrophage, rather than an extensive infection of blood monocytes.

## Pathogenicity

Field isolates and laboratory strains of EIAV differ markedly in their pathogenicity, ranging from avirulent to lethal strains of the virus. Little is known about the viral determinants or host factors that influence the course of virus replication and pathogenesis. In other lentiviruses, differences in viral pathogenesis have been mapped to specific changes in viral envelope genes or to changes in gene regulatory sequences in the viral genome. It is likely that variation in EIAV pathogenicity will follow a similar pattern.

## Clinical Features of Infection

The clinical response of horses following artificial inoculation or natural exposure to EIAV is variable and depends in part on host resistance factors, viral virulence factors, and environmental factors (e.g., weather and work load). In general, EIAV infections can be apparent with distinctive clinical symptoms or inapparent without any clinical signs of EIA. The clinical disease is typically described as acute, chronic, or asymptomatic (**Figure 6**).

Acute EIA is most often associated with the first exposure to the virus, with fever and hemorrhages evident from 7 to 30 days after exposure. Acute disease is thought to be associated with massive virus replication in and destruction of infected macrophages. Horses in the initial phase of acute EIA will be seronegative, because the immune system has had insufficient time to respond to the viral antigens. During the peak of the febrile response in acute EIA, viremia of greater than $10^6$ horse-infectious doses per ml of whole blood is often observed. The initial acute phase of EIA infection may not be seen by the veterinarian unless there is an epizootic of the infection in a group of horses. Even then, the horses must be under close supervision before the initial fever and anorexia are detected. Neither anemia nor edema is seen at this stage of disease.

The more classic clinical signs of EIA such as loss of weight, anemia, diarrhea, and edema are seen later during recurring cycles of the illness, which appear at irregular intervals ranging from a couple of weeks to several months. The frequency and severity of clinical episodes in horses with chronic EIA usually decline with time, about 90% occurring within 1 year of infection. Horses with chronic EIA are seropositive and have variable viremia levels which are the highest during the periodic febrile episodes. Although a small percentage of chronic EIA cases may result in death, the predominant clinical course of infection is a cessation of detectable clinical symptoms by the end of the first year post infection and the establishment of a lifelong inapparent carrier stage. However, animals can experience a recrudescence

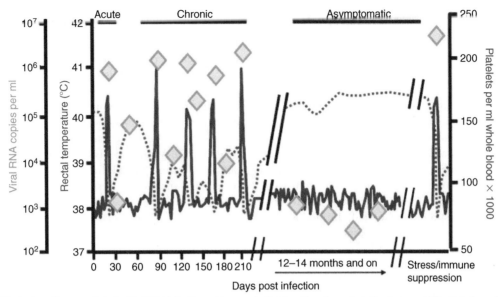

**Figure 6** Clinical profile associated with EIAV infection of horses indicating the characteristic stages of EIA. Febrile episodes are defined as rectal temperatures above 39 °C (103 °F), and thrombocytopenia is defined as platelet levels below 105 000 µl⁻¹ of blood.

of viremia and disease due to stress or immune suppression from a contemporous bacterial or viral infection.

The highest percentage of EIAV-infected horses in the field are in fact inapparent carriers. These horses have no clinical illness associated with the viral infection, and viremia is usually undetectable. However, these inapparent carriers maintain high levels of EIAV-specific antibodies, suggesting a chronic low level of virus replication. Inapparent carriers can be shown to harbor infectious EIAV by transfusions of whole blood (200 ml) to recipient horses that become seropositive to EIAV within 3–6 weeks post inoculation. In addition, treatment of certain inapparent carriers with immunosuppressive drugs or exposure to extreme stress can cause the recrudescence of chronic EIA, even in some horses that have been free of clinical symptoms for years.

## Pathology and Histopathology

Gross and histopathological lesions in EIAV-infected horses are variable and closely associated with levels of viral replication. In the acute stage of EIA, gross pathological lesions consist of swelling of the parenchymatous organs, and hemorrhages can be observed in most tissues. The most pronounced histopathological lesions are hepatic and lymphoid necrosis in association with large numbers of activated macrophage and Kupffer cells. Hepatic necrosis is most severe near the central vein evidently resulting from degenerative changes in the parenchymal cells. Lesions in the spleen are characterized by degenerative erythrocytes, and small focal hemorrhages are found in

the splenic capsule and adjacent tissue. Lymphocytic infiltrations can be observed in several organs including liver, spleen, lymph node, kidney, heart, and lung. The majority of these lesions are thought to be the combined effect of immune-mediated lysis of virus-infected cells and an immune complex-mediated inflammatory response.

The pathological changes in the chronic form of EIA include a developing immunological control of virus replication. Gross pathological lesions include splenomegaly, lymphadenopathy, and hepatomegaly. Microscopic changes are characterized by infiltration of lymphoid cells in almost all organs and tissues. Anemia has long been considered the hallmark of EIA. The two major causes of anemia, hemolysis and bone marrow depression, are closely associated with replicating virus. Hemolysis is immunologically mediated. Erythrocytes are coated with the viral surface glycoprotein which in the presence of specific antibodies and bound C3 induces erythrophagocytosis and complement-mediated hemolysis. Bone marrow suppression is less well characterized but appears to be associated with iron deficiency. Thrombocytopenia is frequently the earliest pathology observed during chronic EIA and can precede the detection of virus-specific antibodies. The mechanism for the marked reduction in blood platelets is unknown, but has recently been associated with cytokine dysregulation.

## Immune Responses

Horses infected with EIAV typically become seropositive in standard serological assays within 21 days post infection. The humoral immune responses are predominantly against the viral envelope glycoproteins, gp90 and gp45, and the major core protein, p26. All currently approved diagnostic assays for EIAV infection are based on the detection of antibody to the major core antigen, although the antibody response to the envelope glycoproteins is at least tenfold greater than the antibody titer measured against the p26 protein. Significantly lower levels of antibody can be detected against virtually all of the other structural and nonstructural proteins encoded by EIAV. Interestingly, EIAV-specific antibody levels remain relatively constant throughout the course of chronic EIA and even in the unapparent stage of infection.

The immune responses generated during chronic EIA initially mediate significant pathogenesis in the presence of sufficient levels of EIAV antigenimia, but progressively evolve to establish a strict immunologic control over virus replication. Thus, the EIAV system is unique among lentiviruses in that the host immune responses routinely accomplish an effective control of aggressive virus replication and recurring clinical disease to maintain an indefinite inapparent stage of infection. The immune correlates of this protection remain to be defined. However, it has been shown that the neutralizing capacity of serum antibodies elicited to EIAV during the chronic stage of disease progressively increases, indicating an evolution of immune responses to the sequential generation of antigenic variants of virus. In addition, recent studies have demonstrated a lengthy and complex evolution of antibody and cellular immune responses to experimental EIAV infections of horses demonstrating a dynamic maturation process that apparently correlates with the development of protective immunity. The specific humoral or cellular immune correlates of protection have not yet been identified. The ability of the horse immune responses to overcome the array of persistence and escape mechanisms employed by EIAV suggests that a successful vaccine is feasible.

## Prevention and Control

The transmission of EIAV infection has been controlled by improving animal husbandry techniques to prevent the spread of infected blood, by reducing the horsefly population in the vicinity of herds, and primarily by identifying and segregating or sacrificing horses that are seropositive for the virus. In the United States, the most common diagnostic assays are an agar gel immunodiffusion test, the Coggins assay, which was developed in the early 1970s and enzyme-linked immunoassay that was approved by the USDA as an EIA diagnostic assay in the 1980s and 1990s. Both diagnostic assay procedures are based on the detection of serum antibodies to the major viral core protein, p26. The diagnostic enzyme-linked immunosorbent assay (ELISA) assay has been engineered to produce a sensitivity that is equivalent to the previously established Coggins test. More sensitive diagnostic assays based on the detection of antibodies to the EIAV envelope glycoproteins have been developed, but have not yet been approved for commercial use. The most sensitive and specific assay for detecting EIAV infection is horse inoculation tests with 200 ml of whole blood from the horse being tested. The horse inoculation test is used only in rare cases where the standard serological assays may give ambiguous results.

There is currently no effective vaccine for the prevention of EIAV infection and disease. The primary challenge in developing an effective EIAV vaccine is overcoming the antigenic diversity intrinsic to this virus. An important practical requirement in the development of any EIAV vaccine is compatibility with established regulatory policies and diagnostic assays. The ability of EIAV-infected horses to routinely establish immunologic control over virus replication and disease suggests that an effective vaccine can indeed be developed, if the critical natural immune correlates of protection can be elicited by a candidate vaccine. An attenuated live EIAV vaccine with a reported protection efficacy of about 70% has been used in China since the early 1980s, but the effectiveness of this vaccine remains to be confirmed outside of that country. Evaluation of other candidate EIAV vaccines (live-attenuated, inactivated whole virus, subunit vaccines, synthetic peptides, etc.) under experimental conditions has revealed a spectrum of vaccine efficacy that ranges from 'sterile protection' (prevention of infection upon inoculation with EIAV) to severe elevation of EIAV replication, and exacerbation of disease. These results indicate that immune responses to EIAV are a double-edged sword that can either mediate protection or yield vaccine enhancement. Vaccine enhancement has previously been reported for other viral infections (dengue virus, respiratory syncitial virus, feline infectious peritonitis virus) and is of special concern with macrophage-tropic viruses. Similar examples of vaccine protection and enhancement have been reported in studies of experimental vaccines for other lentiviruses, including feline immunodeficiency virus, caprine arthritis-encephalitis virus, and visna-maedi virus. These observations in several diverse animal lentivirus systems suggest that the potential for immune enhancement may be a general property of lentiviruses, including HIV-1. Current efforts in the production of a commercial EIAV vaccine are focused on the development of a vaccine that can achieve sufficient maturation of immune responses to provide protection from virus infection, but allow the serological differentiation between vaccinated and infected horses. In this regard, DNA vaccine strategies appear to be well suited to accomplish these criteria for a commercial EIAV vaccine.

## Future Research

EIAV provides a dynamic system for examining the interaction between virus populations and host immune responses that are evolving in response to each other. In addition, EIAV offers a remarkable model for studying the delicate balance between immune responses to a persistent virus infection that result in disease and those that have beneficial results. A characterization of the nature of protective and enhancing immune responses can provide important information about the mechanisms of lentivirus disease and the type of immune responses to

be elicited or avoided by a vaccine. The results of these studies in the EIAV system should be applicable to other lentiviruses, including HIV-1.

## Further Reading

Cook RF, Issel CJ, and Montelaro RC (1996) Equine infectious anemia virus. In: Studdert R (ed.) *Viral Diseases of Equines*, pp. 295–323. Amsterdam: Elsevier.

Cordes TA and Issel CJ (1996) Equine infectious anemia: A status report on its control. USDA Animal and Plant Health Inspection Service Publication No. APHIS 91–55–032.

Montelaro RC, Ball JM, and Rushlow KE (1992) Equine retroviruses. In: Levy J (ed.) *The Retroviridae*, vol. 2, pp. 257–360. New York: Plenum.

Montelaro RC and Bolognesi DP (1995) Vaccines against retroviruses. In: Levy J (ed.) *The Retroviridae*, vol. 2. New York: Plenum.

Sellon DC, Fuller FJ, and McGuire TC (1994) The immunopathogenesis of equine infectious anemia virus. *Virus Research* 32: 111.

# Flaviviruses of Veterinary Importance

**R Swanepoel,** National Institute for Communicable Diseases, Sandringham, South Africa
**F J Burt,** University of the Free State, Bloemfontein, South Africa

## Glossary

**Argasid** Soft-skinned tick, member of the family *Argasidae*.

**Arthropod** Any member of the phylum Arthropoda, including insects and arachnids (spiders, scorpions, ticks, and mites).

**Culicoid midge** Blood-sucking midge of the genus *Culicoides*.

**Instar** Stage in the life cycle of arthropods, for example, egg, larva, nymph, and adult in mosquitoes; egg, larva, nymph, and adult in ticks.

**Ixodid** Tick with a hardened shell or scutum.

**Microhabitat** The environmental niche in which an organism is found.

**Phlebotomine fly** Blood-sucking sandfly of the genus *Phlebotomous*.

**Phylogenetics** The study of the genetic relatedness of organisms.

**Transovarial transmission of virus** Passage of virus infection through the eggs of arthropods to the succeeding generation, thus ensuring perpetuation of the virus.

**Vectors** Blood-sucking arthropods (mosquitoes, midges, sandflies, and ticks) which transmit viruses from one vertebrate to another.

**Virion** A complete virus particle with its protein coat and core of DNA or RNA nucleic acid.

## Introduction

Approximately 94 viruses are currently assigned to three genera (*Flavivirus, Pestivirus,* and *Hepacivirus*) within the family *Flaviviridae* (L. *flavus* = yellow, from the type species *Yellow fever virus*, which causes jaundice); the number of viruses in the family changes with periodic discovery of new members or revision of the taxonomic status of existing viruses. Diseases of major medical and veterinary importance caused by hepaciviruses and pestiviruses are discussed elsewhere in this encyclopedia, while this article summarizes aspects pertaining only to the veterinary importance of members of the genus *Flavivirus*.

Viruses of the *Flaviviridae* have spherical virions 40–60 nm in diameter, with a tightly applied lipid envelope incorporating envelope (E) protein spikes which are glycosylated in pestiviruses and flaviviruses. The genomes consist of a single, linear molecule of positive-sense, single-stranded RNA (ssRNA), ranging in size from approximately 9.5 kbp in hepaciviruses, to 10.7 kbp in flaviviruses, and 12.5 kbp in pestiviruses. Replication takes place in the cytoplasm, with morphogenesis, transport, and maturation of virions occurring in cell membrane vesicles. A single open reading frame (ORF) in the genome is translated directly into a polyprotein which is cleaved into structural proteins, the RNA-associated internal capsid or core (C) protein, envelope proteins (E1, E2), and a membrane (M) protein, plus seven nonstructural proteins which exhibit viral polymerase and other enzymatic activities. The E proteins mediate binding of virus to host cells, are responsible for the hemagglutinating property exhibited by most flaviviruses, and constitute the major antigenic determinants of protective immunity. Viruses of the three genera are not closely related, with less than 30% nucleotide sequence homology and an absence of antigenic cross-reactivity, but they share genome organization and replication strategies. Viruses of the genera *Hepacivirus* and *Pestivirus* are most closely related structurally, and have in common a lack of arthropod vectors and the tendency to cause persistent infection in their vertebrate hosts.

The 82 recognized or tentative members of the genus *Flavivirus* include two inherent viruses of mosquitoes, cell fusion agent virus (CFAV) and Kamiti River virus (KRV), which have no known medical or veterinary significance and which may be assigned to a new genus, plus Tamana bat virus from Trinidad, which may also be assigned to a new genus. Most recently, there has been molecular identification of a tick-associated agent, Ngoye virus from Senegal, which has not as yet been successfully cultured in a laboratory host system, has no known medical or veterinary significance, and is only distantly related to existing flaviviruses. The remaining flaviviruses are antigenically related to each other and were originally assigned to serogroups on the basis of close antigenic affinities. Recent classification of the viruses based on phylogenetic analyses shows remarkable concordance with antigenic classification, and with the biological properties of the viruses, such as vertebrate host and arthropod vector associations.

About 21% of the members of the genus have been isolated from mammals only and have no known vectors (NKV viruses), a further 51% are usually transmitted by mosquitoes, and the remaining 28% appear to be transmitted principally by ticks, although definitive demonstration of transmission by arthropod vectors has been reported in a proportion of instances only. Depending on which genes are subjected to phylogenetic analysis, different conclusions may be reached with regard to the evolution of the flaviviruses, but from limited analyses of whole genome sequences it appears that NKV viruses diverged from a putative ancestor before mosquitoborne viruses, and that tick transmission is a recently acquired trait within the genus. Many flaviviruses were discovered in the course of surveys conducted on vertebrate and arthropod populations, rather than in the investigation of disease syndromes, and consequently many of the viruses have no known medical or veterinary significance. From the genetic distance which exists between the recently discovered Ngoye virus and other members of the genus, and between existing mosquito-borne viruses, it has been extrapolated that several thousand flaviviruses remain to be discovered.

Various mechanisms are postulated to ensure the persistence of arboviruses through prolonged periods of vector inactivity during winters and dry seasons, including the migration of infected vertebrate hosts, hibernation of infected adult vectors, and passage of virus through the eggs of vectors to infect the succeeding generation, so-called transovarial transmission of infection, which generally occurs with low frequency. Unlike mosquitoes, ticks feed on vertebrates in different stages (instars) of their life cycles, as larvae, nymphs, and adults, so that even in the absence of transovarial transmission of infection the perpetuation of virus can be ensured by the long intervals which intervene between the feeding of successive instars on different hosts.

Viruses transmitted by mosquitoes often cause sporadic infections which may pass unrecognized in endemic areas, but they are capable of causing explosive outbreaks when exceptionally heavy rainfall creates favorable breeding conditions for the vectors, or human manipulation of the environment, such as the building of dams and irrigation schemes, or the implementation of intensive livestock production systems, results in the juxtaposition of susceptible human or farm animal populations with vectors. Tick-borne virus infections tend to occur at endemic level within areas of vector distribution, and larger outbreaks are less immediately linked to climatic events which may favor population explosions of the wild hosts of immature ticks, but human intervention, such as changes in livestock farming systems, can also precipitate epidemics. A few arthropod-borne flaviviruses are named for the disease syndromes with which they are associated, but most are named for the geographic location from which the initial isolate was obtained.

## Mosquito-Borne Flaviviruses Causing Livestock or Wildlife Diseases

### Japanese Encephalitis Virus

Japanese encephalitis virus (JEV) was first isolated in 1935 in Japan as a cause of encephalitis in humans. Severe outbreaks of human disease occur at intervals in India, China, Korea, and Japan, and lesser outbreaks or sporadic cases are recorded in Nepal, Bangladesh, Sri Lanka, Laos, Cambodia, Vietnam, the Far East provinces of the Russian Federation, Thailand, Malaysia, Singapore, Philippines, Indonesia, Papua New Guinea, Taiwan, Guam, Saipan, and Myanmar. There are four genotypes of the virus, but they are all cross-protective. The virus is transmitted by *Culex tritaeniorhyncus* and other culicine mosquitoes and circulates between the mosquitoes, water birds, particularly egrets, herons and ducks, and domestic pigs. Overt outbreaks of disease are associated with rainfall and the irrigation of rice fields. The virus infects a wide range of vertebrates, including donkeys, cattle, and dogs, but most animals do not manifest disease. There is fetal wastage and abortion in sows. Humans and horses are incidental hosts which develop encephalitis, but play no significant role in the circulation of the virus. Tens of thousands of human infections occur each year, and while less than 1% of infected persons develop encephalitis the death rate is high in such patients. Case fatality rates may exceed 50% in horses with encephalitis. The virus is not known to cause disease in wild vertebrates, but bats can circulate virus following experimental infection, and low prevalences of antibody to JEV have been found in reptiles and amphibians.

## St. Louis Encephalitis Virus

St. Louis encephalitis virus (SLEV) was isolated in 1933 from human brain as the causative agent of a large outbreak of encephalitis in St. Louis, Missouri, and was subsequently found to be transmitted by culicine mosquitoes, which are capable of breeding in drainage water in urban settings. The virus is widely distributed in North, Central, and South America, but the disease is seen mainly in the USA where it was considered to be the most important arbovirus pathogen prior to the introduction of West Nile virus (WNV) in 1999. There is some regional variation in the mosquitoes involved, but the main vectors are members of the *Cx. pipiens* complex, plus *Cx. tarsalis* and *Cx. nigripalpus*. Human infection with SLEV is usually asymptomatic but a low proportion of patients develop encephalitis with an approximately 10% case fatality rate. Outbreaks of varying magnitude occur at irregular intervals throughout the USA, but there are regional differences in occurrence of the infection depending on host and breeding-site preferences of the mosquito species concerned. Asymptomatic infection occurs in domestic animals such as horses, cattle, goats, sheep, pigs, cats, dogs and poultry, as well as in wild birds and small mammals including raccoons, opossums, rodents, and bats, but only birds are thought to play a significant role in the circulation of the virus. SLEV was isolated from the brain of a gray fox with encephalitis, and forest mammals including sloths are thought to be involved in transmission cycles in South America.

## West Nile Virus

Following the intial isolation of WNV from a febrile patient in Uganda in 1937, sporadic cases and outbreaks of benign febrile disease were recorded in humans in Africa, the Near East and Asia, with the largest outbreaks occurring in Israel in 1950–54 and 1957, and in South Africa in 1974. It was found that WNV is widely endemic in southern Africa in localities where the vectors, ornithophilic (bird-feeding) culicine mosquitoes, and avian hosts of the virus are present, such as at dam sites with reed beds and heronries. Outbreaks of human infection, which occur when high rainfall or hot weather favors mosquito breeding, are associated with high seroconversion rates in wild birds, and 13 species of birds in South Africa were found to support replication of the virus without developing disease. It was deduced that the widespread dispersal of the virus was associated with migrating birds. Cattle and sheep appeared to undergo inapparent infection and could also theoretically serve as hosts for infection of mosquitoes. Subsequently, limited experimental evidence was obtained to indicate that WNV is capable of causing abortion in pregnant sheep.

The occurrence of meningoencephalitis was first observed in elderly WNV patients in Israel in 1957, and subsequently also in young children in India. The occurrence of horse encephalitis was recognized in Egypt in 1962, and in 1962–66 outbreaks of meningoencephalitis were observed in both humans and horses in France. There was a marked increase in the frequency and severity of outbreaks of human disease during the 1990s, often involving horses as well, and including epidemics in Algeria, Romania, Morocco, Tunisia, Italy, Russia, France, and Israel. Moreover, the outbreaks in Romania and Israel were characterized by concurrent mortality in birds. The vectors of WNV included *Cx. univitattus* and *Cx. antennatus* in Africa and Europe, members of the *Cx. pipiens* complex in Europe and Israel, and members of the *Cx. vishnui* complex plus *Cx. fatigans* in Asia.

The presence of WNV in the Western Hemisphere was first recognized in New York in 1999, and over the next few years it spread rapidly throughout the country and beyond into Canada and South America. Vectors in North America included members of the *Cx. pipiens* complex, plus *Cx. restuans*, *Cx. tarsalis*, and *Cx. nigripalpus*. The virus circulating in the USA was found to be genetically most closely related to a WNV isolate associated with goose mortality in Israel in 1998, suggesting that the virus was imported into America from the Near East, either in an infected bird, mosquito, human, or other animal, although the exact mechanism of the introduction will probably remain unknown.

In North America, WNV infection was confirmed in more than 300 species of birds, with death rates approaching 100% in corvids (crows, magpies, and jays), and with robins constituting important hosts for the infection of the mosquito vectors. It is notable that the virus spared African bird species in the New York zoo where deaths of local species were first observed. Infection was also recorded in 30 species of mammals, reptiles, and amphibians. Approximately 10% of infected horses manifested clinical illness, with a high proportion of these developing fatal encephalitis. Vaccine for horses became available in 2005. Although fatal infections were recorded in dogs and a wolf, infection rates were low in cats and dogs. Fatal disease was observed in farmed alligators in the USA and Mexico, with infection resulting from the feeding of infected horse meat, and also from transmission between alligators in crowded conditions. Serological evidence of infection was also found in small wild animals, such as raccoons, opossums, and squirrels, but the pathogenicity of the virus for these hosts is uncertain. Serological evidence of infection was obtained in farmed Nile crocodiles in Israel in the absence of disease. The Kunjin strain of WNV transmitted by *Cx. annulirostris* mosquitoes in Australia generally causes febrile illness in humans, seldom encephalitis, and was confirmed to be associated with encephalitis in horses on one occasion only.

The increase in the frequency of neurologic infections, and the occurrence of human, horse, and bird fatalities in the Northern Hemisphere, raised the question of whether there had been a change in the pathogenicity of WNV. Phylogenetic analyses revealed that WN isolates fell into two lineages. Lineage 1 included isolates from Africa north of the equator, Europe, Asia, and North America, with Kunjin virus from Australia constituting a subtype within this lineage. Lineage 2 consisted solely of viruses from Africa and Madagascar. The findings were interpreted to support the emergence of exalted virulence in lineage 1, with lineage 2 isolates considered to be associated with endemic infection of low virulence in Africa. However, WNV belonging to lineage 2 has recently been isolated from a goshawk with fatal encephalitis in Hungary, and three additional lineages of the virus have been described from the Czech Republic, Georgia, and India. Moreover, despite the apparently low level of virus activity observed in southern Africa in recent years, WNV was isolated from the brain of a suspected rabid dog in Botswana (initially described as having an infection with Wesselsbron virus), and in South Africa from humans and a foal with encephalitis, plus an ostrich chick in a commercial flock where extensive mortalities occurred. Experiments in mice confirmed that neuroinvasive WNV strains occur within both lineage 1 and 2. Thus, it is possible that the virulence of WNV in southern Africa may previously have been underestimated, while the perceived enhanced virulence of the virus in recent epidemics in the Northern

Hemisphere may partly be due to the emergence or re-emergence of existing strains of WNV in geographic locations with immunologically naive populations, high medical alertness, and active surveillance programs.

## Israel Turkey Meningoencephalomyelitis Virus

A disease caused by Israel turkey meningoencephalomyelitis virus (ITV) infection in turkeys was first observed in Israel in 1958 and the causative virus isolated in 1959. ITV was later found to be transmitted by culicine mosquitoes, but was also isolated from culicoid midges, and phlebotomine sandflies were shown to be capable of transmitting the virus. In 1978 the virus was isolated as a cause of disease of turkeys in South Africa. The virus has not been found in any other country, and disease has only been reported in turkeys. The disease generally occurs seasonally, only in birds older than 10 weeks, and it is characterized by progressive paresis and paralysis, with morbidity and mortality rates ranging from 15% to 80%. Turkey breeder hens exhibit a severe drop in egg production. Vaccines are available.

## Sitiawan Virus

Sitiawan virus (SITV) was recently isolated as a cause of deaths of chick embryos and broiler chickens in Malaysia. It is closely related to the mosquito-borne Tembusu virus, which has no known medical or veterinary significance.

## Wesselsbron virus

Wesselsbron virus (WESSV) was identified in 1955 in South Africa as a cause of deaths of newborn lambs in a flock where a modified live vaccine against the mosquito-borne Rift Valley fever virus (RVFV) (not a flavivirus) had been administered 2 weeks previously. There was concern that the RVFV vaccine may have caused the deaths, but it was concluded that the new virus, which also proved to be transmitted by *Aedes* species mosquitoes of the subgenera *Ochlerotatus* and *Neomelanoconion*, occurred in outbreaks together with RVFV and caused similar disease in sheep, cattle, and goats, namely, deaths of young animals and abortion in pregnant animals. Consequently, an attenuated WESSV vaccine was developed by serial intracerebral passage of virus in infant mice, and this was marketed for use together with RVFV vaccine on nonpregnant animals. During extended outbreaks of RVF in South Africa and Namibia in 1974–76 some 13.9 million doses of the live WESSV vaccine and 22 million doses of live RVFV were used indiscriminately on livestock, with resultant widespread occurrence of abortions and congenital malformations in sheep and cattle. It was confirmed experimentally that both of the vaccines were abortigenic and teratogenic. However, it subsequently became clear that WESSV is more widely endemic in southern Africa than RVFV, and although sporadic isolations of virus have been made from livestock in South Africa and Zimbabwe, mainly in association with disease of newborn lambs and calves, the virus has not been incriminated as the cause of large outbreaks of disease in farm animals, nor has a veterinary problem been described elsewhere. The vaccine, which confers lifelong immunity, continues to be marketed for use in nonpregnant sheep and goats.

Altogether, WESSV has been isolated from livestock and a gerbil in southern Africa, a camel in Nigeria, mosquitoes in South Africa, Zimbabwe, Uganda, Kenya, the Central African Republic (CAR), Cameroon, Ivory Coast, Senegal, Guinea and Thailand, a tick in CAR, naturally infected humans in South Africa, Senegal, and CAR, and from human laboratory infections in South Africa, Uganda, Nigeria, Senegal, CAR, and the USA. In addition, antibody has been found in humans and/or livestock in Malawi, Zambia, Botswana, Namibia, Angola, Mozambique, and Madagascar. The principal vectors of the virus appear to be aedine mosquitoes, and although the virus has been isolated from a tick, there is no evidence that ticks play a significant role in transmission of the virus. The few human infections recorded in South Africa were acquired from contact with infected animal tissues or mosquito bite, while human infections reported in Senegal and CAR seem to be consistently associated with mosquito bite. The virus generally causes benign febrile illness in humans, but a patient who acquired laboratory infection from the splashing of virus into an eye developed encephalitis from which he recovered without sequelae.

It cannot be excluded that WESSV or various other flaviviruses could emerge as important pathogens under particular circumstances, as occurred with WNV in North America in 1999. In this connection it should be noted that Bagaza virus has been isolated from aborted cattle fetuses on three occasions in South Africa, that WNV and Banzi virus were shown to cause abortion in experimentally infected pregnant sheep, and that Usutu virus, initially isolated from mosquitoes, a rodent and birds in the context of surveys in Africa, emerged as a cause of bird deaths in Austria in 2001.

## Yellow Fever Virus

Descriptions of disease compatible with yellow fever date back to 1492. However, many medical conditions were confused in early records, and the name yellow fever was first applied to a fatal disease of humans in the Caribbean region in 1750. Shortly thereafter, the presence of the disease was recognized in South America and West Africa. Over the next 150 years the virus, introduced by infected people on ships, caused epidemics in many port cities in North America and Europe. From 1900 onwards the Walter Reed commission from the USA investigated yellow fever in Cuba and, using American military volunteers, demonstrated that the disease could be transmitted from person-to-person by Ae. aegypti mosquitoes, and that the infection was caused by a filterable agent present in the blood of patients (filtration was an early method used to distinguish viruses from bacteria). It was not until 1927 that yellow fever virus (YFV) was isolated in a laboratory host system, rhesus monkeys. Meanwhile, the identification of the Ae. aegypti vectors, which breed in small volumes of water, had facilitated the implementation of mosquito control methods which virtually eliminated circulation of YFV in urban settings. Initially, there was speculation as to whether YFV had originated in Africa or South America, but it was concluded that the virus and Ae. aegypti mosquitoes had been translocated from Africa in ships centuries ago. The occurrence of outbreaks of the disease on ships was well documented.

Resurgence of urban yellow fever in South America led to the discovery of jungle or sylvatic circulation of the virus in 1932. In South America, YFV circulates in the forest canopy between monkeys and Haemagogus species mosquitoes. Persons who live near or enter forests acquire infection and introduce it into urban environments where epidemics are generated by the circulation of YFV between humans and Ae. aegypti mosquitoes. In Africa, mosquitoes such as Ae. africanus transmit YFV between primates at forest canopy level, while mosquitoes which feed at intermediate levels, including Ae. bromeliae and members of the Ae. furcifer-taylori group, serve as link hosts to spread infection to humans which in turn serve to initiate urban transmission cycles involving Ae. aegypti mosquitoes. South American primates including tamarins, marmosets and howling, squirrel, owl, and spider monkeys undergo severe infection with variable mortality, while African monkeys and apes generally undergo viremic infection without overt illness. This was interpreted to indicate that there had been a longer period of co-evolution of YFV with African primates, but African YFV isolates were found to be of reduced virulence for neotropical monkeys. Asian monkeys are susceptible to severe and fatal YFV infection. Birds, reptiles, and amphibia are resistant to infection, and although several mammals including hedgehogs are capable of developing viremia, it appears that they have limited exposure to known vectors.

Effective vaccines were developed in the 1930s and used extensively in conjunction with mosquito control to reduce the occurrence of the human disease. However, the existence of sylvatic transmission cycles precludes eradication of the virus, and since 1980 there has been a marked resurgence of the disease in Africa with outbreaks being recorded in countries extending from Senegal in the north, to Angola in the south, and eastwards to Sudan, Ethiopia, and Kenya. No recent urban outbreaks have been recorded in South America, but fairly extensive outbreaks involving sylvatic vectors have occurred in Peru and Brazil.

Many of the remaining mosquito-borne flaviviruses are believed to circulate in birds and although a few, including Rocio, Spondweni, and Zika, have been associated with human disease on occasion, they have no known veterinary significance. It should be noted, however, that many of the flaviviruses which are pathogenic for humans produce symptomatic infection in a minority of people, and it can be surmised that infections which produce similar low morbidity in farm animals are likely to pass unrecognized.

## Tick-Borne Flaviviruses

It has emerged from recent phylogenetic analyses that the tick-borne flaviviruses comprise three groups: a seabird group which includes three viruses with no known medical or veterinary significance, a Kadam virus group containing a single virus known only to have been isolated from ticks removed from cattle in Uganda and a camel in Saudi Arabia, but which represents a distinct evolutionary lineage, and the so-called mammalian tick-borne group of viruses. Within the mammalian group Gadgets Gully, Royal Farm, and Karshi viruses and are more distantly related to others and are known only to have been isolated from ticks, while the remaining viruses, which were formerly clustered together in a tick-borne encephalitis antigenic complex, include important pathogens of humans and livestock. However, genetic differences between some of these latter viruses are smaller than those which exist between other flaviviruses, and hence they have been tentatively designated as types and subtypes of a proposed tick-borne encephalitis virus (TBEV) species.

## Powassan Virus and Deer Tick Virus

Powassan virus (POWV) was first isolated as a cause of fatal encephalitis in a child in Ontario, Canada, in 1958. The virus was subsequently found in western Canada, and northeast, north-central and western USA. The principal vector was found to be the tick *Ixodes cookei*, and the main host for the tick and virus is believed to be the woodchuck or groundhog (*Marmota monax*). Other *Ixodes* species and squirrels have also been implicated in the circulation of the virus, and there have been isolations from other ticks including *Dermacentor andersoni*. Twelve human cases of encephalitis with four fatalities have been reported in North America. Antibody has been found in a range of animals, and virus was isolated from two dead foxes, although it was not clear that the virus had caused their deaths. The virus was experimentally shown to be capable of causing encephalitis in horses. Reportedly, POWV was isolated in 1978 from the blood of a person who had been

bitten by a tick in the Maritime Province (Primorsky) in the Far East of the former Soviet Union (currently the Russian Federation), and later the virus was isolated from *Ixodes persulcatus* and other ticks and mosquitoes, and antibodies were found in birds in Primorsky. In 1996, deer tick virus (DTV) was isolated from deer ticks, *Ixodes scapularis*, in the eastern USA and found to be closely related to POWV. The white-footed mouse (*Peromyscus leucopus*) is thought to be the main host for the tick and virus, although other mammals, particularly white-tailed deer, are important hosts for the tick. As yet, no disease associations have been made for DTV. Although POWV and DTV are closely related, the results of recent phylogenetic studies confirm that the viruses circulate independently. However, the studies did not include POWV isolates from the western USA or the Russian Federation.

## Kyasanur Forest Disease Virus

Kyasanur forest disease virus (KFDV) was discovered in 1957 as a cause of fatal febrile disease of humans in Karnataka State, India. The vectors are ticks of the genus *Haemaphysalis*, particularly *H. spinigera*, and two species of *Ixodes* ticks, but the virus has also been isolated from the argasid (soft-skinned) tick *Ornithodoros crossi*. Rodents are suggested to be the main hosts of the virus. About 500 human cases of the disease are recorded each year in Karanataka State, with a mortality rate of 5–10%. Infection occurs mainly in people who enter forests to gather wood, and the disease is seasonal with tick activity. Fatal disease occurs in langur and macaque monkeys in the forests, but no disease manifestations have been recorded in domestic animals. The virus has been isolated from rodents, shrews, and bats.

## Omsk Hemorrhagic Fever Virus

Omsk hemorrhagic fever virus (OHFV) was isolated in 1947 from the blood of a patient with hemorrhagic disease in western Siberia in the former Soviet Union. The disease was first observed in 1941, and large numbers of cases were recorded in 1945–49. Since that time only sporadic cases have been recognized in the Omsk, Novosibirsk, Kurgan, and Tjumen regions of western Siberia. The disease affects mostly muskrat trappers and their families. Muskrats, or musquash (*Ondatra zibethicus*), are large rodents which are trapped for their fur. They are indigenous to North America and were introduced into Siberia in 1925. No equivalent virus or disease has been found in North America. The principal vector of the virus in Siberia was found to be the tick *Dermacentor reticulatus* (syn. *D. pictus*) but the virus was also isolated from *D. marginatus* and other ticks and mites. Muskrats and local voles, some of which undergo benign infection, serve as reservoir hosts for the infection of ticks. Muskrats live in swamps, and virus which is present in the excretions of infected muskrats, or leaches into water from dead muskrats, can infect other muskrats or humans. OHFV was also found in mosquitoes and antibody in water birds, but these do not appear to play a significant role in circulation of the virus. Humans acquire infection mainly from contact with infected muskrat tissues, but also from infected water, or from tick bite.

## Tick-Borne Encephalitis Virus

A human encephalitis syndrome was recognized in the far eastern provinces of the former Soviet Union at least as far back as the late nineteenth century, and has been known under a variety of names including Russian spring–summer encephalitis and Far Eastern tick-borne encephalitis. The causative agent, now named tick-borne encephalitis virus-Far Eastern subtype (TBEV-FE), was isolated from human patients in 1937 and later from its *Ixodes persulcatus* tick vectors. The virus occurs in the Primorsky, Khabarovsk, Krasnoyarsk, Altai, Tomsk, Omsk, Kemerovo, Western Siberia, Ural and Priural regions of the Russian Federation, China, and eastern Europe. After World War II the existence of a similar disease was recognized in several countries in Central Europe and adjacent parts of the Soviet Union, and a second virus, tick-borne encephalitis virus-European subtype (TBEV-Eu), was isolated from humans and *Ix. ricinus* ticks. Slight antigenic differences were shown to occur between the two viruses, and TBEV-Eu had human case fatality rates of 0.5–2.0%, in contrast to 5–20% for TBEV-FE. It has since been established that TBEV-Eu occurs in Albania, Austria, Belarus, Bornholm Island of Denmark, Bosnia, Bulgaria, China, Croatia, Czech Republic, Estonia, Finland, France, Germany, Greece, Hungary, Italy, Kazakhstan, Latvia, Lithuania, Norway, Poland, Romania, Russia, Slovakia, Slovenia, Sweden, Switzerland, Turkey, and Ukraine, although the distribution tends to be focal, dependent on suitable tick habitat. The *Ix. persulcatus* tick vector of TBEV-FE is distributed across nontropical Asia from Japan to eastern Europe, where there is overlap with the distribution of the *Ix. ricinus* vector of TBEV-Eu which extends across western Europe to the British Isles and Ireland. Other tick species play a minor role in transmission of the TBEV viruses. Phylogenetic analyses in the 1990s revealed the existence of a third subtype of virus, tick-borne encephalitis virus-Siberian subtype (TBEV-Sib), which is transmitted by *Ix. persulcatus* in the Irkutsk region of Siberia and has similar virulence for humans as does TBEV-FE. It was deduced that the TBEVs evolved in a cline in a westerly direction across the Eurasian continent over the past few thousand years. However, TBEV-FE and TBEV-Sib infections have recently been detected in Europe.

All three subtypes of TBEVs are believed to circulate between ticks and small vertebrates such as field mice and voles which undergo benign viremic infection. Antibody is also found in larger vertebrates such as squirrels, deer, badgers, and farm animals which develop low-grade viremia and are believed not to constitute a significant source of virus for infection of ticks. About 5000–10 000 cases of human disease are recorded each year, mainly in the Russian Federation, with the lowest incidence occurring in Austria where there is widespread use of vaccine. Humans acquire TBEV infection from tick bite, or from the ingestion of unpasteurized infected milk of sheep, goats, and cows. Less than 5% of humans develop symptomatic infection, but high death rates occur in patients who develop nervous disease. There may be neurological sequelae in those who recover, and a few patients develop chronic infections. A fatal hemorrhagic syndrome of humans has been described in the Novosibirsk region of Siberia in association with TBEV-FE infection. Recently, fatal TBEV-Eu infection was reported in captive monkeys in Germany which were inadvertently exposed to ticks.

## Louping III Virus

Descriptions of a sheep disease conforming to louping ill (Scottish dialect *louping* = leaping) date back more than two centuries in Scotland, but it was not until 1929 that the causative virus was isolated, and shortly thereafter shown to be transmitted by the tick *Ix. ricinus*. Other species of ticks can be infected but do not appear to play a significant role in the transmission of the virus. Louping ill virus (LIV) occurs in hill sheep farming areas of Britain and Ireland where there is suitable microhabitat for the ticks. Phylogenetic evidence suggests that the virus was probably originally introduced into Ireland from western Europe as a result of the livestock trade, and successively evolved as Louping ill virus-Ireland (LIV-Ir), and Louping ill virus-British (LIV-Brit) as it spreads through Wales, England, Scotland, and into Norway.

LIV causes fatal encephalomyelitis in a proportion of sheep depending on age and predisposing factors, including concurrent infection with agents such as the tick-borne parasite *Ehrlichia phagocytophila*. In areas with high challenge rates the disease is seen most frequently in lambs once they have lost their maternal immunity, but in areas with low tick burdens primary infection and disease may be seen in sheep of all ages. Infection is less frequently associated with disease in cattle, horses, pigs, farmed red deer, dogs, red grouse, and humans. Infection also occurs in roe deer, mountain hares, feral goats, voles, shrews, and field mice. The only recognized disease problem in wild vertebrates exists in red grouse (*Lagopus lagopus scotticus*), which have a commercial hunting value, and it has been demonstrated that the chicks can acquire infection from ingesting ticks. Sheep and red grouse are the only hosts which develop sufficiently intense viremia for the infection of ticks. However, it has been shown experimentally that the so-called phenomenon of nonviremic transmission of infection between ticks feeding on the same host, facilitated by factors present in tick saliva, occurs with LIV-infected and noninfected ticks co-feeding on mountain hares, which are important hosts of *Ix. ricinus* ticks. The same phenomenon has been demonstrated with TBEV-Eu, and this implies that there should be reassessment of the role of vertebrate hosts in the circulation of tick-borne viruses.

Spanish sheep encephalitis virus, Turkish sheep encephalitis virus, and Greek goat encephalitis virus are recently recognized subtypes of TBEV analogous to LIV that have been associated with encephalitis in sheep and goats in Spain, Greece, Bulgaria, and Turkey, but their distribution and epidemiology are as yet incompletely understood.

### Negishi Virus

A virus given the name Negishi virus (NEGV) was isolated in 1948 from a cerebrospinal fluid sample from a child near Tokyo with suspected Japanese encephalitis, and was found to be antigenically related to the tick-borne encephalitis group of flaviviruses. There were no further isolations of NEGV in Japan and recently the virus was found to be genetically closely related to LIV. However, in 1993 a virus was isolated from a patient with encephalitis in Hokkaido, the northern island of Japan where

*Ix. persulcatus* ticks occur, and subsequently the virus was also obtained from ticks and blood samples from dogs in Hokkaido. The new isolates proved to be phylogenetically most closely related to TBEV-FE.

### Further Reading

Billoir F, de Chesse R, Tolue H, de Micco P, Gould EA, and de Lamballerie X (2000) Phylogeny of the genus *Flavivirus* using complete coding sequences of arthropod-borne viruses and viruses with no known vector. *Journal of General Virology* 81: 781–790.

Cook S, Bennett SN, Holmes EC, de Chesse R, Moureau G, and de Lamballerie X (2006) Isolation of a new strain of the *Flavivirus* cell fusing agent virus in a natural mosquito population from Puerto Rico. *Journal of General Virology* 87: 735–748.

Cook S and Holmes EC (2006) A multigene analysis of the phylogenetic relationships among the *Flaviviruses* (family: *Flaviviridae*) and the evolution of vector transmission. *Archives of Virology* 151: 309–325.

Fauquet CM, Mayo MA, Maniloff J, Desselberger U, and Ball LA (eds.) (2005) *Virus Taxonomy: Eighth Report of the International Committee on Taxonomy of Viruses*. San Diego, CA: Elsevier Academic Press.

Grard G, Lemasson JJ, Sylla M, et al. (2006) Ngoye virus: A novel evolutionary lineage within the genus *Flavivirus*. *Journal of General Virology* 87: 3273–3277.

Grard G, Moureau G, Charrel RN, et al. (2006) Genetic characterization of tick-borne *Flaviviruses:* New insights into evolution, pathogenetic determinants and taxonomy. *Virology* 361: 80–92.

Kono Y, Tsukamoto K, and Hamid MABD (2001) Encephalitis and retarded growth of chicks caused by Sitiawan virus, a new isolate belonging to the genus *Flavivirus*. *American Journal of Tropical Medicine and Hygiene* 63: 94–101.

Pybus OG, Rambaut A, Holmes EC, and Harvey PH (2002) New inferences from tree shape: Numbers of missing taxa and population growth rates. *Systematic Biology* 51: 881–888.

# Foamy Viruses

**M L Linial,** Fred Hutchinson Cancer Research Center, Seattle, WA, USA

### Glossary

**Provirus** A viral DNA that is incorporated into the genetic material of a host cell.

**Syncytia** Structures in a monolayer cell culture formed by fusion of multiple cells that form a large cell with multiple nuclei.

**Zoonotic infection** An infection of animals that is transmitted to humans.

### Introduction

Foamy viruses (FVs, also known as spumaretroviruses or spumaviruses) have been known for over 50 years as the cause of cytopathic effects in cell cultures derived from monkey tissues. The original name, spumaviruses, is derived from the Latin word *spuma* for the foamy appearance of infected tissue culture cells. A foamy virus was isolated from a human-derived tissue culture in 1971 and called HFV for human foamy virus. The cell culture that yielded virus was obtained from a Kenyan patient with a nasopharyngeal carcinoma. At the time, this isolate was thought to be the first human retrovirus. Isolation of HFV generated a considerable amount of interest because of its possible link with human cancer. However, subsequent work over the past decade has definitively shown that the HFV isolate is a chimpanzee virus derived from the species of chimpanzee present in East Africa. This has led to the suggestion that the Kenyan patient had acquired FV through a zoonotic infection. This chimpanzee isolate is now designated PFV for prototype foamy virus. Unless otherwise indicated, the information in this article refers specifically to PFV.

## Epidemiology

FVs have been isolated from a number of hosts (**Table 1**), including all nonhuman primates (NHPs) that have been examined, as well as cats, cows, and horses. It is interesting that all species naturally infected with lentiviruses are also infected with harbor foamy viruses, although the reverse is not true. FV infection of natural hosts has not been linked to any pathologies. The widespread presence of FV suggests that it is part of the natural host microbial flora. In a small number of cases examined, infection of other species such as mice or rabbits has also failed to yield any manifestation of disease.

A large number of publications have suggested links between FVs and a variety of human diseases. However, ultimately none of these have been verified. Currently, there is no evidence of widespread infection of humans with FV. However, human infections are well documented. All the known cases can be traced to interactions with NHP. Veterinarians, primate center workers, bush meat hunters, pet owners, and people associated with monkey parks and monkey temples in Asia have been found to be infected. The frequency of infection in these high risk groups is about 2–3% of those examined. Humans have been shown to be infected by the presence of specific antibodies, and in some cases by sequencing provirus from peripheral blood cells. In the few cases examined, human-to-human transmission has not been observed. Recent studies have shown that primate FVs can be transmitted to monkeys via blood transfusions from naturally infected animals. Whether or not this would also be true for infected human blood is not known. Limited studies have been made to determine whether humans can be infected by feline FVs from domestic cats. To date, there is no evidence for human infection by these agents.

## Taxonomy and Classification

FVs are clearly retroviruses based on their genomic organization and general life cycle. However, they differ in fundamental ways from other retroviruses. These differences have led to their reclassification into a subfamily of *Retroviridae*. All other groups of retroviruses such as human immunodeficiency virus (HIV) are now called orthoretroviruses, or true retroviruses, while foamy viruses are spumaretroviruses (**Table 2**). Many aspects of their replication place FV closer to the hepadnaviruses such as human hepatitis B virus (HBV) than to orthoretroviruses.

## Viral Infections

Primate FV have been shown to have a very broad host range in tissue culture, with almost all vertebrate cell types being susceptible. In tissue culture, many cell types are lytically infected with virus. Such infected cells fuse to form large multinucleated cells, or syncytia. These syncytia rapidly die. Infected cells become filled with large numbers of vesicles, giving the cell cultures a foamy appearance (hence the name). An example of an FV-infected tissue culture is shown in **Figure 1**, using a hamster-derived indicator cell line in which infected cells stain blue. The arrows indicate multinucleate syncytia. However, some cell types in culture, including some

**Table 1**  Foamy virus isolates

| Host species | Virus isolate |
| --- | --- |
| Feline | FFV |
| Bovine | BFV |
| Equine | EFV |
| Rhesus macaque | SFVmac |
| African green monkey | SFVagm |
| Squirrel monkey | SFVsqu |
| Galago | SFVgal |
| Chimpanzee | SFVcpz |
| Spider monkey | SFVspm |
| Capuchin monkey | SFVcap |
| Baboon | SFVbab |
| Orangutan | SFVora |
| Gorilla | SFVgor |
| Marmoset | SFVmar |
| Human (not a natural host) | PFV (chimpanzee origin) |

**Table 2**  Classification of retroviruses (family *Retroviridae*)

| Subfamily | Genus | Type species |
| --- | --- | --- |
| *Orthoretrovirinae* (Orthoretrovirus) | *Alpharetrovirus* | *Avian leukosis virus* |
| | *Betaretrovirus* | *Mouse mammary tumor virus* |
| | *Gammaretrovirus* | *Murine leukemia virus* |
| | *Deltaretrovirus* | *Bovine leukemia virus* |
| | *Epsilonretrovirus* | *Walleye dermal sarcoma virus* |
| | *Lentivirus* | *Human immunodeficiency virus* |
| *Spumaretrovirinae* (Spumavirus) | *Spumavirus* | *Simian foamy virus* |

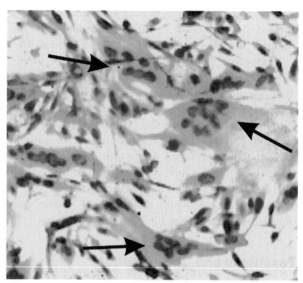

**Figure 1** Baby hamster kidney indicator cells infected with PFV. These cells contain an indicator gene that turns the cell nuclei blue after staining when the viral transactivator Tas is present. The arrows point to multinucleate syncytia formed by PFV infection.

human hematopoietic cell lines, are not killed after infection. Cell lines such as human Jurkat T cells are infected, evidenced by the presence of full-length viral DNA in the chromosomes. Few or no virions are produced from Jurkat cells, and there is no apparent effect on the health of the cells. These cell types are latently infected, and the infection persists indefinitely. The inability of virus to replicate in such persistent cultures may be caused by a transcriptional block. It appears that viral replication in tissue culture cells is invariably associated with cell death. However, it is not known whether or not this is true *in vivo*.

FV infections of organisms are lifelong in all species examined, including humans. There are no documented examples of viral clearance. Antibodies to viral proteins are present at all times after initial infection. Virus is believed to be transmitted between individuals through saliva. NHPs acquire the virus through biting or grooming. Young animals are not infected, and appear to be resistant to virus infection because of acquisition of maternal antibodies. Once such antibodies wane, serum conversion is rapid, and by 3 years of age, most animals are infected. In some populations of NHPs, infection reaches nearly 100% in adult animals. In naturally infected NHPs, viral DNA sequences can be found in most tissues, at very low levels. However, viral replication has only been documented in oral mucosal tissues, and virus is present in saliva. It is likely that FVs are latent in most tissues, and viral replication is confined to a small subset of cells in the oral mucosa. Such infected cells could secreted into saliva and be responsible for viral transmission.

## Virion Properties

FVs resemble other retroviruses in that they are fairly pleotropic in morphology, with large extracellular spikes. One distinct difference is that the FV core is electron lucent rather than condensed into a spherical core as in murine leukemia virus or into a cone-shaped core as in HIV (**Figure 2(a)**, red arrow). The morphology of mature, infectious FV resembles that of immature gammaretroviruses. Foamy virions have a density of about 1.16 gm ml$^{-1}$, as do orthoretroviruses. The infectious particles are surrounded by long spikes, composed of the viral glycoproteins encoded by the *env* gene (**Figure 2(a)**, purple dotted arrow). Like most retroviruses, FV bud from cellular membranes (**Figure 2(b)**, black arrow). Most often budding is from intracellular membranes, and the majority of virions remain cell associated. A cartoon of an FV particle is shown in **Figure 2(c)**. Virions are composed of two large structural proteins (Gag, blue ovals), surrounded by glycoprotein spikes (green). Particles contain the viral enzymes, including reverse transcriptase, encoded in the Pol protein (red). Like orthoretroviruses, FVs package RNA, but unlike orthoretroviruses, the infectious genome of FVs is double-stranded DNA (dsDNA) (depicted by black lines), implying that reverse transcription occurs during assembly and/or budding (see below). Because of the mechanism of Pol synthesis, there are many fewer Pol molecules per foamy virion compared to the orthoretroviruses.

## Genome and Protein Organization and Expression

Foamy viruses are complex retroviruses. Their genomes are greater than 12 kb (**Figure 3(a)**), placing them among the largest retroviruses. They encode the three genes common to all retroviruses (*gag, pol,* and *env*), as well as additional genes (*tas* and *tas/bel2* encoding Bet), whose gene products are not virion associated (**Figure 3(b)**). The Gag, Pol, and Env gene products are all polyproteins that are cleaved by proteases to smaller mature products. The Gag and Pol precursor proteins are cleaved by the viral protease (PR) encoded within the Pol protein (cleavage sites are indicated by the yellow arrows), whereas the Env precursor protein is cleaved by a cellular furin-like protease (indicated by the white arrows). The Gag protein is synthesized from an RNA that is indistinguishable from the viral genome. The Pol and Env proteins are synthesized from spliced mRNAs that utilize the same 5' splice site (5'ss) but different 3' splice sites (**Figure 3(c)**). Synthesis of Env from a spliced mRNA is common to all retroviruses. In contrast, synthesis of Pol from a spliced RNA is unique to FV. Orthoretroviruses synthesize Pol as a Gag–Pol read-through protein from genomic RNA. Since the orthoretrovirus precursor

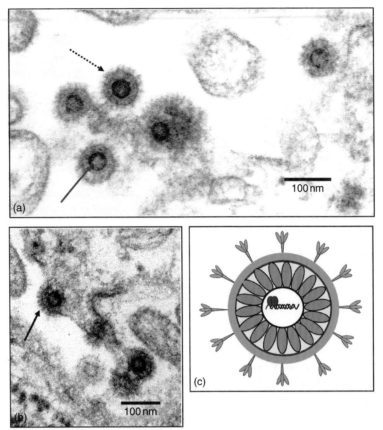

**Figure 2** Morphology of foamy virus particles. (a, b) Negatively stained electron micrographs of tissue culture cells infected with PFV. (a) Intracellular particles; (b) budding particle; (c) depiction of a mature particle. The viral Gag proteins are shown in blue, the Env proteins in green, and the Pol proteins in red. The DNA genome is indicated by the black helix.

Pol protein has Gag determinants, it is co-assembled with Pol into virions. Lack of Gag determinants on FV Pol (**Figure 3(d)**) indicates that Pol encapsidation into virions occurs by a different mechanism. Tas and Bet are synthesized from a second promoter (IP) and Bet is made from a spliced mRNA joining part of *tas* to *bel2* (**Figure 3(c)**).

There are several noticeable differences in organization of the FV Gag, Pol, and Env proteins compared to orthoretroviruses (**Figure 3(b)**). The FV Gag is only cleaved once by PR at a site near the C-terminus and there are no mature cleavage products analogous to the matrix, capsid, or nucleocapsid proteins of orthoretroviruses. FV Gag lacks the hallmarks of other retroviral Gag proteins such as the cysteine–histidine boxes and the major homology region (MHR). The only distinct feature of FV Gag is the presence of three glycine-arginine-rich (GR) boxes near the C-terminus of the protein. These are involved in assembly and/or RNA binding. Most retroviral Gag proteins have a post-translational modification that adds a myristylation signal at the N-terminus. However, this does not occur in foamy viruses. The Pol protein encodes the four enzymatic activities associated with all

retroviruses: PR, reverse transcriptase (RT) with its associated RNase H activity (RH), and integrase (IN). However, only one cleavage occurs in Pol, leading to a PR–RT (RH) fusion protein and an IN protein. The Env protein is composed of three subunits. In addition to the usual surface (SU) and transmembrane (TM) proteins, there is an N-terminal leader peptide (LP). The LP is equivalent to the signal peptide of other retroviruses that is cleaved and discarded. However, in FV, the LP is incorporated into particles with the same stoichiometry as SU and TM. In orthoretroviruses, the signal peptide is not incorporated into particles.

FVs also encode two proteins which are not found in virions, Tas and Bet. They are translated from mRNAs transcribed from the internal promoter located within the *env* coding region (IP; **Figure 3(c)**). Tas is a transcriptional transactivator, which binds to sequences in both the long terminal repeat (LTR) promoter and the IP, although the sites have different sequences. The IP has a higher affinity for Tas, and is activated first after infection. When additional Tas is synthesized from the IP, the level becomes high enough to allow transcription from the LTR and production of the virion proteins Gag, Pol, and Env.

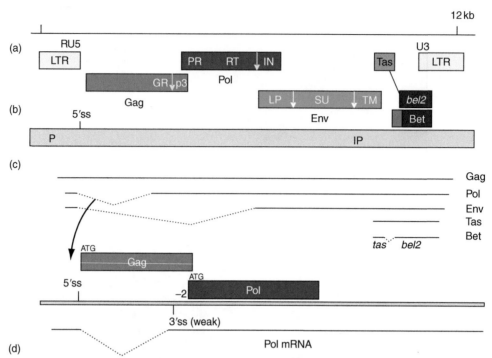

**Figure 3** Viral genome. (a, b) The size of the PFV proviral genome and all of the gene products. The long terminal repeats (LTRs) contain the regulatory elements created by reverse transcription of the viral genomic RNA, duplicating RU5 and U3. The yellow arrows show sites of cleavage by the viral protease, the white arrows show sites of cleavage by a cellular protease. The Gag gene encodes the structural proteins. GR indicates three glycine-arginine-rich regions. One cleavage event occurs releasing a 3 kDa peptide (p3). The Pol gene contains the three enzymatic domains, protease (PR), reverse transcriptase (RT), and integrase (IN). The Env gene contains three domains, leader peptide (LP) unique to foamy viruses, surface (SU), and TM (transmembrane). Tas is the viral transactivator protein, and Bet is made from two exons, Tas and *bel2*. The function of Bet is not completely understood. (c) The location of the two viral promoters; The canonical retroviral promoter (P) in the LTR and the unique internal promoter (IP) encoded within the *env* gene. 5′ss indicates the major splice site. Indicated below are the major mRNAs. (d) The unique spliced mRNA that gives rise to the Pol protein. ATG indicates the start sites for translation. Adapted from Linial ML (1999) Foamy viruses are unconventional retroviruses. *Journal of Virology* 73: 1747–1755, with permission from American Society for Microbiology.

A block at the transcriptional level, preventing sufficient Tas to be synthesized to allow LTR transcription, is thought to occur in latent infections. Some latently infected cells can be activated by protein kinase C pathway activators, leading to viral production and ultimately to cell death. The second nonstructural protein, Bet, is an approximately 60 kDa protein with no obvious functional domains. Although all foamy virus Bet proteins have some similarities, there are no other proteins encoded by any organism with homology. Although the function of Bet is unknown, there are many tantalizing findings. Bet is both nuclear and cytoplasmic, and is also released from cells. It can be taken up by uninfected cells and there is some evidence that it can prevent infection. Although primate foamy virus Bet has not been found to be required for viral infectivity, it does appear to be required for replication of feline FV in some tissue culture cells. The role of Bet in infections of animals has not been assessed. Overexpression of Bet appears to have some effect on activation of the LTR promoter by Tas. Most recently, a number of groups have shown that Bet can inhibit the antiretroviral

effects of the host protein APOBEC3, which is also an inhibitor of HIV and other retroviruses. However, the exact function(s) of Bet in viral replication *in vitro* and *in vivo* remains to be determined.

## Viral Life Cycle

An overview of the FV life cycle is depicted in **Figure 4**. The steps in viral replication that differ in some aspects from those of orthoretroviruses are shown in red text. Some aspects of the viral life cycle are similar to that of the Hepadnaviruses such as hepatitis B virus (HBV), as indicated below.

1. *Viral entry.* The receptor(s) have not been identified for any foamy viruses. Identification is made difficult by the lack of cells that are resistant which could be used for selection. FV entry has been shown to use a pH-dependent endocytic pathway that is resistant to chloroquine, showing that the details of entry differ from that of the well-studied vesicular stomatitis virus.

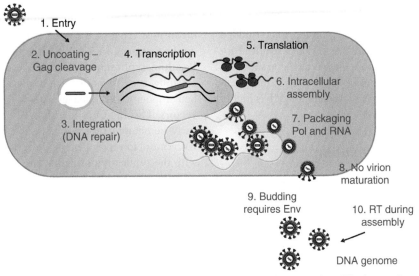

**Figure 4** Viral life cycle. The major events in FV replication are indicated, with the steps that differ from orthoretroviruses indicated in red. For details, see text.

*2. Uncoating.* FV Gag proteins are only cleaved once upon assembly/release by the viral protease PR. However, during viral entry, at least one additional PR cleavage occurs, which is required for infectivity. Presumably, this cleavage is important for uncoating of the viral capsid to release viral nucleic acid. Incoming particles traffic to the cellular microtubule organizing center (MTOC).

*3. Integration.* Although virions contain both RNA and DNA, the infectious genome is double-stranded linear DNA, reverse transcription having occurred late in the replication cycle (step 10, below). FVs share the property of packaging RNA but having DNA genomes with HBV. FV integration appears to occur in a manner similar to orthoretroviruses, although some repair of the dsDNA may occur at this step. The viral integrase (IN) is required for productive infection.

*4 and 5. Transcription and translation.* These occur as in other retroviruses using cellular machinery. As noted above, FV transcription from the two promoters requires the viral DNA binding protein Tas. Unlike other complex retroviruses in the genera *Deltaretrovirus* and *Lentivirus*, no viral proteins have been shown to be involved in RNA splicing and/or export of unspliced RNA from the nucleus. A region in the LTR which is present in both *gag* and subgenomic RNAs is necessary for efficient translation of Gag and Pol proteins.

*6–8. FV assembly and Pol and RNA packaging.* FV assembly occurs intracellularly, rather than at the plasma membrane, in a manner similar to that of Mason–Pfizer monkey virus (MPMV), a type D simian retrovirus. Like MPMV, FV Gag contains a cytoplasmic targeting and retention signal (CTRS) that is required for viral assembly. Newly synthesized Gag traffics to the MTOC which appears to be involved at some stage of viral assembly. RNA is

incorporated into particles through a specific region of the RNA that interacts with one or more of the arginine-rich GR boxes. The RNA sequence is not exclusively located near the $5'$ of the RNA where orthoretroviral packaging sequences (psi) are located. The FV psi sequence is more complex, and appears to include additional sequences encoded within the *pol* gene. The FV Pol protein is synthesized from a spliced mRNA and lacks Gag sequences. Thus, encapsidation is not through Gag assembly domains. Instead, viral RNA is required for Pol packaging. The Pol encapsidation sequences, like psi, are complex and involve both the U5 region of the LTR as well as sequences at the $3'$ end of the *pol* gene. Protein–protein interactions of Gag and Pol may be required for Pol encapsidation. Because of the requirement for RNA sequences for binding, fewer Pol particles are packaged than in orthoretroviruses. As described above, cleavage of Gag into smaller subunits does not occur. This probably is responsible for the morphology of infectious virions that resemble immature retroviruses lacking a condensed core.

*9. Budding.* Orthoretroviral particles can bud from cells in the absence of the envelope glycoproteins, although the presence of Env can increase the efficiency of their release. In contrast, FVs absolutely require Env proteins to bud from cells, reminiscent of HBV. The component of FV Env that is required for particle egress has been mapped to the N-terminus of the LP protein. In the absence of LP intracellular particles accumulate. In general, FV budding is quite inefficient with a vast majority of infectivity remaining cell associated. It is likely that transmission from infected to naive animals occurs via cell-associated virus, rather than free virus.

*10. Reverse transcription.* Unlike orthoretroviruses but similar to HBVs, reverse transcription of the FV RNA genome occurs during assembly. The mechanism of reverse transcription appears to be identical to that of orthoretroviruses, using a $tRNA_{lys1,2}$ as a primer. Budded virions contain full-length dsDNA that it is required for infectivity. DNA extracted from virions has been shown to be infectious when fused into cells. The RT is unique in that it also contains the protease domain. FV RT is highly active and processive *in vitro*.

## Viral Genetics and Evolution

FVs are the most ancient of retroviruses, and of all RNA viruses. It is estimated that they have been present in NHP populations for over 60 million years and in Old World primates for over 30 million years. They appear to have cospeciated with their hosts. The lack of significant homologies to orthoretroviruses in their Gag proteins, suggest that they may have evolved separately from orthoretroviruses. FV viral genomes are very stable and there is much less sequence diversity than seen with other retroviruses, either within or between species. The viral RT appears to be as error prone as that of other retroviruses, so the low sequence diversity may reflect the lower total viral load per animal, as replication is confined to the oral mucosa. It is assumed that FVs undergo recombination and reassortment as seen in the other genera, but this has not been studied.

## Viral Vectors

Orthoretroviruses, including murine leukemia virus and HIV, have been developed into vectors for gene therapy applications. The large genome size, the broad host range, and especially the nonpathogenic nature of FV, have made them excellent candidates for gene therapy vector development. While simian and feline FVs have been developed as vectors, most work has been concentrated on PFV. Vector development has been the impetus for much of the present information about the replication and infection by FVs. FVs are rather stable. They cannot complete replication in nondividing tissue culture cells. If nondividing cells are infected, FVs can apparently persist in the quiescent cells until the cells become activated. At that time, viral infection proceeds and the FV genome integrates into the host chromosome. Viral integrations into normal human cells do not occur preferentially within genes although there is a significant preference for GC-rich regions of the genome.

Thus far, it has not been possible to create stable packaging cell lines which contain all of the viral gene products. Instead, as in the case of HIV, cells are transfected with three vectors encoding separately the *gag, pol,* or *env* genes, and a fourth vector encoding the gene of interest embedded in an RNA containing the RNA and Pol packaging sequences. FV cannot be pseudotyped with vesicular stomatis virus glycoproteins (VSV G), so the cognate FV Env protein is used. This has an equally broad host range as VSV G. The vectors do not use the viral promoters, so the Tas gene product is not required. Resulting replication-defective FV vectors have been successfully used in both mice and dogs to repopulate all hematopoeitic cell lineages with the gene encoded by the vectors. This indicates that the vectors can integrate into early hematopoietic stem cells. Work proceeds on using FV vectors to repair genetic defects, and also to interfere with the replication of pathogens, such as HIV. Thus far, no human trials with FV vectors have been reported.

## Future Perspectives

There are currently two major foci of current foamy virus research. The first is the continued development and refinement of vectors for a variety of applications. The published results thus far have been encouraging and human trials are probably not far away. The second area is surveillance of human populations at risk for FV infection. The progenitors of HIV are apparently not pathogenic in their natural hosts, and the human pathogen arose by recombination between two monkey viruses with a chimpanzee intermediate host. There are obvious parallels with FVs, where humans are increasingly in contact with NHP harboring a variety of FV. Future studies need to determine whether or not humans shed virus in saliva, and if human-to-human transmission can be documented. But many other interesting questions remain to be determined. It is not known how FVs have adapted so perfectly to their hosts, while maintaining the ability to be highly cytopathic, at least *in vitro*. The intricate control mechanisms could reveal new strategies for dealing with other cytopathic retroviruses such as HIV. There are many unanswered questions about the unique FV replication pathway. How is Pol packaged into virions? Why is FV RT activated during assembly whereas HIV RT is not activated until after infection of new cells? What is the FV receptor? Where do the interactions between Gag and Env occur and how do they allow viruses to bud from cells? We have just begun to scratch the surface in unraveling the replication of these fascinating retroviruses.

*See also:* Feline Leukemia and Sarcoma Viruses; Simian Retrovirus D; Vesicular Stomatitis Virus.

## Further Reading

Lecellier C-H and Saïb A (2000) Foamy viruses: Between retroviruses and pararetroviruses. *Virology* 271: 1–8.
Linial ML (1999) Foamy viruses are unconventional retroviruses. *Journal of Virology* 73: 1747–1755.

Linial ML (2007) Foamy viruses. In: Knipe DM and Howley PM (eds.) *Fields Virology*, 5th edn., ch. 60, pp. 2245–2262. Philadelphia: Lippincott Williams and Wilkins.

Meiering CD and Linial ML (2001) Historical perspective of foamy virus epidemiology and infection. *Clinical Microbiology Reviews* 14: 165–176.

Murray SM and Linial ML (2006) Foamy virus infections in primates. Review. *Journal of Medical Primatology* 35: 225–235.

Trobridge G, Vassilopoulos G, Josephson N, and Russell DW (2002) Gene transfer with foamy virus vectors. *Methods in Enzymology* 346: 628–648.

# Foot and Mouth Disease Viruses

**D J Rowlands**, University of Leeds, Leeds, UK

## Glossary

**Serotype** Animals recovered from infection with a virus belonging to a given serotype are resistant to subsequent infection with viruses belonging to that serotype but are still susceptible to infection with viruses belonging to any of the other serotypes.

## History

The earliest account that clearly describes foot-and-mouth disease (FMD) was made by Fracastorius in 1546 and it is still today one of the most important diseases of domestic livestock.

It was the first animal disease demonstrated to be caused by a filterable agent in 1897 by Loeffler and Frosch, who also demonstrated the presence of neutralizing antibody in serum. It is also the first virus for which serotype differences were recognized. Further milestones were the demonstration by Waldemann and Pope in 1921 that guinea pigs could be infected and by Skinner in 1951 that it caused a lethal infection in suckling mice. Subsequently, cultivation of the virus in tissue culture cells has enabled studies of viral structure and replication and also the large-scale production of vaccines.

## Taxonomy and Classification

Foot-and-mouth disease viruses (FMDVs) are a species within the genus *Aphthovirus* of the family *Picornaviridae*. The nature and organization of the genome, mode of replication, and structure of the virion are, in general, similar to other viruses in the family. The subdivision of the *Picornaviridae* into four genera, *Enterovirus*, *Rhinovirus*, *Cardiovirus*, and *Aphthovirus*, was originally based on physicochemical properties such as susceptibility to acid inactivation, buoyant density of CsCl solution, and the nucleotide composition. Analyses of evolutionary relationships by nucleotide sequence comparisons have largely endorsed the original classifications; however, the family has now expanded to include nine genera. Of special note is the recent inclusion of equine rhinitis A virus (ERAV) in the genus *Aphthovirus*. Properties which distinguish the FMDVs are: (1) extreme sensitivity to acid inactivation ($<$ pH 6.8 in low ionic strength buffer); (2) high buoyant density in CsCl ($1.43–1.50 \, g \, cm^{-3}$); (3) possession of a poly (C) tract in the 5' untranslated region (UTR) of the RNA (a property shared with some cardioviruses); (4) three separately encoded VPg proteins; (5) the use of two alternative in-frame protein translation initiation sites; and (6) a leader protease protein located in the N-terminal region of the polyprotein.

## Properties of the Virion

As for other picornaviruses, FMDV particles are non-enveloped icosahedrons comprising 60 copies each of four structural proteins, VP1–VP4, encapsidating a single copy of the single-stranded positive-sense genomic RNA. The crystallographic structure of the virus (**Figure 1**) has shown that the three larger proteins (VP1–VP3) have the eight-stranded antiparallel β-barrel folding motif seen in other picornaviruses and some plant viruses. VP4 is disposed on the inner surface of the particle. In common with other picornaviruses, VP1 molecules are located around the axes of fivefold symmetry whereas VP2 and VP3 alternate around the two- and threefold symmetry axes. Heat or acid degradation of the particles results in dissociation into pentameric subunits, consisting of five copies each of VP1–VP3, with release of the RNA and VP4.

Several features of the structure are unique to FMDV. The protein shell is generally thinner and the external surface is smoother than in other picornaviruses. This is a result of the smaller sizes of VP1–VP3 (VP1 213, VP2 218, VP3 220 amino acids for serotype O1 virus) compared to other picornaviruses. The truncations are in the

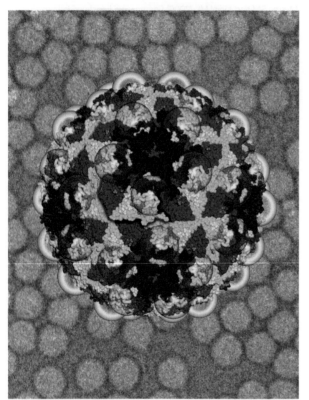

**Figure 1** CPK rendition of reduced FMDV, serotype O superimposed on a cryoelectron micrograph of particles. Color codes: VP1, blue; VP2, green; VP3, red (VP4 is internal and not visible in these views). The VP1 G–H loop is shown as a worm in cyan with the Arg-Gly-Asp residues in orange CPK. Antigenic residues are color-coded according to their classification into sites: sites 1 and 5 (mid-blue), site 2 (pale yellow), site 3 (light blue), site 4 (magenta). The potential occupancy of the mobile VP1 G–H loop is modeled by a transparent sphere centered at the midpoint between the two ends of the loop. A protomeric subunit is outlined in black. Courtesy of E. Fry and D. Stuart.

loop regions linking the core elements of the β barrels, which in other picornaviruses form prominent features at the outer surface. The deep grooves or pits encircling the fivefold axes of many picornaviruses are not present in FMDV and the position equivalent to these invaginations is occupied by the C-terminal portion of VP1. An important exception to the generally smooth contours of the surface of FMDV is provided by the G–H loop of VP1 (**Figure 1**). This large loop extends from about residue 130 to 160 of which residues around 135–158 are too disordered to be visible in electron density maps. In serotype O1 viruses, the disorder of the VP1 G–H loop is induced by a disulfide bond between the cystine residues VP2 130 and VP1 134. Under reducing conditions this bond is broken and the G–H loop collapses onto the surface of the virus in an ordered configuration. This feature includes an immuno-dominant antigenic site to which a high proportion of virus-neutralizing antibodies are directed. Also, synthetic peptides representing sequences from this region are immunogenic and can induce protective immunity. The sequence of this region is variable both in composition and length between different viruses with the exception of a highly conserved receptor binding motif which includes the triplet, Arg, Gly, Asp (see the section titled 'Cell attachment and entry').

## Properties of the Genome

The genome consists of a single molecule of single-stranded positive-sense RNA, which is infectious. The order of the gene products on the genome is basically similar to other picornaviruses but there are some unique features (**Figure 2**). The genomic RNA terminates at the

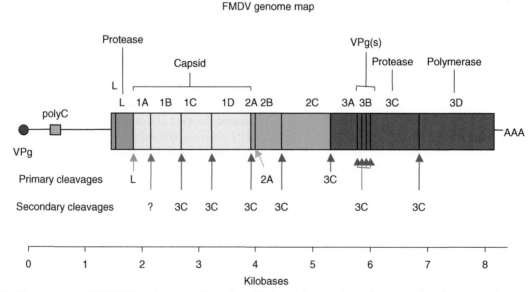

**Figure 2** Genome map of FMDV. Boxed region is the polyprotein translation product with processing sites arrowed.

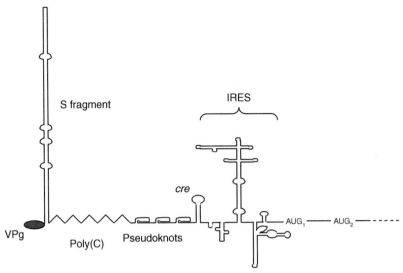

Structure of the 5′ end of FMDV RNA

**Figure 3** Secondary structure prediction for the 5′ UTR of FMDV RNA with major functional motifs individually labeled.

5′ untranslated end with a small protein, VPg, linked by a phosphodiester bond through a Tyr. There is a variable length of poly(A) tract at the 3′ end. Uniquely, the FMDV genome encodes three distinct VPgs, which are used with equal efficiency. The reasons for this gene triplication are unknown. In fact, virus derived from an infectious cDNA clone from which one or two of the VPg copies had been deleted is still infectious, although RNA synthesis is reduced. The 5′ UTR is exceptionally long (*c.* 1300 nt), even by picornavirus standards (**Figure 3**). There is an uninterrupted poly(C) tract of 100–200 residues, depending on the virus isolate, located *c.* 400 nt from the 5′ end. The function of the poly(C) tract is unknown and it is not present in ERAV. There is evidence from FMDV and mengovirus (a cardiovirus) that the length of poly(C) is related to pathogenicity.

The sequence between the 5′ end and the poly(C) tract has a high degree of secondary structure and is predicted to fold into an almost complete hairpin. Its function is unknown but by analogy to the highly structured 5′ sequence of poliovirus RNA it is likely to be involved in the control of RNA replication. To the 3′ side of the poly(C) tract there are a variable number of repeat domains that are predicted to fold as pseudoknot structures. The 3′ 435 nucleotides of the 5′ UTR fold into a series of stem/loop structures similar to those present in the equivalent region of cardiovirus 5′ UTRs and function as an internal ribosome entry site (IRES) to initiate protein synthesis. A stem/loop structure (*cre – cis*-active replication element), located between the pseudoknots and the IRES, functions as a template for the uridylation of VPg, which is an essential step in the initiation of viral RNA synthesis.

## Protein Products

The protein-coding region is a continuous open reading frame of 6999 or 6915 nt for FMDV serotype A[10], depending on which of two functional in-frame initiation codons is used. The order of the gene products is shown in **Figure 2**.

*Leader protein.* The leader protein(s), Lab and Lb, which precede the structural proteins, have a proteolytic function which cleaves at the L–P1 junction and also affects the cell translation machinery (see the section titled 'Translation'). Lb can perform all of the known functions of L and the significance of Lab is unknown, although presence of two polyprotein initiation sites is completely conserved. The L proteins are not essential for virus viability since virus derived from an infectious clone with deleted L domain can replicate. However, it has an attenuated phenotype and has been proposed as a candidate live vaccine.

*P1 region.* The P1 region consists of the structural proteins 1A, 1B, 1C, and 1D, which are equivalent to VP4, VP2, VP3, and VP1, respectively.

*P2 region.* The 2A protein is vestigial in size compared to other picornaviruses, being only 18 amino acids long, but it enables the nascent separation of the polyprotein at the 2A–2B junction. 2C has a nucleoside triphosphate binding motif and it appears to have a role in RNA replication since amino acid changes in this protein can relieve the inhibition of RNA synthesis seen in the presence of guanidine. The precursor protein 2BC influences membrane trafficking in infected cells, a role performed by 3A in poliovirus.

*P3 region.* The role of 3A in FMDV is unclear but it does not seem to function in a similar manner to the 3A protein of poliovirus, which serves as a membrane-bound donor of VPg during viral RNA synthesis.

3B or VPg occurs as three tandem copies of 23, 24, and 24 amino acids. Although differing in sequence, each is rich in Pro, Arg, and Lys residues and has a single Tyr at position 3. Each of the individual VPg molecules is highly conserved between the A, O, and C serotype viruses. The VPg molecules are post-translationally modified to function as primers in RNA synthesis (see next section). All encapsidated RNA molecules terminate with a VPg molecule and each of the three forms is found in equal abundance. Actively translating viral RNA lacks VPg, and cell extracts contain an enzyme that cleaves the phosphodiester bond to produce RNA terminating with a 5′-monophosphate. The observation that all virion-associated RNA terminates in VPg suggests that it may have a role in the selection of molecules for encapsidation. Mutagenesis experiments with an infectious cDNA clone have provided some support for this conclusion.

$3C^{pro}$ is the protease responsible for the majority of the processing cleavages. In common with other picornaviruses, sequence analysis suggests that the catalytic site of $3C^{pro}$ is related to trypsin, a serine protease, but with the replacement of the nucleophilic serine residue with cysteine.

$3D^{pol}$ is the RNA-dependent RNA polymerase responsible for RNA replication and VPg uridylation (see next section). The crystal structure has been solved in the apo form and in complex with primer and template.

The 3CD precursor has a distinct function as a catalyst for the $3D^{pol}$-mediated uridylation of VPg.

The molecular structures of virus particles, $L^{pro}$, $3C^{pro}$, $3D^{pro}$, and precursor 3CD have all been determined by X-ray crystallography.

## RNA Replication

RNA of infecting virus functions as a template for the synthesis of a negative-sense complementary strand, which serves, in turn, as template for the synthesis of positive-sense strands, identical to the original infecting molecule. Positive strands are synthesized in a complex structure (replicative intermediate (RI)) consisting of a single negative-strand template and several (around six) nascent positive strands. RNA synthesis is asymmetrical in favor of positive strands. A proportion of the negative-strand templates occur as full-length double-stranded hybrids (replicative form (RF)) and appear to take no further part in RNA synthesis. RF molecules accumulate in the cell during viral replication. Each RNA replication event is initiated by priming with a uridylated VPg molecule.

A single molecule of viral RNA is sufficient to initiate infection, which implies that it can function sequentially as a template for translation, to produce the polymerase enzyme(s), and as a template for RNA replication.

Single-stranded viral RNA is infectious in the presence of inhibitors of host cell DNA-dependent RNA polymerase. Double-stranded viral RNA is also infectious but not in the presence of inhibitors of the cellular polymerases.

## Translation

FMDV RNA is efficiently translated in a cell-free system (rabbit reticulocyte lysate) to produce protein products similar to those found in infected cells. The 435 nucleotides upstream of the first AUG initiation codon are folded into a complex structure similar to that of the equivalent region of cardiovirus RNAs. This sequence acts as an IRES, allowing initiation of translation in the absence of the host cell cap-binding complex. The rate of total protein synthesis in virus-infected cells does not change until its decline toward the end of the growth cycle, when cytopathic effects (CPEs) are apparent. There is, however, a marked change in the profile of proteins produced. When viral replication is maximal, virtually no host cell proteins are produced. This 'swapover' of translation from host to viral products is similar to the situation in cardiovirus-infected cells and differs from the kinetics of translation following infection of cells with entero- or rhinoviruses. In the latter, infection results in a rapid shutdown of host cell protein translation, which is followed later by a resumption of protein synthesis due to the increasing production of viral proteins. The shutdown induced by entero- and rhinoviruses is largely, if not entirely, due to a virus-induced cleavage of a host protein, p220 or eIF4G, an important component of the cap-binding complex required for the initiation of translation of host mRNAs. In these viruses, eIF4G cleavage is indirectly induced by $2A^{pro}$ protease. Cardioviruses do not induce eIF4G cleavage and appear to simply outcompete host mRNAs for utilization of the translation machinery. Although the kinetics of protein translation in FMDV-infected cells resemble those of cardiovirus-infected cells, eIF4G is cleaved. In contrast to entero- and rhinoviruses, FMDV cleavage of eIF4G is not induced by 2A but by L. $3C^{pro}$ can also cleave eIF4G but at a different site from $L^{pro}$ and later in the infection cycle. Inhibition of host cell protein synthesis is likely to be of advantage to the virus both by removing competition for access to the translation machinery and also by inhibiting the expression of innate immunity response genes in infected cells.

## Post-Translation Processing

The polyprotein translation product of FMDV RNA is proteolytically processed by three of four virus-encoded enzyme activities (**Figure 2**). Three of the cleavages occur nascently on the growing polypeptide chain. The first separates L from P1, the structural protein precursor, and is carried out by leader protein. The cleavage is within a Lys-Gly dipeptide and probably occurs normally in *cis* but can also occur in *trans*. L–P1 cleavage is the only processing step which is inhibited by the tripeptide D-Val-Phe-Lys-CH$_2$Cl. Both Lb and Lab are proteolytically active.

The second primary cleavage occurs at the junction of 2A and 2B and is catalyzed by the 18-amino-acid 2A sequence. There is good evidence that the mechanism of 'cleavage' at the 2A/2B junction involves a novel process of interrupted translation, referred to as ribosomal skipping, rather than proteolytic cleavage.

The third primary cleavage is between 2C and 3A and is catalyzed by 3C$^{pro}$ protease. This protease is responsible for all other processing cleavages, apart from that which generates VP2 (1B) and VP4 (1A) from the precursor VP0 (1AB). Many cleavages catalyzed by 3C$^{pro}$ protease occur at Glu-Gly junctions but other dipeptides are recognized and 3C$^{pro}$ of FMDV is the most promiscuous of the picornavirus proteases. The cleavage event to produce VP2 and VP4 from the precursor, VP0, occurs in the final stages of virus maturation. The mechanism of this cleavage is not known.

## Virus Assembly and Release

A variety of assembly intermediates containing equimolar amounts of VP1, VP2, and VP0 are detected in infected cells. These correspond to monomer and pentamer subunits of the icosahedral capsid and 75S empty particles, which lack viral RNA but possess antigenic properties similar to mature viral particles. Following pulse-labeling experiments, empty particles can be 'chased' into viral particles, but it has not been shown that they are on the direct morphogenetic pathway. All encapsidated RNA terminates with VPg, suggesting that this plays a role in selection. Altered VPg molecules within an infectious cDNA clone are less efficiently encapsidated.

Paracrystalline arrays of virus are visible in infected cells and are released by lysis of the cell. There is evidence that some viral particles are secreted prior to cell disruption.

## Cell Attachment and Entry

The large mobile G–H loop of VP1 located at the surface of FMDV particles mediates their binding to susceptible cells. The sequence of the loop contains a highly conserved motif, Arg, Gly, Asp, which is the hallmark of ligands for a number of heterodimeric cell surface molecules called integrins. Synthetic peptides including this

sequence can compete with virus for cell attachment and treatment of the virus with proteolytic enzymes such as trypsin, which cleave within the G–H loop, also prevents virus binding. Although the virus can bind to a number of integrins there is good evidence that $\alpha_v\beta_6$ is the preferred receptor *in vivo*.

Following attachment the virus is internalized by endocytosis and release of the RNA is triggered by acidification in early endosomes. Reduction of the pH below ~6.8 seems to be all that is required to initiate the infection process and the mechanism by which the genome is delivered to the cytoplasm is unknown. Many tissue-culture-adapted strains of the virus have evolved *in vitro* to use heparin sulfate at cell surface as an alternative receptor.

## Geographic Distribution

FMD occurs widely and is endemic in many countries, especially in tropical regions (**Figures 4** and **5**). North America, Australia, New Zealand, and Japan are free of the disease and maintain this status by rigorous application of import controls and quarantine. Mass vaccination campaigns have virtually eliminated the virus from some areas, for example, Europe, but have been less effective in others, largely due to logistical problems of vaccine distribution and the techniques of animal husbandry employed. The global distribution of the serotypes is shown in **Figures 4** and **5**.

## Host Range and Viral Propagation

The virus typically infects cloven-hoofed species with domestic cattle being the most susceptible. Domestic pigs are also important hosts and are particularly effective in propagating the disease, since they secrete large quantities of virus in the form of aerosols. In sheep and goats, the clinical manifestations of infection are usually less severe than those seen in cattle and pigs. Natural infection of Indian elephants and of camels has been reported. Many wild species of deer and antelope are susceptible to infection, and in African Cape buffalo infection is asymptomatic. Persistent infection with prolonged shedding of virus for months or years has been reported in wild and domestic species. A wide range of animals, including Australian marsupials and birds, have been infected under laboratory conditions and, very rarely, infection of human has been demonstrated.

The most important small animals for laboratory investigations are the guinea pig and the suckling mouse. In the former, injection of virus intradermally into plantar pads results in the formation of vesicular lesions both at the site of injection and in the mouth and the remaining feet, and so resembles the lesion distribution in naturally

Eurasian serotypes, 2000–06

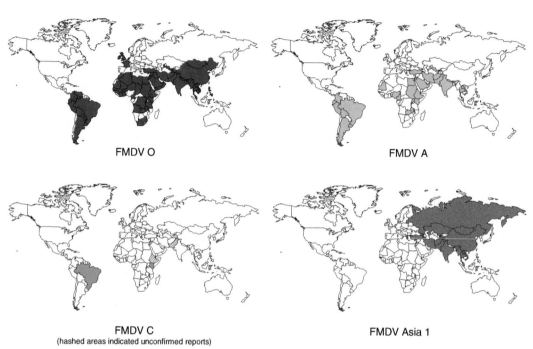

**Figure 4**   Global distribution of FMDV serotypes O, A, C, and Asia 1 between 2000 and 2006. Courtesy of N. Knowles.

SAT serotypes, 2000–06

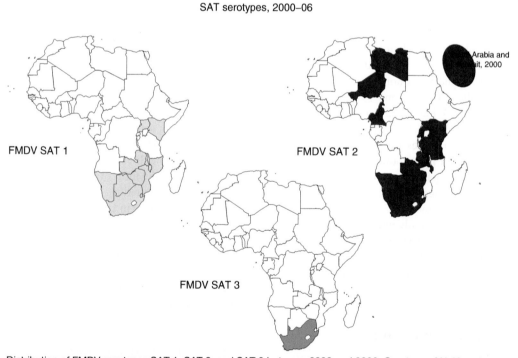

**Figure 5**   Distribution of FMDV serotypes SAT 1, SAT 2, and SAT 3 between 2000 and 2006. Courtesy of N. Knowles.

infected susceptible species. Intraperitoneal infection of suckling mice results in rapid death. The viruses can be propagated in primary cells and cell lines of bovine or porcine origin. Cells derived from the BHK-21 line are most widely used for research or vaccine production purposes. The virus can be titrated by plaque assay in cultured cell monolayers or by cytopathic end point dilution assay in microtiter plates.

## Genetics and Evolution

In common with other RNA viruses, the mutation rate is extremely high and virus populations exist as quasispecies in which each individual genome is likely to differ from every other. Antigenic sites on the viral particle are tolerant of sequence variation, and antigenic diversity is a significant property of the virus.

In addition to evolution by the accumulation of point mutation, genomic recombination occurs at a high rate *in vitro*. The frequency and genomic location of recombinatorial events mirror the genetic relatedness of the parental viruses.

## Serological Relationships and Variability

Seven serotypes of FMDV are recognized, the distinction of serotypes being that an animal convalescent from infection by virus of one serotype is fully susceptible to viruses of any of the remaining six. In addition to the major serotype differences, there is considerable antigenic variation between viruses within serotypes. The serological relationships between FMDV isolates are paralleled by genetic relationships as evidenced by RNA sequence analyses (**Figure 6**).

For epidemiological studies and vaccine strain selection, the serological relationships between field virus isolates or laboratory strains are expressed as *r* values, that is, the ratio of the neutralizing titers of immune sera against heterologous and homologous viruses. The serological relationships between virus isolates are frequently nonreciprocal, showing that closely related viruses may induce broadly cross-reactive or narrowly specific immune responses. Complement fixation assay and enzyme-linked immunosorbent assay (ELISA) using polyclonal sera or monoclonal antibodies are also used for epidemiological studies.

## Epidemiology

In regions endemic for FMD, the virus is most likely maintained in persistently infected animals. It has been shown experimentally that infected bovines can secrete virus for long periods after the initial episode of disease. In some areas the wild animal population may act as a

Genetic relationships between the seven serotypes of
foot-and-mouth disease virus

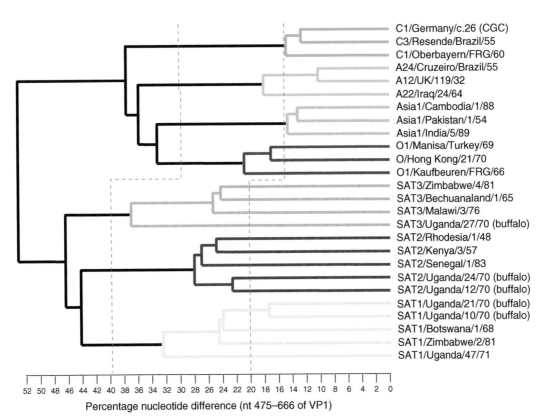

C1/Germany/c.26 (CGC)
C3/Resende/Brazil/55
C1/Oberbayern/FRG/60
A24/Cruzeiro/Brazil/55
A12/UK/119/32
A22/Iraq/24/64
Asia1/Cambodia/1/88
Asia1/Pakistan/1/54
Asia1/India/5/89
O1/Manisa/Turkey/69
O/Hong Kong/21/70
O1/Kaufbeuren/FRG/66
SAT3/Zimbabwe/4/81
SAT3/Bechuanaland/1/65
SAT3/Malawi/3/76
SAT3/Uganda/27/70 (buffalo)
SAT2/Rhodesia/1/48
SAT2/Kenya/3/57
SAT2/Senegal/1/83
SAT2/Uganda/24/70 (buffalo)
SAT2/Uganda/12/70 (buffalo)
SAT1/Uganda/21/70 (buffalo)
SAT1/Uganda/10/70 (buffalo)
SAT1/Botswana/1/68
SAT1/Zimbabwe/2/81
SAT1/Uganda/47/71

52 50 48 46 44 42 40 38 36 34 32 30 28 26 24 22 20 18 16 14 12 10 8 6 4 2 0

Percentage nucleotide difference (nt 475–666 of VP1)

**Figure 6**  Genetic relatedness of FMDV strains and serotypes based on sequences within the VP1 gene. Courtesy of N. Knowles.

reservoir for infection (e.g., Cape buffalo in Africa). In nonendemic areas, infection may be introduced from a variety of sources such as the importation of infected livestock, contaminated animal products such as carcasses containing bone (in contrast to meat, the postmortem acidification of bone marrow and other nonmuscular tissues is insufficient to inactivate the virus), or contaminated materials. More locally, transmission of infection is by direct transport of contaminated animals or materials or by wind-borne carriage of infectious aerosols. It is also suspected that the virus can be passively transmitted by migrating birds.

## Transmission and Tissue Tropism

The principal route of infection appears to be via aerosol impinging on the pharynx and respiratory tract. Aerosols may be produced locally during feeding on contaminated foodstuff or may be transmitted over considerable distances under appropriate meteorological conditions. Pigs secrete particularly high levels of virus-contaminated aerosols. In addition to mucosal secretion, high levels of virus are found in milk. Pasture may be contaminated with virus from urine and feces.

Vesicular lesions appear in the mouth on the tongue, gums, and cheeks and later on interdigital mucosa and coronary bands of the feet. Virus can be isolated from many tissues in the body. The onset of clinical disease is usually very rapid and lesions can develop as early as 1–2 days after infection, depending on the virus strain and level of exposure.

## Pathogenicity

The pathogenicity of FMDV varies according to the virus strain, host species, and age. The factors that govern the virulence of FMDVs are poorly understood and as with most viruses are probably multifactoral. Domestic cattle are usually the most susceptible species and morbidity is usually *c.* 100% in nonvaccinated animals. Wild bovines, such as African Cape buffalo, may produce no clinical manifestations. Although the disease is rarely fatal in adult domestic animals (<5%), significant mortality may occur in young animals (*c.* 50%).

## Clinical Features of Infection

Infection typically produces a rapidly progressing febrile illness and the development of often massive vesicular lesions in the mouth and on the feet. The lesions rupture with considerable loss of epithelial tissue (**Figure 7**). The resulting discomfort discourages feeding until the lesions heal by the infiltration of fibrous tissue. The severity of

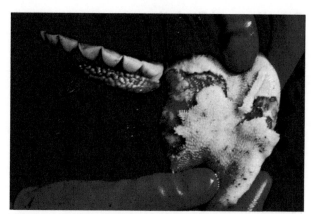

**Figure 7**    Severe symptoms of FMD showing extensive sloughing of linguinal epithelium. Crown copyright. Reproduced from ''Foot and mouth disease: Ageing of lesions'' (Defra, 2005) by permission of the Controller of HMSO.

the disease results in long-term loss of productivity in terms of meat and milk yield, and lameness may be a serious consequence for draught animals. Abortion and chronic subfertility are also common. Other organs infected include mammary glands, pancreas, and heart.

## Immune Response

Infection elicits a vigorous humoral antibody response and, after recovery, immunity to reinfection with viruses of the same serotype is prolonged. The role of cytolytic T cells in recovery is unclear.

Four antigenic sites recognized by antibodies capable of neutralizing the virus have been described. One of these is an immunodominant linear sequence comprising the G–H loop of VP1, and synthetic peptides representing this tract are effective in inducing high levels of virus-neutralizing antibody and can protect animals from infection.

Antibody responses to several of the nonstructural proteins are induced during infection and these are being developed as markers to distinguish vaccinated from infected animals.

## Prevention and Control

In disease-free regions, natural protection afforded by geographical barriers is rigorously reinforced by strict controls on the importation of susceptible animals and potentially contaminated materials. Where outbreaks occur sporadically, due to occasional introduction from external sources, embargoes on animal movement and slaughter of infected herds have been successful in maintaining a disease-free national herd. In endemic areas, control is by mass vaccination. Ring or barrier vaccination is also used to limit the spread of infection.

Dramatic demonstrations of the vulnerability of naive livestock to large-scale epidemics of FMD were provided by the outbreaks of serotype O virus in the UK and of serotype A virus in South America in 2001. The outbreak in the UK resulted in the slaughter of over 10 million animals (most of which were uninfected) to control spread of the disease and the cost to the country was several billions of pounds. In South America, the outbreak was controlled by the resumption of blanket vaccination of all livestock.

The first vaccines against FMD were produced by formalin inactivation of lymph drawn from lesions on the tongues of infected cattle. This source of immunizing virus was replaced by the Frenkel method of culture in fragments of epithelium stripped from the tongues of slaughtered cattle. Most vaccine in use today is produced by growing the virus in suspensions of BHK-21 cells in fermentation vessels of up to 10 000 l capacity. Approximately $2 \times 10^9$ monovalent doses of vaccine are administered annually. Aziridines have largely replaced formalin as the inactivant, since the inactivation kinetics of the latter are nonlinear and residual live virus in vaccines has occasionally been the source of outbreaks of disease. The serotype and strain composition of vaccines have to be tailored for local requirements. Inactivated virus is usually adjuvanted by adsorption onto aluminum hydroxide gel, and saponin may also be added to enhance potency. In pigs, such vaccines elicit only immunoglobulin M responses, and for this species vaccines are formulated with oil adjuvants. The use of oil-adjuvanted vaccines are now being extended to cattle.

Solid protection requires high levels of neutralizing antibodies, and, to achieve this with inactivated vaccines, immunization is repeated two to three times a year. The development of live-attenuated vaccines has largely been abandoned mainly due to the complexity of antigenic diversity and the fear of reversion to a virulent phenotype.

## Future Perspectives

There is scope for developments in FMD vaccines to improve stability, cross-protective efficacy, and duration of immunity. Peptide vaccines, recombinant viral capsids, and rationally designed nonreverting attenuated viruses are potential routes by which these goals may be achieved. The production of non-biodegradable peptides and the creation of an attenuated L protein deletion mutant may be important developments. Since the massive outbreaks in the UK and in South America in 2001, there is increased interest in the development of drugs to halt the rapid spread of infection. Improved rapid diagnostic methods are being explored as is the ability to accurately distinguish infected from vaccinated animals.

As to the molecular properties of the virus, both the determination of the crystallographic structure of the particle and several of the nonstructural proteins and the cloning and manipulation of full-length infectious cDNA molecules are important steps toward understanding the unique features of the virus.

## Further Reading

Barteling SJ and Vreeswijk J (1991) Developments in foot and mouth disease vaccines. *Vaccine* 9: 75–88.

Brooksby JB (1982) Portraits of viruses: Foot and mouth disease virus. *Intervirology* 18: 1–23.

Brown F (1989) The development of chemically synthesised vaccines. *Advances in Veterinary Science and Comparative Medicine* 33: 173.

Defra (2005) Foot and Mouth Disease – Ageing of Lesions. http://www.defra.gov.uk/footandmouth/pdf/ageing-lesions.pdf (accessed January 2008).

Fry E, Logan D, Fox G, Rowlands D, Brown F, and Stuart D (1990) Architecture and topography of an aphthovirus. *Seminars in Virology* 1: 439–451.

Mahy BWJ (ed.) (2005) *Foot-and-Mouth Disease Virus.* Heidelberg: Springer.

Rowlands DJ (ed.) (2003) Special issue: Foot-and-mouth disease virus. *Virus Research* 91: 1–161.

Sobrino F and Domingo E (eds.) (2004) *Foot-and-Mouth Disease – Current Perspectives.* Norfolk, UK: Horizon Bioscience.

# Herpesviruses of Horses

**D J O'Callaghan,** Louisiana State University Health Sciences Center, Shreveport, LA, USA

**N Osterrieder,** Cornell University, Ithaca, NY, USA

## History

The first disease attributed to an equine herpesvirus (EHV), the agent that is now referred to as equid herpesvirus 1 (EHV-1, equine abortion virus; equine rhinopneumonitis virus), was documented at the University of Kentucky Agricultural Experiment Station in Lexington, KY. EHV-1 was first shown to be associated with spontaneous abortions in pregnant mares in 1932. In 1941, equine abortions were found to be associated with mild respiratory disease with clinical signs similar to those associated with equine influenza virus infections. EHV-1 was also shown to be the etiological agent of epizootic respiratory disease in young horses. Based on these investigations, the disease was termed viral rhinopneumonitis, and the agent was called equine rhinopneumonitis virus. In the 1980s, however, the two disease manifestations, viral abortion and viral rhinopneumonitis, were shown to be caused by two closely related but clearly distinct viruses now classified as EHV-1 (equine abortion virus) and EHV-4 (equine rhinopneumonitis virus).

Equid herpesvirus 2 (EHV-2) was first isolated from horses in 1963. The cytopathology caused by this virus closely resembled that of cytomegalovirus infections, which were first described in 1921 in humans. EHV-2 is a ubiquitous, slow-growing virus that infects horses at a very young age (<2 years) and establishes a lifelong chronic infection such that the horse becomes a continuous shedder of the virus. To date, no major disease has been attributed to EHV-2. However, an association of EHV-2 with chronic throat infections (the 'lumpy bumpies') or recurrent eye disease has been established by some investigators, although the causal relationships have not been proved unequivocally. Also, EHV-2 may be a cofactor in EHV-1 and/or EHV-4 infections in that it is able to modulate EHV-1 and EHV-4 replication by immunosuppression, causing general malaise, or by modulation of EHV-1 gene expression through EHV-2-specific transcriptional transactivators.

Equid herpesvirus 3 (EHV-3; equine coital exanthema virus, ECE virus) was first isolated independently in 1968 in Canada, Australia, and the USA. EHV-3 is the etiological agent of equine coital exanthema, a generally mild genital infection of mares and stallions that is transmitted venereally and has been largely eradicated.

Equid herpesvirus 4 (EHV-4) is associated mainly with respiratory disease and has also been associated occasionally with equine abortions. On the other hand, EHV-1 is associated primarily with equine abortions, but frequently causes respiratory disease in young animals, highly fatal neurological disease, fulminating neonatal pneumonitis, and, very rarely, an exanthematous condition involving the external genitalia of the mare.

Equid herpesvirus 5 (EHV-5) is closely related to EHV-2 and no information on possible disease(s) caused by this virus is currently available.

Equid herpesvirus 9 (EHV-9), previously referred to as gazelle herpesvirus 1, was described very recently. It has been shown to be closely related to EHV-1 (and asinine herpesvirus 1) and exhibits a broad host range *in vivo*. While clinical signs in horses seem to be relatively mild, EHV-9 can cause lethal encephalitides in other animals, such as gazelles and goats.

## Taxonomy and Classification

Eight of the nine EHVs have been classified as species in the family *Herpesviridae*. The species names are *Equid herpesvirus 1* through *Equid herpesvirus 9*, with the exception of *Equid herpesvirus 6*, which is not yet in existence as EHV-6 has not yet been fully assigned to a species. EHV-6, EHV-7, and EHV-8 are donkey herpesviruses that are also referred to as asinine herpesviruses 1, 2, and 3, respectively, and will not be discussed in detail in this article. The morphology of all six members is typical of the herpesviruses in that they are enveloped, contain an icosadeltahedral capsid, and have a proteinaceous coat, the so-called tegument, which surrounds the nucleocapsid. EHVs are composed of six distinct species: (1) EHV-1 is the major equine pathogen causing fetal abortions, respiratory illness, and neurological disease; (2) EHV-2 (and perhaps EHV-5) establish mainly asymptomatic, long-term persistent infections; (3) EHV-3 is the causative agent of mild progenital exanthema; (4) EHV-4 is a major respiratory pathogen that differs significantly from EHV-1 at the DNA level and is associated occasionally with equine abortions; and (5) EHV-9 can cause mostly subclinical encephalitides in horses, while infections of other hosts are often lethal. In the latter respect, EHV-9 possesses biological properties very akin to an alphaherpesvirus of pigs, pseudorabies virus (PRV). EHV-1, EHV-3, EHV-4, and EHV-9 are members of subfamily *Alphaherpesvirinae*, genus *Varicellovirus*. EHV-2 and EHV-5 are members of subfamily *Gammaherpesvirinae*, genus *Rhadinovirus*.

## Geographic and Seasonal Distribution

EHV-1 and EHV-4 are distributed worldwide, and infections can occur year-round. Over the past 30 years in the USA, EHV-1 'abortion storms' have occurred in many areas. Major outbreaks have also been reported in Australia and England. Due to the nature of the disease manifestation, viral abortions caused by EHV-1 exhibit a seasonal cumulation in the spring on broodmare farms, whereas EHV-1 and EHV-4 infections of the upper respiratory tract (rhinopneumonitis), as well as the neurological form of EHV-1 disease, are observed mainly on race tracks and after crowding of large numbers of animals.

EHV-2 has also been isolated in many countries, including England, Switzerland, Germany, the USA, and South Africa. The existence of the closely related EHV-5 was described for England and Australia. More thorough studies, however, have led to the assumption that both EHV-2 and EHV-5 are distributed worldwide.

To date, EHV-3 has been isolated in five countries: Germany, USA, Australia, Canada, and England. EHV-9 so far has only been described in captive gazelles in Japan, although zoo animals in other parts of the world have been shown to harbor antibodies against the agent.

## Host Range and Virus Propagation

Although the horse is the natural host of the EHVs, a variety of animals and tissue culture systems can be used to propagate the viruses. Regarding the major equine pathogen, EHV-1, experimental animals include Syrian hamsters and baby hamsters, chick embryos, baby mice and adult mice, and kittens. Primary tissue culture systems used to propagate EHV-1 include cells from a variety of equine tissues such as fetal lung, dermis, spleen, and kidney, as well as cells from domestic cats, dogs, hamsters, rabbits, mice, sheep, and swine. In the laboratory, permanent tissue culture systems commonly used to cultivate EHV-1 include primate HeLa, Vero, and CV-1 cells, rabbit kidney (RK) cells, mouse L–M cells, and equine NBL-6 and Edmin337 cells.

The host range for EHV-2, EHV-3, EHV-4, and EHV-5 is more restrictive than that for EHV-1. Except for RK cells and primary cat cells, EHV-2 and EHV-5 growth appears to be restricted to cells of equine origin. The host range for EHV-3 and EHV-4 is limited to cells of equine origin, although Vero cell culture-adapted EHV-4 strains have been described. EHV-9 is a notable exception of the rule of narrow host range of EHVs *in vivo*. As mentioned above, this virus was first isolated from an outbreak of fatal encephalitis in zoo gazelles and was later characterized in detail and shown to be most closely related to EHV-1. EHV-9 has a wide host range *in vivo* and *in vitro*.

## Genetics

All six EHVs contain a linear, double-stranded DNA genome ranging between 140 and 184 kbp. The reported sizes of the genome are: EHV-1, 150 kbp; EHV-2, 184 kbp; EHV-3, 144 kbp; EHV-4, 145 kbp; and EHV-5, 179 kbp. The size of the EHV-9 genome has not yet been determined, but is likely to be close to that of EHV-1. The genomes of EHV-1, EHV-3, EHV-4, and probably EHV-9 exist in two isomeric forms, since the short region (S) can invert relative to the fixed orientation of the unique long region ($U_L$). The S region is composed of a central segment of unique sequences ($U_S$) bracketed by a pair of inverted sequences (IRs). In the case of the Kentucky A (KyA) tissue culture-adapted strain of EHV-1, each IR is 12.8 kbp. In contrast, the genomes of EHV-2 and EHV-5 exist as one isomer and are comprised of a large (149 kbp)

central segment of unique sequences that is bracketed by a pair of direct repeat sequences. Each of the terminal direct repeat segments is 18 kbp, and the total genome size is 179–184 kbp. Other characteristics of the genomes are shown in **Table 1**.

There are varying degrees of homology at the DNA level among the six EHVs. The sequences shared by EHV-1, EHV-3, EHV-4, and EHV-9 appear to be arranged collinearly and are dispersed throughout the genome. EHV-1 and EHV-4 exhibit 55–84% identity at the DNA level and are antigenically very closely related, and antibodies can cross-neutralize. Levels of identity between EHV-1 and EHV-9 are even higher than those between EHV-1 and EHV-4. EHV-1 and EHV-2 show negligible identity, as do EHV-2 and EHV-3. EHV-1 and EHV-3 exhibit approximately 10% identity at the DNA level. Lastly, EHV-2 and EHV-5 show approximately 60% identity at both the DNA and protein levels.

The cloning of the genomes of a number of EHV-1 strains, among them the attenuated KyA and pathogenic RacL11 strains, as bacterial artificial chromosomes (BACs) has been achieved. These clones are infectious and provide a basis for rapid and efficient mutagenesis of the EHV-1 genome in prokaryotic cells. A variety of recombinant viruses that lack nonessential genes or portions of an essential gene have been generated and used in experiments to elucidate the functions of these genes in virus replication and/or pathogenesis.

## Genome Structure

The entire genomes of EHV-1 strains, Ab4 and V592, EHV-4 strain NS80567, and EHV-2 strain 86/67 have been sequenced. The EHV-1 strain Ab4 genome is 150 224 bp in size, while that of EHV-4 is 145 597 bp. Both genomes contain 76 open reading frames (ORFs) potentially encoding proteins, with 4 duplicated in repeated regions in EHV-1 and -3 in EHV-4, giving a total of 80 ORFs in EHV-1 and -79 in EHV-4. The 63 ORFs in the $U_L$ region are arranged colinearly between EHV-1 and EHV-4 and with those of herpes simplex virus (HSV) and varicella-zoster virus (VZV). Several genes

**Table 1** Properties of equine herpesvirus genomes

| Member | Subfamily | Isomers | S value | G+C content | Clinical manifestations |
|--------|-----------|---------|---------|-------------|-------------------------|
| EHV-1 | Alpha | 2 | 49–55 | 56% | Abortion, respiratory infection, paralysis |
| EHV-2 | Gamma | 1 | 61.8 | 57% | Chronic throat infection; perhaps recurrent eye infection |
| EHV-3 | Alpha | 2 | 55.4 | 66% | Equine coital exanthema |
| EHV-4 | Alpha | 2 | ND[a] | 50% | Respiratory infections |
| EHV-5 | Gamma | 1 | ND | ND | Not known; possibly pneumonia |
| EHV-9 | Alpha | 2 | ND | ND | Mild infections in horses; encephalitis in other animals (e.g., gazelles and goats) |

[a]ND, not determined.

mapping within IR and U$_S$ of the S region differ in arrangement from those of other alphaherpesviruses. In addition, EHV-1 and EHV-4 contain a limited number of unique genes that are present in neither HSV-1 nor VZV and which might represent the viruses' gene repertoire involved in determining host specificity.

Each identical IR of the S region of the KyA tissue culture-adapted strain of EHV-1 is composed of 12 777 nucleotides. Six genes and the origin of DNA replication (ORI) have been mapped to IR: (1) the IR1 gene (gene 64) is an immediate-early (IE) gene encoding a spliced 6.0 kbp mRNA and a major phosphoprotein (1487 amino acid residues) with an apparent molecular mass of 203 kDa; (2) the IR2 gene is an early gene that is embedded within the IR1 gene, and its 4.4 kbp mRNA encodes a 130 kDa polypeptide (1165 amino acid residues) – the protein product of the IR2 gene represents a truncated form of the IE polypeptide; (3) the IR3 gene is a delayed-early gene encoding a 0.9 kbp mRNA that overlaps the IE promoter region on the opposite DNA strand; (4) the EHV-1 ORI maps downstream of IR3 and exhibits 60% identity to the corresponding ORI of HSV-1 and HSV-2; (5) the IR4 gene (gene 65) is a homolog of the ICP22 gene of HSV-1 and is differentially regulated to encode a 1.4 kbp early mRNA and a 1.7 kbp late mRNA; (6) the IR5 gene (gene 66) is a homolog of the US10 gene of HSV-1; and (7) the EHV-1 unique IR6 gene (gene 67) is a 'very early' gene encoding a 1.2 kbp mRNA and a 31/33 kDa phosphoprotein that has been shown to be a capsid constituent and a major determinant of virulence in some EHV-1 strains.

Additional EHV-1 genes in the S region map in the U$_S$ segment and include homologs of the HSV-1 US2 gene, the protein kinase gene, the US9 gene, and genes that encode the glycoproteins (g) gG, gD, gI, and gE. In addition, a unique gene (EUS4 or gene 71) was mapped in U$_S$. This gene encodes a highly O-glycosylated protein referred to as gp2. Some size variations of gp2 were documented for EHV-1 strains KyA, Ab4, RacL11, and an EUS4 gp2 null mutant was apathogenic in a murine model of EHV-1 infection. Replacement of the truncated EUS4 gene of the apathogenic KyA strain with the EUS4 gene of the pathogenic RacL11 strain, which encodes the full size gp2 of 791 amino acid residues, resulted in a 'transfer' of pathogenic properties, indicating that gp2 is a major determinant of virulence. While gD is essential for virus replication in cultured cells, gI and gE are not, but do play a role in virulence. Restoration of the gI and gE sequences to a gI/gE deletion mutant or to vaccine strain KyA, which has an attenuated phenotype, restores virulence in the equine and murine models of infection.

Functional analyses of genes encoded in U$_L$ have also been performed. Among the genes investigated are those encoding thymidine kinase, gB, gC, and gM, which show strong homology to their HSV-1 and VZV counterparts. Functional homology between HSV-1 and EHV-1 genes has been demonstrated for gM and gB.

The genomic sequences of EHV-2 and EHV-4 have been determined, but intensive research on gene functions has not yet been performed. Nothing is known about EHV-3 or EHV-9 gene functions.

## Replication

The receptor for EHV-1 entry has not been identified, but recent studies showed that the virus utilizes a unique entry receptor, as it efficiently entered and replicated in cells that lack the entry receptors HveA, HveB, and HveC used for entry by other alphaherpesviruses, such as HSV-1, HSV-2, and PRV. As with other alphaherpesviruses, EHV-1 entry is mediated by gD.

The genes of the tissue culture-adapted KyA strain of EHV-1 are regulated at the transcriptional and translational levels in a temporal fashion, and three kinetic classes of genes designated IE, early, and late have been described (see **Table 2**). The sole IE gene (IR1) maps in both IR segments and gives rise to a spliced 6.0 kbp mRNA. Multiple IE polypeptide species have been observed, and the major IE protein (IE1, 203 kDa) is a nuclear-localized phosphoprotein that is capable of trans-activating other viral genes and autoregulating its own transcription. The transactivation domain (residues

**Table 2**    Regulatory genes of EHV-1

| Gene | Temporal class | Gene product | Function in replication |
|------|----------------|--------------|-------------------------|
| IE (gene 64) | Immediate early | 1487 aa[a] | Transactivates early genes and activates some late genes |
| IR4 (gene 65) | Early | 293 aa | Enhances IE protein DNA-binding and binds TBP |
| UL5 (gene 5) | Early | 470 aa | Binds the IE protein, TFIIB, and TBP |
| EICP0 (gene 63) | Early | 419 aa | Promiscuous transactivator, which antagonizes IE protein function; binds IE protein, TFIIB, TBP |
| IR2 | Early | 1165 aa | Dominant negative regulator, which blocks IE protein binding to promoters |
| IR3 | Early | 0.9 kb RNA | Antisense to IE mRNA; possible precursor of microRNA |
| ETIF (gene 12) | Late | 479 aa | Transactivates the IE promoter; essential for virus egress |

[a]aa, amino acid residues in the primary translation product.

3–89), the DNA-binding domain (residues 422–597), and the nuclear localization domain (PPAPKRRV; residues 963–970) of the IE protein have been mapped. Recent studies have revealed that the IE protein harbors domains for binding general transcription factors, such as TFIIB and TATA-binding protein (TBP), and thus serves to promote the formation of pre-initiation complexes that mediate viral transcription.

Following IE polypeptide synthesis, approximately 45 early transcripts can be detected. Four of the early proteins serve as regulatory proteins and are designated IR4 (EICP22), UL5 (EICP27), EICP0 (UL63), and IR2. The IR4 protein interacts physically with the IE protein and serves to enhance the DNA binding of the IE protein to its target sequence (ATCGT) present within the promoters of EHV-1 genes characterized to date. The IR4 protein also binds to TBP and is present at viral early promoters in association with the IE protein and TBP. These interactions explain the synergistic effect on the transactivation of viral genes mediated by the IE and IR4 proteins. The EHV-1 UL5 protein exhibits limited identity to HSV-1 ICP27, and is essential for virus replication in cell culture. It acts synergistically with either the IE protein or the EICP0 early regulatory protein to activate expression of both early and late viral gene expression. This early regulatory protein also interacts physically with both the IE protein and TBP, and serves to enhance formation of transcriptional complexes on viral promoters. The third early regulatory protein is EICP0, which is a powerful and promiscuous transactivator that can independently activate expression of viral genes of all three temporal classes. Ironically, EICP0 cannot activate its own promoter, possibly due to a 28 bp negative regulatory element that maps at nucleotides (nt) −204 to −177 within the EICP0 promoter. The EICP0 protein binds to the IE protein and to cellular TFIIB and TBP, but is not a DNA-binding protein. The EICP0 and IE proteins have an antagonistic relationship that may result from their physical interaction in the nucleus and/or from competition for binding to TFIIB and TBP. Both viral proteins bind to the same domain in TFIIB. Deletion of the EICP0 gene greatly impairs virus replication and severely retards late gene expression, suggesting that this regulatory protein is important in the switch from early to late transcription. The fourth early regulatory protein is the IR2 protein, which is a truncated form of the IE protein lacking its essential transactivation and serine-rich domains. The IR2 protein serves a negative regulatory role as it downregulates viral gene expression by acting as a dominant negative protein that blocks IE protein binding to viral promoters and/or by squelching the limited supply of TFIIB and TBP. In addition to these four early auxiliary regulatory proteins, the EHV-1 unique IR3 gene contributes a regulatory role as it encodes a small transcript that is antisense to a portion of the IE transcript.

In transient transfection assays, the IR3 transcript downregulates IE gene expression and is only minimally expressed as a protein. Initial studies suggest that the IR3 transcript is processed to a microRNA, and this indicates that the IR3 gene may use novel mechanisms to downregulate IE gene expression at late times of infection.

Early gene expression is followed by viral DNA replication and the production of approximately 29 late transcripts has been detected. Although these transcripts have been positioned on the viral genome, only a small number of protein products have been identified and characterized (see above).

Viral DNA replication initiates at approximately 4 h post infection and requires the virus-encoded DNA polymerase. DNA replication is thought to occur by the rolling circle mechanism whereby long concatemers of the viral genome are generated, cleaved, and then packaged into the maturing virions. The UL15 homolog of HSV-1, one of the two spliced EHV-1 genes known to date, appears to be essentially involved in the generation of unit length genomes and their packaging into mature capsids. Sequences at the L terminus of the EHV-1 genome are composed of direct repeats (DR1 = 18 bp and DR4 = 16 bp) as well as unique sequences (Uc = 60 bp), while sequences at the terminus of the S region contain a 54 bp region designated Ub. Thus, the sequence arrangement at the concatameric junction following replication of the EHV-1 genome is Ub-DR1-Uc-DR4, which represents a functional cleavage/packaging signal, similar, but not identical, to that of HSV-1.

The start of viral DNA synthesis initiates late gene expression and the synthesis of the late regulatory protein EHV transinducing factor (ETIF), a counterpart to the alpha-transinducing factor of HSV-1. This 60 kDa protein is multifunctional and plays at least three roles in EHV-1 replication. First, ETIF is present in several molecular sizes in the tegument and contributes to overall virion structure. Second, after virus entry and uncoating, ETIF serves to transactivate the IE promoter by binding to cellular factors that mediate its association with the TAATGARATT sequence at nt−630 to −620 in the IE promoter. This transactivation function to initiate viral gene programming is important but not essential, as EHV-1 DNA is infectious and virus progeny are produced in cells transfected with plasmids carrying the EHV-1 genome. The activation of a viral promoter by ETIF is specific for the IE promoter as ETIF has not been shown to transactivate any early or late promoter tested to date. Recent experiments with an ETIF-deleted virus and an ETIF-complementing cell line revealed a third function for ETIF, and one that is essential for virus replication. Ultrastructural studies of cells infected with ETIF-deleted virus showed a marked defect in secondary envelopment of viral nucleocapsids at cytoplasmic membranes, such that few enveloped virions are produced. Thus, this transactivator protein also plays a key role in secondary envelopment.

Three different EHV-1 capsid species have been identified and probably correspond to the forms found in HSV-1, which are designated type A, B, and C capsids. The EHV-1 capsid species were designated: (1) L capsids, which appear to be empty; (2) I capsids which possess an electron-lucent, immature core structure in the shape of a cross; and (3) H capsids, which contain an electron-dense, mature core. All three capsids appear at approximately 6 h post infection. I capsids are believed to be a major precursor in the formation of mature capsids. The major capsid protein has an apparent size of 148 kDa, and other structural proteins have also been identified. As reported for other herpesviruses, EHV-1 maturation occurs by interaction of mature nucleocapsids with the inner portion of the nuclear membrane resulting in the formation of enveloped particles. As noted above, recent studies with ETIF-deleted EHV-1 support the model of the sequential envelopment/de-envelopment/re-envelopment pathway for egress of EHV-1 from the cell.

Infectious EHV-1 particles contain an envelope whose protein component is composed mainly of glycoproteins. To date, 12 EHV-1 glycoproteins have been identified and an association of gB, gC, gD, gG, gH, gL, gM, gp2, and the tegument protein VP13/14 with purified virions has been demonstrated. The glycoproteins have been shown in other alphaherpesviruses to be involved in virus binding, virus penetration, and cell-to-cell spread of infection. In the case of EHV-1, these functions were confirmed for gB, gD, gM, and gp2, and the latter two proteins were shown to be nonessential for virus growth. In contrast, gB- or gD-deleted EHV-1 mutants are unable to grow in cell culture. The defect in replication of gB- and gD-negative viruses is caused by an entry defect and the inability to spread from infected to uninfected cells. Detailed functional analyses for the other glycoproteins have not been performed, but are now facilitated by the use of engineered virus mutants produced by targeted gene deletion or disruption using infectious DNA clones of the virus. Even less is known for proteins that make up the third component of the mature virion, the tegument. Only one protein that is related to an HSV-1 tegument protein has been analyzed in detail. As discussed above, recent studies have shown that ETIF is essential for virus maturation and egress.

## Defective Interfering Particles and Persistent Infection

EHV-1, EHV-2, and EHV-5 have been shown to mediate persistent infection. In the case of EHV-1, defective interfering particles (DIPs) have been shown to initiate and maintain this outcome. EHV-1 DIPs have been generated *in vivo* in the Syrian hamster model, and therefore may be relevant during EHV-1 infection of the natural host. DIPs are replication defective and require standard EHV-1 as a helper. The overwhelming majority of EHV-1 DNA sequences are absent from DIPs. The packaged DIP DNA molecule is a concatamer of EHV-1 sequences ranging in size from 5.9 to 7.3 kbp, repeated head to tail until it is approximately the size of the standard viral genome. DNA sequencing has revealed that sequences from three regions of the EHV-1 genome are conserved in DIPs: (1) the L terminus, including genes UL3, UL4 and the 3' portion of UL5; (2) the junction between $U_L$ and the internal IR; and (3) the central portion of IR, including ORI and the 5' portion of gene IR4. The UL3 and UL4 genes in DIP genomes are 100% identical to those of infectious virus, but their functions in virus replication remain to be elucidated. The DIP genome also contains a perfectly conserved cleavage/packaging signal. The sequences at the L terminus and IR are joined by a homologous recombination event mediated by a conserved 8 bp sequence present at both the L terminus and within the IR4 gene to generate a unique ORF present only in DIPs. This ORF is expressed as a 31 kDa 'hybrid protein' comprising the N-terminal 196 amino acid residues of the IR4 protein (the homolog of HSV-1 ICP22) linked in frame to the C-terminal 68 amino acids of the UL5 protein (the homolog of HSV-1 ICP27). Unique to EHV-1 persistently infected cells (not detected in EHV-1 cytolytic infection) is a 2.2 kbp transcript that maps to the $U_L$/IR junction and is antisense to the IE mRNA. Interestingly, this transcript exhibits significant homology to the latency associated transcripts of HSV-1, which appear to be associated with HSV-1 reactivation rather than establishment of latency.

Lastly, in EHV-1 persistently infected cells, transcription of certain viral genes appears delayed compared with cytolytically infected cells. Recent findings reveal that expression of the 31 kDa IR4/UL5 hybrid protein downregulates expression of specific EHV-1 promoters. Moreover, altered forms of the EHV-1 IE polypeptides have been observed only in persistently infected cells. Taken together, these studies indicate that altered or aberrant viral regulatory mechanisms may be involved in establishing or maintaining persistent infection. Ongoing studies with recombinant forms of the DIP genome indicate that the hybrid gene is not essential for DIP replication, but is important in the ability of EHV-1 DIPs to establish persistent infection.

## Evolution

The six EHVs are biologically distinct. Initial DNA sequence analyses have revealed that genes identified to date are collinearly arranged in the genomes of EHV-1,

EHV-3, and EHV-4, all of which possess a two-isomer genomic structure. Evolutionary relationships have become more apparent now that EHV-1, EHV-2, and EHV-4 have been sequenced and data on EHV-5 sequences and genomic organization are available. It is clear that EHV-1, EHV-4, and EHV-9 are closely related and may have arisen from the same ancestor. The same is true for EHV-2 and EHV-5. However, it is not possible to determine precise details of the EHV ancestor since additional sequence data (especially on EHV-3) are not available.

## Serological Relationship and Variability

The six EHVs share certain antigens, but are antigenically distinct. EHV-1, EHV-4, and EHV-9 are closely related antigenically, such that cross-neutralizing antibodies are generated. Also, EHV-2 and EHV-5 are closely related. Almost no data are available on the relationship of EHV-3 to other members of the EHVs. However, all of the EHVs are believed to share complement-fixing antigens.

## Epidemiology

Rhinopneumonitis caused by EHV-1 and EHV-4 is spread by direct or indirect contact (ingestion and inhalation). The viruses are most commonly shed in nasal droplets for up to 3 weeks after initial infection and are present in large amounts in aborted fetuses and the placenta.

EHV-1 infection can also result in spontaneous abortions in pregnant mares. Horses are most susceptible to EHV-1 infection between the eighth and eleventh months of pregnancy. The peak incidence is in the ninth and tenth months, at which time approximately 70% of abortions occur.

EHV-2 and EHV-5 have been isolated from the respiratory tract, kidneys, spleen, testicles, genital tract, and rectum. Once infected, the horse is a lifelong carrier and excreter of the virus. The exact modes of spread of EHV-2 and EHV-5 are unknown.

EHV-3 causes a mild coital exanthema that is spread by genital contact and – rarely – the respiratory route. An EHV-3 infection is usually cleared after 14 days and is not associated with equine abortions.

## Transmission and Tissue Tropism

EHV-1, EHV-4, and EHV-9 are spread mainly by nasal discharge. EHV-2 and EHV-5 establish a chronic infection and may be spread by the respiratory route. EHV-3 is spread by genital contact. EHV-1 has a wide host range *in vitro* as described above, while EHV-4 is more limited. EHV-2, EHV-3, and EHV-5 are restricted mainly to cells of equine origin.

## Pathogenicity

EHV-1 and EHV-4 cause rhinopneumonitis, which is often transient and mild but can be complicated by secondary bacterial infections and become more severe and long lasting. EHV-1 is also associated with spontaneous abortions as well as neurological disease. Although EHV-1 and EHV-4 respiratory infections are clinically indistinguishable, their pathogenesis is quite different. EHV-1 infection results in a systemic viremia that can lead to abortion and/or neurological disease. Alternatively, EHV-4 infection usually remains restricted to tissues of the upper respiratory tract. EHV-2 and also EHV-5 infections are acquired horizontally early in life usually by inhalation. EHV-2 and EHV-5 establish a chronic lifelong infection in peripheral blood mononuclear cells. EHV-3 causes an acute coital exanthema in both the mare and the stallion, and infection remains localized to the genitalia.

## Clinical Features of Infection

EHV-1 and EHV-4 cause outbreaks of upper respiratory disease ('common cold') in young horses (mainly EHV-4 in adult horses) with no previous exposure to the viruses. Infection is characterized by a short incubation time (<1 day) followed by fever (39–41 °C), which can last between 1 and 4 days, sometimes with a second spike approximately 1 week after the primary pyrexia, and animals suffer from serous nasal discharge and congestion of the nasal mucosa and conjuctiva. Less frequently, one can detect a transitory period of anorexia, enlargement of the submandibular lymph nodes, and edematous swelling of the lower parts of the body and the extremities. An initial leukopenia is followed by leukocytosis before the temperature falls. Recovery is usually uneventful and occurs within 1 week. Older horses show few or no clinical signs, although increased sensitivity is seen in stressed horses. Death is not uncommon from natural acquired infection resulting in neurological disease.

Equine abortions induced by EHV-1 usually occur late in gestation (8–11 months). The foals are usually born dead, but, if alive, often succumb to pneumonia within the first few days. Clinical signs of neurological disease caused by EHV-1 are highly variable and include head pressing, ataxia, and paralysis with complete recumbence. Both EHV-1 and EHV-4 have been isolated from the central nervous system (CNS) of infected horses, but EHV-1 is by far the leading cause of EHV-induced neurological disease. The virus strains do not invade the extravascular nervous tissue and are not neurotropic *per se*. Rather, the virus spreads from the respiratory tract to the CNS via infected leukocytes and infects endothelial cells of the blood vessels supplying the spinal cord. While the neurological form of the disease is usually lethal, some horses have fully recovered from it with no permanent neurological sequelae.

The roles of EHV-2 and EHV-5 in clinical disease are virtually unknown. However, the viruses have been associated occasionally with chronic throat infections and have been isolated from the respiratory tract of horses with respiratory disease.

An incubation period as long as 10 days can be observed following natural infection with EHV-3. The initial lesions are small (1–2 mm), raised, reddened papules. The lesions then progress rapidly to the pustular form, and there is a general reddening of the vaginal mucosa in the mare. The number of lesions increases in the first few days, and by day six, many of the lesions form ulcers up to 20 mm in diameter and 5 mm deep. Lesions can also be seen on the vulva, perineal skin, as well as on the penis and prepuce of the stallion. The disease is usually mild, with temperature, pulse, appetite, and respiration remaining close to normal. The severity of the disease can be increased by secondary bacterial infections; however, uneventful cases are usually cleared within 2 weeks. Lastly, EHV-3 is not abortigenic and does not lead to infertility.

Infections with EHV-9 lead to encephalitis in horses, but, more severely, in other species as well. Among the susceptible hosts are gazelles and goats, and also carnivores such as dogs and cats.

## Pathology and Histopathology

Respiratory disease caused by EHV-1 and EHV-4 results in inflammation, congestion, and sometimes necrosis of the tissues of the upper respiratory tract. Extensive swelling of the nasal mucosa may occur and, in later stages, the lungs may become involved. One can find typical herpesvirus inclusion bodies in the nuclei of the respiratory epithelium. The respiratory infection can become more serious if followed by a secondary bacterial infection, which may lead to bacterial pneumonia.

Fetuses that are aborted as a consequence of EHV-1 infection present with widespread hemorrhages and edema, as well as a yellowish discoloration of the fetal conjunctiva and splenomegaly – if virus is transmitted from mother to animal. However, abortions without infection of the fetus also occur, and the pathogenesis in the uterine vasculature largely resembles that of the vasculitis observed in the neurological form of the disease. The classic histopathology includes the presence of eosinophilic intranuclear inclusion bodies in various organs of the aborted fetuses. Gross pathological and histopathological alterations are sometimes not as obvious, and only sensitive methods (virus isolation or PCR) are able to confirm the EHV-1 abortion. Classically, features associated with EHV-1-induced abortions differ in those fetuses aborted during the first 6 months of gestation as compared with those aborted after 6 months. Those before 6 months present with widespread cell necrosis and inclusion bodies in the liver and lung. Those after 6 months exhibit jaundice, subcutaneous edema, excessive pleural fluid, pulmonary edema, splenomegaly, and necrosis of the liver.

In experimental EHV-1 infections, a severe hepatitis is observed following intraperitoneal infection of the Syrian hamster, and a model of respiratory infection is also available in the hamster. Intranasal infection of mice with EHV-1 results in respiratory disease and subsequent cell-associated viremia, thus serving as a model that somewhat mimics the disease in equines. The murine model of EHV-1 infection is widely used in virulence and immunogenicity studies. Recent studies with a library of EHV-1 mutants reveal the importance of full-size gp2 in respiratory disease. DNA-array analyses of lung tissues confirmed earlier findings from RNase protection assays and showed that the massive influx of inflammatory cells into the lung is preceded by 2–13-fold increases in >30 inflammatory genes. Expression of these genes increased as early as 8–12 h post infection, and they encode major cytokines and chemokines, including interleukin-1β (IL-1β), IL-6, tumor necrosis factor alpha, macrophage inflammatory protein 1α (MIP-1α), MIP-1β, and MIP-2. Future investigations should give insight into specific domains of gp2 that activate this constellation of inflammatory genes and the signal transduction pathways that are involved.

EHV-2 (and also EHV-5) infection becomes widespread throughout the body, and the viruses have been isolated from a variety of tissues. The infected animal becomes a lifelong carrier, and the viruses remain highly cell associated.

Tissues affected following an infection with EHV-3 include the vaginal and vestibular mucosa, penis, prepuce, and the skin of the perineal region. One of the characteristics of an infection with EHV-3 is the sloughing of the surface epithelial cells. On occasion, the skin of the lips and mucus membranes of the respiratory tract may become involved, but the exanthema is usually mild.

## Immune Response

Neutralizing antibodies are detected in the serum soon after an EHV-1 or EHV-4 infection. The antibodies can first be detected from a week following infection and are most abundant after several weeks. However, the immunity is short lived, in that horses can be re-infected and exhibit respiratory symptoms just 3 months after the initial infection. Multiple exposures to either EHV-1 or EHV-4 will result in the development of neutralizing, cross-reactive antibodies. However, cell-mediated immune responses are likely to be primarily responsible for induction of a sustainable immunity.

Immunity to EHV-2, EHV-3, and EHV-5 is poorly understood. However, virtually all horses have antibodies to EHV-2 and EHV-5, confirming the general apathogenicity of these viruses.

## Prevention and Control

A number of vaccine approaches are followed to combat EHV-1 infections; among them are modified live vaccines (e.g., Rhinomune and Prevaccinol), inactivated vaccines (e.g., Pneumabort K and Prestige), inactivated combination vaccines, which – among others – also contain EHV-4 (e.g., Innovator, Resequin, and Duvaxyn1,4), and subunit vaccines also covering both viruses (e.g., Cavalon IR). Unfortunately, many EHV vaccines cause undesirable side effects in the form of massive local reactions while not affording acceptable levels of protection, especially when inactivated combination vaccines are considered. All vaccines are given repeatedly to pregnant mares usually in the third, fifth, seventh, and ninth months of pregnancy, since, to ensure protection, a good level of population immunity is imperative. To protect against viral rhinopneumonitis outbreaks, the vaccine is usually given to all horses every 3–6 months. There is considerable ongoing discussion as to proper vaccination against the neurological disease, which has become more prevalent during past years. Recent studies seem to suggest that modified live virus vaccines are superior, especially to multivalent inactivated vaccines, with respect to duration of fever, virus excretion from the nasal mucosa, and development of neurological symptoms. These studies, however, need to be corroborated by further comparative studies and/or larger numbers of animals in experimental groups.

Clinical management often involves the use of antibiotics to prevent severe bacterial complications following the viral rhinopneumonitis. Control of EHV-1 and EHV-4 infections involves isolation and quarantine of infected horses (for at least 3 weeks) and sound hygiene for prevention of viral infection, since the viruses are highly contagious. Quarantine procedures are required more often with EHV-1 infections, since EHV-1 can lead to more serious diseases of the CNS. Since many of the EHV vaccines provide unacceptable levels of protection, the first step in the prevention and control of EHV-1 and EHV-4 infections involves specific management practices and adequate day-to-day care of the animals. The viruses can be spread easily in contaminated feed and water. In addition, minimizing stress and close contact of large groups of horses can prevent the spread of disease.

## Future Perspectives

Considerable progress in unraveling the nucleotide sequences of EHV-1, EHV-2, EHV-4, and EHV-5 has been made during recent years, and EHV-1, EHV-2, and EHV-4 have been entirely sequenced. With this information in hand, it will be possible to pursue studies on gene expression and on those proteins that are involved in virulence of EHV. These studies will in turn open the possibility for a rational design of anti-EHV vaccines, especially against the most important pathogens, EHV-1 and EHV-4. These goals may be achieved by the use of viral deletion mutants that carry targeted gene deletions, which is greatly facilitated by the advent of a number of infectious DNA clones during the past years. Using novel molecular approaches, a better understanding of EHV biology will be possible and in the future will open new perspectives in the understanding of diseases caused by EHVs.

*See also:* Pseudorabies Virus; Retroviruses of Birds.

## Further Reading

Albrecht RA, Kim SK, and O'Callaghan DJ (2005) The EICP27 protein of equine herpesvirus 1 is recruited to viral promoters by its interaction with the immediate-early protein. *Virology* 333: 74–87.

Buczynski KA, Kim SK, and O'Callaghan DJ (2005) Initial characterization of 17 viruses harboring mutant forms of the immediate early gene of equine herpesvirus 1. *Virus Genes* 31: 229–239.

Goodman LB, Wagner B, Flaminio MJBF, et al. (2006) Comparison of the efficacy of inactivated combination and modified-live virus vaccines against challenge infection with neuropathogenic equine herpesvirus type 1 (EHV-1). *Vaccine* 24: 3636–3645.

Kim SK, Albrecht RA, and O'Callaghan DJ (2004) A negative regulatory element (bp −204 to −177) of the EICP0 promoter of equine herpesvirus 1 abrogates the EICP0 protein's *trans*-activation of its own promoter. *Journal of Virology* 78: 11696–11706.

Pagamjay O, Sakata T, Matsumura T, Yamaguchi T, and Fukushi H (2005) Natural recombinant between equine herpesvirus 1 and 4 in the ICP4 gene. *Microbiology and Immunology* 49: 167–179.

Paillot R, Ellis SS, Daly JM, et al. (2006) Characterisation of CTL and IFN-gamma synthesis in ponies following vaccination with a NYVAC-based construct coding for EHV-1 immediate early gene, followed by challenge infection. *Vaccine* 24: 1490–1500.

Rudolph J, O'Callaghan DJ, and Osterrieder N (2002) Cloning of the genomes of equine herpesvirus type 1 (EHV-1) strains KyA and RacL11 as bacterial artificial chromosomes (BAC). *Journal of Veterinary Medicine. B, Infectious Diseases and Veterinary Public Health* 49: 31–36.

Smith PM, Kahan SM, Rorex CB, von Einem J, Osterrieder N, and O'Callaghan DJ (2005) Expression of the full length form of gp2 of equine herpesvirus 1 (EHV-1) completely restores respiratory virulence to the attenuated EHV-1 strain KyA in CBA mice. *Journal of Virology* 79: 5105–5115.

Soboll G, Whalley JM, Koen MT, et al. (2003) Identification of equine herpesvirus-1 antigens recognized by cytotoxic T lymphocytes. *Journal of General Virology* 84: 2625–2634.

Telford EAR, Studdert MJ, Agius CT, Watson MS, Aird HC, and Davison AJ (1993) Equine herpesviruses 2 and 5 are γ-herpesviruses. *Virology* 195: 492–499.

Telford EAR, Watson MS, Aird HC, Perry J, and Davison AJ (1995) The DNA sequence of equine herpesvirus 2. *Journal of Molecular Biology* 249: 520–528.

Telford EAR, Watson MS, McBride K, and Davison AJ (1992) The DNA sequence of equine herpesvirus-1. *Virology* 189: 304–316.

# Jaagsiekte Sheep Retrovirus

**J M Sharp,** Veterinary Laboratories Agency, Penicuik, UK
**M de las Heras,** University of Glasgow Veterinary School, Glasgow, UK
**T E Spencer,** Texas A&M University, College Station, TX, USA
**M Palmarini,** University of Glasgow Veterinary School, Glasgow, UK

## History

Jaagsiekte sheep retrovirus (JSRV) is the causative agent of a naturally occurring lung adenocarcinoma of sheep known as ovine pulmonary adenocarcinoma (OPA, also known as jaagsiekte or sheep pulmonary adenomatosis). OPA was recognized for the first time in South Africa in the nineteenth century as a cause of dyspnea in herded sheep, hence the origin of the Afrikaans name 'jaagsiekte', meaning driving (=jaagt) sickness (=ziekte). OPA is one of the original 'slow diseases' of sheep (along with scrapie, maedi-visna and paratuberculosis) originally described in the 1930s by the Icelandic physician Björn Sigurdsson. The slow diseases of sheep were of great biological importance as they allowed, for the first time, the recognition that an infectious agent could cause clinical disease many months or years after the initial infection of the host.

Studies on JSRV were hampered for years by the lack of a suitable tissue culture system for the cultivation of JSRV. The isolation of full-length JSRV molecular clones (JSRV$_{21}$ and JS$_7$) allowed the *in vitro* generation of infectious viral particles by a transient transfection system, which has sparked a variety of studies that have elucidated many aspects of the molecular biology of JSRV. JSRV is a remarkable virus in many respects. It is the only known virus that induces a naturally occurring lung adenocarcinoma. In addition, the JSRV envelope glycoprotein is an oncoprotein. This is a unique example among retroviruses and oncogenic viruses in general in which a structural protein functions also as a dominant oncoprotein.

## Classification

JSRV belongs to the genus *Betaretrovirus* within the family of the *Retroviridae*. Retroviruses are divided on the basis of their modality of transmission as 'exogenous' and 'endogenous' viruses. Exogenous retroviruses are horizontally transmitted between infected and uninfected hosts. Endogenous retroviruses are stably integrated in the genome of the host species from which they derive, are usually defective, and are transmitted vertically like any other Mendelian gene. JSRV is an exogenous retrovirus and it is highly related to enzootic nasal tumor virus (ENTV) of sheep (ENTV-1) and goats (ENTV-2). JSRV and ENTV have common pathogenic characteristics, and both cause

low-grade adenocarcinomas of secretory cells in different portions of the respiratory tract of small ruminants. Interestingly, sheep, goats, and other members of the *Caprinae* have several copies of nonpathogenic JSRV-related 'endogenous' retroviruses (commonly referred as enJSRVs) stably integrated in their genome. The phylogenetic relationship between JSRV, ENTV, and enJSRVs is indicated in **Figure 1**.

## Genetic Organization and Virion Proteins

The JSRV virions are enveloped particles of approximately 100 nm in diameter and a density by isopycnic centrifugation in sucrose gradients of $1.15 \, \mathrm{g \, ml^{-1}}$ for particles obtained from cell cultures. Virions purified from lung secretions of OPA-affected sheep have a slightly higher density ($1.16-1.18 \, \mathrm{g \, ml^{-1}}$).

JSRV has the typical genomic organization of a simple retrovirus; the genomic RNA of 7455 nt (in the JSRV$_{21}$ infectious molecular clone) contains the canonical retroviral genes *gag, pro, pol,* and *env* (**Figure 2**). Apart from Env, few studies have been undertaken to assign functions to

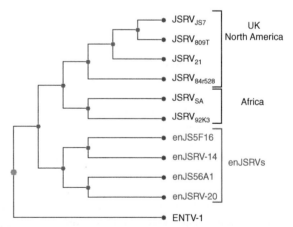

**Figure 1** Phylogenetic analysis of sheep betaretroviruses. A phylogenetic tree of representative small ruminant betaretroviruses was derived by the neighbor-joining method using JSRV, ENTV-1, and enJSRVs *env* aligned using Clustal W. JSRV, enJSRVs, and ENTV-1 cluster in three distinct phylogenetic groups. Note that JSRV isolates from Africa cluster in separate branches from European and North American isolates.

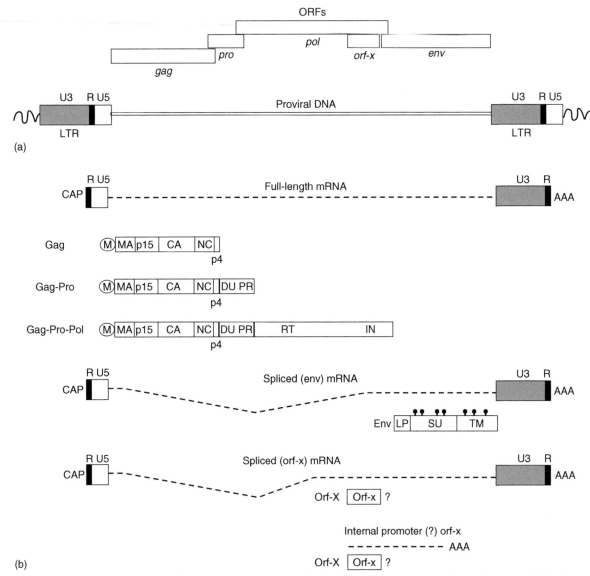

**Figure 2** Genomic organization, mRNAs and viral proteins of JSRV. (a) Schematic organization of the JSRV open reading frames (ORFs) and their relative position in the JSRV provirus. The JSRV LTR, repeated at both ends of the provirus genome, is divided into U3, R and U5. (b) Major JSRV RNAs and proteins. The JSRV provirus transcribes various mRNAs. A full-length mRNA encodes for the Gag, Pro and Pol proteins and serves as genome for the newly synthesized viral particles. A spliced mRNA encodes the viral Env. The Env glycoprotein is glycosylated , and putative glycosylated sites are indicated by full circles. Two additional mRNAs have been detected and encompass the *orf-x* reading frame, but their biological significance is unknown at present. MA, matrix; CA, capsid; NC, nucleocapsid; DU, dUTPase; PR, protease; RT, reverse transcriptase; IN, integrase; LP, leader peptide; SU, surface; TM, transmembrane.

the JSRV proteins and these are assumed to be the same as other retroviruses. The *gag* gene encodes the structural proteins of the viral core. Gag is expressed as an immature polyprotein that is cleaved upon exit by the viral protease. The JSRV Gag is cleaved into at least five proteins: MA (p23), p15, CA (p26), NC, and p4. MA is myristoylated and presumably interacts with the cell membrane during viral egress. CA is the major capsid protein, while NC interacts tightly with the genomic RNA although no specific studies have been conducted on the JSRV NC. The *pro* gene overlaps *gag* and encodes most probably a

dUTPase (DU, deoxyuridine tryphosphatase) and the viral protease (PR). The main function of DU is to avoid misincorporation of uracil into DNA during reverse transcription (see below). As mentioned above, PR cleaves the Gag polyprotein upon exit and it is absolutely required in order to obtain mature infectious viral particles. The *pol* gene overlaps *pro* and is predicted to encode the viral reverse transcriptase (RT) and integrase (IN). Both RT and IN are virion-associated enzymes; RT copies the viral single-stranded RNA genome into double-stranded DNA, while IN serves to join the proviral DNA into the host genome. RNaseH is a subdomain of RT and serves to degrade the viral genomic RNA once has been copied into DNA.

An additional open reading frame (*orf-x*) overlaps *pol* and has some unusual features, including a codon usage different from other genes within JSRV, and a very hydrophobic predicted amino-acid sequence that shows no strong similarities to any known protein and only weak homology to a member of the G protein coupled receptor family. The role of this open reading frame is unknown. Orf-x is conserved among all of the exogenous JSRVs examined to date, but it does not seem to be required for JSRV replication *in vitro* nor for cell transformation either *in vitro* or *in vivo*.

The *env* gene encodes the glycoproteins of the viral envelope (Env). The JSRV Env is formed by two subunits, the surface domain (SU) which interacts with the cellular receptor and mediates viral entry, and the transmembrane domain (TM), which fixes SU to the lipid bilayer. A unique feature of the JSRV *env* is that it functions essentially as a dominant oncogene, and its sole expression is sufficient to induce cell transformation *in vitro* and *in vivo* (see below).

Noncoding regions are present at the 5' and 3' end of the genome. The R region is repeated at the 5' and 3' end of the genome. U5 is present uniquely at the 5' end, and the U3 is present at the 3' end of the genome. The viral promoter and enhancer regions are present in the U3 (see below).

Genomic sequence variability among JSRV strains is very low. For instance, the infectious molecular clones $JSRV_{21}$ and $JSRV_{JS7}$ are 99.3% identical along the entire genomic sequence, and they were derived from naturally occurring OPA cases from Scotland collected many years apart. $JSRV_{21}$ and $JSRV_{JS7}$ Env proteins are 100% identical. JSRV isolates from Africa can be distinguished phylogenetically from the UK and North American isolates, although there is still a high degree of homology (~93% along the entire nucleotide genomic sequence) among the two groups.

## Replication Cycle

In general, the replication cycle of JSRV is not thought to be markedly different from other betaretroviruses. The lack of a suitable tissue culture system for the propagation of JSRV has not allowed detailed studies on the replication of this virus.

JSRV interacts with a specific cellular receptor to enter the cell. The use of retroviral pseudotypes identified hyaluronidase 2 (HYAL2) as the cellular receptor for JSRV entry. HYAL2 is a glycosylphosphatidylinositol (GPI) linked membrane protein with a low hyaluronidase activity and is widely expressed on many different cell types. Besides ovine HYAL2, the human ortholog also

allows JSRV entry, while mouse and rat Hyal2 do not. Detailed steps of JSRV entry and post-entry, such as membrane fusion and the dependence or independence from acidic pH have not been investigated, but are likely to be similar to those of other retroviruses including uncoating, reverse transcription of the viral genome into double-stranded DNA, entry into the nucleus of the pre-integration complex, and stable integration of the proviral DNA into the host DNA. During the process of reverse transcription, the noncoding regions at the 5' and 3' ends of the genome (R, U5, and U3) are duplicated and give origin to the viral long terminal repeats (LTRs).

The retroviral LTRs are major determinants of retrovirus tropism, as the 5' LTR of the provirus initiates transcription and the U3 region contains the majority of *cis*-acting sequences interacting with the cellular RNA polymerase II and with cellular transcription factors. The exogenous JSRV LTRs are particularly active in reporter assays using type II pneumocytes/Clara cell lines and interact with lung-specific transcription factors such as forkhead box A2 (FOXA2; alias HNF-3β). These features may explain the preferential expression of exogenous JSRV in the transformed cells of the lungs, which have phenotypic characteristics of type II pneumocytes and Clara cells.

The expression of JSRV, as in all retroviruses, is believed to follow the basic transcriptional events of cellular mRNAs including capping of the 5' end and polyadenylation at the 3' end. JSRV encodes a full-length mRNA that serves as genome of the viral progeny and is also translated into the Gag polyprotein and the proteins encoded by *pro* and *pol*. The latter are expressed as fusion proteins with Gag. As in all betaretroviruses, *pro* and *pol* are in different open reading frames to *gag* and are expressed by ribosomal frameshifting. The viral Env is produced from a mRNA which is spliced using the splice donor in the untranslated *gag* region and a splice acceptor immediately before *env*.

Another spliced mRNA has been found to use the same splice donor of the *env* mRNA and a splice acceptor before the *orf-x* reading frame. This mRNA presumably expresses a protein encoded by *orf-x*, but there are no published data supporting this assumption. A possible mRNA expressing *orf-x* has been found to lack the R-U5 regions (typical of all other mRNAs starting from the U3) and is thought to derive from the expression of an internal promoter that has not been characterized. Other mRNAs deriving from the use of secondary splice acceptors and non-conventional polyadenylated sites have been detected but their biological significance, if any, is unknown.

JSRV assembles in the cytoplasm (**Figures 3(a)** and **3(b)**) like all betaretroviruses, most likely in the pericentriolar region (**Figures 3(c)–3(e)**). Other retroviruses such as lentiviruses and gammaretroviruses assemble instead mostly at the cell membrane. The JSRV intracellular particles interact with Env at the cell membrane or in a cellular compartment not yet fully identified and egress

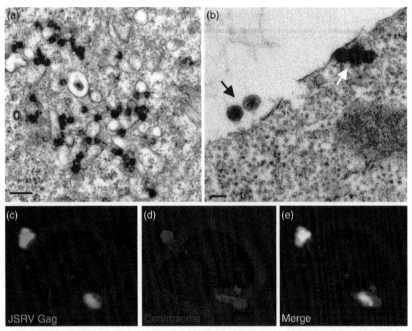

**Figure 3** Electron and confocal microscopy of cells expressing JSRV. Electron microscopy in 293T cells transiently transfected with the $JSRV_{21}$ infectious molecular clone showing intracytoplasmic particles (a; scale = 200 µm). In panel b, intracellular particles in the vicinity of the cell membrane (white arrow) and extracellular particles complete with viral envelope (black arrow) are also visible (scale = 100 µm). (c–e) Confocal microscopy in HeLa cells transiently transfected with JSRV and probed with an antiserum towards the JSRV matrix (c) and γ-tubulin (d). The JSRV Gag concentrates in the pericentrosomal area (e).

from the cell. Upon exit, the Gag polyprotein is cleaved by the viral protease into the mature proteins described above. A more detailed description of the replication cycle of retroviruses is discussed elsewhere in this encyclopedia.

## enJSRVs

The sheep genome contains at least 27 copies of endogenous retroviruses highly related to JSRV (hence the name enJSRVs). Endogenous retroviruses are believed to derive from integration events of ancestral exogenous retroviruses into the germline of the host. enJSRVs have a high degree of homology with JSRV. For example, $JSRV_{21}$ and enJS56A1 are 92% identical at the nucleotide level along the entire genome. Major differences are located in the U3 region, in two regions in Gag (termed variable regions 1 and 2), and in the cytoplasmic tail of the transmembrane domain of the Env (termed variable region 3). At least some of these highly divergent regions are the basis of important biological differences between JSRV and enJSRVs.

enJSRV transcripts have been detected in most tissues by sensitive reverse transcriptase polymerase chain reaction (RT-PCR) assays. However, high levels of enJSRVs (both mRNA and proteins) are found specifically in the epithelia of the genital tract of the ewe and, particularly, in the epithelia of the uterus (**Figure 4**). In the placenta, enJSRVs are expressed in the mononuclear

trophectoderm cells of the conceptus (embryo/fetus and associated extra-embryonic membranes), but are most abundant in the trophoblast giant binucleate cells (BNCs) and multinucleated syncytial plaques of the placentomes. The temporal expression of enJSRVs envelope (*env*) gene in the trophectoderm is coincident with key events in the development of the sheep conceptus. Indeed, using a morpholino antisense oligonucleotide to induce loss-of-function *in utero*, enJSRVs Env knockdown caused a reduction in trophoblast outgrowth and inhibited/prevented trophoblast giant binucleate cell differentiation during blastocyst elongation and formation of the conceptus. Thus, enJSRVs have been proposed to be essential in sheep for peri-implantion growth and differentiation.

enJSRVs expression appears to be regulated by progesterone and expression of the progesterone receptor. However, the specific enJSRV loci that are transcriptionally active are not known at present. enJSRVs are also expressed in the sheep fetus, supporting the idea that sheep are tolerized toward JSRV. Indeed, JSRV-infected naïve sheep (with or without lung adenocarcinoma) have no detectable specific humoral or cellular immune responses, although recombinant JSRV CA, in the presence of adjuvants, can induce antibody production and specific T-cell responses in vaccinated sheep.

Three full-length enJSRV loci have been cloned and characterized (enJS56A1, enJS5F16, and enJS59A1). All three loci have deletions or stop codons that make

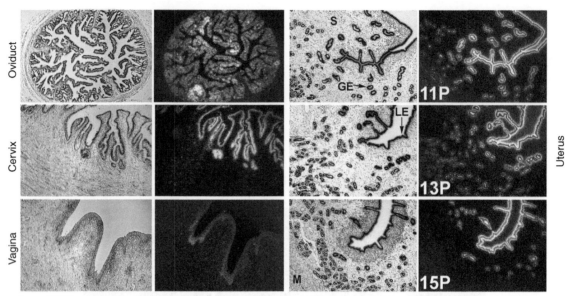

**Figure 4** enJSRVs are highly expressed in epithelia of the genital tract of the ewe. *In situ* hybridization analysis of enJSRVs *env* mRNA in the oviduct, uterus, cervix, and vagina. Note the specific expression of enJSRVs *env* mRNA in the epithelia lining the oviduct, cervix, and vagina of the cycling ewe. During the estrous cycle and pregnancy (P), enJSRVs mRNA is particularly abundant in the luminal and glandular epithelia of the uterus. LE, luminal epithelium; GE, glandular epithelium; M, myometrium; S, stroma. Modified from Palmarini M, Gray CA, Carpenter K, Fan H, Bazer FW, and Spencer TE (2001) Expression of endogenous betaretroviruses in the ovine uterus: Effects of neonatal age, estrous cycle, pregnancy, and progesterone. *Journal of Virology* 75(23): 11319–11327.

them replication incompetent. However, enJS56A1 and enJS5F16 maintain intact ORFs for *gag* and *env*. By using retroviral vectors pseudotyped by the enJSRVs Env, it was found that they too use HYAL2 as a cellular receptor and interfere by receptor competition with JSRV entry.

One of the enJSRVs loci, enJS56A1, is defective for viral exit when overexpressed in transfected cells, although abundant intracytoplasmic Gag is detected and intracytoplasmic viral particles are visible by electron microscopy. The replication defect of enJS56A1 is determined by its Gag protein, which is *trans*-dominant over the exogenous JSRV Gag if co-expressed in the same cell. A tryptophan residue in position 21 of the enJS56A1 Gag (replacing an arginine in JSRV) is the main determinant for the block induced by enJS56A1. Thus, enJS56A1 exerts a unique mechanism of retroviral interference, which occurs at a late step of the replication cycle. The mechanism and timing of the block induced by enJS56A1 are not yet understood. However, the observation of viral particles by electron microscopy in cells expressing enJS56A1 (or co-expressing enJS56A1 and JSRV) suggests that enJS56A1-induced interference depends on a defect in Gag trafficking. Recent studies suggest that enJS56A1 appears to block JSRV, most likely in *trans*, by hampering the ability of the latter to reach the centrosome, the proposed site of assembly for betaretroviruses.

enJSRVs are not expressed in the differentiated epithelial cells of the lungs but are expressed in the epithelium of the genital tract. As mentioned above, enhancer regions are located in the U3 and indeed enJSRVs transcription is regulated by progesterone via the progesterone receptor. Interestingly, the enJSRVs LTRs do not respond to lung transcription factors (such as FOXA2) unlike the exogenous JSRV LTRs. Thus, the LTR appears to be a major contributor to the different tropisms (genital tract vs. respiratory tract) shown by enJSRVs and JSRV.

The enJSRVs Env (or at least the Env of those enJSRVs loci cloned so far) is not able to transform cells *in vitro*, unlike the highly related JSRV Env. Indeed, the cytoplasmic tail of the JSRV Env is where major determinants of transformation are located. In particular, an SH2 binding domain is present in the exogenous JSRV Env, but is absent in the enJSRVs Env sequenced to date. It is hypothesized that enJSRVs have been selected in the sheep for their ability to confer resistance to infection of the host by the related exogenous betaretroviruses. This innate resistance could have provided a selection pressure for betaretroviruses with tropism towards the respiratory tract (i.e., the current JSRV) rather than the genital tract.

## Ovine Pulmonary Adenocarcinoma

OPA is a naturally occurring lung cancer of sheep that has been reported in most sheep-rearing countries. It is absent from Australia and New Zealand and has been eradicated from Iceland. The disease is characterized by a progressive respiratory condition caused by the growth of the lung

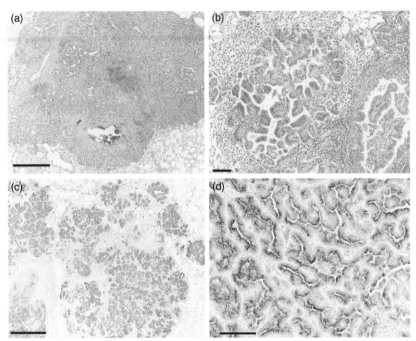

**Figure 5**   JSRV-induced tumours *in vivo*. (a, b) Histology from a lung tumor section of a naturally occurring case of OPA. Sections were stained with hematoxylin and eosin. Note the presence of papillary to acinar neoplastic lesions that replace the normal alveolar structure of the lungs. (c, d) Immunohistochemistry in lung sections from a JSRV experimentally inoculated lamb show expression of the viral Env in tumor cells (characterized by the intracytoplasmic brown color). Scale = 500 μm (a, c); 100 μm (b, d).

adenocarcinoma. The tumor appears to originate from two types of differentiated epithelial secretory cells of the distal respiratory tract, the type II pneumocyte and the Clara cell, which retain their phenotype (**Figure 5**). OPA is invariably fatal once the disease is diagnosed, and affected sheep die as a result of compromised respiratory function caused by tumor enlargement or from secondary bacterial infections. The incubation period of the naturally occurring disease can be very long lasting several months to years.

Susceptibility/resistance to JSRV of some breeds has been suggested but not proved. OPA can be transmitted experimentally only with material that contains JSRV, such as lung secretions collected from affected animals or virions obtained by transiently transfecting cells with JSRV infectious molecular clones. The experimental OPA model is highly reproducible. JSRV infection can be induced in most, if not all, inoculated lambs aged 1–6 months at the time of inoculation and a high proportion of them develop clinical signs and OPA lesions. Neonatal lambs are most susceptible and, in contrast to naturally occurring OPA, the incubation period for experimentally induced OPA can be as short as a few weeks.

Although most experimentally inoculated lambs develop clinical signs and OPA lesions, under natural conditions the majority of JSRV-infected sheep do not develop OPA during their commercial lifespan. Within an endemically infected flock, lambs appear to become infected at a very early age although the routes of transmission have not been

determined yet. Interestingly, most infected animals harbor the virus as a disseminated infection of their lymphoid tissues and do not show detectable pulmonary lesions. Although lymphoreticular cells appear to serve as the principal reservoir of virus infection, viral antigens are detected only rarely in this compartment where sensitive PCR assays are necessary to detect viral RNA or proviral DNA.

The short incubation period in young lambs experimentally infected with JSRV may be explained by the combination of high virus infectious doses present in the inoculum and the higher abundance of the permissive target cells (type 2 pneumocytes and Clara cells) in lambs compared to adult animals. In natural infections, the mechanisms involved in converting the stable persistent lymphoid infection in peripheral tissues to a progressive pulmonary epithelial tumor are not clear. In addition, it is not known whether and how efficiently sheep infected by JSRV, but with no neoplastic lesions, are able to transmit the virus to uninfected sheep. In an affected flock, control of OPA is very difficult as no vaccines or effective diagnostic tests are available.

## Mechanisms of Virus-Induced Cell Transformation

The mechanisms used by JSRV to induce cell transformation are different from those followed by the majority of oncogenic retroviruses. Most of the tumors caused by retroviruses are due to insertional activation of cellular oncogenes nearby the integrated proviruses. As a result, tumors originated by retroviral insertional activation are monoclonal or oligoclonal and common proviral integration sites are detected in tumors from different animals. Another mechanism of retrovirus transformation is transduction of cellular proto-oncogenes by the retroviral genome that are transmitted as a mixture of replication competent 'helper' viruses and replication defective viruses that have captured the oncogene. Tumors caused by retroviral transduction are in general multiclonal.

In contrast, JSRV follows neither of the mechanisms mentioned above. OPA tumors are multiclonal, and common proviral integration sites have been rarely observed. However, no cellular oncogenes have been found to be transduced by JSRV. The oncogenic properties of JSRV are due directly to one of its structural proteins.

Transfection of a variety of fibroblast and epithelial cell lines with expression plasmids for the JSRV Env leads to efficient cell transformation (**Figure 6**). Moreover, experimental infection of mice and lambs, with replication incompetent vectors expressing JSRV Env, induced tumors in the inoculated animals. Thus, the JSRV Env is a dominant oncoprotein both *in vitro* and *in vivo* and viral spread is not necessary for tumorigenesis.

The mechanisms involved in JSRV Env-induced transformation have not been fully elucidated; however, signal transduction involving the PI3K-Akt and H/N Ras-MEK-MAPK pathways are important. Conflicting reports are available on the involvement of other cellular oncogenes such as the Stk/Ron tyrosine kinase in the onset of JSRV Env-induced cell transformation.

One of the major determinants of JSRV Env transformation is the transmembrane domain (TM), although other regions may be important. In particular, a putative docking site (Y-X-X-M) for phosphatidylinositol 3-kinase (PI-3K) is critical for JSRV-Env induced cell transformation. Within this motif, Y590 is crucial for JSRV Env-induced cell transformation, although Y590 mutants maintain a reduced ability to induce cell transformation in some cell lines. In summary, the JSRV Env acts as a dominant oncogene *in vitro* and *in vivo* and its expression is sufficient to induce lung adenocarcinoma in the target species.

## Enzootic Nasal Tumor Virus

ENTVs of sheep and goats are distinct betaretroviruses highly related to each other and JSRV. ENTV causes a contagious tumor of the mucosal nasal glands, as well as respiratory and olfactory mucosa, in their respective target species known as enzootic nasal adenocarcinoma (ENT). Clinically, ENT is characterized by respiratory distress caused by the enlargement of the tumor, nasal

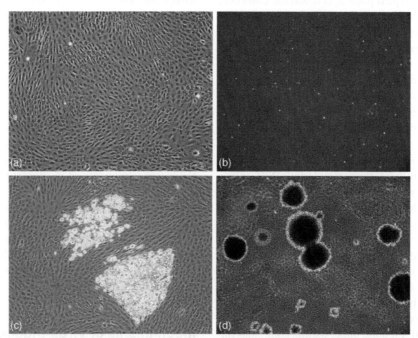

**Figure 6** Expression of the JSRV Env transforms cells *in vitro*. Transformation of the rat fibroblast cell line 208F by the JSRV envelope glycoprotein. 208F cells were mock-transfected (a) or transfected with an expression plasmid for the JSRV Env (c). Mock-transfected 208F cells are morphologically flat, possess a strong contact-inhibition and do not grow in soft agar (b). On the other hand, 208F cells transfected with an expression plasmid for the JSRV Env show the onset of foci of transformed cells (c), which are able to form colonies in soft agar (d).

discharge, and skull deformation. Like OPA, ENT has a long incubation period.

The molecular biology of ENTV has not been studied in great detail, but the virus displays many features in common with JSRV. The cellular receptor for ENTV is also HYAL2 and the ENTV Env, like its JSRV counterpart, is a dominant oncogene that appears to follow the same mechanisms of cell transformation used by JSRV. The main differences between the ENTVs and JSRV appear to be concentrated in the U3 region of the viral LTRs. The ENTV LTR, unlike the JSRV LTR, does not bind lung-specific transcription factors such as FOXA2, which is likely the basis of tropism differences between the two viruses.

## Future Perspectives

Small ruminant betaretroviruses are a fascinating group of viruses with unique characteristics that are of broad interest through their veterinary, comparative medical and biological importance. The veterinary importance arises from the economic impact in many sheep rearing countries of the diseases induced by JSRV and ENTV combined with the absence of any effective control tools or mechanisms. Their comparative medical interest stems from the striking similarity of some forms of human lung adenocarcinoma to OPA, which is considered an excellent outbred large animal model for these tumors with opportunities to investigate issues that are not available from other systems. Lung cancer is the main cause of death among cancer patients and effective therapeutic strategies are greatly needed to improve patient survival and well-being. OPA is a large animal model that can identify and test the efficacy of new therapeutic interventions in a highly reproducible system.

enJSRVs are an especially active group of endogenous retroviruses and offer insights into several areas of general biological interest, such as viral replication, interference, and reproductive biology. Understanding the mechanisms of the enJS56A1-induced block could inspire the design of novel anti-retroviral strategies and shed light on early events in retroviral assembly and/or trafficking. In particular, this unique viral block provides additional clues on the variety of mechanisms shaping co-evolution of endogenous/exogenous retroviruses and their hosts.

enJSRVs are highly expressed in the genital tract of the ewe and are intimately involved in early placental development in this animal species. The sheep/enJSRVs model can be useful to experimentally address the hypothesis that endogenous retroviruses have shaped and are essential for mammalian biology.

*See also:* Simian Retrovirus D.

## Further Reading

Fan H (ed.) (2003) *Jaagsiekte Sheep Retrovirus and Lung Cancer.* Berlin: Springer.

Maeda N, Palmarini M, Murgia C, and Fan H (2001) Direct transformation of rodent fibroblasts by jaagsiekte sheep retrovirus DNA. *Proceedings of the National Academy of Sciences, USA* 98: 4449–4454.

Palmarini M, Gray CA, Carpenter K, Fan H, Bazer FW, and Spencer TE (2001) Expression of endogenous betaretroviruses in the ovine uterus: Effects of neonatal age, estrous cycle, pregnancy, and progesterone. *Journal of Virology* 75(23): 11319–11327.

Palmarini M, Sharp JM, De las Heras M, and Fan H (1999) Jaagsiekte sheep retrovirus is necessary and sufficient to induce a contagious lung cancer in sheep. *Journal of Virology* 73: 6964–6972.

Wootton SK, Halbert CL, and Miller AD (2005) Sheep retrovirus structural protein induces lung tumours. *Nature* 434: 904–907.

# Leporipoviruses and Suipoxviruses

**G McFadden,** University of Florida, Gainesville, FL, USA

## History

Poxviruses of leporids and swine cause a broad range of symptoms varying from mild lesions of the skin right up to the lethal systemic diseases (**Table 1**). The agent of myxomatosis, a virulent disease of domestic rabbits described originally by G. Sanarelli in 1896, was in fact the first viral pathogen discovered for a laboratory animal. The close similarity of myxoma virus (MYX) with other members of the poxvirus family, such as variola and

fowlpox viruses, was first recognized by Aragão in 1927. MYX is notable because, although it causes rather benign lesions in the native *Sylvilagus* rabbit (the brush rabbit in North America and the tropical forest rabbit in South America), when introduced to the European (*Oryctolagus*) rabbit it causes an invasive disease syndrome called myxomatosis with up to 100% mortality. MYX was the first viral agent ever introduced into the wild for the purpose of eradicating a vertebrate pest, namely the feral European rabbit population in Australia in 1950 and, 2 years

**Table 1**   Members of the genera *Leporipoxvirus* and *Suipoxvirus*

| Member | Abbreviation | Natural host | Major arthropod vector | Natural host disease | Disease in domesticated European rabbit (Oryctolagus cuniculus) |
|---|---|---|---|---|---|
| *Leporipoxvirus* | | | | | |
| Myxoma | MYX | California brush rabbit[a], S. American tapeti[b] (*Sylvilagus* sp.) | Mosquito, flea | Localized benign fibroma | Systemic lethal myxomatosis |
| Rabbit fibroma (Shope fibroma) | SFV | N. American cottontail rabbit (*Sylvilagus floridans*) | Mosquito, flea | Localized benign fibroma | Localized benign fibroma |
| Malignant rabbit fibroma[c] | MRV | Lab. rabbit[d] (*Oryctolagus cuniculus*) | | Not observed in wild | Systemic lethal syndrome similar to myxomatosis |
| Squirrel fibroma | SqFV | Gray squirrel (*Sciurus* sp.) | Probably mosquito | Localized or multiple fibromas | Occasional nodular dermal lesions |
| Hare fibroma | HFV | Wild hares (*Lepus* sp.) | Probably mosquito | Localized benign fibroma | Localized benign fibroma |
| *Suipoxvirus* | | | | | |
| Swinepox | SPV | Domestic pigs (Suidae sp.) | Hog lice | Localized cutaneous lesions | Intradermal lesions but no serial propagation |

[a]Also called Marshall–Regnery myxoma.
[b]Also called Aragão's (or Brazilian) myxoma.
[c]Laboratory recombinant between MYX and SFV.
[d]MRV has been propagated only by serial inoculation of laboratory rabbits and in cultured cells.

later, in Europe. The resulting genetic selection of virus isolates with lesser pathogenicity and upsurgence of rabbits with greater resistance to the viral disease was studied intensively by Frank Fenner and his colleagues as a model system to investigate the ecological consequences of virus/host evolution in an outbred population.

Also, of interest to the history of animal virology is the fact that the first DNA virus associated with transmissible tumors was Shope fibroma virus (SFV), described in 1932 by Richard Shope as an infectious agent of fibroma-like hyperplasia in cottontail rabbits (*Sylvilagus floridanus*) in the eastern USA. It is likely that the agent of 'hare sarcoma', described first in Germany in 1909, was also a poxvirus, now called hare fibroma virus (HFV). HFV remains the only leporipoxvirus to have arisen outside the Americas but its biology closely resembles that of SFV.

Very little is known about the remaining leporipoxviruses. Subcutaneous fibromatosis in gray squirrels of the eastern USA and western gray squirrels in California, caused by poxviruses now collectively called squirrel fibroma virus (SqFV), has been observed since 1936, but their rigorous classification with the MYX–SFV group was not made until 1951 by L. Kilham. Similarly, HFV, described first in 1959 in the European hare (*Lepus europaeus*), was also shown to be a closely related poxvirus in 1961. In 1983, an outbreak of a disease resembling myxomatosis in laboratory rabbits in San Diego was caused by a novel leporipoxvirus later shown to be a

genetic recombinant between SFV and a still-undefined strain of MYX. This virus, called malignant rabbit fibroma virus (MRV), has never been observed in wild rabbit populations but is of interest as an experimental model for poxvirus-induced immunosuppression and tumorigenesis. In most respects, MRV can be considered to be a substrain of MYX.

Based on landmark experiments with pneumococcus in the 1920s, the very first example of what was believed to be genetic interaction between viruses was reported in 1936 with the discovery that heat-inactivated myxoma could be reactivated with live SFV (Berry–Dedrick transformation), but later work showed this to be a genome rescue phenomenon rather than true recombination.

The only known member of the *Suipoxvirus* genus, swinepox virus (SPV), has been observed sporadically in pig populations throughout the world, but is not considered a serious pathogen because infected animals usually have only moderate symptoms and recover completely.

## Taxonomy and Classification

The genera *Leporipoxvirus* and *Suipoxvirus* are in the subfamily *Chordopoxvirinae* of the family *Poxviridae*. The prefix 'lepori' comes from Latin *lepus* or *leporis* ('hare') and 'sui' from Latin *sus* ('swine'), to denote the relatively restricted host range of these viruses. All the viruses in the genus *Leporipoxvirus* can be shown to be closely related to each other by serology, immunodiffusion, and fluorescent antibody tests, although antigenic differences can be detected in strains of MYX. SPV (genus *Suipoxvirus*) is antigenically unique and is not known to have any closely related members. In terms of broad features, all are typical poxviruses, with characteristic brick-shaped virions containing a double-stranded DNA (dsDNA) genome with covalently closed hairpin termini and terminal inverted repeat (TIR) sequences. Like other poxviruses, viral macromolecular synthesis takes place exclusively in the cytoplasm of infected cells.

## Properties of the Virion

As for all other members of the poxvirus family, the virions have a characteristic brick-shaped morphology with dimensions of approximately 250–300 nm × 250 nm × 200 nm. The leporipoxviruses are uniquely sensitive to ether and chloroform but otherwise the virions are very stable at ambient temperatures and in skin lesions. In all other respects, such as chemical composition and physical properties, the virus particles are very similar to those of vaccinia virus (VACV).

## Properties of the Viral DNA and Protein

Complete genomic sequences are available for SFV, MYX, and SPV. The leporipoxviruses have dsDNA genomes of 160–163 kbp, with hairpin termini and TIR sequences of 10–13 kbp. SPV DNA is somewhat smaller (146.5 kbp) but otherwise the genome has similar characteristics. Each virus encodes from 150 to 160 proteins. A web-based resource is available that records the predicted proteins expressed by these three poxviruses (see 'Relevant website' section). Viral DNA of leporipoxviruses cross-hybridize at moderate stringencies only with other members of the genus and SPV DNA is unique and is not known to cross-hybridize with any other poxvirus DNA. The MRV DNA genome is 95% identical to that of MYX, except that it possesses five genes derived from SFV plus three SFV/MYX fusion genes.

The nucleotide composition of the leporipoxviruses (44% G + C for MYX) is higher than that of the orthopoxviruses (35% for VACV) but there is evidence that many of the viral genes important for virus replication, gene expression, and viral assembly are conserved between the genera. These conserved genes are clustered near the central regions of the viral genome. In contrast, viral genes mapping near the genomic termini show considerable variability, and are believed to encode many of the specific determinants of pathogenesis, host range, and disease characteristics.

The protein complexities of these viruses are comparable to those of most poxviruses, although the profiles are unique for each member. In general, about 80–90 poxvirus genes are relatively well conserved among the various member poxviruses, whereas the remainder (usually in excess of 50–60 genes) are more diverged and specify the unique features of virus–host interactions, such as host tropism, immunomodulation, and virulence.

## DNA Replication, Transcription, and Translation

All of the major features of macromolecular synthesis by these viruses are very similar to those deduced for the prototype poxvirus, VACV. Viral DNA synthesis is restricted to cytoplasmic sites, although replication for leporipoxviruses tends to be initiated somewhat more slowly than for VACV. The virus-encoded transcriptional apparatus is well conserved between the poxvirus genera, and many of the important regulatory signals that are utilized by VACV, such as promoters and transcription termination sequences, are also utilized with comparable efficiency in the leporipoxviruses. Thus, viral genes from one genus can be introduced to another by recombination or by DNA transfection technologies to generate chimeric virus constructs that maintain the correct regulation of the new genetic information. As in the case of VACV, transcriptional units can be of different kinetic classes (early/intermediate/late) and there is no splicing of viral mRNA.

The leporipoxviruses replicate in cytoplasmic factories that appear by microscopic analysis as eosinophilic B-type inclusion bodies. These factories, also called virosomes, can be visualized by Feulgen, Giemsa, or fluorescent antibody staining. SPV produces nuclear inclusions and vacuolations in addition to cytoplasmic bodies but these nuclear alterations are not believed to be sites of viral replication.

## Molecular Mechanisms of Pathogenesis

Since these viruses are of only minor veterinary importance, recent research has focused on the elucidation of the determinants for viral virulence, particularly with respect to the strategies that these viruses employ to subvert the immune system of the infected host. Particular attention has been paid to the mechanism(s) underlying the immune dysfunction caused by MYX infection in *Oryctolagus* rabbits. To date, at least two classes of viral gene products have been directly implicated in the immunomodulation induced by these viruses:

1. 'Virokines' are secreted virus-encoded proteins that are targeted to host-specific pathways outside the infected cell. For example, SFV and MYX encode growth factors related to epidermal growth factor and transforming growth factor α that participate in stimulating fibroblastic proliferation at primary and secondary tumors.

2. 'Viroceptors' are viral proteins that mimic cellular receptors and function by sequestering important host cytokines that normally participate in the antiviral immune response. Leporipoxviral-encoded receptor-like molecules have been discovered for tumor necrosis factor (TNF) and interferon γ (IFN-γ), and may exist for other antiviral lymphokines as well. SPV encodes a novel homolog of cellular chemokine receptors, and the leporipoxviruses express secreted chemokine-binding proteins that are important for virus pathogenesis.

Interference with antigen presentation by MYX is also believed to play a role in circumventing T-cell recognition during early stages of virus infection. One MYX gene product responsible for evading immune clearance, designated Serp1, is an extracellular inhibitor of cellular serine proteinases, and the purified protein exhibits potent anti-inflammatory properties in a variety of animal model systems of inflammatory disease.

## Geographic and Seasonal Distribution

All three major species of *Sylvilagus* rabbits in the Americas have endemic fibroma-like poxviruses, and myxomatosis is now established in wild *Oryctolagus* rabbit populations of South America, Europe, and Australia. SqFV and HFV have been reported to date only in North America and Europe, respectively. The leporipoxviruses in the wild undergo seasonal fluctuations that correlate well with increased populations of arthropod vectors in summer and autumn, most prominently mosquitoes. An exception to this is found in Britain, where the major vector of MYX is the flea, which is not as seasonally variable.

In the case of SPV, outbreaks are not tied to seasonal cycles but are generally associated with the degree of hog lice infestation.

## Host Range and Virus Propagation

These viruses demonstrate a very restricted host range in terms of ability to cause disease, although viral replication can also occur in cultured cells from some nonsusceptible hosts as well. In some cases, viral replication in tissue culture monolayers or chicken chorioallantoic membranes produces 'foci' in which infected cells manifest minimal cytopathic effects, thus permitting macroscopic cell aggregations to develop. The extent of cytopathology is markedly influenced by both the cell type and the virus strain, and in some instances the infected cells may detach from the monolayer to produce visible plaques. When viral replication is relatively slow and the toxicity to the target cell sufficiently moderate, a chronically infected carrier culture can be established in which progeny virus production persists for extended passages. Although poxviruses cannot permanently transform primary cells into an immortalized state, cells persistently infected with the fibroma-inducing leporipoxviruses can assume many of the phenotypic characteristics associated with the transformed phenotype, such as novel morphology, growth in reduced serum, and ability to form colonies in soft agar. It is likely that some of these phenotypic characteristics are facilitated by secreted poxviral proteins (virokines) that mimic cellular mitogens, such as epidermal growth factor, and trigger neighboring cells into excessive proliferation.

In the cases of the benign leporipoxviruses and SPV, replication is restricted to dermal and subcutaneous sites, with occasional involvement of draining lymph nodes. However, MYX and MRV are unique in that they also replicate efficiently in lymphoid cells, such as macrophages, B cells, and T cells. MYX, like human immunodeficiency virus type 1, replicates in either resting or stimulated T cells, and can be readily isolated from splenocyte cultures. The molecular basis for the uniquely permissive nature of MYX replication in lymphocytes is unknown, but is unquestionably an important factor in the extreme virulence of myxomatosis. Several MYX genes have been identified (e.g., M-T2, M-T4, M-T5, and M11L) that express host range determinants that block the cellular apoptosis response to infection of lymphocytes.

## Evolution and Genetic Variability

The deliberate release of MYX into rabbit populations of Australia, France, and Britain in the early 1950s provided a unique opportunity to study the natural selection pressures exerted on a particularly virulent virus/host interaction. There is an extensive literature on the ecological consequences of the feral rabbit eradication program, and the rapid evolution of myxomatosis in the wild is well documented. Although the original South American MYX virus strain that was introduced left very few survivors in selected populations, within a few years attenuated viral strains with reduced virulence took over and more resistant rabbits became predominant.

In terms of the categories of viral virulence, some strains of MYX are classified as highly virulent (e.g., Moses and Lausanne), and attenuated variants exist down to relatively nonpathogenic (e.g., neuromyxoma and the Nottingham strains). Little is known about the extent of genetic variation in other leporipoxviruses, although different isolates of SFV show marked variations in tumorigenicity. Generally, leporids that recover from infection with one member either become resistant or undergo partial protection from infection by another member.

SPV shares some antigenic crossreactivity with VACV, but neutralizing antibody does not confer cross-protection for secondary infection by members of different genera.

## Transmission and Tissue Tropism

The principal mode of transmission is by biting arthropod vectors, and the major inoculation route is dermal. Since these viruses do not replicate in the vector, the transmission is purely mechanical and hence virus spread can be readily accomplished by alternative routes. Thus, mosquitoes, fleas, blackflies, ticks, lice, mites, and even thistles and the claws of predatory birds have all been implicated in leporipoxvirus transmission. The efficiency of transmission by arthropods is quite variable, and is related to viral titers in skin lesions as well as the size of the vector populations. There are no known respiratory or oral routes of infection with members of either genus, but in some infections, such as MYX in domestic rabbits, the disease can be transmitted by direct contact with ocular discharges or open cutaneous lesions.

The sui- and leporipoxviruses in their native hosts are specific for the epidermis or subdermis and usually do not progress to secondary sites, although draining lymph nodes can be affected. However, in the specific case of MYX infection of the domestic rabbit, the virus can propagate efficiently in lymphocytes and migrate via infected leukocytes through lymphatic channels to establish secondary sites of infection. Recently, it was shown that MYX can productively infect and kill a variety of human cancer cells, likely due to cell signaling changes associated with cellular transformation in the tumor cells.

## Pathogenicity

The leporipoxviruses are restricted to rabbits, squirrels, and hares, and swinepox is found only in domestic pigs. For SFV infection of *Sylvilagus* rabbits, tumors can last for many months before regressing, whereas in *Oryctolagus* rabbits recovery is usually complete within a few weeks. Only MYX manifests dramatic alterations in pathogenicity when the European rabbit is infected. For all of these viruses, the immune status of the host rabbit plays a critical role; for example, in adult rabbits, SFV rarely causes disease symptoms except for the primary fibroblastic lesion, but in newborn or immunocompromised animals the infection can lead to invasive tumors and much higher titers of infectious virus in infected tissues. Agents such as cortisone, X-rays, or immunosuppressants can dramatically increase SFV tumor development, and

chemical promoters like 3,4-benzopyrene or methylcholanthrene can predispose progression to invasive fibromatosis or even metastatic fibrosarcoma.

The ability to cause collapse of the host immune response, replicate in lymphocytes, and spread efficiently to secondary sites is a unique property of MYX in *Oryctolagus* rabbits. The myxomatosis syndrome can be associated with multiple external signs (e.g., South American MYX) or may have relatively fewer gross symptoms (e.g., California MYX) and mortalities can range up to 100%. Supervening Gram-negative bacterial infections in the respiratory tract and conjuctiva are often observed concomitantly during myxomatosis, particularly by the adventitious pathogens *Pasteurella multocida* or *Bordetella bronchoseptica*, and contribute to the lethality of the disease.

SPV is only mildly pathogenic in pigs although it can cause a minor level of mortality, usually associated with milk-feeding reduction in younger animals.

## Clinical Features of Infection

The cutaneous tumors induced by the different leporipoxviruses in their natural hosts are clinically very similar to each other. The fibromas are rarely associated with any other symptoms, such as fever or appetite loss, and invariably regress as long as the animal is not otherwise immunocompromised. In the case of MYX in *Oryctolagus* rabbits, however, the symptoms rapidly become severe as the tumors fail to regress and the concomitant immunosuppression contributes to the lethal myxomatosis syndrome. The clinical features of myxomatosis are influenced by the genetic background of both the virus strain and the rabbit host. In the preacute form of the disease caused by California MYX, the rabbits succumb in less than 1 week, and often have only minor external symptoms, such as inflammation and edema of the eyelids. Skin hemorrhages can be observed in some cases and convulsions often precede death. In the acute form caused by South American strains of MYX, the rabbits survive 1–2 weeks and develop more distinctive symptoms. The primary tumor can be either flat and diffuse or protuberant, and secondary site tumors around the nose, eyes, and ears become prominent by 6–7 days, at which time purulent exudates from the nose and eyes frequently develop. The cutaneous tumors often become necrotic and a generalized immune dysfunction exacerbates the progressive secondary bacterial infestation of the respiratory tract. In the case of the more attenuated MYX isolates, such as neuromyxoma, the disease course is less severe and may be associated with little or no mortality.

The disease course of SPV in pigs is rather different, and resembles that of VACV in humans. Inoculation results in localized dermal papules, which progress to vesicles and pustules, after which the lesions crust and scab over. The only clinical symptom is occasional minor fever and the animals recover within 3 weeks.

## Pathology and Histopathology

The primary tumors caused by leporipoxviruses in *Sylvilagus* rabbits, squirrels, and hares all closely resemble proliferant fibromas. Following inoculation, an acute inflammatory reaction occurs with infiltration of polymorphonuclear and mononuclear cells and proliferation of fibroblast-like cells of uncertain origin. The 'tumor' consists of pleomorphic cells imbedded in a matrix of intercellular fibrils of collagen. Unlike the transformed cells induced by other DNA tumor viruses, cells from poxviral tumors are not immortalized and cannot be propagated independently. Instead they appear to require secreted virus-encoded proteins in order to sustain the hyperproliferative state. Inclusion bodies characteristic of poxviral replication can be observed in the cytoplasms of epithelial and some fibroma cells. As the tumor develops, mononuclear leukocyte cuffing of adjacent vessels is observed and at the base of the tumor there is accumulation of lymphocytes, plasma cells, macrophages, and neutrophils. The ratio between influx of inflammatory cells and fibroblast proliferation is variable but generally there is little or no necrosis. The speed with which immune cells clear the viral infection and reverse the hyperproliferation can range from 1–2 weeks to 6 months, depending on both the virus and the host.

The principal difference between the benign fibroma syndrome described above and the devastating disease caused by MYX in *Oryctolagus* rabbits is that the latter virus efficiently propagates in host lymphocytes and is able to circumvent the cell-mediated immune response to the viral infection. The subcutaneous tumors consist of proliferating undifferentiated mesenchymal cells, which become large and stellate with prominent nuclei ('myxoma' cells). In surrounding tissue there can be extensive proliferation of endothelial cells of the local capillaries and venules, often to the point where complete occusion leads to extensive necrosis of the infected site. The overlying epithelial cells can show hyperplasia or degeneration, depending on the virus strain, and poxviral inclusion bodies are frequently observed in the prickle-cell layer. In some MYX strains, primary and secondary skin tumors can undergo extensive hemorrhage and internal lesions may be found in the stomach, intestines, and heart. The virus readily migrates to secondary sites within infected immune cells and concomitant cellular proliferation can be detected in the reticulum cells of lymph nodes and spleen, as well as the conjunctival and pulmonary alveolar epithelium. The nasal mucosa and conjunctiva overlying secondary tumors undergo squamous metaplasia such that the epithelia become nonciliated and nonkeratizing.

Disruption of the ciliary architecture may be one of the factors that facilitate the extensive Gram-negative bacterial infections of the eyes, nose, and respiratory tract. Varying degrees of inflammatory cell infiltration by polymorphonuclear heterophils occur soon after infection but there is only a limited and ineffective cellular immune response. The lymph nodes and spleen show evidence of aberrant T-cell activation and hyperplasia, and infectious virus can be isolated from all lymphoid organs except the thymus. Death is believed to be caused by a combination of tissue damage from the increasing tumor burden, generalized immunosuppression, and debilitating bacterial colonization of the respiratory tract.

Little is known about SPV pathogenesis but gross features closely resemble those of the noninvasive orthopoxviruses in their native hosts.

## Immune Response

The benign fibromas caused by SFV/SqFV/HFV regress, albeit slowly, due to a combined cellular and humoral immune response. These viruses are excellent antigens, and neutralizing antibody produced during recovery will also cross-react with other members of the genus. All of the leporipoxviruses are strongly cell associated, and cell-mediated immunity is probably the single most important mechanism of viral clearance. Other immune mechanisms are also activated, including interferon production, antibody-mediated cell lysis, sensitized macrophages, and natural killer cells. Neutralizing antibody can last for many months after viral clearance and immunity is usually cross-protective to the other leporipoxviruses.

In the unique case of MYX in *Oryctolagus* rabbits the picture is very different. Although circulating antibody can be detected against virions, as determined by neutralization or agglutination, and against soluble antigens, as determined by complement fixation and precipitin tests, the antibody provides little protection against the disease progression. Instead, cellular immunity is severely compromised, and by day 6–7 lymphocytes (especially splenocytes) are demonstrably dysfunctional in their response to mitogens and lose the ability to secrete critical cytokines such as interleukin-2. Unlike the case of SFV, there is a notable absence of virus-specific T cells in either the spleen or draining lymph nodes. Immune dysfunction is common for viruses that replicate in lymphocytes, but the precise levels at which MYX intervenes in cellular immunity remain to be clarified. There is some evidence that these viruses interfere with the function of cell surface major histocompatibility complex (MHC) class I molecules, which could prevent proper viral antigen presentation and hence interfere with immune recognition of infected cells. Also, several virus-specific gene products have been shown to be secreted homologs of the cellular receptors for TNF and IFN-γ that are believed to bind and sequester these extracellular ligands in the vicinity of virus-infected cells and thus short-circuit immune pathways dependent on TNF and IFN-γ.

SPV-infected pigs generally recover from the infection and become immune to secondary challenge. There are few data on the nature of this immunity, but it bears close resemblance to that of VACV immunization in humans.

## Prevention and Control

Since these viruses are spread principally by biting arthropods, vector control is the single most effective method of disease prevention. The viruses are susceptible to standard anti-poxvirus chemical agents, such as phosphonoacetic acid, arabinosyl cytosine, and rifampicin, but these are of limited utility in infected animals. Immunization against myxomatosis can be accomplished with live SFV or attenuated strains of MYX.

## Future Perspectives

Now that DNA sequencing studies have revealed the genomic repertoire of so many poxviruses, it is likely that more viral proteins which determine the clinical characteristics of their diseases will be characterized. Studies on viral gene products that stimulate fibroblastic and endothelial cells to proliferate will likely provide information on how mitogenesis is regulated by surface receptors on these target cells. Some of the secreted virokines and viroceptors have the potential to be used as drugs to treat inflammatory diseases. The ability of MYX to replicate in lymphocytes offers an important system in which to elucidate the mechanisms of cellular tropism by which these viruses suppress the innate apoptosis response to virus infection. Furthermore, the analysis of virus-induced immunosuppression should shed light on the various immune strategies used by the host to combat viral infections in general. The restricted host ranges of the lepori- and suipoxviruses suggest the potential for the genetic manipulation of these viruses such that heterologous foreign antigen genes can be expressed for the purpose of developing novel vaccines against important pathogens of domestic leporids and swine. Finally, the ability of MYX to infect and kill many human tumor cells offers the potential as a therapy against human cancer.

## Further Reading

Barrett JW, Cao J-X, Hota-Mitchell S, and McFadden G (2001) Immunomodulatory proteins of myxoma virus. *Seminars in Immunology* 13: 73–84.

DiGiacomo RF and Maré CJ (1994) Viral diseases. In: Manning P, Ringler DH,, and Newcomer CE (eds.) *The Biology of the Laboratory Rabbit*, 2nd edn., p. 171. San Diego, CA: Academic Press.

Fenner F and Radcliffe FN (1965) *Myxomatosis*. Cambridge: Cambridge University Press.

Johnston JB and McFadden G (2004) Technical knockout: Understanding poxvirus pathogenesis by selectively deleting viral immunomodulatory genes. *Cellular Microbiology* 6: 695–705.

Kerr PJ and Best SM (1998) Myxoma virus in rabbits. *Revue Scientifique et Technique de l'office International des Épizooties* 17: 256–268.

Kerr P and McFadden G (2002) Immune responses to myxoma virus. *Viral Immunology* 15: 229–246.

Lucas A and McFadden G (2004) Secreted immunomodulatory proteins as novel biotherapeutics. *Journal of Immunology* 173: 4765–4774.

Nazarian SH and McFadden G (2006) Immune evasion by poxviruses. *Future Medicine* 1: 129–132.

Seet BT, Johnston JB, Brunetti CR, *et al.* (2003) Poxviruses and immune evasion. *Annual Review of Immunology* 21: 377–423.

Sypula J, Wang F, Ma Y, Bell J, and McFadden G (2004) Myxoma virus tropism in human tumor cells. *Gene Therapy and Molecular Biology* 8: 103–114.

## Relevant Website

http://www.poxvirus.org – Poxvirus Bioinformatics Resource Center.

# Papillomaviruses of Animals

**A A McBride,** National Institutes of Health, Bethesda, MD, USA

## History

Warts or papillomas have been recognized in animals for centuries. The first description of transmissible animal papillomas was in the ninth century in *Al-Kheyl wal Beytareh*, a book of horse medicine by Ibn Akhi Hazam, the stablemaster for the Caliph of Baghdad. By the late 1800s, there were several examples of experimental transmission of warts in animals such as dogs and horses and in 1907 Ciuffo demonstrated that human warts could be transmitted by sterile filtrates, indicating a viral etiology. Cottontail rabbit or Shope papillomavirus (CRPV) was isolated in 1933 by Richard Shope and this was the first papillomavirus (PV) to be studied in detail.

Papillomas are normally benign, but there are several examples of animal warts undergoing malignant transformation to carcinomas. This was one of the earliest indications that viruses could be involved in the development of cancer and it helped initiate the field of viral oncology. This potential for malignant progression was later important in the recognition that human papillomaviruses (HPVs) were associated with cervical cancer. Relative to other viruses, PV research was hampered because of difficulties in propagating the virus; papillomaviruses (PVs) are species specific and epitheliotrophic and require a stratified and differentiated epithelium for productive infection. In the 1980s, research progressed more rapidly with the advent of molecular cloning because the small viral genomes could be readily propagated, and genetically modified, in a bacterial plasmid. Bovine papillomavirus type 1 (BPV-1) became a very popular prototype because of its unusual ability to transform and maintain its genome in rodent cells in culture. This allowed extensive analysis of the transformation, replication, and transcriptional properties of BPV-1. By the 1990s, several systems had been developed that allowed limited propagation of PVs in culture in artificial skin equivalents or epithelial xenografts in laboratory animals.

Much PV research has centered on the functions of the viral proteins. These small viruses encode only a handful of proteins and most function by interacting with a plethora of cellular proteins. Because viruses target pivotal regulatory functions in the cell, this research has led not only to a detailed understanding of the PV life cycle but has provided great insight into the function of key cellular proteins.

## Taxonomy, Classification, and Evolutionary Relationships

Initially, PVs were grouped with polyomaviruses in the family *Papovaviridae*. However, it was later recognized that these viruses are not closely related and the International Committee on the Taxonomy of Viruses (ICTV) now recognizes the PVs as a new family, the *Papillomaviridae*. The *Papillomaviridae* have been further classified into genera and species based upon phylogenetic clustering of viral capsid protein L1 gene sequences (see **Figure 1**). Different genera have less than 60% and species have 60–70% nucleotide sequence identity. Individual PV types have 71–89% nucleotide identity. Differences of 2–10% identity define a subtype and less than 2%, a variant. Each genus is identified by a Greek letter, for example, *Alphapapillomavirus*. Each PV type is designated according to the host species and sometimes the site of infection, PV for papillomavirus, and finally, if several

PVs have been isolated from the same species, a number. Examples are ROPV (rabbit oral PV) and BPV-1.

PVs have co-evolved with their hosts over millions of years and all types have most likely existed since the speciation of their host. The slow evolution of PVs is probably due to their use of the high-fidelity host DNA polymerase to replicate their genomes. It has been estimated that the most variable parts of PV genomes change at a rate of 0.25% per 10 000–20 000 years and there is no evidence for recombination between different viral types.

## Host Range and Tissue Tropism

PVs are widespread. There are hundreds of different human types and PVs have been isolated from a diverse range of animals. To date, most animal PVs have been isolated from mammals, but viruses have also been identified in birds (see **Table 1**). PVs have been isolated from rodents, such as Syrian hamsters, the European harvest mouse, and the African multimammate rat. Unfortunately, no virus has yet been found that can infect laboratory mice. Multiple viral types have been found in those species that have been examined carefully (e.g., primate, cow, and rabbit) and many subclinical infections have been identified in primates (human and nonhuman). Presumably, more extensive investigation of each host would reveal a number of PV types that might rival the hundreds of PVs found in humans. Therefore, it would not be unreasonable to predict that there might exist over 100 000 different PV types.

All PVs are epitheliotrophic; each virus is species specific and infects and replicates in either cutaneous or mucosal epithelium, often at particular sites in the host. The reason for this tropism is not well understood, but it does not seem to depend on cell surface receptors for the virus and is thought to be due to very precise interactions between viral and host proteins that are required for a successful, productive infection. An exception to this is the fibropapillomaviruses. In addition to the productive infection of the epithelium, these viruses also nonproductively infect the underlying dermal fibroblasts, resulting in a fibroma. Probably because of this, these viruses have a less restricted host range and can nonproductively infect related host species and can transform and nonvegetatively replicate in cells from other hosts. For example, BPV-1 can cause equine sarcoids and can transform rodent cells.

## Transmission, Clinical Features, Pathology, and Pathogenicity

PV-associated disease ranges from clinically inapparent infections, through a variety of benign warts, to malignant

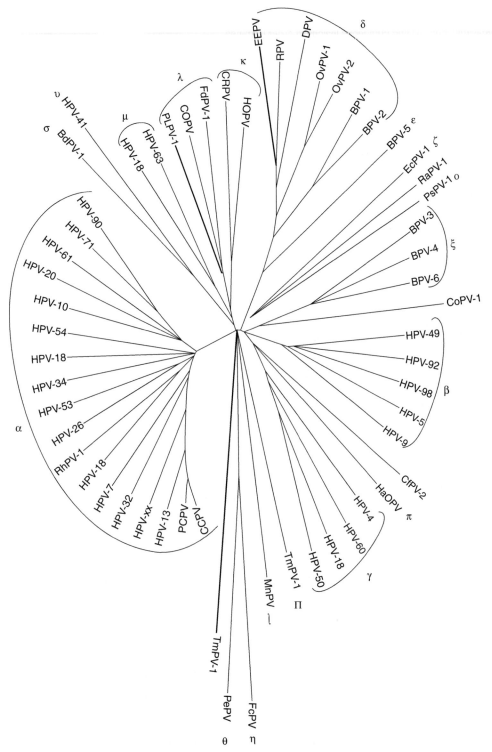

**Figure 1**    The evolutionary relationships between animal and a subset of human papillomaviruses as represented by a phylogenetic tree. Adapted from Van Doorslaer K, Rector A, Vos P, and Van Ranst M (2006) Genetic characterization of the *Capra hircus* papillomavirus: A novel close-to-root artiodactyl papillomavirus. *Virus Research* 118: 164–169, with permission from Elsevier.

carcinoma. These differences in pathology are due to different viral types, different epithelial host cells, and the immune response of the host. The complete viral life cycle requires a stratified, differentiating epithelium

(see **Figure 2**). In normal skin, only the basal cells can divide; after each division, one daughter cell remains in the basal layer and the other is pushed upward to begin the differentiation process. The latter cells withdraw from

**Table 1** Notable animal papillomaviruses (by genus)

*Alphapapillomavirus:* mucosal and cutaneous lesions in order Primates
  PCPV-1: Pygmy chimpanzee (*Pan paniscus*) papillomavirus
  RhPV-1: Rhesus monkey (*Macaca mulatta*) papillomavirus type 1
*Deltapapillomavirus:* fibropapillomas in superorder Ungulata
  BPV-1, BPV-2: Bovine (*Bos taurus*) papillomavirus types 1 and 2
  DPV: Deer (*Cervus*) papillomavirus
  EEPV: European elk (*Alces alces*) papillomavirus
  OvPV-1, OvPV-2: Ovine (*Ovis aries*) papillomavirus types 1 and 2
  RPV: Reindeer (*Rangifer tarandus*) papillomavirus
*Epsilonpapillomavirus:* cutaneous lesions in family *Bovidae*
  BPV-5: Bovine (*Bos taurus*) papillomavirus type 5
*Zetapapillomavirus:* cutaneous lesions in order Perissodactyla
  EcPV-1: Equus caballus (horse) papillomavirus type 1
*Etapapillomavirus:* cutaneous lesions in class Aves (Passeriformes)
  FcPV: Fringilla coelebs (chaffinch) papillomavirus
*Thetapapillomavirus:* cutaneous lesions in class Aves (Psittaciformes)
  PePV: Psittacus erithacus timneh (African grey parrot) papillomavirus
*Iotapapillomavirus:* cutaneous lesions in order Rodentia
  MnPV: Mastomys natalensis (multimammate rat) papillomavirus
*Kappapapillomavirus:* cutaneous and mucosal lesions in order Lagomorpha
  CRPV: Cottontail rabbit (*Sylvilagus*) papillomavirus
  ROPV: Rabbit (*Oryctolagus cuniculus*) oral papillomavirus
*Lambdapapillomavirus:* cutaneous and mucosal lesions in order Carnivora
  COPV: Canine (*Canis familiaris*) oral papillomavirus
  FdPV: Felis domesticus (cat) papillomavirus
*Xipapillomavirus:* cutaneous and mucosal lesions in family *Bovidae*
  BPV-3, BPV-4, BPV-6: Bovine (*Bos taurus*) papillomavirus types 3, 4, and 6
*Omikronpapillomavirus*
  PsPV: Phocoena spinipinnis (porpoise) papillomavirus
*Pipapillomavirus*
  HaOPV: Hamster (*Mesocricetus auratus*) oral papillomavirus
Unassigned
  BPV-7: Bovine (*Bos taurus*) papillomavirus type 7
  CCPV-1: Common chimpanzee (*Pan troglodytes*) papillomavirus type 1
  CfPV-2, CfPV-3: Canine (*Canis familiaris*) papillomavirus types 2 and 3
  CgPV-1, CgPV-2: Colobus monkey (*Colobus guereza*) papillomavirus types 1 and 2
  ChPV-1: Capra hircus (goat) papillomavirus type 1
  EdPV: Erethizon dorsatum ( porcupine) papillomavirus
  MfPV: Macaca fasicularis (long-tailed macaque) papillomavirus
  MmPV: Micromys minutus (European harvest mouse) papillomavirus
  PlPV-1: Procyon lotor (raccoon) papillomavirus type 1
  RaPV-1: Rousettus aegyptiacus (Egyptian fruit bat) papillomavirus type 1
  TmPV-1: Trichechus manatus latirostris (manatee) papillomavirus type 1
  TtPV-1, TtPV-2: Tursiops truncates (bottlenose dolphin) papillomavirus types 1 and 2
  TvPV: Trichosurus vulpecula (brushtall possum) papillomavirus

the cell cycle and begin to synthesize proteins that provide strength and barrier function to the epithelium.

To initiate infection, PVs usually require direct contact with the appropriate epithelia and must access the dividing cells in the basal layer of the epithelium through micro-abrasions or wounds. Viral DNA is established and maintained in the nuclei of dividing basal cells as an extrachromosomal replicating element. The infected basal cells serve as a reservoir of infected cells in the continual, progressive vertical differentiation that occurs in the maturation of the epidermis. Viral genome amplification, capsid protein synthesis, and particle production are restricted to the overlying, terminally differentiated cells. PVs disrupt the normal differentiation process, primarily because they must maintain cells in an S-phase-like state so that DNA replication enzymes are available to amplify the viral genome in differentiated cells. The infectious process is associated with a proliferation of the epidermal layers and in acanthosis (hyperplasia of the spinous layer), parakeratosis (persistence of the nuclei into the stratum corneum), hyperkeratosis (thickened cornified layer), and papillomatosis (undulating epithelium). Koilocytes (large, round, vacuolated cells with pyknotic nuclei) appear in the stratum spinosum and granulosum and abnormal keratohyalin granules are produced.

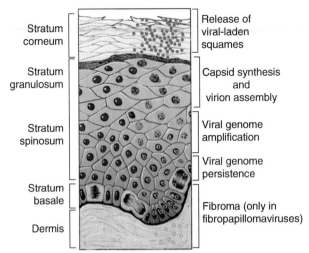

| | |
|---|---|
| Stratum corneum | Release of viral-laden squames |
| Stratum granulosum | Capsid synthesis and virion assembly |
| Stratum spinosum | Viral genome amplification |
| | Viral genome persistence |
| Stratum basale | |
| Dermis | Fibroma (only in fibropapillomaviruses) |

**Figure 2** Life cycle of papillomaviruses. The diagram shows a model of stratified epithelium. The lowermost basal layer provides the germinal cells necessary for regeneration of the epidermis. In the stratum spinosum, desmosomes can be observed between cells giving them a characteristic spiny appearance. The cells of the stratum granulosum accumulate dense basophilic keratohyalin granules that contain lipids, which help form a waterproof barrier function. The outermost layer consists of dead cells filled with mature keratin. The stages of the viral replicative life cycle that occur in each cell layer are indicated. Fibropapillomaviruses also infect fibroblasts in the dermis, resulting in a fibroma.

This process can result in a broad spectrum of papilloma-induced morphologies. For example, BPV-1-induced fibropapillomas in cattle can be sessile or pedunculate and lobate, fungiform, or verrucate. Other BPV types cause flat or filiform teat papillomas or alimentary papillomas. CRPV-induced papillomas occur as dark, highly kerati-nized masses. They range in size from 0.5 to 1 cm in diame-ter and can reach several centimeters in height, resulting in cutaneous 'horns'. In fact, it is thought that these 'horns' inspired the legend of the jackalope, a mythical creature that is a cross between a jackrabbit and an antelope. At the other end of the spectrum, healthy appearing skin from many animals has been found to harbor PVs.

## Replication Cycle

All PVs have similar life cycles, closely linked to kerati-nocyte differentiation, although there are variations in the timing of each stage of infection with respect to differen-tiation that are probably linked to the host cell, the viral type, and the immune response. PVs infect the basal cells and probably use a common cell surface receptor. α6β4 integrin and heparan sulfate proteoglycans are candidate receptors, but there is evidence to suggest that other molecules may be important. In the basal cells, the viral genome is maintained in a low-copy, extrachromosomal

state and is replicated along with cellular DNA in a cell cycle-dependent manner. PV infections are usually long-lived and persistent and these cells must provide a reser-voir of infected cells for the overlying virus producing tissue. As the infected cells differentiate and migrate upward to the stratum spinosum, there are changes in viral gene expression and vegetative viral DNA replication begins. Expression of the viral capsid proteins, L1 and L2, is first detected in cells of the stratum spinosum and virus-specific cytopathic effects are most pronounced in the stratum granulosum. Virions are assembled in the upper differentiated layers of the papilloma and are found throughout the nuclei, frequently organized into paracrys-talline arrays, in cells which are destined to be sloughed from the epidermis. Viral transcription, translation, and replication are regulated through both positive and nega-tive cellular processes that change during terminal differ-entiation. In fibropapillomas, there is also a proliferation of infected fibroblasts in the underlying dermis. Although the viral genome is maintained in the infected fibroblasts, there is no late gene expression or virion production.

## Genome Organization and Expression

All PVs have a double-stranded, circular DNA genome of 7–8 kbp. There is a region of approximately 1 kbp that is called the long control region (LCR), upstream regulatory region (URR), or noncoding region (NCR). This region contains transcriptional enhancers and promoters, the DNA replication origin, and sequences required for genome maintenance (MME; minimal maintenance ele-ment). The viral promoters are regulated by cellular factors and the viral E2 proteins. In most viruses, the genes are organized in the order LCR–E6–E7–E2/ E4–(E5)–SIR–L2–L1, where SIR represents the short intergenic region (see **Figure 3**). The coding region is divided into the early and late regions. The early region is expressed in the lower, more undifferentiated layers of a papilloma and proteins expressed from this region are designated E1 through E8 (see below). The capsid anti-gens, L1 and L2, are encoded by the late region and are expressed in the more superficial, differentiated cells of a papilloma. One exception is the E4 protein, which is encoded by the early region but is expressed abundantly in the upper layers of a wart. All viral RNA species are transcribed from one strand and are extensively processed to give rise to alternatively spliced mRNA species. The early polyadenylation site is located between the early and late regions while the late transcripts use a second site at the end of the late region.

Each viral protein is relatively well conserved from one virus to another. However, proteins from different viral types interact with distinct cellular proteins as well as those common to many viral types, and this likely

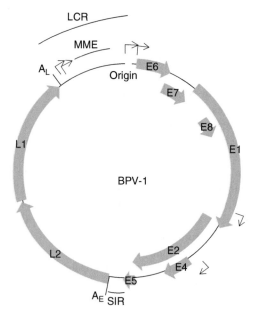

**Figure 3** The BPV-1 genome. E and L designate the early and late open reading frames, respectively; promoters are indicated by arrows. LCR, long control region; SIR, short intragenic region; $A_E$ and $A_L$, early and late polyadenylation sites, respectively; MME, minichromosome maintenance element.

explains their highly selective species and tissue tropism. One exception to the common genomic organization is the E5 gene, which is not present in all viruses. Another is genus *Xipapillomavirus*, which contains certain bovine papillomaviruses (BPV-3, BPV-4, BPV-6), that do not have an E6 gene and instead have a different gene in this position that has been designated E8. E8 is a membrane protein with properties analogous to the E5 proteins of other PVs but there is no evidence that they are evolutionarily related. PePV, the African grey parrot PV, also has two genes at the beginning of the early region that have little similarity with the classical E6 and E7 genes and have instead been designated E8 and E9.

## Functions of Viral Proteins

The functions of the individual viral proteins encoded by animal viruses are somewhat analogous to their HPV counterparts. The E5 protein of BPV-1 is the primary transforming protein and promotes proliferation of infected cells. It is a membrane protein that can transform fibroblasts by inducing constitutive, ligand-independent activation of the β-type platelet-derived growth factor receptor (PDGF-Rβ), and by interfering with Golgi acidification. BPV-4 E5 also transforms fibroblasts and disrupts gap junction-mediated intercellular communication. Many PV E5 proteins downregulate surface expression of major histocompatibility complex (MHC) class I molecules, which helps the virus to evade the host immune system.

The E1 protein is the primary replication protein. It is an ATP-dependent helicase that specifically binds and unwinds the viral DNA replication origin to allow access of the cellular replication proteins. It binds cooperatively to the origin in concert with the E2 protein. The E1 protein then converts to a double hexamer that encircles the DNA and unwinds the origin. The structure and function of the E1 protein is analogous to that of the polyomavirus SV40 T antigen. Much of our understanding about PV replication originates from key studies in BPV-1.

The E2 gene encodes multiple proteins that are the result of expression from multiple promoters and alternative RNA splicing. In BPV-1, there are three E2 proteins (E2TA, E2TR, and E8/E2). They share sequence-specific DNA binding and dimerization activities and the longest protein, E2TA, also contains a transcriptional activating domain. E2TA stimulates viral promoters by binding to multiple 12 bp palindromic sequences in E2-specific enhancers within the LCR. This activity is modulated by the E8/E2 and E2TR proteins which antagonize the functions of E2TA. The E2TA protein also represses transcription from viral promoters when the E2 binding sites overlap essential promoter elements. The E2 protein has an additional role in maintaining and partitioning the genome in the dividing basal cells. The E2 protein is a sequence-specific binding protein that binds to multiple E2 binding sites in the viral genome (in the MME) and tethers them to the cellular mitotic chromosomes through the transactivation activation domain. This has been best characterized for BPV-1, and the cellular bromodomain protein, Brd4, which binds to acetylated histones on chromatin, is an important cellular protein in this tethering complex. E2 also has a role at late stages of infection because expression of BPV-1 E2 proteins is greatly increased in cells that are vegetatively amplifying viral DNA.

Restricting high levels of viral DNA replication and antigens to the more superficial layers of an epithelium and releasing virus by the natural process of desquamation might be important for immune evasion by the virus. However, this means that the virus needs to replicate its DNA in cells that have normally withdrawn from the cell cycle and are undergoing differentiation. One of the main functions of the E6 and E7 proteins seems to be to sustain cells in an S-phase-like state so that the virus has available the enzymes to replicate its own DNA. This aberrant state induces cell cycle sensors that would normally arrest cells and perhaps cause them to undergo apoptosis. The molecular mechanism by which the E6 and E7 proteins of the 'high-risk' HPVs avert this process, by inactivating the retinoblastoma (pRb) and p53 proteins, is well understood. However, it is not yet clear how many of the animal viruses and 'low-risk' HPVs fulfill this function. The BPV-1 E6 protein disrupts the actin cytoskeleton and binds a number of cellular proteins, including ERC-55, the focal adhesion protein paxillin, the E3 ubiquitin ligase E6AP, and the clathrin adaptor complex AP-1. BPV-1 E7 lacks the binding motif that mediates direct binding of the HPV E7 proteins to pRb. However, both BPV and HPV E7 proteins bind a cellular protein, p600, a unique pRb- and calmodulin-binding protein. In the nucleus, p600 and pRB, seem to act as a chromatin scaffold and, in the cytoplasm, p600 forms a meshwork structure with clathrin. Viral-induced hyperplasia is believed to be induced by the viral early gene products, and results from both increased division of the basal cells and delayed maturation of the committed keratinocytes of the spinous layer (acanthosis). An unintended result of this cell cycle deregulation in some viruses is the immortalization of the infected cells and the continual division of cells that have sustained DNA damage, which can lead to a malignant phenotype.

The E4 protein, usually expressed from a spliced mRNA as E1^E4, is expressed at very high levels in the productively infected cells of a wart. It can interfere with the cell cycle, which may be important for deregulation of cell division and differentiation. E4 can also disrupt keratin filaments and induce abnormalities in the cornified envelope. These functions may be important for egress of the virus from the outer layers of a wart.

The L1 protein is the major capsid protein. The minor capsid protein, L2, is important late in infection for packaging the viral genome into the capsid. L2 is also important early in infection to transport the viral DNA to the nucleus and to establish a permissive site within the nucleus to initiate viral transcription and replication.

## Virion Structure and Properties

PV virions form a nonenveloped, icosahedral structure of 55–60 nm diameter (see **Figure 4**). The capsid is composed of the major capsid protein, L1, and the minor capsid protein, L2, which form 72 pentameric capsomeres with an icosahedral symmetry of $T = 7$. The viral genome

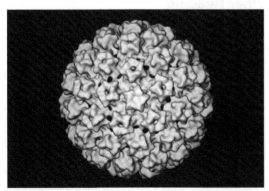

**Figure 4** BPV-1 capsid. Reproduced from Trus BL, Roden RB, Greenstone HL, Vrhel M, Schiller JT, and Booy FP (1997) Novel structural features of bovine papillomavirus capsid revealed by a three-dimensional reconstruction to 9 Å resolution. *Nature Structural Biology* 4: 413–420.

is packed in a nucleohistone complex. The L1 protein can self-assemble into virus-like particles (VLPs); VLPs present the conformational epitopes required for generating high-titer neutralizing antibodies and are the basis of very successful vaccines in humans and animals.

## Virus Propagation

The complete life cycle of PVs requires a stratified, differentiated epithelium because vegetative viral DNA replication and late gene expression can only take place in differentiated keratinocytes. To reproduce this in the laboratory, several xenograft techniques have been developed. Small pieces of epithelial tissue infected with virus and implanted in the renal capsule of an immunocompromised mouse will produce viral particles. Skin from various species can also be grafted onto immunocompromised mice and either infected with virus or transfected with viral DNA. The infected xenograft will form a papilloma-like lesion that will produce virion particles. Artificial skin equivalents (organotypic rafts) can also be established in tissue culture from keratinocytes and fibroblasts of various species. These rafts support the viral life cycle and produce viral particles. Relatively large quantities of infectious virions can also be purified from cells that have been co-transfected with the viral genome along with expression vectors for the L1 and L2 capsid proteins.

## Notable Animal Papillomaviruses

PVs have been isolated and characterized from a multitude of animals including cattle, sheep, deer, horses, rabbits, dogs, mice, birds, and nonhuman primates. Many are listed in **Table 1** and a few of the better-studied viruses are described in detail below.

*BPV-1.* BPV-1 causes fibropapillomas on the cutaneous epithelium of cattle. It is readily transmitted among herd animals through direct contact of abraded skin. BPV-1 belongs to an unusual class of PVs that cause fibropapillomas in ungulates. These viruses have a broader host range than most PVs; BPV-1 can naturally infect horses, giving rise to sarcoids, can cause tumors in hamsters, and can morphologically transform mouse fibroblasts in culture. The infection is nonproductive in each of these cases.

In 1980, Lowy and co-workers demonstrated that cloned BPV-1 DNA could morphologically transform mouse cells in culture. The viral DNA replicated as an extrachromosomal element within these cells. Because of this, BPV-1 became the molecular prototype of the PVs and viral functions responsible for transformation, DNA replication, and transcriptional regulation were first characterized for BPV-1.

*BPV-4.* BPV-4 causes benign papillomas of the alimentary tract in cattle. In certain regions of Scotland, when cattle graze on bracken, these papillomas progress at a high rate to malignant carcinoma. Bracken grown in these regions contains at least one identified co-carcinogen, a flavenoid called quercetin, which promotes malignant progression of the papillomas.

*CRPV.* Cottontail rabbit papillomavirus (CRPV) naturally infects the cutaneous epithelium of wild cottontail rabbits and is also able to infect jackrabbits and snowshoe rabbits. In contrast, experimental infection of domestic rabbits results in nonproductive papillomas that support normal early viral gene expression and genome replication, but are unable to support late gene expression and virus particle production. CRPV-induced papillomas can either persist or regress, depending on host genetic factors, and persistent papillomas can progress to carcinomas in both wild and domestic rabbits. CRPV DNA can induce papillomas on scarified rabbit skin and this has allowed a genetic assessment of which viral functions are required to induce papillomas. The CRPV model has also been used for the development of preventive and therapeutic PV vaccines.

*COPV.* Canine oral PV (COPV) induces warts on the oral mucosa of dogs. Infection is normally followed by spontaneous immune-mediated regression. COPV is a good model for mucosal PV infection and has been very useful in studying the immune response and the development of PV vaccines.

*RhPV-1.* Rhesus papillomavirus type 1 (RhPV-1) is a sexually transmitted PV associated with genital disease that was first isolated from a penile squamous cell carcinoma. RhPV-associated disease progression closely resembles that seen in human genital HPV infections and RhPV-1 is phylogenetically closely related to the 'high-risk' HPVs that are associated with cervical cancer. RhPV-1 will likely become an important model to study human genital PV infections.

## Detection and Diagnosis

Serological tests for PV infection have been unreliable and detection usually relies on testing for viral DNA. Specific viral types can be detected using either hybrid capture or highly sensitive molecular techniques such as nested polymerase chain reaction (PCR) with the use of degenerate primers.

## Immune Response, Prevention, and Control

PV infections can be prolonged and persistent, but usually regress spontaneously. This immune-mediated regression is effected by T-cells while reinfection is prevented by humoral immunity. This phenomenon was noted in 1898 by M'Fadyean and Hobday who concluded after experiments with canine oral papillomas that, "the animal is left in a measure protected against an infection of the same kind." This spontaneous and simultaneous regression of papillomas by systemic immunity has been noted in many animals.

Much of our understanding of the immunology of PV infection comes from studies of animal PVs. Humoral immunity to subsequent infections is due to neutralizing antibodies directed against the capsid antigens. This immunity is type specific and can be bypassed by using viral DNA to induce papillomas in rabbit skin. Effective animal vaccines were produced that consist of crude wart extract, and these have been quite effective in cattle and dogs. The use of highly purified VLPs of COPV, CRPV, BPV, and Equus caballus papillomavirus (EcPV) as effective prophylactic vaccines laid the groundwork for the recently licensed HPV vaccines.

Cellular immunity is crucial for regression of papillomas. Dense infiltrates of T-lymphocytes can be observed in regressing warts in many animal species and immunosuppression can result in severe papillomatosis. The early, noncapsid proteins are important antigens for cell-mediated immunity and these might prove to be effective therapeutic vaccines for existing infections. Vaccination with CRPV early viral gene products has been shown to clear papillomas in rabbits. However, one complication is that PVs encode several functions that enable them to evade the immune system; they are able to inhibit interferon-dependent innate immunity and disrupt viral antigen presentation, which might also interfere with therapeutic vaccination.

*See also:* Papillomaviruses: General Features.

## Further Reading

Campo MS (2002) Animal models of papillomavirus pathogenesis. *Virus Research* 89: 249–261.

de Villiers EM, Fauquet C, Broker TR, Bernard HU, and zur Hausen H (2004) Classification of papillomaviruses. *Virology* 324: 17–27.

Nicholls PK and Stanley MA (2000) The immunology of animal papillomaviruses. *Veterinary Immunology and Immunopathology* 73: 101–127.

Peh WL, Middleton K, Christensen N, *et al.* (2002) Life cycle heterogeneity in animal models of human papillomavirus-associated disease. *Journal of Virology* 76: 10401–10416.

Trus BL, Roden RB, Greenstone HL, Vrhel M, Schiller JT, and Booy FP (1997) Novel structural features of bovine papillomavirus capsid revealed by a three-dimensional reconstruction to 9 Å resolution. *Nature Structural Biology* 4: 413–420.

Van Doorslaer K, Rector A, Vos P, and Van Ranst M (2006) Genetic characterization of the *Capra hircus* papillomavirus: A novel close-to-root artiodactyl papillomavirus. *Virus Research* 118: 164–169.

# Papillomaviruses: General Features

**H U Bernard,** University of California, Irvine, Irvine, CA, USA

## Introduction

Papillomaviruses (PVs) are small DNA viruses that infect mucosal and cutaneous epithelia (skin). More than 100 PV types have been isolated from humans, and one or some few PV types have been found in virtually every carefully studied mammal and bird. PVs are strictly host species specific – human papillomaviruses (HPVs) cannot infect any other mammals, and no animal PV infects humans. Historically, PV research began with certain mammalian PV types (cottontail rabbit papillomavirus and bovine papillomavirus), as the large lesions caused by these viruses were sources for substantial virus preparations. Today's refined techniques led to the isolation and analysis of numerous PV types from a variety of human lesions, notably carcinomas of the cervix uteri (HPV-16), genital (HPV-6), and common warts (HPV-2). PVs cause benign and malignant neoplasia as they express oncoproteins with pleiotropic functions resulting from interactions with numerous cellular proteins. These oncoproteins induce continuing cell divisions in peripheral epithelial layers, while in the absence of PV oncoproteins, cell divisions are restricted to cells of the basal layer of epithelia. The consequence of this deregulation is a localized growth of the epithelium, leading to a papilloma (or wart), which gave this virus family its name. Within the broad spectrum of PV research, most efforts were directed to understand HPV-mediated carcinogenesis. These molecular studies have an increasing impact on medical practice in the form of DNA diagnosis and prophylactic vaccination.

## Papillomavirus Particles and Genomes

PVs have icosahedral, nonenveloped particles (capsids or virions) with a diameter of approximately 55 nm. The particle is composed of 72 capsomers, and each of these capsomers consists of five identical L1 proteins, which are encoded by the PV genome. The virions also contain the minor capsid protein L2, which, however, is not part of the capsomers and is not required to generate a complete virion.

The PV particle contains the circular, double-stranded DNA genome in the form of chromatin. Many important PV types have genome sizes very close to 7900 bp; other viral genomes have sizes of a few hundred basepairs below or above this number. Most PV types encode eight open reading frames (ORFs): E1, E2, E4, E5, E6, E7, L1, and L2

(**Figure 1**). These ORFs are considered genes, as each of them is sufficient to encode a protein, although differential splicing also leads to alternative uses of some ORFs. The exact role and regulation of some alternative splices are still insufficiently understood. PV mRNAs are normally polycistronic (i.e., contain several ORFs), a dramatic deviation from the monocistronic mRNAs typical for eukaryotes and their viruses. The efficient translation of ORFs that are located 3′ of other ORFs is still little understood. Some few PVs lack the E5 or E6 genes. The L1 and E6 genes are separated by a genomic segment constituting about 10% of the PV genome, which contains many *cis*-responsive elements required for viral transcription and replication. This segment is called the long control region (LCR).

## The Most Commonly Studied Papillomaviruses

More than 200 PV types exist in humans, and half of these have been isolated and formally described. The number of additional PV types in mammals is probably unlimited, although so far only a few dozen have been described.

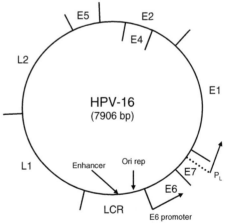

**Figure 1** Genome organization of human papillomavirus type 16 (HPV-16). The genome consists of double-stranded DNA with a size of 7906 bp. LCR: Long control region, containing numerous *cis*-responsive elements for the viral transcription and replication, including the epithelial specific enhancer and the replication origin (ori rep). $P_L$: late promoter; E6 and E7: the two principal oncogenes; E1: replication initiation protein; E2: transcription factor, support of replication, segregation of viral DNA; E4: virion assembly and release; E5: minor oncogene; L2: minor capsid protein, intracellular transport of viral DNA after infection; L1: major capsid protein.

The tremendous diversity of PVs is not such a formidable barrier to understand PV biology as one might fear, as most research was based on only nine HPVs and three PVs from other mammals. Human papillomavirus 1 (HPV-1) induces plantar (foot-sole) warts and HPV-2 common (hand or face) warts. HPV-5 and HPV-8 are associated with epidermodysplasia verruciformis, a skin neoplasia linked to a genetic risk factor. HPV-6 and HPV-11 cause genital and laryngeal warts. HPV-16, HPV-18, and HPV-31 are the most prominent types causally linked to anogenital and some head and neck carcinomas. Bovine papillomavirus 1 (BPV-1) causes fibropapillomas and BPV-4 mucosal lesions in cattle, and the cottontail rabbit papillomavirus (CRPV) cutaneous lesions in rabbits. Owing to its medical importance and high prevalence, HPV-16 has probably been the object of more research than all remaining types together. The information in this article dealing with PV proteins and gene regulation is therefore biased in favor of HPV-16. Many – but clearly not all – functions of this virus are shared with other PVs.

## Taxonomy and Evolution

PVs and polyomaviruses share two properties, namely small circular double-stranded DNA genomes and nonenveloped isosahedral capsids. As a consequence, they had once been lumped into one virus family, *Papovaviridae*. When it became clear that they have different genome organizations and no genomic similarity, they were split into the two families *Papillomaviridae* and *Polyomaviridae*.

The PV literature uses the term 'type' to identify unrelated PV isolates, and the terms 'subtype' and 'serotype' are inappropriate. There are presently more than 100 formally described HPV types. New PV types have been found in all carefully examined mammal species, but so far in only two birds, and none in other animal taxa. Only one or some very few PV types have been detected in each animal host, and it is unclear whether the high number of HPV types has resulted from the more intense study of humans, or whether humans had been a more 'fertile' environment for PV evolution than other mammals.

The taxonomy of PVs was built on the comparison of genomes rather than on amplifiable viruses or on serology, since PVs do not multiply efficiently in cell culture, and since no consistent serology could be established based on natural infections. The genome-based taxonomy of PVs was founded in the 1980s with DNA hybridization data, and was later shifted to nucleotide sequence comparisons. By definition, a PV type is unique when the nucleotide sequence of its L1 gene differs by at least 10% from the L1 sequence of any other PV type. As a consequence, PV types are genotypes and not 'serotypes', although a retrospective study would likely reveal that most PV types are serologically distinct. PV types are designated by one or two capital letters identifying their host, and numbered according to the sequence of isolation, for example, HPV-16 for human papillomavirus type 16.

In order to classify PV types following traditional taxonomic terminology, the term 'type' has been placed in the taxonomic hierarchy below the term 'species'. In other words, phylogenetically closely related PV types with similar or identical biological and pathogenic properties have become lumped into PV species. While this procedure was justified to arrange PVs taxonomically in a manner similar to other virus families, it has created species with potentially confusing numeric designations that may not become generally used in the literature. In order to give an example, HPV types 16, 31, 33, 35, 52, 58, and 67 form the species *Human papillomavirus 16*. At the taxonomic level between species and the family (*Papillomaviridae*), PV species form genera that are designated by Greek prefixes (*Alpha-* through *Pi-papillomavirus*). Most medically important HPV types belong to genus *Alphapapillomavirus*.

Repeated isolates of the same PV type differ by up to 2% of their genomic sequence, and are termed variants of the original prototype isolate. Evidence suggests that this diversity evolved over a period of several hundred thousand years in linkage to the evolution of *Homo sapiens*. The term 'subtype' is used for rare PV isolates that show diversity in between the type and the variant level. PVs do not rapidly diversify like many RNA viruses, and do not form quasi-species.

## Host Range

PVs are host species-specific, with the exception of a few PVs that were found in several different domestic hoofed animals, possibly transmitted by close contact between these animals. It has not been carefully studied whether host specificity is based on the lack of efficient contact or, more likely, on molecular incompatibility between PVs and heterologous hosts.

Within a particular host, notably humans, PVs often have a preferential target tissue. For example, HPV-1 is typically found in flat warts of the foot sole, HPV-2 in common warts of the skin elsewhere, HPV-6 in mucosal but also cutaneous lesions of the genitals, and HPV-16 mostly in anogenital and head and neck mucosal epithelia. This may be based either on molecular restrictions to replication in other types of epithelia, or on the lack of symptoms of established viral infections in inappropriate target epithelia. An example for the latter scenario is the fact that HPV-16 and some related types can cause cancer in women, but infect men normally asymptomatically. This possibility is also supported by the observation of HPV types that cause 'epidermodysplasia verruciformis' in patients with a genetic risk factor, while these same types can be detected in the skin of many individuals of the general human population in the absence of any symptoms.

While nearly all PV types are only found in epithelia, certain PV types replicate in cattle (like BPV-1) and other hoofed animals; also in mesenchymal tissue (fibropapillomaviruses).

## Functions of Papillomavirus Proteins

The PV proteins that participate in viral replication, transcription, and transformation are identified by the letter E (for early), and those found in the capsid by the letter L (for late), each followed by a number according to its size in the first genome characterized (E1 and L1 being the two largest proteins). In the following paragraphs, these proteins will be discussed in the order of their numbers.

The 649-amino-acid residue E1 protein controls the duplication of the PV genome. It initiates DNA replication at the single viral replication origin about 100 bp 5′ of the E6 promoter. By convention, PV genomes are numbered in such a way that the E1 binding site spans the genome position 1. The E1 binding site is only loosely conserved as a 20 bp A+T-rich segment, and is therefore also only poorly recognized by the E1 protein. This failure is compensated by the E2 protein, which has binding sites close to the E1 target. E2 binding sites are much more sequence-specific than those for E1, and by forming a complex with E1, E2 is crucial for binding the replication origin.

E1 binds initially as a dimer and then undergoes polymerizations during the subsequent steps of replication initiation. Central to E1 function is an ATP-dependent helicase, and E1 hexamers melt and unwind the double-stranded DNA of the replication origin and translocate DNA single strands. Beyond these basic E1 functions, PV DNA duplication depends on the host replication machinery. E1 recruits cellular replication proteins to the PV origin of replication, including DNA polymerase α, replication protein A, and topoisomerase I. There is also evidence that E1 is a target for cellular signals that couple PV replication to the cell cycle.

The E2 protein has a size of 365-amino-acid residues and can be divided into three domains, an N-terminal transcription activation domain, a central hinge region, and a C-terminal DNA-binding domain. E2 proteins have at least three functions: stimulation of replication, modulation of transcription, and attachment of PV genomes to cellular chromosomes during mitosis.

All three functions require the DNA-binding domain. E2 proteins form dimers, which bind the palindromic sequence ACCGNNNNCGGT or slightly degenerated targets. The genomes of HPV-16 (and those of many related medically important HPV types) have four E2 binding sites, two of them positioned close to the E6 promoter, one 5′ of the E1 binding site, and one in the center of the LCR. The two E2 binding sites at the E6 promoter overlap with binding sites for TFIID and the Sp1 factor, and E2 represses the promoter by displacing these activators. The E2 binding site 5′ to the E1 binding sites, and one of the two E2 sites at the E6 promoter, lead to cooperation between E1 and E2 in origin function, as described above. The function of the E2 binding site in the center of the LCR is not well understood.

The E2 protein was for the first time studied in BPV-1 and described as an activator of transcription. Occupation of E2 binding sites in the LCR of BPV-1 strongly stimulates the E6 promoter, as these sites form an E2-dependent enhancer. This E2 function depends on the N-terminal transcription activation domain. The N-terminal domain of the HPV-16 E2 protein is homologous to the BPV-1 E2 domain, and the HPV-16 protein functions as a transcriptional activator in the context of BPV-1 genomes. Strangely, however, no enhancer activation function could ever be detected in HPV-16 genomes, and, consequentially, E2 is known only as a repressor of this virus. Many PVs also express shortened transcripts of E2 that solely encode the C-terminal DNA-binding domain and function as repressors by competing with full-size E2 proteins for binding to E2 cis-responsive elements.

The E4 ORF is positioned within the E2 gene, overlapping with the E2 hinge. Its 95-amino-acid residues are translated in a different reading frame from E2. A splice (E1^E4) fuses some N-terminal amino acids of the E1 ORF to E4. Some E4 transcripts terminate downstream of the early genes, while others extend into the late genes and are spliced to L2 or L1. E4 is sometimes considered a late protein due to the resulting co-expression with L2 and L1 and the fact that E4 is highly expressed in differentiating cells. E4 is known to support viral genome amplification in the productive part of the PV life cycle, capsid protein expression, virion assembly, and virion release, although the detailed mechanisms behind these E4 functions are still poorly understood. They include interactions with and reorganization of the cytokeratin network, reorganization of nuclear ND10 domains, and effects on cell cycle regulators.

E5 proteins are small (83-amino-acid residues in HPV-16 and only 44 residues in BPV-1) and do not show inter-type sequence similarities. They have functional homologies, however, as they are highly hydrophobic and thereby localized to the cell membrane and the endoplasmatic reticulum. Cell culture experiments defined E5 proteins as transforming proteins, although they are not expressed in many anogenital carcinomas due to interruption of the viral genome. They are pleiotropic and share at least three functions: (1) association with the 16 kDa subunit of the vacuolar $H^+$-ATPase, influencing the half-life of tyrosine kinase receptors; (2) direct interactions with tyrosine kinase receptors including the platelet-derived growth factor and epidermal growth factor receptors, and (3) downregulation of major histocompatibility complex class I molecules.

E6 and E7 are the two principal transforming proteins of the oncogenic HPV types as judged by cell culture transformation, continued expression in carcinomas, reversion of the transformed phenotype of cancer-derived cell lines after annihilation of E6/E7 expression, and complex pleiotropic molecular functions. They are encoded in the 5' segment of polycistronic mRNAs transcribed from the E6 promoter, although many transcripts lack the ability to translate E6 due to an internal (E6*) splice.

The E6 protein of HPV-16 has a size of 149-amino-acid residues. The position of eight cysteine residues suggests the formation of two zinc fingers, which are larger than zinc fingers reported from cellular proteins. Although one would expect that these would help to induce a strong three-dimensional conformation, there is no information yet about the structure of E6. E6 shares this problem with the E7 protein, which has one single zinc finger with similar sequence properties. The lack of information about the structure of E6 and E7 proteins has remained a major obstacle in efforts to design drugs that would specifically interfere with these important oncoproteins.

More than 20 different cellular targets of E6 proteins have been described, and the contributions of these diverse interactions to the viral life cycle and carcinogenic processes are still much debated. It should be noted that PV oncoprotein functions evolved to support the latent and productive HPV life cycle, that is, the creation of a molecular environment favorable to virus replication. In spite of the medical importance of HPV-induced carcinogenesis, this pathological outcome should be considered an aberration and a fortuitous byproduct of the viral biology.

The most prominent target of E6 is the cell-cycle regulator and tumor suppressor p53. E6 and p53 form a trimeric complex including a protein called E6AP. E6AP is a ubiquitin ligase and the trimeric association results in p53 degradation. As a consequence, p53 is lost as inducer of the cdk inhibitor p21CIP, and the cell cycle of the infected cell is set free to undergo G1/S transition, creating an environment favorable to viral DNA replication, and establishing a prerequisite for oncogenic transformation. p53 is also known to be an inducer of apoptosis, and p53 elimination by E6 protects against this mechanism, which would otherwise eliminate infected cells and terminate PV replication. Yet other functions of E6 include the modulation of transcription by affecting the cofactor CBP/p300, effects on the immune response by interactions with the interferon regulatory factor-3, and alterations of cell shape and signaling by reaction with hDlg in a manner similar to a pathway that is induced by mutations during carcinogenesis of the colon.

The E7 oncoprotein of HPV-16 has a size of only 99 amino acid residues. E7 binds the retinoblastoma (RB) cell cycle regulator and tumor suppressor. In its normal function, RB represses the transcription factor E2F, which, in the absence of RB, induces genes required for G1/S transition of the cell cycle. The normal RB and E2F interactions are controlled by cyclin-dependent kinases. When E7 binds RB, E2F is released from the RB-E2F complex in an uncontrolled manner. Elimination of p53 and RB cell cycle control is a fundamental event in carcinogenesis, as many cancers whose etiology does not depend on viruses carry p53 and RB mutations. E7 is pleiotropic, and its functions include an affinity with the centromere. This leads to chromosomal abnormalities and genomic instability, resulting in a 'mutator phenotype' and promoting establishment of the malignant phenotype.

The 531-amino-acid residue L1 protein is the principal building block of the virion by forming 72 pentamers, which arrange into structurally complete icosahedral capsids in the absence of viral DNA or any other viral protein. This property has led to the production of HPV-6, HPV-11, HPV-16, and HPV-18 particles in heterologous expression systems as prophylactic anti-HPV vaccines. The L1 protein is central to the first step of PV infections by binding to proteoglycans and integrins at the surface of epithelial target cells. The infection does not select specific target cells, and the epithelial specificity of PV infections is established by the transcriptional environment in epithelial cells.

The L2 protein is part of the viral particle, where it forms a complex with the PV DNA. After uptake into endosomes, L2 accompanies the viral DNA by contact to the microtubule network via the motor protein dynein to the nucleus and subsequently to the subnuclear promyelocytic leukemia protein bodies, suggesting that it may be involved in the intracytoplasmic and nuclear transport of the PV DNA.

## Gene Expression

The expression of PV genes, that is, ultimately the availability of each viral protein in the infected cell, is influenced by numerous mechanisms, such as frequency of transcription, recognition of transcription termination sites, differential splicing, mRNA stability, translation efficiency, and protein stability. There are many similarities of these mechanisms among different PVs, notably among the medically important HPV types, but strict generalizations are not possible. An example of exceptions is the transcription factor E2, which is in BPV-1 an enhancer-activating factor, but a negative regulator in HPV-16.

Transcription of all eight PV genes starts a few nucleotides 5' of the ATG of E6 (E6 promoter), and continues unidirectionally around the whole viral genome. The E6 promoter has a TATA box that binds the general transcription factors including TFIID, and a promoter element, bound by Sp1. Among the numerous mRNAs generated from the E6 promoter are those that encode E2. E2 has two binding sites at the E6 promoter, and E2 proteins bound to these sites displace Sp1 and TFIID. Increasing mRNA levels derived from the E6 promoter lead to increased E2 expression and decreased use of this promoter, a perfect negative feedback loop, one of several adaptions of PV genomes to an inefficient (latent) rather than fulminant infection. HPV-16 genomes often recombine with chromosomal DNA in carcinomas such that the E2 gene is disconnected from the E6 promoter, releasing this repression mechanism.

The E6 promoter of HPVs has a low activity and requires activation by an enhancer centered 300 bp upstream of the promoter. This enhancer is only active in epithelial cells and determines the epithelial specificity of PVs. It does not bind E2, but depends on a variety of transcription factors including AP1, NFI, and glucocorticoid and progesterone receptors. Interestingly, the stimulation of PV oncogene expression by progesterone correlates with epidemiological data pointing to a high risk of cancer progression in women with multiple pregnancies and long-term anti-ovulant usage. A second promoter ($p_L$), relevant for the expression of L1 and L2, is positioned within the E7 gene. Activation of the TATA-less $p_L$ is reminiscent of an early-late switch and still little understood.

PV transcription is strongly regulated by epigenetic mechanisms, that is, conformational changes of the PV chromatin, specifically of two nucleosomes that bind the HPV-16 enhancer and promoter. Histone acetylation and deacetylation can permit or restrict transcription. A variety of mechanisms can influence these parameters, notably the antagonistic factors CDP and AP1, which couple PV transcription to epithelial differentiation, and DNA methylation, which may determine whether an infection takes a latent or productive course.

## Transmission and Epidemiology

PV infections are only stable when the pathogen reaches basal layers of an epithelium, for example, in wounds. PV infections result from physical contact between healthy and infected epithelia that peripherally release PV particles (e.g., during desquamation of the skin). As sexual intercourse leads to physical contact between genital epithelia, infections by many HPV types are considered sexually transmitted diseases. Epidemiological data support this mechanistic concept and document a rapid increase of genital PV infections in male and female individuals after commencement of sexual activity. Epidemiological evidence also supports the view that the risk to develop cervical carcinomas increases with young age at the start of sexual activity and with the number of sexual partners per lifetime. Additional risk factors are long-term use of anti-ovulants, multiparity, and tobacco smoking. Epidemiology provided a foundation for the concept of 'high-risk' and 'low-risk' HPV types. Both groups of HPVs are regularly found in exfoliated cells from anogenital sites, but only high-risk HPVs are frequent in cancer. 18 of the roughly 40 HPV types found in anogenital mucosas are considered high-risk types (e.g., HPV-16, HPV-18, and HPV-31), while HPV-6 and HPV-11, the cause of genital warts, are low-risk types, as they are rare in malignancies.

PVs are frequently transferred from mother to child during birth. So far, however, there is no evidence for efficient establishment of infections with high-risk HPV types toward anogenital carcinogenesis by this infection route. It is very possible, however, that the relatively high fraction of juvenile patients affected by laryngeal papillomatosis have acquired their HPV-6 and HPV-11 infections from their mothers.

## Pathogenicity

PVs are well established as the cause of a variety of cutaneous and mucosal neoplastic lesions. As discussed above, the molecular pathology of such lesions is based on changes of epithelial homeostasis affected by the viral oncoproteins. In spite of the detailed knowledge of many molecular mechanisms, many aspects of PV pathogenicity are not as obvious as it is often assumed.

An example is the fact that many PV types have only been found in latent infections, and even those viruses typically associated with benign and malignant neoplasia can regularly be detected in healthy tissue. It is not well understood whether every PV infection leads to neoplasia, unless suppressed by an immune response, or whether the viral biology includes latent stages, maintenance of PV DNA without changes of the infected cell. This is exemplified by the fact that the same HPV types that can induce carcinogenesis of the cervix infect the penis without easily detectable symptoms. While male individuals function efficiently as transient hosts, they are rarely affected by disease. Yet another example is the fact that HPV-associated genital carcinogenesis in women is rare in the vagina, but typically arises from the transformation zone of the cervix, a tissue where adjacent endocervical columnar epithelia and ectocervical squamous epithelia change in a process called squamous metaplasia. As HPV tumors at yet other sites (anal carcinomas and laryngeal papillomas) are also associated with boundaries between different epithelia, one may speculate that yet poorly understood differentiation processes may synergize with PV molecular biology in order to induce neoplastic changes. Lastly, it is well confirmed that progression of precancerous lesions to malignant carcinomas is not just the result of PV-encoded mechanisms, but requires the accumulation of additional genomic changes, which are documented in extensive databases of chromosomal aberrations detected in cervical carcinomas. The molecular identity of these mutations is still a matter of research.

## Diagnosis

HPV infections are diagnosed by the detection of a cutaneous or mucosal neoplasia, that is, a wart. Wart-like lesions, condylomata acuminata, can also occur at the cervix under the influence of the low-risk HPV-6 and HPV-11. High-risk HPVs induce flat condylomas which can be diagnosed by visual inspection through a colposcope. The traditional diagnosis of cervical PV infections is the Papanicolaou test ('pap test'), a technique developed in the 1950s and predating all knowledge about PVs. The Pap test aims to detect and classify dysplasia by microscopic observation of stained cervical exfoliated cells. Diagnostic criteria include a perinuclear halo (believed to result from accumulation of E4 protein) and nuclear enlargement (a consequence of polyploidies). In recent years, Pap tests have become complemented by DNA diagnostic detection of PVs.

## Treatment

The treatment of many benign cutaneous or mucosal PV lesions will typically be a 'wait and see' approach. For those cases where treatment is necessary, surgical procedures can be based on excision by knife, laser, cryotherapy, or caustic substances. The application of concentrated solutions of salicylate is a traditional treatment of common warts, and podophyllin has been used in the treatment of genital warts. Antiviral drugs targeting PVs include interferons and imiquimode. Cervical precancerous lesions are surgically removed by excision of a cone-shaped wedge from the cervix or loop excision of the transformation zone. For information about treatment of malignancies, appropriate handbooks about gynecological oncology, etc., should be consulted.

## Immunology and Vaccination

Anti-PV immune responses can be directed against the viral capsid, that is, targeting the L1 protein, or against virally infected cells, targeting any of the six early proteins.

Particles of HPV-16 and HPV-18 consisting only of L1 protein have been developed as vaccines by Merck and GlaxoSmithKline, the product of the former company also including HPV-6 and HPV-11 capsids. The vaccines became available in 2006/07, and have been cleared by the Food and Drug Administration of the United States for prophylactic vaccination of women aged 9–26. Vaccination during extensive clinical studies efficiently protected PV-uninfected women against *de novo* PV infections over periods exceeding 5 years. The vaccinations led to the stimulation of humoral immune responses by more than an order of magnitude beyond levels found in natural infections. The success of this approach is apparently based on anti-PV immune globulin concentrations in cervical mucus that suffice to neutralize PV particles before they inject the viral DNA into target cells.

Induction of immunity against the early PV proteins could form the basis of therapeutic vaccination, a potentially splendid strategy for anticancer immune therapy. Unfortunately, while scientists are well aware of this possibility, no major success has yet been achieved, and evidence points to numerous major obstacles. Investigations of naturally infected individuals generally showed weak immune responses against early PV proteins, and those humoral or cellular responses that were detectable correlated poorly with pathology or detection of PV DNA. A reason for this fact may be that PV early proteins are poor antigens, as suggested by comparison in animal systems with various other antigens. In addition, many PV proteins are only expressed at low concentrations, notably the oncoprotein E6 present in all cervical carcinomas, and rarely enter the circulation, as they are shed from the epithelium with the infected cell population.

*See also:* Papillomaviruses of Animals.

## Further Reading

Bernard HU (2002) Gene expression of genital human papillomaviruses and potential antiviral approaches. *Antiviral Therapy* 7: 219–237.

Campo MS (ed.) (2006) *Papillomavirus Research: From Natural History to Vaccines and Beyond.* Wymondham, UK: Caister Academic Press.

Davy C and Doorbar J (eds.) (2005) *Human Papillomaviruses, Methods and Protocols.* Totowa, NJ: Humana Press.

de Villiers EM, Fauquet C, Broker TR, Bernard HU, and zur Hausen H (2004) Classification of papillomaviruses. *Virology* 324: 17–27.

Lowy DR and Schiller JT (2006) Prophylactic human papillomavirus vaccines. *Journal of Clinical Investigation* 116: 1167–1173.

Mantovani F and Banks L (2001) The human papillomavirus E6 protein and its contribution to malignant progression. *Oncogene* 20: 7874–7887.

Munger K, Basile JR, Duensing S, et al. (2001) Biological activities and molecular targets of the human papillomavirus E7 oncoprotein. *Oncogene* 20: 7888–7898.

Munoz N, Bosch FX, de Sanjosé S, et al. (2003) Epidemiological classification of human papillomavirus types associated with cervical cancer. *New England Journal of Medicine* 348: 518–527.

zur Hausen H and de Villiers EM (1994) Human papillomaviruses. *Annual Review of Microbiology* 48: 427–447.

# Paramyxoviruses of Animals

**S K Samal,** University of Maryland, College Park, MD, USA

## Glossary

**Emerging virus** A virus that has never before been recognized.
**Phenotype** The collective structural and biological properties of a cell or an organism.
**Reverse genetics** A technique whereby infectious virus is produced entirely from complementary DNA.
**Syncytia** Formation of fused or multinucleated cells.
**Viremia** The presence of a virus in the blood.
**Zoonotic diseases** Diseases that can be transmitted from animals to humans.

## Introduction

The family *Paramyxoviridae* contains a large number of viruses of animals (**Table 1**), including a number of major animal pathogens (such as Newcastle disease virus (NDV), canine distemper virus, and rinderpest virus), zoonotic pathogens (such as Hendra and Nipah viruses), and a number of somewhat obscure viruses whose natural histories are poorly understood. New paramyxoviruses are being isolated on an ongoing basis from a wide variety of animals. For example, new paramyxoviruses have emerged that are pathogenic for marine mammals such as seals, dolphins, and porpoises (e.g., cetacean morbillivirus). Other paramyxoviruses that have been identified from various sources during the last few decades, such as Salem virus, Mossman virus, J-virus, and Beilong virus, are not associated with known diseases and are poorly understood. The recently identified Hendra and Nipah viruses came to light when they crossed species barriers and infected humans, causing severe, often fatal, zoonotic diseases. There are many animal paramyxoviruses, but only a few effective vaccines are currently available. Previously, genetic manipulation of paramyxoviruses was not possible because the genome is not infectious alone and RNA recombination is essentially nonexistent. This posed an impediment to the molecular and biological characterization of these viruses. However, in the last decade, methods of producing virus entirely from cDNA clones (reverse genetics) have been developed and have allowed manipulation of the genome of paramyxoviruses. This has greatly improved our understanding of the functions of each gene in replication and pathogenesis of these viruses. Another important aspect of this new technology is that vaccines can now be designed for some of the animal paramyxoviruses for which either vaccines are not currently available or the available vaccines are not satisfactory.

## Taxonomy and Classification

Paramyxoviruses (some of which are sometimes also called parainfluenza viruses) belong to the family *Paramyxoviridae* of the order *Mononegavirales*. The order contains four families of enveloped viruses possessing linear, nonsegmented, negative-sense, single-stranded RNA genomes. The family *Paramyxoviridae* is further divided into two subfamilies: *Paramyxovirinae* and *Pneumovirinae* (**Table 1**). The two subfamilies differ in several features, most notably: (1) differences in nucleocapsid diameter (18 nm in *Paramyxovirinae* and 13–14 nm in *Pneumovirinae*); (2) possession of six to seven transcriptional units in *Paramyxovirinae*, and eight to ten transcriptional units in *Pneumovirinae*; (3) presence of an additional nucleocapsid-associated protein (M2-1) and an RNA regulatory protein (M2-2) in *Pneumovirinae*; (4) structural differences in the attachment protein; and (5) lack of RNA editing of the P mRNA in *Pneumovirinae*. The subfamily *Paramyxovirinae* comprises five genera, *Rubulavirus*, *Avulavirus*, *Respirovirus*, *Henipavirus*, and *Morbillivirus*, as well as a number of unclassified viruses that might become the basis of one or more additional future genera, in *Paramyxovirinae* (**Table 1**). The division of this subfamily into five genera and the unclassified group is based on: (1) amino acid sequence relationship between the corresponding proteins; (2) the number of transcriptional units; (3) RNA editing products of the P gene; and (4) the presence of neuraminidase and hemagglutinin activities in the attachment protein. The subfamily *Pneumovirinae* contains two genera: *Pneumovirus* and *Metapneumovirus*. These two genera differ by (1) presence of two additional genes, NS1 and NS2, in pneumovirus; (2) the pneumovirus gene order SH–G–F–M2, as opposed to metapneumovirus gene order F–M2–SH–G; and (3) amino acid sequence relationship between the corresponding proteins.

## Host Range and Virus Propagation

Animal paramyxoviruses have been isolated from many different vertebrate animal hosts including mice, rats, bats, dogs, dolphins, seals, birds, cattle, pigs, horses, reptiles, tree shrews, and monkeys. In general, paramyxoviruses

**Table 1**    The genera and species of animal paramyxoviruses

| Subfamily | Genus | Animal virus | Animal host | Disease |
|---|---|---|---|---|
| Paramyxovirinae | Rubulavirus | Parainfluenza virus 5 (formerly simian virus 5) | Dogs, pigs, monkeys | Respiratory disease |
| | | Simian virus 41 | Monkeys | Respiratory disease |
| | | Porcine rubulavirus (La-Piedad-Michoacan-Mexico virus) | Pigs | Encephalitis, reproductive failure, corneal opacity |
| | | Mapuera virus | Bats | Unknown |
| | | Menangle virus (tentative species in the genus) | Pigs, bats | Reproductive failure |
| | | Tioman virus (tentative species in the genus) | Bats | Unknown |
| | Avulavirus | Newcastle disease virus (avian paramyxovirus 1) | Domestic and wild fowl | Respiratory and neurological disease |
| | | Avian paramyxoviruses 2–9 | Domestic and wild fowl | Respiratory disease |
| | Respirovirus | Bovine parainfluenza virus 3 | Cattle, sheep, and other mammals | Respiratory disease |
| | | Sendai virus (murine para influenza virus 1) | Mice, rats, and rabbits | Respiratory disease |
| | | Simian virus 10 | Monkeys | Respiratory disease |
| | Henipavirus | Hendra virus | Bats, horses, humans | Severe respiratory disease |
| | | Nipah virus | Bats, pigs, humans | Encephalitis |
| | Morbillivirus | Canine distemper virus | Carnivora species | Severe generalized and central nervous system disease |
| | | Cetacean morbillivirus | Dolphins and porpoises | Severe respiratory and generalized disease |
| | | Peste des petits ruminants virus | Sheep and goats | Severe generalized disease |
| | | Phocine distemper virus | Seal | Severe generalized and central nervous system disease |
| | | Rinderpest virus | Cattle, wild ruminants | Severe generalized disease |
| | Unclassified | Nariva virus | | Unknown |
| | | J-virus | | Unknown |
| | | Mossman virus | | Unknown |
| | | Tupia paramyxovirus | Tree shrews | Unknown |
| | | Salem virus | Horses | Unknown |
| | | Fer de lance virus | Snakes | Fatal disease |
| | | Beilong virus | Rodents (?) | Unknown |
| Pneumovirinae | Pneumovirus | Bovine respiratory syncytial virus | Cattle | Respiratory disease |
| | | Pneumonia virus of mice | Mice | Respiratory disease |
| | Metapneumovirus | Avian metapneumovirus | Turkeys, chickens | Severe respiratory disease in turkeys |
| | | | | Swollen head syndrome in chickens |

are restricted in host range. However, in recent years, some animal paramyxoviruses have been found to cross species barriers and infect other animal species and humans. In some cases, the animal viruses are highly virulent in the new host, as exemplified by Nipah and Hendra viruses, and pose a major public health concern. Interestingly, fruit bats in the genus *Pteropus* have been implicated as a reservoir of a number of new and emerging zoonotic animal paramyxoviruses. Other paramyxoviruses, such as NDV and bovine parainfluenza virus 3, can experimentally infect a variety of non-natural hosts, including rodents and monkeys, but typically are highly attenuated in these hosts. Many different primary and established cell

cultures are used to grow animal paramyxoviruses. Some viruses do not readily grow in cell culture (e.g., avian metapneumovirus) and require adaptation by several passages in the cell cultures. Cell cultures derived from homologous species are generally used for cultivation of morbilliviruses and pneumoviruses. However, a number of paramyxoviruses grow well in cells of different host origin. For example, avian metapneumoviruses grow well in monkey kidney (Vero) cells, and bovine parainfluenza virus-3 grows well in monkey kidney (LLC-MK2 and Vero) cells and in baby hamster kidney ($BHK_{21}$) cells. Avian paramyxoviruses grow well in embryonated chicken eggs or cells derived from avian species. Some paramyxoviruses require the addition of protease, such as trypsin, α-chymotrypsin, or allantoic fluid (as a source of secreted protease), to the medium for growth in cell culture. This is necessary for cleavage activation of the viral fusion F protein (see below). Characteristic cytopathic effects of paramyxoviruses include the formation of syncytia (multinucleated giant cells) and eosinophilic cytoplasmic inclusion bodies.

## Properties of Virion

The virions are 150–350 nm in diameter, pleomorphic, but usually spherical in shape. They consist of a nucleocapsid surrounded by a lipid envelope. Virion $M_r$ is around $500 \times 10^6$. Virion buoyant density in sucrose is $1.18$–$1.20 \mathrm{g\,cm}^{-3}$. Some viruses (particularly of *Pneumovirinae*) are also produced in long filamentous form. Virions are highly sensitive to dehydration, heat, detergents, lipid solvents, formaldehyde, and oxidizing agents. Virus stability varies from stable (NDV) to very labile (rinderpest, canine distemper, bovine respiratory syncytial virus, and avian metapneumovirus). The schematic of a typical paramyxovirus is shown in **Figure 1**.

## Genome

The genome consists of a single segment of negative-sense RNA (i.e., complementary to mRNA) that is 13–19 kbp in length and contains six to ten genes encoding up to 12

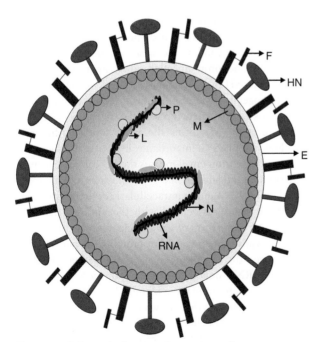

**Figure 1** Schematic diagram of a paramyxovirus. N, nucleocapsid protein; P, phosphoprotein; L, large polymerase protein; M, matrix protein; F, fusion protein; HN, hemagglutinin-neuraminidase protein; E, envelope.

different proteins. The genome contains neither a $5'$ cap nor a $3'$ end poly(A) tail. At the $3'$ and $5'$ ends of the genome are short extragenic (noncoding) regions known as the 'leader' and 'trailer' region, respectively. The length of the leader is approximately 50 nt, whereas the length of the trailer is 23–161 nt. The leader region (*Pneumovirinae*) or the leader region and adjacent upstream end of the adjacent N gene (*Paramyxovirinae*) contains a single genomic promoter that is involved in the synthesis of the mRNAs as well as a complete positive-sense replicative intermediate called the antigenome. Generally, the first 10–12 nt of the leader and trailer are complementary, reflecting a conservation of promoter sequences present at the end of the genome and antigenome. At the beginning and end of each gene are conserved transcriptional control signals involved in initiation and termination/polyadenylation of the mRNAs. These conserved sequences are known as 'gene-start' and 'gene-end' sequences. The genes are separated by short intergenic regions that are not copied into mRNA. There is one exception in bovine respiratory syncytial virus where the L gene-start sequence is located upstream of the gene-end sequence of the upstream M2 gene, resulting in overlapping genes. The intergenic region is a conserved trinucleotide for respiroviruses, morbilliviruses, and henipaviruses, but is variable in length for all other paramyxoviruses. Thus, this might be a potential signal in some viruses, but not in others. The gene map of a representative member of each genus is shown in **Figure 2**. The nucleotide lengths of the genomes of members of subfamily *Paramyxovirinae* are even multiples of six, which is required for efficient RNA replication and is known as the 'rule of six'. However, the rule of six does not apply to the members of the subfamily *Pneumovirinae*. The genome size of a number of animal paramyxoviruses has been determined: 15 384 nt for Sendai virus; 15 456 nt for bovine parainfluenza virus 3; 15 246 nt for simian virus 5; 15 450 nt for simian virus 41; 15 186 nt for NDV; 15 882 nt for rinderpest virus; 15 948 nt for peste des petits ruminants virus; 15 690 nt for canine distemper virus; 15 702 nt for cetacean morbillivirus; 18 234 nt for Hendra virus; 18 246 nt for Nipah virus; 15 140 nt for bovine respiratory syncytial virus; 14 886 nt for pneumonia virus of mice; 15 522 nt for Tioman virus; 16 236 nt for avian paramyxovirus type 6; 13 373 nt for avian metapneumovirus type A; and 14 150 nt for avian metapneumovirus type C.

## Proteins

All paramyxoviruses contain two glycosylated surface envelope proteins, a fusion protein (F) and an attachment protein (G or H or HN). The F protein mediates viral penetration by inducing fusion between the viral envelope and the host cell plasma membrane. In paramyxoviruses,

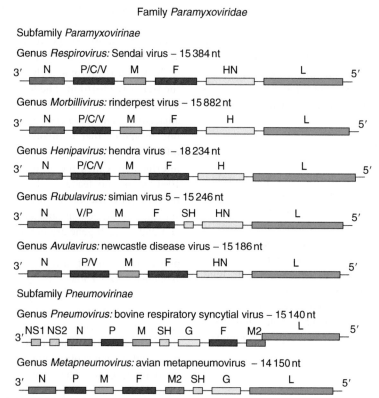

**Figure 2**    Map of genomic RNA (3' to 5') of animal paramyxoviruses representing the seven genera of the family *Paramyxoviridae*. Each box represents a separate gene; multiple distinct open reading frames (ORFs) within a single gene are indicated by slashes. For the P gene, the product encoded by the unedited mRNA is given first. In bovine respiratory syncytial virus of genus *Pneumovirus*, there is a transcriptional overlap at M2 and L genes.

the fusion event occurs at neutral pH. The F protein is synthesized as an inactive precursor ($F_0$), which is activated following cleavage by cellular protease(s) to generate two disulfide-linked $F_1$ and $F_2$ subunits. Some paramyxoviruses have multiple basic residues (arg and lys) at the cleavage site and thus are readily cleaved by furin-like proteases found intracellularly in most tissue types. Other paramyxoviruses have few, or only one, basic residues at the cleavage site and thus are cleaved extracellularly by a trypsin-like protease secreted in the respiratory and intestinal tracts, which limits virus replication. Hence, the number of arg and lys residues at the F protein cleavage site is a major determinant of paramyxovirus virulence. However, other viral proteins also contribute to the virulence of paramyxoviruses. The attachment protein binds to cell surface receptor and facilitates viral penetration. The attachment proteins of rubulaviruses, avulaviruses, and respiroviruses are designated HN since they possesses both hemagglutination activity, which is due to binding to sialic acid, and neuraminidase activity, which cleaves sialic acid on the cell surface and facilitates release. The attachment protein of morbilliviruses is designated H because it possesses hemagglutination activity, which is due to binding to the signaling lymphocyte activation molecule (SLAM) receptor, but not neuraminidase activity. Attachment proteins that generally lack hemagglutination

and neuraminidase activities are designated G (glycoprotein). These occur in members of genera *Henipavirus*, *Pneumovirus*, and *Metapneumovirus*. The envelopes of the genera *Rubulavirus*, *Pneumovirus*, and *Metapneumovirus* contain a third integral membrane protein called small hydrophobic (SH) protein. The SH protein might play a role in cell fusion or in morphogenesis and also has been reported to interfere with cytokine-mediated intracellular signaling. The viral matrix protein (M) forms the inner layer of the virus envelope and plays an important role in virus assembly.

Inside the virion envelope lies the helical nucleocapsid. The genome and antigenome of paramyxoviruses are never found as free RNA either intracellularly or in the virion, but rather are tightly associated with the viral nucleocapsid protein (N) in the form of a ribonucleoprotein core. Virion nucleocapsids contain two other proteins, the phosphoprotein (P) and the large protein (L) that together constitute the viral RNA-dependent RNA polymerase complex. Virion nucleocapsids of the subfamily *Pneumovirinae* contain an additional protein (M2-1), which is a transcription elongation factor. A nonabundant protein (M2-2) is also produced from the second open reading frame (ORF) of the M2 gene and is involved in the balance between genome replication and transcription. The RNA within the nucleocapsid is resistant to nucleases.

Members of subfamily *Paramyxovirinae* encode multiple proteins from the P gene, due in part to a mechanism called 'RNA editing'. The P gene contains an editing site at which nontemplated G residues are added into the P mRNA by stuttering during transcription. The inclusion of additional G residues has the potential to shift the reading frame to access alternate frames, thus creating one or more chimeric proteins in which N-terminal domain is encoded by the P ORF upstream of the editing site and the C-terminal domain is encoded by the alternative ORF downstream of the editing site. In almost all members of the subfamily *Paramyxovirinae*, two of the major products of the P gene are the P and V proteins. For the respiroviruses, morbilliviruses, avulaviruses, and henipaviruses, the unedited mRNA of the P gene produces the P protein. Addition of one G nucleotide at the editing site produces an mRNA that encodes the V protein. In rubulaviruses, the unedited P mRNA encodes the V protein and addition of two G nucleotides produces the P mRNA. The V proteins of respiroviruses and morbilliviruses are nonstructural; whereas, the V proteins of rubulaviruses and avulaviruses are structural components of the virions. The respiroviruses, henipaviruses, and morbilliviruses also encode a third major protein from the P gene, namely the C protein. The C protein is synthesized from a +1 reading frame that overlaps the P and V reading frames. The V and C accessory proteins play important roles counteracting host cell antiviral defense mechanisms, especially the interferon system, and have been reported to be involved in other activities such as RNA synthesis and virion morphogenesis. *Pneumovirinae* lacks RNA editing. The members of genus *Pneumovirus* produce two additional nonstructural proteins (NS1 and NS2) from separate, promoter-proximal genes, which play a role in counteracting host cell antiviral defense mechanisms.

## Replication and Virus Assembly

Paramyxovirus gene expression and RNA replication occur in the cytoplasm of infected cells, and progeny virions bud from the plasma membrane. Various cell surface molecules serve as receptors. Respiroviruses, rubulaviruses, and avulaviruses utilize sialic acid residues on various cellular glycoproteins (e.g., glycophorin) and gangliosides as receptors. Morbilliviruses utilize SLAM (also known as CD150) as a receptor. Infection by respiratory syncytial virus *in vitro* involves glycosaminoglycans, and Hendra and Nipah viruses use ephrin-B2 for infection of human cells. The F protein mediates fusion of the viral envelope and the plasma membrane of the host cell. As a result of the fusion, the viral nucleocapsid is released into the cytoplasm. Once in the cytoplasm, the nucleocapsid initiates transcription. The viral polymerase enters at the promoter located at the 3′-end of the genome.

This promoter serves the dual function of mRNA and antigenome synthesis. Transcription is linear, sequential, and involves a stop-start mechanism guided by the gene-start and gene-end signals. As polymerase molecules progress along the genome, there is some dissociation at each gene junction, leading to a gradient of mRNA abundance that decreases according to distance from the 3′ end of the genome. The viral mRNAs are 5′-capped by the viral polymerase and contain a 3′ poly(A) tail that is produced by stuttering on the gene-end sequence. The intracellular accumulation of viral nucleocapsid-associated proteins results in the initiation of RNA replication. During RNA replication, the gene-start and gene-end signals are ignored and an exact complementary copy of the genome (antigenome) is synthesized. RNA synthesis is tightly linked to encapsidation of the progeny molecule. A promoter located at the 3′ end of the antigenome is used to synthesize genome.

The viral M protein plays a major role in mediating association of the nucleocapsids with patches in the plasma membrane where the viral envelope proteins have accumulated. It is thought that the M protein assembles the virion by forming a bridge between the cytoplasmic tails of envelope proteins and the nucleocapsids. Both the final assembly and budding of the virus occur at the plasma membrane of infected cells.

## Reverse Genetics

Reverse genetics refers to the generation of subviral particles or complete infectious virus entirely by expression of cloned cDNAs. This provides a method for introducing desired changes into the viral genome. A number of animal paramyxoviruses have been recovered from cDNAs using reverse genetics, including simian virus 5, NDV, bovine parainfluenza virus 3, Sendai virus, canine distemper virus, rinderpest virus, bovine respiratory syncytial virus, and avian metapneumovirus. The basic method involves transfecting cultured cells with plasmids encoding the viral N, P, and L proteins, as well as the viral antigenome, all under the control of the T7 promoter. The positive-sense antigenome typically is expressed rather than the negative-sense genome to avoid hybridization with the positive-sense mRNAs, but virus has also been recovered (less efficiently) by expressing the genome. The bacteriophage T7 RNA polymerase is provided either by infection with a recombinant vaccinia virus expressing T7 RNA polymerase or by transfecting into cell lines that constitutively express T7 RNA polymerase. The recovery of bovine respiratory syncytial virus requires expression of an additional plasmid encoding the transcription elongation factor M2-1. Intracellular synthesis of the viral N, P, and L proteins and antigenome RNA results in the assembly of a biologically viral nucleocapsid that launches an infection leading to production of infectious virus. It is now feasible to genetically engineer attenuated viruses for use as live virus vaccines for several animal paramyxoviruses for which effective vaccines are not currently available. Perhaps even more exciting is the potential to use animal paramyxoviruses as vaccine vectors to design multivalent vaccines or to use more stable vectors to express antigens from less stable pathogens. At present, several animal paramyxoviruses, such as Sendai virus, NDV, and bovine parainfluenza virus 3, are being evaluated as vaccine vectors for other animal pathogens and also for use in humans as host-range-restricted vectors expressing antigens of human pathogens.

## Genetic and Serologic Relationships

The relationships among paramyxoviruses can be deduced from nucleotide and amino acid sequence relatedness and serological analysis. Paramyxoviruses show very little amino acid sequence conservation among members of different genera. The sequence relatedness varies greatly within a genus, some members showing higher levels of sequence relatedness than others. The overall sequence conservation of paramyxovirus structural proteins in descending order seems to be L>M>F>N>H/ HN/G>P. The L protein has five short regions of high homology near the center of the protein, which are not only conserved among paramyxoviruses, but are also conserved among all nonsegmented negative-strand RNA viruses. The C-terminal, domain of the V protein, is also conserved among all paramyxoviruses and contains seven invariant cysteine residues. Some animal paramyxoviruses show high levels of relatedness by sequence and serology with human paramyxoviruses. This implies that they have close evolutionary relationships and may have arisen by crossing species boundaries. Examples of pairs of related animal and human viruses include bovine and human parainfluenza virus 3, bovine and human respiratory syncytial virus, Sendai virus and human parainfluenza virus 1, simian virus 5 and human parainfluenza virus 2, and avian and human metapneumoviruses. In addition, all viruses within the genus *Morbillivirus* are related by sequence and serology. Rinderpest virus is more closely related to measles virus than to peste des petits ruminants virus and canine distemper virus. It is thought that the rinderpest virus is the archetype from which the other members of the genus morbillivirus have probably evolved, a process that involved crossing species boundaries.

## Epidemiology

Some paramyxoviruses, such as NDV, canine distemper virus, bovine parainfluenza virus 3, and Sendai virus, have a worldwide distribution. Peste des petits ruminants virus is widespread in all countries lying between the Sahara and the Equator, in the Middle East, and in Southeast Asia. Avian metapneumovirus subtypes A, B, and D are present in Europe, but only subtype C is prevalent in the US. Nipah and Hendra viruses have emerged as new pathogens in Malaysia and Australia, respectively. Outbreaks of Menangle virus infection have been reported only in Australia.

The diseases caused by animal paramyxoviruses depend in part on their tissue tropism: as described below, some remain restricted to the respiratory tract and cause disease at that site, whereas others can disseminate by viremia to other tissues and cause disease that depends on the site of viral replication and pathogenesis. Immunity against viruses whose pathogenesis involves viremia tends to be relatively strong and long-lived, likely reflecting the long life of the serum antibody response. For example, rinderpest virus, which was once present on most continents, has been eradicated from Europe, America, and most of Asia. It remains enzootic only in parts of Asia and Africa. In contrast, immunity against viruses that remain localized in the superficial epithelium of the respiratory tract, such as bovine parainfluenza virus 3 and respiratory syncytial virus, is less effective and long-lived, and reinfection is common.

## Transmission and Pathogenesis

Paramyxoviruses such as NDV and the morbilliviruses are highly infectious. The respiratory tract is the primary portal of entry for most paramyxoviruses and, for many, is the major site of viral replication; a few paramyxoviruses also infect via the enteric tract. Infection occurs by several different routes, including aerosols (NDV, bovine respiratory syncytial virus, avian metapneumovirus) and contaminated feed and water (Newcastle disease, canine distemper, and rinderpest viruses). Transmission of paramyxoviruses from fruit bats to animals is thought to occur by the fecal–oral route. In some viruses, the replication is confined to the respiratory mucosal surface (bovine parainfluenza virus 3, bovine respiratory syncytial virus, avian metapneumovirus), while in others, the initial replication on the respiratory tract is followed by systemic spread. Virulent strains of NDV initially infect the upper respiratory tract and then spread via the blood in the spleen and kidney, producing a secondary viremia. This leads to infection of other target organs, such as lung, intestine, and central nervous systems. In morbilliviruses, after initial replication in the respiratory tract, the virus multiplies further in regional lymph nodes, then enters the bloodstream, carried within lymphocytes, to produce primary viremia that spreads the virus to reticuloendothelial systems. Viruses produced from these sites are carried by lymphocytes to produce secondary viremia, which leads to infection of target tissues, such as lung, intestine, and central nervous systems.

## Diseases

Paramyxoviruses are responsible for a wide variety of diseases in animals. Many paramyxoviruses primarily cause respiratory disease (bovine parainfluenza virus 3, bovine respiratory syncytial virus, avian metapneumovirus), while others cause serious systemic disease (rinderpest, virulent strains of Newcastle disease, canine distemper). Many diseases caused by animal paramyxoviruses also have a neurological component (canine distemper, Newcastle disease, Nipah virus) or a reproductive disease component (parainfluenza virus 5 in pigs and Menangle virus). Interestingly, the type of disease caused by Newcastle disease virus can vary, depending on the strain of the virus. Some strains cause only respiratory tract disease, some cause generalized hemorrhagic lesion, while others cause neurological disease. Most Newcastle disease virus strains replicate in the respiratory tract, while some predominantly replicate in the intestinal tract. Certain members of the genus *Morbillivirus*, canine distemper virus, phocine distemper virus, and cetacean viruses, cause high levels of central nervous system (CNS) diseases in their natural hosts, but CNS diseases are not associated with other members of genus *Morbillivirus*, such as rinderpest and peste des petits ruminant viruses. The severity of clinical disease also varies among animal paramyxoviruses. Some viruses cause asymptomatic or mild respiratory disease (bovine parainfluenza virus 3, simian virus 5, avian paramyxovirus types 2–9), while other viruses can cause severe disease leading to 90–100% mortality in susceptible hosts (rinderpest, Newcastle disease virus, canine distemper virus). There is also extreme variation in the pathogenicity of strains of some paramyxoviruses. For example, Newcastle disease virus strains range from avirulent to highly virulent (causing 100% mortality in chickens).

## Immune Response

Paramyxoviruses induce both local and systemic antibody-mediated and cell-mediated immunity. Secretory IgA and cytotoxic T-lymphocytes play major roles in resolving infection and protecting against reinfection, but are somewhat short-lived, especially following a primary infection. Serum antibodies can also contribute to resolving infection and usually provide durable protection against reinfection. As already noted, serum antibodies are particularly effective against viruses whose pathogenesis involves viremia. Local immune factors play a greater role against viruses that remain localized in the respiratory tract. The envelope glycoproteins, H/HN/G and F, are the major neutralization and protective antigens of paramyxoviruses, although all of the viral proteins have the potential to contain epitopes for cellular immune responses. In some viruses (e.g., bovine parainfluenza virus 3), HN protein is the major protective antigen, while in other viruses (e.g., Newcastle disease virus), F protein is the major protective antigen. Most or all paramyxoviruses have evolved mechanisms that suppress the synthesis of interferon and the establishment of an interferon-mediated antiviral state.

## Prevention and Control

Vaccination is a very effective means of controlling paramyxovirus infections. Both live-attenuated and inactivated vaccines have been developed for major animal paramyxovirus pathogens. Live-attenuated vaccines typically are more effective than the inactivated vaccines. Currently, effective live-attenuated vaccines are available for rinderpest, canine distemper, and Newcastle disease. However, satisfactory live-attenuated or inactivated vaccines are not available for diseases caused by bovine respiratory syncytial virus, Nipah virus, Hendra virus, and avian metapneumoviruses. Although the live-attenuated vaccines for rinderpest, canine distemper, and Newcastle diseases are generally very effective, there have been concerns about their potential safety and reversion to virulence. Furthermore, these vaccines cannot serologically distinguish vaccinated animals from naturally infected animals. Therefore, new and highly effective animal paramyxovirus vaccines are being engineered using reverse genetics techniques.

## Future Perspectives

Some of the animal paramyxoviruses cause devastating diseases of animals, while others appear to be nonpathogenic. Many of the animal paramyxoviruses lack an effective vaccine. Development of reverse genetics systems has not only improved our understanding of the biology of these viruses, but has also provided methods for engineering effective vaccines. It is now possible to adjust the attenuation phenotype of a vaccine, introduce genetic markers into the vaccine viruses for differentiation between vaccine and wild-type strains, and to engineer thermostable vaccines for use in developing countries. The next steps will be to test these vaccines using a large number of animals, and to have them commercially available for vaccination purposes. Another advantage of reverse genetics is the use of animal paramyxoviruses as vectors to express foreign genes. This makes possible the use of one animal paramyxovirus vaccine to protect from multiple animal diseases. Since recombination involving members of *Paramyxoviridae* is essentially nonexistent, they will be particularly valuable as vectors to express the antigens of recombination-prone viruses such as coronaviruses. Some animal paramyxovirus-based vectors can be useful for the development of vaccines against emerging human infections such as H5N1 avian influenza, severe acute respiratory syndrome (SARS), and those caused by Ebola, Marburg, Nipah, and Hendra viruses. Since animal paramyxoviruses can be chosen that are serologically unrelated to common human pathogens, the general human population is susceptible to immunization with animal paramyxovirus-vectored vaccines. Reverse genetics systems are currently available for many but not all animal paramyxoviruses. Therefore, there is a great need to develop reverse genetics systems for the remaining animal paramyxoviruses. Furthermore, it is necessary to develop reverse genetics systems of local paramyxovirus strains for development of effective vaccines against the prevailing virus strains. In addition to vaccine development, it is also important to understand the pathogenesis and determinants of virus virulence and the mechanisms of interspecies transmission of the viruses. Due to the availability of reverse genetics systems for these viruses, we are confident that the next decade will bring a significant improvement in our understanding of their biology and we will witness development of better and safer vaccines against animal diseases.

*See also:* Rinderpest and Distemper Viruses.

## Further Reading

Conzelmann KK (2004) Reverse genetics of mononegavirales. *Current Topics in Microbiology and Immunology* 283: 1–41.

Easton AJ, Domachowske JB, and Rosenberg HF (2004) Animal pneumoviruses: Molecular genetics and pathogenesis. *Clinical Microbiology Reviews* 17: 390–412.

Kurath G, Batts WN, Ahme W, and Winton JR (2004) Complete genome sequence of fer-de-lance virus reveals a novel gene in reptilian paramyxoviruses. *Journal of Virology* 78: 2045–2056.

Lamb RA, Collins PL, Kolakofsky D, *et al.* (2005) *Paramyxoviridae*. In: Fauquet CM, Mayo MA, Maniloff J, Desselberger U,, and Ball LA (eds.) *Virus Taxonomy: Eighth Report of the International Committee on Taxonomy of Viruses*, pp. 655–668. San Diego, CA: Elsevier Academic Press.

Lamb RA and Parks GD (2006) *Paramyxoviridae*: The viruses and their replication. In: Knipe DM, Howley PM, Griffin DE, *et al.* (eds.) *Fields Virology*, 5th edn., pp. 1449–1496. Philadelphia: Lippincott Williams and Wilkins.

Li Z, Yu M, Zhang H, *et al.* (2006) Beilong virus, a novel paramyxovirus with the largest genome of non-segmented negative-stranded RNA viruses. *Virology* 346: 219–228.

Wang LF, Harcourt BH, Yu M, *et al.* (2001) Molecular biology of Hendra and Nipah viruses. *Microbes and Infection* 3: 279–287.

# Parapoxviruses

**D Haig,** Nottingham University, Nottingham, UK
**A A Mercer,** University of Otago, Dunedin, New Zealand

## Introduction

Parapoxviruses (PPVs) are epitheliotropic viruses found worldwide. The individual viruses generally exhibit a narrow host range and infect via scarified or damaged skin and give rise to pustular lesions of the skin and occasionally the buccal mucosa. These lesions are associated with low mortality and high morbidity. In addition to a narrow host range, most of the PPVs can also infect humans.

There are numerous historical references to diseases of domesticated animals such as sheep and cattle that we would now suspect to be the result of infection by PPVs. These references include Jenner's 'spurious' cowpox which is likely to have been caused by the PPV, pseudocowpox virus (PCPV). In the latter part of last century, reports appeared in the scientific literature which recognized the distinct identities of the diseases caused by members of this genus. Following an extensive study of contagious pustular dermatitis of sheep, Aynaud produced a report in 1923 which included the observation that the disease could be transmitted by a 'filterable' agent. The isolation of each of the viruses in cell culture was reported in the period from 1957 to 1963. Detailed reports of the transmission of each disease to humans appeared in 1933 (orf virus (ORFV)), 1963 (PCPV), and 1967 (bovine papular stomatitis virus (BPSV)). The first molecular analyses of PPV genomes appeared in 1979 with publication of restriction endonuclease cleavage site maps and reports of G + C contents. These were followed, in 1989, by the first description of the DNA sequence of a region of a PPV genome and in 2004 with full genome sequence for two strains of ORFV and one of BPSV.

## Taxonomy and Classification

The genus *Parapoxvirus* belongs to the subfamily *Chordopoxvirinae* of the family *Poxviridae*. The type species of the genus is *Orf virus*, and the other species recognized as members are *Bovine papular stomatitis virus, Pseudocowpox virus, Squirrel parapoxvirus*, and a recently identified member, *Parapoxvirus of red deer in New Zealand*. Synonyms for the viruses include contagious pustular dermatitis virus and contagious ecthyma virus for ORFV and milker's nodule virus and paravaccinia virus for PCPV. Tentative species of this genus are Auzduk disease virus (camel contagious ecthyma virus), chamois contagious ecthyma virus, and sealpox virus. A virus that infects red squirrels and induces a pustular skin disease was thought to be a PPV, but recent DNA sequence data suggest that this is not the case.

The three original members of the genus were classified as separate species on the basis of the host animal and/or the pathology of the disease. Likewise, the observation of a parapox-like virus in red deer first suggested that this might represent another species. These separations have been supported by later studies which employed DNA/DNA hybridization, restriction endonuclease profiling, sequence data, or serology.

## Host Range, Epidemiology, and Virus Propagation

Natural infection by ORFV has been reported in domestic, bighorn, and thinhorn sheep, domestic and Rocky Mountain goat, chamois, Himalayan thar, musk-ox, reindeer, steenbok, and humans. Experimental inoculations have shown that monkeys are susceptible to ORFV but a wide range of other animals including mouse, rabbit, dog, cat, and domesticated chicken are resistant. BPSV and PCPV both establish infection in cattle and humans but all other species tested, including sheep, are resistant. The PPV of red deer induces only very mild lesions on sheep and has not been tested in other species. The PPV of seals has been reported in a range of seals and sea lions. PPVs do not produce lesions on the chorioallantoic membrane of the developing chick embryo.

The PPVs of cattle and sheep are found throughout the world, essentially wherever their host animal occurs. The viruses are maintained in populations by a combination of chronic infection, frequent reinfection, and the environmentally resistant nature of the viruses.

ORFV shed in scab material can remain infective under dry conditions for lengthy periods (at least 4 months and possibly years) and infection of naive animals by virus persisting in heavily contaminated areas such as barns, yards, and sheep camps is likely to play a major role in maintaining the disease. One study has shown that if the scab material is ground up so as to release the virus, then exposure to field conditions quickly results in inactivation of ORFV. Several studies have shown that a productive infection can be established in animals which have recovered from a previous infection. Such reinfections result in

lesions that are smaller and resolve more quickly than primary infections. This short-lived immunity is likely to contribute to the persistence of the disease.

In the case of PCPV, it is apparent that infection can be spread within dairy herds by contamination of milking machinery and milkers' hands. The introduction of procedures which reduce damage to teats and improve general hygiene at milking time can control the spread of the disease.

The most widely used cell culture systems have been primary ovine or bovine cells derived from sources such as testis, skin biopsy and embryonic kidney, lung, and muscle. There have also been reports of ORFV isolates adapted to growth in established cell lines. Yields of infectious ORFV from cell culture tend to be 10- to 100-fold lower than those achieved with vaccinia virus.

## Serologic Relationships

PPVs show extensive antigenic cross-reactivity, although monoclonal antibodies have been able to distinguish each of the species. There are also antigens shared with other poxvirus genera but there is no cross-protection between PPVs and either orthopoxviruses or capripoxviruses.

## Clinical Features

PPVs cause proliferative lesions that are confined to the skin and oral mucosa with no evidence of systemic spread (**Figure 1**). Infection is initiated in abrasions and generally proceeds through an afebrile, self-limiting lesion that resolves within 3–9 weeks without leaving a scar. ORFV lesions are most generally seen around the mouth and nares; hence, the infection is commonly referred to as scabby mouth or sore mouth. Lesions are also observed on other parts of the body, for example, the coronet, udder, or vulva. Following experimental inoculation of

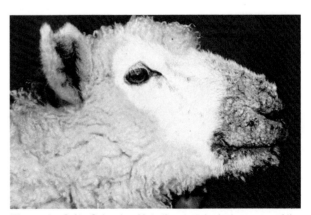

**Figure 1** Orf in *Ovis aries*. Note the pustular lesions around the mouth and nares.

scarified skin, lesions progress through erythema, papule, vesicle, pustule, and scab before resolving. Large, proliferative, tumor-like lesions have been observed. It is likely that these are a result of an immune impairment of the host animal.

Lesions around the mouth can interfere with feeding or suckling and especially in young animals result in failure to thrive. Teat lesions can have similar effects through the inhibition of suckling. Lesions on growing deer antler can affect antler growth and severely affect marketability of the product.

It is probable that all PPVs are able to infect humans, although a human case of the PPV of red deer has not been reported. Transmission to humans occurs readily although there is little evidence of human to human transmission. Progression of the lesions is essentially as seen in sheep and cattle such that the infection is benign and confined to pustular lesions on the skin at the points of infection. More severe progressive disease can occur in immune-compromised individuals. Severe reactions have also been recorded in otherwise normal individuals in cases of burns and in cases of atopic dermatitis. Erythema multiformae reactions in the form of rashes on the backs of the hands and on the legs and ankles are common.

## Properties of the Virion

PPV particles are ovoid in shape and measure 220–300 nm × 147–170 nm (**Figure 2**). In these characteristics they resemble other poxviruses except that PPVs are a little smaller than most other *Chordopoxvirinae*, which are also more commonly described as brick-shaped rather than ovoid. A distinctive feature of PPV virions is their 'ball-of-yarn' appearance when negatively stained specimens are viewed by electron microscopy. This results from a single 10–20 nm wide thread arranged as spiral coil around the particle. This unique morphology has been the basis for confirming a suspected PPV infection. However, this

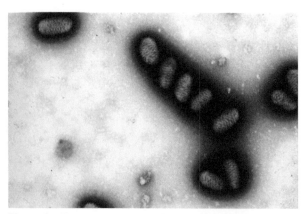

**Figure 2**  Electron micrograph of a cluster of negatively stained orf virus (ORFV) particles.

feature has recently been observed in poxviruses that are not members of the genus *Parapoxvirus* and DNA analysis is required to provide definitive identification.

Analysis of thin sections of virions has revealed a lipoprotein bilayer surrounding a biconcave core and two associated lateral bodies. Some particles have an external membranous structure. It seems likely that this is equivalent to the Golgi-derived membrane which forms the outer layer of the extracellular enveloped form of vaccinia virus.

## Physical Properties

PPVs are resistant to desiccation and, in a dried state within scab material, the viruses retain infectivity for at least 4 months and possibly years. Under laboratory conditions, infectivity may be maintained over many years. UV light, $\gamma$-irradiation, or heating at 56 °C for 1 h will inactivate PPVs.

## PPV Genomes

The PPV genome is a single, linear, double-stranded (ds) DNA molecule of 130–140 kbp with inverted terminal repeats of about 3.5 kbp in the case of ORFV (**Figure 3**). The ends of the genome are cross-linked. The G+C content of the genome is high (average of 64%). Restriction endonuclease cleavage site maps have been produced for each of the PPVs except that infecting red deer. These revealed some variability between isolates of the same species but conserved patterns, consistent with the classification of the genus, were apparent.

Full genome sequences have been obtained for three strains of tissue-culture adapted ORFV (OV-IA82 and NZ2 isolated from sheep and OV-SA00 isolated from a goat) and a tissue-culture-adapted strain of BPSV (BV-AR02). These encode an estimated 133 BPSV or 132 ORFV genes, of which 129 are collinear in the viral genomes and 88 conserved in all *Chordopoxvirinae* studied to date. The majority of these are essential genes involved in virus replication, packaging, and export. There are fewer nucleotide metabolism genes compared with other poxviruses. Seventeen BPSV and eighteen ORFV open reading frames (ORFs) lack amino acid similarity to other poxvirus or cellular proteins. The PPV genomes have some similar features (including three orthologous genes) to that of molluscum contagiosum virus – a skin-tropic poxvirus pathogen of humans. Putative and known pathogenesis-related genes are concentrated in the terminal regions of the genome. In ORFV there are ~25 such genes with unknown structure or function. In one study, the early transcribed genes of ORFV were mapped to identify candidate pathogenesis genes. cDNAs for 38 genes were

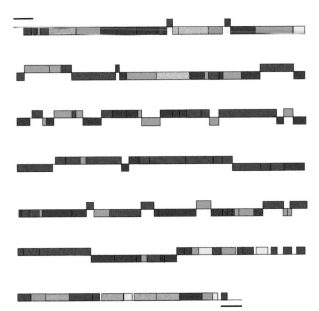

**Figure 3**  Orf virus (ORFV) genetic map. Boxes above the line represent genes transcribed rightward and those below the line genes transcribed leftward. Each line except the last corresponds to 20 kbp. The boxes are colored to indicate predicted functions. Those involved in virion structure or assembly are black, DNA replication or RNA transcription blue, host response modulation yellow, and ankyrin-repeat proteins are indicated with horizontal red lines. Genes of unknown function are further subdivided by their presence in most poxviruses (green), in parapoxviruses only (red), or in parapoxviruses and molluscipoxviruses only (red diagonal stripes).

identified, seven of these unrelated to any poxvirus or cellular gene in public databases.

The identification of transcriptional start points of PPV early genes highlighted adjacent sequences which are very similar to sequences shown to act as transcriptional promoters in vaccinia virus. These observations have been supported by data indicating that A+T-rich transcriptional control sequences characterized in vaccinia virus function in very similar ways in PPVs. Analysis of expression of ORFV antigens expressed from vaccinia virus recombinants carrying large multigene fragments of ORFV DNA suggests that ORFV late genes are also faithfully transcribed from their own promoters by vaccinia virus.

Passage of ORFV in cell culture results in genomic rearrangements. A detailed study of one such rearranged isolate showed that 19.3 kbp from the right end of the genome had been duplicated and replaced 6.6 kbp at the left end, resulting in a net deletion of 3.3 kbp at the left end. This recombination occurred between nonhomologous sequences and caused the deletion of three genes. These alterations to the genome attenuated the growth of the virus in sheep skin. Similar rearrangements have been observed in other isolates.

## Properties of Viral Proteins

SDS-polyacrylamide gel electrophoresis analyses of ORFV and PCPV virions have detected 30–40 polypeptides ranging in size from 10 to 220 kDa. Controlled degradation of the virions into core and surface fractions indicated the presence of 10–13 surface polypeptides. Prominent among these were a polypeptide of 39 kDa (ORFV) or 42–45 kDa (PCPV), which was suggested to be the subunit of the virion surface tubule protein, and a 15 kDa polypeptide. The 39 kDa ORFV polypeptide appears to be a dominant antigen and several independently derived monoclonal antibodies are directed against it.

The genes encoding two major structural proteins of ORFV have been identified. One of these is a 42 kDa protein with strong amino acid sequence similarity to the vaccinia virus protein encoded by gene F13L. This vaccinia virus polypeptide is the major, nonglycosylated, 37 kDa protein specific for the extracellular enveloped form of the virus. Cloning and expression of the ORFV gene has shown that both antibody and T-cell responses are directed against this protein during infection by ORFV. A second ORFV protein, p10k, is a homolog of the vaccinia virus 14 kDa fusion protein encoded by gene A27L. This vaccinia virus protein has a surface location and is associated with intracellular mature virus but is required for the formation of extracellular enveloped virus. The ORFV protein may be involved in the expression of the characteristic basket-weave pattern on the virions. The F1L product of ORFV is a major heparin-binding protein and may be involved in virus binding to cells to initiate the infection cycle.

Pathogenesis-related proteins are discussed in a later section.

## Replication

As with all poxviruses, the replication of PPVs occurs in the cytoplasm of infected cells. Studies in cell culture have shown very similar patterns in the replication of ORFV and PCPV. DNA replication begins 4–8 h post infection (h.p.i.) and reaches a plateau between 25 and 30 h.p.i. The first viral or viral-induced polypeptides appear from 10 h.p.i. Viral particles appear 16–24 h.p.i. and continue to be produced until at least 40 h.p.i. Viral replication is accompanied by inhibition of host DNA and protein synthesis. Some ORFV genes have been shown to be transcribed when infection occurs in the presence of an inhibitor of DNA synthesis and therefore fit the definition of early poxvirus genes. The transition between early and late replication events occurs about 8–10 h.p.i. The presence in ORFV of genes with homology to vaccinia virus intermediate genes encoding late gene transactivators suggests that expression of ORFV genes follows a regulated cascade (early–intermediate–late) similar to that reported for vaccinia virus.

## Pathogenesis and the Host Immune Response to Infection

The histological sequence of events in the skin of sheep after ORFV infection is similar in primary and reinfection lesions, in spite of differences in the magnitude of the lesions and the time taken to resolve. Antibodies to ORFV envelope proteins have been used to detect ORFV antigen in epidermal keratinocytes, particularly those regenerating the damaged skin. Basal keratinocytes at the root of hair follicles can also contain virus. Some infected cells show evidence of a ballooning-like degeneration. There is no evidence that ORFV infects other, nonepithelial cell-types *in vivo*. ORFV lesions often exhibit epidermal downgrowths (rete formation) into the dermis. This is particularly marked in primary lesions. Another characteristic feature is extensive capillary dilation and proliferation.

ORFV lesions contain a dense accumulation of immune and inflammatory cells underneath and adjacent to virus-infected cells. These include neutrophils, lymphocytes (T and B cells), and dendritic cells that stain intensely with major histocompatibility complex class II antigens. This dense network of dendritic cells is characteristic of orf lesions in sheep. The function of these cells is not known. The accumulating cells increase and decrease in number in parallel with the presence of virus in epidermal cells. The histology of human ORFV lesions is generally similar to that described in sheep. A comparison of ORFV and PCPV lesions in humans has not revealed any histopathological differences.

## Immune Response to Infection

PPVs, in common with other poxviruses, stimulate a vigorous immune and inflammatory response in their hosts, and have evolved to replicate in the presence of this response. In sheep experimentally infected with ORFV, studies in the skin and lymph draining into (afferent lymph) and out of (efferent lymph) local lymph nodes have demonstrated that activated CD4+ (helper) and CD8+ (cytotoxic) T cells, B cells, and antibodies are generated as part of the sheep-acquired immune response to infection. The cytokines generated in lymph in response to virus reinfection are typical of type 1 antiviral cell-mediated immune responses and include interleukin (IL)-1β, IL-2, tumor necrosis factor (TNF)-α, granulocyte-macrophage colony-stimulating factor (GM-CSF), interferon (IFN)-α, and IFN-γ. Studies of ORFV reinfection in sheep depleted of specific lymphocyte subsets or treated with the immunosuppressant drug cyclosporin-A indicated that at least CD4+ T cells and interferons are important

components of the host-protective-response against infection. These studies also indicated that the cutaneous damage sustained during ORFV infection is due in large part to the virus rather than host immune-mediated.

Sheep infected with ORFV mount detectable antibody responses to a small number of viral antigens but there is considerable individual qualitative and quantitative variation in the response. There is a lack of neutralizing antibody. There is no apparent correlation between antibody titers and severity of viral lesions and passive transfer of antibody does not confer protection against virus challenge.

## Immunomodulation by ORFV

In general, PPV infection is mild and localized with more severe disease only occurring in stressed or otherwise immune-impaired individuals. An intriguing feature of PPVs is the ability to repeatedly infect animals despite an apparently typical antiviral immune response to infection. This may in part be a result of the action of viral-encoded immune modulators that are a feature of large DNA viruses. There are now several examples of these that have been identified within the terminal regions of the genome of ORFV.

### Viral Vascular Endothelial Growth Factor

The first of these to be reported was a homolog of mammalian vascular endothelial growth factor (VEGF). The viral VEGF is expressed early, shows 16–27% amino acid sequence identity to mammalian VEGFs (VEGF-A,-B, -C,-D) and has been classified as VEGF-E. It is unique among the VEGF family in that it interacts with VEGF receptor 2 (VEGFR-2) but not with either VEGFR-1 or VEGFR-3. VEGFs are specific mitogens for endothelial cells and regulate normal and pathological angiogenesis, including the vascularization of solid tumors. Extensive capillary proliferation and dilation is a feature of ORFV lesions and the viral VEGF plays a major role in generating these features. It may also indirectly enhance proliferation of the epithelium, the target tissue for virus replication, as epidermal proliferation was reduced in lesions with a VEGF gene knock-out virus compared to wild-type virus lesions. A report that human VEGF can inhibit the functional maturation of dendritic cells hints at a possible immune modulating role for the viral VEGF. A VEGF-like gene has not been reported in any other poxvirus.

### Viral Interferon Resistance Protein

ORFV encodes an interferon resistance protein (OVIFNR) produced by the 020 gene early in infection, which inhibits the interferon-induced shutdown of cellular protein translation (via PKR) by binding to viral dsRNA, thus preventing activation of the protein kinase PKR. 020 is a homolog of the vaccinia virus E3L gene (31% predicted amino acid sequence identity) that has the same function.

## Viral IL-10

ORFV IL-10 (vIL-10) is the product of an early viral gene and the predicted protein is very similar to ovine IL-10 over the C-terminal two-thirds of the molecule while differing substantially at the N-terminus (80% amino acid sequence identity overall). The vIL-10 exhibited similar anti-inflammatory and immunostimulatory activities to ovine IL-10. Both cytokines suppressed TNF-$\alpha$ production from macrophages and suppressed IFN-$\gamma$ production from peripheral blood cells. Both vIL-10 and ovine IL-10 stimulated mast cell proliferation provided co-stimulatory cytokines were present (IL-3 or IL-4). vIL-10 is a virulence protein as recombinant virus lacking the vIL-10 gene is attenuated compared to wild-type or vIL-10 gene-reconstituted virus in sheep infection experiments. The ORFV IL-10 may act to suppress elements of the antiviral immune response, thereby delaying virus clearance. IL-10-like genes have been reported in two other poxvirus genera (*Capripoxvirus* and *Yatapoxvirus*) although these proteins show markedly less sequence similarity to mammalian IL-10 than does ORFV IL-10.

## Viral GM-CSF Inhibitory Factor

The protein product of ORFV ORF 117 encodes an early virus protein with novel function. Viral GM-CSF inhibitory Factor (GIF) binds to and inhibits the biological activity of the cytokines GM-CSF and IL-2. Among other properties, GM-CSF regulates the recruitment, differentiation, and activation of macrophages, neutrophils, and dendritic cells. Activated T cells are an important source of GM-CSF during immune responses to pathogens. IL-2 is produced predominantly by T cells and stimulates the expansion and activation of T cells and natural killer cells among other cell types. GIF has probably evolved to perform its dual function from an ancestral type-1 cytokine receptor, as it shares important structure–function features of this receptor family while exhibiting an otherwise divergent primary amino acid sequence. A GIF protein is also expressed in other PPVs, and is conserved in ORFV strains though there is only ~40% amino acid identity between these and BPSV GIF. The role of GIF in ORFV pathogenesis is currently not known.

## Viral Chemokine-Binding Protein

ORFV encodes a chemokine-binding protein, the product of ORF 112, which is expressed early in the virus life cycle. It is structurally and functionally related to the type II CC chemokine-binding proteins of the *Orthopoxvirus* and *Leporipoxvirus* genera. Viral chemokine-binding protein (vCBP) binds CC chemokines, including monocyte-chemotactic protein-1, macrophage inflammatory protein-1$\alpha$ and RANTES (regulated upon activation, normal T-cell-expressed and secreted). These regulate T cell and monocyte/macrophage recruitment to sites of infection. In addition, and uniquely among poxvirus CBPs, vCBP binds to lymphotactin, a C-chemokine that recruits T and B cells, and neutrophils. vCBP may well function to inhibit key aspects of an antiviral immune response.

## PPVs as Vectors and Immunomodulators

ORFV could prove useful as a vector for delivering microbial antigens to the immune system. Proof of concept for this has been obtained with protective immunity generated to pseudorabies virus and Borna disease virus infection of rodents. The restricted host ranges of the PPVs and lack of systemic spread even in immuno-compromised animals make them good viral vector candidates. Furthermore, inactivated ORFV particles have been shown to exhibit nonspecific immuno-modulatory effects that enhance immunity to a variety of pathogens in several species. This is thought to be mediated by IFN and a type 1 immune response that is downregulated at later stages by IL-10, among other cytokines. This feature of ORFV continues to be exploited commercially.

## Prevention and Control

ORFV vaccines have been available for many years and are widely used to protect lambs against the debilitating effects of natural infection. These vaccines consist of live and essentially nonattenuated virus that is applied to a scratch on the skin of a leg. The ensuing infection does not interfere with feeding and provides significant protection against infection for some months. However, the scab derived from vaccination lesions is likely to contaminate the environment and contribute to the perpetuation of the disease. New vaccines that induce protection but do not shed infectious virus are highly desirable. This might be achieved by deleting genes encoding viral virulence determinants or by delivering the protective antigens of the virus in an appropriate way.

Humans may be infected by PPVs following contact with animal lesions or scab. The viruses in scab associated with animal products such as wool or farm equipment can remain infectious for lengthy periods. Care should be taken to avoid contact between any skin wound and potentially contaminated material.

## Future Perspectives

Recent studies with ORFV have raised the possibility of developing a vaccine able to protect animals against infection by this virus without generating significant amounts of infectious virus. Such a vaccine would also be likely to reduce the frequency of human infections.

The use of ORFV and perhaps other PPVs as vaccine vectors is proving a useful and robust strategy. The generation of ORFV recombinants and other PPVs lacking pathogenesis-related genes will continue to advance our understanding of the pathogenesis of PPV diseases. An understanding of PPV pathogenesis and the viral proteins involved, coupled to recombinant virus generation, should lead to improved control strategies for this important group of viruses.

*See also:* Capripoxviruses.

## Further Reading

Delhon G, Tulman ER, Afonso CL, *et al.* (2004) Genomes of the parapoxviruses orf virus and bovine papular stomatitis virus. *Journal of Virology* 78: 168–177.
Haig DM (2006) Orf virus infection and host immunity. *Current Opinion in Infectious Diseases* 19: 127–132.
Haig DM and McInnes CJ (2002) Immunity and counter-immunity during infection with the parapoxvirus orf virus. *Virus Research* 88: 3–16.
Mercer AA, Ueda N, Friederichs SM, *et al.* (2006) Comparative analysis of genome sequences of three isolates of orf virus reveals unexpected sequence variation. *Virus Research* 116: 146–158.

# Pseudorabies Virus

**T C Mettenleiter,** Friedrich-Loeffler-Institut, Greifswald-Insel Riems, Germany

## History

Although its taxonomic species name *Suid herpesvirus 1* testifies that the natural hosts of pseudorabies virus (PrV) are pigs, its symptoms were first described in cattle, and the virus was isolated for the first time from cattle, dogs, and cats. This is due to the fact that PrV infection in swine, particularly in older animals, may produce only innocuous respiratory symptoms or may go unnoticed altogether. However, in other susceptible species productive infection is invariably fatal and characterized by severe central nervous symptoms, a feature that prompted its designation as pseudorabies owing to the rabies-like clinical picture. A typical symptom in these species is extensive pruritus, resulting in the name 'mad itch' to describe the disease in cattle in the USA during the first half of the nineteenth century.

In 1902, the Hungarian physician Aládar Aujeszky reported isolation of the infectious agent from diseased animals (an ox, a dog, and a cat) and differentiated it from rabies. It could be passaged in rabbits, reproducing the typical symptoms. Guinea pigs and mice were also found to be susceptible, whereas chicken and doves were resistant. Thus, the illness has become widely known as Aujeszky's disease (AD). It was not until 1931 that Richard Shope established the identity of the 'mad itch' agent with an infectious agent widely present in domestic pig holdings in the USA. In Germany, Erich Traub was the first to

cultivate PrV *in vitro* in organ explants in 1933. One year later, Albert Sabin published his findings of a serological relationship between PrV and herpes simplex virus (HSV), resulting in the inclusion of PrV in the herpesvirus group.

## Taxonomy

PrV takes the formal species name *Suid herpesvirus 1* and belongs to the subfamily *Alphaherpesvirinae* of the family *Herpesviridae*. Originally on the basis of serological studies, and later confirmed by molecular biological analyses and comparison of the deduced amino acid sequences of homologous proteins, PrV was shown to be most closely related to bovine herpesvirus 1 (BHV-1) and equine herpesvirus 1 (EHV-1), and also to varicella-zoster virus (VZV). This prompted its assignment to the genus *Varicellovirus* within the *Alphaherpesvirinae*. Alphaherpesviruses are characterized by rapid lytic replication, a pronounced neurotropism with establishment of latency in sensory ganglia, and a broad host range. All these features apply to PrV.

## The Virus Particle

PrV particles have a diameter of approximately 180 nm and exhibit the typical herpesvirus morphology. At

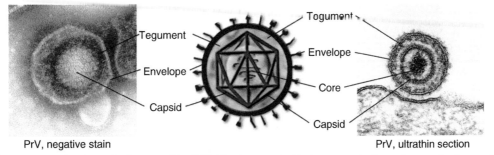

**Figure 1** The PrV virion. A schematic diagram of the PrV virion is presented between an electron micrograph of a negatively stained PrV virion (left) and a thin-sectioned virus particle (right). The locations of the virion subcomponents (core, capsid, tegument, and envelope) are indicated. Spikes at the envelope represent viral glycoproteins.

the center is the genomic DNA enclosed in an icosahedral capsid. The capsid is surrounded by a structure designated the tegument, which is equivalent to the matrix of RNA viruses but significantly more complex. The envelope, which contains virally encoded glycosylated and nonglycosylated proteins anchored in the lipid bilayer, encloses the capsid and tegument (**Figure 1**).

## The Genome

The PrV genome consists of a linear, double-stranded DNA molecule. A complete sequence has recently been assembled from several partial sequences from six different PrV strains. It comprises 143 461 bp with more than 70 protein-coding regions, all of which exhibit homology to genes in related alphaherpesviruses (**Figure 2**). The genome contains a long ($U_L$) and short ($U_S$) unique region with the latter bracketed by inverted repeats ($IR_S$ and $TR_S$), resulting in two isomeric forms of the genome in which $U_S$ is inverted relative to $U_L$. This arrangement has been designated the class D herpesvirus genome structure. So far, three functional origins of DNA replication have been mapped, two in the inverted repeats and one in the middle of $U_L$. A fourth candidate located at the left genome end may not be functional. Compared to the genomes of other alphaherpesviruses, which are generally collinear in their gene arrangement, the PrV genome contains an inversion of approximately 40 kbp that encompasses genes homologous to the UL27 to UL44 genes of HSV (**Figure 2**). A similar inversion is also present in the genome of a distantly related avian alphaherpesvirus, infectious laryngotracheitis virus, but its biological significance is unknown.

A list of identified PrV genes and the functions of the encoded proteins is shown in **Table 1**. Wherever possible, PrV genes have been named after their homologs in HSV. However, the UL3.5 gene of PrV, which has homologs in other alphaherpesviruses such as VZV, BHV-1, and EHV-1, is absent from HSV, as are ORF1 and ORF1.2. PrV does not specify homologs of the UL56, UL45, US5,

US10, US11, and US12 genes of HSV. Approximately half of the total number of PrV genes are considered 'nonessential', a status indicating that they are individually dispensable for viral replication, at least in cell culture. It is estimated that about half of the total number of viral proteins are located in the virion.

## The Capsid

The icosahedral PrV capsid is composed of 162 capsomers. By analogy to the well-analyzed HSV-1 capsid, the capsomers consist of a total of 955 copies of the major capsid protein, the product of the UL19 gene (see below). Homologs of the HSV UL18 and UL38 proteins, which form triplexes connecting and stabilizing the capsomers, as well as the UL35 protein, which is located at the tips of the hexons, have been identified from the genome sequence. Also present are homologs of the UL6 portal protein which forms a dodecameric channel at one vertex for package and release of the viral genome. Several other proteins have been shown to be intimately associated with the capsid, such as the UL17 and UL25 gene products. Whereas the PrV UL17 protein may be present within the capsid shell, the UL25 gene product resides on the outside.

## The Tegument

The herpesvirus tegument is a complex structure which, in the case of PrV, contains in excess of 15 viral proteins. It has become clear that tegument formation is an important step in the morphogenesis of the virion, and requires a network of partially redundant protein–protein interactions. It can be divided into capsid-proximal and envelope-proximal parts. The capsid-proximal tegument is composed of the UL36 gene product, the largest protein in PrV (3084 amino acid residues), which physically interacts with the UL37 gene product. From cryoelectron

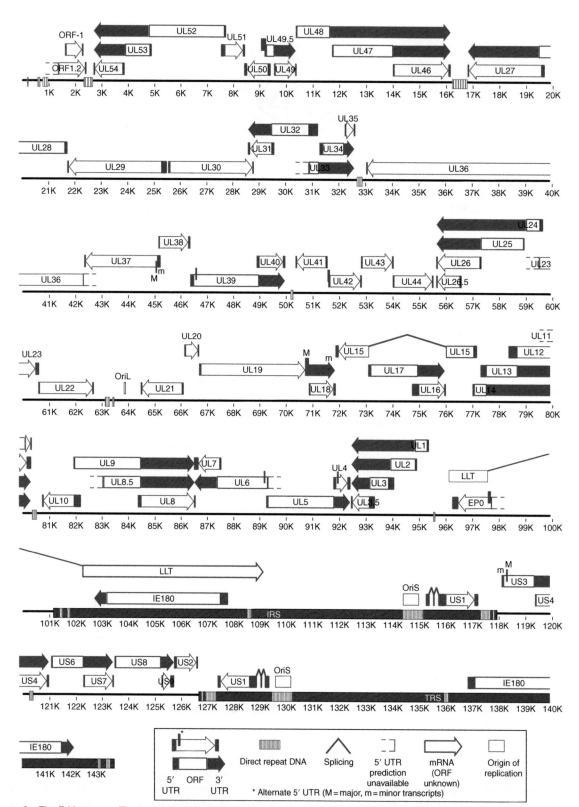

**Figure 2**  The PrV genome. The transcript and gene organization deduced from the complete genomic sequence is shown. The linear form of the PrV genome comprises the unique long sequence (U_L), the internal inverted repeat (IR_S), the unique short sequence (U_S), and the terminal inverted repeat (TR_S). The predicted locations of protein-coding regions (see **Table 1**), 5' and 3' nontranslated regions, DNA repeats, splice sites, and the origins of DNA replication are shown. Reproduced from Klupp BG, Hengartner C, Mettenleiter TC, and Enquist LW (2004) Complete, annotated sequence of the pseudorabies virus genome. *Journal of Virology* 78: 424–440, with permission from the American Society for Microbiology.

**Table 1**  PrV ORFs

| Protein | ORF location[a] | Length (aa) | MW (kDa) | Alias | Function/property[b] | Virion subunit[c] |
|---|---|---|---|---|---|---|
| ORF1.2 | 1252–2259 | 335 | 35.3 | | Unknown | V (?) |
| ORF1 | 1636–2259 | 207 | 21.8 | | Unknown | V (?) |
| UL54 | 3815–2730r | 361 | 40.4 | ICP27 | Gene regulation; early protein | NS |
| UL53 | 4833–3895r | 312 | 33.8 | gK | Viral egress; glycoprotein K; type III membrane protein | V (E) |
| UL52 | 7676–4788r | 962 | 103.3 | | DNA replication; primase subunit of UL5/UL8/UL52 complex | NS |
| UL51 | 7663–8373 | 236 | 25.0 | | Tegument protein | V (T) |
| UL50 | 9333–8527r | 268 | 28.6 | dUTPase | dUTPase | NS |
| UL49.5 | 9257–9553 | 98 | 10.1 | gN | Glycoprotein N; type I membrane protein; complexed with gM | V (E) |
| UL49 | 9591–10340 | 249 | 25.9 | VP22 | Interacts with C-terminal domains of gE and gM; tegument protein | V (T) |
| UL48 | 10404–11645 | 413 | 45.1 | VP16/αTIF | Gene regulation (transactivator); egress (secondary envelopment); tegument protein | V (T) |
| UL47 | 11746–13998 | 750 | 80.4 | VP13/14 | Viral egress (secondary envelopment); tegument protein | V (T) |
| UL46 | 14017–16098 | 693 | 75.5 | VP11/12 | Unknown; tegument protein | V (T) |
| UL27 | 19595–16854r | 913 | 100.2 | gB | Viral entry (fusion); cell-cell spread; glycoprotein B; type I membrane protein | V (E) |
| UL28 | 21640–19466r | 724 | 78.9 | ICP18.5 | DNA cleavage/encapsidation (terminase); associated with UL15, UL33, and UL6 | pC |
| UL29 | 25315–21788r | 1175 | 125.3 | ICP8 | DNA replication/recombination; binds single-stranded DNA | NS |
| UL30 | 25606–28752 | 1048 | 115.3 | | DNA replication; DNA polymerase subunit of UL30/UL42 complex | NS |
| UL31 | 29488–28673r | 271 | 30.4 | | Viral egress (nuclear egress); primary virion tegument protein; interacts with UL34 | pV (T) |
| UL32 | 30893–29481r | 470 | 51.6 | | DNA packaging; efficient localization of capsids to replication compartments | pC |
| UL33 | 30892–31239 | 115 | 12.7 | | DNA cleavage/encapsidation; associated with UL28 and UL15 | NS |
| UL34 | 31398–32186 | 262 | 28.1 | | Viral egress (nuclear egress); primary virion envelope protein; tail-anchored type II nuclear membrane protein; interacts with UL31 | pV (E) |
| UL35 | 32241–32552 | 103 | 11.5 | VP26 | Capsid protein | V (C) |
| UL36 | 42314–33060r | 3084 | 324.4 | VP1/2 | Large tegument protein; interacts with UL37 and UL19 | V (T) |
| UL37 | 45111–42352r | 919 | 98.2 | | Tegument protein; interacts with UL36 | V (T) |
| UL38 | 45168–46274 | 368 | 40.0 | VP19C | Capsid protein; forms triplexes together with UL18 | V (C) |
| UL39 | 46470–48977 | 835 | 91.1 | RR1 | Nucleotide synthesis; large subunit of ribonucleotide reductase | V (?) |
| UL40 | 48987–49898 | 303 | 34.4 | RR2 | Nucleotide synthesis; small subunit of ribonucleotide reductase | NS |
| UL41 | 51498–50401r | 365 | 40.1 | VHS | Gene regulation (inhibitor of gene expression); virion host cell shut off factor | V (T) |
| UL42 | 51628–52782 | 384 | 40.3 | | DNA replication; polymerase accessory subunit of UL30/UL42 complex | NS |
| UL43 | 52842–53963 | 373 | 38.1 | | Unknown; type III membrane protein | V (E) |
| UL44 | 54029–55468 | 479 | 51.2 | gC | Viral entry (virion attachment); glycoprotein C; type I membrane protein; binds to heparan sulfate | V (E) |
| UL26.5 | 56535–55699r | 278 | 28.2 | VP22a | Scaffold protein; substrate for UL26; required for capsid formation and maturation | pC |
| UL26 | 57273–55699r | 524 | 54.6 | VP24 | Scaffold protein; proteinase; required for capsid formation and maturation | V (C) |
| UL25 | 58911–57307r | 534 | 57.4 | | Capsid associated protein; required for DNA packaging and nuclear egress | V (C) |
| UL24 | 59519–59004r | 171 | 19.1 | | Unknown; possible endonuclease | V (*) |
| UL23 | 59512–60474 | 320 | 35.0 | | Nucleotide synthesis; thymidine kinase | NS |
| UL22 | 60610–62670 | 686 | 71.9 | gH | Viral entry (fusion); cell-cell spread; glycoprotein H; type I membrane protein; complexed with gL | V (E) |
| UL21 | 66065–64488r | 525 | 55.2 | | Capsid associated protein; complexed with UL16 | V (?) |
| UL20 | 66172–66657 | 161 | 16.7 | | Viral egress; type III membrane protein | V (?) |
| UL19 | 66744–70736 | 1330 | 146.0 | VP5 | Major capsid protein; forms hexons und pentons | V (C) |
| UL18 | 70896–71783 | 295 | 31.6 | VP23 | Capsid protein; forms triplexes together with UL38 | V (C) |

Continued

**Table 1**    Continued

| Protein | ORF location[a] | Length (aa) | MW (kDa) | Alias | Function/property[b] | Virion subunit[c] |
|---|---|---|---|---|---|---|
| UL15 (Ex2) | 73115–71979r | 735 | 79.1 | | DNA cleavage/encapsidation; terminase subunit; interacts with UL33, UL28, and UL6 | pC |
| UL15 (Ex1) | 77065–75995r | | | | | |
| UL17 | 73166–74959 | 597 | 64.2 | | DNA cleavage/encapsidation | V (C) |
| UL16 | 74986–75972 | 328 | 34.8 | | Tegument protein; complex with UL11 and UL21 | V (T) |
| UL14 | 77064–77543 | 159 | 17.9 | | Unknown | ? |
| UL13 | 77513–78709 | 398 | 41.1 | VP18.8 | Protein-serine/threonine kinase | V (T) |
| UL12 | 78675–80126 | 483 | 51.3 | | DNA recombination; alkaline exonuclease | ? |
| UL11 | 80084–80275 | 63 | 7.0 | | Viral egress (secondary envelopment); membrane-associated tegument protein complex with UL16 | V (T) |
| UL10 | 81935–80754r | 393 | 41.5 | gM | Viral egress (secondary envelopment); glycoprotein M; type III membrane protein; C-terminus interacts with UL49; inhibits membrane fusion in transient assays; complexed with gN | V (E) |
| UL9 | 81934–84465 | 843 | 90.5 | OBP | Sequence specific ori-binding protein | NS |
| UL8.5 | 83053–84465 | 470 | 51.0 | OPBC | C-terminal domain of UL9 | ? |
| UL8 | 84462–86513 | 683 | 71.2 | | DNA replication; part of UL5/UL8/UL52 helicase/primase complex | NS |
| UL7 | 87479–86679r | 266 | 29.0 | | Tegument protein; virion formation and egress | V (T) |
| UL6 | 89301–87370r | 643 | 70.3 | | Capsid protein; portal protein; docking site for terminase | V (C) |
| UL5 | 89300–91804 | 834 | 92.1 | | DNA replication; part of UL5/UL8/UL52 helicase/primase complex; helicase motif | NS |
| UL4 | 91863–92300 | 145 | 15.8 | | Nuclear protein | NS |
| UL3.5 | 93150–92476r | 224 | 24.0 | | Viral egress (secondary envelopment); membrane-associated protein | V (T) |
| UL3 | 93860–93147r | 237 | 25.6 | | Nuclear protein | NS |
| UL2 | 94866–93916r | 316 | 33.0 | UNG | Uracil-DNA glycosylase | NS |
| UL1 | 95314–94844r | 156 | 16.5 | gL | Viral entry; cell–cell spread; glycoprotein L; membrane anchored via complex with gH | V (E) |
| EP0 | 97713–96481r | 410 | 43.8 | ICP0 | Gene regulation (transactivator of viral and cellular genes); early protein | ? |
| IE180 (IRS) | 107511–103171r | 1446 | 148.6 | ICP4 | Gene regulation; immediate-early protein | ? |
| IE180 (TRS) | 137091–141431 | | | | | |
| US1 (IRS) | 115995–117089 | 364 | 39.6 | RSp40/ICP22 | Gene regulation; immediate-early protein | ? |
| US1 (TRS) | 128607–127513r | | | | | |
| US3 (minor) | 118170–119336 | 388 | 42.9 | PK | Minor form of protein kinase (53 kDa mobility) | ? |
| US3 (major) | 118332–119336 | 334 | 36.9 | PK | Viral egress (nuclear egress); major form of protein kinase (41 kDa mobility) | V (T) |
| US4 | 119396–120892 | 498 | 53.7 | gG | Glycoprotein G (secreted) | secreted |
| US6 | 121075–122277 | 400 | 44.3 | gD | Viral entry (cellular receptor binding protein); glycoprotein D; type I membrane protein | V (E) |
| US7 | 122298–123398 | 366 | 38.7 | gI | Cell–cell spread; glycoprotein I; type I membrane protein; complexed with gE | V (E) |
| US8 | 123502–125235 | 577 | 62.4 | gE | Cell–cell spread; glycoprotein E; type I membrane protein; complexed with gI; C-terminus interacts with UL49 | V (E) |
| US9 | 125269–125589 | 106 | 11.3 | 11K | Protein sorting in axons; type II tail-anchored membrane protein | V (E) |
| US2 | 125811–126581 | 256 | 27.7 | 28K | Tegument protein; prenylated | V (T) |

[a]Numbering starts at +1 on the UL end of the genome. r indicates ORF encoded on reverse strand.

[b]Function/property as demonstrated for the PrV and/or HSV-1 homolog.

[c]V (O): virion capsid component; V (T): virion tegument component; V (E): virion envelope component; V (?): virion component of unknown subviral localization; pV: primary enveloped virion precursor component (not found in mature virion); NS: nonstructural protein; pC: present in intranuclear capsid precursor forms but not found in mature virion; ?: unknown.

Reproduced from Klupp BG, Hengartner C, Mettenleiter TC, and Enquist LW (2004) Complete, annotated sequence of the pseudorabies virus genome. *Journal of Virology 78*: 424–440, with permission from the American Society for Microbiology.

image reconstructions of herpesvirus particles, the UL36 gene product is thought to contact the capsid. The UL46, UL47, UL48, and UL49 gene products are easily stripped from the capsid together with the envelope, consistent with a location in the envelope-proximal tegument. Correlating with these findings, the PrV UL49 gene product has been shown to interact with the intracytoplasmic C-termini of the gE and gM envelope proteins. Both parts of the tegument may be connected by the UL48 gene product. Tegument proteins enter the cell after fusion of the virion envelope and the cellular plasma membrane during entry, and prime the cell for virus production. The alphaherpesvirus UL48 gene products are strong transactivators of viral immediate-early (IE) gene expression, whereas the UL41 proteins possess endoribonucleolytic activity to degrade preexisting cellular mRNAs. Cellular proteins have also been detected in the PrV tegument, including actin, annexins, and heat shock proteins. Their biological role is unknown.

## The Envelope

Receptor-binding proteins, as well as major immunogens, are located in the viral envelope. More than 10 envelope constituents have been identified in PrV. Most are modified by the addition of carbohydrate and thus are glycoproteins. Several type I, type II, and type III PrV glycoproteins have been described (**Table 1**). Since the early nomenclature of PrV glycoproteins was somewhat confusing, it has been agreed to name them after their HSV-1 counterparts. Several of these glycoproteins form complexes, such as homooligomeric glycoprotein B (gB) and heterodimeric gE/gI, gH/gL, and gM/gN. The discovery of gN, as well as the gM/gN complex which is conserved throughout the mammalian and avian herpesviruses, was first made in PrV. Nonglycosylated membrane proteins include the US9, UL20, and UL43 gene products (see **Table 1**). The nonstructural gG is proteolytically cleaved and released from infected cells.

## The Replication Cycle

PrV is arguably the most intensively analyzed animal herpesvirus. It has become a major focus of molecular biological research on the basic mechanisms of herpesvirus biology.

In the replication cycle (**Figure 3**), PrV infection of host cells starts with interaction of envelope gC with cell surface heparan sulfate-containing proteoglycans. This interaction is beneficial to, but not essential for, the second step, which involves binding of the essential envelope protein gD to its cellular receptor, nectin. HSV-1 and BHV-1 also use heparan sulfate and nectin for attachment. How-

ever, gD-negative and even gC- and gD-negative infectious PrV mutants have been isolated, which indicates that infection can occur by other routes. These mutants harbor additional mutations in gB and gH.

Penetration (fusion of viral envelope and cellular plasma membrane) requires the essential proteins gB and gH/gL. These glycoproteins are conserved throughout the mammalian and avian herpesviruses, indicating a common mechanism for membrane fusion. After penetration, the capsid is transported via microtubules to the nuclear pore, where it docks and releases the viral genome into the cell nucleus through one vertex. Empty capsids may remain bound to the nuclear pore for a considerable time. The entire entry process can be bypassed *in vitro* by transfection of naked viral DNA.

In the nucleus, transcription of viral genes is initiated by expression of the major IE gene, resulting in the translation of a 180 kDa protein (IE180). Although IE180 has long been considered to be the only IE protein of PrV, studies using specific inhibitors have identified that the US1 (RSp40) mRNA is also expressed with IE kinetics. Like other herpesvirus IE proteins, IE180 is a potent transcriptional activator that transinduces the expression of viral early genes. Early genes encode enzymes involved in nucleotide metabolism (e.g., UL23 = thymidine kinase; UL2 = uracil-DNA glycosylase; UL39/UL40 = ribonucleotide reductase; UL50 = deoxyuridine triphosphatase) and DNA replication (UL30/UL42 = DNA polymerase and an associated factor; UL5/UL8/UL52 = helicase-primase complex; UL29 = single-stranded DNA-binding protein; UL9 = origin-binding protein), as well as two protein kinases (US3, UL13).

DNA replication, whether occurring exclusively via a rolling-circle mechanism or involving intra- and intermolecular recombination and branching, results in the formation of head-to-tail fused concatemers of the genome. Finally, late genes encoding primarily virion structural proteins are expressed and their gene products, after translation in the cytosol, are transported into the nucleus for capsid assembly and DNA packaging. Capsid assembly is morphologically similar in all herpesviruses: capsids containing the major capsid protein UL19, triplex proteins UL18 and UL35, hexon-tip protein UL35, and portal protein UL6 assemble autocatalytically around a protein scaffold consisting of the UL26 and UL26.5 gene products. Packaging occurs via the unique portal at one vertex comprising 12 molecules of the UL6 protein. Genome-length molecules are cleaved from concatemeric replication products during packaging, which requires the UL15, UL28, UL32, and UL33 gene products. The UL17 protein may accompany DNA into the capsid. The UL25 gene product is not required for cleavage/packaging but apparently stabilizes the capsid and is essential for triggering primary envelopment. It is located at the outside of the capsid.

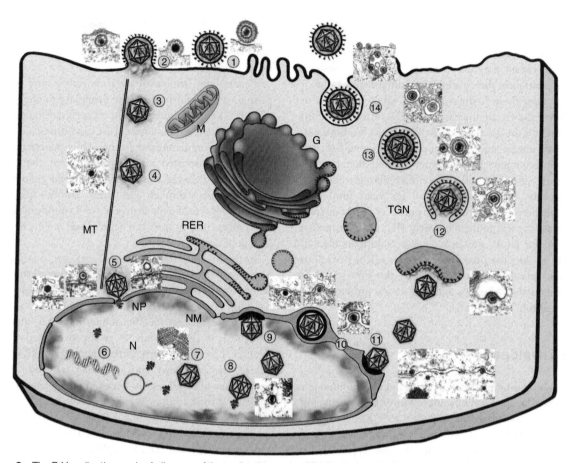

**Figure 3** The PrV replication cycle. A diagram of the replication cycle of PrV is shown together with electron micrographs showing the respective stages. After attachment (1) and penetration (2), capsids are transported to the nucleus N (3) via interaction with microtubuli MT (4), docking at the nuclear pore NP (5) where the viral genome is released into the nucleus. Here, transcription of viral genes and viral genome replication occur (6). Concatemeric replicated viral genomes are cleaved to unit-length molecules during encapsidation (8) into preformed capsids (7), which then leave the nucleus by budding at the inner nuclear membrane NM (9) followed by fusion of the envelope of these primary virions located in the perinuclear cleft (10) with the outer nuclear membrane (11). Final maturation then occurs in the cytoplasm by secondary envelopment of intracytosolic capsids via budding into vesicles of the *trans*-Golgi network TGN (12) containing viral glycoproteins (black spikes), resulting in an enveloped virion within a cellular vesicle. After transport to the cell surface (13), vesicle and plasma membranes fuse, releasing a mature, enveloped PrV particle from the cell (14). RER, rough endoplasmic reticulum; M, mitochondrion; G, Golgi apparatus.

Egress of herpesvirus capsids from the nucleus has been, and still is, a matter of debate. However, numerous findings in recent years, to which studies on PrV contributed significantly, have demonstrated that intranuclear capsids gain access to the cytoplasm by primary envelopment (i.e., budding at the inner leaflet of the nuclear membrane) followed by de-envelopment (fusion) at the outer leaflet. For primary envelopment, the conserved UL31 and UL34 proteins, which form a complex, have been shown to be important, though not always strictly essential, in all three subfamilies of herpesviruses. The UL31/UL34 complex is located in the nuclear membrane and recruits cellular protein kinase C, which phosphorylates and thereby dissociates nuclear lamins, allowing access of nascent capsids to the inner nuclear membrane. Primary enveloped virions in the perinuclear space also contain the UL31/UL34 complex, which

constitutes part of the primary envelope (UL34 is a type II membrane protein) and tegument (UL31). The US3 protein kinase is present in primary and mature virions, whereas the UL31 and UL34 proteins are absent from mature virus particles. The mechanisms of de-envelopment are unclear. However, in the absence of the nonconserved and nonessential US3 kinase, primary enveloped virions accumulate in the perinuclear space, demonstrating the participation of this protein in nuclear egress.

Virion morphogenesis is completed in the cytoplasm by tegumentation, final envelopment, and transport of mature virus particles for release at the plasma membrane. Tegumentation apparently starts at two sites: the capsid and the future envelopment site. At the capsid, the conserved tegument proteins UL36 and UL37 interact. At the future envelopment site (i.e., at vesicles derived from the Golgi apparatus), the C-termini of the type I membrane protein gE and the type III membrane protein gM bind the UL49 tegument protein. Presumably, the UL48 protein links the two parts of the tegument, which drives budding of tegumented virions into the *trans*-Golgi vesicles containing viral glycoproteins to yield mature virions within a vesicle. PrV gM has been shown to relocate other viral and cellular proteins to the *trans*-Golgi and therefore may be involved in assembling the envelope proteins. The conserved UL11 gene product is thought to be involved in directing tegument proteins to the envelopment site. Finally, virion-containing vesicles move to the cell surface, a process in which the UL20 protein is involved, where plasma and vesicle membranes fuse, resulting in release of infectious particles. Apparently, virion gK inhibits an immediate re-fusion of released virions with the cell they just left.

Infectivity can be transmitted via direct cell-to-cell transmission as well as via free virions. Although several of the virion proteins required for penetration (gB, gH/gL) are also required for direct cell-to-cell spread, the mechanism remains enigmatic. In contrast to the situation with other alphaherpesviruses such as HSV, direct cell-to-cell spread of PrV does not require the receptor-binding gD molecule.

## Clinical Features of Infection and Pathology

PrV is able to infect most mammals productively, with the exception of humans and other higher primates. However, primate and human cells are infectable in cell culture, and the reason for the natural resistance is not clear. Equids and goats are also rather resistant but may be infected experimentally. In addition, pseudorabies has been reported in many species of wild mammals, including wild boar, feral pigs, coyotes, raccoons, rats, mice, rabbits, deer, badgers, and coatimundi. It is so far not known whether these animals play a role in farm-to-farm transmission of PrV. In susceptible species other than porcines, infection is fatal and animals die from severe neuronal disorders.

After infection of the natural host, the clinical picture varies depending on the age of the animal, the virulence of the virus, and the route of infection. In nature, infection occurs predominantly oronasally, although genital transmission may also take place, especially in feral pigs. After replication in epithelial cells the virus gains access to neurons innervating the facial and oropharyngeal area, in particular the olfactory, trigeminal, and glossopharyngeal nerves. The virus spreads centripetally by fast axonal retrograde transport and reaches the cell bodies of infected neurons where either lytic or latent infection ensues (see below). PrV is disseminated viremically to many organs, where it replicates in epithelia, vascular endothelium, lymphocytes, and macrophages. In nonporcines, PrV is rather strictly neurotropic.

Neonates become prostrate and die quickly, often without nervous signs. In slightly older piglets, severe central nervous system (CNS) disorders are characterized by incoordination, twitching, paddling, tremors, ataxia, convulsions, and/or paralysis, whereas itching is only rarely present (**Figure 4**). Mortality in piglets up to 2–3 weeks of age may be as high as 100%, resulting in severe losses. Piglets at 3–6 weeks of age may still exhibit neurological signs and high morbidity, but mortality is usually reduced. Infection in older pigs induces primarily respiratory symptoms, such as coughing, sneezing, and heavy breathing, resulting from viral replication in, and destruction of, pulmonary epithelium. Despite the absence of overt nervous signs, virus gains access to neurons and remains latently established in the olfactory bulb, trigeminal ganglia, and brain stem or, after venereal transmission, in the sacral ganglia. PrV infection of pregnant sows may result in abortion or delivery of stillborn or mummified fetuses due to endometritis and necrotizing placentitis with infection of trophoblasts. In susceptible species other than swine, PrV infection is invariably fatal, sometimes after a rapid, peracute course without preceding overt clinical signs. Pruritus is a lead symptom of PrV infection in these species which, particularly in rabbits and rodents, may result in violent itching and automutilation. The

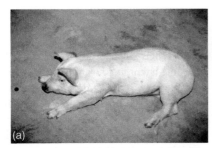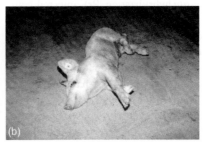

**Figure 4** Neurological symptoms of PrV infection in piglets. The animals show ataxia (a), convulsions and paralysis (b) which ultimately lead to death.

death of mice, rats, cats, or dogs on farms is often a telltale sign of the presence of PrV prior to the appearance of symptoms in pigs.

Transmission occurs via virus-containing body fluids such as nasal and genital secretions, which gain access to epithelial surfaces within the respiratory or genital tract. Airborne transmission is efficient at short range, but long-range transmission covering several kilometers may also occur. Carnivores become infected by ingesting contaminated meat. After primary replication in epithelial cells, the virus enters the endings of sympathetic, parasympathetic or sensory and motor neurons innervating the area of primary replication. Infection probably occurs by the same mechanism as outlined above for cultured cells. Virus is transported in retrograde fashion to the neuronal cell body, where DNA replication and formation of progeny virions ensues. It is not clear whether complete virions or viral subassemblies are then transported to the synapse, or how transsynaptic transfer occurs. Depending on the virulence of the virus and the age and immune status of the host, infection may not proceed beyond the first neuronal level (i.e., ganglia directly innervating the affected peripheral site). However, virus may also spread to the brain resulting in ganglioneuritis and encephalitis. Lymphocytes can also become infected by PrV and this may help viral spread within the body, playing an important role in infection of the fetus. However, the percentage of infected cells in the blood is rather low, even during acute infection, and difficult to detect. A major target organ for latency in swine is the tonsils, and tonsil biopsies allow reliable detection of virus by molecular biological techniques or virus isolation.

There are no pathognomonic, gross lesions of AD. In piglets, there may be necrotizing tonsillitis, rhinotracheitis, or proximal esophagitis. Other lesions commonly seen include pulmonary edema, necrotizing enteritis, and multifocal necrosis of the spleen, lung, liver, lymph nodes, and adrenal glands. Histologically, PrV causes a nonsuppurative meningoencephalitis and paravertebral ganglioneuritis. The gray matter is especially affected, and infected neurons or astrocytes may present acidophilic intranuclear inclusions. The presence of viral antigen can be visualized by immunostaining and viral genomes can be detected by *in situ* hybridization. PrV infected cells usually show more or less extensive degeneration and necrosis due to lytic viral replication. Whether apoptosis induced by PrV infection also plays a role *in vivo* is unclear. A predominantly T-cell-mediated reaction of the immune system induces ganglioneuritis, polio- or panencephalitis with foci of gliosis contributing to the loss of neuronal function. The described extraneural lesions in pigs and acute myocarditis in carnivores might provide additional explanations for the fatal outcome of infections in which virus cannot be recovered from the brain.

## Immunology

Live as well as inactivated vaccines induce efficient protective immunity against AD. Antibodies against a number of viral structural and nonstructural proteins have been detected in infected animals, and virus-neutralizing monoclonal antibodies have been isolated. Antibody responses are primarily directed against the major surface glycoproteins including gB, gC, gD, and gE as well as secreted gG. The most potent complement-independent virus neutralizing antibodies are directed against gC, gD and, to a lesser extent, gB, and subunit vaccines consisting of gB, gC, gD, as well as anti-idiotypic anti-gD antibodies and heterologous vectors expressing gC or gD, elicit protective immunity. In contrast, anti-gE antibodies require complement for neutralization, and anti-gG antibodies have no neutralizing ability at all. Antibodies against whole virus or specific for gB are used in diagnostic assays to detect PrV infection serologically. Major targets for cell-mediated immunity in pigs are primarily gC and, to a lesser extent, gB.

Although the numerous elaborate immune evasion mechanisms of beta- and gammaherpesviruses, including expression of virokines and viroceptors, have not been found in alphaherpesviruses, these viruses still interact with the immune system to evade its activity. Like other alphaherpesvirus gC proteins, PrV gC binds species-specifically to porcine complement component C3, and the gE/gI complex binds the Fc portion of porcine IgG. Secreted gG may bind chemokines, thereby impairing intercellular signaling. Moreover, infection of cells by PrV results in downregulation of major histocompatibility complex class I (MHC-I) antigen presentation, and envelope glycoproteins present at the plasma membrane of infected cells are internalized by as yet unknown factors, resulting in a paucity of antigens presented to the immune system at the cell surface. Recently, the PrV gN protein has been shown to inactivate the transporter which translocates processed peptides for loading onto MHC-I molecules in the endoplasmic reticulum. The combined action of these mechanisms may give the virus an edge over the immune system, facilitating establishment of latency and further virus spread.

## Latency

Like other alphaherpesviruses, PrV has the capacity to become latent in neurons. During latency, the genome persists largely quiescently in a presumably circular form. Expression is restricted to one region, the latency-associated transcript (LAT) gene, which encompasses part of the inverted repeat and adjoining $U_L$ region. The LAT gene, which encodes the large latency transcript (LLT), is located antiparallel to the genes encoding IE180 and

EP0 (see **Figure 2**), and is transcribed into three different RNAs of 8.4, 8.0, and 2.0 kb. The 8.4 and 2.0 kb species are derived by splicing of a larger precursor. During latency, only the 8.4 kb RNA is produced from a separate promotor that is apparently active only under latent conditions, whereas the 8.0 and 2.0 kb species are also transcribed during lytic infection.

PrV encodes proteins which are able to suppress apoptotic cell death as a prerequisite for the establishment of latency. The US3 protein kinase has been demonstrated to mediate this function in porcine fetal trigeminal neurons. PrV establishes latent infections predominantly in neuronal tissues such as the trigeminal or sacral ganglia. However, tonsils have also been identified as sites of latency.

## Epidemiology and Control

In the twentieth century, PrV has become a pathogen distributed worldwide with the exception of Australia, Canada, and the Scandinavian countries. In major swine-producing areas, PrV infection caused significant economic losses amounting to hundreds of millions of dollars, making it one of the most devastating pig diseases. Control and eradication of PrV infection in pigs relied on two strategies. In areas with a low prevalence of infection, serological screening and consequent elimination of seropositive animals resulted in the eradication of AD from countries such as the UK, Denmark, and East Germany. PrV infection can be diagnosed by detecting either the infectious agent (antigen detection by immunofluorescence or virus isolation) or viral DNA using polymerase chain reaction (PCR). The latter method is also suitable for detecting

latent viral genomes. A PrV-specific immune response in live animals can be confirmed using various serological assays (e.g., virus neutralization, latex agglutination, or enzyme-linked immunosorbent assay (ELISA) systems based on complete virus particles or distinct viral antigens such as gB).

To reduce disease prevalence, vaccination with live-attenuated or inactivated vaccines has also been used. However, vaccination does not result in sterile immunity, and vaccinated animals may still be infected with and carry the virus, and these carriers are no longer identifiable by serological analysis. This problem has been solved by the advent of the so-called 'marker' vaccines. This novel concept provided a breakthrough in animal disease control, and serves as a blueprint for control of other infectious diseases. It was based on the finding that several immunogenic envelope glycoproteins of PrV, such as gC, gE, and gG (see above), are not required for productive replication and can be deleted from the viral genome without abolishing virus replication. These gene-deleted strains can be produced easily in conventional cell systems and can be administered as inactivated or modified-live vaccines. In fact, gene-deleted PrV strains were the first genetically engineered live-virus vaccines to be licensed. Thus, PrV has pioneered modern vaccinology. Whereas animals vaccinated with these vaccines do not mount an immune response to the missing gene product, wild-type virus infection results in seroconversion for the differentiating antigen. Serological assays (ELISA) have subsequently been developed that allow easy and sensitive detection of antibodies against these marker proteins, resulting in the identification of animals infected with wild-type virus, regardless of vaccination status (**Figure 5**). Thus, virus circulation can be reduced by vaccination,

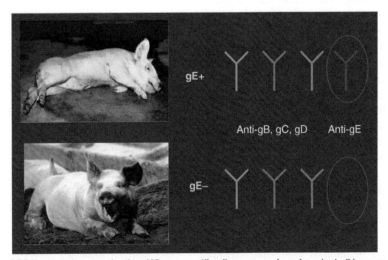

**Figure 5** The principle of DIVA or marker vaccination. Whereas antibodies are produced against all immunogenic viral proteins after wild-type infection, antibodies against the missing gene product (circled) will not be formed after vaccination with a gene-deleted virus. The presence or absence of these antibodies is used to differentiate between infected and vaccinated animals. Reprinted with permission from Mettenleiter TC (2005) Veterinary viruses. *Nova Acta Leopoldina NF92* 344: 221–230.

and infected animals that still harbor field virus can be identified subsequently and eliminated, resulting in cost-efficient eradication.

This breakthrough approach of 'differentiating infected from vaccinated animals' (DIVA) was pioneered in the field with PrV and is now widely accepted and practised with other infectious diseases, such as BHV-1 infection, classical swine fever, and foot-and-mouth disease. Its application resulted in eradication of PrV from heavily infected West Germany within 10 years, and also recently succeeded in eliminating PrV infection from pig herds in New Zealand and the USA. Although European wild boar and American feral pigs also harbor PrV, there is no epidemiological link between PrV in wild boar and domestic pigs in Europe since clearly different viral strains have been isolated from each. However, in the Southern USA infected feral pigs may represent a source of infection to domestic pig holdings.

## PrV as a Tool in Neurobiology

Like other alphaherpesviruses, PrV exhibits a distinct neurotropism, invading the CNS via peripheral nerves. While wild-type strains of PrV may spread within the CNS both laterally and transsynaptically, attenuated PrV mutants have been identified which, under appropriate assay conditions, travel more or less exclusively along nerves and are transported transsynaptically. This property has prompted increasing use of PrV as a transneuronal tracer to label neuronal connections in experimental animal models, and has been useful in elucidating detailed neuroanatomical networks in mice and rats. The virus used most frequently in these studies is the Bartha strain of PrV, a modified-live vaccine strain which had been attenuated by the Hungarian veterinarian Adorján Bartha by multiple passages in embryonated chicken eggs and chicken embryo fibroblasts. Molecular biological analyses demonstrated that this strain carries several lesions compared to wild-type PrV: it lacks the gE, gI, and US9 genes, contains a mutation in the signal sequence for gC, specifies attenuating mutations in the UL21 gene, and expresses a UL10 gene product (gM) that is not glycosylated due to mutation of the N-glycosylation site. The glycoprotein deletion and the UL21 mutation have been shown to be most important for the observed attenuation. Recently, genetically engineered Bartha-derivatives expressing the marker proteins β-galactosidase or green fluorescent protein have been constructed and used in double-tracing studies. Moreover, mutants that express their markers only under specific conditions (e.g., in transgenic cells or animals expressing cre-lox recombinase under control of a tissue-specific promoter) have added further elegant possibilities for tissue-specific labeling.

## Future Perspectives

PrV is a fascinating virus with several interesting properties. The availability of conventional and genetically engineered marker vaccines allows effective and cost-efficient disease control campaigns, which have been shown to result in the eradication of virus and disease from animal populations. Although PrV infection is still widespread, in particular in certain areas in Eastern Europe and Asia, concerted efforts could result in the elimination of the disease on a worldwide scale. Beyond its importance as the causative agent of a relevant animal disease, PrV is an ideal tool to study basic mechanisms of herpesvirus (molecular) biology and has the enormous advantage of an experimentally accessible natural virus–host system by infection of pigs. Moreover, its broad host range allows the use of other well-defined animal models for neuroanatomical, immunological, and molecular biological studies. Since PrV replicates exceedingly well in tissue culture, it is also well suited for detailed analysis of the requirements for (alpha) herpesvirus replication. Thus, PrV will remain under intensive scrutiny for sometime to come.

## Acknowledgments

The author thanks Harald Granzow and Mandy Jörn for **Figures 1** and **3** and Jens Teifke, Thomas Müller, Hanns-Joachim Rziha, and Barbara Kluppa for helpful comments on the manuscript.

*See also:* Bovine Herpesviruses; Herpesviruses of Birds; Herpesviruses of Horses.

## Further Reading

Enquist LW, Husak PJ, Banfield BW, and Smith GA (1999) Infection and spread of alphaherpesviruses in the nervous system. *Advances in Virus Research* 51: 237–347.

Granzow H, Weiland F, Jöns B, Klupp B, Karger A, and Mettenleiter TC (1997) Ultrastructural analysis of pseudorabies virus in cell culture: A reassessment. *Journal of Virology* 71: 2071–2082.

Klupp BG, Hengartner C, Mettenleiter TC, and Enquist LW (2004) Complete, annotated sequence of the pseudorabies virus genome. *Journal of Virology* 78: 424–440.

Mettenleiter TC (2000) Aujeszky's disease (pseudorabies) virus: The virus and molecular pathogenesis. *Veterinary Research* 31: 99–115.

Mettenleiter TC (2005) Veterinary viruses. *Nova Acta Leopoldina NF92* 344: 221–230.

Mettenleiter TC, Klupp BG, and Ganzow H (2006) Herpesvirus assembly: A tale of two membranes. *Current Opinion in Microbiology* 9: 423–429.

Pomeranz L, Reynolds AE, and Hengartner CJ (2006) Molecular biology of pseudorabies virus: Impact on neurovirology and veterinary medicine. *Microbiology and Molecular Biology Reviews* 69: 462–500.

# Retrotransposons of Vertebrates

**A E Peaston,** The Jackson Laboratory, Bar Harbor, ME, USA

## Glossary

**Ancestral retrotransposon** A retrotransposon present in the genome of a common ancestor of two or more host groups. Also referred to as ancestral repeat.

**Apurinic/apyrimidinic** Endonuclease enzyme that catalyzes the cleavage of a phosphodiester bond in a DNA molecule.

**Autonomous retrotransposon** A retrotransposon encoding proteins required for its reverse transcription and transposition.

**Clade** A group of organisms consisting of a single common ancestor and all its descendents.

**DDE transposases** A class of transposase enzymes containing a highly conserved amino acid motif, aspartate–aspartate–glutamate (DDE), required for metal ion coordination in catalyzing integration of retrotransposon cDNA into the host DNA, thus also known as integrase.

**Exaptation** In broad terms, a feature conferring evolutionary fitness on an organism but which was originally nonfunctional or designed for some other function in the organism. Thus, the genes of a retrotransposon newly inserted in the host genome maybe, over evolutionary time, co-opted for function in the host; in this new role they are called exaptations.

**Homoplasy** A structure arising in two or more species as the result of a convergent evolution, and not as a result of common descent which indicates that the feature in one species is homologous to that in the other.

**Lineage-specific retrotransposon** A retrotransposon introduced into the genome of one but not another host grouping after their evolutionary divergence.

**Nucleotide substitution rate** The rate at which single nucleotide mutations occur within regions of a genome not subject to selection. One way to estimate this is by comparison of the consensus sequences of ancestral repeats with their remnant sequences in different host genomes.

**Y-transposase, also known as tyrosine recombinase** A class of transposase enzymes which can use a conserved tyrosine to cut and rejoin its DNA substrates by a 3′ phosphotyrosine linkage; used by some retrotransposons to integrate their cDNA into the host DNA, and thus sometimes called integrase.

## History

Transposable elements are defined segments of DNA which replicate and move to other loci within the genome by a variety of mechanisms. The vast majority of these mobile elements in vertebrates are retrotransposons, which replicate by means of an RNA intermediate that is reverse-transcribed into DNA and inserted in a new location within the genome. Retrotransposons are found in all vertebrate genomes, but have been intensively studied in relatively few.

Retrotransposons were initially detected as discrete fragments of genomic DNA that rapidly reannealed after denaturation, and were recognized to be repetitive sequence elements interspersed within genomic DNA. The advent of DNA analysis by restriction enzyme fragmentation led to the identification of discrete families of repetitive elements whose members shared particular sets of internal restriction sites. The most highly repeated long and short sequences were named long interspersed repetitive elements (LINEs) and short interspersed repetitive elements (SINEs), respectively.

The LTR elements, a third general type of retrotransposon resembling the integrated form of proviruses, was similarly discovered. These endogenous retroviruses and retrovirus-like elements are generally restricted to an intracellular life cycle and vertical transmission through the germline and, unlike 'true' retroviruses, are not infectious. However, notable exceptions blur this distinction.

The advent of whole genome sequencing and sequence analysis is rapidly providing detailed pictures of vertebrate retrotransposon landscapes, such as those of a pufferfish (*Takifugu rubripes*), the chicken (*Gallus gallus*), the laboratory mouse (*Mus musculus*), human (*Homo sapiens*), dog (*Canis lupus familiarus*), and others. New lineage-specific retrotransposons of vertebrates such as primate-specific SVA (SINE-R, VNTR, Alu), are coming to light, as well as the discovery within selected vertebrate lineages of ancient retrotransposons, such as the Penelope-like elements (PLEs) that are present in the genomes of metazoans, fungi, and amoebozoans. Analysis of retroelement phylogenies can assist in disentangling evolutionary relationships of their hosts.

## Nomenclature

Different structural and functional classification schemes for retrotransposable elements have been proposed.

No scheme has been generally accepted by both the virology and the retroelement communities, and at the level of individual elements, nomenclature is frequently based on historical tradition and can be confusing. A simple classification scheme based primarily on genetic structure is used here, with acknowledgment that, with the exception of reverse transcriptase, coding domains are not uniformly retained across different groups. Detailed discussion of classification and individual elements is outside the scope of this article, but the subject can be pursued through references listed in Further Reading.

## Retrotransposon Structural and Functional Features

Retrotransposons are usually subdivided into two structural superfamilies based on the presence or absence of terminal directly repeated sequences of several hundred nucleotides, the LTRs. The LTR-retrotransposon superfamily includes elements resembling integrated or endogenous proviruses, the non-LTR superfamily includes LINEs, SINEs, and SVA elements. In each superfamily, there are autonomous elements, which encode reverse transcriptase (RT) as well as a variable set of other proteins necessary for replication and transposition of the element. The superfamilies also include nonautonomous elements whose open reading frames (ORFs) usually encode no proteins, or putative proteins lacking homology to other transposable element proteins and lacking known function. Nonautonomous elements always have an autonomous partner to provide the necessary proteins *in trans*. A third group of retrotransposable elements, the PLEs, were originally described in invertebrates but have more recently also been reported in vertebrates. PLEs have distinct genomic and transcript structural features which preclude a neat fit in either the LTR or non-LTR superfamilies; consequently, this group will be treated independently in this article.

Fundamental structural features of non-LTR and LTR retrotransposons are illustrated schematically in **Figure 1**. A useful repository of consensus sequences of retrotransposons from different animal species, and their classification is curated by the Genetic Information Research Institute.

## LTR Superfamily

Four major groups of LTR retrotransposons have been identified in vertebrates to date: Ty3/*gypsy*; BEL; the vertebrate retrovirus group; and Ty1/*copia*. The hepadnaviruses, a fifth group encoding RT similar to LTR retrotransposons but which are circular and lack LTRs, are discussed elsewhere in this encyclopedia. The LTR retrotransposon groups are distinguished from one another by amino acid sequence comparison of their homologous

enzymatic domains, primarily RT, and by features specific to one or two groups. Nonautonomous retrotransposon families are distinguished from one another by DNA sequence comparisons of their internal domain and of their LTRs.

The DIRS1 (Dictyostelium repeat sequence 1) subclass LTRs are either inverted repeats, or split direct repeats. In addition, these elements lack the typical integrase and protease coding domains, containing instead a domain encoding a bacteriophage lambda recombinase-like protein also known as tyrosine-recombinase or Y-transposase. These features of DIRS1 make its inclusion in the LTR superfamily problematic, although its RT has homology to the more typical elements of the superfamily.

### Structure

LTR elements are typically constructed as two direct LTRs flanking an internal sequence of variable coding content (**Figure 1**). The LTRs are necessary and sufficient for promoter activity and transcription of the retroelement. Functional features common to LTRs include: 5′ TG and 3′ CA dinucleotides necessary for integration into the host genome; Pol II promoter elements and a transcription start site; and a polyadenylation and cleavage signal.

In typical autonomous LTR retrotransposons, the internal sequence contains a variable but small number of ORFs. Most elements contain an ORF including Gag (group-specific antigen) and Pol (polymerase) domains, and some additionally contain an ORF for Env (envelope). Gag encodes a structural polyprotein integral to the formation of cytoplasmic virus-like particles in which reverse transcription takes place. Pol encodes several enzymatic activities: (1) protease required to cleave the translated products of the gag–pol transcript into their functional forms; (2) RT for transcribing the retrotransposon RNA into double-stranded cDNA; (3) ribonuclease H (RNase H) for processing the RNA template prior to plus strand cDNA synthesis; and (4) integrase incorporating an aspartate (D), aspartate, glutamate (E) (DDE)-type transposase activity. The integrase sequence of the chromovirus genus of the Ty3/*gypsy* group additionally encodes a chromodomain, a domain found in chromatin complex structural proteins or chromatin remodeling proteins. Further information regarding retroviral genes and structure can be found elsewhere in the encyclopedia. The Pol domain order is usually protease, RT, RNase H, integrase, except for the Ty1/Copia group and the Gmr1-like elements of the Ty3/Gypsy group in which integrase is upstream of RT.

In addition to coding sequence, the internal sequence contains a 5′ primer binding site (PBS) for first-strand DNA synthesis and a 3′ polypurine tract which serves as the primer binding site for second-strand DNA synthesis. These two features are conserved in the internal sequence region of nonautonomous LTR retrotransposons.

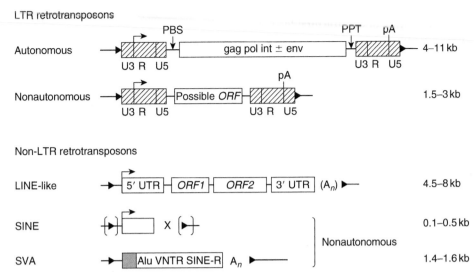

**Figure 1**  General structure of selected retrotransposons. A typical LTR retrotransposon is flanked by target site duplications (black arrowheads) and its LTR domains (hatched) contain a pol II promoter, transcription start site and a polyadenylation and cleavage signal. The internal domain of autonomous elements contains ORFs encoding homologs of retroviral gag and pol genes, and occasionally an additional env gene homolog. The short ORF of nonautonomous elements does not encode these proteins, if any. LINE-like elements terminate in family-specific 3′ UTRs with or without poly (A) tails, the poly (A) tail (A$_n$) indicated here is typical of L1. Flanking target site duplications typical of the L1 clade may or may not be present in other LINE-like clades. The autonomous LINE-like elements contain an internal pol II promoter and ORFs encoding structural and reverse transcriptase (RT) genes required for retrotransposition. SINEs contain an internal pol III promoter but lack an ORF, and may or may not be flanked by target site duplications (in parentheses), depending on their specific LINE-like partner. SVA consists of a 5′ variable number hexameric repeat (gray box), followed by an Alu-like element, a VNTR domain, the SINE-R element derived from the human endogenous retrovirus HERVK10, and a poly (A) tail. SVA elements are thought to be mobilized in trans by L1 proteins, and are flanked by target site duplications typical of L1. Right angled arrow, transcription start site; pA, polyadenylation and cleavage signal; PBS, primer binding site for initiating minus strand cDNA synthesis; PPT, polypurine tract used for initiation of plus strand cDNA synthesis. Element sizes are approximate ranges. The diagrams are not to scale.

Only a few LTR retrotransposons in any genome are intact, a majority of them being inactivated by different mutations. These may be due to intrinsically error-prone, reverse transcription by RT, to mutation associated with the nucleotide substitution rate of the specific genome, to mutation associated with methylation of CpG dinucleotides of the element, to insertional mutation by other transposable elements, or to recombination and deletion. Solitary LTRs usually far outnumber full-length elements in the genome and are understood to be the result of homologous recombination between the 5′ and 3′ LTRs of a full-length element, with excision and loss of the intervening sequence. Over time, older transpositionally active elements of a retrotransposon lineage are inactivated by mutation, becoming functionally extinct. Younger functionally intact members of the lineage continue the retrotransposition activity, or if none exist then that lineage becomes extinct. Transposition-incompetent elements in the genome can be viewed as molecular fossils of past transposition activity.

### Transposition mechanism

Most LTR-retrotransposons are believed to replicate and transpose using a complex process very similar to that of infectious retroviruses, as covered elsewhere in this encyclopedia. In the DIRS1 group, the presence of a

Y-transposase and lack of target site duplications suggests a different mechanism, involving RT-mediated synthesis of a closed circular cDNA, and insertion into the target using Y-mediated recombination.

## Non-LTR Superfamily

Retrotransposons included in this superfamily are the autonomous LINEs and nonautonomous SINEs and SVA elements. One clade of LINEs is the LINE-1 clade (L1), and to minimize confusion, the general category of 'LINE' retrotransposons will be referred to hereafter as LINE-like.

### LINE-like retrotranposon structure

Multiple clades of LINE-like retrotransposons have so far been recognized on the basis of RT and other protein sequence comparisons. At least nine clades are represented in vertebrate genomes. Common structural features of LINE-like retrotransposons include a 5′ untranslated region (UTR) containing a (G+C)-rich promoter region, followed by two nonoverlapping open reading frames (ORF1 and ORF2), and a 3′ UTR.

However, different clades are distinguished by many structural differences. A brief description of the 3′ UTR and ORF differences between the first three identified vertebrate LINE-like clades (LINE-1 (L1), CR1, and RTE) is given below to convey a sense of the structural features distinguishing LINE-like retrotransposons.

Variable-sized target-site duplications flank full-length elements of the L1 and RTE lineages, but not the CR1 lineage. The 3′ UTR of L1 characteristically contains an AATAAA polyadenylation signal and terminates in a 3′ poly (A) tail. In contrast, the 3′ UTR of CRI elements contains no A or AT-rich regions and terminates in a [(CATTCTRT) (GATTCTRT)$_{1-3}$] motif, while the very short 3′ UTRs of the RTE clade are dominated by A/T-rich trimer, tetramer, and/or pentamer repeats.

In the L1 clade, ORF1 encodes a single-stranded, nucleic acid-binding protein with nucleic acid-chaperone activity. A similar activity is proposed for the ORF1 product of CR1, while the 43-amino-acid ORF1 of RTE is thought to be too short to encode these components. In most LINE-like clades, ORF2 encodes a large protein with an N-terminal endonuclease and a C-terminal RT domain. As in most LINE-like clades, the endonuclease is of the apurinic/apyrimidinic type (AP) in L1, CR1, and RTE elements. A site-specific endonuclease typifies a minority of clades. A third domain in the ORF2-encoded protein, a COOH-terminal cysteine-rich domain, is conserved in mammalian L1 elements.

As with LTR retrotransposons, most LINE-like retrotransposons in a genome are transpositionally disabled. For example, of the half million or so L1 copies in the human genome, less than 1% are intact full-length elements. In all LINE-like lineages, 5′ truncation is an exceptionally common mutation, likely reflecting the rarity of successful full-length element reverse transcription and insertion. An interesting speculation is that, by providing opportunity for L1 to acquire novel 5′ ends, 5′ truncation may be an evolutionary strategy for L1 to evade suppression of transcription by the host.

### LINE-like retrotransposon transposition

LINE-like retrotransposons are thought to all use a target-primed mechanism of transposition, reverse transcribing their RNA directly on the new chromosomal integration site, although the details likely vary between the different clades and are not well understood for all. The human L1 is perhaps the best-studied vertebrate LINE-like retrotransposon and is used here to outline the process. Genetic evidence and recent cell culture experiments suggest the following model (**Figure 2**). Following transcription, nuclear export, and translation of the L1 mRNA in the cytoplasm, L1 proteins preferentially associate with their encoding transcript ('*cis* preference') forming a cytoplasmic ribonucleoprotein particle. Upon access of the particle to the nucleus, L1 endonuclease nicks the host DNA at a loose consensus sequence (3′-AA/TTTT-5′) in the minus strand. The L1 transcript poly (A) tail base pairs with the nicked target and the target thus primes first strand syn-

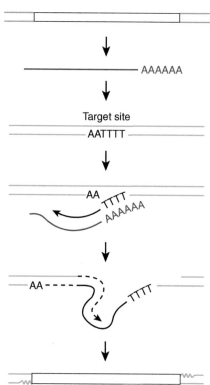

**Figure 2**  Retrotransposition mechanism of L1 elements. Polyadenylated L1 transcripts (red line) are transported to the cytoplasm, packaged in their own translation products, and then transported back to the nucleus. In the nucleus, L1 endonuclease nicks the minus strand of the new insertion site (blue line) at the target consensus sequence 5′ TTTT/AA 3′. The T-rich 3′-OH minus strand primes reverse transcription and first strand synthesis (black line). A nick in the plus strand, staggered in position to the minus strand nick, exposes 3′ plus strand target DNA which is thought to prime L1 second strand transcription (black broken line) using the first strand as template, after RNA degradation by RNase H and strand switching by RT. Finally, host enzymes are thought to participate in repairing the gaps in the host DNA, creating target-site duplications flanking the L1 (zig-zag lines indicate duplicated host DNA).

thesis using L1 RT with L1 mRNA as template. A nick in the target plus strand, offset from the minus-strand nick, is made by an unknown enzyme, possibly L1 endonuclease. Second strand synthesis proceeds using the first strand as template, perhaps primed by microhomology-mediated priming between the first strand and the 3′ end of the plus strand. Host enzymes are thought to be involved in completion of synthesis of both new strands and DNA repair linking them to the host DNA, creating the flanking, perfect target-site duplications typical of L1. L1 uses host ribonuclease H to degrade L1 RNA template, but other clades of LINE-like retrotransposons encode their own RNase H.

### SINE structure

SINEs are small nonautonomous retrotransposons, usually derived from different cellular structural RNAs, such as 7SLRNA or 5S rRNA; however, most eukaryotic SINE families are derived from tRNAs. A SINE generally consists of a 5′ structural RNA-like region containing an internal polymerase III promoter, a region unrelated to structural RNA, and a 3′ end derived from a LINE-like retrotransposon in the same genome. An exception is Alu elements, whose 3′ ends are not shared with L1, their autonomous partner, unless one counts the poly (A) tail. SINEs are usually flanked by target site duplications typical of the element from which their 3′ end is derived.

### SVA structure

SVA elements, exclusively found in hominoid primates, are chimeric elements named for their principal components, SINE-R, VNTR, and Alu. A 5′ (CCCTCT) hexamer repeat is followed by an antisense Alu sequence and then, multiple copies of a variable number tandem repeat (VNTR). The 3′ portion consists of the primate-specific SINE-R, derived from an LTR-retrotransposon thought to be human endogenous retrovirus K-10 (HERVK-10), and finally a polyadenylation and cleavage signal and poly (A) tail.

### Transposition of SINE and SVA

Experimental evidence from several vertebrate species indicates that, as long suspected, the 3′ end of SINE transcripts is recognized *in trans* by the cognate LINE-like machinery for transposition. For example, transcripts of Alu elements, and the mouse SINEs, B1, B2, and ID, are recognized and transposed by L1 machinery, whereas UnaSINE1, an eel SINE, is retrotransposed by UnaL2. Similarly, the characteristics of SVA insertions strongly suggest they use the L1 machinery for retrotransposition.

## Penelope-Like Elements

### Structure

In a few species of vertebrates, a limited number of elements with intact ORFs resembling the Penelope element of *Drosophila virilis* have been described. The elements are flanked by short target site duplications, and usually consist of LTRs flanking anINT. The LTR sequences do not resemble those of LTR retrotransposons, and are thought to represent tandem arrangement of two copies of the element with variable 5′ truncation of the upstream copy. The upstream LTR may be preceded by an inverted LTR fragment. The single ORF includes an N-terminal domain containing a conserved DKG amino acid motif, followed by the RT domain, a variable length linker sequence thought to contain a nuclear localization signal, and an endonuclease domain. The endonuclease is of the GIY-YIG type, otherwise unreported in eukaryotes.

### Transposition

It is not clear how PLEs are transposed. The presence of introns in genomic copies of some PLEs found in invertebrates, and their absence from cDNA of the element, argues against an L1-like 'cis' preference' action of PLE proteins. Other possibilities include unconventional transposition of full-length unspliced mRNA, or use of a DNA template for transposition.

## Evolutionary Features

### Origin

Phylogenetic analyses of autonomous retrotransposable elements have historically relied on amino acid sequence alignments of RT, the only protein coding domain common to all elements. The evidence indicates that LINE-like retrotransposons are divided into 17 or more clades, many of which have wide distribution in eukaryotes. These analyses, and abundant representation of LINE-like retrotransposons in basal eukaryote genomes, support the origin of ancestral LINE-like retrotransposons close to the emergence of the eukaryotic crown group in the Proterozoic eon. Combined analyses of RT, RNaseH, and endonuclease domains suggest that ancestral LINE-like retrotransposons evolved from group II introns in genomes of eubacteria, and fungal and plant organelles, and originally possessed a single ORF for RT and a site-specific endonuclease. Early branching lineages such as L1 acquired a second ORF (ORF1), and the site-specific endonuclease was replaced by a relatively non-site-specific AP endonuclease probably acquired from the host DNA repair machinery. Later branching lineages also acquired an RNaseH domain, most likely from their eukaryotic host, but elements within these lineages have not all retained this domain. Most evidence suggests that LINE-like retrotransposon transmission is strictly vertical through the germline. Evidence supporting horizontal transmission of RTE from snakes to ruminants has been reported, although the mechanism is unknown, and the topic remains controversial.

Phylogenetic studies of LTR elements, together with their absence from some basal eukaryotic genomes, suggest they arose more recently than LINE-like retrotransposons, although this is not a settled topic. It has been speculated that LTR retrotransposons arose as a chimera between a non-LTR retrotransposon carrying RT and RNaseH and a DNA transposon carrying an integrase domain. The acquisition of additional ORFs distinguishes many clades. Evidence suggests the vertebrate retrovirus group acquired a second RNaseH domain, and the primary sequence of the first degenerated, maintaining some structural information but not the catalytic site. The acquisition of Env, enabling infectious transfer is a striking feature of some lineages within the vertebrate retroviral group, although the origin, potentially ancient, of Env in this group is obscure. Strong phylogenetic evidence from invertebrate genomes indicates that other LTR element groups independently acquired different Env-like genes from infectious viruses, but vertebrate representatives of these are yet to be described. The evolutionary success of the Chromovirus clade of the Ty3/*gypsy* group, found in plants and fungi as well as vertebrates, has been attributed to its acquisition of the chromodomain. As with LINE-like retrotransposons, LTR elements have had varying success in colonizing vertebrate genomes, although all major LTR groups are represented by an active element in at least one species of vertebrates (**Table 1**).

New autonomous endogenous LTR elements are acquired through horizontal transfer of exogenous elements, which can then invade the genome and be transmitted through the germline, blurring the distinction between exogenous and endogenous elements. An example of current interest is the ongoing infectious epidemic and endogenization of the Koala retrovirus. However, some genera of the vertebrate retrovirus group, such as the lentiviruses, appear incapable of generating endogenous elements. This appears to be the result of Env

**Table 1** Retrotransposon clades identified in some vertebrate genomes

| Type of retrotransposon | Cartilaginous fish[a,b] | Teleost fish[c] (Tn, Tr, Dr) | Mammals[d] (Hs, Mm, Cf) | Birds (chicken)[e] |
|---|---|---|---|---|
| Non-LTR retrotransposons[f] | 2.15 | 0.78, 1.32, 0.39 | 20.42, 19.2, 16.49 | 6.5 |
| Restriction-enzyme like | | | | |
| NeSL | n.a. | 0.08, 0.01, <0.01 | n.d., n.d., n.d. | n.d. |
| R2 | n.a. | n.d., n.d., <0.01 | n.d., n.d., n.d. | n.d. |
| R4 | n.a. | Fossils,[e] 0.09, n.d. | n.d., n.d., n.d. | n.d. |
| Apurinic/apyrimidinic | | | | |
| R1 | * | n.d., n.d., n.d. | n.d., n.d., n.d. | n.d. |
| L1/TX1 | * | 0.03, 0.06, 0.02 | 16.9, 18.8, 14.5 | n.d. |
| RTE/Rex3[g] | n.a. | 0.18, 0.39, 0.2 | n.d., n.d., n.d. | n.d. |
| L2/Maui | *** | 0.04, 0.53, 0.11 | 3.22, 0.38, 1.84 | 0.1 |
| L3/CR1[h] | *** | n.d., n.d., n.d. | 0.31, 0.05, 0.15 | 6.4 |
| Rex1/Babar | *** | 0.45, 0.25, 0.05 | n.d., n.d., n.d. | n.d. |
| I/Bgr | n.a. | 0.01, fossils, 0.01 | n.d., 0.01, n.d. | n.d. |
| Jockey | * | n.d., n.d., n.d. | n.d., n.d., n.d. | n.d. |
| LOA | * | n.d., n.d., n.d. | n.d., n.d., n.d. | n.d. |
| LTR retrotransposons | 0.1 | 0.12, 0.30, 0.40 | 8.29, 9.87, 3.25 | |
| Vertebrate retroviruses | * | 0.03, 0.09, <0.01 | 8.29, 9.87, 3.25 | 1.3 |
| TY1/Copia | n.a. | 0.02, 0.01, <0.01 | n.d., n.d., n.d. | n.d. |
| TY3/Gypsy[i] | * | 0.06, 0.17, 0.13 | n.d., n.d., n.d. | n.d. |
| BEL | * | Fossils, 0.02, 0.01 | n.d., n.d., n.d. | n.a. |
| DIRS1[h] | n.a. | 0.02, 0.01, 0.25 | n.d., n.d., n.d. | n.a. |
| Penelope-like elements | n.a. | 0.06, 0.09, <0.01 | n.d., n.d., n.d. | n.a. |
| SINEs[h] | 1.36 | | 13.14, 8.22, 9.12 | Fossils |

[a]The estimated percentage of the genome occupied by the respective elements is shown. Where numeric estimates are unavailable, *indicates detected at low frequency, ***indicates detected at high frequency. There are some differences in calculation of the estimates as indicated below.

[b]*Callorhincus milii*. The estimates are based on analysis of 18 Mb of random sequence from this fish; copy number is uncertain and additional retrotransposon clades may be identified when the complete sequence is available. From Venkatesh B, Tay A, Dandona N et al. (2005) A compact cartilaginous fish model genome. *Current Biology* 15: R82–R83.

[c]Teleost fish considered here include *T. nigroviridis*, *T. rubripes*, and *D. rerio* (Tn, Tr, Dr respectively); the percentage is the percentage of RT gene-containing sequence from whole genome shotgun sequences. From Volff JN, Bouneau L, Ozouf-Costas C, and Fischer C (2003). Diversity of retrotransposable elements in compact pufferfish genomes. *Trends in Genetics* 19: 674–678.

[d]Mammals here include human, mouse and domestic dog (Hs, Mm, Cf, respectively) From Waterston RH, Lindblad-Toh K, Birney E, et al. (2002) Initial sequencing and comparative analysis of the mouse genome. *Nature* 420: 520–562; Lander ES, Linton LM, Birren B, et al. (2001) Initial sequencing and analysis of the human genome. *Nature* 409: 860–921; Kirkness EF, Bafna V, Halpern AL, et al. (2003) The dog genome: Survey sequencing and comparative analysis. *Science* 301: 1898–1903.

[e]From Hillier LW, Miller W, Birney E, et al. (2004) Sequence and comparative analysis of chicken genome provide unique perspectives on vertebrate evolution. *Nature* 432: 695–716.

[f]Non-LTR retrotransposons are subdivided into a phylogenetically older group encoding a restriction enzyme-like endonuclease, and a younger group with an apurinic/apyrimidinic endonuclease.

[g]Members of this clade detected in reptiles.

[h]Members of this clade detected in reptiles and amphibians.

[i]Fossils of this clade detected in reptiles, potentially active elements detected in amphibians.

n.a. indicates data not known. n.d. indicates the element was not detected after searching. Fossils are elements deemed to be extinct, having lost the means of retrotransposition or lacking evidence of recent retrotransposition.

mutations that disable their ability to infect germ cells. New nonautonomous elements arise through recombination, and all are transmitted in the germline. In general, LTR elements seem to be active within a genome over short evolutionary scales relative to LINE-like lineages.

As previously mentioned, SINEs appear to have arisen from structural RNA sequences. The primate Alu, mouse B1, and related families were derived from 7SL RNA. However, almost all other SINEs are derived from tRNA, and are placed as an evolutionarily older family than the 7SL-derived group. A new SINE-like family of diverse low-copy-number species- or lineage-specific retrotransposons derived from small nucleolar RNA was recently described in vertebrates.

Construction of a RT-based PLE polygeny is problematic since PLE RT differs from all of other retroelement RTs and more closely resembles telomerase. This, together with their distinct structure, has led to general agreement that PLEs form a separate group from the LTR and non-LTR retrotransposons. A relatively early origin for PLEs is supported by grouping of PLEs found in many eukaryotic genomes. Degenerate, and full-length PLEs have been reported from fungi and a wide range of invertebrates. In vertebrates, they have so far been found in teleost fish, sharks, and amphibia, not always as degenerate molecular fossils. It is possible that some are still active in the fish *Tetraodon nigroviridis* and *Danio rerio*.

## Retrotransposons as Phylogenetic Markers

At any point in time, relatively few copies of a retrotransposon are capable of replication and retrotransposition. As these copies accumulate mutations, the mutations are inherited by subsequent members of the retroelement lineage in the host genome. Once the host lineage splits, new insertions will occur independently in each descendant lineage. Since stably integrated elements are identical by descent, and the probability of parallel independent insertions into a genome is low, retrotransposons can be considered to be homoplasy-free characters, offering unique utility as markers to study evolution of host species. Retrotransposons have been used in several species of fish, mammals, birds, and reptiles, to clarify phylogenetic relationships. As suggested above, these analyses rest on the assumption that, in general, retrotransposons integrate randomly into genomes, with an exceptionally low probability that an element would independently insert in orthologous positions in two species. Another assumption is that, unless removed by segmental deletion, an insertion remains in its locus once fixed in the genome, eventually becoming unrecognizable as a result of accumulated mutations. Evidence that these assumptions do not always hold indicates that, as with analyses based on other genome elements, care is required in the conduct and interpretation of phylogenetic analyses based on retroelements.

## Retrotransposon Effects on the Genome

Transposable elements have profoundly affected the structure and function of vertebrate genomes in many different ways.

### Retrotransposon Content

Vertebrate genomes differ markedly in the total quantity and diversity of retrotransposons they contain, and the evolutionary trajectory of different elements. Genome size has been correlated to the quantity of transposable elements in the genome. Retrotransposons occupy approximately 35–50% or more of mouse, human, and domestic dog genomes. The chicken genome is approximately 39% of the size of mouse and human genomes, but only about 8% of the genome is recognizable retrotransposable elements. In the very compact genomes of smooth pufferfish *T. nigroviridis* and *Takifugu rubripes*, roughly 12% the size of mouse and human genomes, retrotransposable elements occupy less than 5% of the DNA. The enormous retrotransposon copy number accumulation in species with large genomes suggests that these species lack some constraint on retrotransposon activity that is present in animals with small genomes. It has been suggested that retrotransposons physically organize the genome through higher order chromatin structuring, provision of dispersed regulatory units, and other means. Thus, differences in genome retrotransposon content could significantly affect the operation of different genomes.

The pufferfish genomes, considering their small size, contain a remarkable diversity of retrotransposons in comparison with mammals. In mammalian genomes, 4 LINE-like clades have been identified (L1, L2, RTE, and CR1) with L1 the major currently active element, while in pufferfish genomes seven clades have been identified (NeSL, R4, L1, RTE, I, L2, Rex1) most of which have been recently active. Within the L1 clade alone, a single lineage has dominated L1 activity in mouse and human genomes since the mammalian radiation and comprises about 20% of the genome, whereas multiple L1 lineages predating the mammalian L1 emergence are active in several fish species, although present in very low copy numbers. All the major groups of LTR retrotransposons are represented in pufferfish genomes, as are PLEs. In contrast, only the vertebrate retrovirus group (endogenous retroviruses) and a few molecular fossils of the Ty3/Gypsy and DIRS1 groups are present in the mouse and human genomes, and there is no evidence for the presence of PLEs. The zebrafish, *D. rerio*, with a larger genome than the pufferfish, also hosts a great variety of retrotransposons. Whether these obvious differences in retrotransposon evolutionary biology between the three fish genomes and the mouse/human genomes represent the general case between teleosts and mammals is as yet unknown. Birds, as exemplified by the chicken, are different again. A single LINE-like retrotransposon, CR1, comprises about 90% of all identified chicken retrotransposons, L2/MIRs and endogenous retroviruses equally comprise the remainder. Curiously, the chicken genome lacks SINEs although it contains faint remnants of ancient SINEs pre-dating the bird-mammal split. A variety of retrotransposons have been reported from reptile genomes, some revealing lineage-specific retrotransposons such as the Sauria SINE derived from a LINE-like element of the RTE clade.

Mammalian genomes *per se* can differ markedly from one another in their retrotransposon content and activity, reflecting the evolutionary trajectory of different elements. For example, LINE, SINE, and LTR elements occupy similar percentages of mouse and human genomes. However, endogenous retroviruses are almost extinct in humans, while multiple families of endogenous retroviruses are active in rodents. The L1 lineage appears to be still active in most mammalian genomes, but recent evidence indicates its extinction in several tribes of sigmodontine rodents at or after their divergence from the earliest extant genus. As would be predicted, L1 extinction was linked to extinction of B1, a rodent SINE thought to be transposed by L1. Unexpectedly, vigorous expansion of an endogenous retrovirus, MysTR, to very high copy numbers unprecedented in any other endogenous retrovirus group, was also linked to L1 extinction. Whether there is any relationship between L1 activity and endogenous retrovirus activity is unknown.

## Genomic Distribution of Retrotransposons

Diverse patterns of retrotransposon distribution in genomes are dependent on the type of element and the host genome. In the mouse and human, retrotransposons are generally dispersed widely through the genome. In contrast, retroelements strongly cluster in heterochromatic gene-poor regions in *T. nigroviridis*, similar to the distribution in *Drosophila*. Whether this extremely uneven distribution is specific to small genomes, or teleosts, is unknown, and how and why it might arise is the subject for some speculation.

At a smaller scale, much variation is evident within genomes. The density of retrotransposons varies among different chromosomes in individual vertebrate species, and in mammals is usually highest on the X and Y chromosomes. A higher density of L1 on X chromosomes than autosomes is also observed in the Ryuku spiny rat, *Tokudaia osimensis*, in which both males and females have an XO karyotype, arguing against the hypothesis that evolutionary selection of a high density of L1 on X is due to involvement of L1 in X-inactivation. Although LTR elements are distributed more or less uniformly in mouse and human genomes, L1 occurs at much higher density in gene-poor, AT-rich regions and the human SINE, Alu, occurs at high density in GC-rich regions. Closer analysis demonstrates young Alus preferentially occur in AT-rich regions,

whereas in older Alus a stronger bias toward GC-rich regions emerges. One of several possible explanations for this skewed distribution of LINEs and Alus is selective targeting of L1 and Alu to AT-rich regions, and subsequent positive selection for Alus in gene-rich GC-rich regions. A significant antisense bias observed for many older intact LTR elements and solitary LTRs located in mammalian introns, is thought to arise from negative selection of sense-oriented elements bearing strong splice acceptor or donor sites, or strong transcriptional regulatory function.

## Effect on Genes

Through their specific exaptation for use by the host, or through incorporation within genes, retrotransposons significantly contribute to gene evolution, and some examples follow. Sequences from LTR elements alone occupy about 1.5% of mouse and 0.8% of human genes, and genes containing these elements tend to be newly evolved genes. Indeed, LTRs drive developmentally regulated expression of cellular genes in early mouse embryos, perhaps an evolving example fitting with the hypothesis that randomly distributed retrotransposons provide a means to set up, over evolutionary time, co-ordinated transcriptional regulatory circuits. An interesting example of exaptation is the independent selection by sheep, primate, and rodent lineages of Env expression from lineage-specific endogenous retroviruses for function in placental syncytiotrophoblast morphogenesis. At least one ultraconserved sequence in mammalian genomes has proved to be an ancient SINE whose multiple insertions, predating the divergence of amniotes and amphibians, have been exapted for use in transcriptional regulation or as a conserved exon in multiple unrelated genes.

New insertions can also disrupt normal gene function through interference with transcriptional regulation, through physical alteration of transcripts by aberrant splicing or premature termination, and through exon shuffling by inadvertent transduction of non-retrotransposon sequences. While L1 generates processed pseudogenes in the human genome, the paucity of processed pseudogenes in the chicken genome indicates that CR1 does not, suggesting that its retrotransposition machinery does not recognize mRNA. Thus, different vertebrate LINE-like retrotransposons may differ in their effects on different genomes.

Retrotransposons also act as substrates for recombination, fostering genomic instability, and are involved in both duplications and deletions within genomes, and other structural rearrangements. For example, in the human genome, SVA elements are reported to be associated with about 53 kbp of genomic duplications in the human genome, including duplication of entire genes and the creation of new genes. Recently, recombination hot spots in mouse and human genomes were linked with a sequence, CCTCCCT, found in an ancient nonautonomous LTR element (THE1) in humans. The LTR element itself is not recognizable in mouse, likely having been mutated beyond recognition by the higher nucleotide substitution rate in this species. Finally, illegitimate recombination between Alu elements in primate genomes has been linked with occasional genomic deletions. However, the effect of different retrotransposons on genome integrity may vary according to the retrotransposon type and host species. For example, high karyotypic variation in sigmodontine rodent species with extinct L1 compared with those maintaining active L1 supports the notion that L1 proteins may be important for DNA break–repair in these animals. Interestingly, a single L1 element, L1_MM, was enriched in regions of low recombination activity in the mouse, and L1 is underrepresented in human recombination hot-spots.

## Host Responses to Retrotransposons

The inherent tendency of retrotransposons to amplify their copy number creates mutagenic insertions potentially harmful to the host, leading to the view of retrotransposons as genomic parasites. An adaptive response by the host would selectively encourage the evolution of repressive mechanisms directed against retroelements, and this in turn would exert selective pressure on retroelements to resist repression. It has been suggested that evolution of the APOBEC3 family of cytidine deaminases, cellular inhibitors of retrotransposition of LINE-like, SINE and LTR retrotransposons, may have been driven in part as a genome response to invasion of mammalian genomes by retrotransposons. In addition to random mutation of active elements within the genome, other strategies to inhibit retrotransposon proliferation include transcriptional silencing through epigenetic modifications to chromatin and DNA, and post-transcriptional silencing through RNA interference. From time to time, retroelements escape repression and undergo expansion in the affected genome. Thus, continued activity of a retroelement in the genome, such as of endogenous retroviruses in the mouse, may indicate that a host is lagging in the evolutionary race to control the genome invader. Some retrotransposons have been astoundingly successful in certain genomes, for example, there are over $1 \times 10^6$ Alu copies in the human genome, consisting of one family with about 20 subfamilies. This, together with the low frequency of pathogenic effects for many retroelements, and the adoption by hosts of many elements for their own biology, suggest the controversial idea that many retrotransposons have formed or are forming a symbiotic rather than parasitic relationship with their hosts.

## Acknowledgments

This work was supported in part by VSPHS NIH (R01HD037102).

## Further Reading

Aparicio S, Chapman J, Stupka E, et al. (2002) Whole-genome shotgun assembly and analysis of the genome of Fugu rubripes. Science 297: 1301–1310.

Craig NL, Craigie R, Gellert M, and Lambowitz AM (eds.) (2002) Mobile DNA II. Herndon, VA: ASM Press.

Curcio MJ and Derbyshire KM (2003) The outs and ins of transposition: From mu to kangaroo. Nature Reviews Molecular Cell Biology 4: 865–877.

Eickbush TH and Furano AV (2002) Fruit flies and humans respond differently to retrotransposons. Current Opinion in Genetics and Development 12: 669–674.

Furano AV, Duvernell DD, and Boissinot S (2004) L1 (LINE-1) retrotransposon diversity differs dramatically between mammals and fish. Trends in Genetics 20: 9–14.

Goodwin TJ and Poulter RT (2001) The DIRS1 group of retrotransposons. Molecular Biology and Evolution 18: 2067–2082.

Hedges DJ and Deininger PL (2006) Inviting instability: Transposable elements, double-strand breaks, and the maintenance of genome integrity. Mutation Research: Fundamental Mechanisms of Mutagenesis doi:10.1016/j.mrfmmm.2006.11.021.

Hillier LW, Miller W, Birney E, et al. (2004) Sequence and Comparative analysis of chicken genome provide unique perspectives on vertebrate evolution. Nature 432: 695–716.

Kazazian HH, Jr. (2004) Mobile elements: Drivers of genome evolution. Science 303: 1626–1632.

Kordis D (2005) A genomic perspective on the chromodomain-containing retrotransposons: Chromoviruses. Gene 347: 161–173.

Kirkness EF, Bafna V, Halpern AL, et al. (2003) The dog genome: Survey sequencing and comparative analysis. Science 301: 1898–1903.

Lander ES, Linton LM, Birren B, et al. (2001) Initial sequencing and analysis of the human genome. Nature 409: 860–921.

Malik HS and Eickbush TH (2001) Phylogenetic analysis of ribonuclease H domains suggests a late, chimeric origin of LTR retrotransposable elements and retroviruses. Genome Research 11: 1187–1197.

Ostertag EM and Kazazian HH, Jr. (2001) Biology of mammalian L1 retrotransposons. Annual Review of Genetics 35: 501–538.

Piskurek O, Austin CC, and Okada N (2006) Sauria SINEs: Novel short interspersed retroposable elements that are widespread in reptile genomes. Journal of Molecular Evolution 62: 630–644.

Roy-Engel AM, Carroll ML, El-Sawy M, et al. (2002) Non-traditional Alu evolution and primate genomic diversity. Journal of Molecular Biology 316: 1033–1040.

van de Lagemaat LN, Medstrand P, and Mager DL (2006) Multiple effects govern endogenous retrovirus survival patterns in human gene introns. Genome Biology 7: R86.

Venkatesh B, Tay A, Dandona N, et al. (2005) A compact cartilaginous fish model genome. Current Biology 15: R82–R83.

Volff JN (ed.) (2005) Cytogenetic and Genome Research, Vol. 110: Retrotransposable Elements and Genome Evolution. Basel: S Karger AG.

Voff JN, Bouneau L, Ozouf-Costas C, and Fischer C (2003) Diversity of retrotransposable elements in compact Pufferfish genomes. Trends in Genetics 19: 674–678.

Waterston RH, Lindblad-Toh K, Birney E, et al. (2002) Initial sequencing and comparative analysis of the mouse genome. Nature 420: 520–562.

Weber MJ (2006) Mammalian small nucleolar RNAs are mobile genetic elements. Public Library of Science Genetics 2: e205doi:10.1371/journal.pgen.0020205.

## Relevant Website

http://www.girinst.org – Genetic Information Research Institute, Mountain View.

# Retroviral Oncogenes

**P K Vogt and A G Bader,** The Scripps Research Institute, La Jolla, CA, USA

## Glossary

**Chimeric transcript** An mRNA that encodes a fusion protein derived from two individual and originally separate genes.
**Subtractive hybridization** A method to identify differentially expressed mRNAs; the method is based on hybridizing a 'tester' mRNA population with a 'driver' mRNA population and selectively eliminating tester–driver hybrids.

## Historical Perspective

Retroviruses that carry an oncogene induce neoplastic transformation of cells in culture and rapidly cause tumors in the animal. Early studies with Rous sarcoma virus in chicken embryo fibroblasts showed a controlling influence of the retroviral genome on the properties of the transformed cell and suggested that the virus carries oncogenic information. The isolation of temperature-sensitive mutants of Rous sarcoma virus firmly established a dominant role of viral genetic information in the process of virus-induced carcinogenesis. These mutants of Rous sarcoma virus encode an unstable oncoprotein and are able to transform chicken embryo fibroblasts at a low, permissive temperature but fail to induce oncogenic changes at an elevated, nonpermissive temperature. Yet the virus is able to propagate under both permissive and nonpermissive conditions, demonstrating that virus viability and replication are not affected by the mutation and that oncogenicity is governed by genetic information that is distinct from viral replicative genes. Cells transformed by temperature-sensitive Rous sarcoma virus under permissive conditions become normal in morphology and growth behavior if the cell cultures are switched to the nonpermissive temperature. Thus, viral genetic information is required for the initiation as well as for the maintenance of the transformed cellular phenotype. A physical correlate to these genetic experiments was found in studies with transformation-defective Rous sarcoma virus. These spontaneously emerging variants of the virus fail to induce transformation in cell culture but are able to generate viable progeny virus that remains transformation defective. The transformation-defective viruses contain genomes that are about 20% smaller than the genome of oncogenic Rous sarcoma virus. The missing genetic information is of obvious importance for oncogenicity. Subtractive hybridization of DNA transcripts from transformation-defective and transformation-competent viral genomes generates a specific cDNA probe for the oncogenic sequences in Rous sarcoma virus. This probe hybridizes to cellular DNA, revealing the presence of sequences that are homologous to the transforming information of Rous sarcoma virus in the genome of all vertebrate cells. Retroviral oncogenes are therefore derived from the cell genome. The cellular versions of retroviral oncogenes are also referred to as proto-oncogenes or, more commonly, as c-*onc* genes; the corresponding viral versions are called v-*onc* genes. The discovery of oncogenes owes much to the exceptional genetic structure of Rous sarcoma virus. This virus is unique among oncogene-carrying retroviruses in that it is replication competent, containing a full set of viral genes plus the oncogene. Loss of the oncogene in transformation-defective variants still leaves a viable virus, greatly facilitating molecular and genetic analyses.

## Taxonomy of Oncogene-Carrying Retroviruses

Retroviruses are broadly divided into two categories, viruses with simple genomes and viruses with complex genomes. Simple retroviral genomes contain four coding regions with information for virion proteins. These regions are referred to as *gag*, which directs the synthesis of matrix, capsid, and nucleoprotein structures; *pro*, generating the virion protease; *pol*, containing the information for the reverse transcriptase and integrase enzymes; and *env*, which encodes the surface and transmembrane components of the envelope protein. Complex retroviral genomes contain additional information for regulatory nonvirion proteins that are translated from multiply spliced mRNAs.

In taxonomic terms, retroviruses form a family that consists of the subfamilies *Orthoretrovirinae* and *Spumaretrovirinae*. Oncogenes are carried by only two genera of the orthoretroviruses. These are the alpharetroviruses, representing the avian leukosis complex of viruses, and the gammaretroviruses, encompassing murine, feline, and primate leukemia and sarcoma viruses. This restriction of oncogenes to two viral genera probably reflects a set of conditions that have to be met for the acquisition of cellular sequences by a retroviral genome. These conditions include absence of cytotoxicity and efficient viral integration and replication. Complex retroviruses may not tolerate the insertion of cellular sequences into the viral genome because some functions of the regulatory nonvirion proteins that would be displaced by a cellular insert can probably not be complemented in *trans*. These are all hypothetical reasons for the occurrence of oncogenes in just a few retroviruses; mechanistic explanations of these restrictions are currently not available.

## Acquisition of Cellular Sequences by Retroviral Genomes

The acquisition of a cellular oncogene by a retrovirus is a rare event that occurs during viral passage in an animal but is seldom seen in cell culture. Because *de novo* acquisition of cellular sequences cannot be reproduced with significant frequency in cultured cells, the molecular mechanism of acquisition has to be reconstructed using information derived from the structure of viral genomes and from the virus life cycle. The life cycle of retroviruses contains two steps that leads to genetic recombination. (1) Retroviruses are diploid and thus can form heterozygous viral particles. Recombination between distinct but related viral genomes encased in the same particle occurs very frequently and probably results from copy-choice events that occur during reverse transcription. (2) Integration of the provirus into the cellular genome produces a recombinant between virus and cell (**Figure 1**). These two recombinational activities of retroviruses can explain the incorporation of cellular sequences into the viral genome. The first step in this acquisition consists of the integration of a provirus containing a single 5′ (left-hand) long terminal repeat (LTR) into the oncogene proper or into the immediate upstream vicinity of a cellular oncogene. This provirus can then produce a chimeric RNA transcript that starts in the viral LTR, continues by read-through into the cellular gene, and terminates with the poly A stretch of the cellular gene. Alternatively, such a chimeric transcript can be generated by a splicing event that uses a viral splice donor and a cellular splice acceptor in joining upstream viral to downstream cellular sequences. Chimeric RNAs of this type would be incorporated into virions. In the subsequent cycle of infection, reverse transcription could effect a second recombination event, generating a junction between the 3′ region of the cellular sequences and a part of the viral genome carrying the 3′ terminal repeat sequences that are essential for the efficient production of proviral DNA. In this model, the first step of recombination in acquiring cellular sequences is the integration of the provirus, which is DNA-based recombination. The second step occurs during reverse transcription of a heterozygote particle and is RNA-based recombination. It is possible, however, to envisage a second recombination step that is also DNA based. It requires the integration of another provirus immediately downstream of the cellular oncogene

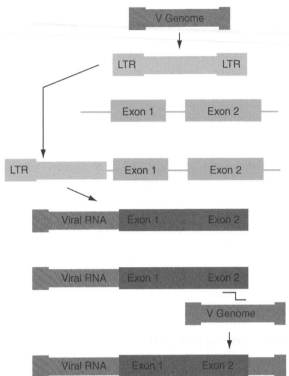

**Figure 1** A hypothetical mechanism for the acquisition of a cellular oncogene by a retroviral genome. The genome of a retrovirus without oncogene is transcribed into DNA and, in a first recombinational event, is integrated upstream of a cellular oncogene containing two exons. The right-hand long terminal repeat (LTR) and adjacent sequences of the viral genome are lost during the integration process. Transcription from the integrated proviral LTR generates a chimeric mRNA by read-through or aberrant splicing. This mRNA contains cell-derived oncogene and viral information. The chimeric mRNA is packaged into viral particles together with wild-type viral genomes. In the next round of infection the second recombinational event occurs during reverse transcription and adds 3′ viral terminal sequences to the DNA transcript, facilitating the production and integration of a functional provirus that contains a cell-derived oncogene. Green: DNA, red and purple: RNA.

to serve as donor of the necessary 3′ (right-hand) LTR for the new provirus that now carries an insertion of cellular sequences. Currently available experimental evidence can be adduced to support either model for the second recombination step in the acquisition of a cellular oncogene. Specific oncogene acquisitions may in fact occur by either mechanism.

## Retroviruses Carrying an Oncogene Are Replication Defective

The incorporation of cellular sequences into the retroviral genome occurs at the expense of viral sequences that are displaced in the process. With one notable exception, Rous sarcoma virus, transducing retroviruses lack one or several essential viral genes. Typical deletions extend from within the viral *gag* gene into the *env* gene, eliminating the 3' portion of *gag*, all of the *pol* gene, and part of *env*. Such defective viruses can infect cells, integrating into the cellular genome, producing the oncoprotein, and inducing neoplastic transformation, but they are unable to synthesize infectious progeny virus. For infectious virus production, they require co-infection of the same cell with a closely related helper retrovirus that in *trans* provides those replicative functions that are missing from the defective transforming virus. Helper retroviruses contain a complete set of viral genes but have not incorporated any cellular oncogenic sequences. They do not induce oncogenic transformation when replicating in cultured cells. In animal infections, they can cause tumors by insertional mutagenesis after extended latent periods. These tumors result from transcriptional upregulation of a cellular oncogene by promoter activities of a provirus integrated nearby.

## Oncoproteins Are Often Fusion Proteins

As a consequence of the initial integration event that leads to oncogene acquisition, viral oncogenes usually code for fusion proteins, consisting of an N-terminal portion derived from the virus and a C-terminal component representing the oncoprotein proper. The viral sequences generally include the N-terminus of the Gag polyprotein. The initial recombination event also often eliminates short lengths from the N-terminus of the cellular oncoprotein, except when viral sequences are spliced onto the cellular gene. Fusion of the cellular oncoproteins to viral *gag* sequences can have important consequences that contribute to the gain of function associated with the viral oncogene. The efficiency of protein translation and the stability of the fusion protein are often increased. Gag sequences also provide an affinity for the plasma membrane which can be critical in activating the oncogenic potential of the protein.

## Functional Classes of Oncogenes

Retroviral oncogenes code for components of cellular growth-regulatory signals (**Table 1**). The major functional categories include growth factors, receptor and nonreceptor tyrosine kinases, serine-threonine and lipid kinases, adaptor proteins, hormone receptors, and a variety of transcriptional regulators. Cellular growth signals are propagated from the cell periphery to the nucleus. Therefore, the nuclear oncoproteins coding for transcriptional regulators are the ultimate effectors of oncogenicity, converting the signal into a pattern of gene expression that is the basis of the oncogenic phenotype of the cell.

Because of this pivotal role of nuclear oncoproteins in specifying neoplastic properties, oncogenic transformation can be viewed as a case of aberrant transcription. However, there is also abundant evidence for a critical role of protein translation in oncogenesis. Oncogenesis induced by the PI3K pathway in particular depends on differential translation of specific growth-promoting proteins.

## Retroviral Transduction of a Cellular Oncogene Results in Gain of Function

Compared to their cellular counterparts, retroviral oncoproteins show an increase in activity. Some of this gain of function is purely quantitative: the viral promoter assures highly efficient transcription of the oncogene. There are several oncogenes for which mere overexpression is sufficient to turn them into effective agents of neoplastic transformation. These code for wild-type oncoproteins that deregulate cellular growth by their virus-mediated abundance. However, many oncoproteins carry specific mutations that are responsible for the gain of function. These mutations remove or inactivate domains of the oncoprotein that effect negative regulation or may enhance specific enzymatic activities of the oncoprotein by other mechanisms including conformational change, improved substrate affinity, or change in cellular localization. They may stabilize the protein or alter the spectrum of downstream targets. Thus both quantitative and qualitative changes resulting from viral transduction and the associated mutation of the oncogene contribute to the gain of function.

## Cooperation of Oncogenes

A few retroviruses carry two oncogenes. These oncogenes are derived from distinct cellular loci situated at distant positions within the host genome. Retroviruses with two oncogenes include Avian erythroblastosis virus R (AEV-R), carrying v-*erbA* and v-*erbB*, Avian myeloblastosis–erythroblastosis virus E26, encoding *myb* and *ets* as a single Gag-myb-ets protein product, and Avian myelocytoma virus MH2, which contains the v-*myc* and v-*mil* (raf) genes. Each of these single oncoproteins can induce neoplastic transformation on its own. However, viruses with two oncogenes are more potent in transformation, indicating that the two oncoproteins cooperate. Whereas primary avian cells can be readily transformed by viruses carrying a single oncogene, in mammalian cells oncogenic transformation generally requires the cooperation of two or more oncogenes. The reasons for this difference in cellular susceptibility to oncogene action are not known.

**Table 1**   Classes of retroviral oncogenes

| Functional groups and oncogenes | Identity and function of cellular homolog | Retrovirus |
|---|---|---|
| **Growth factor** | | |
| sis | Platelet–derived growth factor (PDGF) | Simian sarcoma virus |
| **Receptor tyrosine kinases** | | |
| erbB | Receptor of epithelial growth factor (EGF) | Avian erythroblastosis virus |
| fms | Receptor of colony-stimulating factor 1 (CSF-1) | McDonough feline sarcoma virus |
| sea | Receptor of macrophage-stimulating protein (MSP) | Avian erythroblastosis virus S13 |
| kit | Hematopoietic receptor of stem cell factor (SCF) | Hardy–Zuckerman 4 feline sarcoma virus |
| ros | Orphan receptor tyrosine kinase | Avian sarcoma virus UR2 |
| mpl | Hematopoietic receptor of thrombopoietin | Mouse myeloproliferative leukemia virus |
| eyk | Closest homolog of mammalian c-mer; c-Mer ligands include anticoagulation factor protein S and the growth arrest-specific gene product Gas6 | Avian retrovirus RPL30 |
| **Hormone receptor** | | |
| erbA | Thyroid hormone receptor | Avian erythroblastosis virus |
| **G proteins** | | |
| H-ras | GTPase; MAPK signal transduction | Harvey murine sarcoma virus |
| K-ras | GTPase; MAPK signal transduction | Kirsten murine sarcoma virus |
| **Adaptor protein** | | |
| crk | Adaptor protein containing SH2 and SH3 domains; PI3K/Akt signal transduction | Avian sarcoma virus CT10 |
| **Nonreceptor tyrosine kinases** | | |
| src | MAPK and PI3K/Akt signal transduction | Rous sarcoma virus |
| yes | Src family kinase; signal transduction | Avian sarcoma virus Y73 |
| fps | Cytokine receptor signaling; the fps and fes oncogenes are derived from the same cellular gene | Fujinami poultry sarcoma virus |
| fes | Cytokine receptor signaling; the fps and fes oncogenes are derived from the same cellular gene | Gardner–Arnstein feline sarcoma virus |
| fgr | Src family kinase; signal transduction | Gardner–Rasheed feline sarcoma virus |
| abl | Cytoskeletal signaling and cell cycle regulated transcription | Abelson murine leukemia virus |
| **Serine/threonine kinases** | | |
| mos | Regulator of cell cycle progression; required for germ cell maturation; activates MAPKs | Moloney murine sarcoma virus |
| raf | MAPKKK, MAPK signal transduction | Murine sarcoma virus 3611 |
| akt | PI3K/Akt signal transduction | Murine retrovirus AKT8 |
| **Lipid kinase** | | |
| p3k | PI 3-kinase; PI3K/Akt signal transduction | Avian sarcoma virus 16 |
| **Transcriptional regulators** | | |
| jun | bZIP protein of AP-1 complex; homo- and heterodimer with AP-1 family members; cell cycle progression | Avian sarcoma virus 17 |
| fos | bZIP protein of AP-1 complex; heterodimer with AP-1 family members; cell cycle progression | FBJ murine osteogenic sarcoma virus |
| myc | bHLH-ZIP protein; heterodimer with Max; cell cycle progression | Avian myelocytoma virus MC29 |
| myb | HTH protein; development of hematopoietic system | Avian myeloblastosis virus |

Continued

**Table 1**    Continued

| Functional groups and oncogenes | Identity and function of cellular homolog | Retrovirus |
|---|---|---|
| ets | HTH protein; myeloid and eosinophil differentiation | Avian myeloblastosis–erythroblastosis virus E26 |
| rel | p65 NF-κB subunit; survival pathways | Avian reticuloendotheliosis virus |
| maf | bZIP protein; homo- and heterodimers with various bZIP proteins; differentiation of various tissues | Avian musculoaponeurotic fibrosarcoma virus |
| ski | Adaptor protein for various transcription factors; chromatin-dependent transcriptional regulation; muscle differentiation | Avian Sloan-Kettering retrovirus |
| qin | Avian homolog of mammalian brain factor 1 (BF-1/FoxG1); forkhead/winged helix (FOX) protein; monomer; neuronal differentiation | Avian sarcoma virus 31 |

Abbreviations: Gas6, growth arrest-specific gene 6; MAPK, mitogen-activated protein kinase; MAPKKK, mitogen-activated protein kinase kinase kinase; SH2, Src homology domain 2; SH3, Src homology domain 3; PI3K, phosphoinositide 3-kinase; AP-1, activator protein 1; bZIP, basic region leucine zipper; bHLH-ZIP, basic region helix–loop–helix leucine zipper; HTH, helix–turn–helix; NF-κB, nuclear factor kappa B; FBJ, Finkel–Biskis–Jinkins.

## Coda and Outlook

There are still significant gaps in our knowledge of retroviral oncogenes. We do not know and cannot reproduce the exact mechanism of oncogene acquisition by a retroviral genome. We have only tentative explanations for the failure of some groups of retroviruses to capture cellular sequences. We have no idea why certain growth-promoting cellular genes have not shown up as retroviral oncogenes. Have not enough retroviruses been studied or is there an active mechanism that excludes certain genes? Does some cryptic homology between provirus and oncogene determine the spectrum of genes that can be incorporated? On a more basic level, there is evidence that oncogenes can induce tumors by activating the transcription of specific micro-RNAs. Are there also rapidly oncogenic retroviruses that carry a micro-RNA gene as an oncogene?

Despite these puzzling questions, at a fundamental level the nature and workings of retroviral oncogenes are well understood and have provided important insights into the mechanisms of virus-induced carcinogenesis. The discovery that all retroviral oncogenes are derived from cellular information has greatly expanded the significance of these genes. Originally seen as viral pathogenicity genes, they have become universal effectors of oncogenicity. Viruses have been demoted to just one of several instruments that can activate these genes; mutation, overexpression, and amplification are some of the others. The study of oncogenes, initially a somewhat esoteric part of virology, has grown to determine the course of cancer research during the past three decades and has contributed immensely to our understanding of cancer in general. As targets of specific inhibitors, oncoproteins are now revolutionizing cancer treatment. Gleevec, directed at the BCR-ABL oncoprotein in chronic myelogenous leukemia, and Iressa, inhibiting mutants of the epithelial growth factor receptor in non-small cell lung cancer, have dramatically proven the promise of therapy targeted to oncoproteins.

## Acknowledgments

This work was supported by grants from the National Cancer Institute. This is manuscript number 18 394 of The Scripps Research Institute.

*See also:* Feline Leukemia and Sarcoma Viruses.

## Further Reading

Bister K and Jansen HW (1986) Oncogenes in retroviruses and cells: Biochemistry and molecular genetics. *Advances in Cancer Research* 47: 99–188.

Duesberg PH and Vogt PK (1970) Differences between the ribonucleic acids of transforming and nontransforming avian tumor viruses. *Proceedings of the National Academy of Sciences, USA* 67: 1673–1680.

Hughes SH (1983) Synthesis, integration, and transcription of the retroviral provirus. *Current Topics in Microbiology and Immunology* 103: 23–49.

Land H, Parada LF, and Weinberg RA (1983) Tumorigenic conversion of primary embryo fibroblasts requires at least two cooperating oncogenes. *Nature* 304: 596–602.

Martin GS (1970) Rous sarcoma virus: A function required for the maintenance of the transformed state. *Nature* 227: 1021–1023.

Schwartz JR, Duesberg S, and Duesberg PH (1995) DNA recombination is sufficient for retroviral transduction. *Proceedings of the National Academy of Sciences, USA* 92: 2460–2464.

Stehelin D, Guntaka RV, Varmus HE, and Bishop JM (1976) Purification of DNA complementary to nucleotide sequences required for neoplastic transformation of fibroblasts by avian sarcoma viruses. *Journal of Molecular Biology* 101: 349–365.

Stehelin D, Varmus HE, Bishop JM, and Vogt PK (1976) DNA related to the transforming gene(s) of avian sarcoma viruses is present in normal avian DNA. *Nature* 260: 170–173.

Swanstrom R, Parker RC, Varmus HE, and Bishop JM (1983) Transduction of a cellular oncogene: The genesis of Rous sarcoma virus. *Proceedings of the National Academy of Sciences, USA* 80: 2519–2523.

Tam W, Hughes SH, Hayward WS, and Besmer P (2002) Avian bic, a gene isolated from a common retroviral site in avian leukosis virus-induced lymphomas that encodes a noncoding RNA, cooperates with c-myc in lymphomagenesis and erythroleukemogenesis. *Journal of Virology* 76: 4275–4286.

Temin HM (1960) The control of cellular morphology in embryonic cells infected with Rous sarcoma virus *in vitro*. *Virology* 10: 182–197.

Toyoshima K and Vogt PK (1969) Temperature sensitive mutants of an avian sarcoma virus. *Virology* 39: 930–931.

Varmus HE (1982) Form and function of retroviral proviruses. *Science* 216: 812–820.

Varmus HE (2006) The new era in cancer research. *Science* 312: 1162–1165.

Vogt PK (1971) Genetically stable reassortment of markers during mixed infection with avian tumor viruses. *Virology* 46: 947–952.

Vogt PK (1971) Spontaneous segregation of nontransforming viruses from cloned sarcoma viruses. *Virology* 46: 939–946.

Wang LH (1987) The mechanism of transduction of proto-oncogene c-src by avian retroviruses. *Mutation Research* 186: 135–147.

## Relevant Website

http://www.ncbi.nlm.nih.gov – Virus Databases Online (ICTVdB Index of Viruses), National Center for Biotechnology Information.

# Rift Valley Fever and Other Phleboviruses

**L Nicoletti and M G Ciufolini,** Istituto Superiore di Sanità, Rome, Italy

## Glossary

**Arbovirus** Any virus of vertebrates biologically transmitted by infected hematophagous arthropods.

**Aseptic meningitis** Inflammation of the covering of the brain (meninges) caused by a virus.

**Epizootic** A disease affecting a large number of animals at the same time within a particular region or geographic area.

**Phlebotomus fever viruses or sandfly fever viruses** Viruses that cause disease of brief duration characterized by sudden onset fever, headache, pain in the eyes, malaise, and leukopenia and are transmitted by the bite of infected sandflies.

**Phlebovirus** A genus in the family *Bunyaviridae* containing many viruses, of which the best known are Rift Valley fever virus and sandfly fever viruses.

**Sandfly** Any of various small biting two-winged flies of the families Psychodidae, Simuliidae, and Ceratopogonidae.

**Transovarial transmission** Vertical transmission of a virus from mother to offspring.

**Zoonosis** A disease of animals that can be transmitted to humans.

## Introduction

The genus *Phlebovirus* is one of the five genera of the family *Bunyaviridae*, in which are included more than 300 virus species. The five genera (*Orthobunyavirus, Hantavirus, Nairovirus, Phlebovirus, Tospovirus*) are grouped in one family, primarily because they share structural characteristics, all bear a tripartite RNA genome of negative polarity, and all have a roughly similar protein-coding pattern within each genome segment. It has been demonstrated that Uukuniemi virus, the prototype virus of a group of tick-borne viruses, and its relatives have the same ambisense coding strategy as do phleboviruses. In addition, a high degree of similarity occurs in proteins of Uukuniemi virus and in those of some phleboviruses. As a consequence, all viruses previously included in the genus *Uukuvirus* are now classified in the genus *Phlebovirus*. Therefore, in the genus *Phlebovirus*, viruses previously known as phlebotomus fever viruses and uukuviruses are now placed.

The first description of what was most likely phlebotomus fever occurred at the time of the Napoleonic wars, when a similar disease was reported as 'Mediterranean fever'. The disease was first described with considerable accuracy by Pick in 1886, who termed it 'dog fever' (*hundsfieber*), probably due to the marked signs and symptoms of conjunctivitis, which resembled the eyes of a bloodhound. At the same time in Italy, the disease was already known as pappataci fever, suggesting a possible link with sand flies. In Yugoslavia, epidemics of the disease occurred each summer among newly arrived Austrian troops stationed along the Adriatic coast.

Rift Valley fever virus (RVFV) was first isolated in 1930 during investigation of an epidemic with high mortality rates among sheep on a farm in the Rift Valley in East Africa. In retrospect, epizootics due to this virus had been identified as early as 1912. Epizootics were reported to have occurred in many sub-Saharan countries after 1940 and the vector-borne origin of the disease was definitively proved in 1948.

RVFV is one of the most important viral zoonoses in Africa. Transmission of the virus to humans occurs via arthropod vectors, aerosols of blood or amniotic fluid of infected livestock, or by direct contact with infected animals. RVFV in humans is manifested by a broad spectrum of infections, from asymptomatic infection to a benign febrile illness, to a severe illness (approximately 1–3% of cases) that can include retinitis, encephalitis, and hemorrhagic fever. In addition to the human illness, disability, and suffering, RVFV outbreaks can result in devastating economic losses when livestock in an agricultural society are affected.

RVFV was first confirmed outside Africa in September 2000. An outbreak occurred in southwestern coastal Saudi Arabia and neighboring coastal areas of Yemen. RVFV isolated from the floodwater mosquito *Aedes vexans arabiensis* during the outbreak was closely related to strains from Madagascar (1991) and Kenya (1997), suggesting that the virus was imported through infected mosquitoes or livestock from East Africa.

From blood samples taken during an epidemic occurring in Italy among Allied troops during World War II, Sabin isolated two serologically distinct agents, sandfly fever Sicilian virus and sandfly fever Naples virus. Since then, many distinct viruses have been isolated from sandflies or humans in both the Old World and the New World and, on the basis of serological relationships, classified in the phlebotomus fever group (**Table 1**).

In 1971, in Italy, Toscana virus (TOSV) was isolated from the sandfly, *Phlebotomus perniciosus*. The virus was shown to be antigenically related to sandfly fever Naples virus, and antibody to TOSV was shown to occur at a relatively high prevalence of antibodies in healthy humans. TOSV has since been shown to cause human disease and has been associated with acute neurologic disease.

## Morphology, Structure, and Strategy of Replication

The prototype phlebovirus is RVFV. Similar to other bunyaviruses, the virion is spherical or pleiomorphic, depending on the method used for fixation, with a diameter of 90–100 nm. The virion consists of a core containing the genome and its associated proteins, which are in turn surrounded by an envelope composed of a lipid bilayer containing equivalent numbers of two glycoproteins.

The genome consists of three single-stranded RNA segments: large (L, 6.5–8.5 kbp), medium (M, 3.2–4.3 kbp), and small (S, 1.7–1.9 kbp). Sequence studies demonstrate that the three segments are identical on the 3′-end (UGUGUUUC) and a complementary 5′-end. The S RNA produces many copies of the nucleocapsid protein (20–30 kDa) and the L RNA produces a few copies of the large (L) protein (150–250 kDa), which is a transcriptase.

The glycoproteins, together with a nonstructural protein ($NS_M$), are translated from an mRNA complementary to the M segment as a precursor which is post-translational to $G_N$ and $G_C$ proteins. The S segment codes for two proteins. The N protein is read from a subgenomic mRNA complementary to the 3′-end segment of the viral RNA; the second, a nonstructural protein ($NS_S$, 29–37 kDa), is read from a subgenomic virus-sense mRNA species corresponding to the 5′-half of the viral RNA (**Figure 1**). This strategy of replication is called 'ambisense', and it is utilized also by members of the genus *Tospovirus* as well, and of viruses of the family *Arenaviridae*.

The maturation of phleboviruses occurs in intracellular smooth membranes, principally in the Golgi complex. Exceptionally, RVFV matures on the cell surface of infected rat hepatocytes. The glycoproteins accumulate in the Golgi complex, causing vacuolization, but the Golgi complex remains functional. Virions bud into Golgi vesicles, which are then transported to the cell surface where the particles are released by exocytosis.

## The Agents

### Rift Valley Fever

RVF was first recognized as a viral zoonosis in Kenya in 1930. Since then, several massive epizootics affecting domestic livestock have been reported in widely separated parts of Africa. In 1977–78, RVFV appeared for the first time in Egypt in an epizootic epidemic of unprecedented size. It was estimated that in some areas along the Nile, 25–50% of sheep and cattle were infected, and that there were as

**Table 1**    Viruses of the genus *Phlebovirus*

| Virus species | Viruses |
| --- | --- |
| *Bujaru virus* | Bujaru, Munguba |
| *Candiru virus* | Candiru, Alenquer, Itaituba, Nique, Oriximina, Turuna |
| *Chilibre virus* | Chilibre, Cacao |
| *Frijoles virus* | Frijoles, Joa |
| *Punta Toro virus* | Punta Toro, Buenaventura |
| *Rift Valley fever virus* | Rift Valley fever, Belterra, Icoaraci |
| *Salehebad virus* | Salehebad, Arbia |
| *Sandfly fever Naples virus* | Sandfly fever Naples, Karimabad, Tehran, Toscana |
| *Uukuniemi virus* | Uukuniemi, EgAN 1825–61, Fin V 707, Grand Arbaud, Manawa, Murre, Oceanside, Ponteves, Precarious Point, RML 105355, St. Abbs Head, Tunis, Zaliv Terpeniya |
| Unassigned | Aguacate, Anhanga, Arboledas, Arumowot, Caimito, Chagres, Corfou, Gabek Forest, Gordil, Itaporanga, Odrenisrou, Pacui, Rio Grande, sandfly fever Sicilian, Saint-Floris, Urucuri |

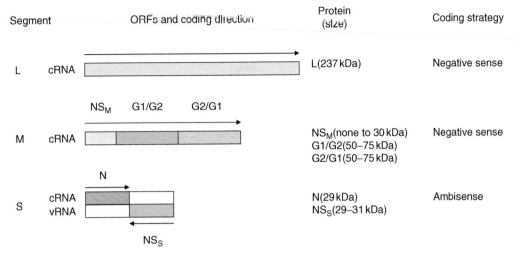

| Segment | | ORFs and coding direction | Protein (size) | Coding strategy |
|---|---|---|---|---|

**Figure 1**    Genome organization and coding strategy of phleboviruses.

many as 200 000 human cases and at least 600 deaths. Several types of severe and sometimes fatal illnesses were observed in humans, including hepatitis with hemorrhagic manifestations, meningoencephalitis, and retinitis. During this epidemic, RVFV was isolated from *Culex pipiens* mosquitoes; however, arthropods of many species have also been shown to be potential vectors.

During epizootics of RVFV, disease occurs first in animals, then in humans. RVFV produces severe disease in domestic animals, sheep being more susceptible than cattle, goats least susceptible. A greater than 90% rate of mortality is observed among infected lambs, and 20–60% among adult sheep. Pregnant ewes (90–100%) abort within a few days after infection.

RVFV can be transmitted to humans by contact with tissues or blood of infected animals during slaughter, autopsy, or disposal of infected animals. The possibility of transmission of the virus via such an airborne route among abattoir or laboratory workers has been recognized. Vector-borne transmission, particularly at the beginning of epizootic phase, is important.

The most common form of illness associated with RVFV infection in humans is the acute febrile disease (see **Table 2**). The febrile period lasts 4–7 days; patients then recover completely within 2 weeks. During the epidemic of RVFV in 1977–78 in Egypt, 5–10% of patients experienced a typical febrile illness, followed by decreased visual acuity after 7–20 days. Hemorrhagic RVFV, which occurs in about 1% of cases, was not documented until a 1975 epizootic in South Africa. Patients infected during this epidemic experienced the sudden onset of a febrile illness, which was followed 2–4 days later by jaundice and hemorrhagic manifestations. Hematemesis, melena, gingival bleeding, and petechial and purpuric skin lesions were common. In fatal cases, death occurred within a week of the onset of jaundice. Shock and hepatic insufficiency represented the most probable cause of death. Mortality rates

range from 0.2% to 14%. The exact incidence of each of the severe clinical syndromes complicating RVFV during the epidemics has not been established. These rates could be influenced by susceptibility of the human population, the virulence of various RVFV strains, and population dynamics of the vector.

## Sandfly Fever Viruses

Classical phlebotomus fevers caused by sandfly fever Naples and sandfly fever Sicilian viruses are mild, self-resolving, flu-like illnesses characterized by sudden onset, fever, frontal headache, low back pain, generalized myalgia, retro-orbital pain, conjunctival injection, photophobia and malaise, and, in some cases, nausea, vomiting, dizziness, and neck stiffness (see **Table 2**). Fever is always present, ranging from 38 to 41 °C. The incubation period is 2–6 days, and the duration of disease varies from a few hours to four days (phlebotomus fever is also known as 'a 3-day fever'). Patients completely recover within 1–2 weeks. No deaths associated with phlebotomus fever have been reported but the large numbers of cases that can occur during epidemics, particularly during wars, make these illnesses potentially incapacitating to entire populations, and therefore are important.

## Toscana Virus

TOSV was initially isolated from *P. perniciosus* in central Italy in 1971. The virus was subsequently isolated from *Phlebotomus perfiliewi* (but never from *Phlebotomus papatasi*) in other areas of Italy and from the brains of Kuhl's Pipistrelle bats (*Pipistrellus kuhlii*) captured in areas where the insect vectors were present. The virus also has been isolated from humans. Transovarial transmission has been demonstrated experimentally by viral isolation from

**Table 2**    Phleboviruses infecting humans

| Virus | Evidence of infection | Isolation from humans | Geographic distribution | Arthropod association |
|---|---|---|---|---|
| Alenquer | Febrile illness | Blood | Brazil | Unknown |
| Arboledas | Antibody | | Colombia | Lutzomyia spp. |
| Arumowot | Antibody | | Africa | Culex antennatus, Culex rubinotus, Mansonia uniformis |
| Bujaru | Antibody | | Brazil | Unknown |
| Cacao | Antibody | | Panama | Lutzomyia trapidoi |
| Candiru | Febrile illness | Blood | Brazil | Unknown |
| Chagres | Febrile illness | Blood | Panama, Colombia | Lutzomyia trapidoi, Lutzomyia ylephiletor |
| Corfou | Antibody | | Greece | Phlebotomus major |
| Gabek Forest | Antibody | | Africa | Unknown |
| Gordil | Antibody | | Africa | Unknown |
| Karimabad | Antibody | | Iran | Phlebotomus spp. |
| Punta Toro | Febrile illness | Blood | Panama | Lutzomyia trapidoi, L. ylephiletor |
| Rift Valley fever | Febrile illness Hemorrhagic fever | Blood, CSF | Africa, Arabian peninsula | Aedes caballus, Aedes circumluteolus, Aedes lineatopennis, Aedes vexans arabiensis, Culex theileri, Culicoides spp., Eretmapodites chrysogaster, Mansonia africana |
| Saint-Floris | Antibody | | Africa | Unknown |
| Salehabad | Antibody | | Iran | Phlebotomus spp. |
| Sandfly fever Sicilian | Febrile illness | Blood | North Africa, South Europe, Central Asia | Phlebotomus spp. |
| Sandfly fever Naples | Febrile illness | Blood | North Africa, South Europe, Central Asia | P. papatasi, P. perfiliewi |
| Toscana | Febrile illness Meningitis | CSF | Italy, Spain, Portugal, Cyprus, France, Greece | P. perniciosus, P. perfiliewi |

male *Phlebotomus* spp. Venereal transmission from infected males to uninfected females has also been demonstrated. For many years, the known distribution of TOSV was limited to Italy and Portugal. More recently, the geographic distribution of the virus has been extended to France, Spain, Slovenia, Greece, Cyprus, and Turkey, according to results from viral isolation and serologic surveys.

TOSV is neurovirulent, a characteristic it shares with RVFV. Clinical cases with signs and symptoms ranging from aseptic meningitis to meningoencephalitis caused by TOSV are observed annually during the summers (see **Table 2**). All studies reported that the highest risk of acquiring TOSV is in August, which corresponds with peak sandfly activity.

Seroprevalence studies suggest that a substantial proportion of infections likely result in asymptomatic infections or cause only mild illnesses. Only severe cases, those involving CNS disease, require hospitalization.

After an incubation period ranging from a few days to 2 weeks, disease onset is intense, with headache, fever, nausea, vomiting, and myalgias. Physical examination may show neck rigidity Kernig signs, poor levels of consciousness, tremors, paresis, and nystagmus.

In most cases, cerebrospinal fluid (CSF) contains more than 5–10 cells with normal content of sugar and protein in it, or leukopenia. The mean duration of the disease is 7 days, and the outcome is usually favorable. However, a small number of severe cases with unusual symptoms have been reported. No sequelae have been described.

A study including subjects of a high-risk, professionally exposed population reported a seroprevalence of 70%, but without neurological symptoms. These data confirmed that TOSV infection can occur with either mild or no symptoms and suggest the frequent presence of TOSV infection in regions where the vector occurs.

## Diagnostic Procedures

Diagnosis of phlebovirus infections has been classically attempted by isolating the agent or demonstrating seroconversion in paired acute- and convalescent-phase serum samples. Several molecular techniques have been developed and used to demonstrate the presence of the virus or viral RNA in patient samples.

## Virus Recovery and Detection

The recovery of phleboviruses from acutely ill phlebotomus fever patients is rare, given that viremias associated with disease are transient (24–36 h) and most patients do not seek medical care within this period.

The most common method of phlebovirus isolation is intracranial inoculation of suckling mice. However, several studies have demonstrated that Vero cells (from kidney tissue of an African green monkey) are more sensitive than are newborn mice for isolation of phleboviruses from wild-caught sandflies. Similar results have been obtained with RVFV.

Identification of isolates can be made with serological methods, such as immunofluorescence, neutralization in mice, or by plaque reduction (PRNT) using hyperimmune sera. Identification can also be performed by complement fixation (CF) or hemagglutination-inhibition (HI); however, care should be taken in areas where more than one phlebovirus circulates, as these latter tests do not discriminate between certain antigenically related viruses. For example, sandfly fever Naples, Toscana, and Tehran viruses are indistinguishable by CF, yet easily identified by PRNT.

Notable diagnostic success in TOSV infections was achieved through molecular reverse transcription-polymerase chain reaction (RT-PCR) techniques. This approach has shown the occurrence of different TOSV variants.

## Serologic Tests

Serologic diagnosis can be performed with many different methods. Most of the work in the past has been done with HI. PRNT provides more clear-cut results, but this test is time consuming, and is not more useful for diagnosis than are other tests when a single serum sample is available. However, the PRNT is the most common assay for assessing antibody titer.

Enzyme-linked immunosorbent assays for IgG and IgM antibodies have been established in the case of many phleboviruses; diagnosis is obtained in most cases by detection of specific IgM antibody. The use of immunoenzymatic techniques has been very useful in the developing tests in which the recombinant nucleoprotein expressed in *Escherichia coli* is used as the specific antigen.

## Epidemiology

Epizootics of RVFV have been reported in many African countries. Prior to 1977, it was believed that the infection was confined to sub-Saharan Africa. However, the epizootic/epidemic in Egypt in 1977–78 occurred in areas outside the recognized range of the virus. Retrospective studies indicated that RVFV had not been endemic in Egypt prior to the epidemic. The epidemic occurred after the progressive implementation of the Aswan dam project, which regulated the irrigation of the Nile delta. The dam resulted in an increase in the number of breeding places of mosquitoes and also facilitated the transport of animals from Sudan to northern Egypt. From 1973 to 1976, an epizootic outbreak of RVFV occurred in Sudan, which extended from south to north and possibly reached Egypt in 1977.

RVFV was firstly detected outside Africa in September 2000. In southwestern coastal Saudi Arabia and neighboring coastal areas of Yemen, an epizootic occurred with >120 human deaths and major losses in livestock populations from disease and required slaughter. Most RVF activity was associated with flooded wadi agricultural systems; no cases were reported in the mountains or in dry sandy regions, where surface water does not accumulate long enough to sustain mosquito breeding.

Representative phleboviruses have been isolated in Southern Europe, Africa, Central Asia, and the Americas. Many phleboviruses occur in tropical and subtropical regions, but some important ones are active in temperate areas (e.g., sandfly fever Naples virus, sandfly fever Sicilian virus, and TOSV in Southern Europe and in the Middle East). Most phleboviruses (66%) have been isolated in Central and Southern America and are associated with sandflies of the genus *Lutzomyia*. On the contrary, the majority of sandfly fever viruses isolated in the Old World always are associated with *Phlebotomus* spp. sandflies.

In general, each serotype has a unique distribution, with limited geographical overlap. However, there are indications of simultaneous circulation of different phleboviruses in the same sandfly population. Sandfly fever Naples and sandfly fever Sicilian viruses have the largest geographical distributions, paralleling that of their vector *P. papatasi*. Reported isolations as well as results of serologic studies indicate that sandfly fever Naples and sandfly fever Sicilian viruses are present in the Mediterranean coastal regions of Europe and North Africa, the Nile valley, most of southwest Asia, areas adjacent to the Black and Caspian Seas, and Central Asia as far as Bangladesh.

Despite the preponderance of phleboviruses in the New World, the incidence of phlebotomus fever, and in general of human infections, in the Americas is relatively low. On the contrary, the Old World phleboviruses, such as sandfly fever Naples virus, sandfly fever Sicilian virus, and TOSV, are relatively widely distributed and are well-known causes of epidemics of human infections. In some rural human communities in endemic areas of the Old World, the prevalence of phlebovirus infection is quite high among the indigenous population. For example, results of serosurveys aimed at defining the extent and prevalence of infection with different serotypes among indigenous human populations indicated prevalences as high as 62% for Karimabad virus in some provinces of Iran and 59% for sandfly fever Sicilian and 56% for sandfly fever Naples viruses in Egypt.

A similar serosurvey for the presence of antibodies to sandfly fever Sicilian virus, sandfly fever Naples virus, and TOSV was done in 1977 in Italy. These seroepidemiological studies indicated that both sandfly fever Sicilian and sandfly fever Naples viral infections decreased after the 1940s, probably as the result of insecticide spraying during malaria eradication campaigns. On the contrary, age-specific antibody rates suggested that TOSV, which is transmitted by *P. perniciosus* and *P. perfiliewi*, is endemic in Italy. A high infection rate (24.8%) was observed among residents of the region where the virus was first isolated. Similar results have been found in other Mediterranean countries (Spain, France, Greece, Cyprus).

Because illnesses due to phlebotomus fevers have been of considerable military and historical interest, much of the early research on phlebotomus fevers was performed by military physicians and epidemiologists. In 1984, cases of sandfly fever Sicilian virus infections were documented in Cyprus among Swedish United Nations soldiers. A follow-up study revealed that 11 of 298 soldiers seroconverted to sandfly fever viruses (mostly Sicilian) during a 6 month stay in Cyprus in the summer of 1985. Infection due to sandfly fever viruses (mostly sandfly fever Sicilian virus) was diagnosed in Swedish tourists contracting a febrile illness associated with their travel during 1986–88 to the Mediterranean region. In contrast, a serological survey among Cypriots revealed a higher antibody prevalence to the sandfly fever Naples virus than to sandfly fever Sicilian virus and TOSV.

Clinical cases with signs and symptoms ranging from aseptic meningitis to meningoencephalitis caused by TOSV are observed annually in central Italy during the summer. The incidence of cases of meningitis due to TOSV is directly related to yearly differences in the density of the vector sandflies, which is greatly influenced by variations of climatic conditions. Most cases have been reported in residents or travellers in central Italy or Spain, and sporadically from other Mediterranean countries, such as Portugal, Cyprus, France, and Greece.

In Spain, TOSV is one of the three leading causes of meningitis. A large study conducted in different regions of Spain showed the presence of IgG antibodies to TOSV (26.2%), sandfly fever Naples virus (2.2%), and sandfly fever Sicilian virus (11.9%).

Studies of people living on the Ionian Islands and on the western mainland of Greece showed a seroprevalence for TOSV of 60% and 35%, respectively. It is also reported that in Cyprus 20% of the healthy population had IgG antibody to TOSV.

## Therapy

The mild nature of phlebotomus fevers has not encouraged studies on the possibility of treating the disease with specific antiviral compounds. Rather, treatment of phlebotomus fever patients is symptomatic. Due to the severity of the disease, several studies have been done both *in vitro* and *in vivo* in an effort to devise possible treatments of RVFV infections. Two different approaches have been evaluated: the use of an antiviral compound such as ribavirin or its derivatives, or the use of interferon or interferon inducers.

High doses of ribavirin have been used successfully to treat experimental infections with RVFV in several strains of mice. However, at low drug doses, treatment failures occur, resulting in death due to either hepatitis or subsequent encephalitis. Better results have been obtained when animals were treated with liposome-encapsulated ribavirin.

Experimental data and epidemiological experience suggest that the major utility of interferon in RVFV infections could most likely be in early postexposure prophylaxis (e.g., laboratory accidents, high-risk exposures). The success of interferon treatment initiated after the appearance of clinical symptoms has not been assessed. However, if maximal levels of circulating interferon in humans are obtained before early viremia, as is seen in rhesus monkeys, it is possible that interferon treatment begun at the first appearance of symptoms could affect the course of illness by limiting the incidence of future complications, particularly hemorrhagic fever. In addition, laboratory data and anecdotal information suggest that ribavirin and convalescent plasma may be beneficial in treating hemorrhagic fevers due to RVFV.

## Prevention and Control

### Vaccines

To date, there are no vaccines available against phlebotomus fever viruses. Given the large number of serotypes that can infect humans, and the lack of cross-immunity between them, to be practical a phlebotomus fever vaccine would have to be polyvalent. Moreover, in view of the relatively benign nature of the disease, vaccination against phlebotomus fever is not cost-effective or advisable as a general public health policy.

As RVFV is primarily of veterinary importance and human epidemics follow livestock epizootics, the immunization of susceptible animals is the most effective means of controlling RVFV infection.

Formalin-inactivated RVFV vaccines have been used for many years in South Africa, Egypt, and Israel to immunize sheep and cattle but they require multiple inoculations to ensure lasting protection. This type of vaccine is recommended for nonendemic areas as well as for livestock to be exported from enzootic areas.

An inactivated RVFV vaccine, developed for human use, is recommended for use to immunize at-risk laboratory and field researchers, or other people at high risk of infection. No clinical cases have been reported after vaccination; however, a few subclinical infections have been detected.

Two live RVFV vaccine candidates have been developed. One is a minute plaque variant and the other is an extensively mutagenized strain, MP-12, passaged in the diploid human lung cell line, MRC-5. Experimental studies in animals have demonstrated that a single dose of MP-12 RVFV vaccine is immunogenic and non-abortogenic in pregnant ewes. It can, therefore, be used safely to protect pregnant ewes and newborn lambs during an RVFV outbreak without increasing mortality due to vaccination.

RVFV MP12 vaccine was developed in cells certified for human vaccine production, and this vaccine may be employed for protecting both humans and livestock against epizootic RVFV infection. Because it is attenuated, this vaccine may be used to prevent an impending RVFV outbreak in an area where the virus is nonendemic, without the risk of spread to the environment.

## Prevention of Transmission

During the Egyptian epidemic of RVFV in 1977–78, insecticides were used both inside and outside human and animal shelters to reduce the adult populations of mosquito vectors. However, it was not demonstrated that the use of these chemicals actually decreased the incidence of the disease. In sub-Saharan Africa, where RVFV outbreaks are thought to occur following flooding of vector mosquito breeding habitats, the possibility of using encapsulated formulations of insecticides to control the larval stages has been considered.

Measurements of green leaf vegetation dynamics recorded by advanced very high resolution radiometer instruments on polar-orbiting, meteorological satellites were used to derive ground moisture and rainfall patterns in Kenya and monitor resulting flooding of mosquito larval habitats likely to support RVFV vector mosquitoes (*Aedes* spp. and *Culex* spp.). These data could be used by local authorities for implementations of specific mosquito control measures to prevent transmission of RVFV to susceptible vertebrate hosts.

At present, the only method effective in controlling phlebotomus fevers is to reduce human contact with the vectors that carry their etiologic agents. Insecticides are extremely effective in the control of peridomestic sandfly species, but are of little value for sylvan species. Mechanical means (e.g., protective clothing, bed nets and screening of windows) and use of repellents, such as diethyltoluamide, can also be used to prevent human–vector contact.

## Further Reading

Baldelli F, Ciufolini MG, Francisci D, *et al.* (2004) Unusual presentation of life-threatening TOSV meningoencephalitis. *Clinical Infectious Diseases* 38: 515–520.

Balkhy HH and Memish ZA (2003) Rift Valley fever: An uninvited zoonosis in the Arabian peninsula. *International Journal of Antimicrobial Agents* 21: 153–157.

Braito A, Corbisiero R, Corradini S, *et al.* (1997) Evidence of Toscana virus infections without central nervous system involvement: A serological study. *European Journal of Epidemiology* 13: 761–764.

Charrel RN, Gallian P, Navarro-Mari JM, *et al.* (2005) Emergence of Toscana virus in Europe. *Emerging Infectious Diseases* 11(11): 1657–1663.

Ciufolini MG, Maroli M, Guandalini E, Marchi A, and Verani P (1989) Experimental studies on the maintenance of Toscana and Arbia viruses (*Bunyaviridae: Phlebovirus*). *American Journal of Tropical Medicine and Hygiene* 40: 669–675.

Flick R and Bouloy M (2005) Rift Valley fever virus. *Current Molecular Medicine* 5: 827–834.

Geisbert TW and Jahrling PB (2004) Exotic emerging viral diseases: Progress and challenges. *Nature Medicine* 10: S110–S121.

Nicoletti L, Verani P, Caciolli S, *et al.* (1991) Central nervous system involvement during infection by the phlebovirus Toscana of residents in natural foci in central Italy (1977–1988). *American Journal of Tropical Medicine and Hygiene* 45: 429–434.

Nicoletti L, Ciufolini MG, and Verani P (1996) Sandfly fever viruses in Italy. *Archives of Virology Supplement* 11: 41–47.

Sánchez Seco MP, Echevarría JM, Hernández L, Estévez D, Navarro-Marí JM, and Tenorio A (2003) Detection and identification of Toscana and other phleboviruses by RT-PCR assays with degenerated primers. *Journal of Medical Virology* 71: 140–149.

Torres-Velez F and Brown C (2004) Emerging infections in animals – potential new zoonoses? *Clinics in Laboratory Medicine* 24: 825–838.

Weaver SC (2005) Host range, amplification and arboviral disease emergence. *Archives of Virology Supplement* 19: 33–44.

## Relevant Website

http://www.cdc.gov – CDC Special Pathogens Branch, Centers for Disease Control and Prevention.

# Rinderpest and Distemper Viruses

**T Barrett,** Institute for Animal Health, Pirbright, UK

## Glossary

**Cytopathic effect** Alterations in the microscopic appearance of cultured cells following virus infection.
**Enzootic** A disease constantly present in an animal community in a defined geographic region.
**Epizootiology** The study of disease epidemics in animal populations.
**Hemagglutinin** Any substance that causes red blood cells to agglutinate; many viruses possess a hemagglutinin protein in the outer envelope.

## History

Rinderpest and its related viruses form a distinct group of paramyxoviruses, the genus *Morbillivirus*. In addition to measles virus (MV), the type virus of the genus, they include important animal pathogens: rinderpest virus (RPV), which infects many species of large ruminant; peste des petits ruminants virus (PPRV), a similar disease of small ruminants; canine distemper virus (CDV), found mainly in carnivores; phocid distemper virus (PDV), in seals; and the cetacean morbillivirus (CeMV), which is found in whales, dolphins, and porpoises. Of the animal viruses, rinderpest is the most important economically. It was also known as cattle plague in the past because of the high mortality associated with infections and the speed with which it spreads in naive cattle populations, which made it an easily recognizable disease. It is one of the oldest documented plagues of domestic livestock. Aristotle (384–322 BC) described a disease in cattle, *struma*, that had all the characteristics of rinderpest and other descriptions date to the fourth century when invasion by Huns into Europe resulted in outbreak of highly contagious disease which had all the characteristics of rinderpest. Steppe cattle of Central Asia are thought to be the original source of rinderpest and 'steepe murrain' was the old English name for the disease. Panzootics of rinderpest were also brought to western Europe with the Mongol invasions in the thirteenth century. In 1709, the disease again entered Europe through Venetian trade with the east and by 1714 had spread as far west as Britain. The economic and social consequences which followed in the wake of these plagues led to the establishment of the first veterinary schools – the first at Lyon, France, in 1762. Other European countries followed France's example and set up their own veterinary schools. Subsequent

brief reintroductions into Europe in the early twentieth century, and into South America and Australia through the import of infected cattle led to the establishment of the Office Internationale des Epizooties (OIE), a body that functions as the World Organisation for Animal Health, to deal specifically with animal diseases in relation to international trade.

Rinderpest was introduced into Africa with disastrous consequences in the late 1880s with cattle imported from India to feed Italian troops in fighting a colonial war in Abyssinia (now Ethiopia). The subsequent panzootic spread to nearly all parts of the African continent within a period of 10 years, reaching South Africa by 1897. The devastation that followed its path as it swept across the African continent wiped out 90% of the domestic cattle and wild buffalo (*Syncerus caffer*). A number of other large wild ruminant species were also highly susceptible to the virus and died in large numbers during this so-called 'Great African Pandemic'.

A similar plague of small ruminants, peste des petits ruminants (PPR), was first scientifically documented in West Africa in the early 1940s and is also known as *kata* in that region. At first, it was thought that PPRV was a variant of RPV adapted to small ruminants but it was subsequently shown to be a genetically distinct virus with an independent epizootiology in areas where both viruses co-circulated.

Canine distemper, which infects many terrestrial carnivore species, is also a disease with a long history. In the eighteenth century, Edward Jenner studied its neurological effects following infection in dogs. In 1988, a distinct but closely related virus, phocine distemper virus (PDV), was isolated from seals found dying in large numbers along the beaches of Northern Europe and which showed clinical signs similar to distemper in dogs. Both harbor (*Phoca vitulina*) and gray (*Halichoerus grypus*) seals were affected and the epizootic resulted in the deaths of more than 20 000 seals. In 1990, large numbers of striped dolphins (*Stenella coeruleoalba*) in the Mediterranean Sea were found dying from a similar infection and a virus was isolated from sick animals. This virus has since been associated with mass die-offs among whales, porpoises, and dolphins (order *Cetacea*) and a fatal epizootic in bottlenose dolphins (*Tursiops truncatus*) from the northwestern Atlantic Ocean in the 1980s. A morbillivirus was also isolated from diseased porpoises (*Phocoena phocoena*) found along the coasts of Ireland and the Netherlands between 1988 and 1990 during the epizootic of PDV in seals. This virus was later found to be very closely related to the dolphin virus and genetically quite distinct from all other morbilliviruses. The dolphin and porpoise virus isolates are now commonly referred to as CeMV, and these virus infections have the potential to cause severe disease and threaten the ecology of many marine mammal species.

## Taxonomy and Classification

As indicated above, these antigenically closely related viruses are classified in the genus *Morbillivirus* within order *Mononegavirales*, family *Paramyxoviridae*, subfamily *Paramyxovirinae*. The name is derived from the diminutive (*morbilli*) of the Latin word *morbus* meaning 'little plague', to distinguish measles from deadlier diseases such as smallpox. The paramyxoviruses are large enveloped pleimorphic particles which bud from the surface of infected cells and the different species are indistinguishable in the electron microscope. They vary in diameter from 300 to 500 nm. The lipid envelope is derived from the host cell membrane as the virions bud from the cell and it encloses a ribonucleoprotein (RNP) core which contains the genome encapsidated by the nucleocapsid protein giving it a characteristic 'herring bone' appearance. Unlike other paramyxoviruses, the morbilliviruses generally lack neuraminidase but a highly substrate-specific neuraminidase activity has been reported for PPRV and RPV. Only MV and PPRV viruses can hemagglutinate red blood cells reproducibly.

## Geographic Distribution

Until the mid-1980s, rinderpest was found in much of tropical Africa and in western and southern Asia. Control and eradication program were established in the mid-1980s and this effort, based on mass vaccination campaigns in the endemic regions, has succeeded in eliminating the disease from Asia and the Middle East; the virus is now almost certainly confined to a defined region of eastern Africa known as the southern Somali ecosystem, a region in eastern Africa comprising southeast Ethiopia, southern Somalia, and northeast Kenya.

PPR is enzootic in West Africa and on the Indian subcontinent and is now spreading from Afghanistan into Central Asia (**Figure 1**). It first appeared as a recognized disease in India in 1988 and has subsequently been found as far east as Bangladesh and north as far as Nepal. Epizootics regularly occur in the Middle East and Turkey through import of infected animals. Turkey's proximity to Southern Europe poses a threat to small ruminants in that region. The widespread distribution of PPRV in southwest Asia suggests that the virus had been present on the continent for some considerable time before it was identified in India. Its presence was most likely masked by

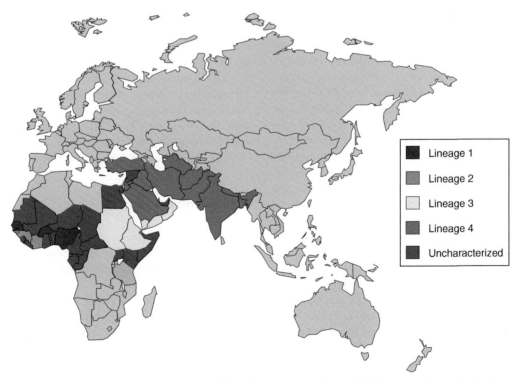

**Figure 1**   The distribution of PPRV. Where known, the different lineages are color-coded. There are only serological or capture enzyme-linked immunosorbent assay (ELISA) data available for countries shown in red.

rinderpest since all morbillivirus-like diseases in small ruminants in India before 1988 were considered to be caused by rinderpest infections. With the subsequent elimination of rinderpest from Asia and the development of more accurate diagnostic techniques it has now become easier to chart the spread of PPRV in the region.

CDV is found in all but the hottest and most arid regions of the globe. The development of attenuated live vaccines in the late 1950s greatly reduced the incidence of the disease in domestic dogs in developed countries. However, many wildlife species are susceptible to CDV infection and can act as reservoirs for the virus. CDV has also been found in Lake Baikal seals (*Phoca sibirica*) and Caspian Sea seals (*Phoca caspica*) and it poses a threat to the survival of the latter species which is highly endangered. There is also serological evidence for infection in Antarctic seals and, as there are no native carnivores on that continent, unvaccinated sledge dogs are blamed for introducing the virus.

The geographic distribution of PDV is not fully defined but, based on serological evidence, it appears to be an endemic infection in some species of seal in the northern Atlantic and Arctic oceans. These are considered to be the most likely source of PDV for the European seal epizootics. The CeMV appears to have a worldwide distribution and there is serological evidence for the presence of this virus in diverse species from all of the world's major oceans.

## Host Range Virus

Each morbillivirus is generally able to cause serious disease only in one order of mammals, the exception being CDV. All cloven-hoofed animals (Artiodactyla) are thought to be susceptible to infection with RPV but the disease is not manifest in all. In the case of cattle, Indian and African breeds (*Bos indicus*, zebu) are more resistant than European (*Bos taurus*). The virus can also infect a range of wild ungulates but disease progression depends on the innate resistance of the species concerned. Some, such as kudu (*Tragelaphus imberbis*), eland (*Taurotragus* spp.), giraffe (*Giraffa* spp.), and wildebeest (*Connochaetes* spp.), are highly susceptible to the virus and died in large numbers during the first African pandemic. Others, mainly small antelope species, proved to be more resistant (**Table 1**).

The full host range of PPRV is unknown but, in addition to sheep and goats, several species of antelope have been fatally infected by contact with infected sheep. Outbreaks of PPRV have been reported in game reserves and zoos where the mortality was 100% in some species. Goats are generally considered to be more sensitive to PPRV infection than sheep. Indian buffaloes (*Bulbalus bulbalis*) have also been reported to have died from

**Table 1**    Susceptibility of wildlife to rinderpest

| Very high | Buffalo, eland, kudu, wart hog |
|---|---|
| High | Giraffe, bushbuck, bush pig, sitatunga, Uganda cob, bongo, wildebeest |
| Moderate | Reedbuck, topi, gemsbok, blesbok, bontbok, oribi, impala, springbok |
| Low | Waterbuck, dukier, orynx, Grant's gazelle, dikdik, hartebeest |
| Very low | Thomson's gazelle, hippopotamus, gerenuk |

Based on data from Plowright W (1982) The effects of rinderpest and rinderpest control on wildlife in Africa. In: Edwards MA and McDonald U (eds.) *Symposia of the Zoological Society of London, No. 50: Animal Diseases in Relation to Animal Conservation*, p. 1. London: Academic Press.

PPRV infections. Cattle have been found in West Africa which were seropositive for PPRV, with up to 80% prevalence in some herds, but there is no evidence that it can cause disease in cattle.

CDV can infect most carnivores but in some it may result in only a mild or subclinical infection, for example, in domestic cats. It causes severe disease in all members of the Canidae (dog, wolf, fox), Mustelidae (ferret, weasel, mink), Procyonidae (raccoon, panda), as well as in collared peccaries (*Tayassu tajacu*, order Artiodactyla). More recently, CDV has been shown to be responsible for high mortalities in both wild and captive big cats and in hyenas (*Crocuta crocuta*). Failure to recognise the disease earlier in these species may have been due to a lack of awareness of a possible viral etiology and/or the availability of diagnostic tools to detect the virus. Outbreaks of CDV in Siberian and Caspian seals have extended its host range to include these species. PDV is known to infect many species of seal in the North Atlantic and Arctic oceans but its full host range is unknown. There is also serological evidence that terrestrial carnivores in Canada, including polar bear (*Ursus maritimus*), lynx (*Fellis lynx*), and wolves (*Canis lupus*), have been infected with the virus and also with CeMV. CeMV infections have been described in a variety of cetaceans and there are serological data indicating infection in many more.

## Virus Propagation

All known morbilliviruses can be propagated on Vero cells, which lack the ability to produce interferon, but it generally requires several blind passages to adapt the virus to these cells. This adaptation can alter the receptor-binding characteristics of the virus and often attenuates it for the natural host. Clinical isolates of rinderpest that retain their pathogenicity can best be grown on primary bovine kidney cells or transformed lymphoid cell lines such as B95a cells. PPRV is normally grown on lamb kidney cells and primary mitogen-stimulated dog or ferret macrophages are the most suitable cells for the isolation of CDV. Alternatively, Madin–Darby canine kidney (MDCK) cells have been shown to be useful for CDV isolation from infected tissues. Primary seal kidney cells were initially used to isolate PDV. Virus is most readily obtained from tissues such as mucosal lesions, lymph nodes, or by co-cultivation of washed buffy coat from infected animals with suitable tissue culture cells. Lung tissue is also a good source of virus for PPRV, CDV, and PDV isolation. Typical cytopathic effects such as cell elongation, cell rounding, the formation of stellate cells, and syncytia can be observed 3–12 days post infection of the cell cultures although several blind passages may sometimes be necessary before cytopathic changes are observed.

Host range is to some extent, but not completely, determined by the expression of a suitable receptor on the host cell. The CD150 molecule, also known as signal lymphocyte activating molecule or SLAM, is thought to be the main cellular receptor for wild-type RPV, CDV, and MV isolates. SLAMs specific to their respective host species may be general morbillivirus receptors. CDV replicates better and causes extensive cell fusion in Vero cells expressing dog SLAM (Vero DST) compared to normal Vero cells and these are a better cell line for propagation and titration of CDV isolates. The expression of SLAM on cells of lymphoid origin, activated lymphocytes, immature thymocytes, macrophages, and mature dendritic cells explains the strong lymphotropism of these viruses. Tissue culture-adapted viruses can use other receptors such as CD46. Alterations in receptor recognition could possibly be a means whereby these viruses could widen their host range in future.

## Properties of the Genome

The morbillivirus genomes consist of a single strand of negative-sense RNA just under 16 kbp in length. They are organized into six contiguous, nonoverlapping, transcription units which encode the six structural proteins, namely the nucleocapsid (N), the phospho (P), the matrix (M), the fusion (F), the hemagglutinin (H), and the large (L) proteins, the latter being the viral RNA-dependent RNA polymerase. They have highly conserved sequences at their 3′ (leader) and 5′ (trailer) terminal extremities that act as promoters for transcription and replication (**Figure 2**). The complete promoter elements include sequences that extend into the untranslated region at the start of the N gene open reading frame (ORF) and the untranslated region at the end of the L gene ORF. These regions contain all the *cis*-acting signals necessary for primary transcription as well as for the production of a full-length positive-sense RNA genome copy required for the production of new genome RNA. There are semi-conserved start–stop sequence motifs at the start and end

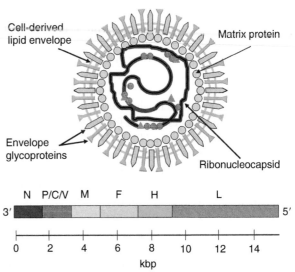

**Figure 2** Cartoon showing the structure of morbillivirus virions. The outer envelope is shown with two projecting glycoproteins (H and F) and the inner helical nucleocapsid containing the genome RNA encapsidated with the N protein and the P and L proteins associated with it. The matrix protein is shown as a ring of circles underneath the virus envelope. The linear order of genes in the genome RNA from 3′ to 5′ is also shown.

of each mRNA transcription unit: (UCCU/C) at each transcription start; and a sequence rich in U residues, which signals the polyadenylation of the mRNAs, at the end. Between the end of one transcription unit and the start of the next is an intergenic triplet (usually GAA) which is not translated into mRNA. Downstream mRNA synthesis depends on termination of the upstream mRNA. The N, P, and L proteins, along with the genome RNA, constitute the transcription/replication unit of the virus, the RNP core. The F and H glycoproteins are embedded in a lipid envelope which is derived from the host cell during the budding process. The nonglycosylated M interacts with cytoplasmic domains of the membrane-associated F and H proteins and also with the nucleocapsid RNPs formed in the cytoplasm during replication and brings together the two components that make up the budded virion. The M protein is essential for efficient virus budding to occur.

Morbilliviruses also produce two nonstructural proteins (C and V) encoded in the P gene transcription unit. The first of these, the C protein, is translated by ribosomes that scan past the first AUG codon and start at the second which is located about 20 nt downstream. This protein is in a different reading frame to the P protein and bears no antigenic relationship to it. The second nonstructural protein, the V protein, in derived by alternative transcription of an mRNA from the P transcription unit by which a nontemplated G residue added to approximately 50% of the P mRNAs. The extra Gs are inserted at a specific, highly conserved, sequence

(5′ UUAAAAAGGG[G]CACAG), known as the editing site, positioned about halfway along the P protein ORF. This so-called editing process is a property of the virus polymerase as it does not occur in artificial transcription systems. Translation of this mRNA produces the V protein which is a chimeric protein consisting of the N-terminus of the P protein with a new, shorter C-terminus rich in cysteine residues derived from template sequence in the third reading frame. The V mRNA is also capable of translating the C protein as its coding region is located before the editing site in P. The nonstructural proteins have functions in controlling transcription and replication and also are involved in virus evasion of the host's innate immune responses.

Morbilliviruses, like some other paramyxoviruses, have a strict genome length requirement in that they should be divisible by 6 (the 'rule of six'). This requirement can be explained by the fact that each N protein monomer associates with exactly 6 nt and that efficient transcription and/or replication can only occur if the RNA genome is encapsidated by the N protein in its entirety. Reverse genetics systems have been established for MV, RPV, and CDV. This enables virus to be 'rescued' from a DNA copy of its genome and this copy can be manipulated to make virus mutants which can then be used to determine the functions of various proteins and sequence motifs and to study the molecular basis of host range and pathogenicity.

## Evolution

The close antigenic relationship and sequence similarity of morbilliviruses indicate that they all evolved from a common ancestor; however, the details of their evolutionary history are unclear. The phylogenetic relationship between the different morbilliviruses, based on the sequence of the P proteins, is shown in **Figure 3**. RPV, PPRV, CDV, and CeMV are equidistant from each other. It appears, therefore, that no existing morbillivirus represents the ancestral virus. MV is genetically more closely related to RPV and PDV to CDV, suggesting that they evolved more recently from their respective common ancestors. A factor that must be considered in their evolutionary history is that animals which have recovered from morbillivirus infections are immune for life and so fairly large populations are required to ensure a constant supply of naive hosts needed to maintain these viruses in circulation. The minimum population size that satisfies this requirement has been estimated to be about 300 000 for MV, and so this virus could not have existed before settled human populations became large enough. Herds of ruminants roaming the steppes of Central Asia, the historic source of rinderpest, would, however, have been able to maintain a morbillivirus in circulation. It is

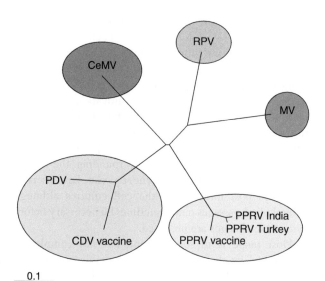

**Figure 3**   Radial tree showing the morbillivirus phylogenetic relationships based on their P protein sequences. The P proteins were aligned using ClustalW (BLOSUM) matrix program. A neighbor-joining radial tree was then generated from this alignment using ClustalX v1.83 and TreeView v1.6.6. Three different PPRV sequences were included to show the extent of variation within each morbillivirus type. The PPRV vaccine and PPRV Turkey are the most distant viruses in the group. Access numbers: RPV (X98291); PPRV (AY560591, X74443, AJ849636); CDV (AF305419); PDV (D10371); DMV (AJ608288); MV (AB012948).

probable that when human communities became large enough, rinderpest, or a rinderpest-like infection, was passed to them from their domesticated cattle. RPV and PPRV are equidistant from the putative ancestral virus and so PPRV did not evolve directly from RPV and must have had a long independent evolutionary history in small ruminants.

Carnivores preying on infected ruminants may similarly have become infected with the progenitor morbillivirus which subsequently evolved in these species to become CDV. CDV infects a wide variety of carnivores and so there is potentially a large reservoir of virus in susceptible wildlife species. PDV most probably evolved quite recently from CDV. Seals have many opportunities to become infected with CDV by contact with terrestrial carnivores such as wolves, foxes, dogs, and polar bears. Arctic seals populations, unlike European seal populations, are large enough to enable a morbillivirus to be maintained and subsequent evolution would select a virus more adapted to replicate efficiently in seals.

The two CeMVs that have been isolated from dolphins and porpoises are very closely related to each other, as related as different lineages of either RPV or PPRV, and can be considered to constitute one virus species. CeMV is antigenically closest to PPRV but is equidistant for the putative ancestral virus by sequence analysis and so this virus also has had a long independent evolutional history.

## Serological Relationships and Variability

All the morbilliviruses are antigenically related, the F, M, and N proteins being the most highly conserved across the group. The two virus-coded glycoproteins, the H and F, are embedded in the virus envelope and neutralizing antibody responses are generated to both of these proteins. The H protein, responsible for attachment of the virions to the host cell surface receptor molecule and is therefore a determinant of host range, is the least cross-reactive of the morbillivirus proteins. While it is possible to differentiate strains of each morbillivirus by monoclonal antibody and sequence analysis, these variations do not result in different serotypes and for vaccination purposes each morbillivirus has only one serotype.

## Epizootiology

Rinderpest and PPR are normally introduced into new regions by importation of live animals. Transmission through infected meat and meat products is considered to be a very low risk due to the highly labile nature of the viruses. Historically, rinderpest outbreaks have been associated with wars and civil conflict when there is uncontrolled movement of people and troops, often bringing live animals from enzootic regions as food. Sheep and goats, and possibly other ruminants, may show only mild disease or subclinical infection with RPV but nevertheless they can then pass the infection to in-contact cattle. Trade in live animals is also another factor that has been responsible for long-distance spread of rinderpest.

Epizootics of rinderpest in naive populations are generally very severe and mortality rates can exceed 90% and affect all age groups, the classic characteristics of cattle plague. The last outbreak of this nature occurred in Pakistan in 1994. In endemic areas, disease is less severe and most often affects animals less than 2 years of age as older animals are generally immune due to previous exposure or vaccination. Newborns are protected for up to 9 months by maternal antibody. The rinderpest virus strain in circulation in the last enzootic focus in Africa belongs to African lineage 2 (**Figure 4(a)**) and is unusual in that it causes only mild disease in cattle. It becomes clinically apparent when it spreads to highly susceptible wildlife species such as buffalo, eland, and kudu. These have suffered very high mortalities when infected with this strain of virus during outbreaks in Kenyan national parks and because of this wildlife are considered excellent sentinels for incursions of rinderpest. They are closely monitored for evidence of reintroduction of the virus from its only known enzootic focus in the southern Somali ecosystem.

PPRV shows a similar epizootiology and can also cause very high mortalities in naive populations of sheep and goats. Introductions into disease-free areas are usually traceable to movement of infected animals from enzootic regions. Phylogenetic analysis on PPRV strains reveals that there are four distinct lineages in circulation (**Figure 4(b)**). PPRV infections in wildlife have not been studied in any detail but the severity of disease when it occurs in captive small ruminants infected by contact with domestic livestock makes it unlikely that there is a significant wildlife reservoir of the virus.

CDV causes periodic epizootics in domesticated dogs and wild carnivores and it remains a problem in poor urban areas where there are many stray dogs and vaccination is not carried out rigorously. In enzootic areas, the density of the susceptible population is an important factor in determining the frequency of epizootics and can also affect its maintenance and spread. Again, disease is most often seen in young animals after maternal antibody has waned. A variety of wild carnivore species are highly susceptible to CDV infections and presence of the virus can be a high-risk factor for some endangered species.

The source of PDV in the two epizootics that occurred in European seals is thought to have been either Canadian harp seals (*Phoca groenlandica*) or Arctic ringed seals (*Phoca hispida*). Retrospective analysis of seal sera from Canada dating back to the early 1980s showed that they were positive for virus-specific antibodies. The two European PDV epizootics, in 1988 and 2002, were remarkably similar and this may be explained by the susceptibility, migratory patterns, and/or breeding habits of the seals. The gray seal is the most likely candidate to act as the vector in the transmission of PDV between Arctic and European seals and between colonies of harbor seals as they are known to move much greater distances between haulout sites. Another important factor is the relative resistance of gray seals to the disease, possibly enabling PDV to circulate in that population without necessarily causing high mortality.

The pilot whale (*Globicephala* spp.) is considered to be the most likely endemic source of CeMV and also the vector for its transmission to other species. Pilot whale populations have the characteristics required for both; they move in large groups (pods), have a widespread pelagic distribution, and are known to associate with many different cetacean species. A high proportion of pilot whales sampled in the mid-1990s showed evidence of infection and over 90% of pilot whales that were involved in mass strandings between 1982 and 1993 were seropositive for morbillivirus.

## Transmission

All morbilliviruses are extremely labile in the environment and are inactivated by heat, ultraviolet (UV) light, and chemicals that alter pH or destroy their lipid envelopes.

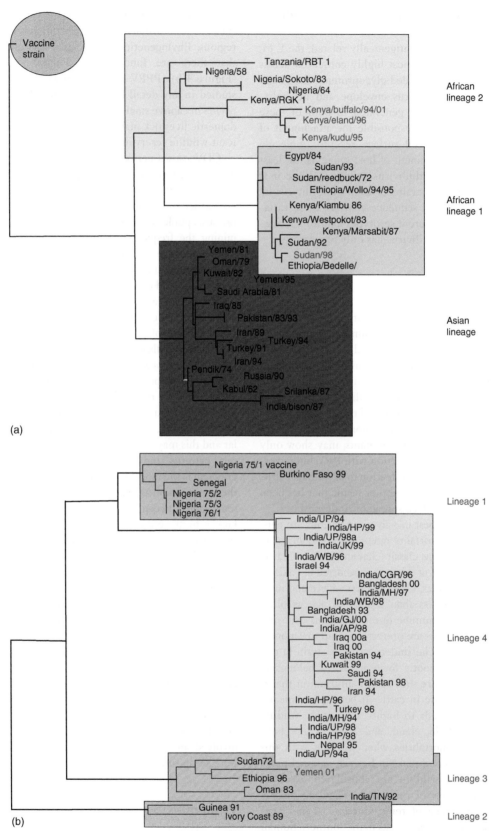

**Figure 4** A computer-generated tree showing the relationship between (a) the African and Asian lineages of rinderpest virus and (b) the currently circulating PPRV lineages. The trees were generated using the PHYLIP program using partial sequence data from the F protein gene. Only RPV African lineage 2 remains extant and the outbreaks in Kenya since 1994 are highlighted in red. The vaccine strain of rinderpest dates to the early part of the twentieth century and was used as the outgroup in the rinderpest and PPRV analysis.

Therefore, although highly contagious, they require close contact between infected and susceptible animals for their transmission which normally occurs via infected air droplets. All secretions and excretions potentially harbor virus and, along with fomites, can also be a source of infection. In the case of seals, contact at haulout sites allows the proximity required for aerosol transmission.

## Clinical Features of Infection

Morbillivirus infections begin in the upper respiratory tract and, after a variable incubation period spread from the local draining lymph nodes via the lymph and blood to other lymphatic tissues and then to the upper and lower respiratory tracts, gastrointestinal mucosa and in some cases the brain. With virulent strains, there is a marked leucopenia leading to a deficiency in the immune system. The incubation period ranges from 3 to 6 days in natural infections or following experimental parenteral inoculation. With less virulent strains of RPV, the incubation period can extend to 15 days and in many cases there may be no clinical signs but the animals seroconvert. The cell (epithelial and lymphoid) tropisms explain the pathological signs most associated with morbillivirus-induced disease: mucocutaneous lesions, severe infection in the gastrointestinal tract; and destruction of the lymphoid organs and consequent immunosuppression. In some cases, skin lesions can be associated with RPV infection but this is not a common finding. Hyperkeratosis of the cornea leading to blindness is a striking feature seen in kudu. Pneumonia is less marked in RPV than in PPRV and other morbillivirus infections.

In CDV infections, the incubation period can range from 1 to 6 weeks. Animals then show an initial febrile response and develop clinical signs commonly seen in other morbillivirus infections: mucopurulent nasal and ocular discharges, vomiting, diarrhoea, and pneumonia. Neurological signs such as convulsions, tremors, and seizures or behavioral changes are seen and they can develop acutely or weeks or months later or they may follow a subclinical infection. Recovered dogs frequently show persistent nervous tics or involuntary movements of one or more legs. In some cases, a hyperkeratosis (hard pad) develops on the foot pads.

Seals infected with either CDV or PDV also show the usual signs associated with a morbillivirus infection, fever, serous or mucopurulent oculonasal discharge, conjunctivitis, dyspnea, diarrhea, lethargy, and abortion in pregnant females. Bronchopneumonia is the most marked pathological feature in aquatic and marine mammal infections (CDV, PDV, and CeMV) which severely affects the animal's ability to dive and forage for food and quickly results in loss of body condition and a reduced blubber thickness. During the epizootic in the Mediterranean in 1990–91, many striped dolphins (*Stenella coeruleoalba*) were also found to be in poor body condition and loss of fat stores led to decreased buoyancy. Skin lesions, necrosis of the buccal mucosa, lymphodepletion, and hemoconcentration were commonly observed. Neurological signs similar to those found in CDV infections are a feature of both PDV and CeMV infections.

## Pathology and Histopathology

The severity of gross pathological lesions observed in RPV and PPRV infections, like the clinical signs observed, is related to the virulence of the virus strain involved. Erosions and ulcerations are found in the upper respiratory, urinogenital, and digestive tracts. In the small intestine there is necrosis and destruction of Peyer's patches. Destruction of the epithelial lining of the gut is responsible for the severe bloody diarrhea seen in acute cases and the packed cell volume can be increased by 40–65%. In the cecum, colon, and rectum of animals infected with RPV and PPRV, so-called 'zebra' or 'tiger' stripes are often found and result from the distension of blood vessels packed with erythrocytes. Dehydration also causes changes in hematology and blood chemistry. A nonsuppurative encephalitis with central nervous system (CNS) degeneration occurs during infections with CDV, PDV, and CeMV, but no CNS involvement has ever been reported in ruminants infected with either RPV or PPRV. Immunosuppression associated with morbillivirus infections can lead secondary bacterial infections which may complicate both the clinical and pathological findings and latent or concurrent infections can be activated.

Histologically, the morbilliviruses show a strong tropism for epithelial and lymphoid cells and all lymphoid organs are affected with damage to the mesenteric lymph nodes, the gut-associated lymphoid tissue, the lymphoid follicles of tonsils, lymph nodes, spleen, and mucosa-associated lymphoid tissues, where severe destruction of the B- and T-cell areas is seen in infections with virulent strains. Mild strains induce less extensive lymphoid destruction and mucosal lesions and in these animals tissue samples show unremarkable histopathological changes in the gastrointestinal tract and the lymphoid tissues and this may account for the reduced ability for these strains to transmit by contact.

## Immune Response

There is a strong cell-mediated component in the response to morbillivirus infection and immunosuppressed individuals are known to be at extreme risk from MV. Neutralizing antibodies are generated only in response to the H and F glycoproteins and vaccines containing purified

H or F proteins are effective only if administered with a strong cytotoxic T-cell-stimulating adjuvant, for example, Quil A (ISCOM vaccines). Inactivated whole virus vaccines give only a poor and short-lived protection. Both the H or F proteins can confer immunity to disease as poxvirus recombinant vaccines expressing either of these glycoproteins can confer fairly long-term (up to 3 years) immunity to clinical disease. In addition, RPV recombinants can also confer cross-immunity to PPR disease in the absence of cross-neutralizing antibodies. All morbillivirus infections appear to give lifelong protection against disease but it is not clear if subclinical reinfection can occur.

## Prevention and Control

In 1711, during a prolonged epizootic of rinderpest in Italy, the Pope's physician, Giovani Lancisi, promulgated rules to deal with the disease in cattle. He insisted on movement controls on all animals in the areas affected, the slaughter of diseased and in-contact cattle, and their burial in lime. He also introduced the idea of quarantine and his policies were backed by strong legal enforcement with severe punishments for transgressors, principles which are still applied today to control animal diseases. This approach, along with import restrictions on cattle from the East, succeeded in controlling the disease in Europe and by the beginning of the twentieth century western Europe was free of enzootic rinderpest. However, these conditions are not always easy to impose in developing countries.

The existence of only one serotype for each of the morbilliviruses, the absence of persistence of infectious virus, and lifelong immunity after recovery from the initial acute infection suggest that outbreaks of these viruses should be easy to control. In addition, the morbilliviruses need close contact for infection to occur, are labile and do not survive long in the environment, and disinfection of infected premises is fairly straightforward. These characteristics of the virus, and the availability of a safe and effective vaccine, were the main drivers for the decision to try to control rinderpest following its resurgence in the early 1980s. International rinderpest control campaigns were begun in the late 1980s, and in 1992 the United Nations Food and Agriculture Organisation (FAO) recommended the global eradication of rinderpest as an internationally coordinated program. In 1994, this became the Global Rinderpest Eradication Programme (GREP), a time-bound program to eliminate rinderpest from the world by the year 2010.

All this effort has succeeded in eradicating the virus from Asia and has eliminated it from most of Africa. The last outbreak of rinderpest occurred in India in 1995 and in Pakistan in 2000. In Africa, the last confirmed case caused by African lineage 1 virus was in southern Sudan in 1998 and so this has probably been eliminated in the field, while the last confirmed case of African lineage 2 was in buffalo in Meru National Park in 2001. Meru is in northeastern Kenya, within the southern Somalia ecosystem, and the major obstacle to completing the GREP by the projected date of 2010 is the continuation of conflict in Somalia.

It was feared that even if rinderpest were eliminated from the domestic cattle populations wild ruminants might act as a reservoir of infection, but history shows that when the disease is eliminated from cattle it disappears from surrounding wildlife, as evidenced by its disappearance from Tanzania, South Africa, and southern Kenya, areas of the continent with many wildlife species. Nevertheless, during outbreaks, rinderpest-infected wildlife can help spread the disease over large distances.

In contrast, only limited resources have been directed to solving the problem of PPRV although a very effective live-attenuated vaccine is also available. From an economic and social perspective, PPR is now considered to be of great importance as it threatens small-ruminant production, the mainstay of many subsistence farmers in much of the developing world.

CDV vaccines have been very effective in controlling infections in domestic dogs; however, not much can be done to prevent infections in wild carnivores, seals, dolphins, and whales. Even if good vaccines were available, vaccination of wild animal populations is logistically very difficult. There are also ethical issues to take into account, such as the potential for uncontrolled spread of vaccine, which may not be attenuated for all species, and the disturbance caused to the animals which may also be harmful.

## Diagnosis

Rapid and accurate diagnosis is the key to success in controlling morbillivirus outbreaks in domestic livestock. Clinical signs, however, are not always clear enough to make a confirmatory diagnosis, even when severe clinical signs are evident, as other viruses can mimic those commonly seen in morbillivirus infections. For example, rinderpest and bovine viral diarrhea viruses are often confused and PPRV can be mistaken for pasteurellosis or other microbial pneumonias. Confirmatory laboratory diagnosis is therefore essential.

Simple and rapid diagnostic tests such as capture enzyme-linked immunosorbent assay (ELISA) and reverse-transcriptase polymerase chain reaction (RT-PCR) have been developed for RPV and PPRV in recent years, and, since these are easy to use for analyzing large numbers of samples, these are now favored for virus detection. With RT-PCR, the DNA product can be sequenced and used for phylogenetic analysis that can be used to identify the strain of virus involved and the potential source of virus entering a new region.

For serological detection of morbillivirus antibodies, the ELISA format is favored and the success of the rinderpest eradication campaign depended to a large extent on the ability to seromonitor large herds following vaccination. The test is based on the use of a highly specific monoclonal antibody directed against the H protein of RPV in a competitive ELISA format. A companion test for the detection of PPRV antibodies is also available.

## Vaccination

The first attenuated rinderpest vaccines were produced in the 1930s when the virus was adapted to replicate in goats (caprinized) and rabbits (lapinized). In the 1940s, a chick embryo-(avianized) adapted vaccine was produced. These vaccines were widely used but they had drawbacks in that they were not fully attenuated and could cause disease in more susceptible breeds. In the early1960s, a tissue culture-adapted strain of RPV, the 'Plowright vaccine', was developed by multiple passage of the virus in primary bovine kidney cells. The vaccine is relatively easy to produce, safe for use in all cattle breeds, and does not spread by contact. It is highly effective in preventing disease and the immunity induced in vaccinated cattle proved to be lifelong. This vaccine has been used successfully since the early 1960s for the control of rinderpest. A similar vaccine to control PPR was produced in the late 1980s by multiple passages of the virus on Vero cells and this is now being used to control the disease in parts of Africa and Asia.

Egg-adapted (Onderstepoort vaccine) and canine tissue culture-attenuated (Rockborn) vaccines for CDV were produced in the 1950s and are still widely used to vaccinate dogs against distemper. Immunity lasts for several years following vaccination of dogs with either vaccine. The distemper vaccines are not attenuated for all carnivores; for example, some species of ferret are extremely susceptible to CDV and develop disease on vaccination.

All morbillivirus vaccines, like their wild-type progenitors, are extremely fragile and heat-labile and so it is expensive and logistically difficult to store and use them in hot climates. The establishment of an effective cold chain for the delivery of vaccine was an essential feature of the success of the rinderpest eradication campaign as was follow-up seromonitoring studies to determine the level of herd immunity and the effectiveness of vaccination teams.

## Future Prospects

Rinderpest is currently on the verge of global eradication and if successful it will be the first veterinary virus disease to have been eradicated globally and the second after smallpox. This goal must not be forgotten and the mild strain of the disease which may still persist in Somalia is of great concern. The worst case scenario is that such a clinically mild strain could move unnoticed into other regions of Africa where, since mass vaccination has ceased, there is a vast naive cattle and wildlife population which could become reinfected. This would provide an excellent opportunity for the virus to evolve to become more pathogenic for cattle. There is a high probability that this could happen as the virus most closely related to this strain was isolated from a giraffe in Kenya in 1962 and is highly pathogenic in cattle.

There is also a major gap in our understanding of the ecology of morbillivirus disease in wild animals, especially in marine and aquatic mammals, and this is an area of research which should be encouraged.

Many questions also remain concerning the host range determinants, biology, molecular biology, and pathogenesis of the morbilliviruses which hopefully can be addressed using reverse genetics.

*See also:* Bovine Viral Diarrhea Virus; Paramyxoviruses of Animals.

## Further Reading

Appel M (1987) Canine distemper virus. In: Apple MJ (ed.) *Virus Infections of Carnivores*, p. 133. Amsterdam: Elsevier.

Barrett T (2001) Morbilliviruses: Dangers old and new. In: Smith GL, McCauley JW,, and Rowlands DJ (eds.) *Society for General Microbiology, Symposium No. 60: New Challenges to Health – Threat of Virus Infection*, 155pp. Cambridge: Cambridge University Press.

Barrett T, Pastoret P-P,, and Taylor WP (eds.) (2005) *Biology of Animal Infections: Rinderpest and Peste des Petits Ruminants Virus*, 341pp. London: Elsevier.

Barrett T and Rima BK (2002) Molecular biology of morbillivirus diseases of marine mammals. In: Pfeiffer CJ (ed.) *Molecular and Cell Biology of Marine Mammals*, pp. 161–172. Melbourne, FL: Krieger Publishing Company.

Kock RA, Wambua JM, Mwanzia J, *et al.* (1999) Rinderpest epidemic in wild ruminants in Kenya 1993–97. *Veterinary Record* 145: 275–283.

Plowright W (1982) The effects of rinderpest and rinderpest control on wildlife in Africa. In: Edwards MA and McDonald U (eds.) *Symposia of the Zoological society of London, No. 50: Animal Diseases in Relation to Animal Conservation*, 1pp. London: Academic Press.

# Vector Transmission of Animal Viruses

**W K Reisen,** University of California, Davis, CA, USA

## Glossary

**Anthroponosis** Virus transmitted among human hosts.

**Arbovirus** Virus transmitted by blood-feeding arthropods among vertebrates.

**Diapause** Arthropod hibernation.

**Gonotrophic cycle** Cycle of blood feeding and egg deposition.

**Transmission** Distribution of virus usually by the bite of an infectious vector.

**Vector** Animal (usually an arthropod) that distributes viruses among hosts.

**Vector competence** Ability of vector to become infected with and transmit a virus.

**Vectorial capacity** Mathematical measure of case distribution or the force of transmission.

**Viremia** The presence of viruses within the vertebrate host peripheral circulatory system.

**Zoonosis** Virus transmitted mainly among animal hosts with incidental transmission to humans.

## Vector Transmission

This article describes how vectors (usually arthropods and especially insects) distribute or transmit viruses among vertebrate hosts. Although occasional instances of mechanical transmission by contaminated mouthparts of the feeding arthropod have been documented and nonviremic transmission among blood-feeding vectors has been demonstrated in the laboratory and occurs in nature, virus transmission generally is biological and propagative (**Figure 1**). This type of transmission demonstrates that the virus infects and multiplies within the tissues of both arthropod and vertebrate hosts before transmission can occur. Viruses transmitted by arthropods have been lumped into a loose assemblage termed 'arboviruses' that includes viruses within the families *Bunyaviridae, Flaviviridae, Rhabdoviridae,* and *Togaviridae.* Transmission rates and therefore the numbers of cases typically remain at low levels, unless there is a disruption in system balance such as a climate anomaly, virus mutation to a virulent form, or an ecological disturbance, or large-scale host movement that enables virus amplification to epidemic levels.

## Horizontal Transmission

Arthropod vectors, such as mosquitoes, feed on vertebrates to obtain blood which is used as a dietary supplement to stimulate and support egg development. If the vertebrate host is circulating a sufficient quantity of virus within its peripheral blood (i.e., is viremic) and if the arthropod is susceptible to infection, then the arthropod may become infected soon after blood feeding. After the blood meal is digested and the eggs are laid, completing the gonotrophic cycle, the surviving arthropods will then seek a subsequent blood meal to initiate the maturation of the next batch of eggs. The duration of the gonotrophic cycle essentially delineates the frequency of vector–host contact and therefore the number of opportunities for transmission by an arthropod during its lifetime. Horizontal arbovirus transmission occurs after the arthropod becomes infectious and is capable of expectorating virus when it feeds to obtain the next and subsequent blood meals. All arthropods expectorate salivary secretions while blood feeding, and this provides a mechanism to deliver the virus to the host thus completing horizontal transmission. After becoming infectious, most arthropods continue transmitting virus throughout the remainder of their lifetime. West Nile virus (WNV) is an example of a virus maintained by horizontal transmission from bird to mosquito to bird.

## Vertical Transmission

Some arboviruses acquired by the arthropod host are transmitted vertically to the next blood-feeding life stage. In ticks that feed once per life stage, transmission is trans-stadial (across life stages) from the larvae or nymphs that acquire the virus, molt, and then pass the virus to nymphs and/or adults that transmit their acquired infection to vertebrate hosts during the next blood meal. Tick-borne encephalitis virus (TBEV) is an example of a virus that is vertically maintained and transmitted within populations of the tick vectors, *Ixodes persulcatus* or *Ixodes ricinus.* In Diptera, acquisition of virus by the host-seeking female may be followed by passage of virus through the egg, larval, and pupal stages to adults in the next generation when transmission to vertebrate hosts is facilitated by infectious females. LaCrosse virus (LACV) is an example of a virus that is maintained vertically by efficient vertical transmission by its primary

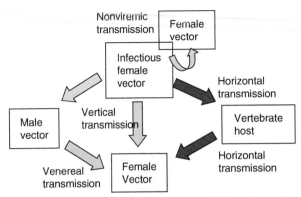

**Figure 1** Types of arbovirus transmission within arthropod vectors and between arthropod vectors and vertebrate hosts. Vertical transmission can be trans-stadial, as in ticks, or transgenerational, as in mosquitoes.

mosquito host, *Aedes triseriatus*, but is also transmitted horizontally to chipmunk reservoir hosts and occasionally to humans. In contrast, vertical passage of WNV occurs occasionally, but still may be important in virus amplification and persistence. In most arthropods vertical transmission is not 100% efficient, and therefore for a virus to be maintained, amplification by horizontal transmission is necessary to increase the number of infected individuals within the vector population.

## Venereal Transmission

Although male mosquitoes and other arthropods may become infected vertically, they usually do not blood-feed and therefore generally are 'dead end' hosts for the viruses that infect them. However, in some instances infected males are able to transmit virus venereally to uninfected females during mating. These females may become infective and then transmit virus horizontally as well as vertically. LACV is also an example of a virus that may be transmitted venereally and then horizontally and vertically by infected females. In contrast, all male tick life stages require a blood meal for molting and therefore can become infected orally. In some instances these males, orally infected as immatures, can transmit virus venereally.

## Nonviremic Transmission

When multiple vectors feed in close proximity, virus may be transmitted from infectious to uninfected arthropods without the host developing a viremia. This method of transmission initially was described for TBEV among *Ixodes* ticks that often attach near to one another on the host and require 4–5 days to blood-feed. Recently, however,

nonviremic transmission has also been demonstrated for *Culicoides* flies as well as mosquitoes in laboratory experiments.

## Types of Transmission Cycles

Epidemiologists have classified virus transmission cycles by the types of vertebrate hosts, with zoonoses maintained by transmission among animal hosts with occasional tangential involvement of humans, and anthroponoses maintained by direct transmission among humans (**Figure 2**).

### Zoonoses

Many arboviruses are zoonoses that are maintained and amplified in transmission cycles involving one or more vectors and a variety of animal hosts. When amplification progresses to elevated levels, transmission may spill over to tangentially include domestic animals and/or humans. St. Louis encephalitis virus is an example of a zoonosis that is maintained and amplified by horizontal transmission by mosquitoes among birds, but spills over to tangentially infect humans (**Figure 2**). In this instance, birds serve as maintenance reservoir and/or amplification hosts, because they are susceptible and capable of producing viremias of sufficient titer to infect blood-feeding mosquitoes. Humans are 'dead end' hosts, because they do not produce sufficient viremias to infect additional mosquitoes. Vectors that participate in the basic zoonotic cycle are termed maintenance vectors, whereas those that carry the virus from the enzootic cycle (among animals) to domestic animals or humans are termed 'bridge' vectors. Bridge vectors may not be able to maintain transmission in the absence of more susceptible and effective maintenance vectors. Although in many zoonoses humans are 'dead end hosts', humans still become infected and may develop serious disease.

### Anthroponoses

In some circumstances, humans produce a viremia sufficiently elevated to infect vectors and maintain a vector–human transmission cycle independent of animal hosts. Dengue viruses (DENVs) are examples of anthroponotic viruses maintained by human–mosquito–human transmission (**Figure 2**). Although there have been reports of horizontal enzootic and vertical transmission of DENV, these events rarely have been associated with or have led to major epidemics (transmission to or among humans). The distinction between zoonoses and anthroponoses becomes blurred with viruses such as yellow fever virus, in which there is a distinct enzootic primate–mosquito–primate maintenance cycle in jungle habitats and then an epidemic human–mosquito–human cycle in urban habitats.

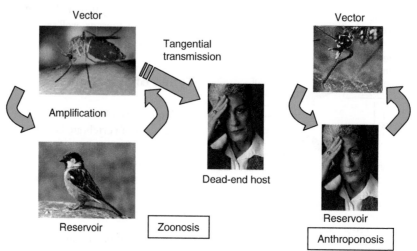

**Figure 2** Comparison between a bird-maintained zoonotic virus (such as the St. Louis encephalitis virus) and an anthroponotic virus (such as dengue virus). Activities to decrease or interrupt virus amplification and thereby prevent human cases.

## Factors Enabling Transmission

The efficiency of arbovirus transmission depends upon genetic factors that encode for susceptibility to infection and for biological traits that enable vector survival and repeated susceptible host contact. These properties may be summarized, respectively, as vector competence and vectorial capacity.

## Vector Competence

The innate ability of an arthropod to acquire and transmit an arbovirus is termed vector competence. Infection occurs when the ingested virus binds to receptor sites in the lumen of the midgut of the vector and then enters the midgut cells. Susceptibility to infection typically relates to the number of receptor sites and to the affinity of the infecting virus to bind with these sites. Many arthropods lack suitable binding sites, do not get infected, and have what is termed a midgut infection barrier. Others allow midgut infection and perhaps low-level virus replication, but the infection remains midgut-limited and does not disseminate to infect the salivary glands. Post-transcriptional gene silencing by RNA interference (RNAi) is a natural antiviral response in mosquitoes. As a countermeasure, some arboviruses evade RNAi or produce RNAi suppressors that limit antiviral defense. These viruses replicate to high levels and escape the midgut; however, not all infect the salivary glands or they infect the salivary glands but are not transmitted. These salivary gland barriers may be similar to midgut infection and escape barriers and are referred to as salivary gland infection and escape barriers. Still other less-known vector

attributes may downregulate infections after or during dissemination, also limiting transmission. In these vectors, transmission peaks soon after infection, but then decreases over time, so that older vectors have lower transmission rates than younger vectors. In general, however, competent vectors frequently become infected and efficiently transmit co-evolved viruses. The risk of infection and transmission by competent vectors increases as a function of vector–host contact which may be measured by the vector's reproductive age.

## Vectorial Capacity

In general, vector competence defines the ability of a vector to become infected with and transmit an arbovirus, usually under laboratory conditions. By comparison, vectorial capacity ($C$) is an epidemiological measure of the force of transmission or the daily case dissemination rate, and combines ecological factors relating to the frequency of reservoir host contact ($ma$, daily vector density in relation to host abundance, squared to account for refeeding), daily vector survival ($P$), the duration of the extrinsic incubation period ($e$), and vector competence ($V$):

$$C = \frac{ma^2 V(P^e)}{-\ln P}$$

Although originally developed to describe the rate of malaria transmission, this formula has been used to describe arbovirus transmission dynamics or to compare the importance of different vector species. For a zoonosis such as WNV, $ma^2$ becomes bites per bird per night. Frequently, measures of vector abundance ($m$, originally the man-biting rate) are combined with measures of vector host selection (*a*, the anthropophagic index or frequency of feeding on humans) to estimate bites per host per day. For zoonoses these terms must be changed to reflect the maintenance host species and the frequency with which they are fed upon by maintenance vector species. Vector blood-meal host-selection patterns determine the vertebrate hosts most frequently infected, and their susceptibility and viremia response then determines the effectiveness of transmission. In general, vectors with a narrow host range that includes susceptible host species will more effectively and rapidly amplify viruses than those with a broad host range that includes both susceptible and nonsusceptible host species. The latter vector species may be important as bridge vectors; for example, *A. aegypti* is a very effective vector of DENV because it feeds almost entirely on humans, whereas *A. albopictus* is less efficient because of its broad host range.

Daily survival (*P*) typically is measured by examination of host-seeking female reproductive age or from mark–release–recapture studies. In the current formula, *P* is considered to be constant throughout the life of the vector; however, some studies indicate that mortality rates may actually decrease as a function of vector age, thereby increasing vectorial capacity. The extrinsic incubation period (*e*) is discussed in detail below, but essentially is the time from infection to transmission by the vector. Vector competence (*V*) is the same as defined above and measures the ability of the vector to become infected and transmit virus.

## Extrinsic Incubation Period

Early in arthropod-transmitted viral epidemics, there are distinct time periods between episodes of new cases that delineate the 'extrinsic incubation period' or virus development outside of the vertebrate or human host. In reality, this measure of transmission dynamics is related to the time from virus acquisition by the vector until the transmission leads to new cases. Because arthropod body temperature approximates ambient conditions and because virus replication is both temperature limited and dependent, the duration of the extrinsic incubation period changes with latitude and as a function of climate variation, being shortest during summer. Degree–day models can be generated in the laboratory by incubating infected females at different temperatures and measuring the time until they are capable of transmission. Transmission is temperature limited, because viruses have threshold below which they will not replicate. This lower threshold delineates viral distribution in time and space. Theoretically, viruses with a lower (i.e., cool) temperature threshold are expected to have a wider geographic distribution

and can be transmitted more effectively at northern latitudes than those with a higher (warm) threshold. Above this lower limit, the rate of viral replication within the vector is dependent upon the temperature of the vector environment and typically increases as an exponential function of ambient temperature. Vector behavior may modify the temperature environment in comparison with ambient conditions, especially during cool periods of the year or day. Species that rest in houses, for example, have a more ameliorated temperature than those that rest outdoors. Nocturnal species that rest in burrows during the day and come out to seek blood-meal hosts at night always enter a warmer environment and therefore their body temperatures may slightly exceed ambient conditions. Both examples of insect behavioral change of body temperature can alter virus replication, transmission rates, and therefore virus amplification.

## Phases of Transmission

Transmission dynamics vary over time and space and may be grouped into three phases: introduction or maintenance, amplification or epidemic, and subsidence.

## Maintenance

Seasonal changes in vector abundance or the autumnal cessation of blood-feeding behavior limit or interrupt arbovirus maintenance transmission. In general, viruses either persist within host populations or become regionally extinct and require reintroduction. At southern latitudes with sufficient vector abundance and warm temperatures, viruses may be transmitted continually during winter. In southern areas with alternating dry and wet seasons, vector abundance changes related to precipitation also dictate the extent and timing of the transmission season. At northern latitudes mechanisms for local maintenance may include persistent infections within either vector or vertebrate host populations that are acquired during fall and then relapse during the following spring. Alternatively, viruses may become regionally extinct and are reintroduced the following spring. Unfortunately, data supporting most overwintering mechanisms are fairly fragmentary despite years of investigation. Recent studies of the molecular genetics of multiple viral isolations made over time and space show patterns of change indicating mutation or extinction, followed by the introduction and persistence of new genotypes. Often, rather small changes in the viral genome can result in marked changes in virulence that affect fitness and therefore amplification. The changes enhancing virulence may be associated with increased host and geographical range.

WNV is an example of a virus that has changed genetically, extended its distribution markedly, and has caused serious epidemics throughout northern latitudes in Europe and North America.

## Amplification

After maintenance or introduction at low levels, arboviruses undergo seasonal amplification (or increase in the numbers of infected hosts) during favorable weather periods. The rate of amplification is dependent upon vector competence and vectorial capacity factors, but may be limited by vertebrate host immunity and climate. Acquired immunity or depopulation of the primary vertebrate host population during the previous season or seasons may affect transmission during the subsequent season, because a large percentage of infected vectors transmit virus to immune hosts that do not become infective to other vectors. In short-lived vertebrate hosts, such as house sparrows, population turnover rates are high and elevated herd immunity levels short-lived. However, elevated immunity rates in long-lived hosts, such as humans, may limit infection to younger, nonimmune cohorts. A second factor that may constrain transmission is the effect of climate on vector abundance. Arthropod populations tend to vary markedly in response to climate variation. During years when climate is unfavorable, abundance may remain low and below thresholds necessary to effectively amplify virus. During these years maintenance transmission remains at very low levels or virus may disappear during the current and subsequent seasons. In contrast, rapid vector population increases and longer survivorship during favorable weather periods frequently are accompanied by concurrent increases in virus amplification to epidemic levels.

## Subsidence

Epizootic and/or epidemic-level transmission may be relatively short-lived and generally is followed by subsidence. Typically, the amplification curve attains asymptotic epidemic levels and then begins to subside due to decreasing numbers of susceptible hosts, seasonal changes in day length or climate, and/or focused intervention measures. In general, the more intensive and extensive the epidemic transmission, the faster and more widespread the seroconversion or depopulation rates within the primary host population, and the more rapid the focal subsidence. During years with low-level transmission, sufficient naive hosts may remain and provide a source for viral amplification during the following season. Eventually, the numbers of susceptible hosts decrease, slowing the force of transmission and decreasing the numbers of new cases.

Seasonal changes in day length and weather can produce comparable dramatic decreases in epidemic transmission without exhausting the number of available hosts which will remain available for amplification during the following season. At temperate latitudes, the onset of cold weather and shortening photoperiod may induce diapause in the primary vector(s), terminate blood feeding, and interrupt transmission, leading to rapid subsidence. At lower latitudes, comparable seasonality of transmission can be induced by variation in rainfall. Amplification the following season may be dependent upon the intensity of transmission during the end of the previous season and the amount of virus present in the overwintering host populations.

## Risk Factors

The risk of infection and disease in vertebrates is related directly to the degree of exposure to host-seeking infectious arthropods and to the vertebrate hosts' immune response to infection.

## Residence

Undoubtedly, place of residence markedly affects the risk of infection. Mostly due to the ecology of the arthropod vectors and vertebrate hosts, most arboviruses tend to be focal in their distribution and associated with particular landscapes. Humans often become infected by zoonotic viruses when housing areas are constructed within transmission foci or when human alteration of the landscape creates environments that bring vector and maintenance host together. Rural housing within or adjacent to wooded areas supporting the mosquito *A. triseriatus* has been found to be a critical risk factor for LACV infection in children. In contrast, urban *Culex* populations produced in municipal wastewater systems interfacing with periurban communally roosting American crow populations have led the spatial aggregation of WNV infection risk in humans.

## Climate

Climate variation affects temperature and precipitation patterns, mosquito abundance and survival, and therefore arbovirus transmission patterns. These changes often vary at different temporal scales. At temperate latitudes seasonal changes in temperature and photoperiod drive transmission cycles, whereas at tropical latitudes seasonal changes may relate more to wet and dry seasons. The magnitude of annual temperature and precipitation changes may have decadal or shorter cycles based on changes in sea surface temperature, such as the El Niño/southern oscillation change in the Pacific sea surface temperature that markedly alters precipitation and temperature patterns in parts of the Americas. These cycles alter storm tracks that affect mosquito and avian abundance, the intensity and frequency of rainfall events, and groundwater depth.

## Age

In the absence of acquired immunity, different viruses seem to exhibit a predilection to cause disease in different host age classes. This may be related to differential biting rates by vector mosquitoes on different host age groups or due to age-related differences in innate immunity. Host-seeking mosquitoes seem to feed more readily on adult than on nestling birds of the same species. With regard to illness, for example, western equine encephalomyelitis virus (WEEV) tends to cause more frequent and severe disease in infants (<1 year), whereas SLEV causes more severe illness in the elderly (>65 years). For endemic viruses, the prevalence of previous infection increases as a function of age, and therefore older cohorts tend to be protected by a greater prevalence of acquired immunity than younger cohorts. This age-related pattern of acquired immunity can change the apparent-to-inapparent ratio of clinical disease for endemic viruses.

## Occupation

Different occupations place workers in different environments at different times, and therefore vary their risk for mosquito and arbovirus exposure. For example, farm workers who pick and pack vegetables outdoors at night in southern California were found to have an 11% seroprevalence rate against SLEV, whereas persons residing within Los Angeles were found to have a lower 1.7% exposure rate. In contrast, persons sitting at home in late afternoon in Thailand have a high attack rate by *A. aegypti* and a high exposure rate to dengue viruses, compared to persons working outdoors from morning to night in agricultural professions.

## Socioeconomic Status

Historically, socioeconomic status has been related closely to the distribution of cases during urban epidemics. Homes and municipal drainage systems frequently are not well maintained in low-income neighborhoods, and this has shown to be related to the distribution of human cases. In the tropics, lack of a municipal water system and domestic water storage has been linked strongly to *A. aegypti* abundance and to disease risk.

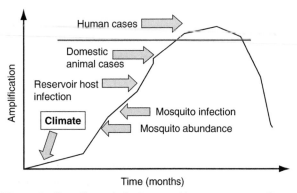

**Figure 3** Surveillance indicators used to measure enzootic virus amplification and forecast the risk of human infection. Climate variation can provide the earliest indication of pending risk and may drive the rate of viral amplification.

## Forecasting Risk

The cascade of different surveillance measures becoming positive over time as virus amplifies can be used to forecast the risk of human infection, especially for endemic zoonoses. **Figure 3** shows the approximate relative times when surveillance measures might become positive along the enzootic amplification curve for a virus such as WEEV. Usually, human cases are the last factor to be detected and tangential transmission occurs only after considerable WEEV amplification in the mosquito–bird cycle. These surveillance data can be used to focus on mosquito control.

*See also:* Animal Rhabdoviruses.

## Further Reading

Black WC, IV and Moore CG (2006) Population biology as a tool for studying vector-borne diseases. In: Beaty BJ and Marquardt WC (eds.) *The Biology of Disease Vectors*, pp. 393–416. Niwot, CO: University Press of Colorado.

Edman JD (2000) Arthropod transmission of vertebrate parasites. In: Eldridge BF and Edman JD (eds.) *Medical Entomology*, pp. 151–164. Dordrecht, The Netherlands: Kluwer.

Eldridge BF (2000) The epidemiology of arthropodborne diseases. In: Eldridge BF and Edman JD (eds.) *Medical Entomology*, pp. 165–186. Dordrecht, The Netherlands: Kluwer.

Hardy JL, Houk EJ, Kramer LD, and Reeves WC (1983) Intrinsic factors affecting vector competence of mosquitoes for arboviruses. *Annual Review of Entomology* 28: 229–262.

Reisen WK (2002) Epidemiology of vector-borne diseases. In: Mullen GR and Durden LA (eds.) *Medical and Veterinary Entomology*, pp. 16–27. New York, NY: Academic Press.

# Vesicular Stomatitis Virus

**S P J Whelan,** Harvard Medical School, Boston, MA, USA

## Historical Perspective

Vesicular stomatitis viruses (VSVs) are transmitted naturally by arthropods to a broad range of animal species. A clinically significant acute disease is manifest in domesticated animals, notably cattle, horses, and pigs, and it is characterized by fever and the appearance of vesicular lesions in the mouth, tongue, udder teats, and hoof coronary bands. Symptoms are therefore similar to those following infection with the apthovirus, foot-and-mouth disease virus (FMDV) and, consequently, rapid diagnosis is important in livestock. VSV infection was first described in the USA in 1916, following an epidemic in cattle and horses. However, reports from 1862 describe a clinically similar disease in army horses during the American Civil War. Today the virus is distributed throughout the Americas and is enzootic in Central America. In Panama, estimates suggest that up to 29% of the human population has been exposed to the virus as judged by the presence of neutralizing antibodies. Infection of humans can result in a mild febrile illness, but is generally asymptomatic. VSVs have been described rarely outside the Western Hemisphere.

## Taxonomy and Classification

VSVs have a nonsegmented negative-sense RNA genome and are assigned to the order *Mononegavirales*. Within this order, they are assigned to the family *Rhabdoviridae*, based upon their characteristic 'bullet' shape. Within the rhabdovirus family, they are further assigned to the genus *Vesiculovirus*. A list of the nine currently recognized species assigned to the genus is provided in **Table 1**, along with their geographic distribution and sources of the virus in nature. The *Eighth Report of the International Committee on the Taxonomy of Viruses* lists an additional 19 members tentatively assigned to this genus. The type species is *Vesicular stomatitis Indiana virus*. Vesicular stomatitis Indiana virus (VSIV) has been widely studied in laboratories as a prototype of all the *Mononegavirales* and will be the primary focus of this article. Much is known about the replication and molecular biology of VSIV. VSIV was isolated following an outbreak of a vesicular disease of cattle in Richmond, Indiana, in 1925. The infectious agent was maintained by serial passage in animals and eventually became the Indiana serotype of VSV. *Vesicular stomatitis New Jersey virus* is also classified as a species in the genus *Vesiculovirus*. It was isolated following an outbreak in cattle in 1926 and is serologically and genetically distinct from VSIV. Vesicular stomatitis Alagoas virus (VSAV) was isolated from domesticated animals in Alagoas Brazil during an outbreak of VSV.

## Structure of VSV

### Particles

A schematic of VSIV is shown in **Figure 1** along with an electron micrograph showing virus particles. The particles appear bullet-shaped and are approximately 180 nm long and 70 nm in diameter. The particles comprise 74% protein, 20% lipid, 3% RNA, and 3% carbohydrate. The virus possesses a lipid envelope that is decorated with trimeric spikes of the 67 kDa attachment glycoprotein (G). The interior of the particle contains a ribonucleoprotein (RNP) core of the genomic RNA complexed with the viral nucleocapsid (N) protein. This N-RNA core is associated with the RNA-dependent RNA polymerase (RdRp), the viral components of which are a 241 kDa large (L) protein and a tetramer of a 29 kDa accessory

**Table 1** Geographic distribution and sources of natural isolation of viruses representing the nine recognized species in the genus *Vesiculovirus*

| Virus | Geographic distribution | Source |
|---|---|---|
| Carajas virus (CJSV) | Brazil | Phlebotomine sandflies |
| Chandipura virus (CHPV) | India, Nigeria | Mammals, sandflies |
| Cocal virus (COCV) | Argentina, Brazil, Trinidad | Mammals, mosquitoes, mites |
| Isfahan virus (ISFV) | Iran, Turkmenistan | Sandflies, ticks |
| Maraba virus (MARAV) | Brazil | Phlebotomine sandflies |
| Piry virus (PIRYV) | Brazil | Mammals |
| Vesicular stomatitis Alagoas virus (VSAV) | Brazil, Columbia | Mammals, sandflies |
| Vesicular stomatitis Indiana virus (VSIV) | Americas | Mammals, mosquitoes, sandflies |
| Vesicular stomatitis New Jersey virus (VSNJV) | Americas | Mammals, mosquitoes, midges, blackflies, houseflies |

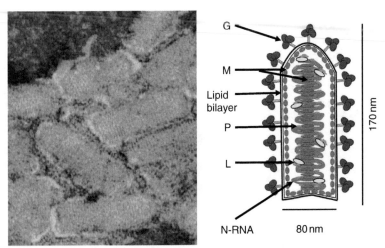

**Figure 1**   Electron micrograph of VSIV particles and a schematic illustration of the virion. At left, a negative-stained image of a group of virus particles is shown. At right, a schematic illustration of the virion is shown along with the dimensions of a viral particle. N-RNA, nucleocapsid protein coated RNA; P, phosphoprotein; M, matrix protein; G, attachment glycoprotein; L, large polymerase subunit. Kindly provided by David Cureton, Harvard Medical School.

phosphoprotein (P). Together, these form the internal helical nucleocapsid. Another major structural component of the virus particles is the 26 kDa matrix (M) protein, which is located below the membrane and associated with the nucleocapsid. The approximate composition of the particle is one molecule of RNA, 1200 copies of N, 500 copies of P, 1800 copies of M, 1200 copies of G, and 50 copies of L. The role of these proteins in viral replication is described in more detail below.

## Genome

VSIV has a nonsegmented, negative-sense RNA genome of 11 161 nt. The genome comprises a 50 nt 3′ leader region (le), five genes that encode in order the N, P, M, G, and L proteins, and a 59 nt 5′ trailer region (**Figure 2**). The 5′ and 3′ ends of the genome are not modified and contain a 5′ triphosphate and 3′ hydroxyl. A key feature of all mononegaviruses is that the RNA genome is not found naked within infected cells. Instead, it is present as a ribonucleoprotein complex, in which it is completely covered by the viral nucleocapsid protein. This N-RNA template, associated with the viral L and P proteins, comprises the transcription-competent core of the virus, and delivery of this complex is required to initiate the infectious cycle. Consequently, in contrast to positive-sense RNA viruses, the naked RNA is not infectious.

## Viral Replication Cycle

The replication cycle (**Figure 3**) should be considered a continuum of events. However, it is convenient to divide the cycle into the following three stages.

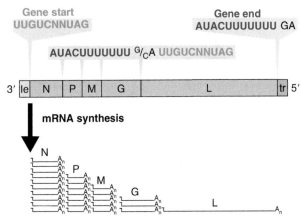

**Figure 2**   A schematic illustration of the VSIV genome highlighting the polymerase regulatory elements. The genome is represented 3′–5′ as a series of boxes, comprising le = leader region, N = nucleocapsid, P = phospho, M = matrix, G = glyco, L = large polymerase, and tr = trailer region. The conserved *cis*-acting elements that regulate polymerase activity during mRNA synthesis are shown for emphasis. Colors: green, the conserved residues of the gene-start sequence; red, the conserved residues of the gene-end sequence; and black, the nontranscribed residues of the gene junction. The leader and trailer regions also contain key elements that regulate polymerase activity and serve as promoters as described in the text.

## Attachment, Entry, and Uncoating

Attachment of VSV to host cells is mediated by the glycoprotein which binds to the surface of cells. Given that VSV G can mediate infection of almost all cells in culture, either the receptor for VSV must be widely distributed, or the virus may be able to utilize multiple surface molecules for attachment. Phosphatidylserine

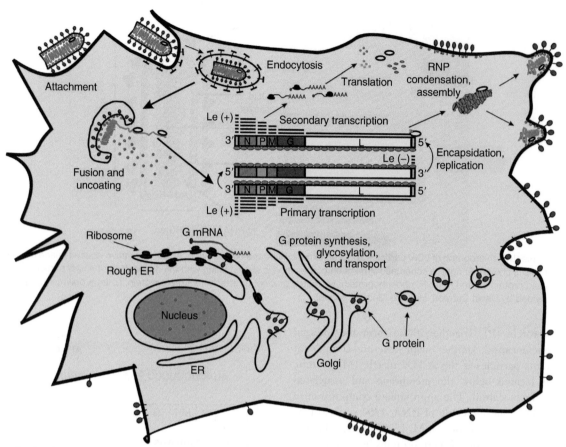

**Figure 3** A schematic illustration of the replication cycle of VSV. The replication cycle (described in the text) is depicted showing attachment of virus to the cell, internalization, release of the viral core into the cytoplasm, primary viral mRNA synthesis, mRNA translation, genomic replication, secondary viral mRNA synthesis, assembly, and budding of infectious particles. Kindly provided by David Cureton, Harvard Medical School.

(PS) was long thought to be the receptor for VSV but recent studies have questioned this finding. Importantly, the PS binding site in VSV G is internal to the trimer in its prefusion form. Following attachment to the cell, the virus is internalized via clathrin-dependent endocytosis and delivered to an early endosome. The pH threshold necessary to trigger the conformational alterations in VSIV G that promote fusion of the viral and cellular membranes is approximately 6.2. This pH is reached in the early endosome, and viral and cellular membranes fuse to release the transcription-competent RNP core into the cytoplasm of the cell. Recent work has called into question this conventional view of the VSV entry pathway and has posited a new model for viral entry. In this model, fusion and RNP release are spatially and temporally separated. Specifically, the low pH encountered during endocytic transport triggers fusion and the delivery of the RNP core into an intralumenal vesicle within an endosomal carrier vesicle. A subsequent (cell-mediated) fusion event is then required to fuse the membrane of the intralumenal

vesicle with the limiting membrane of the cell and deliver the RNP into the cytoplasm to initiate the infectious process. Irrespective of the precise route by which virus enters the cell, the end result is the delivery of the transcription-competent core into the cytoplasm. This is accompanied by the release of M protein, which can migrate to the nucleus where it plays a role in inhibiting host gene expression.

## Gene Expression

Following the delivery of the transcription-competent core into the cytoplasm, RNA synthesis can begin. The replication cycle of VSV is entirely cytoplasmic, occurring efficiently in enucleated cells. The demonstration that purified VSV particles contain a functional RdRp that is active *in vitro* has led to major advances in our understanding of viral gene expression. During RNA synthesis, the polymerase uses the encapsidated genomic RNA as template in two distinct reactions: (1) transcription of five mRNAs that encode the N, P, M, G, and L proteins; and (2) replication to yield full-length anti-genomic, and then genomic RNA strands. Our current understanding of gene expression is summarized as follows. In response to a specific promoter element that is provided by sequences within the 3' leader region and the conserved residues of the first (N) gene-start (3'-UUGUCNNUAG-5') sequence, the RdRp initiates mRNA synthesis. Synthesis commences at the N gene-start sequence and generates an mRNA that is capped, methylated, and polyadenylated, each of these reactions occurring co-transcriptionally. Termination at the end of the N gene is achieved by the polymerase recognizing a highly conserved sequence element referred to as the gene-end 3'-AUACUUUUUUG/C-5'. This sequence signals the polymerase to stutter on the $U_7$ tract to generate the polyA tail, and leads to termination of mRNA synthesis. Termination at the end of the N gene is essential for the polymerase to be able to transcribe the P gene. A poorly understood event that is localized to a short region at the N–P gene junction results in the synthesis of approximately 30% less P mRNA than N mRNA. This sequential and polar synthesis of the viral mRNAs continues through the entire genome and provides a gradient of viral mRNA synthesis such that N > P > M > G > L. These products of mRNA synthesis are illustrated in **Figure 2**.

Among the notable steps of mRNA synthesis are the unusual mechanisms by which the 5' and 3' ends of the RNA are formed. Each stage of mRNA cap formation is distinct from those employed in other systems. Specifically, the 5' end of the pppApApCpApG mRNA is capped by an unusual ribonucleotidyltransferase activity that transfers the monophosphate RNA onto GDP derived from GTP to form the GpppApApCpApG mRNA cap structure. In contrast, all other capping reactions are catalyzed by an RNA guanylyltransferase that transfers GMP onto the 5' end of a diphosphate RNA through a reaction that involves a covalent enzyme GMP intermediate. The VSV L protein is responsible for this novel reaction, which appears to involve a covalent intermediate between L and the viral mRNA. The resulting GpppApApCpApG cap structure is then methylated at guanine N-7 and ribose 2'-O positions to yield 7mGpppAmpApCpApG. These activities are also provided by the L protein, and again differ from conventional mRNA cap methylation reactions. For VSIV, the two enzymatic activities have been shown to share a single binding site for the methyl donor, S-adenosyl-L-methionine (SAM). In contrast, other cap methylation reactions are normally executed by two distinct proteins with separate binding sites for the methyl donor SAM. Formation of the 3' end of the RNA is also unusual. Specifically, polyadenylation occurs in a pseudo-templated fashion in which the polymerase complex reiteratively transcribes the conserved U tract present at the end of each VSV gene.

The viral mRNAs are efficiently translated by the host translation machinery, but how they compete with cellular mRNAs for translation is not well understood. Viral protein synthesis is essential for replication of the genomic RNA. Ongoing translation provides a continuous supply of soluble N protein that drives the encapsidation of the nascent RNA chain. This process is intimately linked to genomic RNA replication which first results in the production of a full-length encapsidated complementary antigenome RNA. This antigenome can then serve as template to produce more progeny genomic RNAs for use as templates for further mRNA synthesis in a process referred to as secondary transcription.

Precisely how the different polymerase activities are regulated in infected cells remains poorly understood. Two functionally distinct pools of polymerase have been purified from cells. One initiates internally at the N gene-start sequence and functions as the viral transcriptase. A second complex initiates at the 3' end of the genome and functions as the viral replicase. These complexes are reported to differ in their composition such that the transcriptase comprises the viral P and L proteins, together with several cellular proteins including translation elongation factor-1α, heat shock protein 60, and the host cell RNA guanylyltransferase. In contrast, the replicase is reported to comprise the viral N, P, and L proteins.

In addition to the species of RNA described above, two short leader RNAs are generated during RNA synthesis: a 47 nt Le+ from the 3' end of the genomic RNA and a 45 nt Le− from the 3' end of the antigenomic RNA. The function of these RNAs is poorly understood, although a role for the Le+ in the shutoff of host gene expression has been described. A long-standing model for the regulation of RNA synthesis in VSV postulates that polymerase initiates all RNA synthesis at position 1 of the genome, and during synthesis of Le+ a crucial regulatory decision is made to either terminate leader and initiate mRNA synthesis at the N gene start, or alternatively to read through the leader–N gene junction and synthesize the full-length antigenome. The obligatory requirement for protein synthesis to provide a source of N protein to encapsidate the nascent RNA during genome replication led to the suggestion that N protein availability switches polymerase activity from transcriptase to replicase.

In recent years, there has been an accumulation of evidence that conflicts with this model. Specifically, a VSV mutant containing a single amino acid change in the template-associated N protein produces an excess of N mRNA over Le+ *in vitro*, suggesting that polymerase can synthesize N independently of Le+. In another series of experiments, recombinant VSVs, containing a 60 nt gene inserted between the leader region and the N gene, were employed.

The recombinant viruses were examined to determine the effect of altering the potential number of ultraviolet (UV)-induced dimers between adjacent uracil residues. Such dimers block progression of the polymerase. These experiments showed that changing the UV sensitivity of the Le+ had no effect on the sensitivity of the 60 nt mRNA in infected cells, suggesting that polymerase can initiate synthesis internally at the first gene start. In addition, two separate pools of polymerase can be isolated from infected cells, one that initiates internally at the N gene start and the second that initiates at the 3′ end of the genome. These findings support the hypothesis that mRNA synthesis can initiate independently of leader synthesis, and show that polymerase function is not simply switched by N protein levels. However, viral gene expression is controlled, it results in the exponential amplification of the input genomic RNA, yielding progeny genomes that can be assembled into infectious particles, the next phase of the viral replication cycle.

## Assembly and Budding

Assembly of infectious virus particles involves many critical interactions. Our current understanding of this intricate process is that the matrix (M) protein complexes with the RNP core and represses transcription of viral mRNAs. This condensed RNP complex acquires a lipid envelope that has been modified by the insertion of an externally oriented glycoprotein. Details of how the RNP is transported to the site of budding and how the matrix interacts with and condenses the RNP are poorly understood. The M protein is only found associated with RNPs at sites of viral budding, and how genomic RNPs (rather than antigenomic RNPs) are specifically selected for budding is unclear. The M protein contains two 'late domains' (PTAP and PPPY motifs) that appear to be critical in the late phase of the assembly-release pathway. Amino acid substitutions in the PPPY motif result in the accumulation of bullet-shaped virions that are stalled at a late stage of virus budding. This motif, and similar motifs in proteins from other enveloped viruses, target virus for budding through interaction with components of the endosomal sorting complex required for transport or ESCRT pathway. The release of infectious particles completes the replication cycle and provides progeny virions for infection of the next cell.

The kinetics of the viral replication cycle are rapid. In mammalian cells in culture, one infectious particle can produce 10 000 infectious progeny within 8 h. While much remains to be explored about the biology of VSV, it is one of the best understood animal viruses. Studies on VSV should continue to prove informative in understanding how enveloped viruses enter and bud from their host cells, and how nonsegmented negative-strand RNA viruses (mononegaviruses) express their genetic information.

## Functions of the Viral Proteins

### Nucleocapsid protein

The N protein coats the viral genomic RNA and the positive-sense antigenomic replicative intermediate to form ribonucleoprotein (RNP) complexes. The interaction with the N protein renders the RNA resistant to cleavage by ribonucleases. It is in this form that the RNA is presented to the polymerase to serve as template. The N protein comprises 422 amino acids and has a molecular weight of approximately 48 kDa. The crystal structure of a complex of 10 molecules of N protein bound to 90 nt of RNA has been solved, revealing that N has a bilobed structure with RNA bound between the lobes. The structure indicates that N protein must be either transiently displaced or substantially remodeled during copying of the RNA genome by the viral polymerase.

### Phosphoprotein

P is a multiply phosphorylated acidic protein of 265 amino acids that functions as an essential polymerase cofactor and plays an additional role in maintaining N protein in a soluble form necessary for RNA encapsidation. Sequence analysis has identified three domains of P. An acidic N-terminal domain (domain I) of 150 amino acids contains phosphorylation sites at Ser 60, Thr 62, and Ser 64. Phosphorylation of these residues by the host casein kinase II leads to the oligomerization of P protein and together with the large polymerase protein L, assembly of the polymerase complex. Domain I is separated from domain II by a highly variable hinge region comprising residues 150–210. Domain II (residues 210–244) contains additional phosphorylation sites at Ser 226, Ser 227, and Ser 233 that appear to be important for RNA replication. Domain III is basic and comprises the C-terminal 21 amino acids. A crystal structure of a fragment comprising amino acids 107–177 of the P protein has been solved, providing evidence that P protein functions as a tetramer. In addition to P, two proteins (C and C′) are produced from the P gene. These proteins are small (55 and 65 amino acids, respectively), are highly basic, and have not been detected in virus particles. Recombinant viruses that are unable to produce C and C′ replicate normally in cultured mammalian cells. The role of these proteins is unclear but may be important for infections in insects and/or mammalian hosts *in vivo*.

### Matrix protein

The matrix (M) protein is the major structural component of virus particles. M is a small 229-amino-acid multifunctional protein. It condenses viral RNPs and drives budding of virus particles from the host plasma membrane. In addition, M downregulates host gene expression by directly interacting with Rae 1, thus inhibiting nuclear transport. The crystal structure of amino acids 48–229 of the matrix protein has been solved and reveals regions of M that may be required for membrane association. Two N-terminal truncations of M are generated in infected cells by initiation of translation at methionines 33 and 51. A recombinant virus engineered to ablate the expression of these two alternate forms of M shows a modest reduction in cytopathic effect in culture cells.

### Glycoprotein

The attachment glycoprotein (G) is a trimer present on the surface of the virion. It is responsible for attachment of virus to cells and promotes fusion of the viral and cellular membranes during endocytosis. The protein is synthesized as a 511-amino-acid polypeptide that is co-translationally inserted into membranes in the endoplasmic reticulum (ER). An N-terminal 16-amino-acid signal sequence is cleaved from the nascent polypeptide upon insertion. A 20-amino-acid hydrophobic sequence acts as the membrane anchor and serves as a stop-transfer signal during ER translocation. The remaining 29 amino acids of G remain as a cytoplasmic tail. Co- and post-translational modifications result in N-glycosylation of two asparagine residues in the ectodomain, and palmitoylation of a cysteine in the cytoplasmic domain. The role of palmitoylation in infection is unclear as some VSV strains lack this modification. However, glycosylation permits association of G with calnexin, an ER-resident chaperone, and mutations that prevent glycosylation result in G protein aggregation. Mature G protein is selectively transported to the basolateral surface of polarized epithelial cells. At the plasma membrane, VSV G clusters in microdomains that are the sites of virus assembly and budding. The determination of the crystal structure of a fragment of the G protein in both pre- and postfusion conformations has provided new insight into the entry process. The structures show that each G protein monomer contains two hydrophobic fusion loops that insert into the target cell membrane. Substantial rearrangements of the G protein that are driven by the low pH environment encountered in the endocytic pathway drive fusion of the viral and cellular membranes.

### Large polymerase protein

The large polymerase protein (L) comprises 2109 amino acids. This 241 kDa multifunctional protein is responsible for template binding, ribonucleotide polymerization, and the co-transcriptional modification of the 5′ and 3′ terminus of the viral mRNAs so that they are capped and methylated. To date, structures are not available for any portion of the L protein. Amino acid sequence alignments of the L genes of representative members of the families *Rhabdoviridae*, *Paramyxoviridae*, and *Filoviridae* have led to the identification of six regions of sequence conservation (CRI–CRVI), separated by regions of no or low sequence homology. These conserved regions are thought to

represent the functional domains of L protein. CRIII contains clearly identifiable motifs found in all polymerases and in which alterations to a universally conserved aspartic acid residue eliminate polymerase activity in reconstructed RNA synthesis assays. CRVI functions as a messenger RNA cap-modifying enzyme. Amino acid substitutions to this region disrupt mRNA cap methylation at both the guanine N-7 and ribose 2′-O positions of the cap structure. The regions of L involved in other modifications have not yet been assigned. As described above, L protein has been reported to associate with a number of host proteins, including translation elongation factor-1α, heat shock protein 60, and the host RNA guanylyltransferase. However, the functional significance of these interactions is not yet certain.

## Host Range and Transmission

In nature, VSVs can infect a broad range of animals including mammals and invertebrates. Overt disease is typically only seen in cattle, horses, and swine, but there is evidence of natural infection in a range of wild ruminants, ungulates, carnivores, marsupials, and rodents. Infection can be transmitted directly from animal to animal, but this requires an abrasion or a means of introducing the virus below the skin. Humans can also be infected by contact with vesicular lesions or the saliva of infected animals, resulting in an influenza-like illness. Aerosol transmission has also been reported in humans. Insect vectors appear to be important in natural transmission of the virus. VSVs have been isolated on more than 40 occasions from hematophagous insects including mosquitoes, biting midges (*Culicoides* spp.), phlebotomine sand flies (*Lutzomyia* spp.), and black flies (*Simulium* spp.). In addition, VSV has been experimentally transmitted to mice from infected mosquitoes and between insects through co-feeding. Susceptible insect hosts are also capable of transovarial transmission and these infected progeny have been shown to infect mammalian hosts. Recovery of vesicular stomatitis New Jersey virus (VSNJV) from nonbiting flies suggests that mechanical transmission may occur. There is also evidence that grasshoppers (*Melanoplus sanguinipes*) can be infected experimentally, and cattle that ingest infected grasshoppers can develop disease.

Consistent with the ability to infect a broad range of experimental animals, VSV replicates efficiently in a variety of cell lines of vertebrate and invertebrate origin. The Syrian hamster kidney cell line, BHK-21, is commonly used to generate viral stocks of high titer ($10^9$–$10^{10}$ pfu ml$^{-1}$). VSV can also infect and replicate to high titers in cultured cells derived from insects, reptiles, and fish, and replication can occur in several insect cell lines. Infection of mammalian, avian, and some insect cells results in a cytopathic effect (CPE). In fibroblasts, this is seen as an increase of membrane blebbing followed by extensive cell rounding. The M protein is responsible for these changes in infected cells. A noncytopathic infection occurs in some insect cells including lines derived from *Aedes aegypti*, *Aedes albopictus* (C6/36), and *Drosophila melanogaster*. Experimentally, the virus has been shown to express its genetic information in spheroblasts derived from the yeast, *Saccharamoyces cerevisae*, and to produce infectious virions in embryonic cells derived from the nematode *Caenorhabditis elegans*. Thus, the host requirements for viral replication are provided by an extremely broad range of eukaryotes.

## Evolution

Several principles of evolutionary biology have been explored using VSV as a model system. The viral polymerase has an error rate of $10^{-3}$ to $10^{-5}$ per nucleotide per round of replication. Given the genome size is 11 161 nt, each time the genome is copied, on average, at least one nucleotide change is introduced. These mutations are typically deleterious, others will be neutral, and some may offer a selective advantage. Consequently, this high mutation rate contributes to VSV's ability to rapidly evolve and adapt to environmental changes. The high mutation rate also begs the question as to why VSV does not mutate itself out of existence. Rather than existing as a single defined sequence, the virus exists as a swarm of mutant sequences around a consensus sequence or a viral quasispecies. Critically, it is this quasispecies that is the biologically relevant target for selection.

Experiments in which the diversity of the viral population is artificially restricted by performing serial plaque-to-plaque transfers (thus restricting the infectious virus population to 1 on each transfer), rapidly result in fitness losses. Such an accumulation of deleterious mutations in populations of asexual organisms lacking compensatory mechanisms such as sex or recombination was predicted by Muller in a concept referred to as Muller's ratchet. This principle has been nicely illustrated in studies of VSV, which is not known to undergo homologous recombination. Studies with VSV have also illustrated other fundamental principles of population genetics. Work by the laboratory of John Holland demonstrated that VSVs of equal fitness could coexist for several generations, but one population would then rapidly outgrow the other. This demonstrated that populations accumulate mutations and, infrequently, mutations provide a selective advantage which leads to its outgrowth. Importantly, the mutation rates in both populations were the same, reflecting an intrinsic property of the viral polymerase. This is referred to as the Red Queen effect. This is a hypothesis proposed by the evolutionary biologist Leigh van Valen in reference to Lewis Carroll's book *Through the Looking Glass*, in which

the Red Queen comments to Alice that "it takes all the running you can do, to keep in the same place."

Despite the intrinsically high polymerase error rate, VSVs isolated in nature can show a remarkable genetic stability. For example, sequence analysis of viruses from different hosts and different years has shown that those isolated from multiple hosts within the same region over a period of decades were more closely related than viruses isolated in the same year, but from a different ecological zone. This suggests that ecological factors are a major driving force in the evolution of VSV. Consistent with this, viruses from similar ecological zones 800 km apart were found to be more closely related than viruses from different ecological zones 25 km apart. VSV evolution is unusual in this apparent lack of a 'molecular clock' in which the genome sequence does not show a clear relationship with year of isolation.

The evolutionary origins of VSVs are uncertain but the conservation of gene order and sequence similarity to other members of the *Mononegavirales* indicate they diverged from a common ancestor. Although the number of genes differ, their order is maintained across the *Mononegavirales* as 3' N–P–M–G–L 5'. The significance of this gene order has been elegantly tested in engineered VSIV recombinants by shuffling the order of the three central genes (P, M, and G), and by moving the N and G genes. Remarkably, all gene orders yield infectious virus, and the replication kinetics of several recombinant viruses in which the P, M, and G genes were shuffled were similar to those of the wild-type parent virus. Consistent with its critical role in driving RNA encapsidation during genome replication, moving the N gene from its promoter proximal position diminished viral replication. These experiments suggest that the conserved gene order may reflect an ancestral gene order that has remained frozen because of the lack of a mechanism for homologous recombination in the *Mononegavirales*.

## Geographic and Seasonal Distribution

VSVs are typically restricted to the Americas. Within this region, VSIV and VSNJV are the two most commonly isolated serotypes and have the broadest geographic distribution ranging from Peru to Canada. Vesicular stomatitis Alagoas virus (VSAV) is the major serotype that is isolated in Brazil. Both VSIV and VSNJV are seen in the United States although most outbreaks are associated with VSNJV. In the US, the last outbreak was from 2004 to 2006. In this outbreak, viral infection was reported in Texas, New Mexico, and Colorado in 2004, and the outbreak spread to include Arizona, Utah, Wyoming, Nebraska, Montana, and Idaho in 2005, with a small number of cases reported in Wyoming in 2006. Overall some 1000 animals were affected, representing the most significant outbreak of disease in the US for almost 10 years. Vesicular stomatitis is endemic in many Latin American countries. In 2002, VSNJV and VSIV were reported in Panama, Costa Rica, Nicaragua, El Salvador, and Mexico, and VSNJV was reported in Honduras, Guatemala, and Belize. In 2004, VSNJV and VSIV were isolated in Columbia, Venezuela, Ecuador, and Peru, and VSIV in Brazil and Bolivia. Although infection is reported throughout the Americas, the highest incidence usually is in tropical regions with more sporadic outbreaks in temperate regions. In temperate regions, outbreaks typically peak in late summer and end by the first frost. In tropical regions, peak incidence typically coincides with the end of the rainy season. These peaks correlate with high insect population levels and, consistent with the role of insect vectors in disease spread, outbreaks tend to spread along waterways. Although, on occasion, VSV has been reported in parts of Europe and Africa, such reports are rare and are probably linked to importation of infected animals.

## Pathogenesis and Pathology

Following exposure of animals to VSV, the incubation period is usually 2–4 days. Prior to the development of lesions, animals can show signs of depression, lameness, a fever of up to 41.5 °C, and excessive salivation. In infected cattle, swine and horses, pink to white papules appear in the mouth, lips, gums, nose, teats, and feet. In these regions, the epithelium separates from the basal layer forming a vesicle that fills with clear yellowish fluid that contains very high titers of infectious virus. These vesicles combine and readily rupture. In some cases, lesions appear at a secondary site relative to the initial point of inoculation. The development of secondary lesions is suggestive of a viremia, but virus has not been isolated from the blood of experimentally inoculated natural hosts. Infection results in significant losses for the livestock industry as weight loss can be significant (up to 135 kg in beef cattle), and dairy cattle usually cease milk production. In the absence of secondary infections, the vesicular lesions typically heal in 1–2 weeks and the animals start to regain weight. Viral RNA has been isolated from animals several months after infection although infectious virus has not been recovered.

## Immune Response

Our understanding of the immune response to VSV in natural hosts is limited. However, in experimental animals, notably mice, the immune response to VSV has been characterized. Interferon plays an important role in the resistance of older mice to VSV infection and,

consistent with this, adult mice that are unable to produce interferon succumb to infection. Different strains of VSV induce different levels of interferon, but there is no clear correlation between levels of interferon *in vitro* and pathogenesis in animals. Neutralizing antibody has also been shown to play a role in the defense against VSV infection in experimentally infected swine and mice. The target of these neutralizing antibodies is the viral attachment protein G, and adoptive transfer experiments have shown that they are sufficient to protect young mice against infection. In endemic areas, susceptible hosts often have detectable neutralizing antibody responses to VSV. However, these responses are not protective, perhaps reflecting the fact that viral replication is largely confined to the epithelium. Experimental infection of mice with VSV also induces a strong cytotoxic T-lymphocyte (CTL) response. The N protein is the predominant antigen recognized and the resulting CTLs are not serotype specific. However, the functional significance of these CTLs in protection against infection is uncertain as mice incapable of mounting such a response survive VSV infection.

## Diagnosis, Prevention, and Control

The similarity of symptoms between VSV and FMDV make rapid diagnosis important, especially in countries that are free of FMDV. Diagnosis is achieved typically by analysis of samples of fluid from vesicular lesions using reverse transcription-polymerase chain reaction (RT-PCR), enzyme-linked immunosorbent assay (ELISA), or growth of virus in cell culture. VSV is listed as a notifiable disease by the World Organisation for Animal Health (OIE) and a positive diagnosis results in quarantine of the affected area. To control spread of disease, farm equipment is disinfected using a 2% bleach solution to interrupt animal-to-animal spread, and insect control measures can be introduced. Vaccines against VSIV and VSNJV have been used to control outbreaks in Central and South America. Although vaccination is not routinely practiced throughout the Americas, experiments demonstrate a substantive decrease in clinical infections in vaccinated animals.

## Future Perspectives

VSVs will continue to serve as an important prototype of the nonsegmented negative-strand RNA viruses. The advantages of VSV as a model for these viruses are: (1) its relative safety, in that the virus is not a significant human pathogen; (2) abundant viral replication in a broad range of cultured cells yielding up to 10 000 pfu cell$^{-1}$ 8–12 h post inoculation of mammalian cells; (3) a robust reverse genetic system which permits the generation of helper-dependent viruses; (4) crystal structures of the N-RNA template, a portion of the P and M proteins, and the pre- and postfusion forms of the G protein; and (5) an *in vitro* system for viral mRNA synthesis using purified recombinant polymerase. Capitalizing on these advantages will continue to provide new mechanistic insights into the molecular details of viral entry, gene expression, and assembly. Among the key questions to address are understanding: (1) how and where the viral RNP core enters a cell; (2) how and where the N-RNA serves as template for gene expression; (3) how the large multifunctional polymerase serves to initiate, cap, methylate, polyadenylate, and terminate mRNA synthesis in response to specific sequence elements; (4) how the activities of the polymerase are controlled between mRNA synthesis and genome replication; and (5) how the nucleocapsid templates are selected for assembly and budding from the cell. In addition to the fundamental questions regarding the molecular biology of these viruses, the future holds promise for unraveling the significance of the different host species and vectors in the biology of infection. Genomic approaches will likely yield clues as to how VSV interacts with host cells of insect and mammalian origin, and how these cells respond to infection. Many questions remain to be answered regarding the ecology of the virus including the maintenance of the virus, its transmission, and its relative genetic stability in nature. Such studies are not only warranted in understanding VSV as a model virus, but also for the prospects of using VSV as an oncolytic virus and a live-attenuated vaccine vector for human disease. These potential applications should only add to the urgency with which studies on this prototypic virus are pursued.

## Further Reading

Eigen M (1993) Viral quasispecies. *Scientific American* 269: 42–49.

Gaudier M, Gaudin Y, and Knossow M (2002) Crystal structure of the vesicular stomatitis virus matrix protein. *EMBO Journal* 21: 2886–2892.

Green TJ, Zhang X, Wertz GW, and Luo M (2006) Structure of the vesicular stomatitis virus nucleoprotein-RNA complex. *Science* 313: 357–360.

Lyles DS and Rupprecht CE (2006) In: Knipe DM, Howley PM, Griffin DE, Lamb RA, and Martin MA (eds.) *Fields Virology,* 5th edn., p. 1364. Philadelphia: Lippincott Williams and Wilkins.

Novella IS (2003) Contributions of vesicular stomatitis virus to the understanding of RNA virus evolution. *Current Opinion in Microbiology* 6: 399–405.

Ogino T and Banerjee AK (2007) Unconventional mechanism of mRNA capping by the RNA-dependent RNA polymerase of vesicular stomatitis virus. *Molecular Cell* 25: 85–97.

Roche S, Bressanelli S, Rey FA, and Gaudin Y (2006) Crystal structure of the low-pH form of the vesicular stomatitis virus glycoprotein G. *Science* 313: 187–191.

Roche S, Rey FA, Gaudin Y, and Bressanelli S (2007) Structure of the prefusion form of the vesicular stomatitis virus glycoprotein G. *Science* 315: 843–848.

Rodriguez LL, Fitch WM, and Nichol ST (1996) Ecological factors rather than temporal factors dominate the evolution of vesicular stomatitis virus. *Proceedings of the National Academy of Sciences, USA* 93: 13030–13035.

Wertz GW, Perepelista VP, and Ball LA (1998) Gene rearrangement attenuates expression and lethality of a nonsegmented negative strand RNA virus. *Proceedings of the National Academy of Sciences, USA* 95: 3501.

Whelan SPJ, Barr JN, and Wertz GW (2004) Transcription and replication of non-segmented negative-strand RNA viruses. *Current Topics in Microbiology and Immunology* 283: 61–119.

# Visna-Maedi Viruses

**B A Blacklaws,** University of Cambridge, Cambridge, UK

## Glossary

**Dyspnea** Shortness of breath.

**Endocytosis** Where a particle is enveloped by the cell membrane and internalized into a vacuole, an endosome.

**Germinal center** Area where B cells undergo proliferation after encountering their specific antigen with helper T lymphocytes.

**Glomerulonephritis** Inflammation of the glomeruli.

**Hyperplasia** Increase in the number of cells.

**Leukoencephalitis** Inflammation of the brain caused by leukocytes.

**Lymphoid follicle** Organized lymphocyte clusters.

**Pneumonitis** Inflammation of the lung.

## Introduction

Visna-maedi virus (VMV) is a retrovirus in the genus *Lentivirus.* Other lentiviruses are human (HIV), simian (SIV), feline (FIV), and bovine (BIV) immunodeficiency viruses, caprine arthritis encephalitis virus (CAEV), and equine infectious anemia virus (EIAV). VMV causes a persistent infection of sheep leading to pneumonitis, demyelinating leukoencephalitis, mastitis, and arthritis, eventually killing the host. VMV originally came to prominence during an epidemic of lung and a separate wasting disease in sheep in Iceland from the 1930s to the 1950s. It was isolated from cases of interstitial pneumonitis (*maedi* = shortness of breath in Icelandic) and demyelinating leukoencephalomyelitis (causes *visna* = wasting in Icelandic) and was the first lentivirus isolated in 1957. Study of the Icelandic epidemic, with scrapie and ovine pulmonary adenomatosis (caused by another retrovirus, Jaagsiekte sheep retrovirus), allowed Björn Sigurdsson to introduce the concept of slow viral infections in 1954. These infections are typified by long incubation periods with pathology developing slowly and progressively, eventually leading to death of the host. The derivation of the genus name, *lenti* (Latin for slow), comes from this.

Clinical lung disease typical of maedi, and in many cases now known to be caused by VMV viruses, has been described since the early 1900s in other countries. Maedi is therefore also known as ovine progressive pneumonia or Montana sheep disease (USA), Graaf Reinet disease (South Africa), zwoegerziekte (the Netherlands), and la bouhite (France). VMV (and/or CAEV) is present in most countries worldwide apart from Iceland (eradicated during the 1940s and the 1950s), Australia, and New Zealand. Where infections are present, economic losses due to loss of milk production, failure to thrive, early culling, and death of animals are seen.

The major target cells for VMV are macrophages and dendritic cells. These are also common target cells for all the other lentiviruses. Aspects of lentivirus infection such as early infection and sites of persistence in accessory cells of the immune system may therefore be studied with VMV without the complication of lymphocyte infection.

## Small Ruminant Lentiviruses

Historically, when a lentivirus was isolated from sheep, it was classified as VMV and from goats as CAEV. Although it was known that experimentally VMV could infect goats and CAEV infect sheep, it was not until recently that the natural interspecies transmission of the viruses was shown by molecular epidemiology. Sequencing data from geographically distant countries and from incidences of interspecies transmission into previously uninfected populations shows that VMV and CAEV are able to infect either species as well as other wild small ruminant species. The viruses have therefore now been grouped together as the small ruminant lentiviruses (SRLVs) although the terms VMV and CAEV are also in common use. This article focuses on studies using 'classical' VMV strains in sheep but also draws on data from CAEV and goats.

## Visna-Maedi Virus

### Virion and Genome

The virion is enveloped with a spherical or coffin-shaped core like other lentiviruses. The virion packages a diploid RNA genome of 9189–9256 bp. Several strains and molecular clones have been fully sequenced. It is a complex retrovirus with three structural genes, *gag*, *pol*, and *env*, and three auxilliary genes, *vif*, *tat* (or *vpr*), and *rev* (**Figure 1**). The functions of the different gene products have been deduced by direct study of VMV and CAEV and also by comparison to HIV and other lentiviruses (**Table 1**).

### Replication Cycle

Replication of the virus occurs in a manner similar to that of other retroviruses. Virus binds directly to the cellular receptor or via Fc receptors if coated in antibody. The virion core is released into the cytoplasm by fusion of the envelope with the plasma membrane or, if the particle has been taken up by endocytosis, with the endosomal membrane. The RNA genome is reverse-transcribed to a double-stranded DNA (dsDNA) intermediate (provirus). The process of DNA replication duplicates the RNA termini forming the long terminal repeats (LTRs) of the provirus which contain the virus promoter, mRNA start site, and polyadenylation signals. The provirus integrates into the host cell genome with no apparent preferred site for integration. It is this integrated provirus that serves as template for viral mRNA and genome

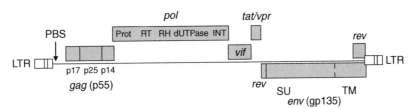

**Figure 1** Proviral map of VMV. The provirus structure of VMV is shown with the position of open reading frames indicated. The proviral long terminal repeats (LTRs) contain the U3, R, and U5 regions (in this order) made during reverse transcription. The viral RNA genome contains R/U5 and U3/R at the 5′ and 3′ termini, respectively, where R is a short direct repeat. The primer binding site (PBS) for initiation of reverse transcription is indicated (binds tRNA lysine). The open reading frames are *gag*, *pol*, *vif*, *tat/vpr*, *env*, and *rev*, which contains two exons.

**Table 1** Gene products of VMV

| ORF | mRNA | Products | Function |
|-----|------|----------|----------|
| gag | Full-length unspliced | Precursor Gag p55 cleaved to:<br>  Matrix p17<br>  Capsid p25<br>  Nucleoprotein p14 | Major core proteins of virion |
| pol | Full-length unspliced | Precursor Gag/Pol polyprotein made by ribosomal frameshift, cleaved to: | |
| | | Protease | Aspartic protease cleaves Gag and Pol |
| | | Reverse transcriptase | Synthesizes proviral cDNA |
| | | RNase H | Degrades genomic RNA to allow second-strand cDNA synthesis |
| | | dUTPase | Reduces dUTP incorporation and so A-to-G mutation in second-strand synthesis. Mutants attenuated *in vitro* and *in vivo* |
| | | Integrase | Integrates provirus into host genome |
| env | Singly spliced | Precursor Env gp135 cleaved to: | |
| | | Surface subunit, SU gp110 | Binds to cellular receptor |
| | | Transmembrane subunit, TM gp41 | Fuses viral envelope to cellular membrane (plasma or endosomal) to release virion core into cytoplasm |
| vif | Singly spliced | VIF | Assumed to be like HIV-1 VIF: inhibits incorporation of cytidine deaminases into virion and so stops new cDNA degradation or G-to-A mutations. Mutants attenuated *in vitro* and *in vivo* |
| tat/vpr | Doubly spliced | TAT/VPR | Historically called TAT but little evidence to support TAT function, more similar to VPR: LTR has no TAR element, high promoter activity without TAT, and TAT increases promoter activity by two- to threefold; cellular location nuclear; not secreted; packaged in virion; arrests cells in G2 phase of cell cycle. Mutants viable *in vivo* and *in vitro* |
| rev | Doubly spliced | REV | Interacts with rev-responsive element (RRE) in *env* coding region to allow export of unspliced and singly spliced mRNA species from the nucleus |

production. VMV has a complex mRNA expression pattern. *In vitro*, during productive replication of fibroblast cells, there is early synthesis and transport of *tat/vpr* and *rev* doubly spliced mRNA to the cytoplasm. Once REV is expressed, late synthesis and transport of *gag*, *pol*, *env*, and *vif* single or unspliced mRNAs or genomic RNA are mediated. This allows expression of the viral structural proteins, virion assembly (by budding through the plasma membrane or into vacuoles), and thus productive replication.

## Target Cells

Monocyte/macrophages and dendritic cells are the major target cell type infected *in vivo* although other cell types have also been shown to either harbor viral nucleic acid or express viral protein, for example, lung, gut, and mammary gland epithelial cells. The frequency of infected cells *in vivo* is very low with often less than 1% of the

macrophage population being infected. There is no productive infection of lymphocytes unlike the primate lentiviruses. The range of cells that VMV infect *in vitro* is wider than macrophages with fibroblasts, an important resource for growing virus in the laboratory, and epithelial, endothelial, and smooth muscle cells all reported to replicate virus.

Replication in the monocyte/macrophage lineage is tightly linked to the maturation stage of the macrophage. Three replication states have been suggested: latent, restricted, and productive. Latent is where cells contain provirus but do not express viral products. In productive infection *in vitro* and *in vivo*, cells express approximately 5000 copies of viral RNA per cell, contain viral proteins, and produce virions. *In vivo* however, most infected cells express low quantities (approximately 5–200 copies) of viral RNA but no protein. This is called restricted replication and is seen in immature macrophages, for example, blood monocytes. It is only when macrophages mature in tissues that productive viral replication is found. Thus macrophages have been called 'Trojan horses' in SRLV infection in that they silently deliver the virus to tissues where virus replication can occur.

The cellular receptors for SRLV have not been identified although VMV strains K1514 and EV1 use a receptor(s) widely expressed on different cells and species. For K1514 this has been mapped to sheep chromosome 3p and the syntenic region of human chromosome 2 (2p25 > q13), and for EV1 to mouse chromosomes 2 and/or 4. If a one-component receptor is assumed, this excludes ovine major histocompatibility complex (MHC) class II (previously identified as a possible receptor by Env binding) and many of the cellular proteins used as co-receptors by other lentiviruses, for example, CXCR4 and CCR5. Studies using viral binding to cellular blots have identified possible candidate receptor proteins that have not yet been fully identified although a membrane proteoglycan is implicated. CAEV strains 63 or Cork may use a receptor which is much more restricted in expression in different species and although it has not been identified, is known, from interference and inhibition assays, to be different from the receptor for VMV strain K1514.

The cellular tropism of VMV is also affected by the ability of the virus to express the provirus. Different promoter activities are the consequence of LTR sequence and its ability to bind different transcription factors. Unlike the primate lentiviruses, SRLV LTRs have no NF-κB binding sites, but interact with AP-1 (only K1514), AP-4, and the AML/PEBP2/CBF family of transcription factors. Nothing is known about the changes that occur in maturing macrophages to allow viral expression although replication is known to be dependent on activation of the extracellular signal-related kinase/p38 mitogen-activated protein (ERK/MAP) kinase pathways.

## Transmission

There are two important routes of transmission for VMV. The first is respiratory by aerosolized lung exudates between animals that are closely housed and/or in contact for long periods of time. The second is oral by colostrum/milk from infected dams to offspring.

As VMV is usually cell associated *in vivo* (there are few reports of cell-free virus), it has commonly been thought that the infective moiety in lung exudates and colostrum/milk was virus-infected macrophages or epithelial cells. However, recent data suggest that cell-free virus may be important in respiratory transmission. The presence of cell-free virus in the lining fluid of lungs with severe lesions has been shown and the lower lung is a more efficient point of infection than the trachea. Aerosolized particles small enough to reach the lower lung could contain free virus but infected cells would be too large. Once in the lower lung, a variety of possible target cells

are present: macrophages (both alveolar and interstitial), dendritic cells, and lung epithelial cells, all of which may allow virus replication.

It is less clear in studies looking at oral transmission of VMV to lambs using colostrum/milk whether cell-free virus or virus-infected cells are important. Induction of lactation corresponds to virus expression in mammary tissue and colostrum contains cell-free virus as well as infected macrophages and epithelial cells. In a transmission study in lambs infected naturally by colostrum, ileal epithelial cells at the tips of the villi were important in early viral replication with virus antigen expression also seen in mononuclear cells in the lamina propria (macrophages), Peyer's patches, and mesenteric lymph nodes (macrophages and dendritic cells). Cell-free virus in colostrum may infect epithelial cells, but these cells could also transcytose viral particles. Similarly infected cells, especially macrophages in colostrum/milk, could transcytose into the lamina propria or beyond to infect the lamb. The appearance of infected mononuclear cells in the lamina propria within 10 h suggests that this route of infection also occurs. Therefore both cell-free and cell-associated virus could infect lambs via colostrum.

## Immunity

### Acute Infection Cannulation Model

Immune responses to VMV are slow to be detected in blood after natural infection. Seroconversion may take 6 months to 2 years to occur and sporadic T-cell reactivities in peripheral blood lymphocytes are often reported. However, when infection is studied in an acute infection cannulation model (**Figure 2**), immune responses are detected much earlier. The induction of antibody specific for Gag p25 can be shown within 4 days by enzyme-linked immunosorbent assay (ELISA) and neutralizing antibody (presumably specific for Env) within 10 days in efferent lymph. T-cell reactivity (by proliferation to Gag antigen and VMV-specific cytotoxic T-lymphocyte precursors (pCTLs)) is detected within 7–15 days. A low percentage of sheep also show directly active cytotoxic T lymphocytes (CTLs) in efferent lymphocytes. Therefore the kinetics of the immune response to VMV are within normal ranges seen to other viruses. However, it takes much more time for this immune reactivity to be detected systemically. The slow replication rate of VMV and low frequencies of virus-infected cells may be responsible for this weak systemic immune response.

### Antibody Responses

In blood, the antibody response is first seen to Gag antigens, in particular capsid antigen p25 (usually 1 month after experimental infection). The anti-Env response

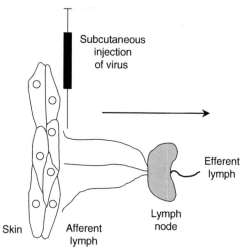

**Figure 2** Lymphatic drainage diagram. The acute infection cannulation model for VMV infection of sheep uses subcutaneous injection of virus. The cellular drainage from the site of infection may be collected by cannulation of the lymphatic vessels draining the area. The lymph node directly draining the site of infection may also be biopsied. Lymphatic drainage flows from the tissue through the afferent lymph to the lymph node and then to the efferent lymph (indicated by an arrow). Virus in lymph cells (detectable by 1–4 days) or plasma (none detected) may be quantified, cells carrying virus identified (macrophages and dendritic cells), and immune reactivity monitored (see text). Even using this model, infected cells are at very low frequency, for example, 1 in $10^5$–$10^6$ cells, although increased levels of infected cells rise to a peak by approximately 10–14 days and then decrease to low persistent levels.

develops slowly, but as disease develops it eventually predominates. Other viral proteins also induce antibody responses. Neutralizing antibody responses are targeted to Env and develop very slowly (usually 2–3 months after experimental infection). Virus neutralization causes inhibition of viral binding to the cell (using fibroblasts as target cells) or inhibition of viral reverse transcription and/or integration (using macrophages as target cells). At least five epitopes have been defined in Env by monoclonal antibody reactivity and one immunodominant region is found in transmembrane (TM) Env. There are regions of hypervariability in Env sequences linked to antibody reactivity and escape (see below). VMV-specific antibodies are also detectable in colostrum and milk, cerebrospinal fluid (CSF), and synovial fluid.

Good IgM and IgG1 responses to VMV are induced but in natural infection, sheep do not make an IgG2-isotype response to viral proteins. Persistently infected sheep are able to make an IgG2 response to viral proteins immunized in adjuvant, and it is therefore thought that there may be abnormalities in the antigen-presenting function or T-cell help to B cells during natural infection. This isotype restriction is not seen in goats infected with CAEV; indeed, the predominant isotype induced is an indicator of whether pathology may develop, with strong

IgG1 responses to Env SU associated with development of arthritis. The antiviral antibodies induced precipitate viral antigen in agar gel immunodiffusion tests and activate complement but the lack of an IgG2 response is associated with the lack of measurable antiviral antibody-dependent cellular cytotoxicity (ADCC) reactivity in antibody from infected sheep.

## T-Lymphocyte Responses

Peripheral blood T-lymphocyte (PBL) proliferative responses to virus antigens are often intermittent with reactivity induced by 1–6 weeks post infection or later, depending on route and amount of virus challenge. Proliferating cells respond to Gag and Env although other viral antigens have not been tested. The response to Gag is mediated by CD4+ T cells. Proliferative T-cell responses to VMV have been detected in CSF by 3 weeks post infection and this reactivity coincides with the initiation of lesion development. Directly active CD8+ CTLs are seen in a low proportion of infected sheep (<20%) but all sheep develop pCTLs (CD8+ T lymphocytes) in their PBL by 3 months after experimental infection. These are induced by day 12 in lymph nodes draining the site of infection and are detectable in lymph nodes and efferent lymph of persistently infected sheep. Infected macrophages can present antigen via MHC class II to stimulate CD4+ T lymphocytes and MHC class I to act as targets for CD8+ CTL as well as to stimulate effector CTL function. Infected macrophages in lesions may therefore present antigen to lymphocytes.

## Protective Immune Responses

Protective immune mechanisms have not been defined against VMV. After experimental infection, viral-infected cell frequencies peak, usually 1–2 weeks post infection, and then drop to levels maintained during persistent infection, suggesting that immune mechanisms are induced which control the level of infection. However, experiments to define protective T-lymphocyte subset(s) by *in vivo* antibody depletion of lymphocytes have not been successful at defining protective cell types. Indeed the experiments showed that CD4+ T lymphocytes are required for efficient infection of sheep by VMV although this lymphocyte subset is not infected. In contrast to the immunodeficiency viruses, no role was detected for CD8+ T cells in control of virus replication. However, the low levels of VMV replication and the return of CD8+ T lymphocytes to the peripheral circulation within 14 days of the start of depletion may mean that sufficient CTL function remained to control the infection. Further work therefore needs to be carried out to investigate protective immune mechanisms against VMV.

## Immune Abnormalities

There is no gross immunodeficiency after infection by SRLV; however, there are conflicting reports of immune abnormalities in SRLV-infected animals including changes in total immunoglobulin levels, CD4/CD8 T-cell ratios, decreased suppressor cell activity, and reduced delayed-type hypersensitivity (DTH) responses in skin and increased responses to certain bacterial infections which may be traced to macrophage dysfunction. The specific clinical state of animals is hard to normalize between studies and this may lead to the differing results.

## Pathogenesis

### Viral Entry

Cell-free virus or virus-infected cells enter the body where they may infect dendritic cells or macrophages in the primary infection site. These cells carry virus to the lymph node where infection is established and then macrophages leaving the lymph node disseminate virus throughout the body leading to a persistent infection. An important tissue for persistent infection of the animal is the bone marrow. Small foci of cells showing restricted replication of VMV have been identified which also express macrophage markers. These are probably myeloid stem cells although no study has defined these well. Infected stem cells may act as a continual source of infected monocyte/macrophages and/or dendritic cells which constantly seed the periphery and tissues. Where the cells mature and express viral antigen, the immune response to the infected cells then causes pathology. Recent molecular data question this theory as very few bone marrow samples from CAEV-infected goats assayed by polymerase chain reaction (PCR) for both proviral DNA and RNA were positive for virus. However, the levels of infection in bone marrow have not been defined well and may be below the detection limit of the assays used. Further work must be done to clarify this point. If bone marrow is not a constant source of infected cells, the virus must be maintained in infected tissues, perhaps lymph nodes and spleen. *In vivo* VMV may be isolated from many tissues including lung, mammary gland, joints, CNS, lymph nodes, spleen, and bone marrow. However, Kupffer cells of the liver are not permissive for virus infection and liver is not involved in pathology of the infection.

### Clinical Signs

Infection by VMV does not cause obvious clinical signs for many months and sometimes years (2–5 years). Once clinical signs occur there is a progressive increase in the severity of the clinical signs with time. The diseases caused by SRLV are all typified by chronic active inflammatory processes. Within tissues, there is lymphocyte infiltration and proliferation, and the formation of organized lymphoid follicles and germinal centers. Lesions consist mostly of lymphocytes, macrophages, and plasma cells, often with CD8+ T lymphocytes predominating. This is overlaid with tissue-specific pathology (see **Table 2** for affected organs). Rarely, more acute disease may be seen in younger animals, usually leukoencephalitis, arthritis, or pneumonitis with high mortality.

## Viral Cytopathic Effect or Immunopathology?

What causes the gradual buildup of pathology is not clear but it has two contributing factors: the effect of virus infection on infected cell and tissue function and the immune response to the virus. Little is known about the direct effect of virus on tissues although peptide analogs of the *tat/vpr* gene product are neurotoxic in rats and mice transgenic for the *tat/vpr* gene show lymphoproliferative disorders. Indeed, the number of virus-infected cells in lesions is low, so direct viral damage may be minimal.

There is a major immunopathological component to lesion formation. Early studies using immunosuppression reduced the number of CNS lesions seen in sheep infected intracerebrally, although the extent of infection within the CNS was the same, suggesting that direct viral toxicity was not a mediator of pathology. Similarly immunization with viral antigen before or after infection or superinfection with virus often increases the level of pathology seen. There is a positive correlation between virus load and pathology, and it is thought the immune response to viral antigen drives lesion formation. This is difficult to comprehend in early lesions where little virus antigen is detectable but once started, a positive-feedback loop of inflammation and increased virus expression drives progressive damage.

Both lymphocytes and macrophages taken from tissues with pathology show an activated phenotype: for example, they upregulate MHC class I and II, and adhesion molecule expression. However, there is variability in findings with functional assays and cytokine expression as to whether cells are activated or inhibited. Alveolar macrophages from lungs with pneumonitis show increased production of granulocyte monocyte colony stimulating factor (GM-CSF), interleukin (IL)-8, and fibronectin but not IL-6, IL-10, or transforming growth factor (TGF) β. Phenotypic changes seen *in vivo* may be caused by immune activation during the inflammatory reaction; however, some studies on infected macrophages *in vitro* suggest direct viral effects on cytokine expression and function. VMV infection of macrophages causes increased expression of IL-8 mRNA but decreased phagocytic and chemotactic activity. MHC class I and II, and LFA-1 and -3 expression are unaffected by infection. CAEV-infected macrophages show a decreased response to

**Table 2**    Diseases caused by SRLV

| Clinical sign (name) | Age of animal infected | Pathology | Infected cells |
|---|---|---|---|
| Dyspnea/ pneumonia (maedi) | Adult sheep, 2–5 years old Goats, 1–6 months old | Interstitial pneumonitis with perivascular infiltrates; lymphofollicular hyperplasia (some with germinal centers) around vessels, bronchi, and bronchioles; smooth muscle hyperplasia near terminal bronchioles and alveolar ducts | Type I and II pneumocytes, interstitial and alveolar macrophages, endothelial cells and fibroblast-like cells Cell-free virus in lung lining fluid |
| Wasting and ascending paralysis (visna) | Adult sheep, 2–5 years old Goats 1–6 months old | Periventricular encephalitis (white matter) with perivascular cuffing and infiltration of the parenchyma by mononuclear cells; focal demyelination in brain and spinal cord; meningitis; areas of necrosis; raised cell numbers in CSF; intrathecal antibody production | Interstitial macrophages, microglial cells, rare endothelial, choroidal epithelial cells and fibroblasts of choroid plexus, astrocytes Cell-free virus in CSF rare |
| Enlarged, hardened udder ('hard bag') | Adult ewes and does | Indurative mastitis with lymphoid hyperplasia, and plasma cells in glandular interstitium, occasional infiltrates into ductal walls and lumens; periductal proliferation and follicle formation; gradual loss of epithelium; diffuse fibrosis; increased numbers of cells and cellular debris in lumen causing increased somatic cell count in milk | Epithelial cells, macrophages, endothelial cells and fibroblast-like cells infected Cell-free virus in colostrum/milk |
| Swollen joints, lameness ('big knee') | Goats, 1–2 years old Rare in sheep | Chronic arthritis with hyperplastic synovial membrane; subsynovial mononuclear cell infiltrates (follicle formation with germinal centers); increased synovial fluid with raised numbers of lymphocytes (some macrophages and synovial cells) and IgG1 levels (produced *in situ*); angiogenesis in villi and subintima; areas of cellular necrosis; frequent mineralization; increase in fibrous connective tissue around synovial membranes | Synovial membrane cells, macrophages, fibroblasts, endothelial cells. Cell-free virus in synovial fluid |
| *Other affected organs* | | | |
| Lymphadenopathy | | Cortical hyperplasia (increased T cells); germinal center expansions and increased B-lymphocyte areas | Macrophages (and dendritic cells) |
| Kidney | | Glomerulonephritis and interstitial nephritis; medulla and corticomedullary junction lesions; proliferation of mesangial and kidney endothelial cells; lymphatic clusters and follicles | Tubular epithelial cells, macrophages |
| Third eyelid | | Lymphoproliferative inflammation | Macrophages, and glandular, ductal and surface epithelia |
| Skin | | Decreased DTH responses | |

bacterial products: inducible nitric oxide synthase (iNOS), tumor necrosis factor (TNF)-α, IL-1β, IL-6, and IL-12p40 induction are all affected. Infection of cells has also been shown to lead to cell death via apoptosis. Infection of macrophages has a complex effect on function which is also altered by the presence of other cells. Co-culture of VMV-infected macrophages with autologous lymphocytes induces the secretion of lentivirus-induced interferon (lentiferon). This is probably a mixture of interferon (IFN)-α and IFN-γ. Effects of lentiferon include inhibition of proliferation and maturation of monocytes and of virus assembly in infected cells, thus decreasing virus replication, but it also increases MHC class II expression on macrophages which may contribute to lymphoproliferative responses.

The cytokines important in upregulating versus inhibiting VMV expression are poorly understood, partly due to the lack of purified ovine cytokines. Only GM-CSF has been shown to increase VMV transcription and antigen production in macrophages. GM-CSF and

TNF-α treatment of cells increases CAEV LTR promoter activity and so may cause increased virus replication. However, there is mixed evidence as to the role that type I IFN plays against VMV infection: pretreatment of choroid plexus cells with a source of ovine type I IFN does not inhibit VMV replication, while pretreatment of cells with human IFN-α does block replication. *In vivo* treatment of lambs early in infection with IFN-τ reduces virus replication and disease development. Although not a cytokine, NO is also known to inhibit virus replication in macrophages.

## Autoimmunity

The lesions caused by SRLV in the CNS and joints are very similar to those seen in multiple sclerosis and rheumatoid arthritis of humans. These have links to autoimmunity, and indeed autoimmunity would explain the chronic development of pathology seen in these infections. However, there is very little evidence for this as a mechanism of lesion formation with VMV. There is no response to myelin basic protein (lymphocytes or antibody) or lipid antigen (antibody) in sheep with visna although elevated levels of autoimmune antibody (specific for rheumatoid factor, single-stranded DNA (ssDNA), and cardiolipin) in serum have been detected in infected sheep.

## Role of Lymphocytes

CD4+ T lymphocytes are important in promoting infection and lesion formation. At the time of acute infection, CD4+ T lymphocytes are necessary for efficient establishment of infection and later lymphocytes are necessary for lesion development. Therefore, immune responses to unrelated antigens, whether secondary infections or experimental immunizations or vaccinations, may cause increased inflammatory reactions that accelerate lesion development.

## Role of the Host and Virus Genetics

Breed resistance to infection and disease development has been documented in sheep and goats. In sheep, the Icelandic breed was particularly susceptible to VMV infection and development of visna, while the Karakul flock, from which infected animals introduced the disease to Iceland, never showed signs of disease. Border Leicester rams are resistant to visna but develop arthritis. This and agricultural practice (e.g., are animals milked?) may explain, in part, the geographical distribution of clinical signs of VMV infection; for example, Iceland commonly saw pneumonitis and encephalomyelitis, UK usually notes pneumonitis, and Spain has documented pneumonitis and mastitis. With interspecies transmission of SRLV, it is not clear whether strains more closely resembling VMV in goats will cause increased incidences of pneumonic disease or whether it is goat genetics which determines joints as a major site of lesion development. In USA, the VMV strains isolated are more closely related to CAEV than European VMV strains and yet pneumonia is still commonly seen in sheep. In goats with CAEV, where only ∼30% of animals develop arthritis, linkages to certain MHC class I alleles have been associated with development of disease.

Strains of virus that can be differentiated phenotypically *in vitro* can cause different patterns of lesion development. Usually strains growing to high titer and causing cytopathic effects in macrophages are the most virulent *in vivo*. Strains selected for increased neurovirulence grow better in sheep choroid plexus cells than those that cause pneumonia. This is linked to LTR sequence variation. Therefore, both host and viral genetics are important elements in disease progression.

## Immune Evasion

SRLVs persist in the host despite an immune response that includes antibody, CD4+, and CD8+ T lymphocytes. Several mechanisms of viral immune evasion have been noted that may allow this to occur. First, integration into the host genome allows latent infection and persistence in cells without expression of antigen. Similarly, gene expression is tightly regulated with no expression of antigen in immature macrophages. Thus these cells are invisible to the immune system. Second, low-titer neutralizing antibody responses producing low-affinity antibody mean that virus may be able to dissociate from antibody and infect cells. Third, neutralization escape mutants have been shown to emerge during infection. Mutants arise by point mutation in Env, one of the first documented incidences of antigenic drift in viruses. Later, the neutralizing antibody response may broaden to include these mutants. It is thought these mutants have a selective advantage and help the virus to persist in the host. Whether escape mutants are important in VMV pathogenesis is debatable as the original parental virus may be isolated late after infection, showing it has not been cleared from animals and replaced by the mutants. Similarly, neutralization mutants arise when antibody is not present, and their presence is unrelated to severity of pathology. Fourth, the ability of VMV to cause cell fusion means that cell-free virus is not required (and very rarely seen *in vivo*) as virus may pass from cell to cell directly and so is not exposed to antibody. Fifth, antibody-mediated enhancement of infection of macrophages has been shown in which antibody-coated virus is taken up into macrophages via Fc receptors, thus increasing the effective viral dose. Sixth, there is no ADCC response to the virus. Seventh, although technically not immune evasion, the virus uses the CD4+ T-cell response to help replication, either by activation of macrophages or attraction of macrophages to the relevant tissue.

## Control

Because of its insidious nature, control of VMV infection is difficult. Due to the economic losses and animal welfare problems that the disease causes, control programs are in place in many countries. These are based on serological tests, usually ELISAs (often to capsid p25 and TM Env) or agar gel immunodiffusion tests. However, because of the length of time taken for induction of a detectable antibody response in blood, and the possibility of fluctuations in the response, testing regimes involve repeated tests to maintain accreditation of SRLV-free status. PCR has not been used routinely for VMV diagnosis due to the strain variation that is present within SRLV and the low provirus load in blood of persistently infected animals.

Several options are open to try to derive SRLV-free flocks. Iceland eradicated the disease in the 1940s and the 1950s by culling all infected flocks and restocking from SRLV-clean animals. Others have used removal of serologically positive animals (and their progeny) from the flock after each test round until serologically free status is achieved. In the Netherlands, there was a successful policy of re-deriving flocks from 'snatched' lambs. These are lambs taken at birth from their mothers before they suckle infected colostrum. The lambs are then hand-reared on either heat-inactivated or bovine colostrum. Once VMV-free flocks are achieved, careful control of importation of animals into flocks/countries is necessary to maintain this status, as it is importation of infected asymptomatic animals that then live in close contact with the host flock that often leads to spread of infection into previously free areas, for example, Iceland (1933) and Finland (1981). With proof now of interspecies transmission, SRLV-free status will only be maintained if both sheep and goats are kept separate or both species kept SRLV free.

## Treatment and Vaccination

At present, there is no treatment against infection although certain anti-retroviral drugs do have activity against VMV. There have now been several vaccination studies using inactivated virus preparations, live-attenuated viruses, and subunit vaccines administered by a variety of vectors, for example, protein, plasmid, and vaccinia virus, using a variety of routes and different adjuvants or cytokine immunomodulators. None has produced sterilizing immunity and some have increased the levels of pathology seen. Induction of neutralizing antibody by immunization with recombinant Env has proven problematic using baculo- and vaccinia virus-expressed

antigen in sheep. The best result has been with bacterial-expressed Env gp70 but only low titers of antibody were seen using this immunogen. Some vaccines have reduced virus load early in infection but pathology has still developed, although in some cases this is less severe than control animals. The most promising result has come from CAEV in goats using DNA prime and then protein boost with Env in Freund's incomplete adjuvant. There was decreased viral replication in lymph node and synovium, and reduced development of severe arthritis for more than 18 months using this vaccine.

The possibility of inducing antibody that enhances the ability of virus to infect macrophages, the induction of CD4+ T lymphocytes responses that may increase the efficiency of the primary infection, as well as increasing the pathological response are all aspects of the immune response to VMV that needs much further study before a successful vaccine will be released to the field.

## Conclusions

VMV has many features in common with the other lentiviruses including infection of macrophages and dendritic cells. There is now an understanding of the type of lesion VMV induces in many tissues. However, there is still much work to be done with VMV to answer questions on sites of persistence of the virus, triggers of lesion development, protective immune responses, and vaccine control of the infection.

*See also:* Equine Infectious Anemia Virus; Simian Immunodeficiency Virus: Animal Models of Disease; Simian Immunodeficiency Virus: General Features.

## Further Reading

Blacklaws B, Bird P, and McConnell I (1995) Early events in infection of lymphoid tissue by a lentivirus, maedi-visna. *Trends in Microbiology* 3: 434–440.

Blacklaws BA, Berriatua E, Torsteinsdottir S, *et al.* (2004) Transmission of small ruminant lentiviruses. *Veterinary Microbiology* 101: 199–208.

de Andres D, Klein D, Watt NJ, *et al.* (2005) Diagnostic tests for small ruminant lentiviruses. *Veterinary Microbiology* 107: 49–62.

Eriksson K, McInnes E, Ryan S, *et al.* (1999) CD4(+) T-cells are required for the establishment of maedi-visna virus infection in macrophages but not dendritic cells *in vivo*. *Virology* 258: 355–364.

Eriksson K, McInnes E, Ryan S, *et al.* (1999) *In vivo* depletion of CD8+ cells does not affect primary maedi visna virus infection in sheep. *Veterinary Immunology and Immunopathology* 70: 173–187.

Gendelman HE, Narayan O, Kennedy-Stoskopf S, *et al.* (1986) Tropism of sheep lentiviruses for monocytes: Susceptibility to infection and virus gene expression increase during maturation of monocytes to macrophages. *Journal of Virology* 58: 67–74.

Gendelman HE, Narayan O, Molineaux S, *et al.* (1985) Slow, persistent replication of lentiviruses: Role of tissue macrophages and macrophage precursors in bone marrow. *Proceedings of the National Academy of Sciences, USA* 82: 7086–7090.

Georgsson G, Pálsson PA, and Pétursson G (1990) Some comparative aspects of visna and AIDS. In: Racz P, Haase AT, and Gluckman JC (eds.) *Modern Pathology of AIDS and Other Retroviral Infections*, pp. 82–98. Basel: Karger.

Haase AT (1986) Pathogenesis of lentivirus infections. *Nature* 322: 130–136.

Peterhans E, Greenland T, Badiola J, *et al.* (2004) Routes of transmission and consequences of small ruminant lentiviruses (SRLVs) infection and eradication schemes. *Veterinary Research* 35: 257–274.

Ravazzolo AP, Nenci C, Vogt HR, *et al.* (2006) Viral load, organ distribution, histopathological lesions, and cytokine mRNA expression in goats infected with a molecular clone of the caprine arthritis encephalitis virus. *Virology* 350: 116–127.

Ryan S, Tiley L, McConnell I, and Blacklaws B (2000) Infection of dendritic cells by the maedi-visna lentivirus. *Journal of Virology* 74: 10096–10103.

Sigurdsson B (1954) Mædi, a slow progressive pneumonia of sheep: An epizoological and a pathological study. *British Veterinary Journal* 110: 255–270.

Sigurdsson B (1954) Rida: A chronic encephalitis of sheep. With general remarks on infections which develop slowly and some of their special characteristics. *British Veterinary Journal* 110: 341–354.

Thormar H (2005) Maedi-visna virus and its relationship to human immunodeficiency virus. *AIDS Reviews* 7: 233–245.

# OTHER ANIMAL VIRUSES

# Cytomegaloviruses: Murine and Other Nonprimate Cytomegaloviruses

**A J Redwood, L M Smith, and G R Shellam,** The University of Western Australia, Crawley, WA, Australia

## Glossary

**Cytomegalia** From Greek *kytos*, cell, and *megas*, large. Refers to the cellular enlargement or swelling (cytomegalia) seen in cytomegalovirus-infected cells. This swelling is typically accompanied by the presence of intranuclear inclusion bodies, which are sometimes called 'owl eye' inclusion bodies because the dense staining inclusion body is surrounded by a cleared halo.

## Classification of Cytomegaloviruses

Cytomegaloviruses (CMVs) are large, enveloped, double-stranded DNA viruses with an icosahedral capsid that belong to subfamily *Betaherpesvirinae* of the family *Herpesviridae*. There are three genera. Genus *Cytomegalovirus* contains human cytomegalovirus (HCMV; species *Human herpesvirus 5*) and a number of other primate CMVs. Genus *Muromegalovirus* contains murine cytomegalovirus (MCMV; *Murid herpesvirus 1*) and rat cytomegalovirus (RCMV; *Murid herpesvirus 2*). Genus *Roseolovirus* contains human herpesviruses 6 and 7 (HHV-6 and HHV-7; *Human herpesvirus 6* and *Human herpesvirus 7*). Other CMVs that have not yet been fully classified within the *Betaherpesvirinae* are guinea pig cytomegalovirus (GPCMV; *Caviid herpesvirus 2*), tree shrew herpesvirus (THV; *Tupaiid herpesvirus 1*), swine cytomegalovirus (SuHV-2; suid herpesvirus 2), European ground squirrel cytomegalovirus (ScHV-1; sciurid herpesvirus 1), and American ground squirrel cytomegalovirus (ScHV-2; sciurid herpesvirus 2).

The recognized nonprimate CMVs are described in **Table 1**. With the exception of MCMV, RCMV, and GPCMV, little is known about the life cycle and pathogenesis of nonprimate CMVs. Nevertheless, general characteristics include strict species specificity, an ability to induce cytomegalia in infected cells, cell-associated replication in cell culture, a slow replication cycle and the establishment of persistent and latent, lifelong infection in the natural host. Tropism for secretory glands, particularly the salivary gland, is also a common feature. Infection is generally asymptomatic unless the host is immunosuppressed or has an immature immune system. In such hosts, infection may result in morbidity or even mortality.

## Murine Cytomegalovirus

*Murid herpesvirus 1* is the type species of the genus *Muromegalovirus*. The term murine cytomegalovirus (MCMV) is more commonly used for the virus than murid herpesvirus 1. The natural host for MCMV is the house mouse, *Mus musculus domesticus*. Because of the strict species specificity of CMVs, MCMV is widely used as an animal model of HCMV infection. Consequently, more is known about MCMV than any other nonprimate CMV.

## Virion Structure and Morphology

CMV virions are spherical, *c.* 230 nm in diameter, and comprise four morphologically distinct elements: the core, capsid, tegument, and envelope. The core encompasses the double-stranded DNA viral genome, which is packaged as a single linear molecule into the protein capsid.

The viral capsid is composed of 162 capsomers comprising hexons and pentons in a $T = 16$ icosahedral lattice structure. The capsids of CMVs are larger and incorporate a larger genome than other herpesviruses. Unlike other CMVs, MCMV preparations may contain a high proportion of multicapsid virions, which contain a number of capsids enclosed within a common membrane. The capsid of MCMV is composed of five proteins: the major capsid protein (MCP), the minor capsid protein, the minor capsid binding protein, the smallest capsid protein, and an assembly/protease. These are encoded by genes *M86*, *M85*, *M46*, *M48.2*, and *M80*, respectively.

The tegument of MCMV is a proteinaceous layer of material between the capsid and envelope, and resembles the matrix of other viruses. By electron microscopy the tegument is seen to have an ordered structure, particularly proximal to the capsid. The tegument proteins of MCMV have been defined by their homology to known HCMV tegument proteins. In HCMV there are at least 25 proteins associated with the tegument. Typically, tegument proteins are phosphorylated (and have the prefix pp). At least nine MCMV tegument proteins with homologs in HCMV have been detected in MCMV virions. These are the upper and lower matrix phosphoproteins (encoded by *M82* and *M83*), large tegument protein (*M48*), pp150 (*M32*), and the gene products from *M25*, *M47*, *M51*, *M94*, and *M99*. The role of most tegument proteins is unknown, but the function of some can be inferred from the function of HCMV homologs. For example, the upper matrix protein of HCMV, also known as pp71, is a transcriptional transactivator that regulates immediate early gene expression, possibly by inhibiting the effects of the host cell transcriptional inhibitor hDaxx. Other tegument phosphoproteins are likely to play similar roles in the transcriptional regulation of viral genes.

**Table 1**     Classification of known and putative nonprimate CMVs by the International Committee on Taxonomy of Viruses

| | | |
|---|---|---|
| Family | 00.031 | *Herpesviridae* |
| Subfamily | 00.031.2 | *Betaherpesvirinae* |
| Genus | 00.031.2.02 | *Muromegalovirus* |
| *Examples* | 00.031.2.02.001 | *Murid herpesvirus 1* (murine cytomegalovirus) |
| | 00.031.2.02.002 | *Murid herpesvirus 2* (rat cytomegalovirus) |
| Unassigned in the subfamily | 00.031.2.00.004 | *Caviid herpesvirus 2* (guinea pig cytomegalovirus) |
| | 00.031.2.00.049 | *Tupaiid herpesvirus 1* (tree shrew herpesvirus) |
| Unassigned in the family | 00.031.0.00.062 | Suid herpesvirus 2 (swine cytomegalovirus) |
| | 00.031.0.00.063 | Sciurid herpesvirus 1 (European ground squirrel cytomegalovirus) |
| | 00.031.0.00.046 | Sciurid herpesvirus 2 (American ground squirrel cytomegalovirus) |

The envelope of MCMV is composed predominantly of lipids obtained from the intracellular membranes of the host cell and contains a considerable number of virus-encoded glycoproteins. The envelope of CMVs is more pleiomorphic, and contains more glycoproteins, than envelopes of other herpesviruses. The major envelope glycoprotein, a product of the *M55* gene, is the highly conserved glycoprotein B (gB) and is a dominant B-cell antigen in CMV-infected animals and humans. It has been found in every mammalian herpesvirus and is one of the most highly conserved herpesvirus proteins. The glycoproteins of CMVs form three distinct complexes that mediate viral attachment and entry into host cells (**Table 2**).

## Genome Architecture and Coding Potential

The MCMV genome comprises a single unique sequence with short terminal direct repeats and several short internal repeats. Unlike that of HCMV, the linear genome of MCMV does not have an isomeric structure because it lacks internal repeat sequences related to the terminal repeats. The nomenclature devised for MCMV genes numbers them left to right along the genome. MCMV genes with homologs in HCMV are assigned the uppercase prefix '*M*', while genes with no sequence identity with HCMV genes are identified by the lowercase prefix '*m*'.

The genome of the Smith strain of MCMV is 230 278 bp in size, and has a coding potential estimated to be between 170 and 204 open reading frames (ORFs), including newly defined splice variants of previously described ORFs. MCMV shares with other members of the herpesvirus family a number of evolutionarily conserved proteins, which are involved in processes such as DNA replication and virion maturation and structure, and are located within

**Table 2**     Structural glycoproteins of MCMV

| Glycoprotein (gene) | Complex | Essential | Function |
|---|---|---|---|
| gB (*M55*) | gCI | Yes | Binds to cellular receptors (e.g., EGFR) and triggers intracellular signaling. *May activate host TLR2. Major B-cell epitope* |
| gN (*M73*) | gCII | Yes | With gM binds HSPG |
| gM (*M100*) | gCII | Yes | With gN binds HSPG |
| gH (*M75*) | gCIII | Yes | As a component of the gCIII complex is involved in binding and membrane fusion. *May activate host TLR2* |
| gL (*M115*) | gCIII | Yes | Required for transport of gH to the gCIII complex. As a component of the gCIII complex is involved in binding and membrane fusion |
| gO (*m74*) | gCIII | No; deletion virus has small plaque size | Enhances cell-to-cell spread of MCMV. As a component of the gCIII complex is involved in binding and membrane fusion |
| gp24 (*m73.5*) | | Unknown | Unknown |

The data are a compilation of information from HCMV and MCMV. Text in italics denotes the host response to glycoproteins. In HCMV, gB forms the disulfide-linked homodimeric gCI complex. The gCII complex is a disulfide-linked heterodimer between gM (*UL100*) and gN (*UL73*). The HCMV glycoproteins gL, gH, and gO (encoded by the genes *UL115, UL75,* and *UL74,* respectively) form the noncovalently associated heterotrimeric complex gCIII. All three complexes are essential for viral replication. MCMV homologs are believed to serve a similar function, although gN has only been demonstrated in the virions of HCMV. Note that gp24 has only been demonstrated in MCMV. In HCMV, gB and gH appear to bind TLR2, but this has not been demonstrated for MCMV.

the central region of the genome. The two terminal regions of the genome contain genes that are unique to MCMV and include the *m02* and *m145* gene families, respectively (**Figure 1**). Many of the genes in these unique regions encode proteins that are involved in modulation of the host's immune response.

## Replication

Viral replication is initiated when infectious virions enter a susceptible host cell (**Figure 2**). A series of receptors have been implicated in the binding, fusion, and entry of CMVs. Most information has come from studies of

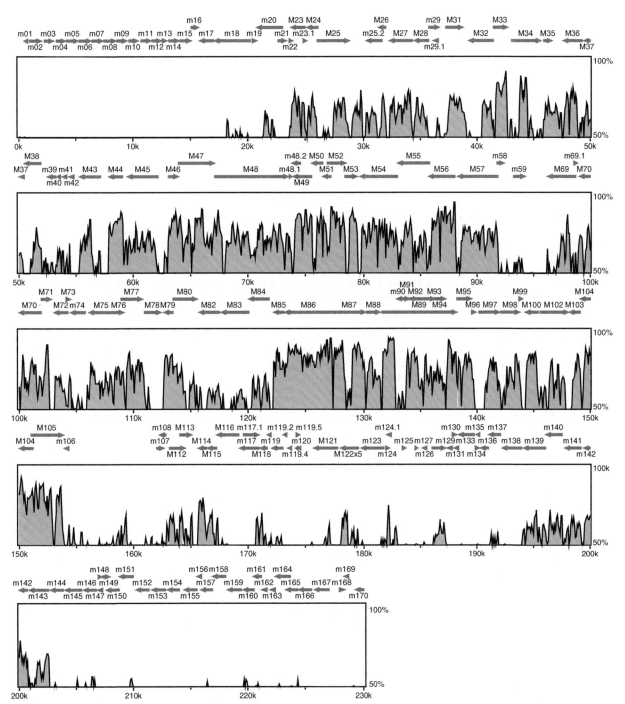

**Figure 1** Moving window comparison of the sequence similarity (shown from 50% to 100%) of the MCMV and RCMV genomes. Selected MCMV genes are marked with an arrow above the plot. The central regions of the genome are highly conserved and represent the herpesvirus-conserved genes. The left and right terminal sequences contain species-specific genes and therefore show little or no sequence similarity. Image created using LAGAN and VISTA (http://genome.lbl.gov/vista/index.shtml).

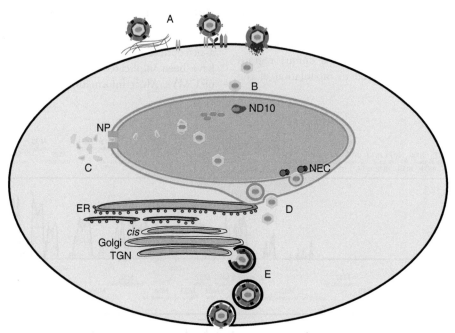

**Figure 2** CMV life cycle. (A) Virus is loosely tethered to the host cell by binding to HSPG via either gB (gCI complex) or gM/gN (gCII complex). Virus is bound more tightly by association with cell receptors such as EGFR (HCMV). Binding causes receptor clustering and the interaction of other receptors such as host cell integrins. The interaction between host receptors and viral glycoproteins induces membrane fusion and the delivery of viral capsid and tegument proteins into the host cell cytoplasm. (B) Viral capsid is transported to the nucleus and, by a process that is not understood, the viral DNA enters the nucleus. Viral DNA is localized at ND10 complexes where viral gene expression is initiated. (C) Viral proteins, including capsid proteins, are produced in the cytoplasm. DNA encapsidation and capsid assembly occur in the nucleus. Capsid proteins either diffuse into the nucleus via nuclear pores or are transported due to the presence of nuclear localization motifs. Large capsid proteins, such as MCP, which lack these motifs, are transported to the nucleus in association with capsid proteins that possess them. (D) Viral capsids acquire a primary envelope as they migrate through the inner nuclear membrane (INM). Viral proteins p35 and p38 (*M50* and *M53*) form the nuclear egress complex (NEC) and serve to disassociate the INM. Transport of the capsid through the outer nuclear membrane results in de-envelopment. (E) The final viral envelope is derived from cytoplasmic organelles, possibly in the *trans*-Golgi network (TGN). Fully formed virions enter the secretory pathway and exit the cell by exocytosis.

HCMV, in which infection is initiated by loose tethering of the virus via viral gCI and gCII complexes and heparan sulfate proteoglycans (HSPGs) on the cell surface. Tethering promotes a stronger binding reaction between the viral gCI complex and host cellular receptors. These receptors have not been fully defined, although for HCMV the epidermal growth factor receptor (EGFR) is thought to be one of the host receptors important in viral binding. This receptor binding promotes receptor co-localization with other host proteins, in particular integrins, into lipid rafts. The β1 and β3 chains of integrins have been implicated in the entry of MCMV into host cells. Integrin-binding domains have been localized to the N-terminus of gB in all betaherpesviruses and most gammaherpesviruses. Finally, receptor binding and/or co-localization triggers intracellular signaling and fusion between the host cell and viral membranes. Cellular signaling appears important for translocation of the capsids to the nucleus.

The exact mechanism by which viral DNA enters the nucleus is unknown. However, it is believed that viral DNA migrates to nuclear domain 10 (ND10) complexes within the nucleus where viral gene transcription occurs. All betaherpesviruses have three gene sets, α, β, and γ, that are temporally regulated. These genes are expressed in the immediate early (IE), early (E), and late (L) phases of viral replication, respectively. The IE phase occurs immediately after viral DNA enters the nucleus and is controlled by the major IE promoter (MIEP) in MCMV. The MIEP controls expression of the transcriptional activator genes *ie1* (*m123*) and *ie3* (*M122*). While both the *ie1* and *ie3* genes are essential for replication, the former is required specifically at low multiplicities of infection. A third IE gene, *ie2*, not present in HCMV, is transcribed from a different promoter and in the opposite direction. The *ie2* gene is not essential for MCMV replication either *in vitro* or *in vivo*.

There is an absolute requirement for IE gene expression prior to E gene expression. Genes transcribed during the E phase of viral replication include those required for entry into the L phase of viral replication, and other genes, such as the immune evasion genes. L phase genes mostly encode structural proteins and are expressed after the start of viral DNA replication, which occurs in the nucleus approximately 16 h after infection. During DNA replication, the sequences at the genomic termini fuse via a 3′ nucleotide extension to form the intermediates for MCMV replication, which occurs by a rolling-circle mechanism. Maturation of the MCMV genome involves the processing and cleavage of newly synthesized concatemeric viral DNA into genome-length monomers prior to packaging into preformed nucleocapsids in the cell nucleus. Herpesvirus-conserved *pac1* and *pac2* DNA sequence motifs are required for cleavage and packaging of the MCMV genome.

The origin of DNA replication of MCMV is the *ori* Lyt region between *M57* and *M69* (**Figure 1**), which extends over 1.7 kbp and is extremely rich in repeat sequences that act as binding elements for various transcription factors. MCMV-encoded proteins required for origin-dependent replication include the DNA polymerase (*M54*), a polymerase accessory protein (*M44*), the single-stranded DNA-binding protein (*M57*), and a helicase-primase complex encoded by *M70*, *M102*, and *M105*. All of these proteins have been detected within purified MCMV virions.

The formation of capsids and the packaging of viral DNA occur in the nucleus of infected cells. Capsid proteins are produced in the cytoplasm and are transported back to the nucleus across the nuclear membrane. The transport of capsid proteins is a result of either their small size, which allows diffusion across the nuclear pore complex, or the presence of nuclear localization signals. Large capsid proteins such as the MCP, which do not contain nuclear localization signals, are transported in association with those that do. Viral DNA is packaged into complete capsids and transported to the cytoplasm via the nuclear membrane where the capsids acquire their primary envelope as they bud through the inner nuclear membrane (INM) as shown in **Figure 2**. In MCMV infection, the virus penetrates the INM with the aid of *M50*/p35 and a partner gene, *M53*/p38. The proteins p35 and p38 form the nuclear egress complex (NEC) and recruit cellular kinases to the INM, specifically to the nuclear lamina. Recruitment of cellular kinases results in phosphorylation and degradation of the lamina, and facilitates egress of the virus from the nucleus.

The mechanism of egress of CMVs from infected cells is incompletely understood. Studies from other herpesviruses suggest that there are two phases of envelopment. A primary envelopment involving the host's INM precedes a final secondary envelopment from another host compartment, possibly the *trans*-Golgi network (TGN), where the virions also gain their tegument. The mature enveloped virions, now present in secretory vesicles, are transported to the plasma membrane, where they are released into the extracellular space by exocytosis (**Figure 2**).

## Pathogenesis

During acute experimental intraperitoneal infection, MCMV replicates predominantly in the spleen and liver and to a lesser extent in the lungs. However, the virus persists in the lungs for longer than in the spleen or liver. Other organs infected during the acute phase include the adrenal glands, kidneys, heart, and ovaries. During the chronic or persistent phase, the virus replicates predominantly in the salivary gland. Intranasal inoculation, which may mimic natural infection, results in viral replication predominantly in the lungs and salivary gland. Histologically, MCMV-infected cells exhibit typical swelling or cytomegalia (from which the virus derives its name) with intranuclear inclusion bodies. In MCMV-infected mice, mononuclear cell infiltration may be observed in inflammatory responses in the heart, lung, adrenals, and other organs.

The seroprevalence of MCMV in free-living mice can be up to 100%, particularly when mouse population densities are high. Transmission of the virus is presumed to be via saliva, possibly as a result of biting and grooming. However, MCMV is found in urine and breast milk, as well as the reproductive tract of male and female mice. This suggests additional modes of transmission, such as from mother to pup during feeding and by sexual activity. Interestingly, infection with multiple strains of MCMV is common, suggesting that mice are either infected simultaneously with multiple MCMV strains or that the lack of sterilizing immunity allows sequential reinfection of mice.

A number of diseases induced by HCMV in humans have been modeled with MCMV in mice. These include myocarditis, hepatitis, adrenalitis, and interstitial pneumonitis. However, natural congenital infection has not been modeled in mice, since MCMV, unlike HCMV, does not cross the placenta in immunocompetent hosts. Mice have also been used to investigate host resistance to CMV. A number of factors affect the capacity of MCMV to cause disease in mice. These include the dose and route of inoculation of the virus as well as the age and genetic constitution of the host. Several genetically linked innate resistance mechanisms have been identified in mice, including *Cmv1*, *Cmv3*, and *Cmv4*. These loci control resistance to MCMV via innate immune responses. Other genetic resistance mechanisms have been demonstrated in New Zealand white mice (*Cmv2*) and in a mouse strain carrying an *N*-ethyl-*N*-nitrosourea-induced mutation of the protein Unc93b1 in which signaling via Toll-like-receptors (TLRs) 3, 7, and 9 is deficient. TLRs 3, 7, and 9 recognize single-stranded RNA, double-stranded RNA (dsRNA), and unmethylated DNA, respectively. Previous studies have highlighted the importance of TLRs 2, 3, and 9 in resistance to MCMV.

## Latency

Persistent infection is a common feature of the betaherpesviruses. The infection may be either chronic, in which infectious virus is produced at very low levels for long periods in particular organs or tissues such as the salivary gland, or latent, in which infectious virus is no longer detected, although the viral genome is present in certain cells in the body. Reactivation from latency usually occurs during immunosuppression to yield infectious virus, which may induce disease and be transmitted to susceptible hosts.

Regulation of transcription is tightly controlled during latency. In MCMV, regulation of IE gene expression is an early checkpoint on the way from latency to recurrence. The IE1/3 transcriptional unit gives rise to IE1 and IE3 mRNAs by differential splicing, which is driven by the $P^{1/3}$ promoter with a strong upstream enhancer that serves as a molecular switch, connecting IE1/3 transcription to the cellular environment. External stimuli, such as the pro-inflammatory cytokine tumor necrosis factor alpha (TNF-$\alpha$), act as the first signal in the reactivation pathway, inducing transcription factors which activate the enhancer by binding to defined sequence motifs. IE3 is believed to be the major transactivator of E gene expression. MCMV latency is controlled after the initiation of IE1/3

transcription and this is the second checkpoint in the pathway of molecular reactivation. The full mechanism of reactivation has not been elucidated, but models postulate a multistep system of MCMV reactivation involving many checkpoints before the production of infectious virus.

## Host Immune Responses and Viral Evasion Strategies

The host immune response to MCMV and the many countermeasures employed by MCMV reflect a dynamic host and pathogen interaction and co-evolution. A range of host immune responses involving antibody, CD4$^+$ T cells, CD8$^+$ T cells, and natural killer (NK) cells help control MCMV infection, and are summarized in **Table 3**.

Innate intracellular defense mechanisms, such as interferon production (see below), apoptosis, and the dsRNA-dependent protein kinase R (PKR)-mediated shutdown of protein synthesis, are all targets of MCMV genes. There are three genes encoded by MCMV whose products inhibit apoptosis and facilitate tropism in specific cell types: apoptosis is inhibited in macrophages by the product of *M36*, in endothelial cells and fibroblasts by the product of *M45*, and in endothelial cells by the product

**Table 3**    Immune evasion strategies of MCMV

| Host control | Effect | MCMV immune subversion | | |
| | | Gene | Function | Mechanism |
|---|---|---|---|---|
| *Innate immunity* | | | | |
| NK cells | Control of MCMV replication in acute infection | *m145* | Inhibits NK cell killing | Downregulates MULT-1, a ligand for the NK cell activating receptor, NKG2D, on infected cells |
| | Cytokine production enhances later immune responses such as T-cell activation and may affect DC/NK cell cross talk | *m152* | Inhibits NK cell killing | Downregulates RAE-1, a ligand for the NK cell activating receptor, NKG2D, on infected cells |
| | | *m155* | Inhibits NK cell killing | Downregulates H60, a ligand for the NK cell activating receptor, NKG2D, on infected cells |
| | | *m144* | Inhibits NK cell killing | MHC homolog, ligand unknown |
| | | *m138* | Inhibits NK cell killing | Downregulates MULT-1 and H60 ligands for the NK cell activating receptor, NKG2D, on infected cells |
| | | *m157* | Activates NK cells | Binds the NK cell activating receptor Ly49H (Cmv1) |
| Monocyte/ macrophages | Phagocytosis of infected cells and cytokine production | Nil | MCMV infects monocytes and macrophages, increasing IL-10 expression and reducing MHC class II expression | Infected monocytes disseminate virus to other organs such as the salivary gland. Differentiation in the tissues to macrophages allows for productive infection |

Continued

**Table 3** Continued

| Host control | Effect | MCMV immune subversion | | |
| | | Gene | Function | Mechanism |
| --- | --- | --- | --- | --- |
| Cytokines | Various effects on both innate and acquired immune responses | M27 | Inhibits innate intracellular resistance to MCMV | Downregulates STAT-2, induces type I and type II IFN resistance |
| | | M33 | Migration of cells, including smooth muscle cells | Agonist independent GPCR, functional homolog of HCMV US28 |
| | | m129/131 | Promotes inflammation | Chemokine homolog, macrophage chemoattractant. May aid dissemination of MCMV to the salivary gland within macrophages |
| *Acquired immunity* | | | | |
| DCs | Priming of T cells Cytokine production Activation of NK cells | m147.5 and other unidentified genes | Inhibition of T-cell priming Inhibits NK cell function Reduction in IL-2 and IL-12 production | Failure of DC maturation, possibly due to multiple MCMV genes affecting MHC expression, co-stimulatory molecule expression, and cytokine production. m147.5 specifically downregulates CD86 |
| CD8 T cells | Direct killing of infected cells | m04 | Blocks CTL function | Binds MHC class I and remains associated on cell surface |
| | Control of reactivation from latency | m06 | Blocks CTL function | Targets MHC class I to lysosome for degradation |
| | | m152 | Blocks CTL function | Retains MHC class I in ERGIC |
| CD4 T cells | Control of viral replication in the salivary gland | Nil | | |
| Antibody | Reduces viral dissemination Reduces MCMV titer after reactivation Passive transfer protects mice from MCMV | m138 | Fc receptor homolog (fcr-1). No known role in evasion of antibody responses | |

MCMV has multiple mechanisms for evading host control. NK cells and CD8$^+$ CTLs are the primary effector cells in host control and this is reflected in the number of immune evasion strategies MCMV employs to evade these mechanisms. Dendritic cells (DCs) also play a major role in the acquired immune systems control of MCMV infection by priming MHC class I and II restricted responses and, in the innate response, by cytokine release and by activation of NK cells. MCMV causes functional paralysis of DC and inhibits the expression of MHC and co-stimulatory molecules on the surface of DCs. These effects presumably serve to reduce T-cell priming as well as the activation of NK cells and may alter the type of immune response generated by perturbing cytokine responses. Macrophages are a major host control mechanism, but MCMV subverts this role by infecting monocytes and using the cells as a means of dissemination to other organs such as the salivary gland. Once in the tissues, monocytes differentiate into macrophages and become permissive for MCMV production. MCMV-encoded chemokine (MCK-2) and chemokine receptor (M33) may serve to recruit inflammatory cells to the site of infection to aid viral dissemination.

of *m41*. An additional gene, *m38.5*, appears to be a homolog of the HCMV viral mitochondria-localized inhibitor of apoptosis (vMIA) encoded by *UL37*. Finally, the products of MCMV genes *m142* and *m143* form a dsRNA-binding complex that inhibits host PKR-mediated shutdown of protein synthesis.

NK cells are the primary host cell involved in the early innate response to MCMV. NK cells limit the severity, extent, and duration of acute infection and also affect the subsequent acquired immune response. MCMV infection can be lethal in their absence. NK cell control of MCMV infection is mediated by direct lysis of infected cells

and by the production of cytokines. Direct NK cell killing is mediated predominantly by perforin, particularly in the spleen. Cytokine contol of infection is most evident in the liver and is predominantly mediated by interferon gamma (IFN-γ). MCMV encodes at least six genes that affect NK cell responses (**Table 3**). The complexity of this interaction is demonstrated in **Figure 3**.

CD8$^+$ cytotoxic T lymphocytes (CTLs) are crucial for the resolution of acute MCMV infection in BALB/c mice. CTLs lyse MCMV-infected fibroblasts *in vitro* and are found in the spleen of infected mice within 3 days. Sensitized CTLs recognize both structural and nonstructural

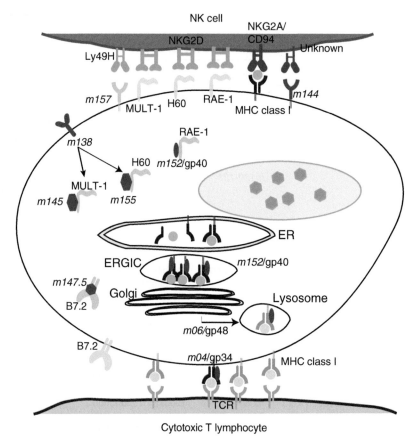

**Figure 3**   MCMV NK cell and CD8$^+$ CTL immune evasion strategies. MCMV has multiple methods of moderating host immune responses. Receptors or genes that inhibit immune responses are shown in red; those that activate immune responses are shown in green. The MHC class I molecules activate immune responses when ligated by host TCR (T-cell receptor) but inhibit responses when ligated by host NK cell NKG2A/CD94 heterodimer and are therefore shown in blue. When downregulated by an MCMV gene, host proteins are shown on the surface of the cell with reduced shading. MCMV targets NK cells by multiple mechanisms. MCMV downregulates host stress ligands that activate NK cells via the NK cell activating receptor NKG2D. MCMV genes *m138*, *m145*, *m152*, and *m155* affect the host proteins MULT-I and H60, MULT-1, H60, and RAE-1, respectively. These interactions have been depicted to occur in the cytoplasm because their actual locations are unknown. MCMV *m144* is an MHC homolog and inhibits NK cells by interaction with an unknown ligand, presumably an NK cell inhibitory receptor. Host CTL responses are avoided by interference with MHC class I expression. The gp48 (*m06*) protein targets MHC class I for degradation in the lysosome, gp40 (*m152*) retains MHC class I in the endoplasmic reticulum-Golgi intermediate compartment (ERGIC), and gp34 (*m04*) binds to MHC class I and inhibits CTL function (and possibly NK cell function). The gene product from *m147.5* downregulates the co-stimulatory molecule B7.2 and functions with other unidentified genes to inhibit DC function and reduce T-cell priming and NK cell function. Note, NKG2D is also found on T cells as a co-stimulatory receptor, but the role of *m138*, *m145*, *m152*, and *m155*, if any, on T-cell response to MCMV has not been explored.

viral antigens. This has been best studied in BALB/c mice where almost 50% of CTLs are directed against the nonstructural pp89 (*IE1*) protein of the Smith strain of MCMV. Epitope mapping has identified the immunodominant H-2L$^d$-restricted pp89 peptide as the nonomer YPHFMPTNL. Other peptides recognized in BALB/c mice are encoded by genes *m04*, *M45*, *m164*, *M83*, and *M84*. Recent studies in C57BL/6 mice have also identified a broad range of CD8 T-cell epitopes.

MCMV encodes a number of genes that are believed to affect CTL-mediated control of infection. Some, such as *m04*/gp34, *m06*/gp48, and *m152*/gp40, affect major histocompatibility complex (MHC) class I molecule expression on the surface of infected cells and/or inhibit CTL

recognition and killing (**Table 3** and **Figure 3**). Their role *in vivo* is yet to be fully explained, but MCMV mutants in which all three genes are deleted exhibit reduced growth in the salivary glands of mice. MCMV also inhibits T-cell priming by causing functional paralysis of dendritic cells (DCs). The MCMV genes responsible for this effect are largely unknown, although *m147.5* is known to downregulate the co-stimulatory molecule B7.2 on the surface of infected DCs.

Antibody and CD4$^+$ T cells play lesser roles in the resistance of mice to MCMV infection. Antibody reduces dissemination of the virus within the host and reduces viral loads after reactivation from latency. As yet, there are no known MCMV genes that target antibody function directly. The MCMV-encoded (*m138*) Fc receptor inhibits NK cell function but does not appear to play a role in inhibiting host-antibody-mediated protection. Similarly, no MCMV-encoded gene has been identified that directly targets host CD4$^+$ T-cell responses. This perhaps reflects the moderate role of host CD4$^+$ T cells in resistance to MCMV, although CD4$^+$ T cells are important in the control of MCMV replication in the salivary gland.

Cytokine responses are also crucial to the resolution of MCMV infection in mice. This is exemplified by the increased sensitivity of interferon-$\alpha\beta$ receptor 1 chain (IFNAR1) and IFN-$\gamma$R1 knockout mice to MCMV. IFNAR1/IFN-$\gamma$R1 double-knockout mice are exquisitely sensitive to MCMV infection. This increased sensitivity is probably due to the combined effects of defective cellular innate and acquired immune responses due to loss of IFN-$\gamma$ (type II IFN) signaling as well as the loss of innate intracellular responses resulting from a loss of type I IFN signaling. As a countermeasure to host type I and II IFNs, MCMV induces a state of type I and II IFN resistance by *M27*-mediated downregulation of STAT2. In addition, infection is enhanced by an MCMV-encoded chemokine and chemokine receptor. *M33* encodes a G protein-coupled receptor (GPCR) homolog that is constitutively active in an agonist-independent manner and promotes dissemination of the virus to the salivary gland, possibly by recruitment of macrophages. The MCMV-encoded (*m129/131*) chemokine MCK-2 serves a similar function in that it increases inflammation, and deletion of *m129/131* reduces viral titers in the salivary gland (**Table 3**).

## Rat Cytomegalovirus

CMVs have been identified in, and isolated from, several species of rat. The Maastricht strain of RCMV is the most widely studied and was isolated from the brown rat, *Rattus norvegicus*. Another strain of RCMV, the English strain, was isolated from *R. norvegicus*; however, its classification as a CMV has been questioned. Recently, more putative strains of RCMV have been isolated from *R. norvegicus*, *Rattus rattus* (black rat), and *Rattus argentiventer* (rice field rat). This article focuses on the Maastricht strain of RCMV.

The Maastricht strain of RCMV was isolated from a wild brown rat in 1982, and has been maintained *in vitro* and *in vivo* in inbred laboratory strains of *R. norvegicus*. The genome has been fully sequenced and consists of a unique region bounded by terminal repeats. Its genome is 230 138 bp in length and is collinear with that of MCMV, encoding at least 170 ORFs, approximately two-thirds of which share significant sequence homology with genes found in MCMV (**Figure 1**). One RCMV gene, *r127*, appears to be unique among CMVs, encoding a homolog of the parvovirus *rep* gene. As with MCMV, RCMV encodes

several genes (e.g., the GPCRs *R33* and *R78*, the MHC class I homolog *r144*, and the CC chemokine homologs *r129* and *r131*) which are homologs of cellular genes and which have therefore presumably been appropriated by the virus during evolution.

As is the case with other CMVs, RCMV is able to modulate and subvert host immune responses. RCMV downregulates the level of MHC class I molecules on the surface of infected cells. However, unlike MCMV, this effect is short-lived and does not result in proteolytic degradation of MHC class I molecules, rather in their delayed exit from the endoplasmic reticulum (ER). The RCMV gene *r131* is a pro-inflammatory CC-chemokine homolog, and appears to act similarly to the MCMV gene *m129/131* in that deletion of these genes results in decreased inflammation at the site of inoculation. This *r131*-mediated inflammation may recruit susceptible target cells to the site of infection, allowing virus dissemination throughout the body. *R33* has been shown to promote smooth muscle cell migration; however, it may play other roles in viral disease.

## Pathogenesis

Following intraperitoneal inoculation of RCMV into rats, low levels of virus can be found in the visceral organs and bone marrow at 4 days post infection (p.i.). Virus can be detected in the salivary gland, in the striated duct cells, from 10 days p.i., with virus titers peaking at 28 days p.i., before gradually decreasing over several months. Interestingly, although at 6 months p.i. viral DNA can occasionally be detected in the visceral organs, infectious virus can only ever be isolated from the salivary gland at this time point. RCMV is capable of entering latency within the infected rat, although the major sites of latent infection are unknown. Virus can be reactivated from latency following immunological stress, such as immunosuppression or stimulation with allogeneic cells, resulting in virus replication.

As is the case with other CMVs, RCMV infection does not result in overt disease in immunocompetent hosts. However, in the immunocompromised animal, it may cause considerable morbidity and mortality. In immunocompetent rats, RCMV is capable of causing vascular injury, such as endothelial cell damage and leukocyte adherence to the aortic endothelium. RCMV infection may also lead to an influx of macrophages and lymphocytes and loosening of endothelial cells from the basement membrane. Inoculation of virus into immunocompromised animals, however, produces a different scale of pathology. Extensive cell necrosis results in organ damage, with multiple hemorrhages in lung, liver, spleen, and kidney. Virus also induces damage to the microvascular epithelium, vasculitis, and thrombotic occlusions.

The tendency of RCMV to induce vascular disease has made it a good model for studying the role of HCMV in these diseases in humans. Atherosclerosis is a chronic inflammatory disorder of large- and medium-sized arteries, and seroepidemiological and histopathological studies have implicated HCMV in the pathogenesis of this disease. RCMV induces vascular lesions with endothelial cell damage and leukocyte presence in the subendothelium, the presence of subendothelial foam cells, and morphological changes to the large blood vessels of infected rats. It has been suggested that RCMV induces smooth muscle cell migration, promotes leukocyte influx, and increases cellular expression of adhesion molecules, inflammatory cytokines, and chemokines, all components of the atherosclerotic process. Infection of rats with RCMV has also been shown to be a suitable model for arterial restenosis and transplant vascular sclerosis (chronic rejection). Both conditions have been linked to infection with HCMV in humans.

## Guinea Pig Cytomegalovirus

Classic viral inclusions were first seen in the salivary gland of guinea pigs in the 1920s. However, GPCMV was not isolated until 1957. Since this time, almost all research conducted on GPCMV has used the Hartley strain of the virus.

The genome of GPCMV, while not fully sequenced, is approximately 230 kbp in length and is collinear with those of other CMVs, sharing genes with HCMV, MCMV, and RCMV within the central two-thirds of its genome but having GPCMV-specific genes near the termini. Several genes have been fully sequenced, particularly those with significant homology to potential HCMV vaccine targets. Again, as with other CMVs, gene expression is temporally regulated with IE, E, and L kinetics, although expression in the latter categories has been less well studied.

Following inoculation with GPCMV, viremia occurs for approximately 10 days, with infectious virus being detectable, and disease evident, in lungs, spleen, liver, kidney, thymus, pancreas, and brain for about another 3 weeks. Virus may be detected in the salivary gland for up to 10 weeks p.i.

GPCMV is unique among rodent CMVs in its ability to cross the placenta and infect the fetus. Hence, it is widely used as a model of congenital infection with HCMV. The guinea pig placenta consists of a single trophoblast layer separating maternal and fetal circulation, and is histologically similar to the human placenta. Infection during early pregnancy leads to pup resorption, while infection late in pregnancy generally leads to pup mortality. Following infection mid-gestation, GPCMV can be detected in placental tissue, even in the face of maternal anti-GPCMV antibodies. However, even in this case, only a proportion of pups attached to infected placentas are infected with GPCMV. These infected pups exhibit CMV disease in the brain, visceral organs, and inner ear, analogous to congenital infection with HCMV. GPCMV has been extensively used in studies of vaccination against congenital CMV infection. Vaccines against both gB and GP83 have been shown to protect against congenital GPCMV infection, although protection against pup mortality was dependent on maternal antibody titer.

## Other Nonprimate Cytomegaloviruses

Swine cytomegalovirus is endemic in swine herds worldwide, and has also been shown to reactivate from pig-to-baboon xenotransplants. It causes rhinitis in young swine and is able to cross the placenta, resulting in generalized disease, runting, and fetal death. Initial sequence analysis of the DNA polymerase complex genes suggests that this virus is more closely related to HHV-6 than to CMVs. Tree shrew herpesvirus has been sequenced and has been found to resemble MCMV and other betaherpesviruses. A CMV has been isolated from deer mice (*Peromyscus maniculatas*) in North America, and has been characterized as a CMV based on physical and biological properties and genetic homology with several genes of other CMVs. CMVs have also been isolated from European and American ground squirrels, and designated as sciurid herpesvirus 1 and sciurid herpesvirus 2, respectively.

Agents resembling CMVs have also been described in hamsters, moles, voles, field mice, the Australian native rodent antechinus, cats, and dogs. These agents have not been characterized further and may not actually be CMVs.

*See also:* Cytomegaloviruses: Simian Cytomegaloviruses.

## Further Reading

Mocarski ES, Jr. (2004) Immune escape and exploitation strategies of cytomegaloviruses: Impact on and imitation of the major histocompatibility system. *Cellular Microbiology* 6: 707–717.

Rawlinson WD, Farrell HE, and Barrell BG (1996) Analysis of the complete DNA sequence of murine cytomegalovirus. *Journal of Virology* 70: 8833–8849.

Reddehase MJ (ed.) (2006) *Cytomegaloviruses Molecular Biology and Immunology.* Wymondham, UK: Caister Academic Press.

Schleiss MR (2002) Animal models of congenital cytomegalovirus infection: An overview of progress in the characterization of guinea pig cytomegalovirus (GPCMV). *Journal of Clinical Virology* 25: S37–S49.

Shellam GR, Redwood AJ, Smith LM, and Gorman S (2007) Mouse cytomegalovirus and other herpesviruses. In: Fox JG, Barthold SW, Davisson MT, Newcomer CE, Quimby FW,, and Smith AL (eds.) *The Mouse in Biomedical Research, Vol. 2: Diseases,* 2nd edn., pp. 1–48. Amsterdam: Academic Press.

Vink C, Beuken E, and Bruggeman CA (2000) Complete DNA sequence of the rat cytomegalovirus genome. *Journal of Virology* 74: 7656–7665.

# Cytomegaloviruses: Simian Cytomegaloviruses

**D J Alcendor and G S Hayward,** Johns Hopkins School of Medicine, Baltimore, MD, USA

## Glossary

**Paralogs** Genes that share homology through gene duplication and often have diverged functions or expression patterns.

**Stealth virus** An unproven chimeric virus that lacks or suppresses genes that trigger immune responses and is thereby able to go undetected by the immune system.

## Introduction

In addition to the well-studied cytomegaloviruses (CMVs) of human (HCMV; salivary gland virus) and mouse (MCMV), related agents with typical CMV-like characteristics have been described in rats (RCMV), guinea pigs (GpCMV), pigs (PCMV), elephants (EEHV, elephant endotheliotropic herpesvirus), Old and New World primates (collectively known as simian CMVs and represented by viruses such as RhCMV), and tree shrews (HVTupaia) (**Table 1**). GpCMV was originally recognized in 1920 and served as a model system for the biology and pathogenicity of HCMV disease for many years.

Most natural nonhuman primate populations studied harbor persistent or latent infections with host-specific simian CMVs. Isolates have been reported from almost all major primate groups, including gorilla, chimpanzee, bonobo, drill, baboon, rhesus and other macaques, African green monkey, spider monkey, owl monkey, capuchin, and marmoset. Infection is also common in captive breeding populations and, even when infection is usually inapparent in the absence of immunsuppression, virus is shed intermittently in urine and saliva. Indeed, simian CMVs are potential contaminants in primary cell cultures obtained from primate sources. Also, all simian CMVs can be adapted to grow in human fibroblasts. For research purposes, the main value of simian CMVs is for genome evolutionary comparisons and as animal models for HCMV disease, in which they are potentially superior to rodent CMVs. The genomes of primate CMVs differ among themselves and from HCMV to a surprisingly large degree, but nonetheless are more closely related to HCMV than are their equivalents in nonprimates.

## Classification and Evolution

CMVs are members of the family *Herpesviridae* and belong to subfamily *Betaherpesvirinae* (**Table 1**). Formally, this subfamily is divided into three genera, namely *Cytomegalovirus* (HCMV-like viruses from primates), *Muromegalovirus* (MCMV-like viruses from rodents), and *Roseolovirus* (HHV-6-like viruses, so far only from great apes). There is one genus pending, *Proboscivirus* (EEHV). Based on the relatively high $G + C$ content of their genomes and their adaptability to grow in fibroblasts in cell culture, most traditionally recognized 'CMVs' are likely to be evolutionarily more similar to genera *Cytomegalovirus* or *Muromegalovirus* than to the $(A + T)$-rich genus *Roseolovirus*. The taxonomy of the *Betaherpesvirinae* will be shaped further with the continuing addition of members that are currently not fully classified , such as GpCMV, PCMV, and HVTupaia.

The genomes of nine betaherpesviruses are currently available, namely those of HCMV (strain AD169 in 1990, 229 354 bp; strain Merlin in 2004, 235 645 bp), CzCMV (in 2003, 241 087 bp), RhCMV (strain 68-1 in 2003, 221 459 bp; strain CMV 180.92 in 2006, 215 678 bp), MCMV (strain Smith, in 1996, 230 278 bp), RCMV (strain Maastricht in 2000, 229 896 bp), HHV6A (strain U1102 in 1995, 159 321 bp), HHV-6B (strain Z29 in 1999, 162 114 bp), HHV-7 (strain JI in, 1996, 144 861 bp; strain RK in, 1998, 153 080 bp), and HVTupaia (in 2001, 195 857 bp). The first complete betaherpesvirus genome sequenced was that of the AD169 isolate of HCMV. However, AD169 is a highly passaged laboratory strain that had suffered deletions and duplications during passaging in culture. Five more HCMV genomes have now been sequenced in the form of bacterial artificial chromosomes, and AD169 has been replaced by strains Merlin and FIX as the prototype HCMV genomes. Two strains of AgmCMV have now also been sequenced (GR2715 and Colburn), and work is in progress on EEHV as well as several other nonhuman primate CMV species.

All formally recognized and probable betaherpesviruses are listed in **Table 1**, with their common and official names and the RefSeq accession numbers of their complete sequences. Two very different muromegaloviruses (with somewhat different gene contents) are both known as RCMV, and are represented by the Maastricht (M) and English (E) strains as RCMV1 and RCMV2, respectively. CMV-like viruses have been associated with fatal hemorrhagic disease in young African and Asian elephants. Ongoing genetic analysis indicates that they are very distinct from members of the three recognized genera, and this has resulted in proposal of a new genus, *Proboscivirus*. An unusual herpesvirus isolate, referred to as 'stealth virus', was reported to have been

**Table 1**    Primate and other viruses classified in or potentially belonging to the subfamily *Betaherpesvirinae*

| Genus | Host group | Host species | Common abbreviation | Formal name | RefSeq accession |
|---|---|---|---|---|---|
| *Cytomegalovirus* | Old World primate | Human | HCMV | *Human herpesvirus 5* | NC_001347; NC_006273 |
| | | African green monkey | AgmCMV | *Cercopithecine herpesvirus 5* | |
| | | Rhesus macaque | RhCMV | *Cercopithecine herpesvirus 8* | NC_006150 |
| | | Chimpanzee | CzCMV | *Pongine herpesvirus 4* | NC_003521 |
| Possible members | | Bonobo | BoCMV | | |
| | | Baboon | BaCMV | | |
| | | Vervet | SA6 | Cercopithecine herpesvirus 3 | |
| | | Vervet | SA15 | Cercopithecine herpesvirus 4 | |
| | New World primate | Marmoset | MaCMV | Callitrichine herpesvirus 2 | |
| | | Owl monkey | HVAotus type 1 | Aotine herpesvirus 1 | |
| | | Owl monkey | HVAotus type 3 | Aotine herpesvirus 3 | |
| | | Cebus | CeCMV | | |
| | | Capuchin | AL-5 | Cebine herpesvirus 1 | |
| | | Capuchin | AP-18 | Cebine herpesvirus 2 | |
| *Muromegalovirus* | Rodent | Mouse | MCMV | *Murid herpesvirus 1* | NC_004065 |
| | | Rat | RCMV1 | *Murid herpesvirus 2* | NC_002512 |
| Possible member | | Rat | RCMV2 | | |
| *Roseolovirus* | Old World Primate | Human | HHV-6A | *Human herpesvirus 6* | NC_001664 |
| | | Human | HHV-6B | *Human herpesvirus 6* | NC_000898 |
| | | Human | HHV-7 | *Human herpesvirus 7* | NC_001716 |
| Possible member | | Chimpanzee | PaHV-6 | | |
| *Proboscivirus* (proposed) | Elephant | African elephant | EEHV | Elephantid herpesvirus 1 | |
| Unassigned | Various | Guinea pig | GpCMV | *Caviid herpesvirus 2* | |
| | | European ground squirrel | SqCMV1 | Sciurid herpesvirus 1 | |
| | | American ground squirrel | SqCMV2 | Sciurid herpesvirus 2 | |
| | | Pig | PCMV | Suid herpesvirus 2 | |
| | | Tree shrew | HVTupaia | *Tupaiid herpesvirus 2* | NC_002794 |

recovered from a human patient with central nervous system (CNS) neuropathy, but genetic analysis has revealed that this virus is virtually identical to several characterized simian CMV isolates from African green and vervet monkeys (AgmCMV). Another AgmCMV isolate, 'Colburn', was also originally thought to have been of human origin, but it is unclear whether it is truly a human isolate rather than a contaminant from primary monkey cell cultures. Based on genome analyses, the bovine herpesvirus BHV-4 and two equine herpesviruses EHV-2 and EHV-5 were originally thought to be CMVs, but were reclassified into the genus *Rhadinovirus* in subfamily *Gammaherpesvirinae*.

Typically, betaherpesviruses have no more than 40 of their 110–165 genes in common with alpha- and gammaherpesviruses. Another 35 genes appear to be betaherpesvirus specific and are likely to be shared by all CMV and HHV-6-like viruses, whereas most of the remaining genes are unique to different virus genera or individual species. As judged by the presence of several large families of related genes in HCMV, AgmCMV, and RhCMV, it appears that the CMVs, which possess the largest of all mammalian herpesvirus genomes, underwent a rapid genomic expansion in the early stages of mammalian evolutionary radiation. In contrast, the roseoloviruses (HHV-6 and HHV-7) and HVTupaia can be considered to be mini-CMVs lacking most of the repeated gene families and the entire S segment of the genome. Unlike other herpesviruses, betaherpesviruses in general do not encode either thymidine kinase or the small subunit of ribonucleotide reductase, although EEHV has both of these. However, probably all betaherpesviruses encode a phosphotransferase (UL97) activity that is the target for the effective anti-CMV agent ganciclovir and its derivatives. Like all other known herpesviruses, primate CMVs encode the typical set of six core DNA replication proteins including DNA polymerase (POL), DNA primase (PRI), helicase (HEL), single-stranded DNA-binding protein (SSB), polymerase processivity factor (PPF), and primase accessory factor (PAF). In contrast to the CMVs and muromegaloviruses, the roseoloviruses and EEHV encode a homolog of the HSV UL9 origin-binding protein (OBP).

## Virion Structure

Primate CMV virions are structurally similar to those of other members of the *Herpesviridae*, and are essentially indistinguishable from those of HCMV in the electron microscope. However, many of the virion proteins of each species display characteristic size variations by polyacrylamide gel electrophoresis (PAGE) analysis. Large nuclear and cytoplasmic inclusion bodies detectable in lytically infected cells by light microscopy are a hallmark of all betaherpesviruses.

## Genome Structure

The genomes of all known CMV DNA molecules are *c.* 210–240 kbp in size, and most have a G + C content of around 58%, in contrast to the 145–166 kbp and 46% G + C content of HHV-6 and HHV-7. Structurally, two distinct CMV genome types can be discerned. The genomes of New World primate CMVs (HVAotus types 1 and 3), HCMV, and CzCMV represent one type, having internal inverted repeats flanking two unique regions (the L segment consisting of unique region $U_L$ flanked by inverted repeats $TR_L/IR_L$, and the S segment consisting of unique region $U_S$ flanked by inverted repeats $TR_S/IR_S$), which generate four isomeric arrangements of the segments, similar to the pattern observed in herpes simplex virus. On the other hand, AgmCMV, RhCMV, HVTupaia, and several rodent CMVs (MCMV, RCMV, and GpCMV) have noninverting DNA molecules. HHV-6 and HHV-7 lack the entire 40 kbp S segment of HCMV and the L segment is bounded by large direct terminal repeats of 5–10 kbp. MCMV has a similarly sized gene block in place of the S segment, but the region has very little organizational resemblance or similarity to the S segment of HCMV. Large blocks of genes at the left and right ends of the L segment of each genome are also unique to each of the three genera for which complete sequence data are available, including the segments mapping to the right of and adjacent to the major immediate-early (MIE) genes in nonhuman primate simian CMV genomes, which differ dramatically from each other as well as from the equivalent regions in HCMV.

DNA and amino acid sequence analysis indicates that species from different mammalian hosts are diverged in accordance with their host phylogeny, with different genes having diverged at different rates. For example, in a region that is highly conserved between HCMV and AgmCMV, the major single-stranded DNA-binding proteins (UL57) have 72% overall amino acid sequence identity, whereas a group of three adjacent betaherpesvirus-specific glycoproteins mapping to the left of the MIE region (UL118, UL120, and UL121) vary from as much as 35% identity overall to as little as 15% in one region. Similarly, the betaherpesvirus-specific IE2 (UL122) immediate-early (IE) regulatory proteins of HCMV and AgmCMV have 58% amino acid sequence identity, but only over the C-terminal half of the protein, and both are equally diverged from RhCMV in this region. Amino acid sequence differences between homologous CMV genes from even the most closely related host species, such as HCMV and CzCMV, are frequently at least 20–30%.

Even the DNA molecules of individual isolates of a single primate CMV species are often distinguishable on the basis of multiple restriction fragment length polymorphisms stemming from overall intraspecies nucleotide variations of up to 3–4%. In fact, different isolates or strains of HCMV and simian CMVs display a number of significant genomic differences. First, so-called laboratory strains of HCMV (such as AD169 and Towne), AgmCMV (Colburn), and RhCMV (68-1) have all undergone deletions and rearrangements. They have also accumulated frameshift or truncation mutations in a number of genes that appear to be critical for preserving natural tropism for endothelial and macrophage cell types, but are evidently selected against during adaptation to fibroblast cells. These changes particularly affect a set of three small genes (UL128, UL130, and UL131A). Even the less passaged HCMV (strain Toledo) has undergone a large inversion that affects UL128.

A second type of strain sequence difference has been documented in HCMV for many years within a subset of 'variable' genes, which include gB (UL55), gN (UL73), gO (UL74), exon 3 of UL37 (UL37ex3), UL9, RL12, RL13, UL144, UL146, and UL147. In each case, even when analyzed directly by polymerase chain reaction (PCR) sequencing of clinical samples, the proteins from different genomes can display up to 30–60% divergence at the amino acid level, with collections of isolates examined falling into clusters of 3, 5, 8, or even 15 subtypes, depending on the locus. The subtype patterns in different 'variable' gene loci are unlinked, and this is indicative of high levels of mixed infections, recombination, and chimerism in HCMV samples. The origin and biological significance of subtype patterns are not well understood, but are most likely related to founder and bottleneck effects during the recent evolutionary spread and migration of humans. Isolates of CMV from nonhuman primate host species also display similar patterns of variability.

The sequenced prototype betaherpesviruses contain several interesting, and in some cases genus-specific, genes that are related to cellular genes and appear to be used primarily for evasion of immune responses. For example, HCMV encodes four viral G protein-coupled receptors (vGPCRs; UL33, UL78, US27, and US28), at least one of which (US28) functions as a broad-spectrum chemokine receptor that promotes migration of smooth muscle cells, and three glycoproteins (US3, US10, and US11) that together function to destabilize or inhibit cellular HLA-mediated responses. HHV-6 and MCMV each encode two GPCR proteins. HCMV and MCMV also each encode diverged homologs of HLA-I (at different locations in their genomes), and HCMV also possesses two separate anti-apoptotic proteins known as vMIA (UL37) and vICA (UL36). Spliced genes in MCMV and RCMV encode two functional β-chemokines, whereas HCMV encodes two α-chemokines (UL146 and UL147). HHV-6 (but not HHV-7) encodes an REP protein apparently captured from adeno-associated virus, and both HHV-6 and HHV-7, as well as RCMV but not MCMV, encode different OX-2-related proteins. RhCMV and AgmCMV, but not HCMV or CzCMV, encode a highly spliced COX2 gene, and HCMV, RhCMV, and AgmCMV encode a spliced vIL-10 gene, whereas CzCMV does not.

The total genome contents of the two 'great ape' CMVs (HCMV and CzCMV) differ by at most a half dozen out of 165 clearly defined genes. However, differences between HCMV and the 'Old World primate' CMVs (RhCMV and AgmCMV) are numerous. One

manifestation is the presence of either five or six tandemly repeated but highly diverged paralogs of the paired US27/US28 vGPCR genes of HCMV in multiple strains of RhCMV and AgmCMV, and the presence of either seven or eight tandemly repeated but highly diverged paralogs of the paired UL146/UL147 α-chemokine genes of HCMV in different strains of AgmCMV (**Figure 1**). Also, there are three, rather than two, of the α-chemokine genes in this cluster in CzCMV and at least three in RhCMV. Both the vGPCR and α-chemokine gene clusters appear to be undergoing highly dynamic evolution in Old World primate CMVs.

## Epidemiology and Physical Properties

Features of host range, virus propagation, virus transmission, tissue tropism, pathogenicity, histopathology, and immune responses of primate CMVs, together with the physical properties and assembly pathways of the virions, and a number of biochemical properties of their structural proteins, closely resemble those of HCMV and MCMV. In general, long-term persistent asymptomatic infection is nearly universal among natural primate populations in the wild, with primary infections occurring in infants and juveniles. Even captive colony-borne animals are rarely free of these viruses, which can be shed intermittently in saliva and urine throughout the host's lifespan. Like all other herpesviruses, primate CMVs have enveloped icosahedral capsids and replicate in the

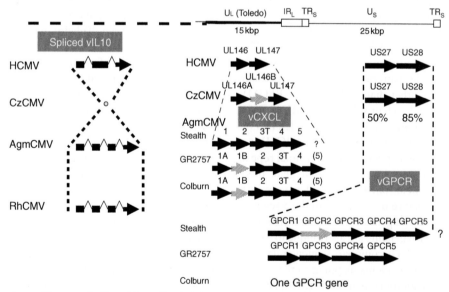

**Figure 1** Comparison of the organization of the spliced vIL10 genes, the UL146 vCXCL α-chemokine ligand gene cluster, and the US28 vGPCR chemokine gene cluster in CMV genomes. Amino acid sequence identity between HCMV and CzCMV is indicated for the US27 and US28 proteins. Stealth, GR2757, and Colburn are distinct isolates of AgmCMV. The position of the additional (but inverted) 15 kbp segment in HCMV strain Toledo U_L compared to strain AD169 is indicated by the solid line. The spliced vIL10 gene is present in HCMV, AgmCMV, and RhCMV but absent from CzCMV. Another spliced gene (the COX2 gene) is present (at another location) in AgmCMV and RhCMV, but not in HCMV or CzCMV.

nucleus. Infection of humans with simian CMVs via prolonged contact with seropositive monkeys or apes, or from vaccines grown in unscreened primary cell cultures from primate sources, is plausible, but has not been documented unambiguously. Laboratory-adapted strains such as AgmCMV Colburn grow vigorously in human fibroblast cell culture (**Figure 2**) and have been known to outgrow HCMV in cell culture. However, primary isolates grow slowly in both human and simian fibroblasts.

## Replication Strategies

The lytic cycle pathway of gene expression for primate CMVs follows the typical herpesvirus cascade of IE mRNAs and proteins followed by activation of delayed-early (DE) then late (L) class genes, with synthesis of viral DNA. In cell culture, fully permissive host cell types for HCMV are restricted almost exclusively to diploid cells, including human fibroblasts, vascular endothelial cells (and the U373 astrocytoma cell line), smooth muscle cells, and differentiated macrophages. Fresh clinical HCMV isolates usually need to be adapted for efficient growth in fibroblasts by multiple rounds of passaging, which is accompanied by selection of inactivating point mutations (or deletions) in certain 'cell tropism' genes and a loss of ability to grow in endothelial cells or macrophages.

Laboratory strains of HCMV replicate their DNA efficiently by 72 h in human fibroblasts, but express only the MIE proteins and fail to synthesize any viral DNA in rodent or monkey fibroblasts. AgmCMV, RhCMV, BaCMV, and CzCMV replicate their DNA and form plaques in both human and simian fibroblasts (**Figure 2**). In contrast, MCMV carries out viral DNA synthesis in

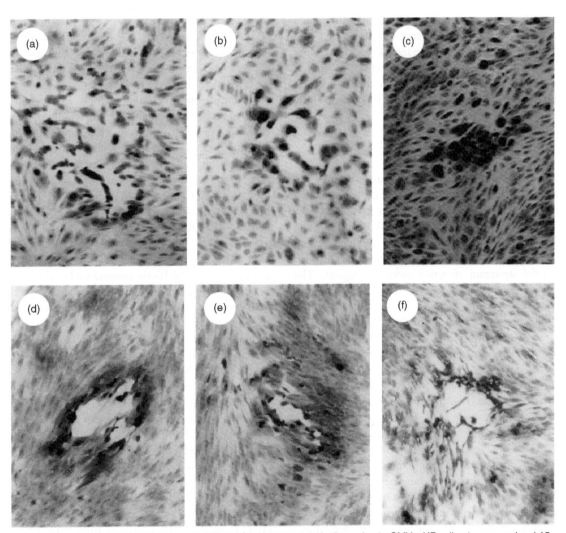

**Figure 2** Infection of human diploid fibroblasts (HF cells) with human and other primate CMVs. HF cells at passage level 15 were infected and examined daily for cytopathic effects. All infections produced characteristic cytomegalic cells in culture. (a) HCMV (Towne strain) plaque at 7 days after infection; (b) AgmCMV plaque at 8 days after infection; (c) BaCMV plaque at 11 days after infection; (d) CzCMV plaque at 14 days after infection; (e) RhCMV plaque at 14 days after infection; (f) CeCMV plaque at 8 days after infection.

human, monkey, and rodent fibroblasts. Most transformed human cell types are nonpermissive for HCMV replication, with the block occurring between DNA entry and synthesis of MIE mRNA. However, some differences between HCMV and AgmCMV have been observed at this stage. For example, HCMV fails to synthesize MIE proteins in infected human (NTera) or mouse (F9) teratocarcinoma stem cells, in human 293 or NBE cells, or in mouse L-cells. In contrast, AgmCMV produces MIE proteins in infected NTera, 293, and NBE cells, but not in F9 or L-cells. After differentiation with retinoic acid (RA), NTera stem cells can become permissive for HCMV MIE expression and infectious virus production. Similarly, F9 cells treated with RA induce AgmCMV, but not HCMV, MIE expression. These biological differences among the different species of Old World primate CMVs appear to coincide with structural differences in the organization of *cis*-acting transcriptional control elements and adjacent accessory domains located both upstream of and within the large first intron of the MIE genes. Although a major site *in vivo* for quiescent inactive infection for HCMV and MCMV is believed to involve monocytes, many other sites of inapparent noncytopathic infection occur, but whether any of these can be defined as the true site of reactivatable latent state infection has not yet been resolved.

## Control of Gene Expression

Similarly organized MIE transcription units, which encode regulatory proteins that trigger the lytic cycle, have been described for HCMV, CzCMV, AgmCMV, RhCMV, BaCMV, GpCMV, RCMV, MCMV, HHV-6, and HHV-7. In each case, these transcription units produce several multiply spliced mRNAs whose expression is controlled by powerful upstream *cis*-acting enhancer regions. The predominant viral mRNAs synthesized after infection of permissive cells in the presence of cycloheximide (an inhibitor of protein synthesis) are the MIE mRNAs, and these are also the only HCMV or AgmCMV mRNAs and proteins produced after infection of nonpermissive rodent fibroblasts. At least two types of phosphorylated nuclear regulatory proteins are encoded by the MIE transcription unit. These include the highly abundant, acidic IE1 (UL122) nuclear protein and the less abundant IE2 (UL123) DNA-binding transactivator/repressor protein. The IE2 DNA-binding transcription factor proteins are not only essential for stimulating transcription of downstream DE and L HCMV promoters, but they also specifically downregulate their own MIE promoters (negative autoregulation) and are probably also engaged in control of viral DNA replication, altering cell cycle function and blocking interferon and apoptotic responses. In particular, both the IE1 and IE2 proteins target to subnuclear domains known as PODs (protein oncogenic domains), which contain the

PML proto-oncoprotein, and appear to modify these sites (also known as ND10 (nuclear domain 10)) for utilization by the viral genomes to initiate viral IE transcription and viral DNA synthesis.

In contrast to the rest of the viral genome, the IE1 and the IE2 coding regions of the MIE transcription units in HCMV, CzCMV, AgmCMV, MCMV, RCMV, HHV-6, and HHV-7 (and probably all other betaherpesviruses) are highly CpG-suppressed, which suggests that they are accessible to cellular methylation events at some stage of the viral life cycle during which all other viral genes are transcriptionally silent. The 490-amino-acid residue HCMV IE1 protein has only 15% amino acid sequence identity with AgmCMV or RhCMV IE1, and much less still is conserved between the primate and MCMV and RCMV versions, although all of the betaherpesvirus IE1 proteins (except for those of HHV-6 and HHV-7) have a highly acidic, Glu-rich C-terminus. In contrast, the 579-amino-acid residue IE2 proteins of HCMV, AgmCMV, RhCMV, MCMV, RCMV, and their much larger counterparts in HHV-6 and HHV-7, exhibit between 25% and 58% sequence identity over the C-terminal 270-residue conserved DNA-binding domain. As expected, the CzCMV IE1 and IE2 proteins are much more similar to the HCMV versions.

The upstream MIE promoter/enhancer regions, which serve to sense the intranuclear environment and control entry into or out of the lytic cycle, are large, complex, noncoding DNA sequence domains that consist of often multicopy, high-affinity binding sites for numerous constitutive or inducible cellular transcription factors. In HCMV, CzCMV, AgmCMV, RhCMV, BaCMV, GpCMV, and MCMV, these sites include response elements for cyclic AMP (CRE, PKA), phorbol esters (TPA, PKC), and RA, together with recognition motifs for SRF/ETS, CREB, SP-1, AP-1, and nuclear factor kappa B (NFκB). Even among the five Old World primate CMVs that have been examined in detail, the organization of these sites within the MIE enhancer regions differs significantly, and the number and pattern of the adjacent tandemly repeated 15 and 30 bp high-affinity NFI/YY1 motifs also differ greatly (**Figure 3**). Overall, the MIE control region in AgmCMV encompassing the BENT, NFI, ENH, and INTRON segments totals 2.3 kbp in size, much more than the approximately 1.1 kbp MIE control region in HCMV.

Other specific regulatory proteins common to HCMV and HHV-6, such as the UL36 and UL37 proteins, members of the US22 family, the UL82 and UL83 matrix phosphoproteins, and the UL84 replication-associated protein, are all conserved in primate CMVs. However, the second immediate early promoter (IES) and its novel, complex NFκB-containing enhancer is found in HCMV and CzCMV upstream from gene US3, and is not conserved in RhCMV or AgmCMV.

The CMV lytic cycle origin of DNA replication (Ori-Lyt) is located to the right of and adjacent to the

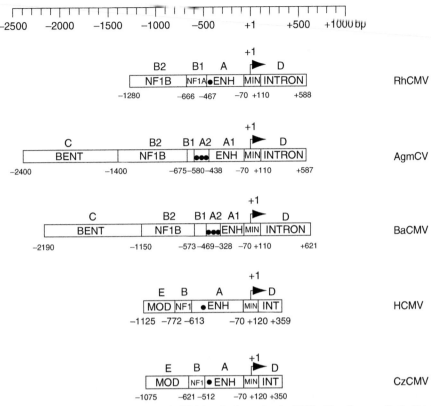

**Figure 3** Upstream control regions in the MIE genes of HCMV and other primate CMVs. The diagram illustrates the respective size and organization of domains containing specific transcription factor-binding motif patterns. These include clusters of nuclear factor 1 (NF1) and YY1 sites, the distal enhancer containing multiple CRE, SRE, and NFκB sites (ENH), the proximal promoter and TATATAA box region (MIN) that includes the start site of transcription at +1 (arrowed), and the 5′ half of the large first intron (INTRON). Where appropriate, additional upstream AT-rich (BENT) and modulatory (MOD) regions are also included. Domain boundaries are designated as + or − nucleotide positions with reference to the start site of transcription and given in bp. The domains have also been designated A–E with subcategories 1 or 2 in the case of the NF1 and ENH block. Adapted from Chan YJ, Chiou CJ, Huang Q, and Hayward GS (1996) Synergistic interactions between overlapping binding sites for the serum response factor and ELK-1 proteins mediate both basel enhancement and phorbal ester responsiveness of primate cytomegalovirus major immediate-early promoters in monocyte and T-lymphocyte cell types. *Journal of Virology* 70: 8590–8605, with permission from American Society for Microbiology.

single-stranded DNA-binding protein gene (UL57), near the center of the HCMV, CzCMV, AgmCMV, RhCMV, and MCMV genomes. It differs significantly from virus to virus in structural organization and apparently cannot be complemented by the protein replication machinery from another virus within this group. Although Ori-Lyt is located at the equivalent site in the genomes of HHV-6 and HHV-7 (and presumably also EEHV), it differs in structure and in its UL9-dependent mode of DNA replication from that in CMVs. It is still not known whether any betaherpesviruses utilize a latent cycle origin of DNA replication, such as that found among gammaherpesviruses.

## Future Perspectives

Persistent, inapparent infection with CMVs is probably virtually ubiquitous in most individuals of all mammalian species. However, the biological and pathological properties of primate CMVs have attracted the interest of herpesvirologists and clinicians interested in HCMV disease in acquired immune deficiency syndrome (AIDS) and organ transplant patients, not so much because of the serious morbidity or economic consequences of these infections in their own hosts, but more often as models for latency and pathogenesis or immunological responses in HCMV. MCMV, RCMV, GpCMV, RhCMV, and BaCMV have all been investigated as models for virus reactivation, and for control of acute and chronic disease by anti-CMV agents (such as ganciclovir, a nucleotide analog that specifically inhibits CMV DNA replication) in association with allografted organ transplants or immunosuppression. There is also interest in questions related to whether different CMVs can cross host species barriers with possible pathological consequences, which is of concern with BaCMV and PCMV for xenografted organ transplants. Primate CMVs also have comparative value in molecular genetics and biochemical analysis because of their similarities to and differences from HCMV or HHV-6 and HHV-7. Current basic scientific interest in genomic evolution (made possible by large-scale DNA sequencing), as well as the role of transcriptional gene regulation mechanisms in determining cell tropism and the switching between latent and lytic cycle virus–cell interaction pathways, and the many novel mechanisms used by betaherpesviruses for immune evasion, should lead to an expansion of these types of studies with nonhuman primate CMVs over the next several years.

*See also:* Cytomegaloviruses: Murine and Other Non-primate Cytomegaloviruses; Simian Alphaherpesviruses; Simian Gammaherpesviruses.

## Further Reading

Bahr U and Darai G (2001) Analysis and characterization of the complete genome of tupaia (tree shrew) herpesvirus. *Journal of Virology* 75: 4354–4370.

Bankier AT, Beck S, Bohni R, *et al.* (1991) The DNA sequence of the human cytomegalovirus genome. *DNA Sequence* 2: 1–12.

Chan YJ, Chiou CJ, Huang Q, and Hayward GS (1996) Synergistic interactions between overlapping binding sites for the serum response factor and ELK-1 proteins mediate both basal enhancement and phorbal ester responsiveness of primate cytomegalovirus major immediate-early promoters in monocyte and T-lymphocyte cell types. *Journal of Virology* 70: 8590–8605.

Chee MS, Bankier AT, Beck S, *et al.* (1990) Analysis of the protein-coding content of the sequence of human cytomegalovirus strain AD169. *Current Topics in Microbiology and Immunology* 154: 125–169.

Davison AJ, Dolan A, Akter P, *et al.* (2003) The human cytomegalovirus genome revisited: Comparison with the chimpanzee cytomegalovirus genome. *Journal of General Virology* 84: 17–28.

Dolan A, Cunningham C, Hector RD, *et al.* (2004) Genetic content of wild-type human cytomegalovirus. *Journal of General Virology* 85: 1301–1312.

Dominguez G, Dambaugh TR, Stamey FR, Dewhurst S, Inoue N, and Pellett PE (1999) Human herpesvirus 6B genome sequence: Coding content and comparison with human herpesvirus 6A. *Journal of Virology* 73: 8040–8052.

Gibson W (1983) Protein counterparts of human and simian cytomegaloviruses. *Virology* 128: 391–406.

Gompels UA, Nicholas J, Lawrence G, *et al.* (1995) The DNA sequence of human herpesvirus-6: Structure, coding content, and genome evolution. *Virology* 209: 29–51.

Hansen SG, Strelow LI, Franchi DC, Anders DG, and Wong SW (2003) Complete sequence and genomic analysis of rhesus cytomegalovirus. *Journal of Virology* 77: 6620–6636.

Kaplan AS (1973) *The Herpesviruses,* chs. 12 and 13. New York: Academic Press.

Megaw AG, Rapaport D, Avidor B, Frenkel N, and Davison AJ (1998) The DNA sequence of the RK strain of human herpesvirus 7. *Virology* 244: 119–132.

Nicholas J (1996) Determination and analysis of the complete nucleotide sequence of human herpesvirus 7. *Journal of Virology* 70: 5975–5989.

Rawlinson WD, Farrell HE, and Barrell BG (1996) Analysis of the complete DNA sequence of murine cytomegalovirus. *Journal of Virology* 70: 8833–8849.

Richman LK, Montali RJ, Garber RL, *et al.* (1999) Novel endotheliotropic herpesviruses fatal for Asian and African elephants. *Science* 283: 1171–1176.

Rivailler P, Kaur A, Johnson RP, and Wang F (2006) Genomic sequence of rhesus cytomegalovirus 180.92: Insights into the coding potential of rhesus cytomegalovirus. *Journal of Virology* 80: 4179–4182.

Staczek J (1990) Primate cytomegaloviruses. *Microbiological Reviews* 54: 247.

Vink C, Beuken E, and Bruggeman CA (2000) Complete DNA sequence of the rat cytomegalovirus genome. *Journal of Virology* 74: 7656–7665.

# Endogenous Retroviruses

**W E Johnson,** New England Primate Research Center, Southborough, MA, USA

## Glossary

**Metazoan** A multicellular animal.
**Monophyletic** A taxonomic grouping comprised exclusively of an ancestor and its descendants.
**Phylogenetic tree** A diagram of the evolutionary relationships between entities descended from a common ancestor.
**Proto-oncogene** A gene whose normal function is to control cell growth or differentiation, but which can be converted into a cancer-causing gene (oncogene) by mutation or disregulation.

## Introduction

At the heart of the retrovirus replication cycle is a stage in which the viral genome, having been converted from single-stranded RNA into double-stranded DNA by the viral reverse transcriptase, is inserted at random into a chromosome of the infected cell. The resulting DNA 'provirus' directs expression and assembly of progeny virions. The integrated provirus itself is contiguous with the rest of the host-cell chromosome, just like any other stretch of genomic DNA sequence. Consequently, if a cell harboring a provirus continues to divide and multiply, the provirus will be inherited by daughter cells during subsequent rounds of cell division like any other cellular gene. If retroviral integration occurs in a cell belonging to germline tissue of a host organism (e.g., in an oocyte or in an embryonic cell destined to develop into germline tissue), the resulting provirus constitutes an insertional mutation, and the new allele can potentially be passed on to the next generation like any other chromosomal locus. As a new allele, the proviral locus will be subject to the processes of random genetic drift and selection and, as a result, many such events may quickly be lost. But some will spread in the population and, given enough time, may eventually become fixed. In fact, this scenario has played out many millions of times over the course of metazoan evolution, such that the genomes of almost all animal species contain numerous sequences resembling proviruses. These elements are referred to as endogenous retroviruses (ERVs). While exogenous retroviruses spread from individual to individual by infection (horizontal transmission), endogenous retroviruses, as components of the germline, are inherited in the same fashion as other genes. The two modes are not mutually exclusive, and virions expressed from ERVs can give rise to spreading infections within the host and may also be transmitted to other individuals.

## Structure

The typical retroviral provirus consists of *gag, pro, pol,* and *env* open reading frames, which encode the viral structural and nonstructural proteins, bookended by two identical regulatory regions called long terminal repeats (LTRs). No chromosomal DNA is lost as a consequence of integration; however, a short stretch of host-cell DNA (typically around 4–6 bp) is duplicated, resulting in direct repeats (DRs) of cellular sequence flanking the provirus. Important *cis*-acting sequences for replication are located within the LTRs, and primer recognition sequences for reverse transcription are located at the junctions between the 5′ LTR and *gag* (first-strand synthesis), and between *env* and the 3′ LTR (second-strand synthesis). Retroviruses use a cellular transfer RNA molecule (tRNA) as the primer for the first step in reverse transcription; thus, the primer binding site (PBS) is complementary to the 3′ end of a cellular tRNA. The second primer is derived from a purine-rich stretch of the viral RNA itself (polypurine tract or PPT). The generic structure of a provirus is therefore:

$$DR\text{-}5'LTR\text{-}PBS\text{-}gag\text{-}pro\text{-}pol\text{-}env\text{-}PPT\text{-}3'LTR\text{-}DR$$

In general, ERVs can be recognized as genomic loci conforming to this basic arrangement, even though in many cases significant portions of the original provirus may be missing (**Figure 1**). There are no viral or cellular mechanisms for precise deletion of integrated proviruses, but ERV sequences can be lost or rearranged, in whole or in part, by the same general processes affecting all chromosomal DNA. For example, homologous recombination can occur between the two LTRs of an ERV, resulting in deletion of the intervening proviral sequences and leaving behind a single LTR (or solo-LTR). Solo-LTRs are abundant in animal genomes, and in many cases may significantly outnumber intact proviruses.

## Discovery and Distribution

Even prior to the discovery of reverse transcriptase in 1970 (and confirmation that retroviruses replicate through

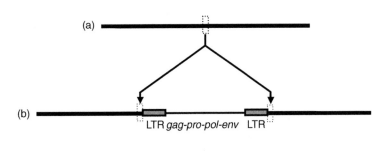
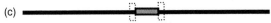

**Figure 1** Structure of an ERV. Thick black line represents a segment of a host-cell chromosome. Thin line (labeled *gag-pro-pol-env*) and gray boxes (LTR) represent integrated viral sequences. Small boxes (dashed line) indicate short segment of chromosomal DNA duplicated (arrowheads) at the time of proviral integration. (a) Chromosomal segment prior to integration of a provirus. (b) Same chromosomal locus, but containing an integrated provirus. No chromosomal DNA is lost due to integration, and a short segment (~4–6 bp) is duplicated. When this structure occurs in the germline, it constitutes an ERV. At the time of integration, the LTRs of the ERV are identical, but these sequences will thereafter diverge due to the accumulation of random mutations; thus, the degree of divergence between the LTRs of an ancient ERV are a reflection of the age of the provirus. (c) Same locus, after recombination between the two LTRs, has resulted in loss of the intervening proviral sequence. Only a single copy of the LTR sequence remains, along with the flanking repeats.

a proviral intermediate), there was some phenotypic evidence for the existence of ERV loci. Then beginning in the early 1970s, the widespread existence of ERVs was quickly revealed using genomic DNA samples and nucleic acid hybridization techniques. Novel ERV sequences were cloned initially using probes derived from existing retroviruses, by accident during the cloning and characterization of unrelated genes, and later by using a variety of polymerase chain reaction (PCR)-based approaches. By far the richest vein of new ERV sequences has come from mining the human genome databases and subsequent whole-genome sequences of other organisms.

The distribution of ERV among modern species speaks of their age. ERV families or specific ERV loci are often shared among the genomes of related species, indicating that the integration events occurred in the genomes of ancestors shared by those species. For example, a large number of ERVs are located in identical positions in humans and closely related primates, such as chimpanzees, bonobos, and gorillas. Thus, these loci must have originated in a common ancestor of these species. This also provides a lower bound to the estimated time of integration based on the approximate time of divergence of these lineages. In the case of an ERV locus shared exclusively by humans and chimpanzees, for example, the provirus will be no less than about 5 million years old, whereas a locus shared by humans, apes, and Old World monkeys will be greater than 25 million years old. In general, the wider spread an ERV-sequence family is among extant species, the more ancient that family is. More modern ERVs are found among a smaller subset of species or are even confined to a single species. (This is a generalization because viruses have the potential for horizontal, cross-species transmission; ERV sequences derived from a modern retrovirus could appear in the genomes of more than one lineage.) Modern ERVs are also more likely to be intact (and capable of expressing virus), and are often closely related to known exogenous retroviruses.

## Origins

There are at least four possible scenarios to explain the presence of multicopy ERV families in the germline: (1) repeated, *de novo* infection of germline tissue by an exogenous retrovirus; (2) expression of an existing endogenous provirus with subsequent reinfections of germline tissue; (3) intracellular retro-transposition from an existing ERV; and (4) duplication of genomic DNA fragments already containing an integrated ERV (however, even in this case, the original ERV sequence must have arisen via one of the first three mechanisms). Although there is experimental proof-in-principle for all four processes, it is generally believed that scenarios involving extracellular replication and infection (i.e., the first two mechanisms) predominate in nature.

Whatever the mechanism, presence in the germline requires that integration, takes place either in cells of germline tissue or, because the provirus is maintained during cell division, in a cell lineage destined to develop into germline tissue. Once integrated, the selective forces that work on the proviral sequences will depend on a number of factors, including the state of the provirus at the time of integration. For example, did the viral genome suffer attenuating or debilitating mutations during reverse transcription? Was it intact and capable of expression at the time of provirus formation? Did integration occur in junk DNA, close to a gene, or in a gene? Was the provirus silenced after integration (e.g., by methylation), and in what developmental stages and in which tissues was the provirus expressed? In other words, whether or not a newly formed provirus will persist as an endogenous retrovirus is determined in part by its immediate effect on the survival of the infected cell and its ultimate effect on reproductive fitness of the host organism. ERVs that are strongly counterselected due to pathogenic or detrimental effects on the host are likely to be lost from the gene pool.

Although the bulk of integrations may occur in junk DNA, experimental evidence suggests that integration may occur preferentially into transcriptionally active areas, which increases the likelihood of insertion in and near genes. Insertional inactivation of critical genes can be immediately deleterious to the host, or may only be lethal in the homozygous state (in the latter case, an ERV-containing locus could persist for many generations as a minor allele). Integration can also lead to activation or aberrant regulation of genes near the site of integration. For example, activation of proto-oncogenes in the vicinity of integrated proviruses has been detected many times in experimental animal models of retroviral pathogenesis; it is possible that similar scenarios could also occur during formation of an ERV. Expression of the ERV can potentially be a source of pathogenic virus or can contribute to pathogenecity by recombination with other retroviruses.

ERV sequences may also have beneficial consequences for the host. Laboratory studies with both chickens and inbred mice have identified several ERV-derived genes that now function to reduce or prevent exogenous retroviral infection. ERV sequences also have the potential to provide new cellular functions during the course of evolution. The human Syncytin protein may be a striking example of the latter; this protein is in fact the envelope protein of an ancient endogenous provirus that appears to have been co-opted during evolution to function in human placental morphogenesis.

Stochastic factors will also influence the persistence of an ERV locus in the genome. Proviruses in the germline are subject to the same processes that affect all genomic sequences, including substitutions, deletions, insertions, recombination, gene conversion, random assortment, and genetic drift. Even in the absence of selective pressures, a newly formed ERV represents a minor allele and stands a good chance of being lost by chance. In the absence of positive selection, random accumulation of mutations over time will eventually degrade the viral open reading frames and the *cis*-acting elements required for expression. Thus, the interplay between random processes, as well as the nature and extent of selective forces acting on the ERV, will affect the way in which these sequences evolve during their residence in the germline.

## Taxonomy and Classification

The term 'endogenous retrovirus' does not refer to a biological entity distinct from other retroviruses, but simply describes any DNA provirus, retroviral in origin, that has found its way into an organismal germline. This is true regardless of whether the provirus is still capable of expressing infectious virions. In fact, even highly degraded proviruses containing large deletions, insertions, and substitutions are often referred to as ERVs, as long as they are still clearly derived from a retrovirus.

Phylogenetic trees incorporating multiple genera of retroviruses are typically constructed using amino acid alignments corresponding to conserved domains in the reverse transcriptase gene. When representatives of multiple ERV families are included in such analyses, they do not form a monophyletic cluster, but rather are scattered within and between the various genera of exogenous retroviruses (**Figure 2**). Moreover, modern ERVs may have very closely related, exogenous counterparts. Thus,

ERVs do not constitute a separate taxonomic division from exogenous retroviruses (this refers to ERVs as a whole; any individual ERV locus or family may still represent a novel (and possibly extinct) retroviral genus).

Although there are exceptions, the vast majority of ERVs (particularly the ancient ERVs) is not closely related to known exogenous retroviruses, is no longer capable of expressing virus, and has no other associated biological or phenotypic properties to facilitate classification. The interleaving of ancient ERV sequences with extant retroviruses in phylogenetic trees, along with similarities to modern viruses in provirus organization, indicates that ancient ERVs are not ancestral stages in the evolutionary pathway leading to retroviruses (i.e., they are not protoretroviruses), but rather represent fully evolved (albeit extinct) sibling species to modern retroviruses.

There is as yet no officially recognized nomenclature for endogenous retroviruses, and a variety of naming conventions exist. In general, these represent myriad naming practices coined by various investigators at the time each novel ERV was discovered. For ERVs originally identified in the human genome, the practice has been adopted of using the acronym HERV (for human endogenous retrovirus) followed by a single letter that specifies the most likely tRNA primer (based on complementarity to the putative PBS sequence). Thus, HERV-K refers to endogenous proviruses with a PBS sequence complementary to a lysine tRNA. This convention has made the HERV literature much more accessible, but in practice it still leads to some ambiguity, because: (1) otherwise unrelated retroviruses may share the same

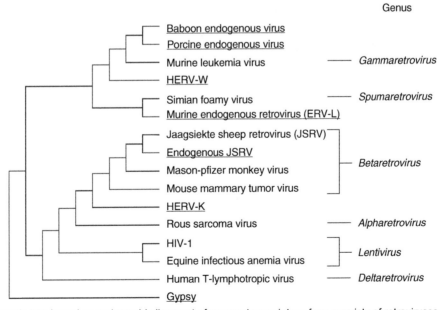

**Figure 2** Phylogenetic tree based on amino acid alignment of reverse transcriptase from a variety of retroviruses. ERVs are underlined. Viruses representing genera in the family *Retroviridae* are indicated. Gypsy is an endogenous retroviral element from the invertebrate species *Drosophila melanogaster*. Tree was generated by maximum parsimony and represents one of five equally parsimonious trees. Note that ERV sequences are interleaved with exogenous sequences and do not represent a separate lineage.

or similar tRNAs; (2) many ERV loci may not contain a recognizable PBS element; and (3) in some cases, the PBS will be sufficiently degraded by substitutions that unambiguous prediction of tRNA specificity is not possible. Despite the name, the vast majority of HERV loci is not unique to humans but is shared with other, closely related primates (having first appeared in a common ancestor); thus, HERV loci should not be thought of as human specific, but rather as human orthologs of loci found in other primate species. Because some HERV families have hundreds or thousands of members, when a specific HERV locus is being described in reference to the chromosomal location, database accession number or cosmid clone is sometimes used for clarity (e.g., HERV-K6p22 refers to a provirus of the HERV-K family found at band 22 on the short arm of chromosome 6). However, this practice is recent and many of the original clone names are still in use.

## Conclusion

Given the sheer number and ubiquity of ERVs among extant species, it is likely that retroviruses have made major contributions to both the content and structure of animal genomes for hundreds of millions of years. Retroviruses can give rise to new DNA content via proviral integration as well as by retro-transposition or transduction of nonviral sequences. Because many ERVs constitute multilocus families of closely related sequences, they can mediate intergenic recombination events leading to large-scale deletions, duplications, interchromosomal translocations, and inversions of chromosomal sequence. All of these processes are also mutagenic, and therefore provide sources of variation upon which selective forces may operate. ERVs can also recombine with exogenous retroviruses during infection, providing additional sources of viral variation and giving rise to retroviruses with altered or novel properties. In modern times, the advent of xenotransplantation (using appropriate animals as organ donors for human transplantation) has raised concerns that ERVs expressed in the donor organs could introduce new retroviruses into the human population. Finally, because of the vast archive of retroviral sequences present in animal genomes in the form of ERVs, the deep evolutionary past of the *Retroviridae* is amenable to scientific exploration in a way that other viral families are not.

*See also:* Bovine and Feline Immunodeficiency Viruses; Equine Infectious Anemia Virus; Feline Leukemia and Sarcoma Viruses; Fish Retroviruses; Foamy Viruses; Host Resistance to Retroviruses; Jaagsiekte Sheep Retrovirus; Mouse Mammary Tumor Virus; Retrotransponsons of Vertebrates; Retroviral Oncogenes; Retroviruses of Birds; Simian Immunodeficiency Virus: Natural Infection; Simian Retrovirus D; Visna-Maedi Viruses.

## Further Reading

Best S, Le Tissier PR, and Stoye JP (1997) Endogenous retroviruses and the evolution of resistance to retroviral infection. *Trends in Microbiology* 5: 313–318.

Boeke JD and Stoye JP (1997) Retrotransposons, endogenous retroviruses, and the evolution of retroelements. In: Coffin JM, Hughes SH,, and Varmus H (eds.) *Retroviruses*, pp. 343–435. New York: Cold Spring Harbor Laboratory Press.

Gifford R and Tristem M (2003) The evolution, distribution and diversity of endogenous retroviruses. *Virus Genes* 26: 291–315.

Jern P, Sperber GO, and Blomberg J (2005) Use of endogenous retroviral sequences (ERVs) and structural markers for retroviral phylogenetic inference and taxonomy. *Retrovirology* 2: 50.

Lower R, Lower J, and Kurth R (1996) The viruses in all of us: Characteristics and biological significance of human endogenous retrovirus sequences. *Proceedings of the National Academy of Sciences, USA* 93: 5177–5184.

Mager DL and Freeman JD (1995) HERV-H endogenous retroviruses: Presence in the New World branch but amplification in the Old World primate lineage. *Virology* 213: 395–404.

Mi S, Lee X, Li X, *et al.* (2000) Syncytin is a captive retroviral envelope protein involved in human placental morphogenesis. *Nature* 403: 785–789.

Sverdlov ED (2000) Retroviruses and primate evolution. *BioEssays* 22: 161–171.

Turner G, Barbulescu M, Su M, Jensen-Seaman MI, Kidd KK, and Lenz J (2001) Insertional polymorphisms of full-length endogenous retroviruses in humans. *Current Biology* 11: 1531–1535.

Weiss RA (2006) The discovery of endogenous retroviruses. *Retrovirology* 3: 67.

# Entomopoxviruses

**M N Becker and R W Moyer**, University of Florida, Gainesville, FL, USA

## Introduction

The entomopoxviruses (EVs) comprise the *Entomopoxvirinae*, one of the two subfamilies of the family *Poxviridae*. EVs infect insect hosts and were first described in 1963. These viruses are found in a number of insect species but are particularly well characterized within the butterflies and moths. The other subfamily of poxviruses is the *Chordopoxvirinae*, which contains the well-known variola virus, the causative agent for smallpox, and vaccinia virus (VV), the vaccine strain for smallpox. The EVs possess a number of the same features as the chordopoxviruses (CVs); however, there are striking differences between the two subfamilies. The similarities include general virion morphology, a double-stranded DNA genome, and a cytoplasmic life cycle. The differences include the host range of the viruses, the presence of occluded virus in EVs, the composition and organization of the DNA genome, differences in gene regulation, and the optimal temperature for growth, which is 27 °C for EVs versus 37 °C for CVs. Although a large number of EVs have been identified, very little is known about most of them with the exception of the *Amsacta moorei* EV (AMEV), which is amenable to growth in culture.

## Phylogeny

Within the subfamily *Chordopoxvirinae* are eight genera. The causative agent of smallpox (variola virus) and the virus used for vaccination against smallpox (VV) are members of the genus *Orthopoxvirus*. Other CVs that cause human disease are cowpox virus and monkeypox virus within this same genus and molluscum contagiosum virus in the genus *Molluscipoxvirus*.

Within the subfamily *Entomopoxvirinae* are three genera, recently renamed by the International Committee on Taxonomy of Viruses: *Alphaentomopoxvirus*, *Betaentomopoxvirus*, and *Gammaentomopoxvirus*. The genera are defined predominantly by the host range of the viruses and by the morphology of the virus particle. The genus *Alphaentomopoxvirus* contains members that infect beetles (coleopterans), and the type species is *Melolontha melolontha entomopoxvirus*. Little is known about the molecular biology of the members of this genus. The genus *Betaentomopoxvirus* contains the best-studied members of the EVs. Betaentomopoxviruses infect either butterflies and moths (Lepidoptera) or grasshoppers and locusts (Orthoptera). The type species is *Amsacta moorei entomopoxvirus*. The host of AMEV is the red hairy caterpillar from India, a member of the tiger moths. Members of the genus *Gammaentomopoxvirus* infect flies, mosquitoes, or midges (Dipterans), and the type species is *Chironomus luridus entomopoxvirus*. There are also a number of unclassified EVs. Included in this group is the well-studied virus from the grasshopper, *Melanoplus sanguinipes* (MSEV). Formerly classified as a betaentomopoxvirus owing to its host range, this virus has been reclassified based on genomic sequencing data and comparison to the genomic sequence of AMEV. Evolutionary trees based on the DNA polymerase sequence indicate not only that the EVs are distinct and evolutionarily separated from the CVs, but that AMEV and MSEV are also highly divergent from each other. There are other unclassified EVs that infect Hymenoptera (bees and wasps). The best studied of these is *Diachasmimorpha* EV, whose host is the parasitic wasp, *Diachasmimorpha longicaudata*.

## Virion Structure

The general virion structure is similar to that of the orthopoxviruses in that it consists of an inner core of electron-dense material surrounded by one or two lateral bodies (**Figure 1**). Within the core are the double-stranded DNA genome and a number of proteins required for the cytoplasmic life cycle of the virus. The entire virion is enveloped by a membrane. **Table 1** indicates the differences in virion size and shape of the lateral bodies of virions from different genera.

One of the unique features of EVs in comparison to CVs is that in nature they exist in an occluded form (**Figure 1**). A variable number of virions are embedded within a paracrystalline protein matrix consisting almost exclusively of a single protein, spheroidin. This is a large protein of 100–115 kDa that is abundant at late times during infection. Spheroidins from different viruses infecting hosts of the same insect order have greater than 80% identity to each other; however, spheroidins from viruses that infect hosts from different orders, such as coleopterans versus lepidopterans, have little similarity. The baculoviruses are another family of double-stranded DNA insect viruses that also produce occluded virus. In baculoviruses, it is the polyhedrin

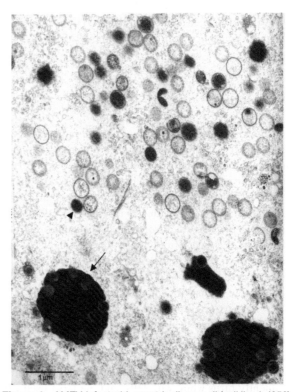

**Figure 1** AMEV-infected *Lymantria dispar* cell (cell line Ld652). Different stages of virion development are seen, including mature virions indicated by an arrowhead and OBs indicated by an arrow.

**Table 1**    Properties of EV virions

|  | Alphaentomopoxvirus | Betaentomopoxvirus | Gammaentomopoxvirus |
|---|---|---|---|
| Size | $450 \times 250\,nm$ | $350 \times 250\,nm$ | $320 \times 230 \times 110\,nm$ |
| Core | Unilateral concave core | Cylindrical | Biconcave |
| Lateral body | Single | Sleeve shaped | Two |
| Virion shape | Ovoid | Ovoid | Brick |

protein that forms the occlusion bodies (OBs). Despite a similar function, spheroidin has little similarity to the baculovirus polyhedrin protein. A large number of cysteines are present with the spheroidin protein, leading to the hypothesis that the OB structure is held together by disulfide bonds.

The function of the OBs is to provide stability for the virus in the environment until ingested by another caterpillar. OBs contain a variable number of virion particles and only mature virions are occluded. OBs are alkaline sensitive, consistent with the high pH of the insect gut. Spheroidin is not required for virulence and the gene is nonessential in tissue culture. Nonoccluded virus is poorly infectious in caterpillars when ingested, but quite virulent when injected. OBs can be induced to form in the absence of virions by the expression of spheroidin protein in cell culture. An alkaline protease is associated with some preparations of EV OBs, and may be useful for dissolution of the OB in the insect gut. AMEV OBs are associated with an alkaline protease when isolated from insects, but not when the virus is grown in culture.

## Pathology

EVs infect primarily the larvae of insects rather than the adult insects. There are reports of infections of adult insects within laboratory settings, however. Most EVs have a restricted host range, although MSEV does infect several grasshopper species. Infection occurs primarily through an oral route with the ingestion of OBs. Once in the gut, the OBs are dissolved by the alkaline environment. The released virions attach to the midgut epithelium and then appear to fuse with the cell membrane. The virus then infects the fat body of the insect and this becomes the primary site of replication for the virus.

EVs are reported to infect the hemocytes and AMEV does infect primary hemocytes in culture. Some researchers argue that the presence of virus in the hemocytes *in vivo* represents phagocytosis rather than infection. As the disease progresses within the insect, the hemolymph frequently turns white with OBs, and the larva itself can take on a whitish or white spotted appearance. The fat body disintegrates and the virus is disseminated throughout the body.

Infected larvae are lethargic and uncoordinated and exhibit a decrease in feeding. The duration of the instar phase is increased before progression to the next instar and few infected larvae continue through pupation. In some EV infections, this is thought to be due to the increased levels of juvenile hormone. There are reports of regurgitation and defecation of AMEV particles by infected *Estigmene acrea* larvae. The time to death of an infected insect is dependent both on the dose of virus received and the larval instar stage. Younger larvae appear to be more susceptible to lower doses of virus and die more quickly than older larvae. The lowest reported $LD_{50}$ is 2.4 spheroids. *Melanoplus sanguinipes* larvae succumbing to an MSEV infection within less than 12 days are reported to lack OBs, although infections of greater than 14 days do possess OBs. The shorter time to death is the result of larger doses of virus.

## Fusolin/Spindles

In addition to spheroidin, some, but not all, members of the alphaentomopoxviruses and many of the lepidopteran members of the betaentomopoxviruses produce another protein termed fusolin that forms crystalline spindles. Among the viruses known to produce spindles are *Melolontha melolontha* EV, *Heliothis armigera* EV, *Choristoneura fumiferana* EV, *Choristoneura biennis* EV, *Pseudaletia separata* EV, and *Anomala cuprea* EV (ACEV). Spindles do not contain virions, though spindles are occasionally found within the OBs of these viruses. Similar to spheroidin, fusolin is highly expressed at late times during infection and is a smaller protein of 38 kDa.

Spindles purified from EV infections enhance the infectivity of a number of baculoviruses. One proposed mechanism of this enhancement is through dissolution of the noncellular peritrophic membrane found within the insect gut. An alternate hypothesis is that the spindles increase the amount of baculovirus-to-cell fusion. Spindles from ACEV have also been demonstrated to enhance the infectivity of ACEV. Clearly, spindles are not required for pathogenicity as evidenced by their absence from most members of the gammaentomopoxviruses and the orthopteran betaentomopoxviruses. It should be noted that although AMEV is a lepidopteran virus it does not produce spindles or encode a gene for fusolin.

## Genome Organization

Genome sizes of the EVs are larger than that of the best-studied CV, VV. The estimated sizes for EV genomes range from 200 to 390 kbp. Two EV genomes have been sequenced, those of AMEV and MSEV. The genome size of AMEV is 232 kbp and of MSEV is 236 kbp. Both genomes are highly A + T-rich, with an A + T content for each genome of approximately 82%, which is in line with DNA melting experiments for EV genomes. In comparison, VV has a genome that is 67% A + T. Both the MSEV and AMEV genomes contain inverted terminal repeats at the ends of the genome.

The organization of the AMEV and MSEV genomes is surprisingly unlike that of the orthopoxviruses. Within the orthopoxviruses there is a core of conserved genes flanked by variable genes involved in pathogenesis and host range. Although many of the same genes are present in EVs, the collinear core is not conserved in either MSEV or AMEV. In fact, it is the lack of conservation of genome organization between AMEV and MSEV, both originally classified as betaentomopoxviruses, that resulted in MSEV being removed from this genus and listed as an unclassified virus.

The available sequence data from the EVs has been included in recent bioinformatics analysis of all available poxvirus sequences. From this analysis, 49 gene families were identified that are conserved across all species of poxviruses. Homologs of the VV G3L gene have recently been identified in AMEV and MSEV, bringing the total of conserved gene families to 50. These 50 genes presumably comprise the minimal complement of genes required for poxvirus function. These conserved gene families include proteins necessary for DNA replication and transcription, polyadenylation of mRNA, and the major structural proteins found within the virion core. An analysis of CVs alone increases the number of conserved genes from 50 to 90. Clearly, the inclusion of the EVs in this type of analysis refines the minimal core of proteins required by a poxvirus.

## Replication

Like other poxviruses, EVs complete their life cycle entirely within the cytoplasm of the cell. A number of enzymes required for DNA synthesis and for temporal regulation of RNA expression are encoded by EVs. These include DNA polymerase, RNA polymerase, poly(A) polymerase, topoisomerase, and a number of transcription factors. Replication within the insect host occurs primarily within the fat body. Many EVs then proceed to infect the hemocytes and other tissues. In cell culture, DNA replication occurs between 6 and 12 h post infection (hpi). At the optimum temperature of 27 °C, the life cycle takes approximately 18–24 h. By 9 hpi, host-cell protein synthesis is shut off. The sites of DNA replication and virion assembly are known as viroplasms or viral factories. Although many virions are packaged into OBs, some are not. Those virions that are not occluded proceed to bud through the cell membrane into the hemocoel of the insect or the cell culture medium *in vitro*. These nonoccluded virus particles are infectious and are thought to be responsible for virus spread with the organism.

RNA production occurs in a temporal fashion with early gene expression occurring from 0 to 6 hpi. Included in the early gene products are transcription factors required for intermediate and late gene production. No intermediate genes have been studied in the EVs, but homologs of several VV intermediate genes are present within both the AMEV and MSEV genomes. Late gene expression appears to follow DNA replication and begins at 9 hpi. The DNA regulatory elements that are present in VV to control this temporal gene expression are present in both AMEV and MSEV, although the functionality of these elements during an EV infection has not been explored. Among the conserved regulatory elements are the TTTTTNT termination sequence at the end of early genes, and the consensus late promoter TAAATG. Similar to the CVs, there is no RNA splicing of EV transcripts.

A unique discovery within the late genes of AMEV is the presence of discrete late transcripts. The late transcripts of VV lack specific 3′ termini, resulting in polydisperse 3′ ends. The rare exceptions to this are several genes that have been identified as having discrete 3′ RNA termini that are formed via cleavage of polydisperse transcripts. A number of major late transcripts of AMEV are discrete in length, unlike what is observed in VV. These include the transcripts for the structural proteins p4a and p4b, the superoxide dismutase, and RAP94, a component of the early RNA polymerase. The spheroidin transcript is also discrete.

## Molecular Biology

Since the sequencing of two EV genomes, a number of interesting features of the EVs have come to light. One of these is the apparent absence of some members of the RNA polymerase complex. There are eight components of the RNA polymerase complex in VV and these are conserved among all sequenced CVs. Three of these proteins have no obvious homologs in AMEV and MSEV. Whether these subunits are not required in an insect cell environment or whether their roles are fulfilled by other nonhomologous proteins is not yet clear. Several transcription factor homologs are also missing from the EVs. Together, this might indicate that the EVs regulate transcription in a different fashion from their orthopoxvirus relatives.

*In vitro* transcription catalyzed by permeabilized AMEV virions requires different conditions from those needed for transcription from VV virions. Unlike VV reactions, which use low levels of detergent and reducing agent, AMEV transcription requires higher levels of reducing agent and the requirement for detergent is less stringent, as transcription can occur in the absence of detergent but not in the absence of reducing agent. AMEV reactions are optimal when an ATP-generating system is present. Such a system is not required for VV virion-mediated transcription. This indicates that the structure of the AMEV virion is different in its response to both reducing agents and detergents. Our attempts to isolate AMEV cores with methodology optimized for the preparation of VV cores has also indicated that key AMEV core proteins partition differently from their VV counterparts.

The transcripts of AMEV are polyadenylated at the 3′ termini, but the composition of the poly(A) polymerase complex appears to be different from that of VV. In VV, poly(A) polymerase is a heterodimer. AMEV has two homologs of the small VV subunit in addition to one homolog of the large subunit. This raises the question of whether both small subunits are involved in polyadenylation or whether there might be tissue or temporal specificity conferred on the complex by the different subunits. It is not clear how common two small poly(A) polymerase subunits are among EVs, since the only other fully sequenced EV (MSEV) only has one small subunit. Spheroidin and other transcripts from EVs have been shown to contain a nonencoded 5′ poly(A) head similar to that reported for a number of VV transcripts.

Protein gel analysis of $^{35}$S-labeled virions indicates that AMEV contains 36–37 structural proteins and MSEV contains 39–45. The proteolytic processing of the large structural proteins that is detected in VV infections has not been found in EV infections. The enzymes thought to be responsible for this proteolytic cleavage in VV are the products of the I7L and G1L genes. These genes are conserved in AMEV and MSEV, indicating that protein processing may occur even though it is as yet undetected.

Both AMEV and MSEV encode an NAD$^+$-dependent DNA ligase. In contrast, VV encodes an ATP-dependent DNA ligase. The AMEV DNA ligase is capable of joining singly nicked DNA fragments. These are the first examples of an NAD$^+$-dependent DNA ligase outside of the eubacteria. The recently sequenced crocodile poxvirus has also been reported to encode an NAD$^+$-dependent DNA ligase.

Poxviruses are known for the wide variety of proteins that they encode to evade the host immunomodulatory response. VV and other orthopoxviruses encode serine protease inhibitors as well as chemokine binding molecules and decoy receptor molecules. Due to the host range of the

EVs, they encode other types of defense molecules. Among these are the *inhibitor of apoptosis* (*iap*) genes. The *iap* of AMEV has been well characterized and functionally inhibits apoptosis. A related AMEV gene that functions to inhibit apoptosis is a homolog of the baculovirus pan-caspase inhibitor, p35.

Another novel protein expressed by AMEV is a Cu–Zn superoxide dismutase (SOD). Although a number of the orthopoxviruses encode genes with homology to this class of SODs, neither the VV or myxoma virus proteins are functional in that capacity, although they are present within the virion. The SOD expressed by AMEV is functional as an SOD but is not essential for virus growth in culture. The deletion of the *sod* gene from AMEV appears to have no effect on the growth of the virus in gypsy moth larvae.

## Summary

It is clear that this large subfamily of the family *Poxviridae* provides a wealth of possible information about the basic mechanisms of the poxvirus lifecycle. There appear to be a number of interesting variations on the molecular details which define this overall family of viruses. There are clear similarities to the vertebrate poxviruses in virion morphology, double-stranded DNA genome, cytoplasmic life cycle, and RNA expression. Yet the differences between the CVs and EVs are significant and represent an area of research that has not been fully explored. The data that have been obtained from genomic sequencing has been essential to identifying some of the different proteins that are present in the EVs, as well as identifying potentially missing homologs of VV proteins. It is important to note that there are large differences at the DNA level between the two sequenced EVs, indicating that there is probably a wide variety of unique features within the EVs as a group. As more sequence information becomes available, the diversity of this family of viruses may become more evident.

## Further Reading

Afonso CL, Tulman ER, Lu Z, *et al.* (1999) The genome of *Melanoplus sanguinipes* entomopoxvirus. *Journal of Virology* 73: 533–552.

Arif BM and Kurstak E (1991) The entomopoxviruses. In: Kurstak E (ed.) *Viruses of Invertebrates* pp. 179–195. New York: Marcel Dekker.

Bawden AL, Glassberg KJ, Diggans J, *et al.* (2000) Complete genomic sequence of the *Amsacta moorei* entomopoxvirus: Analysis and comparison with other poxviruses. *Virology* 274: 120–139.

Becker MN, Greenleaf WB, Ostrov DA, and Moyer RW (2004) *Amsacta moorei* entomopoxvirus expresses an active superoxide dismutase. *Journal of Virology* 78: 10265–10275.

Becker MN and Moyer RW (2007) Subfamily *Entomopoxvirinae*. In: Mercer A, Schmidt A,, and Weber O (eds.) *Poxviruses*, pp. 251–269. Basel: Birkhäuser.

Gubser C, Hue S, Kellam P, and Smith GL (2004) Poxvirus genomes: A phylogenetic analysis. *Journal of General Virology* 85: 105–117.

Li QJ, Liston P, and Moyer RW (2005) Functional analysis of the *inhibitor of apoptosis (iap)* gene carried by the entomopoxvirus of *Amsacta moorei*. *Journal of Virology* 79: 2335–2345.

Li QJ, Liston P, Schokman N, Ho JM, and Moyer RW (2005) *Amsacta moorei* entomopoxvirus inhibitor of apoptosis suppresses cell death by binding grim and hid. *Journal of Virology* 79: 3684–3691.

Miller LK and Ball LA (1998) *The Insect Viruses.* New York: Plenum.

Moss B (2001) *Poxviridae*: The viruses and their replication. In: Knipe DM and Howley PM (eds.) *Fields Virology*, 4th edn., pp. 2849–2883. Philadelphia: Lippincott Williams & Wilkins.

Upton C, Slack S, Hunter AL, Ehlers A, and Roper RL (2003) Poxvirus orthologous clusters: Toward defining the minimum essential poxvirus genome. *Journal of Virology* 77: 7590–7600.

Winter J, Hall RL, and Moyer RW (1995) The effect of inhibitors on the growth of the entomopoxvirus from *Amsacta moorei* in *Lymantria dispar* (gypsy moth) cells. *Virology* 211: 462–473.

# Feline Leukemia and Sarcoma Viruses

**J C Neil,** University of Glasgow, Glasgow, UK

## History

The description of murine leukemia viruses by Moloney and others stimulated an intensive search for similar viruses in other species. William Jarrett made the perceptive observation that lymphomas (lymphosarcomas) in cats often occurred at particularly high incidence in certain households, and in 1964 he showed that typical type C retroviruses could be demonstrated in the tumor cells by electron microscopy. He went on to show that these feline leukemia viruses (FeLVs) could be transmitted to cats where they induced lymphosarcomas and a range of degenerative diseases, including anemias and thymic atrophy.

Following these studies, Snyder and Theilen isolated a retrovirus from a feline fibrosarcoma that rapidly reproduced this tumor on inoculation into experimental cats. It is now recognized that feline sarcoma viruses (FeSVs) arise by recombination between FeLV and cellular protooncogenes and that, in contrast to FeLV, these viruses are not transmitted from cat to cat.

In clinical veterinary medicine, FeLV remains one of the most important viruses affecting the cat, despite advances in control of this infection. As a naturally occurring disease in an outbred host, FeLV has served as a paradigm for the natural history and molecular pathogenesis of the $\gamma$-retrovirus subfamily. It also played a foundational role in cancer genetics as a transducing agent which led to the discovery of novel cellular transforming genes.

## Taxonomy and Classification

FeLVs are RNA viruses and belong to the family *Retroviridae*. They are further classified in the genus *Gammaretroviruses*.

## Virion and Genome Structure

The virion particles are around 100 nm in diameter and consist of an outer membrane derived from the host cell surrounding a spherical core particle. The core encapsidates the viral genome which, as in other members of this viral family, is present as two linear single-stranded RNA molecules linked as a dimer. The virion RNA is positive-stranded and resembles cellular RNA having a 5′ cap and a 3′ poly(A) tract. As deduced from sequencing of proviral forms, the FeLV genome is around 8 kb long with a 67 base terminal redundancy and the gene order gag-pol-env.

The particles have surface spikes composed of multimers of the two env-coded proteins, the gp70 surface glycoprotein (SU), and the p15E transmembrane anchor protein (TM). Inside the envelope are the structural *gag* gene products which form a spherical core particle composed of p27, the major capsid protein (CA), with an outer layer formed by the p15 matrix protein (MA). Another gag product, the p10 nucleocapsid (NC), is associated with the virion RNA. Other minor virion proteins encoded by the *pol* gene comprise the protease (PR), reverse transcriptase (RT), and integrase (IN) enzymes.

## Replication

Virus replication proceeds, following binding to specific host cell-surface receptors, internalization, and uncoating. The virion RNA is converted to a double-stranded DNA form by the virion RT which uses a proline tRNA primer and carries a ribonuclease H function that degrades the virion RNA. After nuclear translocation, viral integration is catalyzed by the IN protein and involves the creation of a staggered cut in cellular DNA with a consequent 4 bp duplication of host DNA at the insertion site.

As illustrated in **Figure 1**, the proviral form is flanked by long terminal repeats (LTRs) of 480–560 bp. These are generated during reverse transcription by duplication of unique sequences at the 3′ (U3) and 5′ (U5) ends of the RNA genome. The LTRs contain promoters and enhancers that drive transcription of viral RNA and also

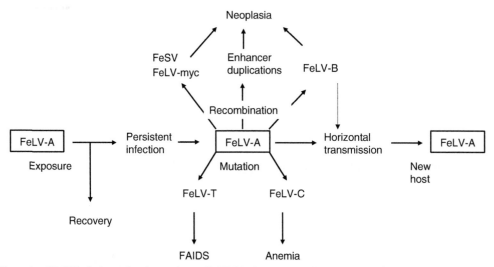

**Figure 1**   Life cycle of FeLV in its host, the domestic cat. FeLV-A is the most readily transmitted form and is found in 100% of isolates. In cats which become persistently viremic, this prototypic virus may evolve by recombination or point mutations to generate pathogenic variants that can lead to the rapid demise of the infected host animal. Multiple variants can arise in a single host. Few of these variants show any capacity for horizontal transmission to new hosts with the exception of FeLV-B. In this way, FeLV inflicts a substantial disease burden without significant reducing host numbers.

processing signals for cleavage and polyadenylation of the RNA transcripts. The 5′ LTR functions to initiate transcription while the 3′ LTR acts primarily as an RNA processing signal.

The virion RNA can function as a messenger RNA for Gag and Pol products, while a spliced subgenomic mRNA of around 3 kb encodes the Env products. Most full-length RNA translation products terminate at the 3′ end of *gag* to produce the Pr65gag precursor, while a small percentage read through into *pol* by misreading of an UAG termination codon, generating the Pr180Gag-pol precursor. During and after the budding process, the virion aspartyl PR catalyzes the cleavage of both precursor proteins to their mature forms. The envelope gene products are synthesized as a Pr80env precursor and processed by cellular PRs to the mature, disulfide-linked gp70 and p15E envelope proteins. The *gag* gene is also abundantly expressed in an alternative, glycosylated form via an upstream AUG codon. This product is expressed on the cell surface and shed after cleavage by cellular PRs. It is dispensable for *in vitro* virus replication but is highly conserved and may play a role *in vivo*.

Assembly of virus particles occurs at the cell surface by extrusion of cores which form at the budding site, concomitantly acquiring a host cell-derived outer membrane with virus-coded surface spikes. Virus replication and release is often noncytopathic.

## Geographic Distribution

FeLV occurs worldwide in domestic cat populations although prevalence varies significantly and has declined in pet cats in areas where active control measures have

been instigated. FeLV has also been isolated from the European wild cat (*Felis sylvestris*). Endogenous retroviral sequences closely matched to FeLV are found in the same species and in related small felids such as the sand cat (*F. margarita*) and the jungle cat (*F. chaus*). Although not a direct source of disease, these endogenous sequences can participate in recombination with exogenous FeLV to generate variant viruses with altered host range.

## Epidemiology

The outcomes of FeLV infection fall into several categories, which vary in likelihood according to the age and immune status of the exposed host. The majority of cats undergo a transient infection lasting up to 3 months, during which they are viremic and shed virus. They then develop neutralizing antibody and concomitantly clear infectious virus and a little later, virus antigen from the blood stream. Some cats appear to clear virus infection successfully, while others may harbor latent virus in the bone marrow for some years. A recent study based on analysis of virus loads by polymerase chain reaction (PCR) suggests that animals that control viremia may be further subdivided into abortive, regressive, or latent infection. Even where latent infection persists, reactivation is not a frequent event and the vast majority of these cats do not develop an FeLV-related disease. However, at this stage virus can be reactivated by immunosuppression. The final group (persistent or progressive infection) remains actively infected, shedding virus from epithelial surfaces and displaying high titer plasma viremia. Such cats may remain apparently healthy for 2–3 years before succumbing to an FeLV-related disease.

The proportion of cases falling into these groups differs between multicat households and those households containing one or two free-ranging cats. In the former case, the introduction of an FeLV carrier results in repeated exposure of susceptible cats, often at a young age so that up to 30–40% become persistently viremic and at risk of disease. Approximately 50% of free-ranging urban and suburban cats have serological evidence of exposure to FeLV but only 1–5% of these cats are actively infected and the disease incidence is correspondingly lower.

Dual infection with FeLV and feline immunodeficiency virus (FIV) occurs and is associated with rapid disease onset, particularly if cats with preexisting FeLV infection encounter FIV. Rapid death of dually infected animals may reduce the apparent overlap of these agents in the field, but the populations at risk of infection also differ. FIV infection rates increase directly with age while persistent FeLV infection has a peak incidence in young cats.

## FeLV Subgroups and Host Range

FeLV isolates were initially classified as subgroup A, B, C according to their viral interference properties in feline fibroblast cells in vitro. Viruses of a given subgroup prevent superinfection (interfere) with other viruses of the same subgroup (**Table 1**). This property is based on the use of three different host cell-surface receptors by FeLV-A, B, and C, and the blockade of these receptors in persistently infected cells by viral Env glycoproteins. The lymphotropic variant FeLV-T has more complex entry requirements, and does not replicate well in fibroblast cells. It appears that this isolate requires the FeLV-A receptor and an auxiliary mechanism in which a truncated env gene product encoded by endogenous FeLV sequences (FeLIX) is used as a co-receptor through binding to the FeLV-B receptor. Primary receptors for subgroups A, B, and C have been identified and shown to be transmembrane transporter molecules which the virus has subverted to gain entry to the host cell.

Natural isolates contain either subgroup A alone, or mixtures of subgroups A + B, A + C, or A + B + C. FeLV isolates of subgroup A are generally restricted to growth in feline cells, whereas subgroups B and C have a greatly expanded host range, infecting cat, human, mink, and canine cells. FeLV infection is generally noncytopathic and persistent and the virus is commonly propagated in long-term cultures of embryo-derived fibroblasts. Some strains such as FeLV-T or FeLV-C are cytopathic or induce apoptosis in lymphoid cells in vitro, reflecting their in vivo pathogenic properties.

## Clinical Features and Pathology

Of those cats which become persistently viremic following FeLV exposure, over 80% die within 3.5 years. Most young cats infected with FeLV die from degenerative diseases rather than from tumors. Profound immunosuppression associated with thymic atrophy is a common finding in kittens. Other diseases seen in FeLV-infected cats include enteritis, immune complex glomerulonephritis, pancytopenia, and hemolytic anemia. Erythroid hypoplasia, an acute disease involving failure of red cell development past the burst-forming unit (BFU) stage, is specifically associated with FeLV subgroup C.

The most common neoplasm induced by FeLV is lymphosarcoma of T-cell origin, usually restricted to the thymus or sometimes occurring as a multicentric tumor in lymph nodes. The tumors often develop between 1 and 3 years after infection and the first signs may be chronic wasting and anemia. At presentation, the normal architecture of the lymphoid organ has usually been destroyed by a monomorphic infiltrate of lymphoblastic cells. The thymic tumors frequently display a rearrangement of the T-cell antigen receptor β-chain gene and may also express the co-receptor molecules CD4+ and/or CD8+. FeLV is also commonly associated with myeloid leukemias and a myelodysplastic syndrome-like disease, as well as with other forms of hematopoietic malignancy. Multicentric fibrosarcoma is a rare sequel to FeLV infection but these tumors are

**Table 1** Properties of feline leukemia virus subgroups

| Subgroup | Origin | Receptor | Function | Pathogenesis |
|---|---|---|---|---|
| A | Exogenous | feTHTR1? | Thiamine transport? | Minimally pathogenic to acute immunosuppression |
| B | Recombination FeLV-A × endogenous FeLV | Pit-1 (Pit-2) | Phosphate transport | More common in leukemic cats |
| | | | | Some isolate-specific diseases, e.g., FeLV-GM1 myeloid leukemia |
| C | Mutation of FeLV-A (Env vrA) | FLVCR | Heme export | Erythroid hypoplasia |
| T | Mutation of FeLV-A (outside RBD) | ? FeLV-A receptor +FeLIX, Pit-1 | | Acute immunosuppression |

often associated with the *de novo* generation of a FeSV. FeLV is also found in association with 35% of alimentary tumors, primarily of B cell origin, but the virus is not always clonally integrated in these tumors and the role of the virus is, therefore, unclear. FIV can also increase the frequency of malignant diseases in cats, and some rare cases arise on a background of dual infection.

## Envelope Gene Variation and Pathogenicity

The common infectious form of FeLV is FeLV-A which is a remarkably highly conserved virus as shown by sequence analysis of several strains and serotypic analysis of a much larger number. FeLV variants frequently arise from FeLV-A by mutation and recombination, and such variants are often implicated in the acute diseases which develop in persistently infected cats. The variant viruses generated from FeLV-A are generally dependent on the continued presence of the prototype for their propagation *in vivo*. However, as the variants are less efficiently transmitted and are in some cases rapidly fatal, they tend to die out with the host while the prototypic FeLV-A continues to colonize new hosts (**Figure 1**).

The most commonly isolated FeLV recombinants are subgroup B viruses (**Table 1**). These are derived by recombination between FeLV-A and endogenous FeLV-related proviruses which are found in the genome of the domestic cat and related small feline species. Although the endogenous FeLV-related proviruses all appear to be replication defective, their envelope genes can be rescued by the recombination process leading to the generation of FeLV-B viruses. FeLV-B can infect cells refractory to, or already containing, FeLV-A by virtue of their distinctive receptor specificity.

The anemia-inducing FeLV-C isolates are rarer and appear to be derived from FeLV-A by mutation of a single variable domain (VRA) of the *env* gene. The acute disease properties of these variants appear to be due to compromised viability of erythroid progenitor cells due to downregulation of the FeLV-C receptor, a vital heme exporter.

Minor *env* mutations also appear to give rise to the acutely immunosuppressive FeLV-FAIDS variants. The prevalence of acutely immunosuppressive viruses in nature is unknown, but immunosuppressive disease is a common manifestation of FeLV infection.

The relationship of subgroup variation to oncogenesis is complex. FeLV-B recombinants are more common in tumor bearing than in infected asymptomatic cats. This higher frequency might reflect merely longer-standing infection, but some FeLV-B-containing isolates have an altered spectrum of neoplastic disease. For example, FeLV-GM1, which contains a replication-defective FeLV-B component, induces mainly myeloid leukemia.

## FeLV Oncogenesis: Virus Evolution and Mutagenesis of Cellular Oncogenes

Two modes of virus-induced host gene mutation have been described in FeLV-associated cancers. The first is 'transduction', where recombination leads to the generation of an acutely oncogenic variant in which viral gene sequences are replaced by a host-derived insert. Such viruses are replication defective and are found in nature in association with a replication-component FeLV helper virus.

Multicentric fibrosarcomas of young cats are relatively rare, but are generally FeLV positive and frequently involve a novel sarcoma virus. Similarly, transduction of c-*myc* has been observed in up to 20% of naturally occurring thymic lymphosarcomas in FeLV positive cats. In all, nine different host cell genes have been shown to be transduced by FeLV (**Table 2a**). The transducing viruses induce tumors with short latency in cats and in the case of FeSVs may transform cells in tissue culture.

Alternatively, host genes can be affected by proviral 'insertional mutagenesis' (*cis*-activation). Four known oncogenes and an uncharacterized novel integration locus have been identified as common tumor-specific insertion

**Table 2a**    FeLV gene transduction in neoplasia

| Gene | Normal function of host gene product | Associated tumor | Examples[a] |
|---|---|---|---|
| *abl* | Plasmamembrane protein kinase | Fibrosarcoma | FeSV-HZ2 |
| *fes* | Plasmamembrane protein kinase | Fibrosarcoma | FeSV-GA,-HZ1,-ST |
| *fgr* | Plasmamembrane protein kinase | Fibrosarcoma | FeLV-GR,-TP1 |
| *fms* | Receptor protein kinase (CSF-1 receptor) | Fibrosarcoma | FeSV-SM,-HZ5 |
| *kit* | Receptor protein kinase (SCF receptor) | Fibrosarcoma | FeSV-HZ4 |
| *myc* | Transcription factor | T-cell lymphoma | FeLV (T3, T17, FTT) |
| *Notch2* | Transmembrane receptor | T-cell lymphoma | (Inoculum FeLV-61E)[a] |
| *sis* | Growth factor (B chain PDGF) | Fibrosarcoma | FeSV-PI |
| *tcr* | T-cell antigen receptor (β-chain) | T-cell lymphoma | FeLV-T17 |

[a]Isolated from naturally occurring tumors apart from the indicated exception.

**Table 2b** Insertional mutagenesis and FeLV oncogenesis

| Common integration site | Gene function | Tumor |
| --- | --- | --- |
| fit-1 | Transcription factor (c-myb) | T-cell lymphoma |
| flvi-1 | Unknown | non-T, non-B lymphoma |
| flvi-2 (bmi-1) | Transcription factor | T-cell lymphoma |
| c-myc | Transcription factor | T-cell lymphoma |
| pim-1 | Protein kinase | T-cell lymphoma |

sites for FeLV in thymic lymphosarcomas (**Table 2b**). In this respect FeLV oncogenesis appears remarkably similar to that of the murine γ-retroviruses, and most studies of this process have been conducted recently in the laboratory mouse which has the advantages of complete genome sequence and the opportunity to manipulate the germline.

Changes within the LTR are also a feature of tumor-associated FeLV. In thymic lymphosarcomas, sequence duplications of the core enhancer domain are frequently found, and have been shown to arise *de novo* from infection with molecularly cloned FeLV isolate lacking such features. By analogy with the murine oncoretroviruses, the duplications are likely to increase the oncogenicity of the virus and reduce the latent period for tumor formation, possibly by increasing the potency of viral enhancer activity on nearby cellular promoters. There is evidence that these adaptive changes to the LTR operate tissue-specifically and proviruses carrying different duplications of LTR regions 5' and 3' to the core-enhancer region have been identified in myeloid leukemias and non-T, non-B splenic lymphomas, respectively. Chimeric murine retroviruses carrying the FeLV enhancer region have been generated, confirming that the tissue specificity is carried by this structure.

## Immune Response

Unlike infection with the lentiviruses HIV and FIV, FeLV infection of cats may lead to recovery. There is evidence that both virus-specific cytotoxic T cells (CTLs) and neutralizing antibodies play a role in resistance as either can be used to prevent or limit infection by passive transfer. In natural infection, CTLs to virus structural protein epitopes can be detected as early as a week after infection and may be the primary means of control of infection as neutralizing antbodies are not detected until around 6 weeks post infection.

In the early literature on FeLV a distinction was made between antiviral immunity and antitumor immunity. Cats with antitumor (FOCMA) antibody were thought to be protected from tumor development. This antibody response is now believed to be directed to endogenous FeLV *env* proteins and its role in modulating tumor development is uncertain.

## Transmission

Cats persistently infected with FeLV shed virus in their saliva, urine, and feces but, as the virus is fragile, close contact is required for transmission. The most frequent routes involve saliva and transplacental spread. Kittens infected *in utero* become persistently infected, but the consequences of infection in older cats depend on a number of factors. There is an age-related resistance to infection such that cats up to 12 weeks of age are highly susceptible, but above 16 weeks they are difficult to infect either naturally or experimentally.

FeLV subgroup A is always found in field isolates and about half also contain FeLV-B, whereas FeLV-C is present in only 1–2% of isolates. Although FeLV-B can arise *de novo* by recombination, it may also be transmitted between cats. This occurrence is dependent on pseudotype formation in which the genome of the B virus becomes enclosed in an envelope containing glycoproteins of the A subgroup.

## Prevention and Control

Successful control measures can be adopted in multicat households by removing or isolating persistently infected animals. Productively infected cats are detected by virus isolation from plasma or more usually by enzyme-linked immunosorbent assay (ELISA) for virus antigen in the blood. A few cats remain persistently antigenemic but nonviremic. These cats do not usually transmit the virus unless they are shedding virus in the milk or saliva. Assays are conducted twice, 3 months apart to exclude cats that are transiently viremic.

Numerous vaccine strategies have been shown to offer protection against FeLV in laboratory conditions (**Table 3**) and FeLV was the first retrovirus for which commercial vaccines were developed. Vaccines in current use include whole inactivated virus preparations, subunit vaccines from recombinant viral Env protein expressed in bacterial cells, and a canarypox recombinant virus expressing Gag and Env. These vaccines offer a measure of protection against experimental challenge and are under evaluation for longer-term efficacy in the field. These vaccines do not generate sterilizing immunity but appear to prime the immune system to favor clearance of virus infection instead of persistent viremia.

**Table 3** FeLV vaccines

| Vaccine | Protection | Commercial use |
|---|---|---|
| Live attenuated FeLV | Yes | No (safety concerns) |
| Inactivated whole virus | Yes | Yes |
| Subunit vaccines | | |
| SU from *E. coli* | Yes | Yes |
| ISCOM-Env (native) | Yes | No |
| Lymphoma cell extract | Yes (poor in some studies) | Withdrawn |
| Live vector vaccine | | |
| Vaccinia-Env | No | No |
| Canarypox-Env-Gag | Yes | Yes |
| Feline herpesvirus-Env | Partial | No |

## Future Perspectives

There is continuing interest in control of FeLV infection due to its importance in veterinary medicine. In the future we can look forward to improvements in vaccine efficacy and further dissection of the host responses that confer protection. While the focus of attention of cancer genetics has moved on to more easily manipulated models, FeLV remains as a useful touchstone for our understanding of retroviral pathogenesis in an outbred, naturally infected host. Also, with the impetus of FIV as a model for human AIDS, the generation of reagents to probe the feline immune system offers new opportunities for comparative study of FeLV.

*See also:* Bovine and Feline Immunodeficiency Viruses.

## Further Reading

Flynn JN, Dunham SP, Watson V, and Jarrett O (2002) Longitudinal analysis of feline leukemia virus-specific cytotoxic T lymphocytes: Correlation with recovery from infection. *Journal of Virology* 76: 2306–2315.

Hanlon L, Barr NI, Blyth K, *et al.* (2003) Long-range effects of retroviral activation on c-myb over-expression may be obscured by silencing during tumor growth *in vitro*. *Journal of Virology* 77: 1059–1068.

Mendoza R, Anderson MM, and Overbaugh J (2006) A putative thiamine transport protein is a receptor for feline leukemia virus subgroup A. *Journal of Virology* 80: 3378–3385.

Miyazawa T (2002) Infections of feline leukemia virus and feline immunodeficiency virus. *Frontiers in Bioscience* 7: D504–D518.

Roca AL, Nash WG, Menninger JC, Murphy WJ, and O'Brien SJ (2005) Insertional polymorphisms of endogenous feline leukemia viruses. *Journal of Virology* 79: 3979–3986.

Sparkes AH (2003) Feline leukaemia virus and vaccination. *Journal of Feline Medicine and Surgery* 5: 97–100.

Torres AN, Mathiason CK, and Hoover EA (2005) Re-examination of feline leukemia virus: Host relationships using real-time PCR. *Virology* 332: 272–283.

Tsatsanis C, Fulton R, Nishigaki K, *et al.* (1994) Genetic determinants of feline leukemia virus-induced lymphoid tumors: Patterns of proviral insertion and gene rearrangement. *Journal of Virology* 68: 8294–8303.

# Host Resistance to Retroviruses

**T Hatziioannou and P D Bieniasz,** Aaron Diamond AIDS Research Center, The Rockefeller University, New York, NY, USA

## Glossary

**APOBECs** A family of cytidine deaminases, the prototypic member is a component of apolipoprotein B editing complex.

**Restriction factor** A cellular protein whose major role is to inhibit retrovirus replication.

**Vif** Virion infectivity factor encoded by many lentiviruses which induces degradation of some APOBEC proteins.

**Vpu** Viral protein U, a small transmembrane protein encoded by HIV-1 and its close relatives.

**Xenotropic** Able to infect cells only from other species.

## Introduction

The evolution of organisms and the viruses that colonize them is, obviously, closely linked. Often, pathogenic viruses impose a negative selection pressure on a host that results in the survival of a subpopulation in which infection is resisted, attenuated, or tolerated. In the case of retroviruses, the evolutionary association of virus and host can be exceptionally close, because of the unusual degree to which retroviral infection persists. Retroviral infection is normally lifelong, in part due to the propensity of retroviral genomes to irreversibly integrate into host DNA. Sometimes the targets of retroviral infection include germline cells, and infection of these cells, which generate so-called endogenous proviruses, enables persistence, not only for the host's own lifetime, but also that of its progeny. This persistence and inextricable association of host and virus may allow retroviruses to impose a uniquely sustained selection pressure and may explain why hosts have evolved unique and specific ways for their cells to resist colonization by retroviruses.

In principle, hosts could evolve resistance to the negative consequences of retroviral infection through changes in components of their innate and adaptive immune systems, but it has also become clear that host factors which directly inhibit the ability of retroviruses to replicate in host cells evolve under pressure of retroviral infection. Host resistance to retroviral infection can be acquired in many forms and be manifested at various stages of the retroviral life cycle (**Figure 1**). Of particular note are a collection of autonomously and constitutively active intracellular proteins, termed restriction factors, whose major function appears to be to provide intrinsic immunity to retroviral infection. As such, they are uniquely capable of actively preventing retrovirus replication at the very earliest stages of host colonization. Naturally, some retroviruses have adapted to cellular host resistance in its various forms. Since exogenous retroviruses evolve much more rapidly than their hosts,

it seems obvious that they would do so. Nevertheless, some of the obstacles that cells have placed in the path of retroviral replication are not easily escaped by simple mutation, and in some cases retroviruses have learned how to avoid or ablate host restriction factors in interesting and unique ways.

## Host Cell Resistance Defined Early in the Retrovirus Life Cycle

### Resistance to Retrovirus Entry

Imagine a cell attempting to thwart an infection event by a retrovirus. Optimal strategies would involve aborting the viral life cycle before integration into the genomic DNA and avoiding permanent residence of the retrovirus in the cell and all of its progeny. This could be achieved in numerous ways, an obvious approach being removal or alteration of the receptors that are exploited by retroviruses to enable entry. Several occurrences of this phenomenon are known. A striking example is the occurrence of endogenous murine leukemia viruses (MLVs) that are termed xenotropic because they are unable to replicate in their

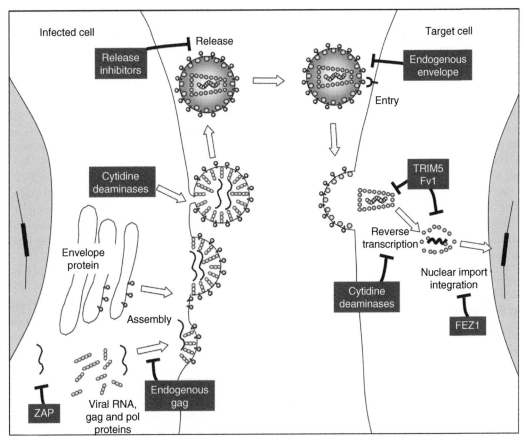

**Figure 1** Overview of the retrovirus life cycle and activities encoded by cells that are known to inhibit retrovirus replication.

own hosts. Xenotropism generally occurs as a consequence of mutations that are acquired in the gene encoding the relevant receptor, presumably after colonization of the germline by the xenotropic MLV. Another important example of a receptor mutation that confers resistance to infection is present in humans. In this case a defective allele of the CCR5 co-receptor (*CCR5Δ32*) for HIV-1 exists at high frequency in certain human populations, and individuals that are homozygous for this mutation are resistant to infection by many strains of HIV-1. Although it is quite unlikely that HIV-1 itself is the source of the original evolutionary pressure that led to the dissemination of the *CCR5Δ32* allele, widespread HIV-1 infection in humans would clearly sustain or even increase the prevalence of the *CCR5Δ32* allele in populations where it is present. Other polymorphisms in the human *CCR5* gene also appear to have more modest effects on the acquisition and consequences of HIV-1 infection.

While receptor inactivation could clearly confer resistance to infection by certain retroviruses, some species have acquired or amplified specific genes that actively inhibit retroviral infection at the level of receptor–envelope interaction. Endogenous retroviruses themselves have proved to be a good source of such inhibitors and a few endogenous retroviral genes can efficiently control infection and inhibit the progression of disease caused by exogenous retroviruses. Certain of these preserved endogenous retroviral gene products, for example, Fv4 and Rmcf in mice, are viral envelope glycoproteins that bind and block the receptors shared by exogenous viruses, and constitute especially effective and specific entry inhibitors. The natural cellular ligands of viral receptors can also provide resistance to infection. For example, the chemokine ligands of CCR5 act as competitive inhibitors of HIV-1 envelope binding and one of the genes encoding a CCR5 ligand (*CCL3-L1*) exists in variable copy numbers in humans. Individuals with higher copy numbers tend to be less likely to acquire HIV-1 infection, and once infected seem less susceptible to its effects. While it is not yet certain that these effects are not immunologically mediated, it seems most likely that the *CCL3-L1* gene product acts as a direct inhibitor of HIV-1 infection and replication in humans.

## Post-Entry Resistance Factors Targeting Incoming Retroviruses

In addition to providing a source of receptor-blocking viral envelope proteins, endogenous retroviruses have provided additional factors that restrict retroviral replication. A particularly intriguing restriction factor of endogenous retroviral origin is Friend virus susceptibility factor 1 (Fv1), a protein with about 60% homology to human and mouse endogenous retroviral Gag proteins. *Fv1* was first characterized as a dominant, heritable trait

in laboratory mice that conferred resistance to infection by particular MLV strains. The two principal alleles of Fv1 are functionally distinguished by the spectrum of MLV strains to which they confer resistance: The $Fv1^n$ allele renders cells permissive to infection by N-tropic MLV but restricts B-tropic MLV infection, whereas $Fv1^b$ renders cells permissive to B-tropic MLV but resistant to N-tropic MLV. Heterozygous animals that carry both *Fv1* alleles are resistant to both N- and B-tropic MLV strains, while certain MLV strains are not susceptible to restriction by either *Fv1* allele and are known as NB-tropic. Additional *Fv1* alleles that induce partly overlapping patterns of sensitivity/resistance exist, as do inactive variants. While Fv1 restriction is not absolute, it can be very substantial at low multiplicities of infection and Fv1 restriction can have extremely dramatic effects on MLV pathogenesis.

An important feature of Fv1-mediated resistance is that it is saturable and infection by any given virus particle is greatly facilitated by the presence of large numbers of additional restricted virus particles, even if they are inactivated. Most interestingly, the Fv1-imposed block in MLV infection occurs after reverse transcription has been completed but before integration of the provirus in the host genome. The viral determinant governing Fv1 sensitivity is the capsid protein and a single-amino-acid change from arginine to glutamate at position 110 is sufficient to convert an N-tropic MLV strain to B-tropism. Other residues in proximal positions can also affect Fv1 sensitivity and together these data suggest that Fv1 is an inhibitor that inactivates incoming MLV capsids in the cytoplasm of target cells.

Several non-murine mammalian cells, including those from humans, African green monkeys (AGMs), and cows, restrict infection by N-tropic, but permit infection by B-tropic, MLV. Remarkably, this occurs despite the absence of an Fv1-like gene in species other than mice. The characteristics of restriction of N-MLV in these cells are similar to those mediated by Fv1 in mouse cells, that is, restriction can be saturated and amino acid 110 of capsid determines restriction sensitivity. However, in most cases of nonmurine mammalian cells, capsid-specific blocks to infection appear to occur before reverse transcription is completed.

In addition, lentiviruses are also subject to a similar type of post-entry restriction in primate cells. Again, dominant saturable factors are responsible and the viral determinant governing restriction is the capsid protein. Cells from different primate species often exhibit distinct retrovirus restriction specificities. For example, human cells restrict infection by equine infectious anaemia virus (EIAV) but not primate lentiviruses. Conversely, AGM cells restrict multiple primate lentiviruses and EIAV but not simian immunodeficiency viruses (SIVs) naturally found in AGMs. Remarkably, in many cases, restriction of one retrovirus can be abolished by saturation with another even if the two viruses are not closely related, provided that both viruses are restricted in the target cell. For example, in AGM cells, which restrict N-tropic MLV as well as HIV-1, HIV-2, SIVmac, and EIAV, saturation with lentivirus particles can completely abrogate restriction of N-tropic MLV infection. These findings demonstrate the divergence in specificity of mammalian restriction factors but also predict the presence of a single restriction factor capable of recognizing retroviruses whose capsids share little sequence homology.

Indeed, recent work shows that the gene that is largely responsible for the retrovirus restriction properties of primate cells is *TRIM5* and that variation in its sequence can account for most of the variation in species-specific retrovirus restriction properties. Unlike Fv1, TRIM5 has no homology with any known retroviral sequences. Rather, *TRIM5* is one member of a family of dozens of cellular genes that share a similar architecture. Indeed, *TRIM5* itself exists as one of a small cluster of closely related *TRIM* genes on human chromosome 11. Each *TRIM* gene encodes a protein with an amino-terminal tripartite motif, comprised of a RING domain, one or two additional zinc-binding or 'B-box' domains, and a coiled-coil domain (**Figure 2**). The TRIM domain can be linked to one of a number of C-terminal domains, and a single *TRIM* gene can encode several variant proteins with different C-terminal domains as a result of alternative splicing. The α-spliced variant of *TRIM5* gene is responsible for retrovirus restriction and encodes a C-terminal SPRY domain, which is related to domains found in other proteins of diverse organization and function, as well as in several other members of the TRIM protein family. Functional dissection of the TRIM5α protein has revealed that the amino-terminal RING and the B-box sequences comprise a so-called effector domain that is required for restriction but not for recognition of incoming capsids. Conversely, the central coiled-coil is necessary for TRIM5 trimerization while the C-terminal SPRY domain

is the principal specificity determinant that governs which retroviruses are inhibited by a given TRIM5α variant. The fact that TRIM5α exists as a trimer suggests a mode of capsid recognition that involves threefold symmetry, since the viral target of TRIM5 consists primarily of a hexameric array of capsid molecules. Moreover, residues on the outer surface of the hexameric capsid lattice of both HIV-1 and MLV have been shown to be important determinants of cell tropism and, in some cases, sensitivity to TRIM5α and Fv1.

The sequences of *TRIM5* genes in various primate species reveal rapid evolution and an excess of nonsynonymous mutations, specifically in the SPRY domain that determines restriction specifically. This finding is consistent with the notion that TRIM5 has been placed under evolutionary pressure by a variable selective force, most likely viral infections. Remarkably, in one particular New World monkey species, namely owl monkeys, a retrotransposition event has resulted in the almost precise replacement of the C-terminal SPRY domain with a cyclophilinA (CypA) domain. The resulting protein, termed TRIMCyp, inhibits HIV-1 and certain other retroviruses whose capsids bind to CypA.

The ability of certain retroviral capsid proteins, particularly that of HIV-1, to bind CypA can influence their sensitivity to TRIM5α as well as TRIMCyp, and there is a complex relationship between CypA:capsid interactions and sensitivity to restriction in various cell types. CypA binds to a flexible loop that is exposed on the surface of the viral capsid and overlaps with viral determinants that govern sensitivity to TRIM5α. The CypA:capsid interaction can be inhibited by drugs such as cyclosporine A (CsA), and treatment of certain human cells with CsA inhibits replication of HIV-1 while lentiviruses whose capsids do not bind CypA are unaffected. While CsA does not appear to render HIV-1 highly sensitive to human TRIM5α, mutations in the CypA-binding site do confer partial sensitivity to it and allow HIV-1 capsids to saturate human TRIM5α. These findings suggest that HIV-1 capsid may have specifically adapted to bind CypA in order to avoid inhibition by restriction factors, like TRIM5α, in humans.

However, the situation is more complex than these findings would suggest. The requirement for CypA for replication in human cells is HIV-1 strain and host cell-type dependent. Indeed, there are several examples of viral strains whose capsid binds CypA but in which disruption of the interaction has no detectable effect on virus replication. This phenotype is conferred by both naturally occurring and *in vitro* selected mutations that occur within the CypA binding loop but do not affect CypA binding. Remarkably, some of these mutations can confer CsA dependence in other human cell types. These differences among human cell types are not due to variation in TRIM5α sequence and suggest the existence of additional capsid-based restriction factors in human cells,

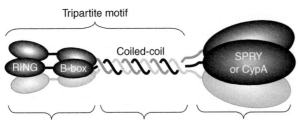

**Figure 2** Domain and functional organization of the TRIM5 class of retrovirus restriction factors that block viral infection by targeting incoming capsids. Three major domains that are required for restriction are the N-terminal effector domain, of unknown function, a cenrtal coiled-coil that mediates trimerization, and a C-terminal domain that is responsible for capsid recognition.

whose activity is actually facilitated by the capsid:CypA interaction. Moreover, it appears that HIV-1 restriction by TRIM5α in Old World monkeys is facilitated by CypA:CA interactions.

Generally, the events immediately following entry of a retrovirus into the target cell are not well understood, complicating efforts to determine molecular details of the mechanism by which Fv1 and TRIM5α prevent retroviral infection. Although the hexameric capsid lattice forms the outer shell of the subviral complex that is delivered into the cell, biochemical studies suggest that the capsid shell may be discarded, in a process known as uncoating, shortly after entry. Therefore, there may be a relatively short time frame in which restriction factors such as TRIM5α and Fv1 can initiate events that inhibit infection. Experimental evidence is partly consistent with this notion, and irreversible TRIM5-mediated restriction events can indeed be initiated very rapidly, within minutes of virus entry into the target cell cytoplasm. TRIM5 can interact specifically with capsid proteins of restricted viruses *in vitro*, and direct binding of TRIM5 to capsids is almost certainly the initiating event in restriction. Ensuing events may involve accelerated capsid uncoating and/or degradation. While restriction by TRIM5 is often manifested as apparent inhibition of reverse transcription, this is not a necessary part of restriction since some TRIM5 variants do not affect viral DNA accumulation, nor does Fv1. The known involvement of RING domains in ubiquitin/sumoylation reactions is suggestive of potential effector mechanisms but neither of these pathways appears to be required for restriction activity, although proteasome inhibition can restore DNA synthesis.

## Other Cellular Inhibitors of Incoming Retroviruses

In addition to the intensively studied TRIM5 and Fv1 proteins, cell-type-dependent effects on the early post-entry event in retroviral replication suggest the existence of additional factors that may inhibit incoming retroviruses. For example, certain HIV-1 and HIV-2 strains appear restricted in particular human cells in a manner that depends on both the envelope and capsid. This finding suggests that the route of retroviral entry may affect the sensitivity to unknown capsid-specific restriction factors, although TRIM5 and Fv1 restriction is clearly independent of entry route. Moreover, studies of chemically mutagenized cell lines have revealed that overexpression of fasciculation and elongation protein zeta-1 can be detrimental to retroviral infection. Whether these additional apparent inhibitors of retroviral infection are physiologically relevant and the mechanisms by which they work has not yet been established. However, it is entirely possible that there remain more, and perhaps many, undiscovered inhibitors of incoming retroviruses.

## Host Resistance to Infectious Virus Generation

Cells have also evolved alternative antiretroviral activities that act after retroviral DNA has integrated into the host genome. Several inhibitors that act at the level of viral genome accumulation, or affect particle assembly, release, or infectivity are known. While such activities cannot preserve the uninfected state of the cell that expresses them, these intrinsic immune functions can attenuate or prevent the spread of infection to subsequent generations of target cells.

## Cellular Cytidine Deaminases as Retrovirus Resistance Factors

One such defense strategy relies on a group of genes, exemplified by *APOBEC3G*, that act primarily by deaminating cytidines in nascent retroviral DNA. *APOBEC3G* is one of a group of genes that exhibit cytidine deamination activity, and other members of this family (e.g., *APOBEC1* and *AID*) are involved in editing of specific cellular mRNAs and genomic loci in order to change their coding potential. APOBEC3G is incorporated into retroviral particles and deaminates nascent viral DNA during reverse transcription in subsequently infected target cells by virtue of its single-stranded DNA-specific deaminase activity (**Figure 3**). Cytidine deamination results in the generation of uracil-containing viral DNA, which likely becomes targeted by DNA repair/degradation enzymes. However, if the viral DNA escapes degradation then uracil is replicated to adenosine during second strand synthesis, resulting in viral DNA with characteristic G-to-A hypermutation. Generally, the burden of G-to-A mutations is high, rendering the proviral DNA incapable of encoding replication-competent progeny.

APOBEC3G is promiscuous with respect to its antiretroviral effect, because it is packaged into diverse retrovirus particles. The mechanism by which this is achieved involves a substantial nonspecific component, whereby APOBEC3G binds in an apparently sequence-independent manner to the RNA that is packaged into virions. Thus, APOBEC3G exploits an essential property of retroviruses to infiltrate particles and therefore makes it difficult for retroviruses to evolve mutations that avoid packaging APOBEC3G into virions. Perhaps because of this difficulty, primate lentiviruses have arrived at an unusual and highly effective solution to the problem imposed on them by APOBEC3G. Indeed, all primate lentiviruses encode an accessory gene, *vif*, whose only function appears to be to counteract APOBEC3G. Vif proteins bind simultaneously to APOBEC3G and to a ubiquitin ligase complex containing Cul5, elongin B, and elongin C to induce ubiquitination of APOBEC3G. Predictably, this leads to proteasome-dependent APOBEC3G

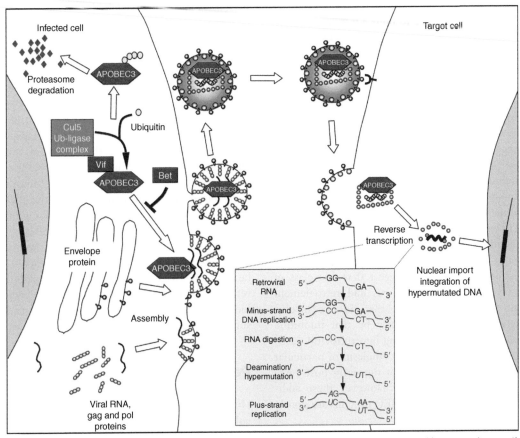

**Figure 3** Major mode of action and alternative fates of APOBEC3 proteins that become incorporated into retrovirus particles and catalyzed cytidine deamination during infection of target cells. Some APOBEC3 proteins can be recruited by lentiviral Vif proteins to a ubiquitin ligase complex and degraded in a proteasome-dependent manner. Alternatively, foamy virus Bet proteins prevent incorporation of APOBEC3 into virus particles by unknown mechanisms.

degradation, effectively depletes APOBEC3G from the cell, and abolishes incorporation into virion particles. Interactions between APOBEC3G and Vif proteins form the basis of additional species tropism restrictions in primate lentiviruses. Although HIV-1 Vif can efficiently bind to and induce the degradation of human APOBEC3G, it is inactive against its rhesus macaque or AGM counterparts. In contrast, rhesus macaque and AGM APOBEC3G can be recognized by Vif proteins from SIVs found in macaques and AGMs. A single-amino-acid difference between human and monkey APOBEC3G proteins (K128D) is responsible for differential sensitivity to Vif proteins and imparts a second barrier to cross-species transmission for at least some primate lentiviruses. Foamy viruses that are also common in primates have also acquired a gene, Bet, whose function is to exclude APOBEC3 proteins from virion particles. Moreover, other retroviruses appear to avoid the APOBEC3 proteins without encoding accessory genes to exclude it from particles. However, in these cases the molecular mechanism of particle exclusion is not clearly defined.

Like *TRIM5*, the locus containing *APOBEC3G* has been under evolutionary pressure during mammalian speciation, most likely as a consequence of viral infections. Indeed, while mice have only one *APOBEC3* gene, humans have no less than seven that have arisen as a result of *APOBEC3* gene duplication and recombination events. Most of the *APOBEC3* genes, like TRIM5, exhibit excess nonsynonymous polymorphisms in primates, again suggesting evolutionary pressure. Several members of the *APOBEC3* gene cluster exhibit varying levels of activity against numerous retroviruses and retroelements, and some are targeted for degradation by primate lentiviral Vif proteins. In some cases, the APOBEC3 proteins are distinguishable by their substrate preference. For example, APOBEC3G-mutated retroviral DNA carries G-to-A changes primarily in the context of GG dinucleotides, while its close relative, APOBEC3F, preferentially targets GA dinucleotides. In the context of HIV-1-infected humans, APOBEC3G and its close relative APOBEC3F appear to be the major contributors to cytidine deamination-based host defense. Indeed, viral DNA carrying G-to-A hypermutation can be found quite easily in some patients, and the context in which the G-to-A changes occur suggests that both APOBEC3G and APOBEC3F are responsible.

While APOBEC3G and its relatives can clearly inhibit retrovirus replication by inducing catastrophic hypermutation, it may be that lentiviruses have turned its cytidine deamination activity to their advantage and are evolved to only partially resist APOBEC3 proteins. Less dramatic changes in viral DNA sequence may result from partial destruction of APOBEC3G by Vif, and infiltration of viral particles by a small number of APOBEC3 molecules. Indeed, Vif proteins with a range of potencies can be found in HIV-1-infected patients. Primate lentiviruses are capable of extremely rapid sequence divergence, and this is probably required to maintain their characteristic high levels of chronic replication in the presence of strong adaptive immune responses. Certainly, the A-rich nature of their genomes suggests that cytidine deaminases have played a role in influencing the rate and direction of sequence divergence in primate lentiviruses.

While cytidine deamination is thought to be the major mechanism by which APOBEC3 proteins inhibit retrovirus replication, some studies suggest that this class of proteins may also inhibit retrovirus and retroelement replication through mechanisms that do not involve hypermutation. In addition, it may be that inhibition does not require APOBEC packing into retroviral particles and that its presence in the cytoplasm of particular target cells is sufficient to inhibit the early post-entry steps of the retrovirus life cycle. However, these additional apparent activities of APOBEC proteins are poorly understood at present.

### Other Host Resistance Factors That Act during Virus Generation

The genomes of retroviruses appear to be the target of a further host defense activity that likely recognizes newly synthesized RNA. Zinc-finger antiviral protein (ZAP) inhibits the cytoplasmic accumulation of the genomes of some retroviruses and, more impressively, alphaviruses. Its mechanism of action may be related to that of the tristetraprolin-like proteins that it resembles, which induce the degradation of cytokine mRNAs by binding to AU-rich sequences in their 3' untranslated regions. By doing so, ZAP may recruit viral RNAs to a collection of ribonucleolytic activities referred to as the exosome. ZAP obviously must distinguish between viral and cellular mRNAs but the molecular basis for this distinction is currently unknown.

It is also possible for cells to interfere with the assembly of retrovirus particles. There exists at least one example where defective Gag proteins encoded by an endogenous retrovirus, namely Jaagsiekte sheep retrovirus, can form heteromultimers with and interfere with the assembly of the Gag protein of its exogenous cousin. Yet another intrinsic immune mechanism targets retrovirus particle release. In some human cells, retrovirus particles are released very inefficiently, unless a protein that is expressed by a subset of primate lentiviruses, termed Vpu, is also present. Vpu is not required for the efficient release of retroviruses from some cell lines, but fusion of cells that do or do not require the presence of Vpu for efficient release results in heterokaryons that exhibit the Vpu-dependent virus release phenotype. While many retroviruses do not encode a Vpu protein, some envelope proteins appear to exhibit a similar activity. These findings suggest the existence of a cellular inhibitor of retrovirus release that is counteracted by Vpu or envelope proteins. Because Vpu can facilitate the release of a number of divergent retroviruses, the presumed release inhibitor must target particle release in a rather nonspecific way. A current model that explains many of the effects of Vpu invokes the existence of a release inhibitor that endows cells and/or nascent virions with an adhesive property. Virion–cell adhesion would result in the retention of viral particles on the cell surface, from where they would be subsequently endocytosed. Consistent with this model, retroviral particles generated by cells in which release is inefficient in the absence of Vpu accumulate at the cell surface and later within intracellular endosomes.

## Perspectives

Historically, the ability or inability of retroviruses to colonize a particular species or cell type was thought to be defined almost entirely by its ability to parasitize host functions present therein that are necessary to complete its life cycle. However, recent findings have shown that evolution has equipped cells with an often robust and multicomponent defense against retroviruses that seek to colonize them. These activities constitute an equally important determinant of retroviral cell tropism. Studies of restriction factors are in their infancy, but these new insights have given a deeper understanding of the evolutionary relationships between retroviruses and their hosts and what governs the ability of retroviruses to engage in zoonosis. Moreover, the discovery of anti-retroviral activities within cells that target pathogenic retroviruses may provide new opportunities for therapeutic intervention.

*See also:* Equine Infectious Anemia Virus; Foamy Viruses; Jaagsiekte Sheep Retrovirus; Simian Immunodeficiency Virus: General Features.

## Further Reading

Best S, Le Tissier P, Towers G, and Stoye JP (1996) Positional cloning of the mouse retrovirus restriction gene Fv1. *Nature* 382: 826–829.
Bieniasz PD (2004) Intrinsic immunity: A front-line defense against viral attack. *Nature Immunology* 5: 1109–1115.
Goff SP (2004) Genetic control of retrovirus susceptibility in mammalian cells. *Annual Review of Genetics* 38: 61–85.

Harris RS, Bishop KN, Sheehy AM, *et al.* (2003) DNA
deamination mediates innate immunity to retroviral infection.
*Cell* 113: 803–809.

Hatziioannou T, Perez-Caballero D, Yang A, Cowan S, and Bieniasz PD
(2004) Retrovirus resistance factors Ref1 and Lv1 are species-
specific variants of TRIM5{alpha}. *Proceedings of the National
Academy of Sciences, USA* 101: 10774–10779.

Sayah DM, Sokolskaja E, Berthoux L, and Luban J (2004) Cyclophilin
A retrotransposition into TRIM5 explains owl monkey resistance to
HIV-1. *Nature* 430: 569–573.

Sheehy AM, Gaddis NC, Choi JD, and Malim MH (2002) Isolation of a
human gene that inhibits HIV-1 infection and is suppressed by the
viral Vif protein. *Nature* 418: 646–650.

Stremlau M, Owens CM, Perron MJ, Kiessling M, Autissier P, and
Sodroski J (2004) The cytoplasmic body component TRIM5alpha
restricts HIV-1 infection in Old World monkeys. *Nature* 427: 848–853.

Towers G, Bock M, Martin S, Takeuchi Y, Stoye JP, and Danos O (2000)
A conserved mechanism of retrovirus restriction in mammals.
*Proceedings of the National Academy of Sciences, USA* 97:
12295–12299.

# Iridoviruses of Vertebrates

**A D Hyatt,** Australian Animal Health Laboratory, Geelong, VIC, Australia
**V G Chinchar,** University of Mississippi Medical Center, Jackson, MS, USA

## Glossary

**Anemia** Reduced number (below normal) of
erythrocytes (red blood cells).

**Ectothemic** Animals whose temperature varies with
the surrounding environment. Also known as
poikliotherms.

**Epitheliotropic** Having a special affinity for epithelial
cells.

**Hyperplasia** Abnormal increase in the volume of a
tissue or organ caused by an increase in the number
of normal cells.

**Karyolysis** Dissolution of a cell nucleus.

**Karyorrhexis** Rupture of the cell nucleus in which
the chromatin disintegrates and is extruded from
the cell.

**Pyknosis** Degeneration of a cell in which the nucleus
shrinks in size and the chromatin appears as a solid,
structureless feature.

**Urodeles** Amphibians belonging to the order
Caudata, including the salamanders and newts, in
which the larval tail persists in adult life.

## Introduction

The family *Iridoviridae* encompasses five recognized
genera, two of which infect invertebrates (*Iridovirus, Chloriridovirus*), and three of which infect ectothermic vertebrates (*Ranavirus, Lymphocystivirus,* and *Megalocytivirus*). In
addition, two other viruses that infect cold-blooded vertebrates (*Erthrocytic necrosis virus* and *White sturgeon iridovirus* (WSIV) remain unassigned members of the family.

Iridoviruses that infect 'cold-blooded' vertebrates (fish,
amphibians, and reptiles) have become the focus of recent
interest. These viruses are being identified and isolated
with increasing frequency and their importance is being
measured in terms of their impact on farmed production
and trade in fish and amphibians. There are also significant impacts of iridoviruses on biodiversity, most notably
the decline of local amphibian populations.

The history of research into these viruses extends back
to the nineteenth century for lymphocystis virus, the
1940s for *Frog virus 3* (FV3, genus *Ranavirus*) and 1980s
for the first description of a highly infectious fresh water
piscine ranavirus, *Epizootic haematopoietic necrosis virus*
(EHNV, genus *Ranavirus*) and saltwater megalocytiviruses
such as red sea bream iridovirus (RSIV, species *Infectious
spleen and kidney necrosis virus*, genus *Megalocystivirus*).
Recent interest in the ranaviruses and megalocytiviruses
is associated with disease epizootics of freshwater and salt
water finfish, die-offs of frogs and salamanders, and illegal
trade in wildlife. Fish, amphibians, and reptiles are being
bought and sold illegally and transported across national
and/or international borders without appropriate certification and quarantine. Increasing reports of disease
involving vertebrate iridoviruses suggests expansion of
the geographic distribution and host range, and, as such,
they are considered to represent a significant group of
emerging viruses.

## Structure

Each of the three recognized genera of chordate iridoviruses shares common structural, replicative, genomic,
and protein characteristics, and each genus contains

several distinct species and isolates/strains. The virions of vertebrate iridoviruses range in size from 100–300 nm. They are comprised of four concentric layers: an outer envelope composed of a lipid bilayer and virus-encoded transmembrane proteins; an icosahedral protein shell comprised of the major capsid protein (MCP), an inner lipid membrane; and a central dsDNA core (approximately 170 kbp) and associated proteins. The outer membrane is acquired as the virus buds through the plasma membrane (**Figure 1(a)**). Lymphocystiviruses and megalocytiviruses differ from the above in that they are seldom observed budding from the host cell plasma membranes. Lymphocystiviruses differ from ranaviruses, megalocytiviruses, and erythrocytic necrosis viruses in that the capsids contain an outer fringe of external, fibril-like protusions (**Figure 1(g)**). Megalocytiviruses also differ from ranaviruses in that assembly sites within cells infected *in vivo* are membrane bound (**Figure 1(e)**).

## Geographical Distribution and Host Range

**Table 1** illustrates the diversity of hosts and geographic locations from which vertebrate iridoviruses have been identified and/or isolated. It is important to note that while many iridoviruses have been observed and isolated, they cannot be assigned to a specific taxonomic group until specific demarcation criteria relating to their molecular, structural, and host-disease characteristics are determined and interpreted as prescribed by the International Committee on Taxonomy of Viruses (ICTV).

Differences in virion size and topography, host range, and geographic locations distribution are generally restricted to specific isolates. Lymphocystis viruses have been reported worldwide and infect both freshwater and marine finfish. Similarly, ranaviruses have been isolated from most continents and have been reported to infect freshwater finfish, anurans (frogs and toads), urodeles (salamanders), and reptiles (turtles and snakes). Megalocytiviruses infect more than 30 species of cultured marine and freshwater finfish belonging mainly to the orders Perciformes and Pleuroneciformes (**Table 1**).

Hosts for vertebrate iridoviruses include all classes of ectothermic vertebrates. However, to date, only one vertebrate iridovirus, namely Bohle iridovirus (BIV), has been shown, under experimental conditions, to infect multiple vertebrate species, genera, and classes. While cross-species/class transmission has been demonstrated following experimental exposure, BIV is yet to be isolated from any epizootic. Moreover, the maximum permissive temperature for vertebrate iridovirus replication (approximately 15–25 °C) precludes replication in mammals or in mammalian cells incubated at 37 °C.

## Phylogeny

At the genomic level, megalocytiviruses, ranaviruses, and lymphocystiviruses differ markedly in genomic organization, GC content, and sequence identity. The GC content of lymphocystiviruses (27–29%) is markedly lower than that of ranaviruses or megalocytiviruses (49–55%). Construction of a phylogenetic tree based on the inferred amino acid sequence of the major capsid protein indicates that three genera of vertebrate iridoviruses form separate clusters that are distinct from each other and from the invertebrate viruses (**Figure 2**). Sequence similarity/identity between different vertebrate iridovirus genera is typically <50%, whereas it is greater than 70% within a genus. Moreover, there is more sequence diversity among ranaviruses, which infect all classes of ectotherms, than among megalocytiviruses, which infect only teleost fish.

## Clinical Features and Pathology

Iridoviruses of fish, amphibians, and reptiles are often highly virulent and can cause fatal infections in their hosts. Epizootics leading to mass mortalities with death rates approaching 100% have been reported in fish and amphibians.

Lymphocystosis in fish is, in the main, chronic and benign and not life-threatening; its impact is mainly cosmetic. Infection causes cellular hypertrophy with individual cells reaching 100 μm to 1 mm in diameter. Infected cells develop a thick hyline capsule, a central, enlarged nucleus and basophilic inclusions which correspond to the comparatively large size (up to 300 nm) of the viruses. Megalocytiviruses, on the other hand, cause a darkening of body color and lethargy which has led to the disease being referred to as 'sleepy disease'. Infected animals also exhibit severe anemia, petechia of the gill, and enlargement of the spleen. Enlarged, inclusion body-bearing cells which function as viral assembly sites are characteristic structures of the spleen, kidney, liver, and other internal organs. WSIV, which is currently an unassigned member of the family, causes significant mortalities among farm-raised juvenile white sturgeon (*Acipenser transmontanus*) in North America. The virus is epitheliotropic, infecting the skin, gills, and upper alimentary tract. Affected tissues display hyperplasia with characteristic amphophilic to basophilic enlarged Malpighian cells filled with virus particles. Erthrocytic necrosis iridoviruses of fish, amphibians, and reptiles are associated with intracytoplasmic inclusion bodies within erythrocytes. Infection is characterized by nuclear degeneration, margination of chromatin, pyknosis, karyorrhexis, and karyolysis. A major clinical feature of such animals is anemia.

The clinical outcome of ranavirus infections varies from benign to fatal. Infections can lead to ulceration

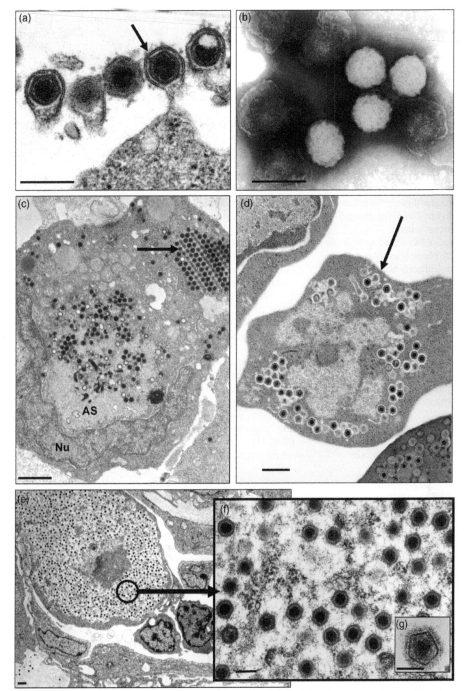

**Figure 1** Electron micrographs of iridoviruses identified within or isolated from fish, amphibians, and reptiles. (a) Transmission electron micrograph of an ultrathin section from an EHNV-infected cell. The host-derived membrane is indicated (arrow). (b) Micrograph of a negatively stained EHNV illustrating the difference in appearance when the whole virus is imaged. (c) Low magnification image of a single cultured cell (Chinook salmon embryo cell) infected with EHNV. The image is from an ultrathin section and illustrates the presence of paracrystalline arrays (arrow), virus assembly sites (AS), and a distorted nucleus (Nu). (d) Image of an ultrathin section of a reptilian erythrocyte (arrow) infected with erythrocytic necrosis iridovirus. Bar represents 1 μm. (e) An ultrathin section of an unknown hypertrophied cell from a dwarf gourami infected with an unknown megalocytivirus. The enlarged cell is apparent. (f) Enlargement of the indicated region from panel (e). Large icosahedral viruses are apparent. (g) Image of a single lymphocystivirus from an ultrathin section of an infected cell. The virus differs from the others due to the presence of surface-associated fibrils (arrow). Scale = 200 nm (a, b, g); 1 μm (c–e); 300 μm (f).

**Table 1**    Vertebrate iridoviruses[a]

| Host | Virus | Country or region where isolated |
| --- | --- | --- |
| *Fish* | | |
| Examples of ranaviruses | | |
| Red-fin perch (*Perca fluviatilis*) and rainbow trout (*Onchorhynchus mykiss*) | Epizootic hemotopoietic necrosis virus (EHNV) | Australia |
| Catfish (*Ictalurus melas*) | European catfish virus (ECV) | Europe (France) |
| Largemouth bass (*Micropterus salmonides*) | Largemouth bass virus (LMBV) | North America (USA) |
| Guppy fish (*Poecilia reticlata*) | Guppy fish iridovirus (GV6) | Southeast Asia |
| Examples of meglacytiviruses | | |
| Red sea bream (*Pagrus major*) | Red seabream iridovirus (RSIV) | Japan |
| Sea bass (*Lateolabrax sp.*) | | Japan |
| Brown spotted grouper (*Epinephelus tauvina*) | Grouper sleepy disease virus (GSIV) | Southeast Asia |
| Cultured mandarin fish (*Siniperca chuatsi*) | Infectious spleen and kidney necrosis virus (ISKNV) | Southeast Asia |
| Examples of lymphocystiviruses | | |
| Infect a large range of fish including flounder (*Platichthys flesus*), plaice (*Pleuronectes platessa*), and dab (*Limanda limanda*) | Lymphocystis disease virus 1 (LCDV-1) (also referred to as Flounder lymphocystis disease virus, FLDV, Dab lymphocystis disease virus (LCDV-2, tentative species of genus *Lymphocystivius*) | Ubiquitous |
| *Amphibians* | | |
| Examples of ranaviruses | | |
| Leopard frog (*Rana pipiens*) | Frog virus 3 | North America (USA) |
| Leopard frog (*Rana pipiens*) | Leopard frog iridoviruses (LT1-LT4) | North America (USA) |
| Red eft (*Diemictylus viridescens*) | T6–20 | North America (USA) |
| North American bullfrog (*Rana catesbeiana*) | Tadpole edema virus (TEV) | North America (USA) |
| Edible frog (*Rana esculenta*) | *Rana esculanta* iridovirus (REIR) | Europe (Croatia) |
| Ornate burrowing frog (*Limnodynastis ornatus*) | Bohle iridovirus (BIV) | Australia |
| Cane toad (*Bufo marinus*) | *Bufo marinus* Venezuelan iridovirus 1 (GV) | South America (Venezuela) |
| Common frog (*Rana temporaria*) | *Rana temporaria* United Kingdom iridovirus 1 (RUK 11)* | Europe (UK) |
| Tiger salamander (*Ambystoma tigrinum stebbensi*) | *Ambystoma tigrinum* iridovirus (ATV) | North America (USA) |
| *Reptiles* | | |
| Examples of ranaviruses | | |
| Box turtle (*Terrapene c. Carolina*) | Tortoise virus 3 (TV3) | North America (USA) |
| Central Asian tortoise (*Testudo horsefieldi*) | Tortoise virus 5 (TV5) | North America (USA) |
| Gopher tortoise (*Gopherus polyphemus*) | | North America (USA) |
| Green tree python (*Morelia viridis*) | Wamena virus (WV)* | Australia (origin Irian Jaya) |

[a]Listed viruses are examples of vertebrate iridoviruses; the list is not exhaustive. Not all listed viruses are included within the *Eighth Report of the International Committee on Taxonomy of Viruses* (Fauquet *et al.*); those which are not assigned to genera are indicated (*).

and/or systemic hematopoietic necrosis in amphibians and fish, and skin polyps, skin sloughing, and systemic hematopoietic necrosis in urodeles. The pathology of vertebrate iridovirus infections is best described for the ranavirus EHNV. The associated disease is referred to as epizootic hemaopoietic necrosis and this designation is applicable to most ranavirus infections. Infection results in the degeneration of hematopoietic cells and damage to the vascular endothelium within most organs. For example, in infected kidneys (**Figure 3**) destruction of the blood-forming cells, termed acute hematopoietic necrosis, occurs. Within the liver and spleen, multifocal necrosis is common. Other organs are also affected, including the pancreas and the vascular endothelium within the liver, spleen, kidney, gill, and heart.

## Emerging Infectious Pathogens

Although lymphocystis disease has been known since the nineteenth century, other vertebrate iridoviruses are more recently recognized and the incidence of reports of ranavirus and meglocytivirus infections has increased in recent years with respect to the number of new hosts and new geographic locations. Ranavirus and megalocytivirus epizootics have been reported in finfish in Asia, North America, South America, the United Kingdom, and Australia. However, long-term declines in finfish populations have been attributed to over-fishing rather than infectious disease. Dramatic fluctuations of amphibian populations due to ranavirus infections have been reported but these have not been recognized as causative agents for reported global

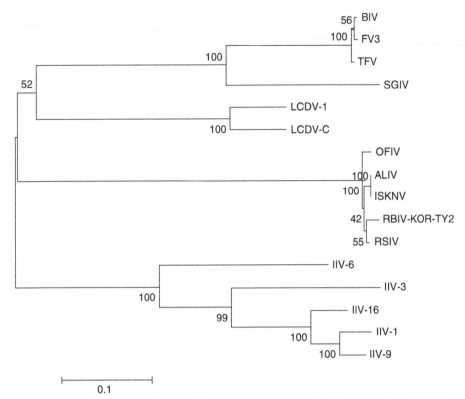

**Figure 2** Phylogenetic relationships among iridoviruses. The inferred amino acid sequences of the MCP of 16 iridoviruses, representing all five currently recognized genera, were aligned using the CLUSTAL W program and used to construct a phylogenetic tree using the Neighbor-Joining algorithm and Poisson correction within MEGA version 3.1. The tree was validated by 1000 bootstrap repetitions. Branch lengths are drawn to scale and a scale bar is shown. The number at each node indicates bootstrapped percentage values. The sequences used to construct the tree were obtained from the following viruses: genus *Megalocytivirus* – ISKNV, infectious skin and kidney necrosis virus (AF370008); ALIV, African lampeye iridovirus (AB109368); OFIV, olive flounder iridovirus (AY661546); RSIV, red sea bream iridovirus (AY310918); RBIV, rock bream iridovirus (AY533035); genus *Ranavirus* – SGIV, Singapore grouper iridovirus (AF364593); TFV, tiger frog virus (AY033630); BIV, Bohle iridovirus (AY187046); FV3, frog virus 3 (U36913); genus *Lymphocystivirus* – LCDV-1, lymphocystis disease virus (L63545); LCDV-C, lymphocystis disease virus – China (AAS47819.1); genus *Iridovirus* – IIV-6, invertebrate iridescent virus 6 (AAK82135.1); IIV-16 (AF025775), IIV-1 (M33542), and IIV-9 (AF025774); genus *Chloriridovirus* – IIV-3 (DQ643392).

amphibian population declines; these are due, in the main, to the fungus Batrachochytrium dendrobatidis.

## Transmission and Control

Lymphocystiviruses are transmitted horizontally via abraded lesions, *Aedes aegypti*, *Aedes albopictus* (C6/36), and *Drosophila melanogaster*. The principal mode of transmission of megalocytiviruses (e.g., RSIV) and ranaviruses is horizontally via virus-containing water. Ranaviruses remain viable in water, as dried culture medium, in frozen carcasses, and at various temperatures ($4\,^{\circ}\text{C}$, $-20\,^{\circ}\text{C}$, and $-70\,^{\circ}\text{C}$) for prolonged periods, indicating that they can exist between epizootics both within and outside their biological host(s). The resistant nature of these viruses also indicates their potential for translocation via fomites such as boots, boat hulls, and fishing tackle, in live fish used for stocking aquaculture ponds, via bait fish, and on the skin surfaces of predatory animals such as birds. The international trade in wildlife, a considerable portion of which is illegally

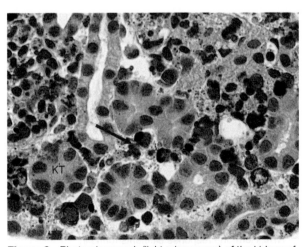

**Figure 3** Photomicrograph (light microscopy) of the kidney of an infected *Bufo marinus* tadpole infected with a South American ranavirus. Extensive necrosis of the hematopoietic cells is indicated by the presence of chromogen (brick-red color) following an immunoperoxidase procedure using a primary antibody against EHNV. KT, kidney tubules. The image was viewed at ×100 magnification.

performed, is also a recognized mechanism for the effective global transport of vertebrate iridoviruses.

To date, vaccines have only been developed against the megalocytiviruses of Asia. For RSIV, a formalin-inactivated vaccine and a DNA vaccine have been used for the protection of finfish including red sea bream, yellowtail, and amberjack. Control of other diseases such as epizootic hematopoietic necrosis is by containment using diagnosis, surveillance, and management strategies documented by the Office Internationale des Epizooties (OIE). No control measures exist for other ranaviruses or erythrocytic necrosis viruses.

## Concluding Remarks

Iridoviruses of fish, amphibians, and reptiles represent a potential health risk to both free-ranging and captured ectothermic vertebrates and are recognized as agents of economical importance by commercial fishing and aquaculture industries; they are not a direct health risk to humans. Over the past two decades, there has been an increase in the number of reported disease incidents involving these large dsDNA viruses. In some reports, surveillance has indicated that these viruses have increased their geographical range and may, therefore, be regarded as emerging viruses. While iridovirus-associated diseases can cause mass mortalities of some species, they are not recognized as a primary cause of the reported global population declines of amphibians or finfish.

The patterns of disease and details on viral structure for the recognized genera are known. However, detailed knowledge of the cellular pathways associated with the pathogenesis of the various diseases is limited.

## Further Reading

Chinchar VG (2002) Ranaviruses (family *Iridoviridae*): Cold-blooded killers. *Archives of Virology* 147: 447–470.

Chinchar VG, Essbauer S, He JG, *et al.* (2005) Family *Iridoviridae*. In: Fauquat C, Mayo MA, Maniloff M, Desselberger U, and Ball LA (eds.) *Virus Taxonomy: Eighth Report of the International Committee on Taxonomy of Viruses*, pp. 145–162. San Diego, CA: Elsevier Academic Press.

Chinchar VG, Hyatt AD, Miyazaki T, and Williams T (in press) Family *Iridoviridae*: Poor viral relations no longer. *Current Topics Microbiology and Immunology* .

Daszak P, Berger L, Cunningham AA, Hyatt AD, Green DE, and Speare R (1999) Emerging infectious diseases and amphibian population declines. *Emerging Infectious Diseases* 5: 735–748.

Daszak P, Cunningham AA, and Hyatt AD (2000) Emerging infectious diseases of wildlife – threats to biodiversity and human health. *Science* 287: 443–449.

Eaton HE, Metcalf J, Penny E, Tcherepanov V, Upton C, and Brunetti CR (2007) Comparative genomic analsis of the family *Iridoviridae*: Re-annotating and defining the core set of iridovirus genes. *Virology Journal* 4: 11.

Fauquet CM, Mayo MA, Maniloff J, Desselberger U, and Ball LA (eds.) (2005) *Virus Taxonomy. Classification and Nomenclature of Viruses. Eighth Report of the International Committee on the Taxonomy of Viruses*, San Diego, CA: Elsevier Academic Press.

Hyatt AD, Gould AR, Zupanovic Z, *et al.* (2000) Comparative studies of piscine and amphibian iridovirues. *Archives of Virology* 145: 301–331.

Office Internationale des Epizooties (2006) Epizootic haematopoietic necrosis. In: *Aquatic Animal Health Code*, p. 2.1.1. Paris: OIE.

Robert J, Morales H, Buck W, Cohen N, Marr S, and Gantress J (2005) Adaptive immunity and histopathology in frog virus 3-infected Xenopus. *Virology* 332: 667–675.

Schock DM, Bollinger TK, Chinchar VG, Jancovich JK, and Collins JP (2008) Experimental evidence that amphibian ranaviruses are multi-host pathogens. *Copeia* 2008: 133–143.

Tan WGH, Barkman TJ, Chinchar VG, and Essani K (2004) Comparative genomic analyses of frog virus 3, type species of the genus *Ranavirus* (family *Iridoviridae*). *Virology* 323: 70–84.

Williams T, Barbosa-Solomieu V, and Chinchar VG (2005) A decade of advances in iridovirus research. *Advances in Virus Research* 65: 173–248.

# Mouse Mammary Tumor Virus

**J P Dudley,** The University of Texas at Austin, Austin, TX, USA

## Glossary

**HRE** Hormone response elements found in several viral genomes that bind the activated forms of steroid hormone receptors to increase transcription in the presence of a steroid ligand.

**Rem** A Rev-like RNA-binding protein that is responsible for efficient nuclear export of unspliced mouse mammary tumor virus RNA.

**Superantigen** A protein that interacts with entire classes of T cells primarily through the variable region of the beta-chain of the T-cell receptor, leading to signal transduction and the release of cytokines.

## History

Mouse mammary tumor virus (MMTV) was first reported in 1933 by the Jackson Memorial Laboratory and by Korteweg in 1934 as an extrachromosomal influence on the incidence of breast cancer in inbred mouse strains. Initial crosses between strains with a high mammary cancer incidence and strains with a low mammary cancer incidence revealed that female progeny invariably had the mammary cancer incidence of the female parent. Subsequently, Bittner showed that an extrachromosomal factor was transmitted through maternal milk, and this factor was later associated with viral particles, called 'B-particles', which caused breast cancer in susceptible mice.

## Taxonomy and Classification

MMTV is a prototype species of the genus *Betaretrovirus* in the family *Retroviridae*. These viruses previously were referred to as type B retroviruses based on their appearance by electron microscopy (a characteristic acentric core within particles of *c.* 100 nm). Milk-borne MMTVs are often named for the inbred mouse strain from which they are derived, for example, C3H MMTV or MMTV (C3H). Multiple double-stranded DNA copies are found in the chromosomal DNA of most commonly used laboratory strains of mice (called integrated or endogenous proviruses). These endogenous proviruses presumably represent viral insertions into chromosomal DNA of germline cells and are referred to as *Mtv* followed by an Arabic number, for example, *Mtv8*. Most endogenous *Mtv*s have defects in one or more genes and, therefore,

these proviruses often fail to produce infectious virus. Currently, MMTV is classified with other betaretroviruses including Mason–Pfizer monkey virus (MPMV), Jaagsiekte sheep retrovirus (JSRV), and human endogenous retrovirus type-K (HERV-K).

## Properties of the Virion

MMTV particles contain a single-stranded positive-sense RNA, which exists as a dimer, and is encapsidated as a helical ribonucleoprotein (RNP) by the nucleocapsid (NC) protein; reverse transcriptase (RT) and integrase (IN) are closely associated with the RNP. The RNP is surrounded by an icosahedral shell (although the exact structure has not been carefully studied) composed of capsid (CA) protein. There is considerable variation in the size of cores, similar to that observed with human immunodeficiency virus 1 (HIV-1). MMTV capsids are bound via the matrix (MA) protein to the viral envelope, a portion of the cellular plasma membrane that has been modified by the insertion of the surface (SU) and transmembrane (TM) proteins.

## Properties of the Genome

The viral RNA is bound at either end by a short direct repeat (R) of 15 bp (**Figure 1**). The R regions are adjacent to unique regions of approximately 120 and 1200 bp, respectively, present at the 5′ (U5) or 3′ (U3) ends of the RNA. A cellular tRNA (tRNA3Lys) is bound through 18 bp of complementarity to each copy of the viral RNA

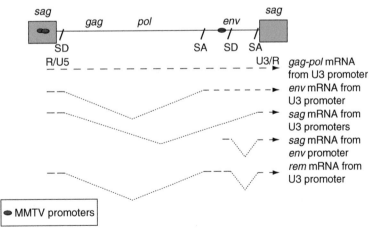

**Figure 1** Diagram of the MMTV proviral genome and structure of viral mRNAs. The boxed regions represent the LTRs with two described promoters. The standard promoter gives unspliced transcripts that start with the first base of the R region in the 5′ LTR and end at the last base of the R region of the 3′ LTR. Unspliced transcripts may be directly exported from the nucleus for Gag, Gag-Pro, and Gag-Pro-Pol translation. Alternatively, such transcripts may be spliced to give two singly spliced mRNAs encoding either envelope or superantigen. A fourth transcript from the LTR promoter gives a doubly spliced mRNA that encodes the RNA export protein, Rem. An internal promoter in the envelope gene also allows production of a singly spliced RNA encoding the superantigen. The positions of known splice donors (SD) and acceptors (SA) are also shown.

at the primer-binding site (PBS) located just downstream of U5. Although the RNA packaging site (often referred to as ψ) has not been defined, this site is likely to include the region between the splice donor (SD) and splice acceptor (SA) sites for the envelope (*env*) mRNA. Packaging of viral mRNAs, other than genomic RNA, is prevented by exclusion of the ψ region. The first SD site precedes the group-specific antigen (*gag*) region that encodes a Gag precursor with the nonglycosylated proteins of the virion in the order NH2-MA-p21-CA-NC-COOH. Interestingly, the virus also encodes two other precursor polypeptides, Gag-Pro and Gag-Pro-Pol, from the genomic RNA by ribosomal frameshifting. Gag-Pro encodes the Gag proteins, a dUTPase (DU), and the viral protease (PR), whereas the Gag-Pro-Pol protein also encodes RT, including a ribonuclease H (RNase H) activity, and IN. Both the DU and RT are trans-frame proteins that contain sequences from the preceding protein, NC and PR, respectively. At the 3′ end of the genome, the envelope (Env) proteins are specified in the order NH2-SU-TM-COOH from a singly spliced mRNA. Recent findings indicate that MMTV encodes another protein called regulator of export of MMTV mRNA or Rem from a doubly spliced mRNA. The *rem* mRNA is translated from the open reading frame that also specifies SU and TM. Such data emphasize the efficiency with which MMTV and other viruses use their genetic information. Furthermore, unlike most other retroviruses, which have multiple stop codons within the long terminal repeat (LTR), the MMTV U3 region has yet another gene that encodes a superantigen (Sag) from one or more singly spliced mRNAs.

## Virus Replication

Recent evidence indicates that MMTV uses the transferrin receptor 1 (Tfr1) to mediate infection. Tfr1 is ubiquitously expressed in many rodent cells, and this observation may explain infection of numerous rat and mouse cell lines in culture. Differences in mouse Tfr1 and primate Tfr1 appear to be sufficient to prevent MMTV infection of monkey and human cells. Despite numerous reports of MMTV sequences in human tumors, failure of human Tfr1 to allow viral entry is one argument against the validity of these data. However, use of other receptors for MMTV entry, particularly in specific cell types, is possible. Entry through Tfr1 appears to occur through adsorptive endocytosis, and receptors are recycled to the cell surface where they allow entry of additional MMTV particles into previously infected cells. Thus, unlike many retroviruses, MMTV is not susceptible to superinfection resistance, and many chronically infected mouse lines have large numbers of integrated proviruses.

Following entry and partial uncoating in the cytoplasm, the virally encoded RT is activated. Using the cellular lysyl-tRNA primer bound to genomic RNA, RT synthesizes a partial minus-strand DNA bound to plus-stranded RNA. Using the RT-associated RNase H activity and several strand transfers, the RNA template is degraded and a double-stranded provirus is synthesized. However, the product of reverse transcription is different from the starting template so that the U5 and U3 sequences present uniquely in viral RNA are duplicated to give longer repeats at each end of the provirus (LTRs). The LTRs have the structure U3-R-U5 (**Figure 1**). Because nuclear entry of the preintegration complex (PIC) containing the provirus is thought to require nuclear envelope breakdown during mitosis, it is generally believed that MMTV must infect dividing cells. However, MMTV encodes DU, a protein found in many nonprimate lentiviruses that infect nondividing cells. DU prevents misincorporation of uracil and mutation of newly synthesized proviruses in nondividing cells where the ratio of dUTP to TTP is high.

After nuclear entry of the PIC, the provirus integrates using the MMTV-encoded IN protein cleaved from the Gag-Pro-Pol precursor. IN protein introduces an asymmetric cut 2 bp from the linear ends of the provirus as well as an asymmetric break exactly 6 bp apart on opposite DNA strands of host DNA. Proviral integrations are not site specific and may occur at transcriptionally active sites, although this idea has not been tested directly. Following the joining reaction, the repair of virus–cell junctions by cellular enzymes generates a 6 bp direct repeat of cell DNA that flanks the viral LTRs. Such a structure resembles those formed by the transposable elements of bacteria, yeast, and *Drosophila*.

The integrated provirus contains all the signals necessary for recognition by RNA polymerase II, and many of these signals are present in the U3 region of the LTR. Transcription from the standard promoter is initiated in the 5′ LTR starting at the U3/R junction and terminating at the R/U5 junction (**Figure 1**). However, several other promoters have been described, including one approximately 500 bp upstream of the U3/R junction and another within the envelope gene. Termination appears to be reasonably inefficient, and some MMTV transcripts probably terminate in the adjacent cellular DNA. A portion of genome-length MMTV RNA is processed into singly spliced *env* and *sag* mRNAs.

Surprisingly, the *sag* gene appears to be expressed by at least two singly spliced mRNAs from independent promoters (**Figure 1**), possibly allowing different levels of Sag in various cell types. MMTV also produces a doubly spliced mRNA that encodes the RNA export protein, Rem. In most cell types, the levels of *gag-pol* and *env* mRNAs greatly exceed *sag* and *rem* mRNAs.

The unspliced RNA (8.7 kb) is translated into Gag, Gag-Pro, and Gag-Pro-Pol precursor proteins. Since *pro* (the viral protease gene) and *pol* (the polymerase/integrase gene) are out of frame with respect to *gag* and each other, one ribosomal frameshift is required for Gag-Pro synthesis, and a second frameshift is necessary to produce Gag-Pro-Pol (**Figure 2**). Because the first frameshift is quite efficient, MMTV RT levels in infected cells are equivalent to those produced by other retroviruses. The *env* mRNA is translated into a precursor protein on membrane-bound polyribosomes. This precursor is modified by glycosylation in both the endoplasmic reticulum and the Golgi, and protein cleavage to SU and TM also occurs in the latter compartment. The *sag* mRNA appears to be translated into a type II transmembrane protein of 36 kDa; this protein is glycosylated and reportedly cleaved to generate a C-terminal fragment of 18 kDa. Sag is associated with major histocompatibility complex (MHC) class II protein at the surface of antigen-presenting cells. Unlike the previously described proteins, Sag is not a known structural component of virions. The Rem protein is translated in the same frame as the envelope protein, including the Env signal peptide (**Figure 2**). The nascent protein escapes signal recognition particle, and the full-length Rem protein (33 kDa) localizes to the nucleolus using motifs found in the signal peptide. Rem synthesis is required for efficient export of unspliced genomic RNA and must precede production of infectious viral particles. The N-terminal one-third of Rem appears to encode all functions necessary for RNA export, and deletion of the C-terminus increases the ability of Rem to function in export assays. These data indicate that unspliced MMTV RNA export and particle production are negatively regulated, at least in some cell types.

The precursors for Gag, Gag-Pro, and Gag-Pro-Pol aggregate within the cell cytoplasm into procapsids called intracytoplasmic A particles. This process is distinct from the maturation of C-type particles that assemble Gag precursors at the cell surface concomitant with the budding process. Presumably, the precursor proteins are folded so that NC and RT proteins are sequestered inside the particle to interact with a dimer of viral RNA and the lysyl tRNA. The viral PR, which is present in a fraction of the Gag precursors, is apparently responsible for the cleavage events that produce the mature virion proteins, MA, p21, p3, p8, CA, and NC. The functions of p21, p3, and p8 are currently unknown. Like HIV, the MMTV Gag precursor contains a P(S/T)AP sequence that likely functions as a late (L) domain; such domains interact with cellular protein complexes (known as ESCRTs) to promote budding. Further cleavages by PR to give functional RT and IN, and mature cores apparently occur after budding.

## Transmission and Tissue Tropism

MMTV is transmitted horizontally through maternal milk (called exogenous or milk-borne virus) or vertically through the germline (endogenous viruses). The exogenous viruses are responsible primarily for the high mammary cancer incidence of mouse strains such as RIII and C3H. However, some strains, such as GR, carry an endogenous virus (in this case, *Mtv2*) that is also transmitted through milk. Although most common inbred mouse strains carry endogenous *Mtvs*, some recently inbred strains lack such proviruses. Interestingly, strains that lack *Mtvs* often show resistance to disease induced by exogenous MMTV regardless of the route of transmission.

MMTV particles ingested by newborn mice in maternal milk survive passage through the stomach during the first weeks of life prior to maturation of the intestinal tract (**Figure 3**). These particles enter the small intestine where they cross the epithelium through M cells. Subsequently, MMTV virions encounter and infect dendritic cells and B cells. Following reverse transcription, integration, and transcription, Sag protein is produced and presented at the surface of such cells in association with MHC class II protein. Sag signaling through the T-cell receptor (TCR) leads to the release of cytokines, leading to a pool of dividing lymphoid cells for MMTV infection as well as division of previously infected cells. Both B and T cells are required for MMTV transmission since knockout or transgenic animals lacking either lymphoid subset cannot be infected efficiently by the milk-borne route. This lymphoid cell reservoir is necessary to preserve MMTV infectivity prior to the onset of puberty in mice when a source of susceptible and dividing mammary cells becomes available. Sag-mediated stimulation of lymphoid cells also improves the efficiency of viral transfer within the mammary gland. MMTV production increases during lactation when hormone levels elevate transcription from the hormone-responsive element (HRE) in the LTR U3 region (**Figure 4**). High virion production during lactation ensures that large amounts of particles will be produced at a time when newborn offspring can be infected.

Horizontal transmission of MMTV by seminal or salivary fluid has been reported. The low infectivity of

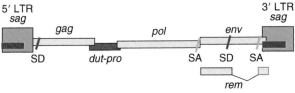

**Figure 2** Positions of the open reading frames within MMTV proviral DNA. The large boxes represent the 5' and 3' LTRs, whereas the smaller elongated boxes represent the reading frames for the genes shown in italics. The *rem* gene is in the same reading frame as the envelope gene, which is altered by splicing (V shape). The *sag* coding sequence at the 5' end of the genome is not expressed because it is located upstream of the viral promoters.

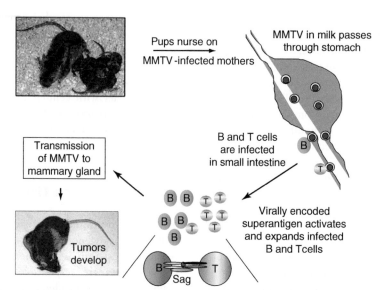

**Figure 3**  The MMTV life cycle. Infected mothers transmit virus to their pups through milk. In the first few weeks of life, the pups ingest the virus, which passes through the stomach into the small intestine. MMTV then transverses the M cells to deliver virus to gut-associated lymphoid cells. B cells in the gut are infected and express Sag protein at the cell surface in conjunction with MHC class II protein. Recognition of the Sag C-terminal amino acids by the variable portion of the β-chain of the T-cell receptor results in signal transduction and the release of cytokines. Cytokines then stimulate the proliferation of adjacent B and T cells, which act as a reservoir for the virus until transmission to mammary epithelial cells occurs during puberty. Virus expression and release is highest during lactation to ensure milk-borne transmission. Mammary tumors arise after multiple rounds of pregnancy and lactation due to insertional mutagenesis.

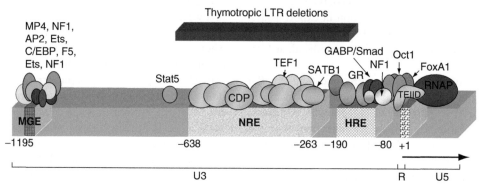

**Figure 4**  Transcriptional control elements in the MMTV LTR. The major transcriptional start site is located at the U3/R border in the 5′ LTR of integrated proviral DNA. The mammary gland enhancer (MGE) is located near the 5′ end of the LTR. The negative regulatory element (NRE) contains binding sites for Cutl1/CDP, SATB1, and TEF1, but different cell types vary in the level of these factors. The hormone response element (HRE) contains multiple binding sites for the activated forms of several steroid receptors, including glucocorticoid receptor (GR). The GR sites appear to be flanked by binding sites for FoxA1. The region spanning deletions found in thymotropic strains of MMTV is shown above the LTR. TFIID, transcription factor IID; RNAP, RNA polymerase II.

most body fluids (other than milk) may be attributable to virally infected lymphoid cells and the absence of large amounts of infectious MMTV particles.

## Genetics and Disease Susceptibility

MMTV causes mammary adenocarcinomas by infection of the mammary epithelium. The genetic factors that influence mammary tumor incidence in mice include

(1) the presence or absence of milk-borne virus, (2) the presence of an infectious endogenous MMTV, (3) cellular factors that determine virus entry and replication, and (4) host factors that may influence the immune response (including the Sag response) or hormonal levels in the animals. The presence of milk-borne virus has been demonstrated in mouse strains with a high mammary cancer incidence by foster nursing experiments as originally described by Bittner. Shortly thereafter, it was shown that such high-cancer-incidence strains (e.g., C3H) permanently

lost this trait if nursed on mothers with a low mammary cancer incidence (e.g., BALB/c). Such strains, known as C3Hf, have a mammary tumor incidence between 38% and 47% (average latency of 600 days) in multiparous animals, whereas C3H strains expressing milk-borne MMTV have a tumor incidence of 88–95% (average latency of 300 days) in breeding females. Mammary tumors appearing in C3Hf mice are the result of expression of a replication-competent endogenous provirus known as *Mtv1*. Strains, such as BALB/c and C57BL, which have a mammary tumor incidence of 1% or less with long latencies, appear to lack a replication-competent MMTV.

A number of cellular and host factors also influence the appearance of mammary tumors in different mouse strains. Most of these factors have not been defined, but many of them appear to directly or indirectly affect the ability of MMTV to replicate. For example, the resistance of C57BL to MMTV infection appears to be the result of failure to express MHC class II I–E molecules, one of two types of class II antigens expressed in mice. Although many MMTV Sag proteins apparently interact with class II I–A proteins, this interaction is less efficient than the Sag/MHC class II I–E complexes in the stimulation of lymphoid cells. Loss of specific class II molecules is not the only defense against MMTV infection. The presence of endogenous MMTV proviruses that express Sag proteins results in the deletion of specific subsets of T cells. If these endogenous viruses encode Sags with the same TCR reactivity as exogenous MMTVs, milk-borne infection is blocked by preventing viral amplification in lymphoid cells (**Figure 3**). For example, endogenous *Mtv7* expresses a Sag protein that reacts with and causes deletion of Vβ6+ T cells; therefore, the milk-borne MMTV (SW) strain that encodes TCR Vβ6-reactive Sag cannot infect mouse strains that carry *Mtv7* because these mice lack the T-cell subset required for MMTV transmission.

Resistance to exogenous MMTV infection is usually a recessive characteristic, which has been used to determine if various mouse strains have the same or different resistance genes. For example, C57BL and I strain mice are both resistant to C3H MMTV infection, yet F1 hybrids of these strains have a high incidence of mammary tumors when infected by C3H virus. This result suggests that I strain mice (H-2$^i$) encode a functional MHC class II I–E molecule that complements the defect in C57BL mice and overcomes resistance to MMTV infection. More recently, disease resistance in I strain mice has been attributed to the development of strong neutralizing antibodies to MMTV. Further, development of neutralizing antibodies appears to be dependent on the MMTV strain. MMTVs with weak Sag activities (e.g., C3H MMTV) appear to elicit few neutralizing antibodies, whereas the opposite applies to MMTVs with strong Sag function (e.g., SW MMTV). Another host

resistance mechanism is mediated by Toll-like receptor 4 (TLR4) signaling, which normally triggers an innate immune response. Wild-type C3H MMTV is lost during passage in C3H/HeJ animals, which lack functional TLR4, but not in related TLR4+ mice. C3H MMTV interactions with TLR4 trigger the immunosuppressive cytokine IL-10, allowing the virus to subvert the innate immunity by elimination of cytotoxic T cells. Further, YBR/Ei mice exhibit a dominant resistance to MMTV that depends on an adaptive T-cell response to the infection. However, not all MMTV resistance mechanisms may depend on the immune response; NH mice are resistant to the virus, perhaps related to hormonal changes that lead to early reproductive difficulties in this strain.

Traditional types of genetic experiments with MMTV have been difficult for two reasons. First, since MMTV does not form plaques or foci in cultured cells, cloning of viral stocks has not been possible. Second, molecular cloning of an intact MMTV provirus has been difficult for some MMTV strains because of selection against a specific part of the *gag* region during growth of proviral clones in *Escherichia coli*. This difficulty has been overcome by combining the 5′ end of an endogenous provirus (e.g., *Mtv1*) with the 3′ end of an exogenous provirus (e.g., C3H MMTV). Such hybrid proviruses have been used to produce infectious virions that retain oncogenicity for the mammary gland and to show that the MMTV *gag* region contributes to development of mammary tumors.

## Pathogenicity

MMTV induces primarily type A and B mammary adenocarcinomas. Insertional mutagenesis is presumed to be the mechanism of MMTV-induced mammary tumors and is consistent with the relatively long latent period for tumor development (6–9 months). However, the MMTV envelope protein may act as a tumor initiator for mammary cells.

Common integration sites can be identified from MMTV-induced tumors. Current data have implicated more than 10 different loci (designated *int* or integration site genes) in MMTV-induced mammary tumors (**Table 1**). Most of these integration sites share the following characteristics:

1. The majority of the MMTV integrations are outside of the gene-coding regions, and the MMTV promoter is rarely used to initiate *int* gene transcription. Thus, an unmodified protein product is produced.
2. The MMTV provirus can activate target gene transcription over considerable distance (in excess of 15 kb). There may be activation of multiple genes in a cluster.
3. Proviruses often are integrated upstream in the opposite transcriptional orientation or downstream in the same orientation as the target gene.

**Table 1**    Common integration sites found in MMTV-induced mammary tumors

| Locus | Gene family/function | Mouse chromosome | Integration frequency |
|---|---|---|---|
| Wnt1 (Int-1) | Wingless/growth factor | 15 | 80% in C3H; 70% in BR6; 30% in GR |
| Wnt3 (Int-4) | Wingless/growth factor | 11 | 10% in GR |
| Wnt10b | Wingless/growth factor | 15 | 23% of Fgf3 transgenic |
| eIF3-p48 (Int-6) | Eukaryotic translation initiation factor | 15 | 6% in Fgf3 transgenic |
| Rspo2 (Int-7) | R-spondin homolog/ growth factor receptor | 15 | 13% in Czech II |
| Fgf3 (Int-2) | Fibroblast growth factor | 7 | 65% in BR6; 5% in C3H; 20% in GR |
| Fgf4 (Fgfk/hst/hst-1/ Hstf-1) | Fibroblast growth factor | 7 | 10% in BR6 |
| Fgf8 (Aigf) | Fibroblast growth factor | 19 | 80% in Wnt1 transgenic |
| Notch1 (Mis6/Tan1) | Notch | 2 | 8% of Erbb2 transgenic |
| Notch4 (Int-3) | Notch | 17 | 20% in Czech II; 8% in BR6 |
| Cyp19a1 (Cyp19/Int-5/ Int-H) | Cytochrome P450/aromatase | 9 | 3 chemically induced BALB/c hyperplasias |

4. Target gene transcription is low or undetectable in normal adult mammary glands.
5. Transcription of the *int* genes is regulated developmentally.
6. The *int* genes appear to be conserved evolutionarily, and a number of these genes encode growth factors or truncated growth factor receptors.

Such observations are consistent with the transcriptional activation of conserved genes in the mammary gland by their proximity to MMTV LTR enhancers. Transgenic animals overexpressing the *int* genes often show mammary hyperplasias and sporadic tumors; this observation confirms the involvement of multiple genes during oncogenesis. Mating of animals with different transgenes accelerates this process, indicating cooperation between *int* genes.

MMTV variants that are expressed preferentially in T cells induce T-cell lymphomas. Interestingly, these thymotropic MMTV appear to activate a different set of oncogenes, for example, c-*myc* and *Rorc*, relative to milk-borne MMTVs as a result of LTR alterations.

## Transcriptional Regulation

Studies of the MMTV HRE have been a paradigm for hormone-regulated gene expression. MMTV RNA levels increase *c.* 10–50-fold in the presence of glucocorticoids, progesterone, or androgens at the level of transcriptional initiation. Hormone inducibility is conferred by multiple binding sites to allow cooperative binding with the consensus TGTTCT in the region from −80 to −190 (**Figure 4**). Glucocorticoids are believed to bind to their receptors (GRs) in the cytoplasm and to subsequently translocate to the nucleus where they exchange rapidly with their binding sites. The integrated MMTV LTR is occupied by six nucleosomes (A–F) (not shown) with the A nucleosome located at the transcription initiation site (+1). The standard MMTV promoter contains a TATA element (−30 bp), which binds transcription factor IID (TFIID). Hormone-bound GR is believed to recruit remodeling factors to increase accessibility at nucleosome B and to allow binding of transcription factors Oct1 and NF1 between the TATA box and the HRE.

The tissue distribution of MMTV expression is tightly linked to viral transcriptional control, yet steroid receptors are present in many tissues in which MMTV transcription is repressed. The importance of negative regulation in MMTV transcription and disease specificity is exemplified by the isolation of MMTV variants, such as type B leukemogenic virus (TBLV), which induce T-cell lymphomas rather than mammary tumors. Such variants lack all or part of the negative regulatory element (NRE) present upstream of the HRE and acquire a T-cell specific enhancer. The NRE binds at least two related homeodomain-containing proteins called special AT-rich binding protein 1 (SATB1) and Cut-like protein1/CCAAT displacement protein (Cutl1/CDP), which have different tissue distributions and act as repressors of MMTV transcription. The highest levels of SATB1 are expressed not only in T cells but also in B cells explaining transcriptional repression in most lymphoid tissues. Mutations of the promoter-proximal SATB1-binding site elevate MMTV expression of LTR-reporter constructs in cultured cells and in lymphoid tissues of transgenic mice. Interestingly, CDP expression is high in undifferentiated B cells and mammary cells and decreases during differentiation. In mammary epithelial cells, where SATB1 is also absent, CDP is cleaved during differentiation to yield a dominant-negative protein that interferes with full-length CDP binding to the MMTV LTR. Therefore, the levels of functional CDP repressor are lowest when MMTV particle production is highest at lactation, the period when virus transmission occurs in milk.

MMTV specifies several enhancer elements, including the HRE and a mammary gland enhancer (MGE) near the 5′ end of the LTR. The MGE contains binding sites for multiple nuclear factors, including MP4, NF1, AP2, Ets, and C/EBP. Synthesis of some factors is inducible by prolactin, epidermal growth factor, or tumor necrosis factor α. The absence of NRE-binding repressors and ligand-bound steroid receptors presumably cooperate with the HRE to maximize virus production in milk.

## Immune Response

Endogenous MMTVs, like exogenous viruses, express Sag proteins, initially known as minor lymphocyte stimulating (Mls) antigens. Unlike conventional antigens where a peptide associates with the groove formed by the MHC class II α- and β-chains, the central portion of Sag binds to class II protein (**Figure 5**). Since Sag is a type II transmembrane protein, the C-terminal portion is available to interact with the variable region of the β-chain (Vβ) of the TCR on a subset of CD4+ or CD4+CD8+ cells. Therefore, Sag recognizes entire classes of T cells (up to 30% of the entire T-cell repertoire), in contrast to conventional antigens that recognize TCR on less than 1 in $10^4$ T cells. Sag stimulation leads to the rapid deletion of reactive cells if Sag is expressed in the thymus, whereas extrathymic deletion appears to occur more slowly.

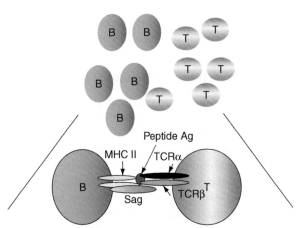

**Figure 5** Interaction of MMTV Sag with the TCR. The α and β chains of the TCR on CD4+ cells combine to recognize a peptide (foreign or self) (small circle) residing in the binding pocket of the MHC class II molecule on MMTV-infected antigen-presenting cells. The C-terminal end of Sag interacts with the variable region of the TCR β-chain, although the TCR α-chain has been reported to affect Sag binding. Accessory molecules such as CD4 probably affect the stability of the Sag–TCR interaction.

Sag is relatively conserved among different MMTV strains, except at the C-terminus, which mediates TCR interactions. C-terminal polymorphisms correlate with reactivity with specific TCR β-chains; for example, C3H MMTV reacts with Vβ14 and 15 chains. Molecular switching experiments have shown that the C-terminal half is sufficient to specify TCR reactivity, and virtually any mutation within this region is sufficient to abolish function. Deletion of specific T-cell subsets in various feral and laboratory mouse strains is believed to provide immunity to specific milk-borne MMTVs, and there is evidence that endogenous *Mtv*s shape the immune response against other pathogens.

## Future Perspectives

MMTV has been valuable for studies of hormone-regulated gene expression, tissue-specific transcription, immune response, and mechanisms of oncogenesis. The recent discovery that MMTV is a complex retrovirus suggests that this virus will provide a useful model for understanding pathogenesis by human retroviruses, such as HTLV and HIV.

## Further Reading

Bhadra S, Lozano MM, and Dudley JP (2005) Conversion of mouse mammary tumor virus to a lymphomagenic virus. *Journal of Virology* 79: 12592–12596.

Callahan R and Smith GH (2000) MMTV-induced mammary tumorigenesis: Gene discovery, progression to malignancy and cellular pathways. *Oncogene* 19: 992–1001.

Czarneski J, Rassa JC, and Ross SR (2003) Mouse mammary tumor virus and the immune system. *Immunologic Research* 27: 469–480.

Golovkina TV, Chervonsky A, Dudley JP, and Ross SR (1992) Transgenic mouse mammary tumor virus superantigen expression prevents viral infection. *Cell* 69: 637–645.

Held W, Waanders GA, Shakhov AN, Scarpellino L, Acha-Orbea H, and MacDonald HR (1993) Superantigen-induced immune stimulation amplifies mouse mammary tumor virus infection and allows virus transmission. *Cell* 74: 529–540.

Jude BA, Pobezinskaya Y, Bishop J, *et al.* (2003) Subversion of the innate immune system by a retrovirus. *Nature Immunology* 4: 573–578.

Kinyamu HK, Chen J, and Archer TK (2005) Linking the ubiquitin-proteasome pathway to chromatin remodeling/modification by nuclear receptors. *Journal of Molecular Endocrinology* 34: 281–297.

Liu J, Bramblett D, Zhu Q, *et al.* (1997) The matrix attachment region-binding protein SATB1 participates in negative regulation of tissue-specific gene expression. *Molecular and Cellular Biology* 17: 5275–5287.

Mertz JA, Simper MS, Lozano MM, Payne SM, and Dudley JP (2005) Mouse mammary tumor virus encodes a self-regulatory RNA export protein and is a complex retrovirus. *Journal of Virology* 79: 14737–14747.

Ross SR, Schofield JJ, Farr CJ, and Bucan M (2002) Mouse transferrin receptor 1 is the cell entry receptor for mouse mammary tumor virus. *Proceedings of the National Academy of Sciences, USA* 99: 12386–12390.

Zhu Q, Maitra U, Johnston D, Lozano M, and Dudley JP (2004) The homeodomain protein CDP regulates mammary-specific gene transcription and tumorigenesis. *Molecular and Cellular Biology* 24: 4810–4823.

# Mousepox and Rabbitpox Viruses

**M Regner, F Fenner, and A Müllbacher,** Australian National University, Canberra, ACT, Australia

## Glossary

**Pyknotic** Exhibiting a degenerate nucleus by contraction of nuclear contents; a sign of cell death.

## Introduction

Ectomelia virus (ECTV), which is the agent of mousepox, and rabbitpox virus (RPXV) share two features; they are both orthopoxviruses and both are known only as infections of laboratory animals, the mouse and rabbit, respectively.

## Ectromelia Virus

### History

ECTV was discovered in 1930 by J. Marchal, as a spontaneous infection of laboratory mice at the National Institute of Medical Research in London. It was called infectious ectromelia because of the frequent occurrence of amputation of a foot in animals that had recovered from infection. Soon after, J. E. Barnard showed, by ultraviolet (UV) microscopy, that it had oval virions about the same size as those of vaccinia virus (VACV). The only other experiments done with the virus at that time involved studies of experimental epidemics by W. W. C. Topley and his colleagues.

In 1946, F. M. Burnet, in Melbourne, showed that ECTV was serologically related to VACV. During experimental epidemics carried out in Burnet's laboratory, F. Fenner found that in animals that did not die of acute hepatitis there was a rash, and he named the disease mousepox. Subsequent studies led to the development of a classical model explaining the spread of virus around the body in generalized viral infections with rash.

In laboratories in Europe and the USA, the virus was regarded as a major menace to colonies of laboratory mice, and stringent steps were taken to prevent its entry to the USA. Only after extensive outbreaks in several cities of that country in 1979 were studies of the virus undertaken in the USA, in high-security laboratories.

### Classification

*Ectromelia virus* is a species within the genus *Orthopoxvirus* of the family *Poxviridae*, as evidenced by the morphology of the virion, cross-protection tests, and restriction endonuclease mapping. Most strains of *Ectromelia virus* (e.g., Moscow, Hampstead) recovered from naturally infected mouse colonies are highly virulent. However, a substrain of Marchal's original strain was attenuated by serial passage on the chorioallantoic membrane of chicken eggs (Hampstead egg).

### Genetics

The ECTV genome is typical for an orthopoxvirus in size and composition. It is A + T-rich and comprises 210 kbp. Almost half of the genome consists of a central region of high homology to other orthopoxviruses and this is flanked by significantly more variable terminal regions. The genome comprises 175 potential genes encoding proteins, including numerous predicated host range proteins and host response modifiers. ECTV does not cluster phylogenetically with any other member of the virus family.

### Host Range and Virus Propagation

ECTV produces disease in *Mus musculus* and several other species of mice, and is considered a natural mouse pathogen. The rabbit, guinea pig, and rat can be infected by intradermal or intranasal inoculation, with the production of small skin lesions or an inapparent infection. ECTV will grow on the chorioallantoic membrane of the developing chick embryo, and also in cell cultures derived from a variety of species. Quantitation of virus stocks is determined by growth on cell culture monolayers (plaque assay).

### Geographic Range and Seasonal Distribution

ECTV has been spread around the world inadvertently by scientists working with laboratory mice, and has been repeatedly reported from laboratories in several countries of Europe and from Japan and China. Mousepox has never been enzootic for prolonged periods in mouse colonies in the USA, but accidental importations sometimes occurred with mice or mouse tissues from European laboratories, with devastating consequences. In contrast, there are extremely limited data regarding the occurrence of ECTV in wild animals.

### Epidemiology

In laboratory mice, ECTV is infectious by all routes of inoculation. It always produces a generalized infection but there are local lesions in the lungs after intranasal inoculation and in the peritoneal cavity after intraperitoneal injection. The response of mice is strongly conditioned by mouse genotype (see below).

The usual source of natural infection is via minor abrasions of the skin, which may occur from contaminated bedding or during manipulations by animal handlers. Infection may also occur by the respiratory route, but probably only between mice in close proximity to each other. A primary lesion usually develops at the site of infection. Since mice are readily infected by inoculation, virus-contaminated mouse serum, ascites fluid or mouse cells, tumors or tissues constitute a risk to laboratory colonies previously free of infection.

## Enzootic Mousepox

Until the introduction of rigorous screening techniques in the 1960s, mousepox was enzootic in many mouse-breeding establishments in Europe and Japan. A variety of mechanisms probably operated to maintain the virus, without disrupting the mouse-breeding program as to make control mandatory. One important factor was probably the high level of genetic resistance and trivial symptomatology exhibited by many mouse genotypes. Another may have been maternal antibody. Another possible mechanism for maintaining enzootic infection is chronic, clinically inapparent infection, which sometimes occurs after oral administration, when some mice show infection of Peyer's patches, excretion of virus in the feces, and lesions in tail skin.

## Susceptibility of Different Strains of Mice

Analysis of spontaneous epizootics and deliberate experiments in the 1980s showed that C57BL/6, 129J, and AKR mice were highly resistant to mousepox, CBA/J and SJL/J intermediate, and BALB/c and A/J mice were highly susceptible. Strain differences are best demonstrated after footpad inoculation or in natural epizootics, since C57BL/6 mice are relatively susceptible by intranasal, intracerebral, or intraperitoneal infection.

## Pathogenesis

Fenner's work in the 1930s to 1940s established mousepox as a model system for the study of generalized viral infections. Müllbacher has more recently used the mousepox model for the analysis of immune effector molecules required for resistance to ECTV infections, using specific gene knockout mutant mouse strains. Mousepox is generally considered an excellent mouse model of human smallpox and is now used increasingly by the bioterrorism defense research community.

Mice are usually infected in the footpad and, after an incubation period of *c.* 7 days (as found in natural infections), a local ('primary') lesion develops at the inoculation site. A few days later some mice die, with no other visible skin lesions but with acute necrosis of the liver and spleen, and in those that survive a rash develops which goes through macular and pustular stages before it scabs.

During the incubation period the virus passes through the mouse body in a stepwise fashion: infection, multiplication and liberation, usually accompanied by cell necrosis, first in the skin and then the regional and possibly the deeper lymph nodes, until it reaches the bloodstream (primary viremia).

C. A. Mims showed in the 1960s that, during the primary viremia, virus is ingested by the phagocytic littoral cells of the liver and spleen. After a day or so, much larger amounts of virus are liberated into the circulation (secondary viremia). Next follows an interval during which the virus multiplies to high titer before visible changes are produced, so that 2 or 3 days usually elapse between the appearance of the primary lesion and the secondary rash. Some animals die before skin lesions appear, but titration experiments and histological examination showed that early skin lesions are present.

## Clinical Features of Infection

Early workers described two forms of the disease, a rapidly fatal form in which apparently healthy mice die within a few hours of the first signs of illness and show extensive necrosis of the liver and spleen at autopsy, and a chronic form characterized by ulcerating lesions of the feet, tail, and snout. Fenner found that in natural infections most mice develop a primary lesion, usually on the snout, feet, or belly. Subsequently, virus multiplies to high titer in the liver and spleen. Some mice die at this stage, but if they survive they almost invariably develop a generalized rash (**Figure 1**).

Age affects the response of genetically susceptible mice. Both virulent and attenuated strains produce higher mortalities in suckling mice and in mice about a year old than in 8-week-old mice.

### Pathology and histopathology

The pathological changes in naturally occurring mousepox in susceptible mice are quite characteristic. Additional lesions in the peritoneal cavity or lung occur after intraperitoneal or intranasal inoculation, respectively; these are important because mousepox sometimes occurs after unwitting passage of ECTV by these routes.

### Intracytoplasmic inclusion bodies

ECTV produces two types of intracytoplasmic inclusion body in infected cells, A-type and B-type. The latter occur in all poxvirus infections and are the sites of viral multiplication; more characteristic of mousepox are the prominent acidophilic inclusion bodies (A-type), which are always found in infected epithelial cells but rarely in liver cells (**Figure 2**).

### Skin lesions

The earliest primary lesions that can be recognized macroscopically are the seat of advanced histological changes, for viral multiplication has then been in progress for several days. There is no macroscopic breach of the skin

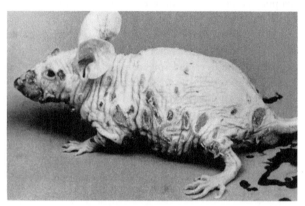

**Figure 1** The rash of mousepox as it appears 14 days after infection, in a naturally infected genetically hairless mouse (not athymic). Similar lesions occur beneath the hair of other strains of susceptible mice and can be clearly demonstrated by epilation. Reproduced from Fenner F (1982) Mousepox. In: Foster HL, Small JD, and Fox JG (eds.) *The Mouse in Biomedical Research*, vol II, pp. 209–330. New York: Academic Press, with permission from Elsevier.

surface, but the dermis and subcutaneous tissue are edematous and there is widespread lymphocytic infiltration of the dermis. Inclusion bodies can be seen in the epidermal cells at the summit of the lesion. Necrosis of these epidermal cells is followed by ulceration of the surface. The exudate forms a scab beneath which healing occurs. Histologically, the changes of the rash are similar to those in the primary lesion.

### Lesions of the liver

The liver and spleen are invariably invaded during the incubation period and virus multiplies to high titer here. The liver remains macroscopically normal until within 24 h of death, when it appears enlarged and studded with minute white foci. The necrotic process extends rapidly and at the time of death the liver is enlarged with many large semiconfluent necrotic foci. In animals that survive, the liver usually returns to its normal macroscopic appearance, but occasionally numerous white foci occur.

Histologically, little change is apparent until macroscopic changes have appeared, although immunofluorescence techniques have shown that infection always occurs first in the littoral cells of the hepatic ducts, from which the virus spreads to contiguous parenchymal cells. Numerous scattered foci of necrosis then appear throughout the liver parenchyma and in fatal cases these rapidly extend until they became semiconfluent. The portal tracts show slight infiltration with lymphoid cells. Liver regeneration commences early and is active, especially in nonfatal cases, and fibrosis does not occur.

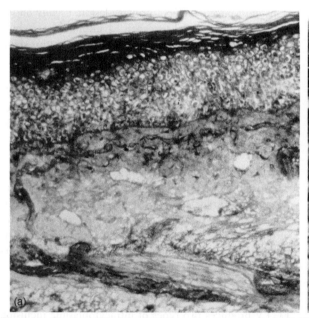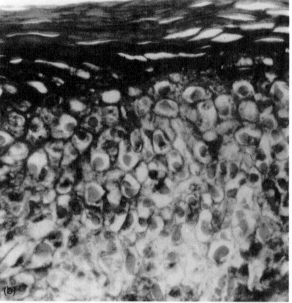

**Figure 2** Section of the skin of the foot of a mouse injected with ECTV in the footpad six days earlier. (a) Low power. (b) High power, Mann's stain. Almost every epithelial cell contains an eosinophilic A-type inclusion body. With most strains of ECTV, these A-type inclusion bodies contain large numbers of mature virions. Reproduced from Fenner F (1982) Mousepox. In: Foster HL, Small JD, and Fox JG (eds.) *The Mouse in Biomedical Research*, vol II, pp. 209–330. New York: Academic Press, with permission from Elsevier.

### Lesions of the spleen

The spleen shows macroscopic changes at least a day earlier than the liver and higher titers of virus are found in the spleen. Virus reaches the spleen in infected lymphocytes, which initiate infection in the substance of the follicles. While infected follicles are destroyed by the spreading infection, neighboring follicles show the proliferative response characteristic of antibody production.

In surviving mice, lesions of the spleen vary from small raised plaques about a millimeter in diameter to areas of fibrous tissue that, after severe attacks, almost completely replace the normal splenic tissue. These changes constitute reliable autopsy evidence that a mouse has recovered from an attack of mousepox.

### Lesions of other organs

The regional lymph nodes draining the site of the primary lesion are enlarged from the time the primary lesions can be detected, and they usually show localized areas of necrosis, with pyknotic nuclear debris in a featureless background. In fatal cases, the gut is often engorged and the lymphoid follicles enlarged. Small necrotic foci with typical inclusion bodies occur in the intestines in most acutely fatal cases of mousepox. Occasionally, especially in very young mice, there are hemorrhagic foci in the kidneys.

### Lesions after intraperitoneal inoculation

There is no primary skin lesion, but in acutely fatal cases the necrosis of the liver and spleen resembles that found after natural infection. In addition, there is usually some increase in intraperitoneal fluid and a considerable amount of pleural fluid, and the pancreas is often grossly edematous. In animals that survive the acute infection there is a great excess of peritoneal and pleural fluid, the peritoneal surfaces of the liver and spleen are covered with a white exudate, the walls of the gut are thickened and rigid, and there is often fat necrosis in the intraperitoneal fat. Extensive adhesions between the abdominal viscera develop later.

### Lesions after intranasal inoculation

When small doses of virus are inoculated intranasally, there is usually little change in the lungs except patchy congestion; the changes in the liver and spleen are those characteristic of naturally acquired mousepox. With larger doses of virus, congestion of the lungs is more pronounced and consolidation may occur, and when very large doses are given death occurs with patchy or complete consolidation of the lungs and little change in the liver and spleen. The apparent pneumotropism is due to the fact that the local reaction, which occurs after the intranasal inoculation of very large doses of virus, kills the animal before there is time for the characteristic changes in the liver and spleen to occur.

## Immune Response

Two weeks after infection mice are solidly immune to reinfection by footpad inoculation of the virus. This immunity declines slowly but even a year after recovery multiplication of the virus after footpad challenge is confined to the local skin lesion.

### Humoral immunity

Antibodies generated by a primary infection protect from subsequent challenge. Newborn mice receive maternal antibody via the placenta and in the milk during the first 7 days after birth. Until titers decline to undetectable levels by the seventh week after birth, this maternal antibody confers protection against death, but not against infection, with moderate doses of ECTV. Furthermore, in the absence of functional B cells, clearance of primary infection with ECTV may be deficient, leading to viral persistence and eventual death.

### Cell-mediated immunity

Work by Blanden in the early 1970s showed that T cells are critical in recovery from primary infection with ECTV, and mice pre-treated with anti-thymocyte serum die from otherwise sublethal doses of virus due to uncontrolled viral growth in target organs. These mice have impaired cell-mediated responses but normal neutralizing antibody responses, elevated interferon levels in the spleen, and unchanged innate resistance in target organs. The active cells in the immune population are cytotoxic T cells, although natural killer cells probably also play an important role early in the infection.

Virus-specific cytotoxic T cells are detectable 4 days after infection and reach peak levels in the spleen 1–2 days later, while delayed hypersensitivity is detectable by the footpad test 5–6 days after inoculation. In contrast, significant neutralizing antibody is not detectable in the circulation until the eighth day.

Cytotoxic T cells employ two different mechanisms to destroy virus-infected cells before the release of viral progeny: one, the granule exocytosis pathway, is mediated by perforin and granzymes that are stored in cytolytic granules and secreted toward, and enter, the infected cell, inducing apoptosis; the other one via triggering of death receptors (e.g., Fas) on the surface of infected cells, inducing a cascade of caspase activation that also leads to apoptosis. However, poxviruses encode inhibitors of the death receptor pathway of killing (e.g., SPI-2, see below), rendering the granule pathway indispensable for recovery. Consequently, mice genetically deficient in perforin or both principal granzymes (A and B) are highly susceptible to ECTV infection.

T-cell-secreted cytokines are also important factors determining the outcome of infection. Whereas interferon-gamma (IFN-γ) critically contributes to viral clearance, an imbalanced cytokine response of the so-called Th2 type, characterized by lack of IFN-γ and excess of interleukin-4 (IL-4), predisposes to greater susceptibility. A recombinant ECTV expressing IL-4 was found to be highly virulent even in resistant strains of mice and those vaccinated with attenuated virus, prompting concerns about the possible creation of recombinant poxviruses with increased virulence in humans for the purpose of bioterrorism.

### Host response modulation

As do other poxviruses, ECTV encodes numerous host-response modifiers in order to evade or suppress the immune response to allow for maximal viral replication. Broadly, these can be divided into inhibitors of the inflammatory response, and anti-apoptotic proteins. Several ECTV-encoded proteins have been shown to neutralize or inhibit key inflammatory cytokine pathways, for example, an IL-18-binding protein and homologs of the IL-1β, tumor necrosis factor (TNF) and IFN receptors. On the other hand, virally encoded inhibitors of components of the caspase cascade inhibit apoptotic pathways. Examples are the ECTV protein p28, a RING finger-domain protein, which is a potent ECTV virulence factor that inhibits UV-induced, but not Fas- or TNF-induced apoptosis; and SPI-2, a serine proteinase inhibitor, which blocks TNF-α-mediated apoptosis via caspase 1/8 inhibition.

## Future

Mousepox is now very rare as a natural infection in laboratory colonies of mice but it is likely that, despite the strict controls necessary to protect mouse colonies, mousepox will be investigated more extensively in the future. Workers in Australia, the USA, and the UK are now using it as a model for studies of problems such as immunocontraception and the role of the many homologs of mammalian host response modifier genes that are found in all poxviruses. In addition, the recognition of mousepox as a good mouse model for human smallpox has, in the light of increased interest in poxvirus immunobiology, seen a resurgence of research into its pathologies, immune evasion strategies, and the mechanisms of recovery from this disease.

## Rabbitpox Virus

### History and Classification

Rabbitpox is a laboratory artifact, due to the infection of laboratory rabbits with VACV, usually with neuro-VACV variants; hence this account of RPXV will omit reference to those aspects that are covered in the article on VACV.

The name rabbitpox was originally given to devastating outbreaks of a generalized disease, likened to smallpox in man, in a colony of laboratory rabbits at the Rockefeller Institute of Medical Research in New York in 1932–34, when other scientists had been working with neuro-VACV in rabbits in an adjacent room prior to the outbreak. The virus recovered from the outbreak was called RPXV and was shown to be very similar to neuro-VACV in its biological properties. Subsequently, the restriction map of the Utrecht strain (see below) was found to be almost identical with that of VACV.

Another outbreak occurred in the Netherlands in 1941. It began among rabbits bought from a dealer a few days after they were introduced into the laboratory colony, and spread among the stock rabbits. The disease was usually lethal, death occurring before there was time for the development of a rash. The virus that caused this outbreak, designated RPXV-Utrecht, caused similar highly lethal epizootics when it 'escaped' in the Institut Pasteur in Paris in 1947; other outbreaks have been described in laboratory rabbits in the USA in the 1960s.

## Epidemiology

In all outbreaks, spread appeared to occur by the respiratory route, and experiments confirmed that infection occurs readily by this route. Rabbits infected by contact are not infectious for other rabbits until the second day of illness, which is usually 5 days after infection. Actual contact is not necessary; transmission can occur across the width of a room, and air sampling revealed the presence of RPXV in the air of rooms housing infected rabbits.

## Genetics

Since 1960, the Utrecht strain of RPXV virus has been used for genetic studies on poxviruses, since it was found to give rise to white pock mutants on the chorioallantoic membrane of chicken eggs and host range mutants in a pig kidney cell line, both of which entail deletions and transpositions of DNA. Recombination experiments with the white pock mutants were used to construct the first crude 'genetic map' produced for an animal virus.

When the complete coding sequence of the Utrecht strain was reported, it was confirmed that it is most closely related to VACV, with more than 95% sequence similarity. It was also established that RPXV is not a direct evolutionary descendant from VACV, as it contains several genes present in smallpox virus but not VACV.

## Pathogenesis

A good deal of experimental work has been carried out on the pathogenesis of rabbitpox as an animal model of smallpox, with results that were largely confirmatory of those obtained with mousepox. In rabbits infected by the intranasal instillation of a small dose of virus, by aerosol, or after intradermal infection or contact infection, there is a stepwise spread of virus through the organs, although the incubation period is shorter than in mousepox and there seems to be little delay at the regional lymph nodes. Viremia is leukocyte associated.

## Clinical Features of Infection

RPXV causes an acute generalized disease in which a rash appears in animals that survive long enough, presenting as pocks on the skin and mucous membranes (**Figure 3**). Rabbits dying of hyperacute infection show no obvious skin lesions, the so-called 'pockless' rabbitpox. Such infections are analogous to acutely lethal cases of mousepox.

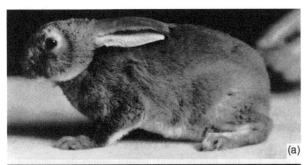

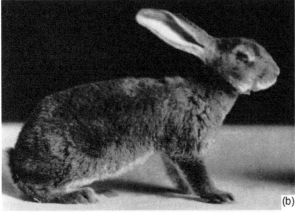

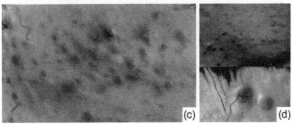

**Figure 3** Rabbitpox. (a) and (b) Littermates with different types of disease. The course of infection was mild in the rabbit shown in (a) and external lesions were limited in the skin; the animal in (b) was seriously ill and its posture is a manifestation of acute respiratory distress resulting from extensive mouth lesions. (c) Cutaneous lesions on the trunk. The coat in this area was loose and easily plucked by hand. (d ) Skin of a pregnant doe self-plucked for nest fur, showing both dry crusted pustules and others in earlier stages of development. Reproduced from Greene HSN (1934) Rabbit pox: I. Clinical manifestations and course of disease *Journal of Experimental Medicine* 60: 427–440. Copyright 1934 The Rockefeller University Press.

and perhaps to early hemorrhagic-type smallpox, in which death occurs before there is time for pustular skin lesions to develop.

## Pathology and Histopathology

The most distinctive lesions are the pocks on the skin and mucous membranes and occasionally small areas of focal necrosis are found in the internal organs (liver, spleen, lung, testes, ovaries, uterus, adrenals, and lymph nodes). In the so-called 'pockless' form, a few pocks may occur around the mouth and they may be visible on the shaved skin. The most prominent gross lesions are pleuritis, focal necrosis of the liver, enlarged spleen, and edema and hemorrhage of the testes.

RPXV, being a strain of VACV, produces B-type inclusions (Guarnieri bodies) in infected cells, but not the prominent A-type inclusions found in cells infected with ECTV.

## Immune Response

Rabbits that have recovered from rabbitpox are immune to infection with VACV, but in very severe infections rabbits die before there is time for an effective immune response. The importance of enveloped virions in the pathogenesis and immunology of orthopoxvirus infections was fist demonstrated in experiments with RPXV. Passive immunization with sera that did not contain antibody to the viral envelope failed to protect rabbits against challenge infection, even though the neutralization titer of the ineffective antiserum (produced by immunization with inactivated VACV) was much higher, as judged by conventional neutralization tests. This work helped explain the failure of inactivated VACV to provide protection against infection with orthopoxviruses.

## Future

Since rabbitpox appears to be a laboratory artifact, due to the introduction of strains of VACV that can spread from one rabbit to another in rabbit colonies, prophylaxis appears to be a matter of preventing such events. These events were rare even when VACV, and especially neuro-VACV, were extensively used in animal experiments several decades ago, and it is unlikely that further episodes will occur now that most research with VACV utilizes cultured cells rather than intact animals. Nevertheless, laboratory managers who use rabbits should be aware of the possibility that some strains of VACV can spread naturally from one rabbit to another.

Because of the higher sensitivity of rabbits to low doses with RPXV compared to that of mice to ECTV, and efficient spread via the aerosol and respiratory routes, RPXV has also been recently revisited as a model for human smallpox.

## Further Reading

Adams MM (2007) Rabbitpox and vaccinia virus infections of rabbits as a model for human smallpox. *Journal of Virology* 81: 11084–11095.

Esteban DJ and Buller RM (2005) Ectromelia virus: The causative agent of mousepox. *Journal of General Virology* 86: 2645–2659.

Fenner F (1982) Mousepox. In: Foster HL, Small JD,, and Fox JG (eds.) *The Mouse in Biomedical Research,* vol. II, pp. 209–230. New York: Academic Press.

Fenner F and Buller RML (1996) *Mousepox.* In: Nathanson N (ed.) *Viral Pathogenesis,* 535pp. Philadelphia: Lippincot-Raven.

Fenner F, Wittek R, and Dumbell KR (1989) *The Orthopoxviruses.* San Diego: Academic Press.

Greene HSN (1934) Rabbit pox. I: Clinical manifestations and course of disease. *Journal of Experimental Medicine* 60: 427–440.

Müllbacher A (2003) Cell-mediated cytotoxicity in recovery from poxvirus infections. *Reviews in Medical Virology* 13: 223–232.

Müllbacher A and Lobigs M (2001) Creation of killer poxvirus could have been predicted. *Journal of Virology* 75: 8353–8355.

# Murine Gammaherpesvirus 68

**A A Nash and B M Dutia,** University of Edinburgh, Edinburgh, UK

## Origins and Ecology

Murine gammaherpesvirus 68 (MHV-68) belongs to species *Murid herpesvirus 4*, genus *Rhadinovirus*, subfamily *Gammaherpesvirinae*, family *Herpesviridae*. It was originally isolated from a bank vole (*Clethrionomys glareolus*) in Slovakia. Two other related herpesviruses (MHV-60 and MHV-72) also came from bank voles and two more (MHV-76 and MHV-78) from wood mice (*Apodemus flavicollis*). The five viruses were originally isolated following the inoculation of diluted suspensions of various tissues (lung, spleen, liver, kidney, and heart) into the brains of newborn mice. Different virus isolates were obtained from the brains of mice following either the first, second, or third intracranial passage from mouse to mouse. These Slovakian viruses developed cytopathic effect in epithelial and fibroblast cell lines from a variety of species ranging from chickens to primates. One other isolate (MHV-Brest) was reported in a shrew (*Crocidura russula*). Subsequently, a number of new isolates have arisen primarily from wood mice following a survey of wild rodents in the Wirrell, Liverpool.

## Virus Structure and Genetic Content

MHV-68 virion structure is similar to that of other herpesviruses. The capsid, tegument, and glycoprotein genes are homologous to those of other herpesviruses and can be predicted to fulfill the same roles in the MHV-68 virion. The composition of the MHV-68 capsid, tegument, and envelope has been investigated, revealing five capsid proteins (encoded by ORF25, ORF62, ORF26, ORF65, and ORF29), three tegument proteins (ORF75c, ORF45, and ORF11), five envelope proteins (ORF8, ORF51, ORF27, ORF28, and ORF22), and four proteins of undetermined locations (ORF20, ORF24, ORF48, and ORF52). The viral tRNA-like RNAs (vtRNAs), which are unique to MHV-68,

are present in the tegument. Other structural proteins are predicted by analogy with other herpesviruses but their presence in the virion is yet to be demonstrated.

The genetic content of MHV-68 is based on the complete DNA sequences of MHV-68 strains g2.4 and WUMS. These are not independent strains, since the latter was derived by limited passage and plaque purification of the former. As a consequence, the two sequences are very similar (g2.4, GenBank accession number AF105037; WUMS, U97553). The proposed gene layout is shown in **Figure 1**.

The linear, double-stranded DNA genome of MHV-68 consists of a single unique region of 118 237 bp flanked by a variable number of 1213 bp terminal repeats. The unique region and terminal repeats have nucleotide compositions of 46 and 77.6% G+C, respectively. Two internal tandem repeats are located within the unique region: a 40 bp repeat located at genome coordinates 26 778–28 191 and a 100 bp repeat located at coordinates 98 981–10 1170.

The unique region of the MHV-68 genome is largely collinear with the genomes of other rhadinoviruses, including Kaposi's sarcoma-associated herpesvirus (KSHV) and herpesvirus saimiri. It contains 73 protein-coding open reading frames (ORFs) and also encodes eight vtRNAs and nine predicted microRNAs (miRNAs). As with other rhadinoviruses, MHV-68 possesses a number of cellular homologs, including a complement regulatory protein (CRP, encoded by ORF4), a Bcl-2 homolog (vBcl-2, M11), a cyclin D homolog (vcyclin, ORF72), and a G protein-coupled receptor (vGPCR, ORF74).

MHV-68 also contains a number of unique genes clustered at the left end of the genome. These include four genes encoding proteins (M1, M2, M3, and M4) and eight genes encoding the vtRNAs and miRNAs. In MHV-76, the first 9.5 kbp of the genome, containing M1–M4 and the vtRNAs and miRNAs, is absent; otherwise the genome is identical to that of MHV-68. MHV-72 is deficient in the first 7 kbp of the genome

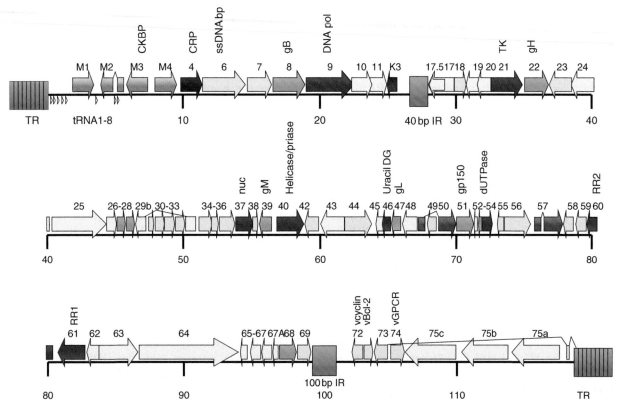

**Figure 1**    Organization of the MHV-68 genome. Yellow color indicates structural proteins; light green, glycoproteins; red, enzymes; violet, transcriptional transactivators; lavender, unique MHV-68 genes ; plum, immunomodulatory proteins; and dark green, repeats. TR, terminal repeat; IR, internal repeat; CKBP, chemokine-binding protein; CRP, complement regulatory protein; TK, thymidine kinase; nuc; alkaline exonuclease; uracil DG, uracil deglycosylase; RR, ribonucleotide reductase; vGPCR, viral G protein-coupled receptor.

and lacks M1–M3 and the vtRNAs and miRNAs; otherwise the genome is identical to that of MHV-68. It is not known whether MHV-76 and MHV-72 are deletion mutants of MHV-68 that arose during isolation or whether they exist naturally. MHV-Brest is closely related to MHV-68 but appears to represent a different virus species. The sequence of the left end region is particularly highly conserved between MHV-Brest and MHV-68, with greatest divergence in M2.

## Infection and Replication

MHV-68 is able to infect and replicate in a range of mammalian epithelial and fibroblast cell lines. A productive infection occurs in the majority of cell lines, but a persistent infection is established in some lymphoid cells. MHV-68 establishes a latent infection in NS0, a myeloma cell line, but not in the thymoma cell line BW5147. The virus is maintained indefinitely in NS0 cells as a latent infection, with approximately 5% of the cells undergoing reactivation and expressing lytic cycle proteins. This scenario is similar to that seen for lymphoblastoid cell lines infected with Epstein–Barr virus (EBV). Other B cell lines can also be infected, including B cell

hybridomas and the commonly used A20 cell line. One latently infected B cell line, S11, has been derived from a lymphoma obtained from a MHV-68-infected mouse.

Many MHV-68 genes have been assigned functions based on their orthology to genes of other herpesviruses whose roles are known. The use of signature-tagged transposon mutagenesis has resulted in the identification of a number of MHV-68 genes that are essential for the replication process, as well as several genes that are not essential but significantly enhance viral replication. So far, 41 genes have been shown to be essential for viral replication, of which 17 are essential for replication in all herpesviruses, including MHV-68 ORF6 (encoding the single-stranded DNA-binding protein, ssDNA bp), ORF8 (glycoprotein B, gB), ORF9 (DNA polymerase, DNA pol), ORF22 (glycoprotein H, gH), and ORF64 (large tegument protein). Some essential genes have homologs only within the gammaherpesviruses, including ORF45, which corresponds to the KSHV IRF7-binding protein.

MHV-68 transcription occurs in a temporal fashion and is detected from 3 h post infection (p.i.) *in vitro*. The replication genes ORF6 (ssDNA bp), ORF9 (DNA pol), ORF60 (ribonucleotide reductase subunit 2, RR2), and ORF61 (RR1) are transcribed with similar kinetics, with a defined early peak of transcription. ORF57, a conserved herpesvirus protein involved in RNA transport and stability that can also act as a transcriptional transactivator, shows similar kinetics. Other genes can be clustered into three general expression patterns. One exhibits a peak in transcript levels at 5 h p.i., followed by a gradual decrease thereafter, and includes ORF50 (Rta), ORF37 (alkaline exonuclease, nuc), and glycoprotein L (gL). The second group has a peak at approximately 8 h p.i., and includes the structural genes ORF25 (major capsid protein), ORF33 (a tegument protein), ORF38 (a tegument-associated membrane protein), and ORF51 (envelope glycoprotein gp150), as well as several genes of unknown function (ORF20 and ORF52). The final group shows a peak of transcription at 12 h p.i., and includes a second group of structural proteins such as ORF19 (a tegument protein), ORF66 (a capsid protein), ORF68 (a glycoprotein), and ORF65 (a capsid protein). From this temporal analysis of viral gene expression, it is possible to build up a profile of the events that take place during MHV-68 replication.

Along with the essential replication proteins, a number of nonessential genes are also expressed during infection *in vitro*. The M4, K3, and ORF73 genes are expressed with immediate early kinetics, while genes with cellular homologs (encoding vcyclin, vBcl-2, and vGPCR) are expressed with early–late kinetics. The early–late group also includes the abundantly expressed M3 gene, which encodes a chemokine-binding protein.

New virions are assembled in a manner similar to that observed for herpes simplex virus type 1. MHV-68 can exit the cell into the extracellular space or can directly infect adjacent cells. ORF51 (encoding gp150) is necessary for viral egress into the extracellular space, whereas ORF27 (gp48) has been identified in the process of egress directly into adjacent cells. gp48 must be localized to the plasma membrane for efficient movement of virions into new cells, a process that requires the ORF58 protein.

## Expression of Unique Viral Genes

The unique MHV-68 genes (M1–M4 and the vtRNA genes) are important determinants of pathogenicity. They are absent from the deletion mutant MHV-76, which replicates with the same efficiency as MHV-68 *in vitro* but is attenuated *in vivo*. The functions of these genes have been the subject of intense study but currently they are not fully understood. The M1, M3, and M4 protein sequences are related to each other, but similar proteins have not been detected in sequence databases. Similarly, the M2 protein is not related to known proteins. The M1, M3, and M4 proteins are secreted from infected cells. Studies with mutant viruses have shown that M1 is involved in reactivation from latent infection and in pathogenesis in the lung. M4 is an immediate early gene

involved in the establishment of latent infection. M3 encodes an abundant protein that is expressed early in the lytic cycle and found during productive infection and establishment of a latent infection. It is an important determinant of pathogenesis during the acute stages of infection but does not appear to be transcribed during long-term latent infection. It is secreted from cells in large quantities and has a high affinity for specific members of the chemokine family, binding to all classes of chemokines (CC, CXC, C, and CX3X) and functionally inhibiting the ability of chemokines to signal through host G protein-coupled receptors.

M2 is a B-cell-specific gene that is involved in acute latent infection. It encodes a membrane-associated protein required for efficient establishment of latency and control of latent infection in B cells. In its absence, there is a defect in memory B-cell latency and increased long-term latency in germinal center B cells. M2 is likely to play a multifunctional role in MHV-68 infection and potentially interacts with a number of cellular proteins. It binds the guanine nucleotide exchange factor vav, altering the normal lymphocyte signaling process and inhibiting B cell receptor-induced cell-cycle arrest and apoptosis. M2 interacts with the DDB1/COP9/cullin repair complex and the ATM DNA damage transducer, blocking DNA damage-induced apoptosis. There is also evidence that M2 inhibits the cellular response to interferon (IFN) by binding to Stat1/Stat2 proteins.

The vtRNAs are predicted to fold into typical cloverleaf structures and, like cellular tRNAs, are thought to be transcribed by RNA polymerase III since the appropriate promoter elements are present within the genes. Following cleavage of excess nucleotides at both the 5′ and 3′ termini, the transcripts are post-transcriptionally modified by the addition of a 3′ CCA sequence, but are not aminoacylated. Only one vtRNA, vtRNA5, contains all the variant or semivariant bases present in mammalian tRNA sequences. The vtRNAs are expressed during lytic and latent infection and have been used widely as a marker for latent infection *in vivo* as their high level of expression means they are readily detectable by *in situ* hybridization. Their function is unknown. The primary vtRNA transcripts also encode miRNAs. The miRNAs are processed and expressed in infected cells, but no information is available on their specificity and function or on their expression *in vivo*. They are currently the only miRNAs known to be transcribed by polymerase III, and their association with the vtRNAs is intriguing.

## Entry and Spread within the Host

The natural route of infection is uncertain, but by analogy with other animal gammaherpesviruses the respiratory tract is likely to be a primary route. Introduction of virus intranasally into inbred mice leads to a productive infection of alveolar epithelial cells, resulting in bronchiolitis. During MHV-68 infection, inflammatory responses in the lung evolve slowly compared to the response seen in MHV-76 infection, where a rapid inflammatory cell infiltrate occurs. This difference could be attributed to the chemokine-binding activity of the M3 protein in MHV-68 delaying the onset of inflammation. During MHV-68 infection, the evolution of the inflammatory response includes an initial wave of macrophages, peaking at day 3, followed by a wave of CD8 T cells peaking at day 7. Inflammation resolves by the second week, although in some mice focal accumulations of mononuclear cells are seen in the lung as late as day 30. In fact, the lung continues to be a site of virus persistence for the life of the infected animal. This indicates a potential role for the lung as a major site for virus transmission.

From the lung, the virus enters the local lymph node (mediastinal lymph node, MLN). Here, dendritic cells and macrophages are initially infected, followed by infection of B cells. Evidence supporting a role for dendritic cells in this process comes from studies using an MHV-68 recombinant expressing green fluorescent protein, in which infected cells are tracked in normal and in B cell-deficient (μMT) mice. In the presence and absence of B cells, virus is detected in CD11c-positive dendritic cells and F4/80-positive macrophages. Infection appears to be transient in the absence of B cells and there is little or no viremic phase. The MLN is considered to be the primary site for B-cell infection and B cells the principal cell population responsible for disseminating virus within the host. Tropism of MHV-68 for B cells may be related to the presence of gp150 on the virion envelope. Experiments using tagged gp150 have demonstrated binding to CD19$^+$ (B cells) and to some CD19$^-$ spleen cells. However, there was no interaction between gp150 and murine epithelial cells. During the first week of infection in the MLN, B cells undergo a rapid expansion accompanied by an increase in the number of latently infected B cells against a background of lymphadenopathy. From the MLN, infected B cells traffic to the spleen and other lymphoid tissues. By the second week of infection, a similar rapid expansion of latently infected B cells is observed in the spleen, concomitant with appearance of splenomegaly. The number of latently infected cells increases from $1/10^7$ to $1/10^4$ spleen cells in the space of a few days, and then the numbers decline to between $1/5 \times 10^5$ and $1/10^6$ by the third or fourth week of infection.

B-cell proliferation, and hence the number of latently infected cells observed during lymphadenopathy and splenomegaly, is controlled by CD4 T cells. This indicates that the virus exploits T–B cell collaboration to its advantage, for example, by utilizing B-cell proliferation as a means to maximize the number of latently infected B cells. However, the virus does not depend completely on this strategy, since in the absence of CD4

T cells a long-term latent infection is still established, suggesting that the virus has the capability directly to manipulate B-cell growth and differentiation in order to establish a latent infection (a possible role for the M2 protein). A remarkable feature of MHV-68 latency is the constant number ($1–2/10^6$ latent cells) found in the spleen for the life of the animal. This number is established whether or not CD4 T cells are present in the host.

The presence of B cells and CD4 T cells is absolutely required for the evolution of splenomegaly, which suggests that cognate interactions occur between these cells similar to those for any other antigenic response. During splenomegaly, there are large increases in both B- and T-cell populations. Germinal centers increase in number and size and act as the principal location for latently infected cells. By the third week of infection there is an increase in the number of circulating lymphocytes, dominated by Vβ4$^+$ CD8 T cells. This phase of infection is similar to the infectious mononucleosis caused by EBV. The mechanism for this selective increase in Vβ4 usage is not known, but indicates a form of super-antigen-driven proliferation. A summary of the processes involved in entry and spread is shown in **Figure 2**.

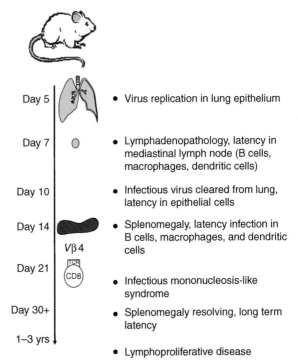

| | |
|---|---|
| Day 5 | • Virus replication in lung epithelium |
| Day 7 | • Lymphadenopathology, latency in mediastinal lymph node (B cells, macrophages, dendritic cells) |
| Day 10 | • Infectious virus cleared from lung, latency in epithelial cells |
| Day 14 | • Splenomegaly, latency infection in B cells, macrophages, and dendritic cells |
| Day 21 | • Infectious mononucleosis-like syndrome |
| Day 30+ | • Splenomegaly resolving, long term latency |
| 1–3 yrs | • Lymphoproliferative disease |

**Figure 2** Pathogenesis of MHV-68 infection following intranasal infection. Virus replicates in lung epithelium before spreading to the mediastinal lymph nodes (MLN) which drain the lung. Latent infection is established in the MLN and the virus trafficks throughout the lymphoid system causing transient splenomegaly and expansion of Vβ4+ CD8 T cells. After about 30 days, asymptomatic long-term latency is established. At later times, infection may lead to lymphoproliferative disease.

## Host Factors Influencing Infection

The age and immunological status of animals influence the spread of infection and tissue tropism. Infection of young (2–3-week old) or immunocompromised mice results in spread of virus via the bloodstream to a number of tissues, resulting in a productive infection. These include the heart, kidney, liver, adrenal gland, and peripheral nervous system (e.g., trigeminal ganglion). The central nervous system can also become infected when virus is introduced intracranially. Both glial and neuronal cells are observed to undergo a productive infection. These data argue in favor of a promiscuous virus infection, which is supported by observations of the infection of peritoneal exudate cells and epithelial cells in the gut.

## Molecular and Cellular Basis of Latency

Viral gene expression changes dramatically from infection in the lung to infection in the spleen. As the virus enters into the latent state, there is a progressive shutdown of gene expression. In MHV-68 infection, this depends to a large extent on the cell type infected. Four cell types have been implicated in maintaining the latent state: B cells, macrophages, dendritic cells, and epithelial cells in the lung. Different populations of B cells are involved in the latent infection. Naive B cells are the initial source of latent virus and, as these cells differentiate following signals from CD4 T cells, they form Germinal Centre B cells (a major site of latency), which may undergo isotype switching and develop into plasma cells and memory B cells, another source of latent infection. Epithelial cells probably represent the main site of persistence, based on the evidence from wood mice where virus is readily isolated from lung tissue, indicating that the respiratory tract may be the principal site of virus shedding.

A number of genes have been linked with MHV-68 latency. These include the vtRNA genes, M2, M3, M4, K3, ORF72 (vcyclin), ORF73, ORF74 (vGPCR), M11 (vBcl-2), and ORF65.

As discussed above, M2 is important for the establishment and maintenance of the initial phases of B cell latency in splenic follicles. However, long-term latency is maintained in the absence of M2 expression. Many of the other genes associated with latency do so by improving the efficiency of the latent infection and/or the reactivation of virus from latency. An exception is ORF73, which is essential for the establishment of MHV-68 latency *in vivo*. The encoded protein is conserved among the gammaherpesviruses and shares with KSHV LANA-1 structural and sequence homology and similar functions such as the ability to tether the viral episome to chromatin to enable the viral genome to be carried to daughter cells during mitosis. Another key function of the ORF73 protein is in inhibiting the activity of Rta, a replication and transcription activator encoded by ORF50, which is a key protein in the reactivation of virus from latency. The balance between the ORF73 protein and Rta is pivotal in defining whether latency or reactivation to a productive infection prevails.

## Pathogenesis

Lymphoproliferative disorders are a feature of gammaherpesvirus infection. In MHV-68 infection, a spectrum of disorders of increasing severity occurs, with splenomegaly at one end and lymphomas at the other. The development of lymphoproliferative disease is dependent on mouse strain and host immune status. Lymphomas have been reported in BALB/c mice infected for periods of 9 months or longer (median 14 months). In one study, approximately 10% of infected mice developed tumors in both lymphoid and nonlymphoid tissue (lung, liver, kidney, and heart), of which 50% were classified as high-grade lymphomas. In a separate investigation, the frequency of mice with tumors increased to over 50% following treatment with the immunosuppressive drug, cyclosporin A. The tumors in both experiments were of mixed cell phenotype with CD3+ T cells interspersed among B220+ B cells. The B cells were either kappa or lambda light chain restricted, suggesting a clonal origin of the B-cell population. MHV-68 DNA-positive lymphocytes were found interspersed in the tumor cell mass or on the fringes of lymphomas. In some animals, the number of virus-positive cells was low, whereas in others there were huge numbers of genome-positive cells. The infected cells were not positive for lytic cycle proteins, suggesting that virus reactivation was not occurring in these mice.

BALB/c mice infected with MHV-72 also develop tumors with a frequency similar to MHV-68. The number of tumor-bearing mice increased following immunosuppression with the antifungal agent, FK-506. In 5 of 13 neoplasia-positive mice, virus was isolated directly from the tumors. Lymphoproliferative disease in BALB/c mice has also been reported for MHV-60 and another Slovakian isolate, MHV-Sumava.

BALB/c mice lacking β2-microglobulin (β2m) develop lymphomas and an atypical lymphoid hyperplasia (ALH), with lymphocytosis resembling EBV-associated post-transplant lymphoproliferative disease at a higher rate than wild type BALB/c mice. A total of 67% of the BALB/c β2m mice developed lymphoproliferative disease compared to 22% of mock-infected controls. MHV-68 infected cells were common in the ALH cells but, again, scarce in the lymphomas, suggesting that, while MHV-68 may instigate lymphomagenesis, continued presence of the virus is not necessary in transformed cells.

A number of B cell lines have been established from MHV-68-infected tumor-positive mice, of which S11 is the best characterized. This immunoglobulin M-positive, major histocompatibility complex class II-positive B cell line harbors the virus in a latent form as demonstrated by the presence of a circular genome, a marker of latent infection. As with lymphoblastoid cell lines derived from EBV infection, S11 has around 2–5% of cells expressing lytic antigens. A transcript analysis of S11 revealed that vtRNA and M2, but not M3, were expressed in virtually all latently infected cells. S11 establishes tumors when transferred to nude mice, and has been used to dissect the immunological mechanisms involved in targeting tumor cell growth. In a series of adoptive transfer experiments of MHV-68-specific CD8 and CD4 T cells into S11 tumor-bearing nude mice, regression of tumor cell growth was effectively achieved by CD4 T cells but surprisingly not with CD8 T cells.

The molecular basis for tumor cell induction is not known. Cell lines adapted from lymphomas in mice have multiple chromosome rearrangements, and in the situation where viral DNA was detected in such cells, it is tempting to speculate that virus could initiate tumorigenesis by a hit-and-run mechanism. A number of candidate viral genes could initiate cell transformation, including ORF72 (encoding vcyclin), ORF74 (vGPCR), and M11 (vBcl-2). Transgenic mice expressing vcyclin under the control of the lck promoter, which is active early in thymocyte development, showed increased numbers of immature thymocytes. High-grade lymphoblastic lymphomas developed in the thymuses of 45% of these mice. These mice also show a decrease in the number of mature T cells and an increase in thymic apoptosis, supporting the notion that vcyclin may require the involvement of other factors to promote cell survival and tumor formation. Transfection of MHV-68 ORF74 into 3T3 cell lines leads to the establishment of stable transformed cells. These cells do not, however, develop into tumors in nude mice. vBcl-2 is expressed during the latent phase and is highly efficient at preventing cell death via such immunological mechanisms as tumor necrosis factor α and Fas–Fas ligand interaction. It therefore seems likely that *in vivo* a number of genes act in concert to promote cellular proliferation, survival, and tumor formation.

MHV-68 is also involved with the genesis of other pathologies. In young or immunologically compromised mice (e.g., deficient in the IFN-γ receptor), the virus is associated with arteritis, where persistently infected macrophages colonize the media of the major blood vessels, leading eventually to rupture of the arterial wall and cardiac arrest. Infection of mice deficient in an IFN-γ response results in fibrosis of lymphoid tissue, liver, and lung, from which the animals recover.

*See also:* Simian Gammaherpesviruses.

## Further Reading

Blaskovic D, Stancekova M, Svobodova J, and Mistrikova J (1980) Isolation of five strains of herpesviruses from two species of free living small rodents [letter]. *Acta Virologica* 24: 468.

Nash AA, Dutia BM, Stewart JP, and Davison A (2001) Natural history of murine gammaherpesvirus infection. *Philosophical Transactions of the Royal Society of London, Series B* 356: 569–579.

Speck SH and Virgin HW (1999) Host and viral genetics of chronic infection: A mouse model of gammaherpesvirus pathogenesis. *Current Opinion in Immunology* 16: 456–462.

Stevenson PG and Efstathiou S (2005) Immune mechanisms in murine gammaherpesvirus-68 infection. *Viral Immunology* 18: 445–456.

Sunil-Chandra NP, Efstathiou S, Arno J, and Nash AA (1992) Virological and pathological features of mice infected with murine gammaherpesvirus 68. *Journal of General Virology* 73: 2347–2356.

Virgin HW, Latreille P, Wamsley P, et al. (1997) Complete sequence and genomic analysis of murine gammaherpesvirus 68. *Journal of Virology* 71: 5894–5904.

# Polyomaviruses of Mice

**B Schaffhausen,** Tufts University School of Medicine, Boston, MA, USA

## Introduction

Murine polyomavirus, the virus that gives the name to the family *Polyomaviridae* and to the single genus (*Polyomavirus*) in the family, was discovered in the 1950s. Gross and Stewart observed that cell-free extracts from leukemic mice could induce neck tumors as well as leukemia in newborn mice. It soon became apparent that the leukemia-inducing activity could be separated from the activity inducing parotid tumors. Because the viral agent was found to induce a variety of solid tumors, the name 'polyoma' became attached to the virus. Epidemiology showed that the virus was widely disseminated in the mouse population.

Polyoviruses have been valuable models for basic eukaryotic processes such as splicing and DNA replication. They have been especially important for studying growth regulation. The viruses require the apparatus of cellular DNA synthesis for their own replication. To meet this need they have evolved many different ways to intervene in cellular growth regulation. This intervention can cause tumors. Interestingly, although polyoma can be an extraordinarily potent tumor virus in certain laboratory strains of mice or in immunocompromised animals, the frequency of tumors in natural mouse populations is low despite the broad dissemination of the virus. Much of this resistance reflects the ability of T-cell immunity to prevent viral oncogenesis.

## Virus Particles

Two major types of particles are found in lysates of infected cells: virions containing viral DNA and protein, and empty capsids that lack DNA and are noninfectious. Early physical characterization determined a molecular weight for virions of approximately 23 million Da with a sedimentation constant of 240S. The viral capsid is approximately 450 Å in diameter and possesses icosahedral symmetry. The viral coat consists of 72 pentameric capsomeres that are made up of VP1, the major viral structural protein. VP2 and VP3, which consists of the C-terminal 204 amino acid residues of VP2, represent the minor capsid proteins (**Table 1**). They appear to be found at the bottom of the central 'hole' in each capsomere. Although not required to assemble capsids, the infectivity of particles lacking VP2 or VP3 is dramatically reduced. The viral DNA is a closed, circular, supercoiled molecule of approximately 5300 bp. In virions, the DNA is associated with the cellular core histones H2A, H2B, H3, and H4, but not H1. Compared to host chromatin, the histones of the viral particle are much more highly acetylated, a modification known to be associated with gene activity.

## Organization of the Viral Genome

The genome (**Figure 1**) is divisible into two almost equal parts. One half is used for the expression of the capsid proteins and the other is used for the expression of the three major early gene products. The early products are

called T antigens (large T, middle T, and small T) because they were discovered using serum from tumor-bearing animals. Between the initiation codons for the late protein VP2 and the T antigens, there is a region of approximately 470 bp that contains control elements and the initiation sites for transcription and replication (**Figure 2**).

Genetic analysis has defined sequences necessary for viral DNA replication. There is a core origin of approximately 70 bp that includes an A + T-rich region on the late side and a highly purine-rich region (on one strand) on the early side. These regions flank a central 34 bp inverted repeat containing four pentanucleotide large T binding sites arranged as two head-to-head pairs. Replication initiated at this core origin requires a functional enhancer in *cis*.

Viral transcription and replication are regulated by the polyoma enhancer. **Figure 2** shows that the enhancer is located on the late side of the origin region. The enhancer has often been subdivided into two elements alpha (or A) and beta (or B) with overlapping function. It represents the binding sites for a series of cellular proteins that support viral transcription and replication. The most prominent binding sites are for PEA1 (AP1), PEA2 (runx), and PEA3 (ets family). Additional factors include polyomavirus enhancer B binding protein 1 (PEB1), EF-C, PED1, and c/EBP. Within the alpha element is a bipartite PEA1/PEA3 site of particular importance. Not surprisingly, given the number of cellular transcription

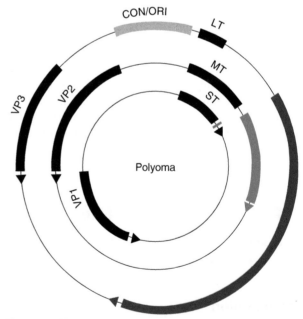

**Figure 1** The organization of the polyoma genome. Early transcription of the T antigens (large T, LT; middle T, MT; small T, ST), late transcription of the capsid proteins (VP1, VP2, and VP3), as well as the origin of viral DNA replication (ORI), are regulated by the control (CON) region. The protein-coding sequences are indicated in colors to emphasize reading frame differences for the T antigens.

**Table 1**    Polyomavirus (A2 strain) proteins and sizes (amino acid residues)

| Early proteins (no of residues) | | Late proteins | |
| --- | --- | --- | --- |
| Large T antigen | 785 | VP1 | 383 |
| Middle T antigen | 421 | VP2 | 319 |
| Small T antigen | 195 | VP3 | 204 |

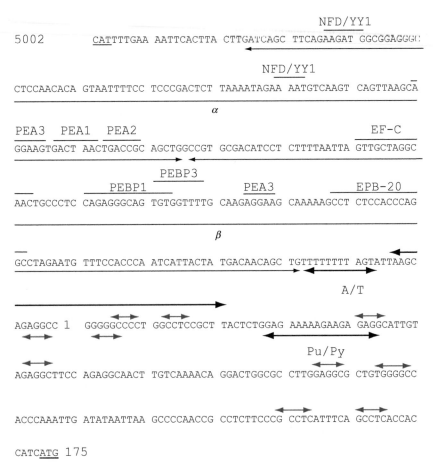

**Figure 2** The origin/control region. The sequence between the initation codons for VP2 and large T is shown. The enhancer region is shown by the light arrows indicating the alpha (A) and beta (B) regions. Some transcription factor binding sites are indicated. The A + T-rich, purine-rich (one strand), and central palindrome regions of the core origin are shown by the thick arrows. Large T-binding sequences are indicated by red arrows.

factors that bind to it, there is redundancy built into the enhancer. The activity of the enhancer varies among cell types. It is clear that the enhancer structure can change in response to cellular environment or viral mutation. Ordinarily, polyoma grows poorly in embryonal carcinoma cell lines such as F9 cells. Viruses selected to grow on these cells were found to have alterations in the enhancer region. Hr-t mutants that lack middle T and small T were found to have enhancer alterations that contribute to their ability to grow. Mutants with deletions in the B enhancer domain grow poorly in neonatal, but almost normally in adult mice.

Not only can alterations in enhancer sequences affect behavior of the virus, but alterations on the early side of the control region can affect the tumor profile as well.

## Virus Infection

Infection by polyoma can have three outcomes: productive infection, which results in the production of more virus; 'abortive transformation' in which the infected cell temporarily assumes the transformed phenotype; and stable transformation, which permanently alters the cell to a transformed phenotype. In mouse cells, which are permissive for the virus, productive infection is the predominant response. In nonpermissive rat or hamster cells, abortive transformation is the most common response. Stable transformation is associated with integration of the viral DNA into host chromosomes, although episomal DNA has been demonstrated in tumors. The frequency of stable transformation is generally low and varies with the cell line.

A brief summary may be useful before dealing with the infectious cycle in more detail. The kinetics of infection depends on the multiplicity. In a high-multiplicity infection, early mRNA can be detected by polymerase chain reaction (PCR) as early as 6 h post infection. Large T can be observed by 8 h. Viral DNA replication begins 12–18 h post infection and continues for approximately 20 h. Late transcription is observed following viral DNA replication. Progeny virions begin to appear in the nucleus between

20 and 25 h post infection. Virus production plateaus around 40–48 h with the appearance of cytopathic effects.

Since the virus uses host DNA and RNA polymerases for its replication, it must enter the cell and reach the nucleus. Different polyomaviruses appear to have different entry processes upon infection. It has been known for 40 years that neuraminidase blocks polyoma infection. Polyoma binds sialic acid residues of glycoproteins and GD1a glycolipids with a critical sialic acid-α2,3-Gal structure. Interestingly, differences in the ability of virus strains to recognize different carbohydrate structures, thereby allowing interactions with 'pseudoreceptors', result in changes in virus spread in the mouse. After binding, the virus is internalized by caveolin-dependent and -independent pathways into the endoplasmic reticulum (ER). Successful infection occurs with conformational changes taking place in the ER determined by ER-localized oxidoreductase ERp29 and protein disulfide isomerase. Recent data indicating a role for Derlin2 in infection suggest that the quality control system of the ER is involved in transferring infecting virus to the cytoplasm. Nuclear localization sequences found in the capsid proteins and cellular histones are available to allow transport into the nucleus.

## RNA Transcription and Processing

Viral transcription is divided into two types, early and late, that proceed in opposite directions from the viral control region. The early transcription unit that encodes the T antigens is active soon after infection begins. Differential splicing produces the three major early proteins, large T, middle T, and small T; a fourth spliced product, tiny T, has been observed, but its significance is uncertain. Late transcripts encoding the viral structural proteins are made early in infection, but they are not processed efficiently and have a short half-life. Late RNA does not accumulate until viral DNA replication proceeds, and late messages are generated for each of the three capsid proteins VP1, VP2, and VP3. Starting at that time, inefficient polyadenylation and termination generates large, multigenome length, heterogeneous late mRNAs. These RNAs are processed by leader-to-leader splicing so that there are tandem repeats of a 57 bp late leader, which is thought to allow accumulation of stable late message. The accumulation of late message means that there are now sequences present that are antisense to the early transcript. Editing of double-stranded RNA (dsRNA) by the ADAR enzyme converts up to 50% of early RNA adenosines to inosines with a resulting decrease in levels of early protein synthesis. The basis for the switch that allows late leader splicing is not yet fully appreciated, but may well involve the organization of polyadenylation sites and a balance of their editing and cleavage.

## Viral Transformation and Tumorigenesis

Investigating polyomavirus transformation has provided repeated insights into normal and abnormal cell behavior. Tyrosine phosphorylation and phosphatidylinositol 3-kinase (PI3-K) are two discoveries that came directly from polyoma middle T studies. The p53 tumor suppressor was discovered using SV40, the monkey polyomavirus. Studies on interactions of large T with the retinoblastoma (Rb) tumor suppressor family (pRb, p107, p130) have led to insights into the E2F family and its regulation. In addition, and in contrast to many oncogenic RNA viruses, polyoma early gene products are also required for productive infection. Large T is required for viral DNA replication. The limited host range of hr-t mutants shows that middle T and small T act to provide a cellular environment that is supportive for viral replication.

Viral transformation is carried out by the early region. As a result of the splicing described above, all four early proteins share a common domain of 79 amino acid residues. This common N-terminus represents a DnaJ domain. Proteins that contain DnaJ domains ordinarily function as cofactors for DnaK proteins that act as molecular chaperones. Small T shares additional 112 amino acid residues with middle T. Each T antigen has unique C-terminal sequences. In the case of small T, the unique C-terminus is only four amino acid residues. The result of this processing is that three proteins, large T, middle T, and small T, have different intracellular localization and different functions. Each of these proteins has the independent ability to affect cell growth and survival. Viral transformation results from T antigen association with, and regulation of, cellular signal-transducing proteins. Only large T is known to have intrinsic enzymatic activity, but even large T binds cellular proteins to regulate host function. Each of the three major T antigens will be discussed in turn. Because important insights have come from comparison studies with SV40, some mention will be made of SV40 small T and large T as well. SV40 has no direct counterpart to middle T.

## Middle T

Middle T is key to polyoma transformation and tumor induction. Middle T is necessary and usually sufficient for transformation in cultured cells. The importance of middle T in tumor induction is clear. Viruses with middle T mutations show decreased tumorigenesis and changes in tumor profile. A number of transgenic models show tumor formation in response to middle T expression in the absence of either small T or large T. A mouse mammary tumor virus (MMTV)-middle T model of breast cancer has been especially well studied. Middle T has been a particularly useful model, because mutations that affect particular associations have usually had clearly identifiable phenotypes. In some instances, both in culture and in animals, middle T requires complementation from other viral oncogenes in order to transform. For example, in primary cells, polyoma middle T needs complementation by large T or nonpolyoma oncogenes for transformation. In REF52 cells, middle T also requires complementation with small T. While the role of middle T in transformation is clear, it is important to remember that middle T also plays an important role in polyoma infection. It can upregulate viral gene expression and viral DNA replication. Middle T has also been shown to regulate phosphorylation of the major capsid protein VP1.

Middle T functions as a kind of adaptor on which cellular signaling proteins are assembled (**Figure 3**). It might be viewed as a kind of constitutively active growth factor receptor. Middle T is associated with membranes; this membrane association is critical for transformation. Middle T binds the major cellular serine/threonine phosphatase PP2A. Cellular PP2A exists as a complex, either as two subunits, A and C, or as three subunits, A, B, and C. The B family is especially diverse, with many members, and appears to be involved in regulating targeting and activity. Both polyoma middle T and small T exist in complexes with the A and C subunits of the enzyme. Interestingly, middle T binds both $A\alpha$ and $A\beta$ forms of PP2A.

Association with PP2A allows middle Ts to bind and activate some of the src family tyrosine kinases (PTKs). C-src, c-yes, and c-fyn, but not c-hck, are all bound by middle T. Curiously, the PP2A does not have to be

catalytically active for the PTK complex to form, suggesting that it may function as some kind of scaffold.

Tyrosine kinase activity is critical for transformation, so middle T mutants lacking associated tyrosine kinase activity are not able to transform. The c-src associated with middle T is activated, presumably, because it is lacking phosphorylation at Y527. In the complexes with PTK, middle T is phosphorylated on tyrosine residues. The major sites of phosphorylation are at residues 250, 315, and 322. These phosphorylations provide docking sites for signaling molecules. The initial picture of interactions was relatively straightforward. Each of the major sites represents a connection to a signal generator: 315 to PI3-K, 250 to Shc, and 322 to PLCγl. The picture is now more complicated from three points of view. First, there must be phosphorylation at minor tyrosines in the C-terminal half of middle T that can contribute to function. Second, there are clearly multiple connections to PI3-K, for example, mediated by more than one phosphotyrosine. Gab 1 protein, for example, binds middle T through its association with grb2 at 250 and can provide a connection to PI3-K. Third, multiple cellular targets seem to be reached through the single phosphotyrosine at 315. One is PI3-K, but the other remains to be identified.

Genetic analysis has been very useful in illuminating some of the signaling pathways of middle T. Mutation of 322, the PLCγ1 site, has modest effects in some transformation assays, but in low serum there is a substantial effect. Association with PLCγ1 is likely to be the basis for increased levels of IP3 observed in middle-T-transformed

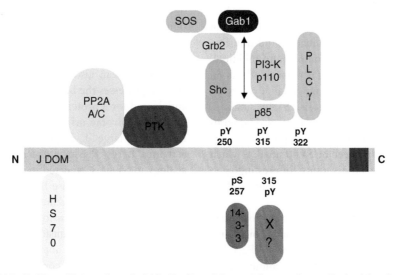

**Figure 3** Polyoma middle T. Sites of interaction of middle T with cellular proteins are shown. Each of the signal transducers shown above the middle T sequence is known to be important for transformation. PP2A, protein phosphatase 2A; PTK, src family tyrosine kinase; PI3-K, phosphatidylinositol 3-kinase; X, missing partner at 315 indicated by genetics; PLCγ phospholipase Cγ1. There is also association between Gab1 and PI3-K. The red block represents the hydrophobic membrane attachment site. Small T shares with middle T the N-terminal 191 amino acid residues that include the J domain and PP2A binding site, but not the PTK binding site T and has only four unique residues at the C-terminus.

cells and for effects on PKC. Mutation of tyrosine 250 affects transforming ability and tumorigenesis, as do mutations just N-terminal to 250 (the NPTY motif). This represents a binding site for the adaptor Shc, and that binding leads to tyrosine phosphorylation of Shc. In turn, Shc binding and tyrosine phosphorylation are responsible for the association of Grb2. This in turn leads to the recruitment of SOS, a ras exchange factor that activates ras. Interestingly, while the 250 phosphorylation site seems to be especially important for transformation either in mouse cells or the transgenic middle T mammary tumor model, virus with a mutation at 250 is relatively efficient at forming tumors. Association with PI3-K, which is abolished by mutation at 315, is profoundly important for transformation in cultured rat fibroblasts and has a dramatic effect on the tumor profile in mice. PI3-Ks are broadly important enzymes that have been strongly linked to cancer. Downstream signaling from PI3-K includes both activation of Akt, a kinase important in preventing apoptosis, and activation of rac1, a G-protein involved in cytoskeletal organization and oxidative signaling.

## Small T

In the past, small T has been studied less intensively than large T and middle T. However, increased attention has recently been focused on small T, since SV40 small T can play a role in transformation of human cells. It cooperates with hTert, SV40 large T, and ras in oncogene complementation assays. Transgenic SV40 small T can also contribute to mammary gland tumorigenesis.

Wild-type small T is not sufficient for transformation. Independent expression of small T in fibroblasts enables them to grow to a high cell density. However, small T can complement middle T for tumor induction and transformation. For example, small T can complement middle T for transformation of REF52 cells through its effects on arf-mediated activation of p53. Polyoma small T can resist the effects of p53-induced apoptosis. SV40 small T opposes apoptosis induced by large T. It also opposes Fas-mediated apoptosis of hepatocytes. Reports have suggested that Akt activity is induced by SV40 small T, which might account for these observations. Interestingly, in some cellular contexts both polyoma and SV40 small T also appear to be able to induce apoptosis.

Small T can be found in the nuclear and cytoplasmic compartments. Both SV40 and polyoma small T bind zinc. Like middle T, small T has been shown to bind PP2A. For SV40, the ability to displace specific B subunit family members such as B56$\gamma$ seems important for its function.

Small T has been connected to a variety of cellular functions. For example, polyoma small T induces the membrane lectin agglutinability that is usually associated with cell transformation. SV40 small T can both disrupt tight junctions and disturb actin structure in epithelial cell monolayers. It has also been reported to perturb centrosome function. Most attention has focused on DNA replication and RNA synthesis. In serum-starved cells, polyoma small T can contribute to S phase induction in conjunction with large T. For example, it regulated the cyclin-cdk inhibitor p27. Small T can also affect viral DNA synthesis. Polyoma small T has also been implicated in virion assembly. For SV40, it has been shown that small T can transactivate or even repress various exogenous promoters. In many instances this has been related to the ability to bind PP2A. For SV40 small T, the interaction with PP2A stimulates the MAP kinase pathway, inducing cell proliferation. To cite just two recent examples of transcriptional activators, SV40 small T activates Sp1 and the FHL2 co-activator in a PP2A-dependent manner.

## Large T

Polyomavirus large Ts have a dual role, acting not only directly in viral DNA replication and transcription, but also functioning to alter host-cell signaling. The role of large T in viral DNA replication has been studied extensively. SV40 provided the major model for establishing the mechanisms of cellular DNA replication, and its replication is still the best understood. In a productive infection, polyoma large T initiates viral DNA replication. It is thought to do this by forming a double hexamer at the two head-to-head pairs of binding sites in the origin region; it then can unwind the origin and recruit factors such as DNA polymerase and RNA polymerase. By analogy to SV40, it is also likely to participate in the elongation phase of DNA synthesis. Its role in replication is important in other contexts as well. In transformation, it is responsible for integration and excision of the viral genome and can also promote recombination. Polyoma large T possesses the biochemical activities that might be anticipated for a protein involved in DNA replication. It binds the polyoma origin region at GAGGC sequences. Like SV40 large T, it possesses helicase and ATPase activities. Large T associates with pol $\alpha$-primase, and by analogy to SV40 is expected to associate with RNA polymerase and topoisomerase I.

Large Ts are directly involved in cell transformation. Large T is the major transforming protein of SV40. Polyoma large T does not transform by itself, and viruses that make only large T do not cause tumors. Much of the difference in phenotype comes from the obvious interaction of SV40 large T with p53. Although there is a recent indication that polyoma large T may interact with p53 phosphorylated on serine 18, polyoma tumors show no evidence of a p53 block seen in SV40 tumors, and cell lines from tumors retain a normal p53 response to DNA damage. Nonetheless, polyoma large T can cooperate with other oncogenes such as middle T or ras in the transformation of primary cells. Similar complementation can also be seen in tumorigenesis.

Polyoma large T has important effects on cell phenotype, presumably to prepare the cellular environment for viral replication. Large T immortalizes primary cells in a manner dependent on the binding site for the retinoblastoma susceptibility (pRb), p107, and p130 gene products. Large T prevents differentiation, either of myoblasts or preadipocytes. The ability of large T to block withdrawal of myoblasts from the cell cycle and to prevent differentiation is dependent on Rb binding. Large T can induce dramatic apoptosis. These effects also involve interactions with the Rb family.

Given these phenotypes, it is not surprising that large T affects cellular DNA and RNA synthesis. Large T induces cellular DNA synthesis, using both Rb-dependent and -independent mechanisms. In the case of SV40 large T, at least four separate functions that contribute to the induction of cellular DNA synthesis have been identified. These functions have been mapped to the binding domains for p53, pRb/p107, p300, and TEF-1, and at least in the case of pRb requires the J domain as well.

Large T is a transcriptional activator of cellular genes. The first target identified was dihydrofolate reductase (DHFR); since then, many others have been identified as targets, such as the thymidine kinase (TK), human heat shock protein 70 (hsp 70), DNA polymerase alpha (pol α), proliferating-cell nuclear antigen (PCNA), thymidylate synthase (TS), and cyclin A genes. Transactivation of the TK, pol α, PCNA, DHFR, and TS genes requires an intact pRb/p107 binding site on polyoma large T and is mediated via the cellular transcription factor E2F. The ability of large T to activate these E2F-responsive genes depends upon an intact N-terminal J domain that binds hsc 70. As shown most clearly for SV40 large T, the role of this chaperone function is to disrupt E2F-Rb family complexes. While Rb binding is one function, transactivation of cellular and viral promoters by polyoma large T can also occur in the absence of pRb/p107 binding. Similarly the cyclin A promoter can be activated, even when the E2F site is mutant. There are certainly multiple mechanisms that require a more complete understanding. In fact, studies on SV40 large T have suggested that it is a somewhat promiscuous activator. Both the nature of the TATA/Inr element and the upstream sequences can contribute to the activation. This has led to a description of SV40 large T as being a TBP-associated factor (TAF)-like protein. A potentially important mechanism is association with histone acetyltransferases. Large T can associate with p300/CBP-associated factor (PCAF), p300, and CREB-binding protein (CBP).

**Figure 4** shows a current view of the anatomy of large T. Large T is a nuclear zinc-containing phosphoprotein of

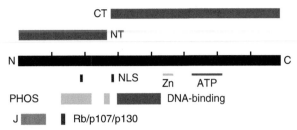

**Figure 4** Large T antigen. The positions of the N-terminal (NT) and C-terminal (CT) domains are shown. The positions of the DNA-binding domain, zinc-binding element, ATP-binding domain, J domain, Rb-binding site, and nuclear localization sequences (NLS) are shown as bars. The regions containing phosphorylation sites are also indicated.

785 amino acid residues. The zinc-binding motif is a C2H2 element that differs from that in middle T and small T. In large T, it promotes self-association. Large T can be divided into two major domains that exhibit independent function. The N-terminal domain primarily functions to stimulate the host cell, while the C-terminal domain functions primarily in DNA replication. There are additional subdomains, for instance, the DNA-binding domain can function autonomously. Large T functions both in self-association through the zinc-binding region and in association with cellular proteins, including members of the Rb family and the DnaK family of proteins. Large T function can clearly be regulated by its phosphorylation. Phosphorylation at threonine 278 by cyclin/cdk kinases is required for viral DNA replication.

## Host Effects on Transformation and the Transformed Phenotype

Although the discussion of viral transformation and tumorigenesis has focused until now on the viral gene products, there are dramatic differences in the response of different inbred mouse strains to polyoma. Some strains such as C57BL/6J are quite resistant to tumor induction. Others such as C3H/BiDa are quite sensitive as neonates but develop resistance as adults. Much of this variation arises from the immune system. High tumor susceptibility can result, for example, from inheritance of a particular super antigen that affects the T-cell repertoire. Other mouse strains such as Ma/MyJ are resistant for reasons apparently related to spread of virus in the animal rather than immune mechanisms.

Transgenic middle T models point to the effects of host background on tumor behavior. The maternal genotype has a striking effect on tumor latency and on the likelihood of metastasis. Gene expression profiles resulting from middle T expression show obvious differences among strains.

## Further Reading

Michael JI and Eugene OM (2007) *Polyomaviruses*. In: Knipe D, Howley P, Griffin DE, *et al.* (eds.) *Fields Virology,* 5th edn., pp. 2263–2298. Philadelphia, PA: Lippincott Williams and Wilkins.

Stephen MD (2002) Polyoma virus middle T antigen and its role in identifying cancer-related molecules. *Nature Reviews Cancer* 2: 951–956.

Thomas LB (2001) Polyoma virus: Old findings and new challenges. *Virology* 289: 167–173.

# Simian Alphaherpesviruses

**J Hilliard,** Georgia State University, Atlanta, GA, USA

## History

Members of the subfamily *Alphaherpesvirinae* in the family *Herpesviridae* have been identified in Old World monkeys and apes and in New World monkeys. It appears that nearly all host species have co-evolved with one or more alphaherpesviruses, and so it comes as no surprise that new agents in this group continue to be discovered. Indeed, the increased use of nonhuman primates in biomedical research has facilitated the discovery and characterization of such viruses. As assays improve, more virus isolates from nonhuman primates have been identified, and subsequently have been differentiated from closely related viruses by molecular and immunological means. The benefit of enhanced techniques for virus differentiation is exemplified by the early reports in the 1970s that simian agent 8 (SA8; *Cercopithecine herpesvirus 2*) was not only found in vervets but also in baboons. It was not until nearly two decades later that the virus isolated from baboons in a captive colony was recognized to be herpesvirus papio 2 (HVP-2; *Cercopithecine herpesvirus 16*). Although improved technology enables differentiation of closely related herpesviruses, it remains a time-consuming task to find species-specific viruses, characterize the associated pathogeneses, and verify the natural hosts. Like human alphaherpesviruses, nonhuman primate alphaherpesviruses fall into the genera *Simplexvirus* and *Varicellovirus*.

Simplexviruses are readily isolated because they replicate rapidly in cell cultures from a variety of mammals. They produce a distinct cytopathology as quickly as 24–48 h following infection. Examples of this cytopathology and some of the differences among simplexviruses are shown in **Figure 1**. The property of rapid growth is one of the initial criteria for establishing that an isolate is an alphaherpesvirus. These viruses are most frequently isolated from mucosal sites or from necropsy samples, and occasionally from fomites. With sequence analysis readily available, they can be differentiated easily from close counterparts endemic in related species of Old and New World monkeys, apes, and humans. The zoonotic potential of these viruses is of particular interest, because at least one, B virus (*Cercopithecine herpesvirus 1*), can be rapidly lethal in humans when antiviral therapy is initiated too late.

Frequently, the identity of the natural host of a virus isolate has been established by the use of seroepidemiological assays. The natural host often shows 80–100% seroprevalence in the wild by the time the animals reach sexual maturity. Most data in this regard have been summarized from studies of vervets, baboons, and macaques in the wild, although there are excellent studies that have focused on apes and New World monkeys. The assays, however, upon which seroprevalence are based are not always uniform, and may utilize antigens that are not necessarily unique to the specific virus for which antibody is reactive, resulting in difficulty identifying the natural host of a particular virus. Nonetheless, the plethora of assays has afforded investigators the opportunity to establish candidates for the natural host, and, as assays improve, the identity of the natural host can be narrowed.

Owing to the close evolutionary relationships between monkeys, most notably within Old World groups and New World groups, the viruses that have co-evolved in each host group share significant similarities genotypically and phenotypically. Although genes are arranged mostly in a collinear layout in viruses from both groups of nonhuman primates, viruses from Old World and New World monkeys differ from each other more than viruses from within each monkey group. This point is best illustrated by studies evaluating immunological cross-reactivity among nonhuman primate alphaherpesviruses between groups and within groups. Within either of the Old World and New World groups, extensive genetic conservation renders classical serological assays using virus or infected cell lysates of relatively limited value in identifying the natural

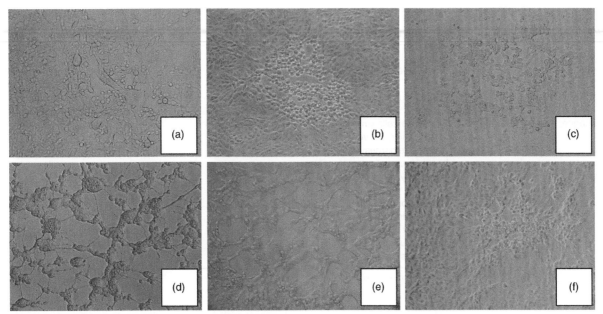

**Figure 1** Vero cells in culture (ATCC-081) 24 h after infection with (a) B virus (E2490), (b) HSV-1 (KOS), (c) HVP-2 (SWF), (d) mangabey herpesvirus (EM-GS), (e) SA8 (Hull), or (f) langur herpesvirus (BZ).

host, due to significant cross-reactivity of immunogenic epitopes. An assay for detection of HVP-2 will cross-react sufficiently strongly with mangabey or langur herpesviruses, such that differentiation of the antibody specificity will be nearly impossible using a virus- or infected cell-based immunoassay. With the advent of recombinant viral proteins, differentiation assays for human alphaherpesviruses have improved, but conservation of the major antigenic proteins can still cloud identification of endemic populations in nonhuman primates. The strategies that differentiate alphaherpesviruses in humans have not proved to be entirely successful when extrapolated to identifying alphaherpesviruses in nonhuman primates. The best example of this is the confusion caused by the finding that SA8 was endemic in baboons as well as vervets, which was still manifest decades after the first publication citing the identification of this agent in baboons. It is now appreciated that the viruses infecting vervets and baboons are distinct alphaherpesviruses, SA8 and HVP-2, respectively. Identification of the natural host of simian varicella virus (SVV) provides a similar example, since both macaques (Asian) and vervets (African) host similar, if not identical, varicelloviruses.

## Classification and Evolution

The current list of nonhuman primate alphaherpesviruses is shown in **Table 1**. Nonhuman primate alphaherpesviruses belong to genus *Simplexvirus* (with human herpes simplex virus (HSV) types 1 (HSV-1) and 2 (HSV-2)), with the exception of SVV (*Cercopithecine herpesvirus 9*), which belongs to genus *Varicellovirus* (with human varicella-zoster virus, VZV). The marked genetic similarities between the nonhuman primate viruses and their counterparts in humans strongly support a co-evolutionary history.

The genomes of the Old World monkey simplexviruses have been shown to exist in four isomeric forms, like those of HSV (type E genome structure). The DNA sequences of B virus, SA8, mangabey herpesvirus, langur herpesvirus, and HVP-2 are similar in size (151–157 kbp) to those of their human counterparts, with somewhat greater G+C contents. The genetic contents of these viruses are very similar to that of HSV-1 and HSV-2, except that they lack the gene encoding the neurovirulence protein ICP34.5. The varicelloviruses have a type D genome structure, and the genetic content of SVV is very similar to that of VZV, differing in only a couple of genes at the left genome terminus.

In accord with the relationships among their hosts, simplexviruses of New World primates are more distantly related to those of Old World primates, and the genomes are smaller in size with relatively less complex isomeric organization. The evolutionary distances are apparent from the fact that antisera prepared against the major HSV proteins cross-react with homologous proteins from Old World, but not New World, simplexviruses. Thus far, no varicelloviruses have been found to be endemic in New World monkeys.

**Table 1**    Nonhuman primate alphaherpesviruses

| Host | Common virus name | Official species name |
|---|---|---|
| *Old World* | | |
| Vervet (African green monkey) | Simian agent 8 (SA8) | *Cercopithecine herpesvirus 2* |
| Baboon | Herpesvirus papio 2 (HVP-2) | *Cercopithecine herpesvirus 16* |
| Macaque | B virus | *Cercopithecine herpesvirus 1* |
| Macaque | Simian varicella virus (SVV) (also known as Patas delta, Liverpool vervet and Medical Lake macaque herpesvirus) | *Cercopithecine herpesvirus 9* |
| Langur | Langur herpesvirus | Currently unnamed |
| Mangabey | Mangabey herpesvirus | Currently unnamed |
| *New World* | | |
| Spider monkey | Spider monkey herpesvirus (also known as herpesvirus ateles) | *Ateline herpesvirus 1* |
| Marmoset | Marmoset herpesvirus (also known as herpesvirus saimiri and, in other platyrrhine monkeys, herpesvirus tamarinus) | *Saimiriine herpesvirus1* |

## Virion Structure

Nonhuman primate alphaherpesviruses are similar in structure to the other members of the subfamily *Alphaherpesvirinae*. By electron microscopy, virus particles consist of capsids sheathed by a tegument and surrounded by an envelope. The icosahedral capsids are assembled in the infected cell nucleus and finally enveloped in the cytoplasm. Unenveloped capsids can be found in both the cytoplasm and nucleus, and are most abundant in the latter. Temporal studies of the kinetics of virus replication suggest that the envelope is acquired in a two-step process, similar to that of HSV. The envelope is rich in virus glycoproteins, which, as judged from antibodies induced during infection, are highly immunogenic. Sequencing and immunological cross-reactivity studies indicate that glycoprotein B is the most highly conserved glycoprotein.

## Physical Properties and Epidemiology

Each of the nonhuman primate alphaherpesviruses has features in common with its human counterparts with respect to host range, replication kinetics, transmission, tissue tropism, pathogenecity, histopathology, and induced immune responses. The exception is B virus, which can infect humans, often resulting in a fatal zoonotic infection when left untreated. Each virus is predominantly found in one type of monkey, and recent experience indicates that antibody cross-reactivity with isolates from other species should be evaluated carefully in order to avoid deducing wrongly that a virus is endemic in multiple monkey types. As mentioned above, this is particularly apparent in the case of SA8 and HVP-2,

but also features in case studies of alphaherpesviruses from Asian and African monkeys, as well as greater and lesser apes. Although apes are likely to have co-evolved with their own respective alphaherpesviruses, investigators have not yet found herpesviruses other than HSV-1 and HSV-2 in these animals.

Transmission of nonhuman primate alphaherpesviruses from animal to animal occurs as a result of biting, scratching, and splashing activities that contaminate susceptible mucosal epithelial cells. Seroprevalence of virus-induced antibodies increases with the onset of sexual maturity, but infected infants have also been identified, albeit infrequently. Infection is associated with few or no apparent symptoms, whether the virus is latent or replicating actively. Periodic reactivations from latency have been associated with virus shedding from mucus membranes, and this is the time period during which transmission is greatest. Except for B virus, none of the nonhuman primate alphaherpesviruses appears to be transmissible to humans under natural circumstances. Evidence for transmission of human viruses to apes has been substantiated in certain circumstances, as mentioned above, but nonhuman primates are not usually found to be infected with human alphaherpesviruses. When transmission of Old World simplex- or varicelloviruses to New World primates occurs, infection is readily apparent with high morbidity and frequent mortality.

## Virus Replication

Nonhuman primate alphaherpesviruses appear to follow the same pattern of biosynthetic activities leading to virus replication and assembly as do their human counterparts, with some exceptions noted. The nonhuman primate simplexviruses replicate in a manner similar to HSV, with a replication cycle of approximately 18 h. Cytopathic effects in cultured cells are also similar, with the exceptions of B virus and mangabey herpesvirus, which induce cell fusion between infected cells and also with neighboring uninfected cells. **Figure 1** shows representative cytopathic effects of B virus versus other alphaherpesviruses in nonhuman primate cells. SVV replicates with kinetics similar to VZV over an interval of 48–72 h in cell culture and, like VZV, remains mostly cell associated.

Following adsorption of a nonhuman primate alphaherpesvirus to a susceptible cell, de-enveloped capsids are released into the cytoplasm and proceed to the nuclear membrane by mechanisms that are poorly understood, but which probably involve the cell's cytoskeleton components. Microarray studies have revealed that host gene remodeling in B virus-infected cells begins within the first hour post infection, and within 3 h post infection the events are clearly distinguishable from those transpiring in HSV-infected cells. Nonetheless, the outcome at the level of the infected cell in culture is the same for both human and nonhuman primate alphaherpesviruses – productive virus replication. The temporal cascade of protein synthesis is conserved, with immediate early, early, and late expression. The major difference between human and nonhuman primate alphaherpesviruses is that the US11 protein is produced as an immediate early protein in the nonhuman primate viruses and as an early protein in HSV-1 and HSV-2. This protein in nonhuman primate viruses prevents phosphorylation of protein kinase R, which in turn prevents phosphorylation of eIF-2$\alpha$, thus blocking apoptosis in the infected cell and enabling virus replication.

## Immune Response to Infection

Nonhuman primates infected by their respective alphaherpesviruses induce humoral antibodies generally within 7–14 days following the onset of acute replication. Antibody titers, however, are not apparent in all animals within this period. Titers can also wax and wane depending on the intervals between reactivated infections. Nonetheless, intermittent virus shedding makes reliance on virus isolation or polymerase chain reaction (PCR) impractical; thus, detection of antibodies is used as the current indicator of whether an animal is infected. Antibodies induced in Old and New World monkeys are cross-reactive with the alphaherpesviruses infecting animals within each group, but there is no apparent cross-reactivity between the two groups. There is little evidence that Old World monkeys can be infected by New World monkey viruses, but New World monkeys generally succumb to viruses from Old World monkeys or humans. Cross-species housing is generally avoided.

The antibodies most commonly produced are against the major glycoprotein (glycoprotein B). There is no clear-cut evolution of the humoral immune response, but the antibodies most observed include those reactive with glycoprotein B, glycoprotein C, glycoprotein D, glycoprotein G, and the major capsid protein. Having said this, antibody profiles from different animals are quite distinct, as in the case of human antibody profiles induced against HSV.

## Future Perspectives

Identification and characterization of simplex- and varicelloviruses from nonhuman primates afford the opportunity to learn more about the origins, evolutionary processes, and pathogenic properties of these viruses. Thus, study of a particular member provides insights on the virus as an individual species and as a representative of a lineage of related agents. Perhaps even more important is the development of understanding on how to approach novel viruses, whether newly discovered or emerging. Knowledge of these viruses in relation to their natural hosts often cannot be extrapolated to their effects in foreign hosts, and the responses of a non-natural host can influence pathogenesis in unexpected ways. This is illustrated by B virus infection of humans, the most dramatic example of cross-species transmission among the herpesviruses. Current attention focused worldwide on emerging viruses and viruses that invade foreign hosts places an emphasis on primate alphaherpesviruses that will teach investigators for decades to come.

*See also:* Simian Gammaherpesviruses.

## Further Reading

Cohen JI, Davenport DS, Stewart JA, *et al.* (2002) Recommendations for prevention of and therapy for exposure to B virus (*Cercopithecine herpesvirus 1*). *Clinical Infectious Diseases* 35: 1191–1203.

Davison AJ and Clements JB (1997) Herpesviruses: General properties. In: Mahy BWJ and Collier LH (eds.) *Topley and Wilson's Microbiology and Microbial Infections*, 9th edn., pp. 309–323. London: Arnold.

Eberle R and Hilliard J (1995) The simian herpesviruses. *Infectious Agents Disease – Reviews Issues and Commentary* 4: 55–70.

Gray WL, Gusick NJ, Ek-Kommonen C, Kempson SE, and Fletcher TM, III (1995) The inverted repeat regions of the simian varicella virus and varicella-zoster virus genomes have a similar genetic organization. *Virus Research* 39: 181–193.

Weigler J (1992) Biology of B virus in macaque and human hosts: A review. *Clinical Infectious Diseases* 14: 555–567.

Whitley RJ and Hilliard J (2007) Cercopithecine herpesvirus 1 (B Virus). In: Knipe DM and Howley PM (eds.) *Fields Virology*, 5th edn., vol. 2, p. 2889. Philadelphia: Lippincott Williams and Wilkins.

# Simian Gammaherpesviruses

**A Ensser,** Virologisches Institut, Universitätsklinikum, Erlangen, Germany

## Introduction

The *Gammaherpesvirinae* is a large subfamily of the family *Herpesviridae*. Although gammaherpesviruses usually cause limited disease upon primary infection of their natural hosts, several are relevant tumor viruses of the hematopoietic system and form an important chapter of viral oncology. The first clearly identified human herpesvirus, Epstein–Barr virus (EBV; species *Human herpesvirus 4*), is the prototype of genus *Lymphocryptovirus* (whose members are referred to as lymphocryptoviruses or γ1-herpesviruses) and the cause of infectious mononucleosis. Homologs of EBV had been recognized for decades in various Old World primates, and have been found recently in several species of American monkeys. They may serve to develop models for pathogenesis or treatment of human lymphoproliferative diseases and cancers that are caused by EBV, such as B-cell lymphomas and other lymphoproliferative syndromes, nasopharyngeal carcinomas, and, possibly, gastric cancer.

The second genus of gammaherpesviruses, *Rhadinovirus* (whose members are referred to as rhadinoviruses or γ2-herpesviruses), is distinct biologically and molecularly. The prototypic member of this group, herpesvirus saimiri (HVS; species *Saimiriine herpesvirus 2*), and herpesvirus ateles (HVA; species *Ateline herpesvirus 2* and ateline herpesvirus 3) were detected as T-lymphotropic viruses in neotropical primates and raised primary interest from the fact that they cause fulminant T-cell lymphomas in numerous primate species as well as in rabbits. The related animal pathogens alcelaphine herpesvirus 1 and ovine herpesvirus 2 cause malignant catarrhal fever, a T lymphoproliferative disease of ruminants. Although no exact correlates of these T-cell tumors exist in human pathology, HVS strains of subgroup C are capable of transforming human and simian T lymphocytes to continuous growth in cell culture. This provided for the first time a reliable means of immortalizing human T lymphocytes in cell culture, a useful tool for T-cell immunology. These viruses have been used as expression vectors for gene transfer in T lymphocytes and have facilitated study of the mechanisms of episomal persistence in the T-cell system. Further interest in the rhadinoviruses arose when the first human member of this genus was recognized. This virus was found to be strongly associated with all forms of Kaposi's sarcoma (KS), as well as with multicentric Castleman's disease and primary effusion lymphoma (PEL). Since DNA from this virus is regularly found in all KS forms, specifically in the spindle cells of KS, it was also termed KS-associated herpesvirus (KSHV; species *Human herpesvirus 8*). Viral membrane-associated oncoproteins Stp and Tip, which act on T-lymphocyte signaling, were defined in HVS, though it is far less clear which of several candidate genes encode the relevant oncoproteins of KSHV.

For many years, research on lymphotropic simian herpesviruses focused on the tumorigenic T-lymphotropic rhadinoviruses, especially HVS. Then the discovery of KSHV prompted research on B-lymphotropic agents and led to the description of rhesus rhadinovirus (RRV; species *Cercopithecine herpesvirus 17*) and several closely related rhadinoviruses in various Old World primates, although these are only loosely associated with pathogenicity or tumor induction. New World primate EBV-like viruses were discovered recently, and an increasing number of DNA sequences from additional, new gammaherpesviruses are being amplified from diverse host species using degenerate polymerase chain reaction (PCR) techniques that target strongly conserved herpesvirus genes, such as that encoding DNA polymerase. A provisional compilation of the better defined primate gammaherpesviruses is represented in **Table 1**, and more extensive information is available in the website of the International Committee on Taxonomy of Viruses (ICTV).

## Herpesvirus Saimiri and Herpesvirus Ateles

This section focuses on the basic biology, gene content, and viral mechanisms of oncogenic transformation of HVS and HVA, and their possible applications as T-cell vectors and in cell-based immunotherapy. These gammaherpesviruses must not be confused with two alphaherpesviruses isolated from the same host species, designated as species *Saimiriine herpesvirus 1* and *Ateline herpesvirus 1*, respectively.

### History, Host Range, Transmission, and Pathology

HVS was originally isolated by Melendez and others from captive monkeys of various species, but it soon became clear that this virus is found regularly only in squirrel monkeys (*Saimiri sciureus*), whose natural habitat is South American rainforests. Squirrel monkeys are usually infected via saliva within the first two years of life. The virus does not cause disease or tumors, and establishes

**Table 1**  Primate gammaherpesviruses

| Species | Common name(s) and abbreviation(s) | Host | Associated pathogenicity |
|---|---|---|---|
| Genus *Rhadinovirus* | | | |
| Human herpesvirus 8 | Kaposi's sarcoma-associated herpesvirus (KSHV) | Human (*Homo sapiens*) | Kaposi's sarcoma, multicentric Castleman's disease, primary effusion lymphoma |
| NA[a] | Chimpanzee rhadinovirus | Chimpanzee (*Pan troglodytes*) | Unknown |
| NA | Gorilla rhadinovirus | Gorilla (*Gorilla gorilla*) | Unknown |
| *Cercopithecine herpesvirus 17* | Rhesus rhadinovirus (RRV), *Macaca mulatta* rhadinovirus | Rhesus macaque (*M. mullata*) | B-cell hyperplasia? |
| NA | Retroperitoneal fibromatosis-associated herpesvirus (RFHV, RFHVMn, RFHVMm) | Southern pig-tailed macaque (*M. nemestrina*), rhesus macaque (*M. mullatta*) | Retroperitoneal fibromatosis? |
| NA | *Macaca nemestrina* rhadinovirus 2 (MnRRV) | Southern pig-tailed macaque (*M. nemestrina*) | Unknown |
| *Saimiriine herpesvirus 2*[b] | Herpesvirus saimiri (HVS) | Squirrel monkey (*Saimiri sciureus*) | T-cell lymphoma in other neotropical monkey species |
| *Ateline herpesvirus 2* | Herpesvirus ateles (HVA) | Spider monkey (*Ateles paniscus*) | T-cell lymphoma in other neotropical monkey species |
| NA | Herpesvirus ateles strain 73 (HVA), ateline herpesvirus 3 | Spider monkey (*A. paniscus*) | T-cell lymphoma in other neotropical monkey species |
| Genus *Lymphocryptovirus* | | | |
| Human herpesvirus 4[b] | Epstein–Barr virus (EBV) | Human (*Homo sapiens*) | B-cell lymphoma, nasopharyngeal lymphoma, Hodgkin's disease |
| *Pongine herpesvirus 1* | Herpesvirus pan, chimpanzee lymphocryptovirus | Chimpanzee (*Pan* sp.) | Unknown |
| *Pongine herpesvirus 2* | Orangutan herpesvirus | Orangutan (*Pongo* sp.) | Unknown |
| *Pongine herpesvirus 3* | Gorilla herpesvirus | Gorilla (*Gorilla* sp.) | Unknown |
| *Cercopithecine herpesvirus 12* | Baboon herpesvirus, herpesvirus papio | Baboon (*Papio* sp.) | Spontaneous B-cell lymphoma (and in immunosuppressed animals) |
| *Cercopithecine herpesvirus 14* | African green monkey EBV-like virus | African green monkey (*Chlorocebus aethiops*) | Unknown |
| *Cercopithecine herpesvirus 15* | Rhesus EBV-like herpesvirus, rhesus lymphocryptovirus | Rhesus macaque (*M. mullatta*) | Spontaneous B-cell lymphoma (and in immunosuppressed animals) |
| NA | Cynomolgus EBV-like virus, *Macaca fascicularis* gammaherpesvirus (herpesvirus MF1, A4, TsB-B6, Si-IIA-EBV) | Cynomolgus monkey (*M. fascicularis*) | Spontaneous B-cell lymphoma (and in immunosuppressed animals) |
| *Callitrichine herpesvirus 3* | Marmoset lymphocryptovirus | Common marmoset (*Callithrix jacchus*) | Spontaneous B-cell lymphoma |
| NA | Gold-handed tamarin lymphocryptovirus (SmiLHV1) | Gold-handed tamarin (*Saguinus midas*) | Unknown |
| NA | Squirrel monkey lymphocryptovirus (SscLHV1) | Squirrel monkey (*S. sciureus*) | Unknown |
| NA | White-faced saki lymphocryptovirus (PpiLHV1) | White-faced saki (*Pithecia pithecia*) | Unknown |

[a]NA, species not assigned by ICTV.
[b]Type species of the genus.

lifelong persistence. In other New World primate species such as tamarins (*Saguinus* spp.), common marmosets (*Callithrix jacchus*), or owl monkeys (*Aotus trivirgatus*), infection with HVS causes acute peripheral T-cell lymphoma within less than 2 months after experimental intramuscular or intravenous infection. Intramuscular injection of purified virion DNA can also cause disease in susceptible primates.

HVS strains are classified into three subgroups (A, B, and C) depending on pathogenic properties and

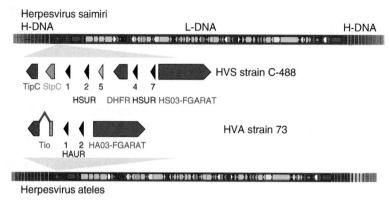

**Figure 1**   Gene arrangements at the left genome end of HVS and HVA. The oncoproteins Stp, Tip, or Tio are encoded at the variable left terminal region of the coding L-DNA. Stp, saimiri transformation-associated protein of the respective subgroup A, B, or C; Tio, two-in-one-protein of HVA; Tip, tyrosine kinase-interacting protein of HVS subgroup C; HSUR or HAUR, HVS or HVA-encoded URNA; HS03-/HA03-FGARAT, formylglycineamide ribotide amidotransferase ORF3.

on sequence divergence in the left-terminal nonrepetitive region of the genome (**Figure 1**). The major representative strains are the prototypic A11 for subgroup A; B S295C and B-SMHI for subgroup B; and C488 and C484 for subgroup C.

Viruses of HVS subgroups B and C are considered to be the least and most oncogenic, respectively. Tamarins are susceptible to viruses of all subgroups, whereas subgroup B viruses are not able to cause disease in adult common marmosets. Strain C488 causes acute peripheral T-cell lymphoma within only a few weeks in common marmosets or cottontop tamarins (*S. oedipus*). A similar fulminant disease is induced in Old World rhesus and cynomolgus monkeys (*Macaca mulatta* and *M. fascicularis*, respectively) by large intravenous doses of C488. Similar to the situation in New World primates, the disease in cynomolgus monkeys is designated as a pleomorphic, peripheral T-cell lymphoma or a pleomorphic, T-lymphoproliferative disorder. A high-titer infection in New Zealand white rabbits results in tumor induction, but pathogenicity has not been reported in rodents. HVS can be isolated from the peripheral blood cells of persistently infected squirrel monkeys or diseased tamarins, presumably from infected T cells, by co-cultivation with permissive owl monkey kidney (OMK) cells. HVS replicates productively in, and induces cell lysis of, OMK cells and some primary mesenchymal cultures established from marmosets, and less efficient replication is possible in Vero (African green monkey) cells.

HVA can be isolated at a high frequency from spider monkeys (*Ateles* spp.). Strain 810 from *A. geoffroyii* is a member of species *Ateline herpesvirus 2*, whereas strain 73 and related strains (87, 93, and 94) from *A. paniscus* are isolates of ateline herpesvirus 3. HVA replicates in OMK cells, but remains mostly cell-associated with syncytia formation. As a result, supernatants of such cultures have low, unstable virus titers.

Like HVS, HVA is not pathogenic in its natural host, but causes acute T-cell lymphomas in various New World primate species, including cottontop tamarins and owl monkeys. The pathological changes are similar to those observed after HVS infection. In addition, HVA transforms T cells of certain New World monkey species (such as cottontop tamarin) in culture, yielding cytotoxic T-cell lines. Human T cells are not susceptible to transformation with various HVA strains, but could be transformed by a recombinant HVS C strain in which the HVS oncogenes were replaced by the HVA oncogene Tio.

Transformed T-cell lines have been derived from HVA-infected tamarins and cultivated continuously for several years. Whereas in most cases virus particles were found initially, virus production was frequently lost after prolonged culture. The episomal DNA is heavily methylated in such nonproductive cell lines, and rearrangements or large deletions are evident in the viral genomes. Marmoset and tamarin T cells can be transformed by HVS to stable T-cell lines *in vitro* and are designated as semipermissive, since virus particles are released, although to lower titers than from OMK cells.

## Genome Properties, Replication, and Gene Content

The term 'rhadino' viruses was coined from the ancient Greek word ραδινοσ for fragile, because the viral genomic DNA breaks upon isopyknic centrifugation in CsCl gradients into two classes of highly differing densities. The L DNA (low density, low G + C content) contains the viral protein-coding genes, and the repetitive H DNA (high density, high G + C content) from the genome termini is noncoding. The intact viral (M) genome has intermediate density. Two strains of HVS, strain A11 and the highly oncogenic subgroup C strain C488, have been sequenced. The A11 H DNA consists of multiple tandem repeats of 1444 bp (70.8% G + C), and the unique L DNA comprises 112 930 bp (34.5% G + C). The size of the M DNA genome is variable owing to different numbers of H DNA repeats attached to both ends of the linear virion genome. In strain C488, the L DNA comprises 113 027 bp, and it is flanked by arrays of two distinct repeat unit types of 1318 and 1458 bp, the shorter representing the longer with 140 bp deleted. The packaged M genome of C488 is approximately 155 kbp in size, with a range of 130–160 kbp owing to variable numbers of terminal H DNA repeats. The HVS L DNA contains at least 76–77 protein-coding open reading frames (ORFs) and encodes 5–7 U RNAs (termed HSURs) (**Figure 1**).

HVA strain 73 has a similar genome structure to HVS, with a slightly shorter L DNA of 108 409 bp (36.6% G + C), and H DNA consisting of multiple tandem repeats of 1582 bp (77.1% G + C). The HVA L DNA contains 73 ORFs and only two genes for U RNA-like transcripts (termed HAURs). HVA does not encode ORF12, vIL17, vCD59, or vFLIP homologs, but the genes encoding superantigen (SAG), cyclin, and G-protein-coupled receptor (GPCR) are conserved. Thus, HVA may be an ancient variant of HVS that has either collected a smaller set of cell-homologous genes or has secondarily lost several genes.

In all gammaherpesviruses, the genes that are conserved among the herpesvirus subfamilies are arranged in blocks. Flanking or interspersed among the blocks are other genes, most of which do not occur in the other subfamilies. Among these are transforming oncogenes and viral homologs of cellular genes, which are described below. Most genes are well conserved between different HVS strains, but there is pronounced sequence variation near the left end of the HVS L DNA and in the region of the R transactivator gene (*orf50*) and the adjacent glycoprotein gene (*orf51*), a region that is also highly variable among other rhadinoviruses.

The replication mechanism of rhadinoviruses has not been investigated in much detail, and is generally considered to follow that of other herpesviruses. The lytic origin of DNA replication (OriLyt) in HVS strain A11 has been mapped to an untranslated region upstream of the thymidylate synthase gene. A putative latent origin of DNA replication (OriP) in the left-terminal region of the L DNA in strain C484 was reported to mediate episomal maintenance, but is not conserved between different HVS strains and is not required for viral replication or episomal persistence. Thus, although HVS persists in transformed human T cells as stable nonintegrated episomes at high copy number, OriP and the viral factors involved remain unidentified. Histone modification of the HVS C488 episome in human T cells has been analyzed, and bears similarities to that of KSHV episomes in B cells.

Infection of tissue culture cells by HVS is asynchronous, and hence the assignment of HVS genes to the immediate early (IE) phase of infection is based mostly on experiments using cycloheximide to inhibit protein synthesis. The IE57 post-transcriptional regulator encoded by *orf57* appears to be the sole regulatory viral IE gene. It codes for a nuclear phosphoprotein of 52 kDa with structural and functional homology to herpes simplex virus ICP27 and EBV BMLF1. IE57 stimulates the expression of unspliced, and represses the expression of spliced, transcripts, has been shown to redistribute nuclear components of the splicing machinery, and is involved in nuclear RNA export. A strong viral transactivator function was mapped to the delayed early gene *orf50*, the homolog of the EBV R transactivator gene. Owing to differential splicing and promoter usage, this gene codes for a full-length protein (ORF50A) and a smaller, C-terminal variant (ORF50B). The transactivation domain resides in the C-terminal region of these proteins and binds to the TATA-binding protein in the basal transcription complex. Although IE57 is highly conserved between subgroups A and C, the *orf50* region is divergent. Neither HVS nor HVA encodes a homolog of bZip/Zta of EBV or KSHV.

The HVS ORF73 protein of strains A11 and C488 localizes to the host cell nucleus, and, like the latent nuclear antigen (LANA) of KSHV, can associate with host cell chromosomal DNA. The A11 ORF73 protein can associate with cellular p32 and binds to GSK-3$\beta$. Although not detectable by northern blotting of RNA from C488-transformed human T cells, *orf73* transcripts are detectable by reverse transcription-polymerase chain reaction (RT-PCR). The C488 ORF73 protein can down-regulate the *orf50A* and *orf50B* promoters, and this prevents ORF50-mediated activation of viral replication gene promoters. This suggests that the HVS ORF73 protein, and its homologs in the other rhadinoviruses, can block initiation of the lytic replication cascade, thereby controlling the transition between latency and lytic replication.

## Sequestered Cellular Genes

Rhadinoviruses such as HVS and KSHV contain several intronless genes that are homologous to cellular genes; in this context, a role for reverse transcription during putative capture of these genes might be speculated upon. A few of these cellular gene homologs are unique to specific viruses, and some are common to several rhadinoviruses (and to lymphocryptoviruses, including EBV). This suggests that successful uptake of cellular genes is a rather infrequent event during herpesvirus evolution. Most of these cellular homologs can be categorized into two major groups: (1) genes related to cellular growth control or nucleotide metabolism, and (2) genes that modulate innate or adaptive immune functions, including apoptosis. For example, HVS *orf72* codes for a functional viral cyclin D, and homologs related to nucleotide metabolism include a dihydrofolate reductase (DHFR; *orf2*) and a functional thymidylate synthase (TS; *orf70*). Both *orf3* and *orf75* encode large tegument proteins that share similarity with formylglycineamide ribotide amidotransferase (FGARAT). It is thought that these enzymes may possibly augment the free nucleotide pools and could thus facilitate DNA synthesis and virus replication.

## Oncogenic Signaling and Transformation

### The Stp Oncoproteins

The HVS oncogenes required for induction of T-cell leukemia and T-cell transformation *in vitro* reside in the variable region at the left end of the L DNA (**Figure 1**). Subgroup A and B strains have a single gene termed *stpA* or *stpB* (saimiri transformation-associated protein of subgroup A or B strains), and subgroup C strains carry *stpC* (*stp* of subgroup C strains) and *tip* (tyrosine kinase-interacting protein). The proteins StpA and StpB share limited sequence homology with StpC, but are structurally unrelated to Tip. Although *stpA* and *stpC/tip* are not required for viral replication, deletion of either *stpA*, *stpC*, or *tip* abolishes transformation by HVS *in vitro* and pathogenicity *in vivo*. *stpA*- or *stpC*-transfected rodent fibroblasts form foci *in vitro* and induced tumors in nude mice. *stpA*-transgenic mice develop polyclonal peripheral T-cell lymphomas, and an *stpC* transgene induces epithelial tumors.

*stpC* and *tip* are transcribed into a single bicistronic mRNA from a common promoter directed toward the left end of the L DNA, with *tip* situated downstream from *stpC*. Transcription of *stpC/tip* is regulated similarly to IE genes in human T cells, and no obvious viral factors seem to be involved. The *stpC/tip* promoter carries euchromatic histone modifications in C488-transformed human T cells.

The 102-residue StpC phosphoprotein has an N terminus of 17 mostly charged residues, and the C terminus contains a hydrophobic region that probably serves as an anchor to perinuclear membranes. In between are 18 collagen tripeptide repeats of the form $(GPX)_n$, which may mediate multimerization of the protein. StpA and the less efficiently transforming StpB bind to, and are phosphorylated by, the nonreceptor tyrosine kinase Src. StpC interacts with the small G-protein Ras and stimulates mitogen-activated protein (MAP) kinase activity. Both StpA and StpC interact with tumor necrosis factor receptor-associated factors (TRAFs), leading to nuclear factor kappa B (NFκB) activation.

### The Tip Oncoprotein

The subgroup C-specific 40 kDa Tip phosphoprotein has been shown to co-precipitate with the T-cell-specific nonreceptor Src family tyrosine kinase p56/Lck in C488-transformed T cells. Tip-transgenic mice develop T-cell proliferations. Tip has an N-terminal glutamate-rich

region, duplicated in some strains, followed by one or two serine-rich regions, a bipartite kinase-interacting domain, and a C-terminal hydrophobic domain that anchors the molecule at the inside of the plasma membrane. The kinase-interacting domain consists of nine residues with homology to the C-terminal regulatory regions of various Src kinases (CSKH), and a proline-rich SH3-domain-binding sequence (SH3B). Several tyrosine residues, three of which are conserved between all strains investigated, are substrates for Lck. Tyrosine residue 127 (Y127) is the major tyrosine phosphorylation site of Tip (strain C488), but this modification does not enhance Lck binding in T cells. Recombinant viruses expressing mutations in Tip show that the strong Lck binding mediated by cooperation of the SH3B and CSKH motifs is essential for transformation of human T cells by C488, whereas Tip Y127 is required for transformation in the absence of exogenous interleukin-2, suggesting its involvement in cytokine signaling pathways.

Tip binding to Lck modulates the kinase activity and could result in an altered substrate specificity, contributing to the abrogation of ZAP70 phosphorylation. This dysregulation may further link Tip-bound Lck to alternative downstream effectors. In addition, the implication of Tip Y114 with constitutively active signal transducers and activators of transcription (STATs), especially STAT3, and the role of STATs in growth regulation and oncogenesis in multiple cell types, suggest a central role for Tip-induced STAT activity in viral T-cell transformation. However, recombinant HVS C488 expressing Tip with a tyrosine-to-phenylalanine mutation at residue 114 was able to transform primary human T lymphocytes in the absence of STAT1 or STAT3 activation. Tip is further associated with lipid rafts, and this is essential for the T-cell receptor (TCR) and CD4 downregulation but not for inhibition of TCR signal transduction and activation of STAT3 transcription factor. The activation of Lck and the inhibition of T-cell signaling by Tip may represent two different aspects of the same function, since the activation of Lck by Tip might trigger negative feedback mechanisms, such as apoptosis, in stably transfected Jurkat cells expressing high levels of Tip.

### The Tio Oncoprotein

A spliced gene with two exons is located at the junction between H DNA and the left-terminal L DNA in HVA strain 73. The encoded protein shares local similarity with StpC and Tip of HVS subgroup C strains, and was therefore termed 'two in one' (Tio). Tio is expressed in HVA-transformed simian T cells, and is bound to, and phosphorylated by, the Src family tyrosine kinases Lck or Src. Phosphorylation of Tio at Y136 is required for successful transformation of human T cells. These cells are also transformed by recombinant HVS C488 in which *stpC* and *tip* has been replaced by a *tio* cDNA transcribed from a heterologous promoter. Furthermore, Tio induces NFκB signaling via direct interaction with TRAF6.

## Growth Transformation of Human T Cells by Rhadinoviruses

Human T-cell growth transformation by HVS subgroup C strains has provided a reproducible technique for generating T-cell lines, and has opened up a new research direction linking T-cell biology, signal transduction pathways, and viral transforming functions. Infection of cord or peripheral blood mononuclear cells, thymocytes, or established human T-cell clones by C488 results in T-cell lines that grow continuously without restimulation by antigen or mitogen and do not require the presence of feeder or antigen-presenting cells. Many HVS subgroup C strains are able to transform human T cells, though to a varying extent; C488 is often preferred, as it achieves dependable growth transformation. Recombinant HVS C488 in which *stpC* and *tip* have been replaced by HVA *tio* can offer increased efficiency of human T-cell transformation along with a decreased requirement for IL-2. HVS C488 carrying mutations in Tip is being investigated for an expanding range of T-cell phenotypes.

The resulting polyclonal T-cell lines display the irregular morphology of T blasts. They carry nonintegrated HVS genomes in high copy numbers, have a normal karyotype, and are not tumorigenic in nude or severe combined immune-deficient (SCID) mice. The phenotype of HVS-transformed T cells is remarkably stable for many months in culture. It corresponds to that of mature, activated CD4+ CD8− or CD4− CD8+ T cells, usually with αβ-type (less frequently γδ-type) T-cell receptors. Transformed lines derived from established T-cell clones show the phenotype and human leukocyte antigen-restricted of the parental T cells. Cellular responses after CD3, CD4, or IL-2 receptor stimulation or antigen contact can be measured by signal transduction parameters, by proliferation, or, most reliably, by interferon-γ production. Transformation of cytotoxic T lymphocytes (CTLs) is rather inefficient, but may be increased by optimized protocols for prestimulation and culture of CTLs.

Transformation by HVS C488 has, in many cases, been the only way to cultivate and amplify T cells from patients with primary human immune deficiencies, including genetic T-cell defects involving the CD3γ chain, IL-2Rγ chain, CD95/Fas, IL-12R, major histocompatibility complex class II, Wiskott–Aldrich syndrome, or CD18/LFA-1. HVS-transformed human CD4+ T cells provide a productive system for T-lymphotropic viruses such as human herpesvirus 6 and human immunodeficiency virus (HIV) types 1 and 2, including primary clinical and macrophage-tropic HIV isolates.

Although most HVS-transformed New World monkey T lymphocytes produce infectious viral particles, HVS-transformed human T-cell lines maintain an intact viral genome but do not shed infectious virus. Production of infectious particles is also not induced by specific or nonspecific stimulation of the cells, using phorbol esters, nucleoside analogues, or other drugs that can reactivate viruses such as EBV or KSHV. Many macaque T-cell lines have been shown to shed very low amounts of virus particles, in contrast to their human counterparts, and the infusion of HVS-transformed autologous T cells into donor macaques did not cause disease. The reinfused T cells persisted for extended periods and the animals were protected against challenge with HVS C488. This is a relevant observation, since macaques are a common model for the situation in humans, and HVS-transformed simian T lymphocytes are similar to their human counterparts in many characteristics, including retained antigen specificity and presentation.

### Alterations

StpC and Tip are the only viral proteins that have been demonstrated regularly in HVS-transformed human T cells, and yet their expression alone or together in a lentiviral background is not sufficient to transform primate T cells. The HSURs are expressed abundantly in a similar way to the small, noncoding RNAs (EBERs) of EBV, but deletion of all the HSUR genes does not influence virus replication or T-cell transformation. Viral transcription other than that of the bicistronic *stpC/tip* genes is rarely detected in human T cells; it is restricted to *ie14/vsag*, and few others at extremely low abundance (*orf57/IE57*, *orf50/RTA*, *orf70/TS*, *orf71/vFLIP*, *orf72/vCyclin*, and *orf73/LANA*). Some of these increased after stimulation with phorbol ester. Many other viral genes, such as the weakly transcribed *orf71* and *orf72*, have been shown by deletion analysis not to be required for T-cell transformation.

Compared to parental, untransformed T cells, a few cellular and biochemical alterations have been detected consistently in HVS-transformed T-cell lines: CD2 and its ligand CD58 are both expressed at high densities on the cell surface and there is hyper-responsiveness to CD2 ligation. Since withdrawal by limiting dilution halts the growth of HVS-infected human T cells, IL-2 induction by CD2–CD58 contact likely contributes to the transformed phenotype of HVS-transformed human T cells. Furthermore, subcloning of HVS-transformed cells is not possible. The Src family protein tyrosine kinase $p53/56^{Lyn}$ is usually expressed in B cells. Lyn is also found in HVS-transformed T-cell lines, similar to HTLV-1-immortalized T cells, but is not activated by HVS Tip. HVS-transformed T cells secrete high amounts of the Th1 cytokine interferon gamma (IFN-γ), and

Th2-skewed T cells or Th2 clones shift toward a Th1 or Th0 profile. Many transformed clones also secrete large amounts of chemokines, such as MIP-1α and MIP-1β, and CCL1/I-309, which may protect HVS-transformed T cells from apoptosis via CCR8. IL-26, a new IL-10 cytokine family member, was discovered due to its over-expression in HVS-transformed T cells. IL-26 may influence T-cell interaction with epithelial cells *in vivo* but seemingly does not contribute to HVS-mediated T-cell transformation.

## Gene Transfer

HVS vectors are attractive for gene transfer into T cells, since the functional phenotype of transformed T lymphocytes is maintained and the T cells can be simultaneously expanded by transformation. They may even be considered for therapeutic redirection of human T-cell antigen specificity, as tools for experimental cancer therapy applications. However, replication-deficient vector variants are necessary, and a number of biosafety aspects remain to be clarified. Remarkably, ganciclovir administration does not prevent pathogenesis by HVS expressing a TK suicide gene, and tumor induction is even more rapid than with a wild-type HVS control.

Genetic alteration of HVS-transformed cells can be achieved by transduction with retroviral or lentiviral vectors, or by using recombinant HVS. Efficient infection and occasionally limited productive replication of HVS have been observed in various human cell types, including human bone marrow stroma cells, primary fibroblasts, and hematopoietic precursors. Although foreign genes were first inserted into the genome of HVS more than two decades ago, the reconstitution of virus from overlapping cosmids and engineering of bacterial artificial chromosomes has greatly facilitated mutational analysis of the HVS genome and expression cloning in HVS. This includes attenuated, nononcogenic vectors deleted in the transformation-associated left-terminal region of L DNA that harbors the HVS oncogenes. Episomally persisting herpesvirus vectors, based either on replication defective viruses or on amplicons, are currently regarded as a promising alternative that can avoid side effects of integration, which is now a major concern in the field of gene transfer.

## Rhesus Rhadinovirus and Related Old World Primate Rhadinoviruses

### Natural Occurrence and Pathology

The discovery of KSHV as the first human rhadinovirus in 1994 greatly stimulated the search for rhadinoviruses in other Old World primates. Serological studies using KSHV-derived antigens indicated that a related herpesvirus may exist in rhesus monkeys. This led to the isolation of RRV by co-cultivation of lymphocytes from seropositive rhesus monkeys with rhesus fibroblasts by Desrosiers and colleagues in 1997. RRV seems to be very widespread in captive monkeys and, in contrast to KSHV, can be propagated efficiently in cell culture. Although there exists no clear disease association for RRV in infected healthy macaques, there is one report concerning rhesus macaques that were immunosuppressed by previous infection with simian immunodeficiency virus (SIV). In this case, RRV infection resulted in a multifocal lymphoproliferative disease resembling multicentric Castleman's disease. However, this had not been noticed previously in numerous studies of SIV-infected macaques of unknown, but presumably mostly positive, RRV infection status.

Using degenerate PCR of the DNA polymerase gene, DNA fragments of rhadinovirus origin have been identified in various Old World primates, including African green monkey, chimpanzee, gorilla, and mandrill. Phylogenetic analysis of short sequences has revealed that Old World primate rhadinoviruses probably segregate into two groups: one that is more closely related to KSHV and another that is more closely related to RRV.

### Genome Structure and Replication

Analysis of the genome sequences of two independent strains has revealed that RRV is indeed more closely related to KSHV than to the prototypic rhadinovirus HVS. The RRV genome organization is essentially collinear with that of KSHV. It has (at least) 79 genes, 67 of which are homologous to genes found in both KSHV and HVS. Of the remaining 12 genes, 8 are similar to KSHV genes (see below). Interestingly, *orf2*/DHFR is in the same position as in HVS, and different from that in KSHV. The RRV OriLyt is located in the same region as in HVS and KSHV, between *orf69* and *orf71*/vFLIP. The functions of viral transactivators and regulatory proteins resemble those of KSHV. The gene content of RRV is similar to that of KSHV, but contains only one *vMIP* gene and lacks *K3* and *K5*. The genes encoding CCPH and vIL-6 are conserved in RRV, and eight genes are present with homology to the family of viral interferon regulatory factors (*vIRF-1* through *vIRF-8*). Several large DNA viruses have been shown to encode micro-RNAs (miRNAs), including EBV and the rhadinoviruses RRV and KSHV, and miRNA genes are evolutionary conserved in at least the lymphocryptoviruses. However, the role of miRNA and RNA interference in the viral context is controversial. Given the specificity of RNA interference, it remains to be determined whether this can have a role in herpesviral transformation of foreign hosts. An interesting speculation is that herpesviral miRNAs may act as specificity factors that initiate heterochromatin assembly of the latent viral genome.

## Rhadinoviruses from Retroperitoneal Fibrosis

In an approach using a degenerate PCR technique, Rose and co-workers identified fragments of a herpesvirus DNA polymerase gene in tissue specimens from retroperitoneal fibromatosis (RF) from macaque species, *M. nemestrina* (six cases) and *M. mulatta* (one case). RF is a rare disease occurring in immunesuppressed macaques that consists of aggressively proliferating fibrous tissue with a high degree of vascularization; thus, it somewhat resembles KS. Earlier transmission studies indicated that an infectious agent may be involved in RF pathogenesis. Sequence comparisons indicate that the DNA polymerase and adjacent genes of these two potentially novel rhadinoviruses, tentatively termed RFHVMm and RFHVMn, are related more closely to KSHV than RRV. Attempts to isolate the viruses on cultured cells have so far been unsuccessful. The possible coexistence of two different rhadinoviruses in the same host animal is also indicated, since in one study all RF-diseased macaques harbored RRV DNA (and all were coinfected with simian retrovirus 2 and/or SIV). In these animals, RFHV DNA was present at significantly higher copy numbers in the RF tumors.

## Lymphocryptoviruses of Old and New World Primates

Gammaherpesviruses closely related to EBV have been recognized in several species of Old World primates from the mid-1970s. The genome of rhesus lymphocryptovirus (abbreviated to rhesus LCV; species *Cercopithecine herpesvirus 15*) has been sequenced. Until recently, the paradigm was that the lymphocryptoviruses are restricted to Old World primates, including humans. However, a virus related to EBV was isolated from common marmosets, both from healthy animals and animals with spontaneous B-cell lymphomas. Related lymphocryptoviruses have also been detected in several other New World primate species (**Table 1**). The new lymphocryptovirus (marmoset LCV; species *Callitrichine herpesvirus 3*) has an EBV-like genome structure, and determination of the genome sequence has shown that several Old World primate lymphocryptovirus-specific genes are absent. Specifically, homologs of EBV BCRF1/vIL10, BARF1/CSF-1R, BARF0, the EBERs, and several other genes of unknown function have not been detected, and marked divergences exist in LMP-1, LMP-2, EBNA-LP, EBNA-2, and the EBNA-3 family. Also, the organization of the putative marmoset LCV OriP-region is clearly distinct from that in Old World primate lymphocryptoviruses.

*In vitro* transformation of B cells by human and simian Old World primate lymphocryptoviruses seems to be mostly restricted to the natural host or closely related species. However, experimental T-cell tumors can be induced in rabbits following infection by cynomolgus LCV or baboon LCV.

## Conclusion and Perspective

Viruses of the gammaherpesvirus genera *Lymphocryptovirus* and *Rhadinovirus* can be found in New World and Old World primates, including humans. Although several members of both genera are closely associated with viral oncogenesis, the simian viruses do not generally provide a straightforward model for multifaceted human diseases. The direct transforming action of viral oncogenes, as well as a chronic inflammatory reaction that may be affected by KSHV-encoded or KSHV-induced cytokines or angiogenic factors, may contribute to the genesis of KS. The KSHV-related simian rhadinoviruses do not provide a corresponding animal model as yet. Historically, interest in the rhadinoviruses has focused on the long-established prototype, HVS. Although a comparable virus-associated, acute, peripheral, pleomorphic T-cell lymphoma is not known yet in humans, this disease, which is induced reproducibly by HVS within weeks, can serve as an experimental model for general tumor development. The ability of certain HVS strains to transform human T lymphocytes to stable proliferation in culture provides a valuable tool for laboratory studies of T-cell immunology, including inherited and acquired immunodeficiency. In addition to their use as an immunological and biochemical T-cell model, HVS-transformed T cells can provide a source for the purification of specifically overexpressed cytokines or chemokines from culture supernatants. A detailed analysis of differential gene expression will lead to identification of signaling pathways that lead to lymphocyte transformation by herpesviral oncoproteins. Those involving STAT, nuclear factor of activated T cells (NFAT), and NFκB may be particularly important, perhaps providing hints to the roles of the respective pathways in human (nonviral) T-cell malignancy. Furthermore, rhadinovirus-transformed T-cell lines can be valuable tools in screening for specific drugs that target these pathways.

The side effects of retroviral integration have shown the requirement for efficient nonintegrating vectors. Recombinant rhadinoviruses can deliver foreign genes into primary human mesenchymal cells and T lymphocytes; this may prepare the ground for future therapeutic applications of persisting rhadinoviral vectors in adoptive immunotherapy. Safety considerations will prevent the use of unconditionally transforming rhadinovirus vectors, and require the development of novel rhadinovirus-based T-lymphotropic episomes, including conditional/attenuated or amplicon vector systems. Analysis of viral genome episomal modification in host T cells and the detection of genomic insulating regions can provide markers for the selection of regions suitable for the insertion of transgenes into the viral backbone.

## Acknowledgments

Original work included in this review article was supported by the Deutsche Forschungsgemeinschaft (SFB643 TP A2, EN423/2-1), the Wilhelm Sander Stiftung, Bavarian International Graduate School of Science (BIGS), and the Interdisciplinary Center for Clinical Research (IZKF) at the University of Erlangen-Nuremberg.

*See also:* Murine Gammaherpesvirus 68; Simian Alpha-herpesviruses.

## Further Reading

Alberter B and Ensser A (2007) Histone modification pattern of the T cellular *Herpesvirus saimiri* genome in latency. *Journal of Virology* 81: 2524–2530.

Bruce AG, Bakke AM, Bielefeldt-Ohmann H, *et al.* (2006) High levels of retroperitoneal fibromatosis (RF)-associated herpesvirus in RF lesions in macaques are associated with ORF73 LANA expression in spindleoid tumour cells. *Journal of General Virology* 87: 3529–3538.

Cai X, Schäfer A, Lu S, *et al.* (2006) Epstein–Barr virus microRNAs are evolutionarily conserved and differentially expressed. *PLoS Pathogens* 2: e23.

Cho NH, Feng P, Lee SH, *et al.* (2004) Inhibition of T-cell receptor signal transduction by tyrosine kinase-interacting protein of herpesvirus saimiri. *Journal of Experimental Medicine* 200: 681–687.

Cullen BR (2006) Viruses and microRNAs. *Nature Genetics* 38: S25–S30.

Damania B (2004) Oncogenic gamma-herpesviruses: Comparison of viral proteins involved in tumorigenesis. *Nature Reviews Microbiology* 2: 656–668.

Ensser A (2006) Transformation by herpesviruses: Focus on T-cells. *Future Virology* 1: 109–121.

Ensser A and Fleckenstein B (2004) Herpesvirus saimiri transformation of human T lymphocytes. In: Coligan JE, Bierer BE, Margulies DH, *et al.* (eds.) *Current Protocols in Immunology*, pp. 7.21.1–7.21.10. New York: Wiley.

Ensser A and Fleckenstein B (2005) T-cell transformation and oncogenesis by γ2-herpesviruses. *Advances in Cancer Research* 93: 91–128.

Ensser A, Thurau M, Wittmann S, *et al.* (2003) The genome of herpesvirus saimiri C488 which is capable of transforming human T cells. *Virology* 314: 471–487.

Heck E, Friedrich U, Gack MU, *et al.* (2006) Growth transformation of human T-cells by herpesvirus saimiri requires multiple Tip–Lck interaction motifs. *Journal of Virology* 80: 9934–9942.

Li HW and Ding SW (2005) Antiviral silencing in animals. *FEBS Letters* 579: 5965–5973.

Pfeffer S, Zavolan M, Grasser FA, *et al.* (2004) Identification of virus-encoded microRNAs. *Science* 304: 734–736.

Searles RP, Bergquam EP, Axthelm MK, *et al.* (1999) Sequence and genomic analysis of a rhesus macaque rhadinovirus with similarity to Kaposi's sarcoma-associated herpesvirus/human herpesvirus 8. *Journal of Virology* 73: 3040–3053.

Schäfer A, Lengenfelder D, Grillhösl C, *et al.* (2003) The latency-associated nuclear antigen homolog of herpesvirus saimiri inhibits lytic virus replication. *Journal of Virology* 77: 5911–5925.

## Relevant Websites

http://en.wikipedia.org – Cebidae; Herpesviridae; Rhadinovirus.
http://www.ncbi.nlm.nih.gov – International Committee on Taxonomy of Viruses, ICTVdb.

# Simian Immunodeficiency Virus: General Features

**M E Laird and R C Desrosiers,** New England Primate Research Center, Southborough, MA, USA

## History

Simian immunodeficiency virus (SIV) was first isolated in 1984 from captive rhesus macaques (*Macaca mulatta*) at the New England Primate Research Center (NEPRC). This virus was originally called STLV-III because it displayed similar morphology, growth characteristics, and antigenic properties to the newly described immunosuppressive virus HTLV-III of humans. When HTLV-III was renamed human immunodeficiency virus (HIV), the name STLV-III was also changed to SIV. Retrospective studies have shown that SIV was introduced to the NEPRC when a group of rhesus macaques with immuosuppressive disease was delivered from another primate center 15 years prior to the initial SIV isolation. The original cohort of rhesus monkeys was most likely accidentally infected with SIV from wild-caught sooty mangabey monkeys at the same institution. SIV has been subsequently isolated from other captive macaque species (*M. fascicularis, M. nemestrina, and M. arctoides*) that were dying of immunosuppression-associated diseases, and from many species of feral asymptomatic African nonhuman primates (**Table 1**).

## Taxonomy and Classification

SIVs belong to the genus *Lentivirus* of the family *Retroviridae.* Related lentiviruses have been isolated from

**Table 1** Detailed listing of primate lentiviruses[a]

| Virus designation | Primate Lentivirus grouping | Species (common) | Species (formal) | Subspecies Isolates |
|---|---|---|---|---|
| HIV-1 | HIV-1/SIVcpz | Humans | *Homo sapiens* | |
| SIVcpz | HIV-1/SIVcpz | Chimpanzees | *Pan troglodytes* | P. t. troglodytes |
| | | | | P. t. schweinfurthi |
| SIVsm | SIVmac/SIVsm/HIV-2 | Sooty mangabeys | *Cercocebus atys* | |
| SIVmac | SIVmac/SIVsm/HIV-2 | Macaques | *Macaca mulatta* | M. arctoides |
| | | | | M. nemestrina |
| | | | | M. fascicularis |
| HIV-2 | SIVmac/SIVsm/HIV-2 | Humans | *Homo sapiens* | |
| SIVagm | SIVagm | African green monkeys | *Chlorocebus aethiops* | C. a. grivet |
| | | | | C. a. tantalus |
| | | | | C. a. sabeus |
| | | | | C. a. alboqularis |
| | | | | C. a. nictitans |
| SIVsyk | SIVsyk | Sykes' monkeys | *Cercopithecus mitis* | |
| SIVgsn | SIVgsn/SIVmon/SIVmus | greater spot-nosed monkey | *Cercopithicus mitis* | |
| SIVmon | SIVgsn/SIVmon/SIVmus | mona monkey | *Cercopithicus mona* | |
| SIVmus | SIVgsn/SIVmon/SIVmus | mustached monkey | *Cercopithicus cephus* | |
| SIVlhoesti | SIVsun/SIVlhoesti | L'hoest monkey | *Cercopithicus lhoesti* | C. l. lhoesti |
| SIVsun | SIVsun/SIVlhoesti | Sun-tailed monkey | *Cercopithicus lhoesti* | C. l. solatus |
| SIVdeb | SIVdeb | DeBrazza monkey | *Cercopithicus neglectus* | |
| SIVden | SIVdeb | Dent's mona monkey | *Cercopithicus mona denti* | C. m. denti |
| SIVrcm | SIVrcm | Red-capped mangabey | *Cercocebus torguatus* | C. t. torguatus |
| SIVmnd | SIVmnd 1 | Mandrill | *Mandrillus sphinx* | |
| SIVmnd | SIVmnd 2 | Mandrill | *Mandrillus sphinx* | |
| SIVdrl | SIVmnd 2 | Drill | *Mandrillus leucophaeus* | |
| SIVcol | SIVcol | Querza colobus | *Colobus querza* | |
| SIVolc | SIVolc | Olive colobus | *ProColobus badius* | |
| SIVwrc | SIVwrc | Western red colobus | *Pilocolobus badius* | |
| SIVtal | SIVtal | Angolia-talapoin monkey | *Miopithicus talapoin* | |
| SIVtal | SIVtal | Gabon talapoin monkey | *Miopithicus ogouensis* | |

[a]Partial pol sequences have also been obtained from a black mangabey (*Loplcocebus aterrimus*) and from a Schmidt's guenon (*Cercopithicus ascanius schmidti*). In addition to the primate lentiviruses listed, serologic surveys for the detection of antibodies to SIV have suggested SIV infection of a variety of other species.

sheep, goats, horses, cattle, cats, and humans. Based on host species and genetic analysis, 14 discrete evolutionary groupings of primate lentiviruses are now recognized (**Figure 1**). Even within a single grouping, discrete sub-groupings are defined based on host subspecies, geography, and genetic distance. Within a specific subgroup whose host range covers an extensive geographical area, discrete genetic sub-subgroups are further defined that correlate with monkey subspecies and precise natural geographic habitat.

The lentiviruses have a common morphogenesis and morphology that distinguish them from other retrovirus subgroups. Lentivirus particles are 80–100 nm in diameter and consist of an RNA genome and viral enzymes enclosed in viral protein core that is encased by a cell-derived membrane spiked with viral envelope glycopro-teins. In lymphocytes, immature lentiviruses bud from the plasma membrane without a preformed nucleoid; mature particles contain a characteristic conical or rod-shaped nucleoid. Classification of lentiviruses by morphology alone is consistent with classification by phylogenetic

analysis of polymerase (*pol*) gene sequences. The *pol* gene exhibits the greatest degree of sequence conserva-tion and viruses classified as lentiviruses have *pol* gene sequences more closely related to one another than to other retroviruses.

Lentiviruses also share similarities in certain biological properties and genome organization. All lentiviruses have a propensity to replicate in macrophages and produce long-term, persistent infections in susceptible hosts. SIVs use CD4 as the first of two receptors used sequen-tially for viral entry into cells. The chronic disease induced by SIV includes immunodeficiency, undoubtedly because of the targeting of CD4+ lymphocytes for infec-tion through the use of CD4 as the primary receptor. In addition to the *gag, pol,* and *env* genes that are found in all simpler retroviruses, lentiviruses have a number of auxiliary genes (**Figure 2** and **Tables 2** and **3**).

The SIVs are named according to the primate species of origin, for example, SIVmac from macaques or SIVsmm from sooty mangabey monkeys. Widespread availability of DNA sequencing has allowed an in-depth understanding

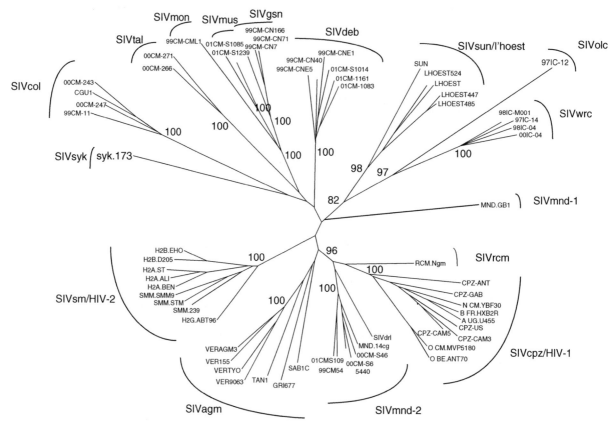

**Figure 1**  Phylogeny of primate lentiviruses. The 14 groupings of primate lentiviruses are shown. Please see **Table 1** for species abbreviations. Adapted from Courgnaud V, Formenty P, Koffi CA, *et al*. (2003) Partial molecular characterization of two simian immunodeficiency viruses (SIV) from African colobids: SIVwrc from Western Red Colobus (*Piliocolobus badius*) and SIVolc from Olive Colobus (*Procolobus verus*). *Journal of Virology* 77(1): 744–748, with permission from American Society for Microbiology.

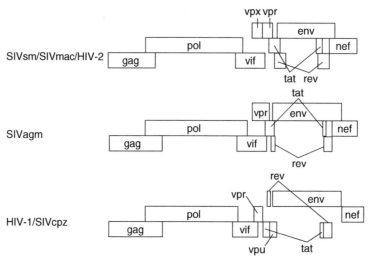

**Figure 2**  Genome organizations of representative primate lentiviruses.

of phylogenetic relationships among SIVs. However, to date, only 39 of the 69 recognized species of nonhuman primates that inhabit sub-Saharan Africa have been surveyed; additional distinct SIV groupings will likely be identified.

## Geographic Distribution and Host Range

Many different species of African nonhuman primates are known to be infected with SIV in their natural habitats. However, few studies have investigated the distribution or

**Table 2**   Presence of auxiliary genes in SIV species

| | SIVsm/SIVmac/HIV-2 | SIVagm | SIVsyk | SIVsun/SIVl'hoesti | HIV-1/SIVcpz | SIVgsn/SIVmon/SIVmus | SIVrcm |
|---|---|---|---|---|---|---|---|
| vif | + | + | + | + | + | + | + |
| vpu | − | − | − | − | + | + | − |
| vpr | + | + | + | + | + | + | + |
| vpx | + | − | − | − | − | − | + |
| tat | + | + | + | + | + | + | + |
| rev | + | + | + | + | + | + | + |
| nef | + | + | + | + | + | + | + |

Different SIV species may vary with respect to the auxiliary genes that they carry. The presence or absence of these auxiliary genes do not always associate with phylogenetic clustering. For example, SIVmnd2 has a *vpx* gene, but SIVmnd1 does not. SIVden from a pet Dent's Mona monkey (*Cercopithecus mona denti*) has a *vpu* gene, although it clusters more closely to the SIV from DeBrazza monkeys, SIVdeb. SIVdeb has a *vpr* gene, but no *vpx* or *vpu* genes.

**Table 3**   Auxiliary gene function in SIV

| Auxiliary gene product | Essential for replication? | Early gene product? | Function |
|---|---|---|---|
| tat | Yes | Yes | Potent activator of viral gene expression; enhances LTR-driven transcription |
| rev | Yes | Yes | Required for efficient transport of unspliced and singly spliced viral RNAs into the cytoplasm |
| nef | No | Yes | Functional activities include CD4 downregulation, MHC downregulation, infectivity enhancement and lymphocyte activation |
| vif | Yes/no[a] | No | Blocks restricting activity of innate cellular proteins, APOBEC-3G and APOBEC-3F |
| vpr | No | No | Involved in $G_2/M$ phase cell-cycle arrest; mediates apoptosis of CD4+ T cells |
| vpx | No | No | Facilitates nuclear import of the preintegration complex in nondividing cells |

[a]SIV strains containing a deletion in *vif* (SIVΔvif) can be grown in a *vif*-complementing cell line; when inoculated into animals no virus or PCR-amplifiable sequences could be recovered from PBMCs; however, monkeys still developed lowlevel antibody titers suggesting highly attenuated infection.

extent of natural SIV infection. There has recently been an effort to overcome this shortfall of information by identifying and assessing the extent of SIV infection in wild primate populations. In 2002, Peeters *et al.*, collected and screened 788 blood samples from wild-caught monkeys for the prevalence of SIV infection in 13 different monkey species in Cameroon. The study examined the rates of SIV infection in monkeys hunted for bushmeat and those captured as pets as possible routes of zoonotic transmission. It was reported that 18.4% of bushmeat samples and 11.6% of pets tested positive for SIV infection. These results identified four species of monkeys not previously known to harbor SIV (*Cercocebus agilis, Lophocebus albigena, C. pogonias,* and *Papio anubis*) and likely underestimate the extent of SIV prevalence as not all native primate species were screened.

The origins of both HIV-2 and HIV-1 in humans are believed to have occurred through cross-species transmission events from SIV-infected simians relatively recently in history. SIVsmm is closely related to HIV-2 with the same genome organization and both viruses group together phylogenetically apart from the other 13 groups of primate lentiviruses. The sooty mangabey monkey is native to the coastal forest regions of western Africa,

where HIV-2 emerged and is now endemic in the human population. Thus, strong circumstantial evidence involving both viral sequences and geographic distribution link the monkey SIVsmm and HIV-2 in western Africa. In 2006, Keele and co-workers examined the wild chimpanzee (*Pan troglodytes troglodytes*) populations of Cameroon to determine the extent of natural SIVcpz infection and to investigate which infected populations may be responsible for the cross-species transmission events that initially introduced HIV-1 into the human population. By measuring the presence of anti-HIV cross-reactive antibodies and the ability to amplify viral gene sequences it was determined that SIV infection was widespread but uneven among the chimpanzee populations, with the prevalence of infection ranging from 23% to 35% in some isolated groups to a 4–5% infection rate in others, while still others had a complete absence of SIV infection. Sequence and phylogenetic analyses of the newly identified wild SIVcpz strains supported that distinct geographical chimpanzee groups acted as the sources of HIV-1 groups M and N in the human population.

Although SIVs naturally infect a variety of African nonhuman primates, a single example of natural infection of Asian Old World monkeys is yet to be reported. SIVsmm and SIVagm, when used to infect macaque monkeys (Asian Old World primates), can persist and cause an AIDS-like disease. Accidental introduction of SIVsmm into macaque monkeys in captive United States colonies occurred and was spread unknowingly into other macaques for more than a decade before it was identified and eliminated. At least one clear case of laboratory-acquired infection of a human with SIVmac has been documented.

## Virus Propagation and Receptor Use

SIVs can be propagated in mitogen-stimulated primary peripheral blood mononuclear cells (PBMCs), in monocytes/macrophages from the primate host, and in many cultured cell lines including human tumor-derived CD4+ T-lymphocyte cell lines. The types of cells that can be infected by different strains of SIV correlate with the receptor(s) that are expressed on the cell surface. Some acutely pathogenic strains are unusual in their ability to replicate in lymphocytes of resting PBMC cultures without prior stimulation. In PBMC cultures and many cell lines, viral infection results in the fusion of cellular membranes producing large syncytial cells. Syncytium formation, which is mediated by *env*, allows the virus to spread directly from cell to cell in addition to direct infection. Several isolates also grow well in cultured macrophages derived from lung, blood, or bone marrow.

As with HIV-1, the SIVs use both CD4 and a chemokine receptor for viral entry. The SIVsmm/SIVmac/HIV-2 and SIVagm groups of viruses are known to use CCR5 as their principal co-receptor. However, a variety of other chemokine receptors, CCR2b, CCR3, STRL33 (Bonzo), GPR15 (Bob), and GPR1, also can be used as the co-receptor, depending on the individual virus isolate. A larger percentage of isolates from the SIVsmm/SIVmac/HIV-2 group of viruses show less dependence on CD4 for entry than do HIV-1 variants. Isolates of SIVsmm/SIVmac appear to use CXCR4 as the principal co-receptor much less frequently than HIV-1 isolates. SIVs from red-capped mangabeys (*Cercocebus torquatus torquatus*) predominantly use CCR2b as the principal co-receptor.

## Genetics

SIV, like other retroviruses, replicates its genome through a proviral DNA intermediate. From the 5' cap to the 3' polyadenylation site, the SIV genome is approximately 9.6 kbp in length. The viral particle contains a diploid genome of single-stranded RNA that is linked noncovalently near the 5' end of the molecules. The 5' end of the viral genome is capped and the 3' end is polyadenylated. DNA synthesis by the viral-encoded reverse transcriptase is primed by host tRNA that is base-paired to viral RNA.

The double-stranded proviral DNA is integrated into the host cell chromosome by a viral-encoded integrase and further replication events of transcription, translation, and particle assembly depend on cellular components. Particles then assemble at and bud through the plasma membrane. Because of this replication strategy, cloned DNA representing the entire proviral genome can yield infectious virus.

All retroviruses contain certain standard features in their genomic organization (**Figure 2**). Sequences regulating DNA synthesis, integration, transcription, and other functions are contained in the long terminal repeat (LTR) region at each end of the provirus. Open reading frames (ORFs) encoding the major structural and nonstructural proteins lie between the LTRs. Genes are encoded in any of three possible ORFs; overlaps between ORFs are common. All retroviruses contain three standard genes called *gag* (group-specific antigen), which encodes the core proteins; *pol* (polymerase), which encodes the viral reverse transcriptase, protease, and integrase; and *env* (envelope), which encodes the envelope glycoproteins.

*Env* is essential for virus replication. The envelope glycoproteins are responsible for binding the receptor and co-receptor on the cell surface and mediating viral entry. The *env* products are the main targets of antibodies that can neutralize infection. In addition, determinants of cell and tissue tropism often map to the *env* gene. Derivatives in which the SIVmac *env* has been replaced by envelope of HIV-1 are replication competent in macaque cells and are capable of infecting rhesus monkeys. These recombinant viruses are known as simian–human immunodeficiency viruses (SHIVs). Serial passage of several SHIV strains has resulted in second-generation SHIVs that are consistently pathogenic in macaques.

In addition to *gag, pol,* and *env,* all lentiviruses, including SIV, encode additional accessory genes not found in other simple retroviruses (**Tables 2** and **3**). Both SIV and HIV encode *tat* (transactivator protein), *rev* (regulator of gene expression), *vif* (viral infectivity factor), *nef* (originally termed negative factor), and *vpr* (viral protein 'r'). SIVagm and SIVsmm/HIV-2/SIVmac encode an additional gene, *vpx* (viral protein 'x'), thought to be a duplicated homolog of *vpr.* The ORF for *vpu,* found in HIV-1/SIVcpz and SIVgsn/SIVmon/SIVmus/SIVden, is not contained in HIV-2 or in other SIVs. These auxiliary genes likely contribute to the complex life cycle of lentiviruses, including persistent viral replication and immune evasion.

Some of the accessory proteins found in SIV can be deleted without abrogating the ability of the virus to replicate *in vivo* and *in vitro,* specifically *nef, vpr,* and *vpx.* However, the presence and the conservation of these genes in several different subgroups of lentiviruses suggest that they contribute to the virus' ability to replicate and persist *in vivo.* Cloned proviral DNAs containing deletions in these auxiliary ORFs have been used to study the contributions to replication and functional activity of the auxiliary genes in the context of experimental animal infection. Auxiliary gene functional data are summarized in **Table 3**.

## Evolution

Comparison of genetic sequences among human and simian immunodeficiency suggests that there are at least 14 discrete groups of primate lentiviruses in existence: HIV-1/SIVcpz; SIVmnd-2; SIVagm; SIVsmm/HIV-2; SIVsyk; SIVcol; SIVtal; SIVmon/SIVmus/SIVgsn; SIVdeb/den; SIVsun/l'hoest; SIVolc; SIVwrc; SIVmnd-1; and SIVrcm (**Figure 1**). It is thought that HIV-1 and HIV-2 evolved from simian viruses that entered the human population through cross-species transmission events relatively recently in human history. Cross-species transmission among non-human primates occurring in nature may have generated further pathogenic variants; however, it is likely that most of the primate immunodeficiency viruses have long been present in the natural host but not recognized until recently. The SIVs and HIVs are more closely related to each other than to any other nonprimate retrovirus, suggesting that they are inherently primate viruses, not derived from nonprimate viruses that were introduced via other cross-species transmission events.

## Serologic Relationships and Genetic Diversity

The *pol* gene generally contains the greatest degree of sequence conservation and therefore is most often used for the comparison of lentiviruses from different groups or subgroups to assess relatedness. *Pol* sequences from one subgroup of SIV (e.g., SIVsmm) will generally contain only a 55–60% amino acid identity when compared to another SIV subgroup (e.g., SIVagm). When different lentivirus groups are compared (e.g., EIAV with SIV) the amino acid identity in *pol* is often 35% or less, and the sequence homology found in other genes is even less. Antiserum to the Gag protein is generally cross-reactive to different strains within a group, whereas antiserum to the envelope is not and can be used to distinguish between isolates within a group.

## Epidemiology

SIV has been found in many species of nonhuman primates throughout sub-Saharan Africa, but in most cases infection does not seem to cause an AIDS-like disease in the natural host. There are only a few examples of immunodeficiency in monkey species naturally infected with SIV. In contrast, though infection does not appear in nature, SIV infection of Asian macaques in captivity induces an AIDS-like disease similar to that observed in HIV-infected humans.

## Transmission

There is little information regarding natural modes of SIV transmission. A study of wild grivet monkeys in Awash National Park in Ethiopia analyzed SIVagm serologic status as compared to age, sex, and risk. Infection was found overwhelmingly in females of reproductive age and was nearly absent among younger female animals. In the male population, infection was only observed in monkeys that were fully adult. These data support a predominantly sexual mode of transmission among the grivet population. SIV transmission through contact with infected blood from aggressive contacts (e.g., bite and scratch wounds) may also be a prominent mode by which SIV may be spread. In addition, maternal–infant transmission of SIV has been observed in captive animals.

Experimental infection of laboratory animals has most commonly been performed by direct needle inoculation. However, mucosal exposure is being used more frequently, especially in vaccine studies, as a model for the most common routes of HIV infection.

## Features of Infection

While SIV infection of the natural host is usually not associated with any disease progression, SIV infection of macaques induces both acute and chronic disease symptoms that are similar to that which HIV-1 causes in human patients. SIV infection of rhesus macaques is generally thought to be the closest model of AIDS in humans.

The main sites of pathogenic SIV replication shortly after infection have been localized to the gastrointestinal (GI) tract, thymus, spleen, and other lymphoid tissues. SIV has been detected at early time points within periarteriolar lymphoid sheaths in the spleen, paracortex of lymph nodes, and medulla of the thymus. SIV infection of rhesus monkeys results in a dramatic and selective depletion of CD4+ T cells in the GI tract within days of infection, before depletion is evident in the peripheral lymphoid tissues. Coincident with the loss of CD4+ T cells in the GI tract is the productive infection of large quantities of mononuclear cells at this site. It is now clear that SIV replicates principally in the CD4+ CCR5+ cells of the memory T-cell phenotype. These cells predominate in the gut and other mucosal sites and are found at much lower levels in peripheral lymphoid tissues. Therefore, the GI tract appears to be a major site of SIV replication and CD4+ memory T-cell depletion early in the course of infection. Within the thymus, marked depletion of thymic progenitor cells has been observed 21 days post infection with pathogenic SIV; this cell depletion is followed by increased cell proliferation in the thymus and a marked increase in thymocyte progenitors. SIV can also be found in the central nervous system (CNS) at early time points following infection. The cells that are targeted in the brain, either early in infection or in late-stage SIV-induced encephalitis, are primarily cells of the monocyte/macrophage lineage.

Viral loads in infected animals decrease with the onset of immune responses, and this decrease correlates with CD8+ T-cell lymphocytosis and the rise of SIV-specific antibodies. Following immune system activation, animals enter an asymptomatic period of infection of variable duration. Viral replication persists during this period, inducing immune abnormalities, including gradual declines in CD4+ T-cell count, CD4/CD8 ratio, and the ability to respond to mitogens. Infected animals can also exhibit chronic diarrhea and wasting resulting in up to a 60% loss of the original body weight. Over the course of disease, dramatic changes, including hyperplasia and/or atrophy, take place in most of the lymphoid tissues. Terminal stages of SIV infection are characterized by a range of diseases that can be grouped into four broad categories: SIV-related inflammatory disease, opportunistic infections associated with SIV-induced immunosuppression, neoplastic diseases, and diseases of unknown pathogenesis. The tropism of SIV strains for monocytes/macrophages correlates with dramatic inflammatory and degenerative changes seen in the CNS, lung, digestive tract, and other organs that are separate from the pathogenesis of opportunistic infections. The characteristics and frequency of inflammatory lesions in SIV-infected macaques closely resembles those seen in HIV-infected patients. SIV-induced encephalitis is frequent, although the appearance of brain lesions is dependent on the infecting SIV strain. At necropsy, 30–50% of SIVmac-infected animals have characteristic multinucleate giant cell encephalitis that closely resembles that seen in HIV-associated encephalitis. The opportunistic infections seen in infected monkeys are also similar to those observed in HIV-infected individuals and include *Pneumocystis carinii*, *Mycobacterium avium*, *Crytposporidia* sp., *Toxoplasma gondii*, rhesus Epstein–Barr virus (rhesus lymphocrytovirus), cytomegalovirus, polyomavirus (SV40), and adenovirus. Neoplastic diseases during SIV infection are primarily limited to lymphomas, the frequency of which varies from study to study. Lymphoma induction in SIV-infected macaques has additionally been associated with the co-infection of rhesus Epstein–Barr virus. Diseases of unknown pathogenesis include generalized lymphoproliferative syndrome, arteritis, and arteriopathy.

Acutely pathogenic strains exist, such as SIVsmPBj14, which can be acutely lethal in infected macaques. SIVsm PBj14 infection causes death in infected monkeys within 14 days. These animals have very high viral loads, severe GI disease, cytokine disregulation, lymphoproliferative disease, and organ system failure. The increased pathogenicity of this virus has been attributed to the creation of an ITAM motif by a tyrosine at residue 17 of the nef protein. This change allows the virus to induce lymphocyte activation and replicate to high titers in PBMC cultures without prior stimulation. However, the disease induced by the majority of SIV infections is typically chronic and manifests itself over the course of 1–3 years post infection.

Several independent research groups have constructed recombinant forms of SIVmac with HIV-1 *env*, *tat*, *rev*, and, in some cases, *nef* and/or *vpu* genes renamed 'SHIV' (for simian–human immunodeficiency virus) that have been passaged in macaques to establish pathogenic virus strains. Although most of the HIV-1 envelopes that were used to construct these SHIVs were dual-tropic, in that they can use either CCR5 or CXCR4 as a co-receptor, the large majority of SHIV viruses appear to target primarily CXCR4-expressing cells when used to infect rhesus macaques. The pathogenic SHIVs consistently, rapidly, and irreversibly deplete CD4+ T cells from the periphery and can be acutely lethal.

## Immune Response and Persistence

SIV-infected macaques typically produce high levels of antiviral antibodies and high-frequency cytotoxic T-lymphocyte (CTL) responses to the infecting virus. These immune responses persist for the lifetime of the infected host in both natural and experimental infection. SIV deletion mutants that are progressively more attenuated based on viral load measurements generate progressively weaker anti-SIV antibody responses. Anti-SIV CTL responses have been demonstrated as being major histocompatibility complex (MHC) restricted. Detailed investigation of CTL responses has been impeded by a lack of information regarding MHC types in different monkey species. However, a considerable amount of new information regarding MHC alleles and their cognate peptides is emerging for rhesus macaques.

The importance of CD8+ lymphocytes in limiting the extent of SIV or SHIV replication has been definitively shown using CD8+ T-cell depletion. Extensive depletion of CD8+ cells was accomplished by intravenous administration of large doses of anti-CD8 monoclonal antibodies. When CD8+ T cells were depleted during primary infection, viral replication continued unabated after the usual peak of viral loads, 10–14 days post infection; this was in stark contrast to undepleted animals, in which intact immune responses typically act to decrease viral loads after 14 days post infection. During chronic infection, elimination of CD8+ lymphocytes through depletion resulted in a rapid and dramatic increase in viremia, which was again suppressed upon removal of anti-CD8 antibody and the return of the SIV-specific CD8+ lymphocytes. Depletion of CD8+ T cells in animals infected with SHIV viruses has facilitated the appearance of the more highly pathogenic, passaged variants.

In macaques developing SIV-induced disease from wild-type strains of SIV, viral-specific, proliferative responses of CD4+ T cells are typically weak or absent all together. However, infection by attenuated SIV mutants containing a deletion of the *nef* gene produces strong, SIV-specific, CD4+ helper cell proliferative responses. This situation recalls that of HIV infection in humans, in which HIV-specific CD4+ proliferative responses in progressing patients are usually weak or absent, but are often very strong in nonprogressors that are able to control their infection. It seems that as CD4+ helper T cells try to respond to SIV at sites of infection, they arrive in the location where they are the ideal target cells for the invading virus. In pathogenic infections, the virus wins the battle between it and the responding CD4+ T cells.

All lentiviruses persist in the infected host through chronic active viral replication. Over the course of the months and years of chronic infection, macaques infected with SIV are producing and turning over millions of viral particles and infected cells every day. Although active replication persists throughout the course of infection,

there are some cells that are most likely infected in a quiescent or latent fashion. The extent of chronic active replication may also differ depending on the infecting virus strain and the host. Consistent with prolonged antigen expression and chronic replication is the long-term persistence of a high level of circulating antibody and viral-specific CTLs. Nonpathogenic SIV derivatives also continue to replicate at low levels over long periods, as demonstrated by accumulated sequence changes in these viral genomes and persistent antibody titers.

The dilemma of all lentiviruses is how to replicate persistently in the face of an apparently strong immune response. The levels of antiviral antibody and the frequency of CTLs in the infected individual have been measured and appear to be consistently high. Several strategies are used by SIV and other lentiviruses to allow persistent replication and evade the immune response. These are summarized in **Figure 3**.

## Prevention and Control

Extensive testing and removal programs have essentially eliminated SIV from captive macaque colonies. However, continued vigilance is required to minimize the chance that breeding colonies may again become accidentally

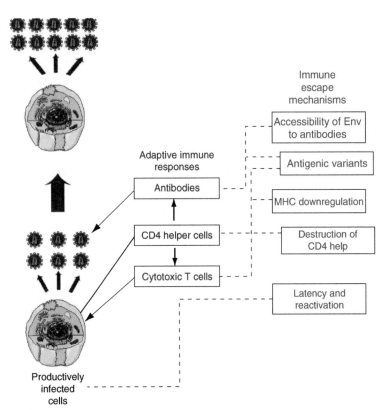

**Figure 3** Simian immunodeficiency virus uses a variety of strategies to avoid recognition and clearance by both the humoral and cellular arms of the immune system.

exposed to the virus. Animals can be easily and conveniently tested serologically for infection. Cases of SIV infection in humans are extremely rare and laboratory personnel that work with SIV follow the same precautions when working with SIV as working with HIV-1. Disposable gloves and surgical gowns are used, all work with live virus is performed in a biosafety hood, procedures creating aerosols are avoided, and any use of glass or needles in conjunction with live virus is minimized.

## Future Perspectives

The development of a safe, effective, affordable vaccine for HIV/AIDS is one of the greatest challenges of our time. SIV will inevitably play an important role in instructing what is needed for protective immunity and how best to make a vaccine. Because SIVs are the closest known relatives of HIVs, the induction of AIDS in macaques by infectious molecular clones of SIV represents the best existing animal model for AIDS. SHIV infections are also extensively used in vaccine development because it allows for the analysis of HIV-1 envelope-containing vaccine products in an established system. Vaccine studies in animal models are vitally important as they provide useful information in several different ways. Head-to-head comparisons of different vaccine approaches can be performed to investigate which approach is more effective, at least within defined experimental conditions. Further, more in-depth analyses of specific vaccine approaches may also provide fundamental insights into what is needed to establish persistent, protective immunity to SIV and/or HIV infection. The worldwide crisis of HIV infection and AIDS has brought attention to the SIV system as a source of information that will shed light on the human condition. SIV as an animal model can contribute to further understanding of the most critical issues for future progress, including better understanding of pathogenesis, improvements in therapy and, most importantly, the development of a safe, effective, and affordable vaccine.

## Further Reading

Campbell RSF and Robinson WF (1998) The comparative pathology of lentiviruses. *Journal of Comparative Pathology* 119: 333–395.

Courgnaud V, Formenty P, Akoua-Koffi C, *et al.* (2003) Partial molecular characterization of two simian immunodeficiency viruses (SIV) from African colobids: SIVwrc from Western Red Colobus (*Piliocolobus badius*) and SIVolc from Olive Colobus (*Procolobus verus*). *Journal of Virology* 77: 744–748.

Daniel MD, Letvin NL, King NW, *et al.* (1985) Isolation of T-cell tropic HTLV-III-like retrovirus from macaques. *Science* 228: 1201–1204.

Desrosiers RC (2001) Nonhuman Lentiviruses. In: Knipe DM and Howley PM (eds.) *Fields Virology*, 4th edn., pp. 2095–2122. Philadelphia, PA: Lippincott Williams and Wilkins.

Desrosiers RC (2004) Prospects for an AIDS vaccine. *Nature Medicine* 5: 723–725.

Johnson WE and Desrosiers RC (2002) Viral persistence: HIV's strategies of immune system evasion. *Annual Review of Medicine* 53: 499–518.

Keele BF, Van Heuverswyn F, Li Y, *et al.* (2006) Chimpanzee reservoirs of pandemic and nonpandemic HIV-1. *Science* 313: 523–526.

Kestler H, Kodama T, Ringler D, *et al.* (1990) Induction of AIDS in rhesus monkeys by molecularly cloned simian immunodeficiency virus. *Science* 248: 1109–1112.

Koff WC, Johnson PR, Watkins DI, *et al.* (2006) HIV vaccine design: Insights from live attenuated SIV vaccines. *Nature Immunology* 7: 19–23.

Peeters M, Courgnaud V, Abela B, *et al.* (2002) Risk to human health from a plethora of simian immunodeficiency viruses in primate bushmeat. *Emerging Infectious Disease* 8: 451–457.

Veazey RS, DeMaria M, Chalifoux LV, *et al.* (1998) Gastrointestinal tract as a major site of CD4+ T cell depletion and viral replication in SIV infection. *Science* 280: 427–431.

# Simian Immunodeficiency Virus: Natural Infection

**I Pandrea,** Tulane National Primate Research Center, Covington, LA, USA
**G Silvestri,** University of Pennsylvania, Philadelphia, PA, USA
**C Apetrei,** Tulane National Primate Research Center, Covington, LA, USA

## Glossary

**APOBEC** Human protein superfamily that interferes with the HIV/SIV replication. This family of proteins has cytidine deaminase activity and has been suggested to play an important role in innate antiviral immunity.

**Catarrhines** Relating to or being any of a division of primates (*Catarrhina*) comprising the Old World monkeys, great apes, and hominids that have nostrils close together and directed downward, 32 teeth, and a tail, when present, which is never prehensile.

**Chemokine receptors** Family of approximately 20 different G-protein-coupled receptors that have seven transmembrane segment polypeptides, and which cause cell activation. Each receptor subtype is capable of binding multiple chemokines within the same family.

**Endemic** (1) Natural to or characteristic of a specific place; native; indigenous. (2) A disease which persists in a given population or locality.

**Giant cell disease** Pathologic condition specific for nonhuman primates with severe immunodeficiency characterized by infiltration with syncytial cells in multiple tissues.

**Guenon** An Old World monkey native to sub-Saharan Africa; possesses a round head with beard, and 'whiskers' at side of face; slender, with long hind legs and tail; some species with colorful coats.

**Sympatric** Of two or more population or taxa, inhabiting the same geographic area.

## Introduction

More than 40 different types of simian immunodeficiency viruses (SIVs) naturally infect different species of monkeys and apes. Two of these, SIVcpz, which naturally infects chimpanzees, and SIVsmm, which naturally infects sooty mangabeys (SMs), are the ancestors of HIV-1 and HIV-2, respectively. Inadvertent cross-species transmission of SIVsmm from naturally infected SMs to different species of macaques resulted in severe immunodeficiency and subsequent development of the animal models for AIDS. Unlike HIV/SIV infection of humans and macaques, which normally progresses to AIDS, natural SIV infection is generally nonpathogenic in African nonhuman primates (NHPs). The mechanisms behind this lack of disease progression are currently under investigation.

## History

The history of SIVs began two decades prior to virus discovery, when two outbreaks of opportunistic infections and lymphoma occurred in rhesus macaques (RMs) (1968) and in stump-tailed macaques (1973) at the California National Primate Research Center (CNPRC). SIVmac was discovered in 1985, during another outbreak of lymphomas in RMs at the New England Primate Research Center from monkeys transferred from CNPRC. However, occurrence of SIV infection in macaques was perplexing since tests carried out on RMs in Asia failed to reveal any evidence of SIV circulation in the wild. In 1986, at the Tulane National Primate Research Center, attempts to transmit leprosy from SMs to RMs resulted in a new AIDS outbreak in RMs, establishing the link between pathogenic SIVs in macaques and an African monkey species. During the following 20 years, more than 40 SIVs were identified in different African NHP species.

SIVsmm is also the ancestor of HIV-2. At least eight cross-species transmissions in West Africa resulted in the emergence of the eight HIV-2 groups (AH). In 1989, the discovery of SIVcpz in chimpanzees from Gabon identified the ancestor of HIV-1. At least three cross-species transmissions were at the origin of HIV-1 groups M, N, and O. Groups M and N resulted from cross-species transmission of SIVcpz from *Pan troglodytes troglodytes* in West-Central Africa. Group O is more closely related to the recently discovered SIVgor from *Gorilla gorilla*.

The arguments to support cross-species transmission from NHPs as the origin of HIVs are: (1) similarities in viral genome organization; (2) phylogenetic relatedness; (3) prevalence in the natural host; (4) geographic coincidence; and (5) plausible routes of transmission. All these criteria are fulfilled by both SIVsmm/HIV-2 and SIVcpz+SIVgor/HIV-1. Therefore, the discovery of SIVs in African species identified the origin of HIVs. However, the events behind HIV emergence are still under debate. Some authors consider that human exposure to SIVs through bush meat consumption is the original source of AIDS ('cut-hunter theory'). Others believe that simian exposure is necessary but insufficient for HIV emergence as a human pathogen, which requires adaptation to the new human host. Reuse of needles and syringes or transfusions may have played a role in triggering SIV adaptation to humans. It is probable that deforestation, political unrest, increase in urbanization and travel in the second half of the twentieth century also acted as cofactors of HIV emergence. Altogether, the action of these factors explain why HIVs only emerged in the second half of the twentieth century while people in sub-Saharan Africa were exposed to SIVs for millennia.

## Virology

Currently, there are 47 fully sequenced SIV genomes from 21 NHP species. Partial genomic sequences are available for 13 additional SIVs, and serological evidence only of SIV infection has been obtained for seven primates (**Table 1**). Asian species of Old World monkeys (colobine and macaques), as well as some African species (such as baboons) do not carry a species-specific SIV, suggesting that the last common ancestor of the catarrhines (Old World monkeys and apes) was not SIV-infected 25 million years ago and that SIV emerged after species radiation, from a nonprimate source.

### Classification and Taxonomy

In most instances, the infected NHP species represents the reservoir of that virus type, which is designated by a three-letter abbreviation of the vernacular name of the host (**Table 1**). When related NHP subspecies are infected,

**Table 1**    African apes and monkeys infected with SIV

| Species/ subspecies | Virus type | Geographic location[a] | Seroprevalence | Pathogenicity | Cross-species transmission |
|---|---|---|---|---|---|
| Common chimp (*Pan troglodytes troglodytes*) | SIVcpz.Ptt | Central Africa (Cameroon, Gabon, Congo) | <10% | Not reported | Humans, HIV-1 groups M and N *P. t. velerosus* |
| Eastern chimp (*Pan troglodytes schweinfurthii*) | SIVcpz.Pts | East Africa (Tanzania, Democratic Republic of Congo-DRC) | <10% | Thrombocytopenia | Not reported |
| Pan troglodytes velerosus | SIVcpz.Ptt[b] | Zoo in Cameroon | | Not reported | |
| Gorilla gorilla | SIVgor | West-Central Africa (Cameroon) | ? | Not reported | Humans, HIV-1 group O |
| Sooty mangabey (*Cercocebus atys*) | SIVsmm | West Africa (Sierra Leone, Liberia, Ivory Coast) | 20–58% | AIDS | Humans, HIV-2 Experimentally to *M. mulatta* (SIVmac), *M. nemestrina* (SIVptm), *M. fascicularis* and *M. arctoides* (SIVstm): AIDS. Accidentally to *L. aterrimus* (AIDS) |
| Red-capped mangabey (*Cercocebus torquatus*) | SIVrcm | West-Central Africa (Gabon, Cameroon, Nigeria) | 10–20% | Not reported | Agile mangabey Experimentally, to *Macaca mulatta* and *M. fascicularis* (no AIDS) |
| Agile mangabey (*Cercocebus agilis*) | SIVagi | West-Central Africa (Cameroon) | 0–10% | Not reported | Not reported |
| White-crowned mangabey (*Cercocebus lunulatus*) | SIVagm.ver[b] | Zoo in Tanzania | | Not reported | |
| Gray-crested mangabey (*Lophocebus albigena*) | ? | Central Africa | ? | ? | ? |
| Black mangabey (*Lophocebus aterrimus*) | SIVbkm | Central Africa (DRC) | Not known | Not reported | Not reported |
| Mandrill (*Mandrillus sphinx*) | SIVmnd-1 | Central Africa (Gabon) | 50% | AIDS in captivity | Not reported |
| | SIVmnd-2 | West-Central Africa (Cameroon, Gabon) | 50% | AIDS in captivity | Experimentally, to *M. mulatta* (transient infection) |
| Drill (*Mandrillus leucophaeus*) | SIVdrl | West-Central Africa (Nigeria, Cameroon, Gabon, Bioko) | Not known | Not reported | Not reported |
| Yellow baboon (*Papio cynocephalus*) | SIVagm.ver[c] | Tanzania | Not known | Not reported | Not reported |
| Chacma baboon (*Papio ursinus*) | SIVagm.ver[c] | South Africa | Not known | Not reported | Not reported |
| Allen's monkey (*Allenopithecus nigroviridis*) | ? | Central Africa | ? | ? | ? |
| Talapoin (*Miopithecus talapoin*, *M. ougouensis*) | SIVtal | Central Africa (Gabon, Angola, Cameroon) | 11% | Not reported | Transient infection in Rh upon experimental transmission |

Continued

**Table 1**    Continued

| Species/ subspecies | Virus type | Geographic location[a] | Seroprevalence | Pathogenicity | Cross-species transmission |
|---|---|---|---|---|---|
| Patas (*Erythrocebus patas*) | SIVagm.ver[c] | West Africa | Not known | Not reported | Not reported |
| Grivet (*Chlorocebus aethiops*) | SIVagm.gri | East Africa | >50% | Not reported | Not reported |
| Vervet (*Chlorocebus pygerythrus*) | SIVagm.ver | East and South Africa | >50% | AIDS in a monkey co-infected with STLV | Naturally, to baboons in the wild and white-crowned mangabeys in captivity; Experimentally, to *M. nemestrina* (AIDS) and *M. mulatta* (transient infection) |
| Tantalus (*Chlorocebus tantalus*) | SIVagm.tan | Central Africa | >50% | Not reported | Not reported |
| Sabaeus (*Chlorocebus sabaeus*) | SIVagm.sab | West Africa | >60% | Not reported | Naturally transmitted to patas (No AIDS); experimentally transmitted to Rh (no AIDS) |
| Diana (*Cercopithecus diana*) | ? | West-Central Africa | ? | ? | ? |
| Greater spot-nosed monkey (*Cercopithecus nictitans*) | SIVgsn | Central Africa | 4–20% | Not reported | Potential source virus for SIVcpz |
| Blue monkey (*Cercopithecus mitis*) | SIVblu | Central-East Africa | >60% | Not reported | Not reported |
| Syke's monkey (*Cercopithecus albogularis*) | SIVsyk | East Africa | 30–60% | Not reported | Experimentally, to *M. mulatta* (transient infection) |
| Mona (*Cercopithecus mona*) | SIVmon | West-Central Africa (Cameroon, Nigeria) | Not known | Not reported | Not reported |
| Dent's mona (*Cercopithecus denti*) | SIVden | Central Africa | 10% | | |
| Crested mona (*Cercopithecus pogonias*) | ? | West Africa | ? | ? | ? |
| Campbell's mona (*Cercopithecus campbelli*) | ? | West Africa | ? | ? | ? |
| Lowe's mona (*Cercopithecus lowei*) | ? | West Africa | ? | ? | ? |
| Mustached monkey (*Cercopithecus cephus*) | SIVmus | Central Africa | 3% | Not reported | Potential source virus for SIVcpz |
| Red-tailed monkey (*Cercopithecus ascanius*) | SIVasc/ SIVschm | Central Africa (DRC) | Not known | Not reported | Not reported |
| Red-eared monkeys (*Cercopithecus erythrotis*) | SIVery | Central Africa (Bioko) | Not known | Not reported | Not reported |

Continued

**Table 1**   Continued

| Species/ subspecies | Virus type | Geographic location[a] | Seroprevalence | Pathogenicity | Cross-species transmission |
|---|---|---|---|---|---|
| De Brazza's monkey (*Cercopithecus neglectus*) | SIVdeb | West-Central and Central Africa | 40% | Not reported | Not reported |
| Owl-faced monkey (*Cercopithecus hamlyni*) | ? | Central Africa | ? | ? | ? |
| L'Hoest's monkey (*Cercopithecus lhoesti*) | SIVlhoest/ SIVlho | East Africa | 50% | Not reported | Experimentally, to *M. nemestrina* (AIDS) |
| Sun-tailed monkey (*Cercopithecus solatus*) | SIVsun | Central Africa | Not known | Not reported | Source virus for SIVmnd-1; Experimentally, to *M. nemestrina* (AIDS); Experimentally, to *M. fascicularis* (transient infection); |
| Preuss's monkey (*Cercopithecus preussi*) | SIVpre | Central Africa (Bioko) | Not known | Not reported | Not reported |
| Mantled colobus (*Colobus guereza*) | SIVcol | Central Africa | 28% | Not reported | Not reported |
| Western Red colobus (*Piliocolobus badius*) | SIVwrc | West Africa | 40% | Not reported | Not reported |
| Olive colobus (*Procolobus verus*) | SIVolc | West Africa | 40% | Not reported | Not reported |

[a]Countries listed correspond to reported evidences of SIV circulation in that NHP species and not to species distribution.
[b]Cross-species transmission in captivity.
[c]Cross-species transmission in the wild.

the subspecies name is included in virus designation. Thus, for chimpanzee subspecies infected by SIVs, the two SIVcpz are identified as SIVcpz.Ptt (from *Pan troglodytes troglodytes*) and SIVcpz.Pts (from *P. t. schwenfurthii*). For individual isolates, nomenclature includes SIV type and the country of origin: SIVrcmGB1 is a red-capped magabey virus isolated from Gabon. The year of sample can also be included: SIVsmmSL92 is an SM virus isolated from Sierra Leone in 1992. This feature is useful in tracking the origin and evolution of viruses.

## Phylogenetic Relationships

SIVs have a starburst phylogenetic pattern, suggesting the evolution from a single ancestor, and a high genetic divergence, forming six SIV lineages with genetic distances of up to 40% in Pol proteins (**Table 2** and **Figure 1**). Each SIV lineage is represented by two or more strains. The l'hoesti lineage is unique in being formed by SIVs circulating in distantly related species. The relationship between SIV lineages and newly characterized SIVs is complicated by sequence diversity and recombination

that results in different clustering patterns when different genomic regions are analyzed.

To better understand SIV phylogenetic relationships, a brief presentation of primate species radiation follows. African NHPs belong to two different groups: Old World monkeys and anthropoid primates (apes). Two ape genera are endemic in Africa: *Pan* (formed by the four subspecies of chimpanzees and bonobo) and *Gorilla*. The Old World monkeys (family *Cercopithecidae*) are divided into two subfamilies (*Cercopithecinae* and *Colobinae*), separated 11 million years ago (**Figure 1**). *Cercopithecinae* are divided into two tribes: Papionini (mangabeys (*Cercocebus* and *Lophocebus*), baboons (*Papio*), mandrills and drills (*Mandrillus*), gelada (*Theropithecus*), and the Asian genus, *Macaca*) and Cercopithecini (25 species in 3 arboreal genera: *Allenopithecus*, *Miopithecus*, and *Cercopithecus*, and three terrestrial genera: *Erythrocebus*, *Chlorocebus*, and *Cercopithecus lhoesti* supergroup).

The approximate equidistance among the major SIV lineages does not always match the relationships among their hosts (**Figure 1**). Thus, terrestrial monkeys form a single clade indicating that the evolutionary transition

**Table 2**    SIV clusters based upon phylogenetic relationships

| Cluster | Species | SIV strain | Comments |
|---------|---------|------------|----------|
| 1 | Arboreal guenons (*Cercopithecus*) | SIVsyk, SIVblu, SIVgsn, SIVdeb, SIVmon, SIVden, SIVmus, SIVasc, SIVtal, SIVery | Ancestral source of SIVcpz/SIVgor/HIV-1 (SIVgsn, SIVmon, SIVmus, and SIVden harbor a *vpu* gene); lineage formed by all arboreal guenons; partial sequences from SIVbkm from the black mangabey cluster in this lineage |
| 2 | Sooty mangabey | SIVsmm | Ancestral virus of SIVmac/HIV-2; SMs from Ivory Coast harbor SIVsmm strains related to the epidemic HIV-2 groups A and B; those from Sierra Leone are the sources of HIV-2 groups C-H |
| 3 | African Green Monkey | SIVagm (SIVagm.ver, SIVagm.tan, SIVrcm.gri, SIVagm.sab) | Four different SIV subtypes described for each species in the genus *Chlorocebus*, suggesting host-dependent evolution; SIVagm.sab is a recombinant between an SIVagm ancestor and a SIVrcm-like virus |
| 4 | L'Hoest supergroup, mandrill | SIVlhoest, SIVsun, SIVmnd-1, SIVpre | Host-dependent evolution for monkeys in the C.l'hoesti supergroup; cross-species transmission from solatus guenon to mandrills |
| 5 | Red-capped Mangabeys | SIVrcm, SIVagi | Originally considered recombinants, now appear to be 'pure' viruses; SIVagi is cross-species transmitted from RCMs |
| 6 | Mantled colobus | SIVcol | First virus isolated from *Colbinae*; other viruses from Western colobus species do not cluster with SIVcol |

between arboreality and terrestriality has occurred only once among the extinct lineages. However, each of the terrestrial genera are infected with specific viral lineages. Arboreal guenons are infected with a cluster of viruses sharing biological properties and structural features. Papionini monkeys are infected with related viruses, though a higher proportion of recombinant viruses can be observed in these monkeys.

## Genome Organization and Composition

SIVs have a complex genomic structure with three structural genes – *gag* (group antigen gene), *pol* (polymerase), and *env* (envelope) – and several accessory genes whose number varies in different SIVs. The accessory genes *vif* (virus infectivity factor), *tat* (transcriptional *trans*-activator), and *rev* are facilitators of viral transcription and activation; *tat* and *rev* each consists of two exons; *nef* induces CD4 and class I downregulation. Three accessory genes are specific for primate lentiviruses: *vpr*, *vpx*, and *vpu*. All primate lentiviruses harbor *vif*, *rev*, *tat*, *vpr*, and *nef*. The presence of *vpx* and *vpu* is variable and defines three patterns of genomic organization (**Figure 2**): (1) SIVsyk, SIVasc, SIVdeb, SIVblu, SIVtal, SIVagm, SIVmnd-1, SIVlhoest, SIVsun, and SIVcol contain no *vpx* or *vpu*; (2) Papionini viruses, SIVsmm, SIVmac, SIVstm, SIVrcm, SIVmnd-2, SIVdrl together with HIV-2 harbor a *vpx* gene, acquired following a nonhomologous recombination and duplication of the *vpr*, and (3) SIVcpz, SIVgor, SIVgsn, SIVmus, SIVmon, SIVden together with HIV-1 encode a *vpu* gene. *vpu* first appeared in cercopithecines, which appear to be the reservoir for viruses in the SIVcpz/HIV-1 lineage. SIVblu, SIVolc, SIVwrc, SIVbkm, SIVery,

and SIVagi have not yet been completely sequenced; therefore, their classifications are pending.

## SIV Recombination

Virus substrain recombination is a hallmark of SIVs and represents an important intrinsic mechanism other than rapidly accumulating point mutations for developing strains adapted to evade host defense mechanisms or for cross-species transmission. The most critical recombination of SIVs appears to be that involving SIVgsn/mon/mus and SIVrcm which resulted in the origin of the chimpanzee SIVcpz. Subsequent cross-species transmission from chimpanzees to humans is the root cause of the HIV/AIDS pandemic. Other recombinant SIVs include SIVagm.sab (containing SIVrcm-like fragments) and SIVmnd-2/SIVdrl (mosaic between SIVrcm and SIVmnd-1).

## Host Range

Typically, SIVs are restricted to their host species (species-specific). However, cross-species transmissions can occur as rare events, the most notable of which were those of SIVrcm and SIVgsn/mon/mus to chimpanzees to generate SIVcpz and those of SIVcpz and SIVsmm to humans to generate HIV-1 and HIV-2, respectively. Macaque exposure to SIVsmm, SIVagm, SIVsun, and SIVlho resulted in persistent infection and induced AIDS. In the wild, SIVagm has been isolated from a yellow baboon (*Papio cynocephalus*), a chacma baboon (*P. ursinus*), and patas monkey (*Erythrocebus patas*). In captivity, in Kenya, SIVagm.ver was transmitted to a white-crowned mangabey (*Cercocebus lunulatus*). None of these recipient

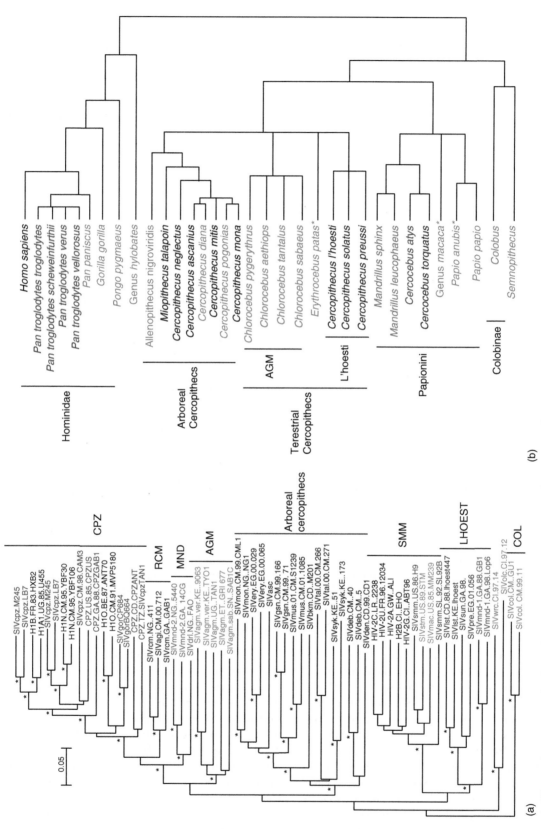

**Figure 1** Comparison between SIV phylogeny (a) and primate phylogeny (b). Neighbor-joining tree constructed from available SIV sequences (a); primate phylogeny is a schematic using relationships cited in the text (b). While general alignment of host vs. virus can be observed, cross-species transmissions and viral recombination events make this correlation less than absolute. Asterisks indicate significant bootstrap values. Adapted from VandeWoude S and Apetrei C (2006) Going wild: Lessons from T-lymphotropic naturally occurring lentiviruses. *Reviews in Clinical Microbiology Reviews* 19: 728–762, with permission from American Society for Microbiology.

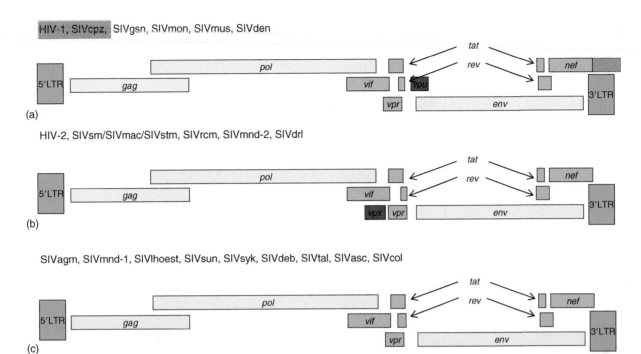

**Figure 2** Genomic organization of the SIV strains belonging to different genomic types. SIV classification based on genomic structures is not superimposable on phylogenetic relationships. For references, see **Table 1**. Adapted from VandeWoude S and Apetrei C (2006) Going wild: Lessons from T-lymphotropic naturally occurring lentiviruses. *Reviews in Clinical Microbiolology Reviews* 19: 728–762, with permission from American Society for Microbiology.

species have been reported to date to carry a specific SIV, which may explain the higher susceptibility to cross-species transmitted infection. It is not known if SIVagm is endemic or pathogenic in these species. SIVmnd-1 also resulted from cross-species transmission of SIVsun from sympatric *Cercopithecus lhoesti solatus*. The reasons for success of cross-species transmission infections, and the factors necessary for infection to result in pathogenicity, have not been clearly delineated.

## Coreceptor Usage

Similar to HIV-1, SIVs use CD4 as the binding receptor, and chemokine co-receptors such as CCR5 and CXCR4. Most of the SIVs naturally infecting African NHPs use CCR5 as the main co-receptor. Different from HIV-1, for which a switch in viral tropism from R5 ('macrophage' tropic) to X4 ('lymphocyte' tropic) occurs with disease progression, no correlation between co-receptor usage and pathogenesis *in vivo* can be established for SIVs. SIVmnd-1, SIVagm.sab and some strains of SIVsmm use CXCR4, with no pathologic consequence. Experimental infection of sabeaus AGMs with SIVagm.sab (an X4/R5 virus) did not show a particular pattern of viral replication or disease progression. SIVrcm uses the CCR2b co-receptor for viral entry as a consequence of a 24-bp deletion in the CCR5 gene. As such, this example illustrates selected viral evolution, similar to CXCR4 infection of humans who possess the delta-32 mutation in the CCR5 gene.

## Diagnosis

### Antibody Detection

Serology is the gold standard for studying the prevalence of SIVs in NHPs. Commercial HIV-1/HIV-2 enzyme-linked immunosorbent assay (ELISA) and Western blot assays can be used for anti-SIV antibody screening in NHPs due to cross-reactivity with other lentiviral lineages. For a more sensitive detection of SIVs, two strategies are available: use of a highly sensitive line assay (INNO-LIA HIV, Innogenetics) as a screening test; more than 10 different new SIV types have been identified using this strategy. Alternatively, the use of SIV-specific synthetic peptides allows for increased sensitivity (Gp41/36 peptide) and specificity (V3 peptides); several SIVs have been discovered using this technique.

### Propagation and Assay in Cell Culture

The efficiency of *in vitro* isolation of SIVs varies widely. The ability to replicate in human PBMC or T-cell lines has been documented for SIVcpz, SIVsm/SIVmac, SIVagm, SIVlhoest, SIVmnd-1, SIVrcm, SIVmnd-2, and SIVdrl and constitutes the major argument for the threat that these viruses may pose for humans (**Table 3**). SIVs' ability to infect human macrophages has also been reported for SIVsmm, SIVagm, and SIVmnd. SIVsun and SIVsyk cannot replicate in human peripheral blood mononuclear cells (PBMCs) or macrophages. SIVagm replication in human

**Table 3**  Host range of *in vitro* replication SIV in different blood subsets and human T-cell lines

| Growth support | Cell description | SIVcpz | SIVsm | SIVmac | SIVagm | SIVlhoest | SIVsun | SIVmnd-1 | SIVsyk | SIVtal | SIVrcm | SIVmnd-2 | SIVdrl |
|---|---|---|---|---|---|---|---|---|---|---|---|---|---|
| human PBMC[a] | | + | + | + | +± | + | − | + | − | − | + | + | + |
| human MDM[b] | | − | + | + | +± | + | − | − | − | − | +± | | |
| macaque PBMC | | | ± | + | | | | | − | − | − | + | + |
| chimpanzee PBMC | | + | − | + | | + | | + | − | | | | |
| MT2 | T-cell line | | | | | − | − | | | | | − | − |
| C8166 | T-cell line | | ± | + | + | + | + | | | − | | | − |
| H9 | Cloned from Hut78 | | + | + | + | − | − | | | − | + | | − |
| MT4 | T-cell line | | | − | − | + | + | | | | + | + | + |
| U937 | Promonocytic cell line | | | − | + | − | − | | | | | | − |
| SupT1 | T-cell line | | +± | + | − | + | + | | + | − | + | + | + |
| PM1 | | | +± | − | | − | − | | | | + | | − |
| Hut78 | T-cell line | | + | | + | − | − | | | | − | | + |
| Molt 4 Clone 8 | T-cell line | ++ | − | | − | + | + | | − | − | | + | ++ |
| CEMss | T-cell line | ++ | | | + | + | + | | | | − | − | ++ |
| CEMx174 | T-cell–B-cell hybrid line | + | + | + | − | + | − | | ++ | + | − | + | + |

[a]PBMC-peripheral blood mononuclear cells.
[b]MDM-monocyte-derived macrophages.

PBMCs is strain specific. SIVmnd-1 was reported to replicate in human PBMCs but not in macrophages. Some SIVs might require special culture conditions.

## Epidemiology

### Prevalence in the Wild

Due to their number, genetic diversity, and large distribution in sub-Saharan Africa, guenons (tribe Cercopithecini) are the largest reservoir species for SIV. SIV prevalence is high (50–60%) in some monkey species (AGMs, SMs, mandrills, l'Hoest and Syke's monkeys) and significantly lower (4–5%) in others (greater spotted nose monkeys, mustached monkeys, or agile mangabeys). Only two chimpanzee subspecies and one of gorilla were reported to carry SIVs at low prevalence levels. Geographical foci of SIVcpz infection were defined within the endemic area. The highest SIVcpz prevalence was observed in Cameroon (10%), in agreement with HIV-1 emergence in that area. The SIVgor strains also originated from Cameroon. No evidence of SIV infection was thus far reported for some African species, most notably baboons and some species of mangabeys.

### Modes of Transmission

Epidemiologic patterns of SIV seroconversion in natural hosts showed the most efficient virus transmission during adult contact, similar to HIV-1, which is spread by sexual contact via primarily mucosal exposure. Horizontal transmission also occurs by biting or aggressive contact for dominance. While maternal to offspring transmission has been reported, it is relatively rare compared to horizontal transmissions.

## Pathogenesis and Pathology

### Pathogenicity of Natural SIV Infection

For 20 years, it was believed that natural SIV infections were nonpathogenic. This was a major paradox given the context of an active viral replication and high prevalence levels. However, occasionally, natural SIV infection of mandrills, AGMs, and SMs may eventually lead to the development of immunodeficiency. Cases of progression to AIDS in African NHP hosts are rare, possibly because host↔virus adaptation has occurred, resulting in a long-term persistent infection with an incubation period that exceeds the normal life span of the naturally infected animal.

AIDS was also reported to develop in African NHPs after infection with heterologous viruses (an SIVsmm-infected black mangabey, HIV-2-infected baboons, and a subset of HIV-1-infected chimpanzees). In these cases, disease progression occurred earlier than in naturally infected African NHP hosts, and the outcome of cross-species transmitted SIV infections varied widely, with some animals clearing the cross-species transmitted SIV, others being persistently infected (albeit without disease progression) and the rest progressing to AIDS.

### Cell and Tissue Tropism

Upon infection, SIVs are disseminated to tissues by the blood. The target cells are CD4+ T lymphocytes and macrophages, with lymphocytes vastly predominating in terms of infected cells. The major sites of SIV replication are the gastrointestinal tract, lymph nodes (LNs), spleen, and other lymphoid tissues. Natural hosts for SIV infection (SMs, AGMs, mandrills, and chimpanzees) express lower levels of CCR5 on CD4+ T cells in blood and mucosal tissues, compared to immunodeficiency-susceptible hosts (macaques, baboons, and humans). Moreover, chimpanzees, which are more recent hosts of SIV, show an intermediate level of CD4+ CCR5+ T cells. As CCR5 is the main co-receptor for SIVs, African species with endemic naturally occurring SIVs may be less susceptible to pathogenic disease because they have fewer receptor-expressing targets for infection, leading to an evolutionary mechanism of 'passive co-existence' between SIV replication and natural host immune system function.

### Virus Replication *In Vivo*

The lack of disease in African NHPs is not associated with effective host containment of viral replication, this is in contrast to HIV/SIV pathogenic infections for which levels of plasma viral loads (VLs) are the best predictor of the disease progression. Experimental SIV infections in natural hosts (SMs, AGMs, and mandrills) showed a consistent pattern of SIV replication with a peak of viremia ($10^6$–$10^9$ copies per ml of plasma) occurring around days 9–11 post infection, followed by a sharp decline (1–2 logs) and attainment of a stable level of VL (set point), which is maintained at high levels ($10^5$–$10^6$ copies per ml of plasma) during chronic infection (**Figure 3**). Experimental data were confirmed in naturally SIV-infected African NHPs, where chronic VLs were higher than in HIV-1 chronically infected asymptomatic patients and remained relatively constant over years. Some species-specific differences in viral replication between different African NHP species can occur without significant pathogenic consequences: SIV VLs are generally lower in AGMs than in other African NHP species. SIV proviral loads in the LNs are also 100-fold lower in AGMs than in naturally infected SMs or MNDs.

### Immune Response and Persistence

Acute SIV infection in the natural host induces massive mucosal CD4+ T-cell depletion, of the same magnitude

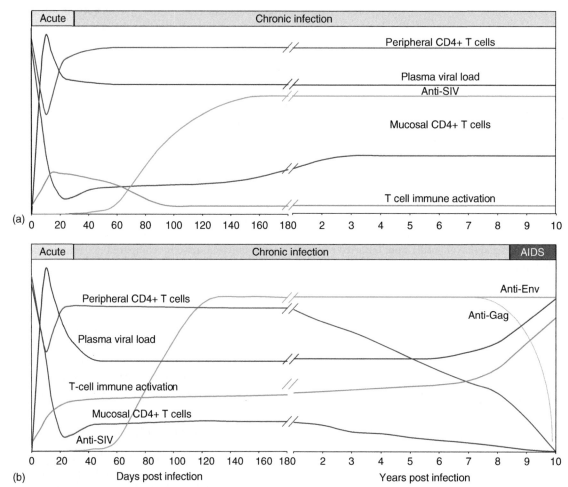

**Figure 3**  Pathogenesis of SIV infection in natural hosts (a) compared to the pathogenesis of HIV-1 infection (b). No significant difference can be observed between the two models during acute infection. During chronic SIV infection, natural hosts harbor higher viral loads, lower antibody titers, lower levels of T-cell immune activation. CD4+ T-cell levels are maintained at near pre-infection levels in natural hosts. Mucosal CD4+ T cells are partially restored during chronic infection, despite high levels of viral replication. Progression to AIDS is absent in most cases, being a rare outcome of SIV natural infection.

as in pathogenic HIV/SIV infection. However, during chronic infection, in spite of persistent high viral replication, there is a partial immune restoration of CD4+ T-cells in natural hosts, probably as a consequence of the preservation of a mucosal immunologic barrier and normal levels of immune activation. In marked contrast to HIV infection, in which a failure of the lymphoid regenerative capacity is an important factor in the pathogenesis of the immunodeficiency, the regenerative capacity of the CD4+ T-cell compartment is fully preserved in natural hosts and may play a key role in determining the lack of disease progression. Interleukin-7 (IL-7) has a critical role in preserving T-cell regeneration and in avoiding CD4+ T-cell depletion and disease progression in natural infections.

The high level of viral replication during chronic SIV infection in natural hosts is associated with low level of immunologic pressure, T-cell activation and proliferation, and apoptosis, resulting in limited bystander pathology. Thus, natural hosts of SIV are not confronted with the massive tissue destruction observed in HIV-1/SIVmac infection. This equilibrium is probably disrupted after cross-species transmission of viruses, when virus penetrates a new ecological niche, inducing a different immune response.

In natural SIV infections, *de novo* immune responses are muted compared to pathogenic HIV/SIVmac infections that induce robust neutralizing and cellular immune responses and continuous immune escape. Therefore, it is believed that natural SIV infections are characterized by tolerance to the virus or to specific antigens or epitopes, or by immune responses that differ qualitatively and quantitatively from those observed in pathogenic infections. Antibody responses are observed in natural SIV infection, but mainly directed to Env rather than Gag, as in SIVmac infection. The intensity of the antibody response is lower in natural hosts: for equivalent VL, antibody titers in SMs are about one log lower than in RMs.

Neutralizing antibodies are rarely detected in SIV-infected SMs, while SIVagm is susceptible to neutralization depending on the cell line used in the assay. In contrast to HIV-1, SIVagm infectivity is enhanced by the addition of soluble CD4 and this enhanced infectivity can be abrogated by SIVagm-specific antibodies. However, very high amounts of passively transferred specific immunoglobulins failed to prevent SIVagm infection suggesting that humoral immune response in AGMs is largely ineffective.

SIV-infected SMs and AGMs develop cytotoxic T-lymphocyte responses that are functional to some degree in controlling viral replication. Moreover, there is evidence of transient but massive expansion of CD8+ T cells in infected AGMs, SMs, and mandrills during acute infection, showing that the immune system of natural hosts is influenced by SIV infection. It is not yet clear if CD8+ T-cell expansion results from active stimulation of the specific immune response or from a nonspecific stimulation of the immune system in general.

SIV-specific T-cell responses can be detected in the majority of naturally SIV-infected NHPs. However, their magnitude is generally lower than in HIV-infected patients. In addition, no correlation was found between breadth or magnitude of SIV-specific T-cell responses and either VLs or CD4+ T-cell counts. Moreover, the magnitude of the SIV-specific cellular responses did not appear to determine the level of T-cell activation and proliferation in SMs and AGMs. Therefore, the presence of a strong and broadly reactive T-cell response to SIV antigens is not a requirement for the lack of disease progression in natural infections; conversely, the complete suppression of SIV-specific T-cell responses (i.e., immunologic tolerance and/or ignorance) is not required for the low levels of T-cell activation that are likely instrumental in avoiding AIDS.

Both acute and chronic natural SIV infections (SMs, AGMs, and mandrills) are associated with lower levels of T-cell activation, pro-inflammatory responses, immunopathology, and bystander apoptosis than pathogenic HIV/SIV infection. In addition, natural hosts of SIV maintain T-cell regenerative capacity, with normal bone marrow morphology and function, normal levels of T-cell receptor excision circle (TREC)-expressing T cells and preserved LN architecture. This downregulation of the immune response favors preservation of CD4+ T-cell homeostasis and is completely different from pathogenic HIV/SIV infections for which chronic immune activation and proliferation drive excessive activation-induced T-cell apoptosis, and ultimately result in the collapse of the immune system and progression to AIDS. Altogether, this is consistent with the hypothesis that chronic immune activation is a major determinant of disease progression during HIV infection.

In AGMs, low immune activation levels are due to a strong anti-inflammatory response (with induction of TGF-β1 and FOXP3, and a significant increase in IL-10 expression), which occurs early in the SIVagm infection. Together with an early increase in the levels of CD4+ CD25+ T cells, this results in the rapid establishment of an anti-inflammatory environment which may prevent damages to the mucosal immunologic barrier, microbial translocation, and thus aberrant chronic T-cell hyperactivation that is correlated with progression to AIDS during HIV-1/SIVmac infection.

## Virulence

Viral factors may be related to a lack of virulence in natural SIV infections. In RMs, SIVmac *nef* gene deletion mutants were reported to replicate poorly *in vivo* and to be nonpathogenic, which corroborates the description of *nef* gene mutations of HIV-1-infected long-term progressors. Nef downregulates CD4, CD28, and the class I major histocompatibility complex, resulting in virus immune evasion. Nef may also enhance the responsiveness of T cells to activation, but this effect is not uniformly observed among SIVs. All SIVs from African monkeys have open reading frames corresponding to a functional Nef, and therefore the *nef* structure cannot account entirely for differences in pathogenicity. Nef proteins from the great majority of primate lentiviruses, including HIV-2, down-modulate T-cell receptor-CD3, which subsequently blocks T-cell activation. In contrast, Nef proteins derived from HIV-1 and closely related SIVs do not induce CD3 downregulation, which may have predisposed the simian precursor of HIV-1 to greater pathogenicity in humans. However, simian counterparts of HIV-1 (SIVcpz and SIVgsn/SIVmon/SIVmus), which do not induce CD3 downregulation, do not typically induce AIDS in their natural hosts. Further, SIVmac, which induces CD3 downregulation, is even more pathogenic in RMs than HIV-1 is in humans, suggesting that this accessory gene does not solely account for virulence.

## Clinical and Pathologic Features

In contrast to macaques in which SIV infection constantly leads to an AIDS-like disease characterized by opportunistic infections and cancers, SIV infection in natural hosts generally does not show any clinical or pathological abnormalities. During progression to AIDS, SIV-infected RMs initially develop lymphadenopathy with confluent follicular hyperplasia, followed by LN atrophy due to lymphoid depletion and fibrosis. In contrast, SIV-infected natural hosts display normal LN morphology without evidence of either hyperplasia or depletion. No follicular trapping or CD8+ T-cell infiltration of the germinal centers and no replacement of the normal LN architecture with connective tissue is observed in chronic SIV infection of natural hosts. Also, no thymic disinvolution, nodular lymphocytic infiltrates, or giant cell disease are seen in SIV-infected natural hosts. The few AIDS cases reported in African NHP hosts presented with the entire range of diseases and pathologic lesions of AIDS.

## Host Genetic Resistance

SIV species specificity has typically been ascribed to factors such as virus–host receptor compatibility and cellular machinery needed to direct viral replication. Specific host factors also prevent SIV cross-species infections *in vitro*.

### Cytidine deaminase and Vif

Vif is involved in species specificity of SIVs. Its cellular target is a member of the cytidine deaminase APOBEC family. The cellular deaminase is incorporated into the virion during the reverse transcription to direct the deamination of cytidine to uridine on the minus strand of viral DNA. Deamination results in catastrophic G-to-A mutations followed by inactivation and/or degradation of the viral genome. At least two primate APOBEC family members (APOBEC3G and APOBEC3F) play a central role in antagonizing viral replication because they are expressed in natural targets of SIVs, including lymphocytes and macrophages. Lentiviruses are able to successfully infect and replicate in host target cells containing APOBEC when host-adapted Vif interferes with this mechanism. Vif activity is species specific: human APOBEC3G is inhibited by HIV-1 Vif but not by SIVagm Vif, whereas AGM APOBEC3G is inhibited by SIVagm Vif, but not by HIV-1 Vif. This specificity relies on a single amino acid change that can alter the ability of *vif* to interfere with APOBEC activity.

### TRIM5-α

The cytoplasmic body component TRIM5-α, previously referred to as REF-1 and LV-1, restricts HIV-1 infection of monkey cells. TRIM5-α interferes with the viral uncoating step that is required to liberate viral nucleic acids into the cytoplasm upon viral binding and fusion with the target cell. Sensitivity to TRIM5-α restriction is dictated by a small region in the viral capsid gene, previously shown to be involved in cyclophilin A binding. Subtle amino acid differences in this region influence the strength of binding to TRIM5-α and, hence, relative sensitivity to its restriction. HIV-2, but not closely related SIVmac, is highly susceptible to RM TRIM5-α. Furthermore, HIV-2 is weakly restricted by human TRIM5-α, which may contribute to the lower pathogenic potential of the HIV-2 vs. HIV-1 in humans. Strategies to exploit TRIM5-α restriction for intervention of HIV-1 replication are under development.

*See also:* Host Resistance to Retroviruses; Simian Immunodeficiency Virus: Animal Models of Disease; Simian Immunodeficiency Virus: General Features.

## Further Reading

Beer BE, Bailes E, Sharp PM, and Hirsch VM (1999) Diversity and evolution of primate lentiviruses. In: Kuiken CL, Foley B, Hahn B, *et al.* (eds.) *Human Retroviruses and AIDS 1999*, pp. 460–474. Los Alamos, NM: Theoretical Biology and Biophysics Group and Los Alamos National Laboratory.

Chakrabarti LA (2004) The paradox of simian immunodeficiency virus infection in sooty mangabeys: Active viral replication without disease progression. *Frontiers in Biosciences* 9: 521–539.

Drucker E, Alcabes PG, and Marx PA (2001) The injection century: Massive unsterile injections and the emergence of human pathogens. *Lancet* 358(9297): 1989–1992.

Gordon S, Pandrea I, Dunham R, Apetrei C, and Silvestri G (2005) The call of the wild: What can be learned from studies of SIV infection of natural hosts? In: Leitner T, Foley B, Hahn B, *et al.* (eds.) *HIV Sequence Compendium 2004*, pp. 2–29. Los Alamos, NM: Theoretical Biology and Biophysics Group and Los Alamos National Laboratory.

Hirsch VM (2004) What can natural infection of African monkeys with simian immunodeficiency virus tell us about the pathogenesis of AIDS? *AIDS Reviews* 6(1): 40–53.

Muller MC and Barre-Sinoussi F (2003) SIVagm: Genetic and biological features associated with replication. *Frontiers in Biosciences* 8: D1170–D1185.

Norley S and Kurth R (2004) The role of the immune response during SIVagm infection of the African green monkey natural host. *Frontiers in Biosciences* 9: 550–564.

Sharp PM, Shaw GM, and Hahn BH (2005) Simian immunodeficiency virus infection of chimpanzees. *Journal of Virology* 79(7): 3891–3902.

VandeWoude S and Apetrei C (2006) Going wild: Lessons from T-lymphotropic naturally occurring lentiviruses. *Clinical Microbiology Reviews* 19: 728–762.

# Simian Immunodeficiency Virus: Animal Models of Disease

**C J Miller and M Marthas,** University of California, Davis, Davis, CA, USA

## Glossary

**Dysplasia** Abnormal growth of tissues, organs, or cells.
**Endemic** Prevalent in a particular group of animals or people.

**Epitope** The part of a macromolecule that is recognized by the immune system.
**Hypergammaglobulinemia** Increased blood levels of gamma globulin (IgG).

**Hyperplasia** An abnormal increase in the number of cells in an organ or a tissue with consequent enlargement.

**MHC-I (major histocompatibility complex I)** T-cell epitopes are presented on the surface of an antigen-presenting cell, where they are bound to MHC molecules. T-cell epitopes presented by MHC class I molecules are typically peptides between 8 and 11 amino acids in length, while MHC class II molecules present longer peptides, and nonclassical MHC molecules.

## Taxonomy and Discovery

Simian immunodeficiency viruses (SIVs) are members of the genus *Lentivirus* and the family *Retroviridae*. The genus *Lentivirus* includes viruses that infect ungulates (maedi-visna virus of sheep; caprine arthritis-encephalitis virus, CAEV), horses (equine infectious anemia virus, EIAV), cows (bovine immunodeficiency virus, BIV), wild and domesticated cats (feline immunodeficiency virus, FIV), nonhuman primates (NHPs; SIV), and humans (human immunodeficiency virus, HIV). All retroviruses are spherical, 80–100 nm in diameter, and have a diploid, single-stranded RNA genome and viral enzymes inside a viral protein case, or core, which is enveloped by a host cell membrane studded with viral glycoproteins. The diploid genome of single-stranded RNA is linked noncovalently near the 5′ end of the molecules. The 5′ end of the viral RNA is capped and the 3′ end is polyadenylated. DNA synthesis by the viral encoded reverse transcriptase (RT) is primed by host tRNA that is base-paired to the viral RNA. The double-stranded DNA provirus is integrated into the host chromosomes by a viral encoded integrase and the remaining events in transcription, translation, and assembly are host cell dependent. Depending on the cell type infected, particles assemble and bud through the plasma membrane or into membrane-lined intracytoplasmic vesicles. The morphological feature that distinguishes lentiviruses from other retroviruses is the cone or rod shape of the viral core protein in a mature virion.

SIV$_{mac}$ was the first member of the group to be identified following isolation of a retrovirus from a captive rhesus macaque housed at a US primate center. Apparently, the virus was introduced into captive macaque populations in the US during experiments into the transmission of kuru and leprosy, at which time material derived from tissue of SIV-infected African monkeys was deliberately introduced into Asian macaques. SIV has been eliminated from captive populations of macaques in the US through a rigorous testing program. Fortunately, serology provides an effective and economical tool for screening for infection. Extended quarantine periods and regular serologic testing programs are rigorously applied to maintain the SIV-free status of captive macaque colonies.

## Nomenclature and Classification of Primate Lentiviruses

Primate lentiviruses are classified as originating in NHPs (SIVs) or humans (HIVs). SIVs are given specific names based on the NHP species from which they are isolated, for example, SIV$_{cpz}$ was isolated from chimpanzees and SIV$_{deb}$ from De Brazza's monkeys.

Recently, a hierarchical nomenclature has been developed to describe the high level of genetic diversity found among the many HIV isolates. HIV is first divided into two broad types, designated HIV-1 and HIV-2. Both HIV types are subdivided into groups consisting of phylogenetically similar viruses that resulted from different nonhuman-primate–human SIV transmission events (**Figures 1** and **2**). Within a group, phylogenetic clusters of viruses are termed subtypes. There is a movement toward a unified, standard nomenclature to describe genetic diversity within and among SIVs in which a three-letter abbreviation of the vernacular name of the NHP species is used (**Figure 3**). For example, the SIV from chimpanzees is termed SIV$_{cpz}$ and subspecies designation is provided a three-letter abbreviation – thus SIV$_{cpz.Ptt}$ is derived from *Pan troglodytes troglodytes*. SIVs of African green monkeys (SIV$_{agm}$) are divided into four subtypes, each named for the African green monkey subspecies from which it was isolated (**Figure 3**).

## Genome Organization

Like all retroviruses, lentivirus genomes contain long terminal repeats (LTRs) at each end and genes encoding three virion structural components: core (*gag*), polymerase (*pol*), and envelope (*env*). In addition, all primate lentivirus genomes also contain five accessory genes: *vif, vpr, rev, tat,* and *nef*. The genomes of a subset of primate lentiviruses have one of two unique genes: *vpr* or *vpu*. Three types of genomic structure are observed for primate lentiviruses (**Figure 4**). Group A includes SIVs only from African NHPs; these SIVs cause no disease in the host species from which the SIV was isolated: SIV$_{agm}$, SIV$_{syk}$, SIV$_{lhoest}$, SIV$_{mnd-1}$, SIV$_{sun}$, and SIV$_{col}$ (A, **Figure 4**). SIVs in group A all have the basic primate lentivirus genome structure, which contains only five accessory genes. Group B includes HIV-2 and SIVs most closely related to HIV-2 (SIV$_{sm}$, SIV$_{mac}$, SIV$_{rcm}$, and SIV$_{mnd-2}$); each group B virus has a *vpx* gene which is absent in the Group A viruses (B, **Figure 4**). Group C viruses include HIV-1, SIV$_{cpz}$, and other SIVs with a *vpu* gene, but lacking *vpx* (SIV$_{gsn}$, SIV$_{mon}$, and SIV$_{mus}$; C, **Figure 4**).

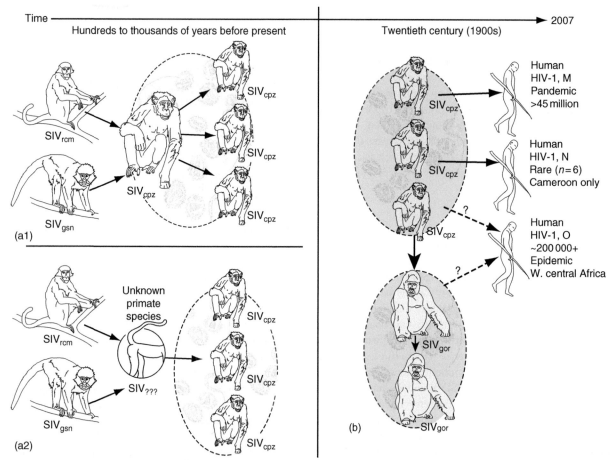

**Figure 1**   Origin of HIV-1 inferred from phylogenetic analyses of SIV and HIV-1 genomes. (a) The earliest event is transmission of SIVs from African monkeys (red-capped mangabey (RCM) infected with SIV ($SIV_{rcm}$) and greater spot nose monkey (GSN) infected with SIV ($SIV_{gsn}$)) to chimpanzees followed by virus recombination that resulted in $SIV_{cpz}$. Two scenarios are consistent with the data: (a1) $SIV_{rcm}$ and $SIV_{gsn}$ initially infected a chimpanzee; or (a2) $SIV_{rcm}$ and $SIV_{gsn}$ first infected an unknown primate species where virus recombination occurred – in either case, a recombinant SIV was transmitted among chimpanzees producing $SIV_{cpz}$. (b) Three separate transmissions of SIVs to humans occurred from distinct populations of chimpanzee ($SIV_{cpz}$) or gorilla ($SIV_{gor}$) in the 1900s producing three HIV-1 groups, M (main), N, and O (outlier). Recent, but limited, phylogenetic data show that HIV-1 group O is most closely related to $SIV_{gor}$. The most likely scenario suggested by the data is that chimpanzees transmitted $SIV_{cpz}$ to gorillas which resulted in $SIV_{gor}$; it is unknown whether HIV-1 group O was transmitted to humans from gorillas or from an as yet unidentified chimpanzee reservoir infected with $SIV_{cpz}$ more closely related to HIV-1 O. Only HIV-1 groups M and O have established efficient human-to-human transmission. Group M HIV-1 is pandemic, infecting over 45 million persons; group O HIV-1 is epidemic having infected an estimated several thousands of persons in Africa. In contrast, only six individuals from Cameroon are known to be infected with HIV-1 group N. Dotted circles indicate distinct populations of a primate species; shading indicates SIV isolated from individuals of this species; solid arrows show inferred transmissions of SIV; dashed arrows indicate where SIV transmission is hypothesized, but there are insufficient data to confirm.

As retroviruses, all lentiviruses also have two complete RNA genomes in a single virion. Therefore, when a host cell is infected with two or more genetically different primate lentiviruses, two different genomic viral RNAs can be packaged into the same virion, generating recombinant viral genomes in the next viral replication cycle. *vpx* shares sequence similarity with *vpr* and is thought to have originated by recombination among SIV genomes. Thus, viral recombination has been a dominant force in the evolution of primate lentiviruses as suggested by the diagrams of primate lentivirus genomes in **Figure 4**. As SIVs are isolated from more primate species and their full genome sequences compared, it was found that some

primates harbored SIV with apparently 'mosaic' genomes which included portions of structural genes derived from SIVs of different primate species. Thus, recombination among SIVs has resulted in novel viruses; for example, the current $SIV_{cpz}$ evolved from a recombinant between two SIVs – $SIV_{rcm}$ from red-capped mangabeys and $SIV_{gsn}$ from greater spot nose monkeys (**Figure 1**).

## Evolution

All primate lentiviruses are more closely related to each other than to lentiviruses from nonprimates. This genetic

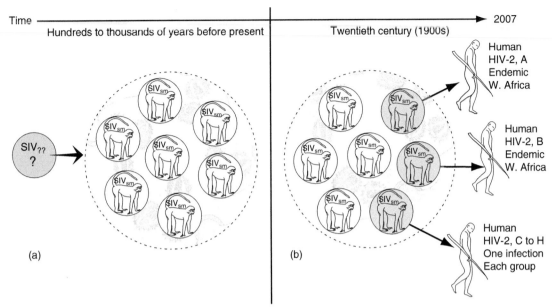

**Figure 2** Origin of HIV-2 inferred from phylogenetic analyses of SIV and HIV-2 genomes. (a) SIV probably infected sooty mangabeys (SMs) thousands of years ago. Multiple separate transmissions of $SIV_{sm}$ from distinct populations of SMs to humans occurred during the 1900s giving rise to eight HIV-2 groups, A–H (b). Only HIV-2 groups A and B have resulted in efficient human transmission and established epidemics; a single person is known to be infected with each of the HIV-2 groups C–H. Dotted circles indicate distinct populations of SMs; shading indicates $SIV_{sm}$ isolated from individual SM in a population; arrows show inferred transmissions of SIVs.

similarity suggests primate lentiviruses co-evolved with their host species and that primates have not been infected by lentiviruses from other mammals, such as ungulates or felines. SIVs have been isolated from many wild African NHP species, but no SIVs have been found to infect any wild Asian or New World NHPs. This suggests that lentiviruses became established in primates sometime after the divergence of Old and New World primate species (~35–40 million years ago). Although they lack an endemic SIV, Asian macaques are susceptible to experimental infection with a variety of SIV isolates and develop acquired immune deficiency syndrome (AIDS), similar to HIV-infected humans. The estimated origin of the macaque genus is ~6 million years ago and emigration of macaques from Africa to Eurasia began ~5 million years ago. Thus, it is probable that lentiviruses were not widespread among African primates 5 million years ago.

Lentiviral replication generates high genetic diversity in two ways: mutation caused by the highly error-prone retroviral polymerase (RT) and recombination between two different viral genomic RNA molecules packaged in a virion. The majority of African NHP species have genetically distinct SIVs. The isolation of more than one distinct SIV from a primate species provides evidence for regular interspecies SIV transmission (**Figures 1** and **3**). A notable example is isolation of two SIVs from mandrills ($SIV_{mnd-1}$ and $SIV_{mnd-2}$; **Figure 4**) that are as genetically different from each other as are HIV-1 and HIV-2.

Thus, genetic diversity of primate lentiviruses has evolved in two ways: (1) within a single host species, and (2) by transmission of SIV from one primate host species to another (cross-species transmission). Cross-species SIV transmission has occurred in both wild and captive primates. The most likely modes of SIV transmission between wild primate species are thought to be fighting among different primates or hunting and eating of one primate species by another; for example, wild chimpanzees are known to kill and eat a variety of monkeys that share the same geographic range. When a cross-species SIV transmission event occurs in an individual already SIV infected, there is the opportunity for viral recombination and, thus, the generation of SIV variants with novel phenotypes, including increased pathogenicity. Such a dual SIV infection is proposed to have been the origin of $SIV_{cpz}$ (**Figure 1**). Dual (or multiple) SIV infection of individuals can also occur when a primate species has genetically distinct SIV variants in one or different populations of animals. Thus, intraspecific SIV recombination increases the genetic diversity within an SIV lineage (**Figure 3**).

## Virology

The life cycle of SIV is similar to all retroviruses; once uncoated from the capsid, the RNA genome is reverse-transcribed into a full-length DNA genome that is transported to the nucleus and integrated into host chromosomes. Once

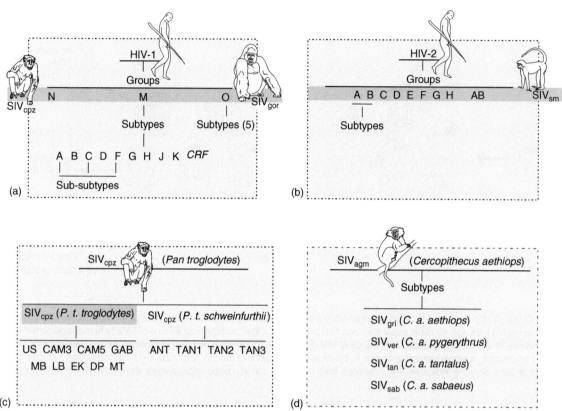

**Figure 3** Classification and phylogenetic relationships of primate lentiviruses. (a) HIV-1 lineage. HIV-1 is divided into three groups: M (main), N (non-M/non-O or 'new'), and O (outlier); based on phylogenetic clustering with SIVs, each group represents a separate chimpanzee- or gorilla-to-human transmission event (see also **Figure 1**). Subtype diversification occurred in humans after each cross-species transmission; CRF indicates inter-subtype recombinants. Clusters of diversity within a subtype are called sub-subtypes. The shaded bar indicates the SIVs which gave rise to the HIV-1 groups. (b) HIV-2 lineage. HIV-2 is divided into eight groups (A–H); based on phylogenetic clustering with SIVs, each group represents a separate sooty mangabey-to-human transmission event (see also **Figure 2**); AB indicates recombinant virus. The shaded bar indicates SIV$_{sm}$ giving rise to the HIV-2 groups. (c) SIV$_{cpz}$ lineage. SIV$_{cpz}$ is designated as one subtype although SIV$_{cpz}$'s have been isolated from two subspecies of chimpanzees, *Pan troglodytes troglodytes* and *Pan troglodytes schweinfurthii*; multiple SIV$_{cpz}$'s from each of these two subspecies have been isolated and sequenced (abbreviations are listed). SIV$_{cpz}$ from *P. t. troglodytes* (shaded bar) is most closely related to HIV-1. (d) SIV$_{agm}$ lineage. There are four subtypes of SIV$_{agm}$, one for each of the four subspecies of African green monkey, *Cercopithecus aethiops*: *C. a. aethiops* (grivet), *C. a. pygerythrus* (vervet), *C. a. tantalus* (tantalus), and *C. a. sabaeus* (sabaeus).

integrated, the provirus produces a variety of RNA species that can be spliced to produce all the proteins required for virion assembly and egress. In T cells the immature virions bud from the plasma membrane into the extracellular space, but in macrophages virions often bud into intracellular vesicles that can eventually fuse with the plasma membrane of the cell releasing the progeny virions.

SIV can be propagated in many human T-cell and macrophage cell lines derived from tumors, mitogen-stimulated peripheral blood mononuclear cells (PBMCs), monocyte-derived macrophages, etc., although the range of permissive cell types varies from isolate to isolate. In PBMC cultures and many cell lines, viral infection results in obvious cytopathic effects including ballooning degeneration and syncytia formation due to fusion of cell membranes. Syncytium formation is mediated by the envelope glycoprotein and allows direct cell-to-cell spread of the infection.

The CD4 molecule is the primary cellular receptor for SIV. As with HIV, infection is primarily mediated by CD4 but interaction with CD4 alone is not sufficient to allow viral entry into the cell. A number of chemokine receptors are required co-receptors for SIV and HIV infection. The SIV envelope glycoprotein (gp120) binds to CD4 resulting in a conformational shift in the glycoprotein that exposes a co-receptor binding site. This secondary binding site interacts with a chemokine receptor on the cell surface, and fusion of cell and virion membranes results. Although various SIV strains can use a variety of chemokine receptors (CCR5, BOB, Bonzo) as a co-receptor *in vitro*, CCR5 is the most important co-receptor for SIV *in vivo* as it widely expressed by target cells (T cells, macrophages, dendritic cells (DCs)) in the body. Chimeric viruses have been constructed using SIV as a backbone for inserting HIV genes. In HIV infection, differential co-receptor

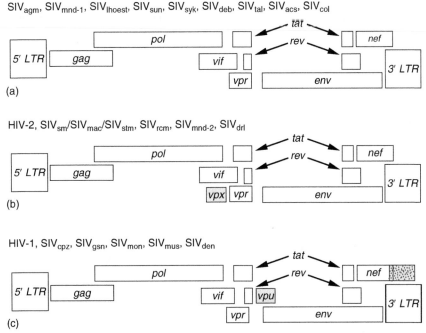

**Figure 4** Genomic structure of primate lentiviruses. Viral genes are represented by rectangles with names inside and arrows show genes with two separate coding regions. Group A includes SIVs only from African NHPs (agm, African green monkey; mnd, mandrill; lhoest, l'Hoest monkey; sun, sun-tailed monkey; syk, Sykes monkey; deb, de Brazza's monkey; tal, talapoin; acs, *ascanius*; col, colobus). Group B includes HIV-2 and SIVs most closely related to HIV-2; each group B virus has a *vpx* gene (shaded box), that is absent in the Group A viruses (sm, sooty mangabey; mac, macaque; stm, stump-tailed macaque; rcm, red-capped mangabey; mnd, mandrill; drl, drill). Group C viruses include HIV-1, SIV$_{cpz}$, and other SIVs with a *vpu* gene, but lacking *vpx* (cpz, chimpanzee; gsn, greater spot nose monkey; mon, mona monkey; mus, mustached guenon; den, Dent's mona monkey). For HIV-1 and SIV$_{cpz}$ genomes only, the *nef* gene (stippled) does not overlap the *env* gene.

usage by HIV variants has been implicated as a determinant in virulence and pathogenesis. Some of the SIV/SHIV (SHIV) viruses have been constructed using the *env* from HIV variants known to preferentially use CxCR4 or CCR5 as co-receptors. Although differential co-receptor usage can be demonstrated by the chimeric viruses *in vitro*, the extent to which altered replication capacity independent of co-receptor usage contributes to observed differences in pathogenesis has been difficult to determine.

Host cellular factors have recently been identified that confer resistance or susceptibility to productive SIV infection. In host cells resistant to another species' lentivirus, the host protein APOBEC3G is incorporated into the virion during particle formation. During reverse transcription, virion-incorporated APOBEC3G deaminates the minus strand of viral DNA and inactivates/degrades the viral genome. In permissive cells, the *vif* gene permits SIV to replicate by targeting APOBEC3G for degradation in the proteosome and preventing its incorporation into the virion. However, the activity of *vif* is species specific. Thus human APOBEC3G is inhibited by HIV-1 Vif but not by SIV$_{agm}$ Vif, and AGM APOBEC3G is inhibited by SIV$_{agm}$ Vif, but not by HIV-1 Vif. TRIM5alpha, a member of the poorly understood tripartite motif (TRIM) family of

proteins, is another host-restriction factor. TRIM5alpha restricts HIV replication in rhesus macaques, by interacting with the virion capsid and blocking the uncoating of HIV-1 after entry but before reverse transcription.

## Transmission and Dissemination

When experimentally inoculated onto intact mucosal surfaces, SIV rapidly infects local DCs, macrophages, and T cells. Although the number of SIV-infected cells is generally higher in the lamina propria adjacent to regions of epithelial damage, SIV-infected DCs and T cells can be found within the intact epithelium of the genital tract, indicating that the virus can cross the intact genital mucosa. Within 24 h of infection, SIV-infected cells can be detected in the lymph nodes that drain a mucosal inoculation site. Initially, there is limited viral replication in local tissues prior to widely disseminated infection in peripheral lymphoid tissues, but by 1 week, post inoculation (PI), viral replication is explosive with dramatic increases in viral RNA levels in all lymphoid tissues. At 10–14 days PI, the peak of viral replication and plasma vRNA levels occurs, and adaptive immune

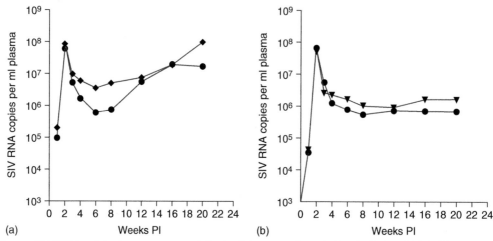

**Figure 5**    Plasma SIV RNA levels in rhesus macaques following intravenous inoculation of pathogenic SIV. (a) Plasma vRNA levels in two macaques inoculated with SIVmac251. (b) Plasma vRNA levels in 2 macaques inoculated with SIVmac239. Note in all four animals there was a peak in plasma vRNA at 2 weeks PI followed by a variable period of declining or stable plasma vRNA. While setpoint vRNA levels remained stable in both SIVmac239 inoculated animals over the period of observation, plasma vRNA had begun increasing by 24 weeks PI in both SIVmac251-infected animals, suggesting that these animals would soon develop clinical AIDS.

responses develop. By day 28–56 PI, plasma vRNA levels decline to moderate levels, where they remain for a variable period of time. Eventually viral replication increases, CD4+ T-cell levels decline further and AIDS develops. Examples of plasma viral levels in rhesus macaques inoculated with two pathogenic SIV variants are provided in **Figure 5**.

## Disease Pathogenesis

While the endemic SIV infections of African monkeys and apes seem to be minimally pathogenic, SIV infections of Asian macaques cause simian AIDS. This disease results from the profound destruction of CD4+ T cells in lymphoid organs throughout the body. To an even greater degree than HIV infection of people, SIV replicates to very high levels in the infected host with as many as $10^9$ vRNA copies per ml of plasma during peak infection. This high replicative capacity coupled with the error-prone viral RT produces viral quasi-species of tremendous genetic diversity in infected individuals. This viral quasi-species makes the virus very adaptable to changing conditions in the host as antiviral immune responses develop or successive waves of target cells are destroyed. As in HIV infection, the level of SIV RNA in plasma is an excellent indicator of clinical prognosis in Asian macaques.

The central feature of AIDS is the destruction of CD4+ T cells and the crippling effect this has on the host's ability to control opportunistic, or latent, infections. The majority of the CD4+ T cells in the body reside in the gastrointestinal (GI) tract and other mucosal sites, and these cells are activated memory and CCR5+ T cells. Thus the

GI tract is a major site for the destruction of CD4+ T cells. As viral replication occurs, the level of immune activation and lymphocyte proliferation dramatically increases as the host attempts to mount an immune response. Many of the transcriptional signals involved in the host's innate and adaptive immune responses are controlled by nuclear factor-kappa B (NF-κB) transcriptional factors. NF-κB is also a key promoter for SIV replication as the viral LTR contains binding sites for NF-κB transcription factors. Thus the host immune response to SIV generates activated T cells with high levels of critical molecules (dNTPs, transcriptional factors) and, paradoxically, these are the cellular targets needed for optimal viral replication.

In addition to the effects of CD4+ T-cell depletion on the host defenses, SIV can directly produce disease. Thus SIV crosses the blood–brain barrier, infecting resident and transient cells of the macrophage lineage, which can result in viral encephalitis. In addition, the high levels of viral antigen and strong antibody responses can produce immune complex glomerulonephritis, while SIV infection of bone marrow macrophages is presumed to be the cause of the anemia and other hematologic abnormalities that SIV infection produces. The above features are also common in HIV infection, but SIV infection of macrophages can produce histiocytic inflammation with syncytial cell formation in the lung, lymphoid tissues, and GI tract.

The above discussion describes the pathogenesis of AIDS in SIV-infected Asian macaques, but in the African primates that are natural hosts of SIV there is little clinical effect of infection. A key difference lies in the response of natural hosts and Asian macaques to SIV infection. Thus SIV-infected African primates mount a complete adaptive immune response but there is little inflammation and no chronic immune activation associated with these immune responses despite continuous high-level viral replication. In marked contrast, SIV infection of macaques, as with HIV infection of humans, produces chronic immune activation and inflammation that is associated with depletion of central memory T-cell pools and loss of effector memory T cells. Thus despite levels of viral replication that are similar to Asian macaques, SIV infection rarely produces AIDS in natural hosts indicating that inflammation and immune activation are necessary for AIDS pathogenesis.

Specific strains of SIV have altered pathogenesis with a number of molecular clones and biologic isolates being attenuated for replication in Asian macaques. Although these variants do not produce disease in the typical time course of viruses with higher replicative capacity, some eventually produce disease in adults or infant macaques, while other attenuated SIV variants (SIVmac1A11) have failed to produce disease in infected macaques after more than 15 years of observation. In addition, some strains of SIV have specific tropism for monocyte/macrophages that are mediated by post-entry events. Infections with these macrophage-tropic SIV strains are more commonly associated with SIV-induced meningoencephalitis than other SIV strains.

## Immune Response to SIV Infection

As SIV infection is lifelong, the host immune response cannot clear the infection but, in some cases, it can exert considerable control on the level to which SIV replicates. Before day 5 after mucosal SIV inoculation, there is little evidence of innate immune responses with only modest increases in type 1 interferon levels and interferon-stimulated gene levels at the site of inoculation. At days 6–7 PI, there is a dramatic and simultaneous increase in innate antiviral immune responses in all lymphoid tissues that coincides with the dramatic explosion of viral replication in these tissues. By days 10–14 PI, SIV-specific CD8+ T-cell responses are present in blood and in the mucosal sites of inoculation, with strong antiviral T-cell responses widespread by day 28 PI. This rapid increase in antiviral effector T cells occurs as viral replication and plasma vRNA levels decline from a peak at 14 days PI. The temporal relationship between the decline in plasma viremia and the appearance of antiviral T cells has been interpreted to be evidence that CD8+ T cells are critical in the control of HIV replication. Further evidence for the control of SIV replication by CD8+ lymphocytes has been obtained by using monoclonal antibodies to the α-chain of the CD8 complex to transiently deplete T cells and natural killer (NK) cells. In chronically infected animals, plasma vRNA levels dramatically increase during the period of CD8+ lymphocyte depletion and then rapidly fall as the lymphocyte population is replenished. Finally, as in HIV infection,

detailed studies of well-characterized MHC-I-restricted T-cell epitopes in infected macaques have shown that as the host T-cell response targets a specific peptide sequence, viral variants with proteins that contain a variant of the targeted epitope become increasingly common. The effect of these mutated epitopes on viral replication is variable. In some cases, these variants are relatively unfit and the virus gains little advantage; however, in other cases, these immune escape variants are relatively fit and viral replication increases dramatically as the escape variants appear in the viral population. Finally, as in humans, specific MHC-I alleles of macaques (i.e., Mamu-A*01) are associated with particularly strong CD8+ T-cell responses, enhanced immune control of viral replication, and increased disease-free survival times after infection. Taken together, these observations argue that CD8+ T-cell responses can play a significant role in controlling viral replication. B-cell responses also have a role in controlling HIV and SIV replication. Thus it has been shown that passive transfer of high-titer SIV-specific gammaglobulin or neutralizing anti-HIV antibodies inhibits SIV and SHIV replication and retards the pace of disease progression. Further, if macaques are prevented from developing anti-SIV IgG antibodies by B-cell depletion prior to infection with highly pathogenic SIV, they rapidly develop uncontrolled viral replication, and progress to AIDS in a few months PI, while most SIV-infected macaques make strong antibody responses and develop AIDS at 10–24 months PI.

## Clinical Features, Pathology, and Histopathology of SIV Infection in Asian Macaques

End-stage disease in SIV infection is indistinguishable from human AIDS and can be divided into four broad categories: (1) opportunistic infections, (2) SIV-mediated inflammatory diseases, (3) neoplastic diseases, and (4) diseases of unknown etiology. The clinical course of SIV varies with the strain involved but rhesus macaques infected with common pathogenic SIV strains develop AIDS within 6–24 months PI. In the first few weeks of infection, all animals initially develop lymphocytosis consisting largely of CD8+ T cells, which resolves in 4–6 weeks. Lymphadenopathy and splenomegaly are apparent by 2–4 weeks PI and these conditions remain manifest until a very late stage of the disease when lymphoid collapse can occur. As in HIV infection, hypergammaglobulinemia due to polyclonal B-cell activation is often a feature of the disease. Anemia can also be a feature of the clinical disease. Weight loss and diarrhea are very common in SIV-infected animals and can be the result of opportunistic infections (*Mycobacterium avium* complex, cytomegalovirus, adenovirus, *Cryptosporidium* sp., *Ameoba* sp., *Balantidium coli*) or an unknown etiology. Often these enteric conditions do not respond to antibiotic therapy. Lymphomas are the only neoplastic condition of significance in SIV-infected macaques. In fact, a B-cell lymphoma arising in a 19-year-old sooty mangabey infected with SIV may represent the best candidate for the case of an SIV-related fatal disease in a naturally infected African primate.

Lymphoid tissues, including the mucosal-associated lymphoid tissues of the GI, reproductive, and respiratory tracts, are the targets of SIV infection, and a range of histopathologic changes occur in these tissues from follicular hyperplasia to dysplasia, followed by follicular collapse and expansion of the paracortex, ultimately ending in lymphoid depletion, collapse, and fibrosis. These changes occur independent of any opportunistic infections. The same pattern of histologic changes occurs in lymphoid tissues of HIV-1-infected humans and these histologic changes accurately reflect the clinical stage of the infection in both SIV and HIV.

## SIV Infections as Animal Models of AIDS

The HIV-1 pandemic continues unabated and developing effective vaccines and therapies is the greatest current public health need. Samples from HIV-infected individuals have provided key insights into AIDS pathogenesis. However, direct experimental testing of specific hypothesis arising from these studies cannot be undertaken in humans for ethical reasons and HIV-1 infection of chimpanzees does not produce AIDS. Thus, SIV infection of Asian macaques is the most widely accepted animal model of HIV pathogenesis. The biology of the macaque immune system, and the key organ systems (gut, lymphoid tissue, and reproductive tract) involved in AIDS pathogenesis and HIV transmission are very similar to humans, and SIV and HIV are closely related phylogenetically. Thus, SIV infection of macaques closely mimics the pathogenesis, virology, immunology, and pathology of HIV infection in the human. The model has been used to show that infection with a molecular clone of SIV is sufficient to cause AIDS, that the GI tract is a major site of CD4$^+$ T-cell depletion, and that some vaccine strategies elicit immune responses that can provide considerable control of viral replication. The macaque monkey model of AIDS has been used to define the molecular determinants of viral pathogenesis, the basis for nonpathogenic infections in natural hosts. These animal models have been particularly valuable for defining the mechanisms of HIV transmission and events in acute infection that are very difficult to study in humans.

Sexual HIV transmission can occur through oral, anal, or vaginal intercourse. Allowing SIV-discordant macaques to mate normally would seem to be most similar to sexual HIV infection. However, sexual SIV transmission occurs at a low or variable rate after natural mating, and, in addition, there is significant biting behavior during mating and thus significant potential for blood-borne SIV transmission. When SIV-discordant juvenile rhesus macaques were housed in groups, SIV transmission most commonly occurred when uninfected, dominant animals bit their SIV-infected, subdominant cagemates as part of social interactions. Thus, once deposited in the mouth of an uninfected macaque SIV-infected blood-transmitted infection therefore biting during mating would confound transmission studies.

A more controlled experimental approach to reliably transmit SIV across the genital mucosa is to intravaginally inoculate female macaques with a known quantity of well-characterized SIV stock. Most studies have used suspensions of cell-free SIV virions, but infection can be transmitted by intravaginal inoculation with SIV-infected cells. In order to reliably transmit SIV to monkeys by a single intravaginal inoculation, relatively high doses of cell-free virus (2–3 log 10 more virus) are used compared to intravenous inoculation. In addition, exogenous progestins have been used to ensure reliable intravaginal SIV transmission, as these hormones thin up the genital mucosa, lower the barrier to transmission, and enhance SIV transmission. Finally, intravaginally inoculating animals with relatively low doses of virus, approximately the same dose needed for IV transmission, repeatedly over the course for several months eventually produced infection in all exposed animals, although the number of exposures needed to acquire infection is variable; this strategy probably best models the level of virus exposure that occurs during HIV sexual transmission.

HIV transmission by sexual, intravenous, and perinatal routes is often associated with the acquisition of a limited distribution of genetic variant. In many instances, the transmitted variant represents a minor variant in the donor's virus population. Given the extent of genetic diversity between HIV isolates, these findings have been interpreted to suggest that HIV transmission may involve selective entry or selective amplification of specific viral variants. However, the inherent limitations of all studies using human samples include small sample sizes and uncertainty as to the genetic identity and the extent of genetic diversity of the virus population in the donor at the time of transmission. Thus, the mechanisms that underlie the sexual transmission of HIV variants are unclear, and are difficult to assess because of the difficulties in establishing the precise time of infection. The SIV macaque model for HIV transmission is particularly valuable for evaluating the role of viral selection during transmission. The model allows access to information that is usually unattainable in human studies, such as: the genotypic and phenotypic properties of the infecting virus; knowledge of the exact time of virus exposure; and the characteristics of viral variants in the infected host immediately after transmission. Both IV and IVAG SIV inoculation transmit genetically diverse populations of SIV env V1–V2 variants to macaques. However, compared to the complex SIV populations in the IV inoculated animals, most IVAG inoculated animals are infected with SIV populations that have relatively low genetic diversity in the env gene. The finding that genetically diverse SIV populations are transmitted to some IVAG inoculated monkeys is consistent with the observation that a more genetically diverse population of viral variants is sexually transmitted from HIV-infected men to women. The model has also been used to show that recombination can occur readily *in vivo* after mucosal SIV exposure and thus viral recombination contributes to the generation of viral genetic diversity and enhancement of viral fitness in the peracute stages of infection. The model has also been used to show that the mucosal barrier of the female genital tract greatly limits the infection of cervicovaginal tissues after intravaginal SIV inoculation, and thus the initial founder populations of infected cells are small. Despite limited foothold, SIV rapidly disseminates to distal sites, and continuous seeding from an infection in the genital tract is likely critical for the later establishment of a productive disseminated systemic infection.

Perinatal HIV transmission can occur at any time during gestation, delivery, or breast-feeding. Allowing female macaques infected with virulent SIV before or during pregnancy is most similar to perinatal HIV infection, because SIV/SHIV transmission can occur any time during gestation, delivery, or breast-feeding. However, mother–infant SIV transmission occurs at a low or variable rate and the timing of virus transmission is unknown. Alternatively, female macaques can be infected with SIV after delivery and the infant allowed to breast-feed normally. This model best mimics natural HIV breast milk transmission by eliminating fetal exposure to virus and transplacental transfer of maternal virus-specific antibodies to the infant. Thus, this approach controls more variables and transmission rates are high; however, a major limitation is that the time at which breast-feeding infants become SIV infected varies substantially (i.e., a few weeks to several months). Finally, direct oral inoculation of infant macaques with SIV or SHIV can be performed without infecting their dams. This approach controls most of the important variables related to the viral inoculum (dose, number, timing, and duration of virus exposure), maternal host immune response (level and quality of anti-HIV-specific maternal/passively transferred antibodies), and infant rearing (by uninfected dams or in a primate nursery). This system has been used to show that after oral inoculation of infant rhesus macaques with virulent SIV-mac251, virus disseminates to distal lymphoid tissues faster than after oral inoculation of juvenile macaques or vaginal inoculation of adult macaques with the same virus.

In addition to helping define critical steps in AIDS pathogenesis, these SIV mucosal transmission models are ideal for testing vaccines and microbicide strategies designed to prevent HIV transmission. The demonstrated utility of the SIV model for vaccine testing contrasts sharply with the inability of models using macaques infected with CxCR4 SHIVs (SHIV 89.6P) to meaningfully segregate HIV-1 vaccine candidates by relative efficacy. Thus the SIVs will continue to be the most valuable model of HIV infection and a critical tool in AIDS research.

*See also:* Bovine and Feline Immunodeficiency Viruses; Simian Immunodeficiency Virus: General Features; Simian Immunodeficiency Virus: Natural Infection.

## Further Reading

Butler IF, Pandrea I, Marx PA, and Apetrei C (2007) HIV genetic diversity: Biological and public health consequences. *Current HIV Research* 5: 23–45.

Gardner MB (2003) Simian AIDS: An historical perspective. *Journal of Medical Primatology* 32: 180–186.

Gordon S, Pandrea I, Dunham R, Apetrei C, and Silvestri G (2005) The call of the wild: What can be learned from studies of SIV infection of natural hosts? In: Leitner T, Foley B, Hahn B, *et al.* (eds.) *HIV Sequence Compendium 2005, LA-UR 06–0680*, pp 2–29. Los Alamos, NM: Los Alamos National Laboratory.

Greenier JL, Miller CJ, Lu D, *et al.* (2001) Route of simian immunodeficiency virus inoculation determines the complexity but not the identity of viral variant populations that infect rhesus macaques. *Journal of Virology* 75: 3753–3765.

Jayaraman P and Haigwood NL (2006) Animal models for perinatal transmission of HIV-1. *Frontiers in Biosciences* 11: 2828–2844.

Kestler H, Kodama T, Ringler D, *et al.* (1990) Induction of AIDS in rhesus monkeys by molecularly cloned simian immunodeficiency virus. *Science* 248: 1109–1112.

Kim EY, Busch M, Abel K, *et al.* (2005) Retroviral recombination *in vivo*: Viral replication patterns and genetic structure of simian immunodeficiency virus (SIV) populations in rhesus macaques after simultaneous or sequential intravaginal inoculation with SIVmac239Deltavpx/Deltavpr and SIVmac239Deltanef. *Journal of Virology* 79: 4886–4895.

Lifson JD and Martin MA (2002) One step forwards, one step back. *Nature* 415: 272–273.

Long EM, Martin HL Jr., Kreiss JK, *et al.* (2000) Gender differences in HIV-1 diversity at time of infection. *Nature Medicine* 6: 71–75.

Marthas ML and Miller CJ (2007) Developing a neonatal HIV vaccine: Insights from macaque models of pediatric HIV/AIDS. *Current Opinion in HIV and AIDS* 2(5): 367–374.

Miller CJ (1994) Mucosal transmission of SIV. In: Desrosiers RC and Letvin NL (eds.) *Current Topics in Microbiology and Immunology*, pp. 107–122. Berlin: Springer.

Miller CJ, Alexander NJ, Sutjipto S, *et al.* (1989) Genital mucosal transmission of simian immunodeficiency virus: Animal model for heterosexual transmission of human immunodeficiency virus. *Journal of Virology* 63: 4277–4284.

Miller CJ, Li Q, Abel K, *et al.* (2005) Propagation and dissemination of infection after vaginal transmission of simian immunodeficiency virus. *Journal of Virology* 79: 9217–9227.

Veazey RS and Lackner AA (2004) Getting to the guts of HIV pathogenesis. *Journal of Experimental Medicine* 200(6): 697–700.

## Relevant Website

http://www.hiv.lanl.gov – HIV Sequence Database: Nomenclature Overview (modified 26 April 2007), HIV Databases by Los Alamos National Laboratory.

# Simian Retrovirus D

**P A Marx,** Tulane University, Covington, LA, USA

## Glossary

**Codon** The basic unit of the genetic code consisting of three consecutive nucleotides in DNA that specify the order of amino acids in a protein.

**Monocistronic mRNA** Messenger RNA that codes for a single protein.

**Monoclonal antibody** Antibody made *in vitro* that reacts with a single protein.

**Pneumocystis carinii** A fungus that causes pneumonia, especially in persons or animals with suppressed immune systems.

**Polyprotein** A precursor protein that is cut after its synthesis into smaller functional proteins.

**Ribosomal frameshifting** A change in the translational reading frame that allows the synthesis of different proteins from a single region of overlapping genes. For example, if the genetic code begins on the first of the three nucleotides of a codon, the out-of-frame code would begin on the second nucleotide. A second frameshift beginning on the third nucleotide is also possible. Frameshifting is an economical way to code for proteins.

**Syncytium** Cell-derived structure in culture or *in vivo* giant cell consisting of fused cells having more than one nucleus.

**Virion** Infectious viral particle containing the genome of the virus and a full complement of viral proteins required for growth and replication.

**Western blot** Nitrocellulose blotting paper containing viral polypeptides sorted by molecular size. The blot is soaked in diluted serum suspected of containing antibodies. A positive test requires binding to polypeptides from at least two different viral genes. More weight is often given to env polypeptide reactions. False results against a single *gag* coded protein commonly occur and are reported as indeterminant.

**Zoonosis** Microbial infection (virus, bacteria, or parasite) acquired directly through animal contact that progresses to a clinical disease.

**Zoonotic infection** Microbial infection (virus, bacteria, or parasite) acquired directly through animal contact that may or may not progress to disease.

## Introduction

Simian type D retroviruses (SRVs) and Mason–Pfizer monkey viruses (MPMVs) are members of the family *Retroviridae* and comprise one species belonging to the genus *Betaretrovirus*. These viruses naturally infect members of the nonhuman primate genus *Macaca*, commonly known as macaque monkeys. SRV appears to be highly species specific, although the virus will replicate in the cells of other primate species, including tissue culture cells of human origin. Betaretroviruses are characterized by their simple genomic structure consisting of 4 genes, *gag, pro, pol,* and *env* (**Figure 1**).

MPMVs and SRVs are exogenous retroviruses, meaning that the virus is acquired from another infected macaque monkey. This transmission mechanism distinguishes SRVs from endogenous D retroviruses that are inherited and are a part of the genome of the host species. Endogenous D retroviruses occur in both New and Old World monkeys, including African baboons as well as Asian langur and South American squirrel monkeys.

Seven distinct isolates are known and each can be distinguished by serum neutralization tests or competitive binding tests between homologous p27 *gag* proteins. They are named SRV serotypes 1–7. Serotype 3 is also known as MPMV. A nomenclature has been devised that is similar to that used for influenza viruses and is an aid for tracking isolates and their origins. For example, D1/rhe/CA/84 represented the D retrovirus that was isolated at the California Primate Center Davis, CA from a rhesus macaque with an acquired immune deficiency syndrome (AIDS)-like disease and was reported in 1984. D2/Cel/OR/85 was a 1985 SRV-2 isolate from a Celebes black macaque with retroperitoneal fibromatosis (RF) at the Oregon Primate Center. MPMV is the prototype of this viral species and retains its original name for historical reasons.

## History

In 1971, the first D retrovirus isolate was reported. The virus was recovered from a rhesus monkey with a mammary carcinoma. The virus was named after the Mason Institute in Worcester, Massachusetts, where the macaque had been housed. The Pfizer Pharmaceutical Company had supported research using this female monkey, hence the name Mason–Pfizer monkey virus (MPMV). The impact of MPMV was greatly enhanced because the virus was isolated directly from cancerous breast tissue. Because of this association with neoplasia, MPMV was classified as an oncornavirus (Onco RNA for cancer-causing RNA virus). This classification persisted for many years.

The finding of MPMV in monkey breast cancer tissue prompted numerous reports in the 1970s of D retroviruses

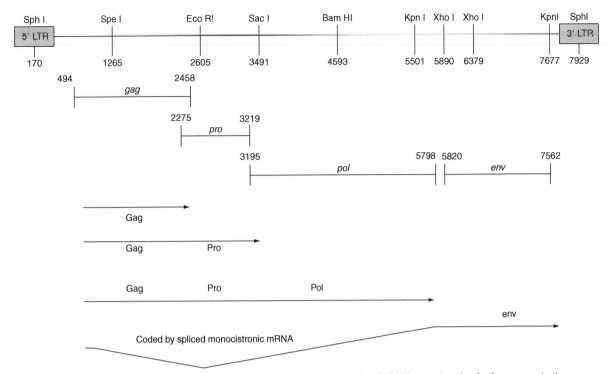

**Figure 1** Map of the genome of primate D retroviruses. Top is the provirus that is 8105 nt and codes for four genes in three separate reading frames, *gag*, *pro*, *pol*, and *env*. The messenger RNAs consist of two forms, a genomic-length mRNA that is translated into the polyprotein Gag. After frameshifting(s), Gag-Pro and Gag-Pro-Pol precursors are made. Polyproteins are cleaved into smaller functional virion proteins. The second mRNA form is a spliced mRNA that encodes the Env proteins, SU (also named gp70) and TM (also named gp20). Reprinted from Marracci GH, Avery NA, Shiigi SM, *et al*. (1999) Molecular cloning and cell-specific growth characterization of polymorphic variants of type D serogroup 2 simian retroviruses. *Virology* 261: 43–58, with permission from Elsevier.

in association with human breast cancer. With the development of sensitive detection techniques along with complete sequencing of the MPMV and SRV genomes, it became apparent that nonhuman primate D retroviral sequences were not causally associated with human tumors. A 1975 report on immune impairment in neonatal monkeys infected with MPMV marked the beginning of our understanding of primate D retroviruses as a causative agent of simian AIDS. The modern era of type D retrovirus research deals with its immunosuppressive properties.

AIDS, the disease, was discovered in 1981 in persons displaying symptoms of a severe and fatal immunodeficiency. The first detailed report consisted of four men with *Pneumocystis carinii* pneumonia, evidence of cytomegalovirus infection (CMV), and Kaposi sarcoma, a skin cancer not commonly seen in young men. Early theories on the cause of AIDS implicated drug-induced impairment of the immune system. Drugs were known to suppress the immune system, but the idea that severe and fatal immune deficiency could be caused by a virus was not yet appreciated. A breeding group of rhesus monkeys that was housed outdoors at the California National Primate Research Center in Davis, CA, played a significant role in changing that perception. This breeding group had a higher mortality rate than monkeys in other outdoor groups only a short distance away. The affected animals

had diarrhea, cytomegalovirus infections, and fibrosarcoma, a tumor that resembled Kaposi sarcoma upon microscopic inspection. A link was made between AIDS in monkeys and AIDS in humans. The study of this group of monkeys resulted in the isolation and characterization of a virus related to MPMV. This distinct D retrovirus was named simian retrovirus (SRV) and was used to prove the retroviral etiology of this fatal immune deficiency disease in monkeys. A similar virus was isolated from rhesus macaques at the New England Primate Research Center.

## Replication

The synthesis of new progeny virus begins with the DNA provirus that is integrated into a host DNA chromosome (**Figure 1**). The provirus is a double-stranded (ds) DNA copy of the virus genome. The provirus is flanked by two repeated sequences called the long terminal repeat (LTR). The order of the coding and noncoding regions are the LTR, *gag* (for group antigen), *pol* (polymerase), *env* (envelope), and a second copy of the LTR. The viral genome is synthesized from the minus DNA strand of the provirus by host cell enzymes. The newly made viral genome is the same sense as messenger RNA (+-stranded) and is exported from the nucleus without being spliced.

The cellular requirement for splicing is bypassed by the interaction of the constitutive transport element (CTE) with cellular proteins. This genomic RNA is translated in the cytoplasm into Gag and Pol viral proteins in a process that involves several steps.

The *gag* gene codes for 654 amino acids that are synthesized as a 78 kDa polyprotein precursor of smaller functional virion proteins. The *gag*-encoded polyprotein is cleaved by a protease enzyme, which in turn is coded by the *pro* gene. This Gag precursor is cleaved into six mature virion proteins, the p10 matrix protein (polypeptide 10 000 Da molecular weight (MW)), pp24 (phosphoprotein), p12 (assembly scaffold domain), p24 major capsid protein, p14 nucleocapsid protein, and p4 (chaperonin binding domain). The major capsid protein, p24 (in M-PMV, p27), is the most abundant protein in the mature virion (**Figures 2(b)** and **3**). The p10 protein is the matrix protein and resides just under the external envelope of the virion (**Figure 3**). The nucleocapsid protein p14 forms a tightly associated complex with the RNA genome. Unlike most other retroviruses, D-type retroviruses form immature capsids that are preassembled in the cytoplasm (**Figure 2** – see arrows). This is facilitated by a cytoplasmic targeting and retention signal in the matrix domain of Gag, which binds to the microtubule motor dynein and targets translating polysomes to the pericentriolar region of the cell where assembly occurs. The p12 region of Gag acts to facilitate this intracytoplasmic assembly process.

The protease (*pro*) gene overlaps the *gag* region by 61 codons (183 nt). The protease is an enzyme that cleaves protein and is highly conserved across the genus with 82.8% and 83.8% identity between SRV-1 and MPMV, respectively. The protease itself is translated from the

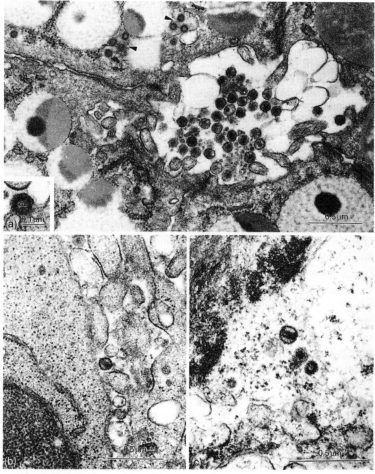

**Figure 2** Electron microscopic demonstration of type D retroviral particles in (a) salivary gland, (b) germinal center of a lymph node, and (c) spleen of rhesus monkeys with AIDS. In the salivary gland (a), numerous mature extracellular particles in a small acinar lumen, as well as immature intracytoplasmic A particles (arrows) and a budding particle (inset) are seen. In the germinal center (b), a single mature virion particle adjacent to a lymphoid cell and numerous cellular processes possibly belonging to follicular dendritic cells are seen. (c) In the spleen, a single mature particle is seen in the extracellular space. Modified from Lackner AA, Rodriguez MH, Bush CE, *et al.* (1988) Distribution of a macaque immunosuppressive type D retrovirus in neural, lymphoid, and salivary tissues. *Journal of Virology* 62: 2134–2142, with permission from American Society for Microbiology.

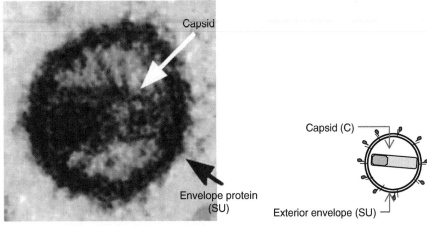

**Figure 3** Mature D retrovirus virion showing the external envelope and the major capsid core. Modified from Marx PA, Maul DH, Osborn KG, *et al.* (1984) Simian AIDS: Isolation of a type D retrovirus and transmission of the disease. *Science* 223: 1083–1086, with permission from AAAS.

genome-length mRNA (**Figure 1**) as two polyproteins (Gag-Pro) and Gag-Pro-Pol. Because the *pro* gene is out of frame with respect to *gag*, the polyprotein that contains the protease results from a ribosomal frameshifting mechanism during translation of genome-length mRNA. The final protease protein is produced by two autocatalytic cuts, one at the N-terminus producing a 17 kDa product and a second cut producing the final 13 kDa protease enzyme. The protease is incorporated into the immature capsids in the cytoplasm (**Figure 2** – see arrows). It functions to cleave the *gag*-coded polyprotein into smaller proteins that make up the internal capsid structure of the virion. The three-dimensional (3-D) structure of the protease has been resolved and this 3-D structure is well conserved across the retrovirus family.

A second ribosomal frameshift within the *pro-pol* overlap region generates a larger polyprotein precursor containing the pol proteins (**Figure 1**). The *pol* gene encodes the reverse transcriptase (RT)-endonuclease and integrase proteins. The gene encoding the integrase of MPMV is located at the 3′ end of the *pol* open reading frame and the RT is encoded by the 5′ end of the gene. The RT, integrase, and endonuclease enzymes function after the progeny virus infects a new cell, and are incorporated into the immature capsids as Gag-Pro and Gag-Pro-Pol precursors. These polyproteins undergo post-translational cleavage during virion maturation to produce separate RT and endonuclease/integrase proteins. They are required to initiate the early steps of replication after the virus enters a host cell to begin a new cycle of replication.

The *env* gene is expressed from the 3′ end of the genome (**Figure 1**). *env* encodes two proteins, the external envelope spike protein (SU for surface) and the transmembrane protein (TM). The mRNA coding of the Env proteins is spliced in the nucleus to remove *gag* and *pol*

coding regions. The mRNA is exported to the cytoplasm and is handled like a monocistronic mRNA. The *env* gene product is cleaved into the SU or gp70 (glycoprotein 70 000 Da) (**Figure 1**) and the TM (or gp20). Both the SU gp70 and TM gp20 proteins have sugar molecules bound to some of the amino acids that make up these two proteins. The SU glycoprotein can potentially contain 22 sugar residues. The TM is a membrane-spanning protein that anchors the complex in the virion membrane. An immunosuppressive motif is present within the TM protein and this protein motif may play a role in immune suppression. A monoclonal antibody is available against the TM-gp20 and this antibody is useful for diagnostic testing. The external glycoprotein is the least conserved among the macaque D retroviruses and is reflected in different serotypes. Neutralizing antibodies are defined by binding to the external glycoprotein. Therefore the major biological differences between SRV-1, SRV-2, MPMV, SRV-4, and SRV-5 are in fact differences in the amino acid sequence of Env.

Immature capsids (see arrows in **Figure 2**) are transported to the plasma membrane where they bud through the membrane (**Figure 2** inset) and acquire the Env proteins. The morphology of the completed D-type virion consists of an envelope and a cylindrical or rod-shaped core (**Figure 3**; a virion grown in tissue culture (**Figure 2**), and virions in the extracellular tissue space of an infected rhesus monkey).

The extracellular infectious virion initiates a new round of replication by attaching itself to a susceptible cell via a specific receptor on the surface membrane of the host cell. The receptor molecule for SRV and MPMV is an amino acid transport protein (ATBo) that is present in human tissues and cell lines, including white blood cells.

After entry in the cell, the RT synthesizes a minus DNA strand from the +-sense incoming SRV RNA genome.

The RT next catalyzes the synthesis of a complementary plus sense DNA strand, making a dsDNA copy of the D retrovirus RNA genome that contains two LTRs. The LTRs flank the viral genes and, through their interaction with the viral integrase, ensure that the genome will integrate in the correct orientation for expression of the viral genes. Usually DNA codes for RNA, but the RT reverses the process by making DNA from an RNA template, hence its name reverse transcriptase. The integrase then enzymatically integrates the linear dsDNA copy of the original RNA genome into host cell DNA. This dsDNA copy of the virus genome is called a provirus. With transcription of the provirus to form full-length genomic mRNA and spliced env mRNA, the replication cycle is completed and begins a new round.

## Natural Hosts

The natural host of SRV and MPMV is the Asian monkey genus *Macaca* or macaques. The known hosts are primarily common laboratory monkeys, such as the rhesus monkey (*M. mulatta*) of northern India, southern China, and geographical areas in between. SRV infection of rhesus macaques in China has been reported. Other macaque species housed at Primate Research Centers are also commonly infected. They include the cynomolgus macaque (*M. fascicularis*), also known as the long-tailed macaque and crab-eating macaque of Southeast (SE) Asia; *M. nemistrina*, the pig-tailed macaque of SE Asia; *M. nigra*, the Sulawesi or Celebes black macaque; and the bonnet macaque, *M. radiata*, of southern India. Feral cynomolgus macaques are infected, showing a natural Asian origin of this virus. Type D retroviruses are a significant problem for laboratory research, since infected animals may develop an AIDS-like disease. The most common SRV isolate in primate centers is SRV-2, followed by SRV-1, SRV-5, and MPMV. SRV-4 is only known from a single outbreak in cynomolgus macaques at a public health laboratory in Berkeley, California.

## Transmission

SRV is present in blood, urine, saliva, lymphoid, and nonlymphoid tissues of infected macaques (**Figure 2**). With the possible exception of brain tissue, infectious SRV is found throughout the body. Inoculation of any of these fluids or tissues to rhesus monkeys will transmit the infection and disease. Although infection is easily transmitted under laboratory conditions, a classic experiment on SRV infections transmitted in outdoor enclosures strongly pointed to natural transmission by bite from infected saliva. In these experiments at the California Primate Center, it was first shown that uninfected monkeys must be in physical contact with infected monkeys for transmission to occur. The need for this contact was proven by keeping uninfected monkeys in the same enclosure with infected monkeys, but separated by two fences creating a 10-foot barrier. The barrier prevented contact between infected and uninfected groups, but allowed birds, rodents, and insects to move freely between the enclosures as well as allowing rainwater to wash back and forth. The result was that only monkeys in physical contact with infected monkeys became SRV infected even after 5 years of testing.

SRV transmission to healthy monkeys was linked to healthy carriers, in particular to female healthy carriers that occupied socially dominant roles in the enclosure. Healthy carriers were infected for as long as 10 years without developing the AIDS-like disease that is characteristic of SRV infections. Repeated testing of the saliva of healthy carriers showed >1 million infectious units of SRV per ml of saliva, hence the likely link between saliva and transmission. Healthy carriers were a major problem for laboratory colonies because they could spread the SRV immune deficiency and themselves remain undetected, compromising the usefulness of these research colonies. The problem is now largely controlled by screening for SRV infection by antibody enzyme-linked immunosorbent assay (ELISA) and polymerase chain reaction (PCR) testing. Infected animals are removed from contact with the rest of the laboratory colony. This test and removal program is a highly successful approach to developing specific pathogen-free colonies for research.

## Broad *In Vitro* and *In Vivo* Cell Tropism

SRV has a broad cellular tropism and infects lymphoid, monocytes, and epithelial cells *in vitro*. SRV readily infects human T-cell lines, HuT-78, CEM-SS, MT-4, and SubT-1. The human B Raji cell line is also infected and SRV induces syncytia formation in this cell line. Adherent mononuclear cells from rhesus macaques were also infected *in vitro*. Peripheral blood mononuclear cells collected from infected animals and separated into CD4+ and CD8+ T-lymphocytes were also infected.

*In vivo* studies carried out on SRV-1-infected rhesus macaques showed infection of epithelial and lymphoid cells in the gut and elsewhere (**Figure 2**). The oral cavity and salivary glands have also been examined. Mucosal epithelia cells were heavily infected as early as 1 month post inoculation. Rarely, Langerhans cells were also shown to be infected using immunohistochemical techniques. Southern blot analyses showed salivary glands and lymphoid tissue to be more heavily infected than brain tissue. The infection of epithelia cells *in vivo* is striking in its widespread nature.

## Pathogenesis

The pathogenesis of SRV, MPMV, and SRV-2 is well described. Inoculation of any of these three grown in rhesus monkey tissue culture will induce an AIDS-like disease in most of the infected macaques. Pathogenesis studies are best carried out using virus grown in cells of the original host. Cultivation of the virus in human cells, especially Raji B cells, may attenuate the virus. The clinical course for SRV-1 is typically one-third developing disease in less than 6 months, one-third developing disease in 6 months to 2 years, and a third recover but remain antibody positive for SRV. Recovered animals may develop AIDS after a long clinically latent normal period. The disease is very similar to AIDS in human beings and includes opportunistic infections such as generalized cytomegalovirus disease and its associated pneumonia, wasting, chronic diarrhea unresponsive to therapy, and severe anemia. Infecting with a molecular clone, ruling out adventitious agents, proved the pathogenesis of SRV-1.

The disease induced by SRV is AIDS, but SRV should not be confused with simian immunodeficiency virus (SIV), a lentivirus related to human immunodeficiency virus 2 (HIV-2) that also causes AIDS in rhesus macaques. Macaques are not the natural hosts of SIV, since SIV naturally occurs in only sub-Saharan African cercopithecine monkeys and apes. The species naturally infected with SRV are all Asian macaque species. These two infections can be easily distinguished by specific Western blot. AIDS caused by SRV and SIV are both severe immunodeficiency syndromes, but differ in that SIV-induced AIDS is frequently associated with pneumocystis pneumonia, atypical tuberculosis, and B-cell lymphomas. In contrast, Kaposi sarcoma-like neoplasias are seen exclusively in type D SRV-induced AIDS.

## Simian RF

A tumor that occurs in the space behind the abdominal cavity (retroperitoneum) is associated with SRV-2 infections and the retroperitoneal fibromatosis herpesvirus (RFHV). RFHV is the macaque homolog of the human rhadinovirus that is associated with the Kaposi's sarcoma herpesvirus (KSHV). This monkey tumor is therefore an excellent model for Kaposi's sarcoma, one of the tumors that commonly occur in AIDS patients. DNA sequence data identified KSHV related herpes viruses in the RF tissue of pig-tailed and rhesus macaques. The basic fibroblast growth factor was found to be associated with RF tissues in SRV-2-infected macaques. The fibrosarcoma associated with SRV-1-induced AIDS is also a Kaposi-like tumor.

## Vaccines

Two types of vaccines have been successfully tested in the SRV AIDS model. The first used a killed-virus formulation. The virus was inactivated with formalin and injected intramuscularly to induce antibody. The SRV challenge virus used to test the efficacy of the vaccine was prepared in isogenic rhesus monkey kidney cells, therefore ruling out induction of anticellular antibody as a protective mechanism. Protection was associated with neutralizing antibody. This was the first vaccine shown to be effective against a primate retrovirus. The second vaccine used a recombinant vaccinia virus vector. The vaccinia virus vector expressed the envelope proteins (gp70 and gp20) of SRV-1 and MPMV. Upon challenge with live SRV-1 by the intravenous route, both MPMV- and SRV-1-immunized animals were protected. The vaccine therefore conferred cross-protection for SRV types 1 and MPMV, demonstrating *in vivo* their close relationship. The neutralizing antibody did not cross-react with the more distant SRV-2.

## Human Infections with SRV and Related Viruses

D-type retroviruses easily infect tissue culture cells derived from humans. Consequentially, several research groups have reported contamination of tissue cell lines. Therefore, there is a strong risk of contaminating cell cultures with this virus in the laboratories. Evidence for human infection that is based only on isolation of a D-type retrovirus from cultured human cells must be viewed with caution.

Human infections with SRV or MPMV have been reported in widely different diseases such as cancer and schizophrenia. Evidence of D-type virus has been reported in children with Burkett's lymphoma and in adult humans with breast cancer. However, direct evidence of SRV as an etiologic agent of human disease is thus far lacking.

An MPMV serological survey of European and African blood donors in Guinea-Bissau revealed 1 of 61 to be weakly positive for the MPMV p27 Gag polypeptide using Western blots. Squirrel monkey retrovirus-specific Western blots also revealed a few additional positive samples. Reaction in a blood donor consisting of only a single polypeptide is usually reported as an indeterminant result and is a false positive reaction. Nevertheless, D virus is widespread in nature and sequences related to the SRVs are found in the genomes of several primate species. Therefore, exposure to the virus is clearly possible. Nevertheless, extensive studies on over 1000 persons with various diseases have failed to find evidence of SRV infections in humans.

Diseases tested included lymphoproliferative disease patients, HIV-1 infected persons, persons with unexplained low CD4 lymphocyte counts, blood donors, and intravenous drug users from the USA and Thailand. Serum samples were screened for antibodies against SRV by an ELISA, and reactive samples were re-tested by Western blot. None of the samples were seropositive.

The most convincing evidence for nonpathogenic SRV infections in humans comes from a serosurvey of workers occupationally exposed to macaque D-type retroviruses at primate centers in the USA. Occupational exposure could come from an accidental bite from infected monkeys during routine care such as cage cleaning or accidental exposure by a contaminated needle stick. Two of 231 persons tested were strongly positive by Western blot. Each person displayed antibody to more than one gene of SRV (**Figure 4**). Lanes 1 and 2 showing a reactive band at the 70, 31, 24, and 20 Da markers indicated reaction with the *pol*, *env*, and *gag* gene products. One individual had neutralizing antibody to SRV-2, providing convincing evidence of an active SRV infection in the past. The most important tests to document active infections were negative. Repeated attempts to amplify the genomic DNA specific for SRV from specimens, as well as attempts to recover infectious virus, were not successful.

These findings are nevertheless important for understanding zoonotic infections and the related but more dangerous outcome of zoonosis. Zoonotic infections are fairly common under the right exposure conditions, but a zoonosis is a rare outcome. Even though SRV may infect human blood cells *in vivo* and grow temporary in the new host, the immune system of the non-natural human host is capable of eliminating the zoonotic infection. The past infection will be evident from trace amounts of specific antibody that was induced during the transient infection. Infection of humans with simian D and other simian retroviruses is well documented, but evidence of zoonosis has not been found.

*See also:* Mouse Mammary Tumor Virus; Simian Immunodeficiency Virus: General Features.

## Further Reading

Colcher D, Spiegelman S, and Schlom J (1974) Sequence homology between the RNA of Mason–Pfizer monkey virus and the RNA of human malignant breast tumors. *Proceedings of National Academy of Sciences, USA* 71(12): 4975–4979.

Daniel MD, King NW, Letvin NL, Hunt RD, Sehgal PK, and Desrosiers RC (1984) A new type D retrovirus isolated from macaques with an immunodeficiency syndrome. *Science* 223: 602–605.

Gardner MB and Marx PA (1985) Simian acquired immunodeficiency syndrome. In: Klein G (ed.) *Advances in Viral Oncology*, vol. 5, pp. 57–81. New York: Raven Press.

Heidecker G, Lerche NW, Lowenstine LJ, *et al.* (1987) Induction of simian acquired immune deficiency syndrome (SAIDS) with a molecular clone of a type D SAIDS retrovirus. *Journal of Virology* 61(10): 3066–3071.

Lackner AA, Rodriguez MH, Bush CE, *et al.* (1988) Distribution of a macaque immunosuppressive type D retrovirus in neural, lymphoid, and salivary tissues. *Journal of Virology* 62: 2134–2142.

Lerche NW, Marx PA, Osborn KG, *et al.* (1987) Natural history of endemic type D retrovirus infection and acquired immune deficiency syndrome in group-housed rhesus monkeys. *Journal of the National Cancer Institute* 79(4): 847–854.

Lerche NW, Switzer WM, Yee JL, *et al.* (2001) Evidence of infection with simian type D retrovirus in persons occupationally exposed to nonhuman primates. *Journal of Virology* 75(4): 1783–1789.

Linial M and Weiss R (2001) Other human and primate retroviruses. In: Knipe DM and Howley PM (eds.) *Fields Virology*, 4th edn., pp. 2123–2139. Philadelphia: Lippincott Williams and Wilkins.

Marracci GH, Avery N, Shiigi S, *et al.* (1999) Molecular cloning and cell-specific growth characterization of polymorphic variants of type D serogroup 2 simian retroviruses. *Virology* 261: 43–58.

Marx PA, Maul DH, Osborn KG, *et al.* (1984) Simian AIDS: Isolation of a type D retrovirus and transmission of the disease. *Science* 223: 1083–1086.

Marx PA, Pedersen NC, Lerche NW, *et al.* (1986) Prevention of simian acquired immune deficiency syndrome with a formalin-inactivated type D retrovirus vaccine. *Journal of Virology* 60(2): 431–435.

Rose TM, Strand KB, Schultz ER, *et al.* (1997) Identification of two homologs of the Kaposi's sarcoma-associated herpesvirus (human herpesvirus 8) in retroperitoneal fibromatosis of different macaque species. *Journal of Virology* 71(5): 4138–4144.

Sonigo P, Barker C, Hunter E, and Wain-Hobson S (1986) Nucleotide sequence of Mason–Pfizer monkey virus: An immunosuppressive D-type retrovirus. *Cell* 45(3): 375–385.

Stromberg K, Benveniste RE, Arthur LO, *et al.* (1984) Characterization of exogenous type D retrovirus from a fibroma of a macaque with simian AIDS and fibromatosis. *Science* 224(4646): 289–292.

Wolfheim JH (ed.) (1983) *Primates of the World*. Washington: University of Washington Press.

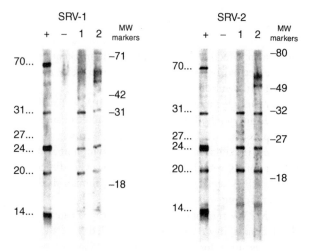

**Figure 4**  WB reactivity against SRV-1 and SRV-2 on initial screening in sera from two persons occupationally exposed to nonhuman primates. Lanes: (+)-lane is known SRV-positive serum from a rhesus monkey; (–)-lane is SRV-negative serum from a known negative rhesus monkey; lane 1, subject 1, lane 2, subject 2. MW, molecular weight (weights are in thousands of daltons). gp70 is the surface spike of SRV. Reproduced from Lerche NW, Switzer WM, Yee JL, *et al.* (2001) Evidence of infection with simian type D retrovirus in persons occupationally exposed to nonhuman primates. *Journal of Virology* 75(4): 1783–1789, with permission from American Society for Microbiology.

# St. Louis Encephalitis

**W K Reisen,** University of California, Davis, CA, USA

## Glossary

**Bridge vector** Vector responsible for carrying virus from the primary cycle to tangential hosts such as humans.

**Diapause** Insect hibernation.

**Gonotrophic cycle** Recurrent cycle of blood feeding and egg laying by female mosquitoes.

**Maintenance vector** Vector responsible for transmission of virus among primary vertebrate host species.

**Neuroinvasive** Ability of virus to invade the central nervous system.

**Vector competence** Ability of an insect to become infected with and transmit a pathogen.

**Viremia** Concentration of virus within peripheral blood.

**Viremogenic** Ability to elicit an elevated viremia response.

## History

St. Louis encephalitis virus (SLEV) probably has been present in the New World within its enzootic cycle for thousands of years. The arrival of European settlers in the 1600s and the extensive agricultural development that followed greatly altered the landscape by clearing and irrigating vast areas of North America and establishing extensive urban centers. These changes probably increased the abundance of peridomestic *Culex* mosquito species and avian hosts such as house finches and mourning doves, introduced new avian hosts such as house sparrows, intensified human–vector mosquito contact, and probably increased the incidence of human infection. However, diagnosis of diseases caused by arbovirus infections such as SLEV assuredly was confounded with other infections causing fever and central nervous system (CNS) disease during summer.

During the summer of 1933, a major encephalitis epidemic with more than 1000 clinical cases occurred in St. Louis, Missouri. These cases occurred during the middle of an exceptionally hot, dry summer and were concentrated within areas of the city adjacent to open storm water and sewage channels that produced a high abundance of *Culex* mosquitoes. A virus, later named St. Louis encephalitis virus, was isolated at autopsy from human brain specimens. Mouse protection assays using convalescent human sera demonstrated that SLEV differed from other viruses causing seasonal CNS disease, such as the equine encephalitides, poliomyelitis, and vesicular stomatitis. The epidemiological features of this epidemic included the late summer occurrence of cases (especially in persons over 50 years of age), exceptionally warm temperatures, and elevated *Culex* mosquito abundance associated with a poorly draining wastewater system. These features remain the hallmark of SLEV epidemics to date.

A multidisciplinary team of entomologists, vertebrate ecologists, epidemiologists, and microbiologists from the University of California subsequently investigated an SLEV epidemic in the Yakima Valley of Washington State during 1941 and 1942 and established the components of the summer transmission cycle, including wild birds as primary vertebrate hosts and *Culex* mosquitoes as vectors. The isolations of SLEV from *Culex tarsalis* and *Culex pipiens* mosquitoes were among the first isolations of any virus from mosquitoes and stimulated the redirection of mosquito control in North America from *Anopheles* malaria vectors and pestiferous *Aedes* to *Culex* encephalitis vectors.

Understanding the basic transmission cycle, an appreciation of the wide range of clinical symptoms, and the development of laboratory diagnostic procedures provided an expanding view of the public health significance of SLEV, with epidemics or clusters of cases recognized annually throughout the US. Wide geographic distribution and consistent annual transmission since 1933 has resulted in >1000 deaths, >10 000 cases of severe illness, and >1 000 000 mild or subclinical infections. The largest documented SLEV epidemic occurred during 1975 in the Ohio River drainage, with >2000 human cases documented. Other substantial human epidemics involving hundreds of cases have occurred in Missouri (1933, 1937), Texas (1954, 1956, 1964, 1966), Mississippi (1975), and Florida (1977, 1990). Smaller outbreaks have been recognized in California (1952), New Jersey (1962), and several other states plus Ontario (1975), Canada. Cases reported annually to the Centers for Disease Control and Prevention (CDC) since 1964 are shown in **Figure 1**.

## Distribution

SLEV is distributed from southern Canada south through Argentina and from the west to the east coasts of North America and into the Caribbean Islands. Historically, human cases have been detected in Ontario and Manitoba, Canada, all of the continental US (except the New England States and South Carolina, **Figure 2**), Mexico, Panama, Brazil, Argentina, and Trinidad. The

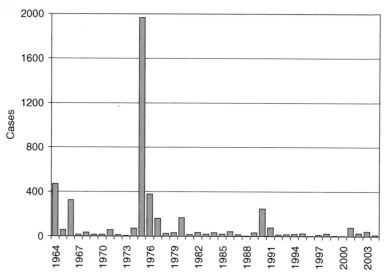

**Figure 1** Number of clinical cases of St. Louis encephalitis reported to the US CDC, 1964–2004. Data provided by ArboNet, Center for Disease Control and Prevention, Ft. Collins, CO, USA.

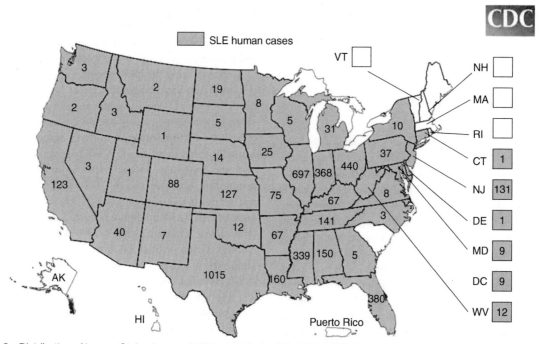

**Figure 2** Distribution of human St. Louis encephalitis cases in the US, 1964–2004. Map provided by ArboNet, Center for Disease Control and Prevention, Ft. Collins, CO, USA.

low number of human cases in Canada probably reflects the warm temperature requirements for SLEV replication in the mosquito host, whereas the low numbers of cases from tropical America may reflect inadequate laboratory diagnosis, the circulation of attenuated virus strains, and/or enzootic cycles involving mosquitoes that feed infrequently on humans. Support for this geographic distribution comes from laboratory-confirmed human cases, SLEV isolations from birds, mammals, and mosquitoes, and serological surveys of mammal and avian populations.

## Classification

Taxonomically, SLEV is classified within the Japanese encephalitis virus (JEV) complex in the genus *Flavivirus* of the family *Flaviviridae*. Related viruses within this group include Japanese encephalitis, Murray Valley encephalitis, West Nile, and Usutu. SLEV consists of a positive-sense, single-stranded RNA enclosed within a capsid composed of a single polypeptide (C) and surrounded by an envelope containing one glycosylated (E) and one nonglycosylated (M) protein. Marked differences in the severity of SLEV epidemics stimulated interest in possible differences among isolates made over time and space. Detailed studies by the CDC during the 1980s clearly demonstrated geographic variation among 43 different SLEV isolates using oligonucleotide finger printing and virulence in model vertebrate hosts. These strains are grouped into six clusters: (1) east central and Atlantic USA, (2) Florida epidemic, (3) Florida enzootic, (4) eastern USA, (5) Central and South America with mixed virulence, and (6) South America with low virulence. Changes in virulence were attributed, in part, to differences in mosquito vector competence and were supported by the historical presence or absence of human cases. Subsequent genetic sequencing studies extended the understanding of SLEV genetics and provided further insight into patterns of geographical variation. Sequences of the envelope gene from SLEV strains isolated in California from 1952 to 1995 varied temporally and spatially, but indicated regional persistence in the Central Valley for at least 25 years as well as sporadic introduction and extinction. Studies in Texas using a single-strand conformation polymorphism technique showed that multiple SLEV strains circulate concurrently and remain highly focal, whereas other strains amplify and disseminate aggressively during some summers, but then disappear. Further analyses of sequences from 62 isolates made throughout the known geographical range of SLEV indicated that there have been seven lineages that overlapped somewhat with the six groups the CDC defined previously using oligonucleotide fingerprinting: (1) western USA, (2) central and eastern USA and three isolates from Mexico and Central America, (3) one mosquito isolate from Argentina, (4) five isolates from Panama mosquitoes, (5) South American strains plus an isolate from Trinidad, (6) one Panama isolate from a chicken, and (7) two isolates from Argentina rodents. Collectively, these data indicated that SLEV strains vary markedly in virulence and that the frequency and intensity of epidemics in the US may be related to genetic selection by different host systems. Interestingly, transmission within the Neotropics appears to have given rise and/or allowed the persistence of less-virulent strains that rarely amplify to produce epidemic-level transmission, a scenario duplicated by West Nile virus in the Americas.

## Host Range

### Arthropods

Although a wide variety of mosquitoes occasionally have been found infected in nature, three avian-feeding species within the genus *Culex* appear to be the most frequently infected and important arthropod hosts: *C. pipiens* (including the subspecies *C. pipiens quinquefasciatus* at southern latitudes, *C. p. pipiens* at northern latitudes,

and intergrades) in urban and periurban environments throughout North and South America, *C. tarsalis* in irrigated agricultural settings in western North America including northern Mexico, and *Culex nigripalpus* in the southeastern US, the Carribean, and parts of the Neotropics. Although these species feed predominantly on birds, they also feed on mammals including humans, and therefore function as both maintenance and bridge vectors. Other *Culex* species such as *stigmatosoma* in the west, *restuans* and *salinarius* in the east, and perhaps species in the subgenus *Melanoconion* in the Neotropics also may be important in local transmission. Ticks have been found naturally infected, but their role in virus epidemiology most likely is minimal.

### Wild Birds

The importance of avian host species appears to be related to vector *Culex* host-selection patterns as well as to avian susceptibility to the virus. Species can be separated into those frequently, sporadically, and never found infected in nature, and these groupings are related directly to their nocturnal roosting/nesting behavior and the questing behavior of *Culex* vectors. Wild birds do not develop apparent illness following experimental infection, but their viremia response varies markedly, depending upon virus strain, bird species, and bird age. Titers sufficient to infect mosquitoes typically are limited to 1–5 days post-infection. Based on serological surveys during or after epidemics, peridomestic passeriforms (including house finches, house sparrows, cardinals, and blue jays) and columbiforms (including mourning oves and rock doves or domestic pigeons) seem to be infected most frequently. In house sparrows, SLEV strains isolated from *C. pipiens* complex mosquitoes from the central and eastern USA produced elevated viremias, whereas strains isolated from *C. tarsalis* from the western USA were weakly viremogenic. Although host competence studies have been limited, the adults of few bird species seem to develop elevated viremias. However, nestling house finches, house sparrows, and mourning doves produce high viremias that readily infect mosquitoes. Therefore, the nesting period of multibrooded species may be critical for virus amplification. Regardless of their viremia response, most experimentally infected birds produce antibody and, although titers typically decay rapidly, these birds remain protected for life.

### Humans

Humans are incidental hosts and do not produce viremias sufficient to infect mosquitoes. Like most arboviruses that cause CNS disease, infection with SLEV does not result in a clear clinical picture in humans and most infections remain unrecognized, unless associated with an epidemic. When presented with such diverse symptoms, few physicians initially suspect SLEV, even in endemic areas. Most SLEV infections, especially in young or middle age groups, fail to produce clinical disease, and infected individuals rarely experience more than a mild malaise of short duration with spontaneous recovery.

## Domestic Animals

Although frequently antibody positive during serosurveys, SLEV infection does not produce elevated viremias or cause clinical illness in domestic animals, including equines, porcines, bovines, or felines. In a single experiment, dogs (purebred beagles) produced a low-level viremia, with only two of eight dogs developing clinical illness. Similar to wild birds, immature fowl <1 month old (including chickens and ducks) consistently developed sufficient viremia to infect mosquitoes, but did not develop clinical illness. Adult chickens (>22 weeks old) usually failed to develop a detectable viremia, and along with immature birds, developed long-lasting antibodies.

## Wild Mammals

The response of wild mammals to natural or experimental infection varies. Serosurveys occasionally have shown higher SLEV prevalence in mammals than in birds, but these data could be confounded because mammalian hosts typically live longer than avian hosts and therefore have a longer history of exposure. Rodents in the genera *Ammospermophilus* and *Dipodomys* were susceptible to infection after subcutaneous (s.c.) inoculation, whereas *Spermophilus, Rattus, Sigmodon,* and *Peromyscus* were refractory. Similarly varied were lagomorphs: *Lepus* was susceptible, whereas four species within *Sylvilagus* ranged from refractory to susceptible. Raccoons and skunks were refractory, whereas opossums and woodchucks were susceptible. Like birds, susceptible mammals produced an immediate viremic response that generally persisted for <1 week, and all species produced detectable antibodies regardless of their viremia response. SLEV frequently has been isolated from bats (*Tadarida, Myotis,* etc.), and many populations exhibit a high prevalence of neutralizing antibody. Overall, the role of mammalian infection in SLEV epidemiology is complex and difficult to interpret. All reputed *Culex* vectors feed most frequently on avian hosts, occasionally on large mammals and lagomorphs, rarely on rodents, and almost never on bats.

## Pathogenicity

In humans, clinical disease due to SLEV infection may be divided into three syndromes in increasing order of severity: (1) 'Febrile headache' with fever, headache possibly associated with nausea or vomiting, and no CNS illness;

(2) 'Aseptic meningitis' with high fever and stiff neck; and (3) 'Encephalitis' (including meningoencephalitis and encephalomyelitis) with high fever, altered consciousness, and/or neurological dysfunction. The onset of illness may be sudden (<4 days after infection) and acute, leading rapidly to encephalitis, or insidious, progressing gradually through all three syndromes. Symptoms may resolve spontaneously during any stage of the illness, with full recovery. Acute illness may be followed by 'convalescent fatigue syndrome' in <50% of patients, with complaints of general weakness, depression, and the inability to concentrate that generally resolve within 3 years. Other sequelae include headache, disturbances in gait, and memory loss.

Pathogensis in SLEV follows a course similar to other flaviviruses in the JEV complex. The extent of illness usually is dependent upon viremia level and duration. Virus replication occurs within the lymphatic system soon after infection, and resulting viremias reflect the balance between virus production and release by the lymphatic system and clearance mediated by phagocytes of the liver and spleen. The probability of CNS involvement is directly correlated with the extent and duration of the viremia, although the mechanism of neuroinvasion remains unclear. Movement from peripheral to central nervous tissue most likely is by passive transport through neuron cytoplasm and then by transport across associated membranes after cell lysis. CNS pathology consists of necrosis of neurons and glia cells and inflammatory changes. Inflammatory changes typically are most important in slowly progressing or sublethal CNS disease and sequelae. Viral clearance is dependent upon a functional immune system and the rapid production of neutralizing antibody, which usually appears within 7 days after infection.

## Epidemiology

Transmission of SLEV is complex and requires that the virus replicate in and avoid the immune responses of alternating insect and vertebrate hosts under temperatures ranging from below 0 °C in diapausing mosquitoes to more than 40 °C in febrile avian hosts. Annual transmission activity may be divided into overwintering, vernal and/or summer amplification, and autumnal subsidence periods.

## Overwintering

Three possible mechanisms may explain the persistence of SLEV at temperate latitudes; however, few supportive field data are available.

### Persistence in mosquito populations

Three mechanisms may explain SLEV overwintering within vector mosquito populations. First, low-level vertical passage of SLEV from infected females to F1 progeny has been demonstrated repeatedly in laboratory experiments. Although not detected for SLEV in nature, vertical transmission has been documented for other viruses in the JEV complex, including JEV and West Nile virus (WNV). Second, *C. p. pipiens* females destined for diapause have been shown to take small blood meals during late summer and early fall without ovarian development. Two isolations of SLEV made from diapausing *C. p. pipiens* females collected resting during winter in Maryland were considered to have been infected by this mechanism, although infection by vertical transmission also was possible. Third, *Culex p. quinquefasciatus* and *C. nigripalpus* do not enter reproductive diapause, remain reproductively active throughout winter at southern latitudes and, depending upon ambient temperature, could maintain SLEV by continued, infrequent transmission among resident birds. Experimentally infected, reproductively active *C. p. quinquefasciatus* females have been shown to survive winter as gravid females and to then transmit SLEV to recipient birds throughout the following spring.

### Persistence in vertebrate populations

SLEVs may also persist over winter within vertebrate host populations. Passeriform birds infrequently develop chronic infections that persist as long as a year following experimental infection. However, attempts to demonstrate natural relapse or to trigger relapse experimentally have not been successful. Flaviviruses, including SLEV, have also been isolated repeatedly from bats, and experimental infections in bats destined for hibernation have been maintained for 20 days at 10 °C. When returned to room temperature, SLEV was detected in the brown fat and at low levels in the blood. These data indicated that bats could function as an overwintering host. However, studies of mosquito host-selection patterns indicated that bats rarely, if ever, were fed upon by host-seeking mosquitoes.

### Reintroduction of virus

An alternative hypothesis to local persistence involves annual or periodic reintroduction of virus into northern latitudes from southern refugia. Long-distance movement of SLEV has been indicated indirectly from genetic evidence as well as by the reappearance of SLEV after years of absence. Two possible hypotheses address reintroduction, but neither is well supported by field evidence. Many species of birds and some bats have long-distance annual migrations that could allow the transport of virus from foci active during winter in southern latitudes or south of the equator to receptive areas north of the equator during spring. These vertebrate migrations typically are very consistent in their summer and winter destinations, and this would allow the same or similar genetic strains to reappear each summer at the same locality. However, molecular genetic studies of North, Central, and South American isolates indicate that they are relatively

distinct, thereby implying infrequent genetic exchange. In addition, migratory birds do not seem to be frequently involved in transmission because they infrequently are found positive for virus or antibody.

### Amplification

Regardless of the persistence mechanism, summer enzootic amplification transmission in North America involves *Culex* mosquitoes and primarily birds in the orders Passeriformes and Columbiformes. Humans become infected tangentially to the primary cycle, do not develop viremias sufficient to infect mosquitoes, and are considered to be 'dead end' hosts (**Figure 3**). Transmission appears to be initiated after the *Culex* vectors resume blood-feeding and reproductive activity, and ambient temperatures warm sufficiently to allow the replication of virus in the mosquito host. Infection is acquired when a female *Culex* blood feeds on a viremic avian host. Virus imbibed within infectious blood meals taken in early in spring when ambient temperatures average <17 °C may lay dormant until warm conditions or changes in mosquito physiology stimulate replication. Under warm temperatures, virus replicates rapidly, disseminates within the mosquito during the ensuing extrinsic incubation period, and then may be transmitted by bite after the female oviposits and attempts to imbibe a subsequent blood meal. The duration of the extrinsic incubation period is temperature dependent and requires >10 days and perhaps two mosquito gonotrophic cycles when temperatures average 22 °C. In contrast, the viremia response in susceptible avian hosts typically is of short duration, lasting 2–4 days.

Four distinct transmission cycles of SLEV are defined by differences in the biology of the primary vector mosquito species and their distribution, and include: (1) rural North America, west of the Mississippi River transmitted by *C. tarsalis*; (2) rural and urban central and eastern North America transmitted by members of the *C. pipiens* complex; (3) Florida, Caribbean, and parts of Central America transmitted by *C. nigripalpus*; and (4) urban and rural South America transmitted by *C. pipiens* complex and mosquitoes of other taxa.

### Subsidence

Intensity of enzootic transmission and occurrence of new human cases always subsides rapidly during autumn. Cool evening temperatures slow the replication of SLEV within infected mosquito hosts, decreasing the efficiency of transmission and, concurrently, the combination of cool water temperature and shortening days during larval development initiates reproductive diapause (*C. tarsalis, C. p. pipiens*) or quiescence (*C. p. quinquefasciatus, C. nigripalpus*) in vector females emerging during fall. The fall mosquito population declines in abundance and divides

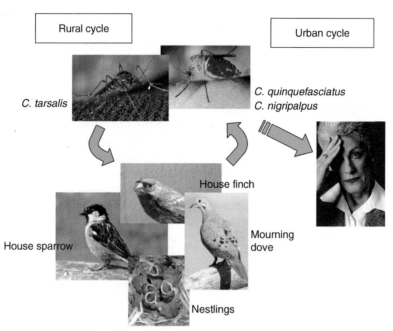

**Figure 3**  Amplification transmission cycle of St. Louis encephalitis virus in North America.

into newly emerged females that do not routinely blood-feed and survive the winter, and remnants of the summer population that continue reproductive activity, but fail to survive winter. The critical day length that triggers the onset of diapause in *C. p. pipiens* may occur in late summer at northern latitudes, markedly shortening the SLEV transmission season. During warm days, however, females may become infected when taking partial blood meals from viremic birds, survive winter, and then transmit the virus after diapause is terminated by warm spring temperatures. *Culex p. quinquefasciatus* does not undergo diapause, so that reproductive activity may continue through winter, albeit at a rate slowed by winter temperatures. Populations exploiting underground storm water systems for resting or for larval development may be exposed to relatively warm temperatures throughout winter.

### Risk Factors for Human Infection

Five factors have been associated with human risk of SLEV infection.

### Residence

Clearly, place of residence markedly affects the risk of infection, with geographic regions in the southern USA having the greatest numbers of human cases and greatest incidence of disease (**Figure 2**). Based on experimental infection patterns in laboratory mice, virus strains from this geographical area also exhibit greater neurovirulence than strains from the western USA or South America. Because of mosquito abundance relative to humans and host-selection patterns, urban residents seem to be at greater risk for SLEV infection than rural residents.

However, these conclusions may be confounded by protective immunity acquired early in life that may be greater among rural residents and by low apparent: inapparent case ratios that require a substantially large population to produce recognizable clusters of human cases.

### Age

In the absence of acquired immunity, clinical illness and fatality rates, but not necessarily infection rates, increase dramatically with age. Infection seems to occur equally among different age classes as indicated by the increase in antibody as a function of age in endemic areas and by cohort seroconversion rates determined after epidemics in previously unexposed populations. For example, using data following the 1964 Houston (Texas) epidemic, seroprevalence rates remained similar among cohorts, whereas the case–incidence rates increased from 8.2 per 100 000 for the 0–9-year-old cohort to 13.5–27.6 for the 10–59-year-old cohorts and to 78.0 for the >60-year-old group; apparent to inapparent ratios decreased concomitantly from 1:806 to 1:490–1:239 and to 1:85, respectively. Case–fatality rates among 2288 cases reported to the CDC from 1971–83 increased from <6.7% for 0–64-year-old age classes to 9.5% for the 65–74-year-old class to 18% for the >75-year-old class.

### Occupation

In the West, where SLE historically was a rural disease, infection risk was greatest among male agricultural workers who frequently lived in suboptimum housing and worked at night. However, infection patterns during recent urban outbreaks indicated that attack rates were highest among elderly women. These data indicated that there may be differences in risk related to vector species, with elderly women infected most readily during urban outbreaks associated with the *C. pipiens* complex, and men working outdoors at greatest risk during rural outbreaks associated with *C. tarsalis*.

### Socioeconomic status

Historically, socioeconomic status has been related closely to the distribution of cases during urban epidemics. Homes and municipal drainage systems frequently were not well maintained in low-income neighborhoods, and this was related to the distribution of human cases, but not necessarily the occurrence of virus within the enzootic transmission cycle. TV and air conditioning ownership that brought people indoors during the evening *Culex* host-seeking period was found to reduce risk.

### Weather

Climate variability affects temperature and precipitation patterns, mosquito abundance and survival, and therefore SLEV transmission. Annual temperature changes based on the El Niño/southern oscillation in the Pacific alter precipitation and temperature patterns over the Americas and cycle with varying intensity at 3–5 year intervals. These cycles alter storm tracks that affect mosquito and avian abundance, the intensity and frequency of rainfall events, and groundwater depth, all related to SLEV risk. Above-normal temperatures have been especially necessary for northern latitude SLEV epidemics, because elevated temperatures are required for effective SLEV replication within the mosquito host.

## Prevention and Control

Effective vector control remains the only approach available to suppress summer virus amplification and prevent human infections. Best results are achieved using an integrated management approach that focuses on mosquito vector population suppression through habitat inspection and larviciding. Failure of larval management can be followed by emergency adult control focusing on reducing the force of transmission and preventing human infection. Protection of the human population by vaccination does not seem cost-effective or prudent, because there is no human-to-human transmission, few human infections produce disease, and infection rates remain relatively low, even during epidemics. However, if regional infection rates were to become high, thereby placing selected cohorts at high risk for disease, then selective vaccination may be warranted. There currently is no approved commercial vaccine for SLEV, although vaccination against other flaviviruses such as JEV may impart some protection. Control of avian hosts such as house sparrows and pigeons in urban situations could be done, but this approach is not generally acceptable to the public. Notification of the public of infection risk through the media and the wide scale use of personal protection through changes in behavior (staying indoors after sunset) and/or repellent application were credited with reducing the number of infections during the 1990 epidemic in Florida.

## Further Reading

Day JF (2001) Predicting St. Louis encephalitis virus epidemics: Lessons from recent, and not so recent, outbreaks. *Annual Review of Entomology* 46: 111–138.

Kramer LD and Chandler LJ (2001) Phylogenetic analysis of the envelope gene of St. Louis encephalitis virus. *Archives of Virology* 146: 2341–2355.

Monath TP (1980) In: *St. Louis Encephalitis*, 680pp. Washington, DC: American Public Health Association.

Monath TP and Tsai TF (1987) St. Louis encephalitis: Lessons from the last decade. *American Journal of Tropical Medicine and Hygiene* 37: 40s–59s.

Reeves WC, Asman SM, Hardy JL, Milby MM, and Reisen WK (eds.) (1990) In: *Epidemiology and Control of Mosquito-Borne Arboviruses in California, 1943–1987*, 508pp. Sacramento, CA: California Mosquito and Vector Control Association.

Reisen WK (2003) Epidemiology of St. Louis encephalitis virus. In: Chambers TJ and Monath TP (eds.) *The Flaviviruses: Detection, Diagnosis and Vaccine Development*, pp. 139–183. San Diego, CA: Elsevier.

# Theiler's Virus

**H L Lipton and S Hertzler,** University of Illinois at Chicago, Chicago, IL, USA
**N Knowles,** Institute for Animal Health, Pirbright, UK

## Glossary

**Cardiovirus** Genus in the family *Picornaviridae*.
**Demyelination** Pathological process of damage to the proteolipid coat around nerve fibers (axons).

**L\*** Virus-encoded protein that is translated in alternative reading frame to that of the polyprotein.
**Theilovirus** Species within the genus *Cardiovirus*.
**Theiler's murine encephalomyelitis viruses (TMEVs)** Abbreviation for mouse Theiler's viruses.

## History, Geographic Distribution, and Host Range

The mouse encephalomyelitis viruses are enteric pathogens of mice. Discovered by Max Theiler in the early 1930s and originally called murine polioviruses, these agents are commonly referred to as Theiler's murine encephalomyelitis viruses (TMEVs). Theiler initially recovered isolates from mice with spontaneous paralysis housed at the time in the animal colony at the Rockefeller Institute; subsequently, TMEVs were found in virtually all nonbarrier mouse colonies, where they caused asymptomatic intestinal infections. While TMEVs are widely distributed in the world, their host range is narrow, including mice and rats. Serological evidence indicates that *Mus musculus*, the feral house mouse, is the natural host, but several other species of voles and possibly rats may also serve as hosts. As is the case for other picornaviruses, following peripheral routes of infection, TMEV spreads to the central nervous system (CNS) producing encephalitis or poliomyelitis (spontaneous paralysis). In the older literature, the incidence of spontaneous paralysis was reported to be approximately one paralyzed animal per 1000–5000 colony-bred mice. Since TMEVs may go undetected unless appropriate serological tests are performed, these agents are a potential hazard for investigators using mice in biomedical research.

In recent years, this group of viruses has assumed additional importance, because TMEV infection in mice provides one of the few available experimental animal models for multiple sclerosis. TMEV-induced demyelinating disease in mice is a relevant model for multiple sclerosis because: (1) chronic pathological involvement is virtually limited to the CNS white matter; (2) myelin breakdown is accompanied by mononuclear cell inflammation; (3) demyelination results in clinical disease, for example, spasticity, from involvement of upper motor neuron pathways; (4) myelin breakdown is in part immune-mediated; and (5) the disease is under multigenic control with a strong linkage to the major histocompatibility complex (MHC) gene H2D.

## Classification and Serologic Relationships

Based on the complete nucleotide sequence and genome organization, TMEVs have been classified in the genus *Cardiovirus* of the family *Picornaviridae* along with encephalomyocarditis virus (EMCV). EMCV and TMEV (or Theilovirus) constitute separate species within the genus *Cardiovirus*. Polyclonal antisera show no cross-neutralization between TMEV and EMCV; however, since the coat proteins of the two *Cardiovirus* species share ~50% identity of their amino acid sequences, cross-reactions

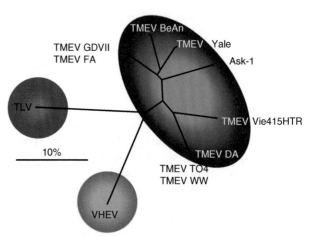

**Figure 1** Phylogenetic analysis of the P1 capsid-coding region of the Theiloviruses showing three clades, presumably representing three distinct serogroups: TMEV, Vilyuisk human encephalomyelitis virus (VHEV), and Theiler's-like virus of rats (TLV).

are observed with antibody binding assays such as enzyme-linked immunosorbent assay (ELISA) and complement fixation. Phylogenetic analysis of the complete P1 capsid-coding region has revealed three major clades: TMEV, Vilyuisk human encephalomyelitis virus (VHEV), and the Theiler's-like virus (TLV) of rats (**Figure 1**). These three clades presumably represent three distinct serotypes of the species *Theilovirus*; however, comprehensive serological studies remain to be performed.

## Physical Properties

Because the TMEVs do not have an envelope they are insensitive to chloroform, ether, nonionic detergents, such as deoxycholate, NP40 and Tween-80, and the ionic detergent sodium dodecyl sulfate, but are inactivated by 0.3% formaldehyde and HCl $0.1 \, \mathrm{mol \, l^{-1}}$. TMEVs are rapidly destroyed at temperatures over 50 °C and lose some infectivity upon lyophilization. Purified virions can be stored for long periods of time at −70 °C without loss of infectivity, but slowly lose infectivity on storage at −20 °C. Enteroviruses require stability at low pH to pass through the acidic conditions of the stomach. TMEVs are stable over the entire pH range from 3 to 9.5, but in contrast to the other cardioviruses, such as EMCV, they are not highly thermolabile in the presence of $0.1 \, \mathrm{mol \, l^{-1}}$ chloride or bromide in the pH range 5–7.

## Virion Structure

Picornavirions have a relative molecular mass of ~8.5 × $10^6$ Da, of which 30% is RNA and 70% protein. Theiler's

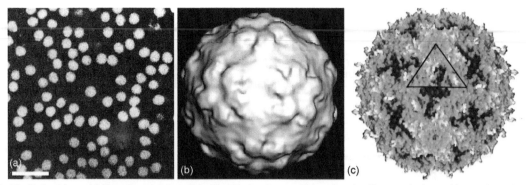

**Figure 2** Theiler's virions. (a) Negative staining of purified BeAn virus particles showing the morphology of featureless virus profiles due to the impermeability of the capsid to the electron dense stain. Scale = 100 μm. (b) Cyroelectron micrograph of a GDVII virion at 20 Å resolution showing the star-shaped profile of the plateau around the fivefold axes. (c) GRASP image of a BeAn virion showing a topographical relief map of the VP1 and VP2 surface loops in white. The superimposed triangle represents a protomer with its apex pointing at the fivefold axis. The darkened area within the outlined iscosahedral unit is a surface depression of the pit or receptor binding site. This depression extends across the twofold axis.

virions are 30 nm in diameter and their structure reveals only a spherical virion by negative staining (**Figure 2(a)**). Virions have a sedimentation coefficient of 150 S by velocity centrifugation in sucrose and a buoyant density of 1.34 g ml$^{-1}$ by isopycnic centrifugation in cesium salts.

The three-dimensional structures of the GDVII, BeAn, and DA strains have been determined at ∼3 Å resolution by X-ray crystallography (**Figures 2(b)** and **2(c)**). The overall architecture is quite similar to that of other picornaviruses and closely resembles that of Mengo virus, another member of the EMCV species. Each virion is composed of 12 pentamers, with each pentamer made up of five protomers, each containing a single copy of the four capsid proteins. Each of the three major capsid proteins VP1, VP2, and VP3 consist of a wedge-shaped eight-stranded antiparallel β-barrel. The N-termini of the capsid proteins form an extensive, intertwined network on the inner surface of the protein shell. The loops connecting the β-strands form the outer surface features of the protein shell and provide surface differences with Mengo virus. A 25 Å depression on the virion surface at the junction between VP1 and VP2 along the twofold axis, termed the pit, is believed to be the viral receptor and is a broad depression. The TMEV surface structures are differentiated from that of Mengo virus in having: (1) a larger VP1 CD double loop, with loop I containing an extra five residues, that is shifted more toward the VP2 EF puff at the twofold axis, while loop II is directed more toward the fivefold axis; (2) an 11-residue insertion in the VP2 EF puff forming a double loop in which the inserted loop interacts with the VP1 FMDV GH loop; and (3) the tip of the VP3 knob (a loop inserted in βE) points directly outward on the rim of the pit.

## Properties of the Genome

The genetic component of the TMEV virion is a single-stranded, positive-polarity RNA molecule 8100 nt in size that has a sedimentation coefficient of 35 S. The virion RNA has a virally encoded 20 amino acid protein, VPg, covalently linked to the 5′ uridine, and a poly(A) tract on the 3′ end. The complete genomes of the GDVII, DA, BeAn strains, as well as TLV have been sequenced. With the notable absence of a poly(C) tract in the 5′ untranslated region, the organization and sequence of the TMEV genome is remarkably similar to that of EMCV. The polyprotein of the prototypic BeAn strain initiates at the AUG codon at nucleotide 1065 and extends for 6909 nt (or 2303 codons), ending at the single UGA termination triplet at base 7972 (**Figure 3**). The polyprotein-coding region is flanked by 5′ and 3′ untranslated sequences of 1064 and 125 nt, respectively. In BeAn the 5′ untranslated region contains a stretch of 11 pyrimidines interrupted by a single purine before the AUG at nucleotide 1065. In picornaviruses, the 5′ untranslated region mediates cap-independent translation and serves as an internal ribosome entry site (IRES). The TMEV 5′ untranslated sequences have been predicted to form stable secondary structures, which in the 500 nt upstream of the authentic AUG (at 1065) are nearly identical to those predicted for EMCV and foot-and-mouth disease virus. In BeAn, eight AUGs precede the initiator AUG, but none of them has an optimum Kozak context sequence. Hence, it could be argued that selection of the authentic initiator AUG after binding of ribosomes to TMEV RNA does not involve internal ribosome binding. However, BeAn nucleotides ∼500–1065 determine a structure that serves as an IRES in bicistronic mRNAs both *in vitro* (BHK-21 cells). A poly(A) tail of indeterminate length is present on the 3′ end of the viral genome.

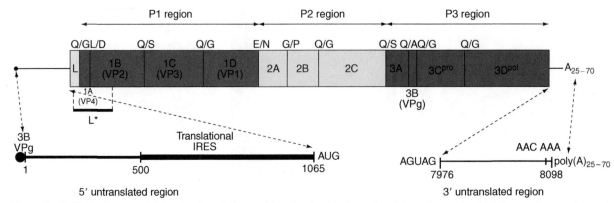

**Figure 3**    TMEV 8 kbp genome showing 5′ and 3′ untranslated regions (enlarged) and the polyprotein which is superimposed over the 7 kbp nucleotide open reading frame (ORF) and contains the final 12 viral gene products. The 5′ end of the viral RNA is not capped but has protein 3B (VPg) covalently attached to the first nucleotide. A ~500 base internal ribosome entry site (IRES) is present in the 5′ untranslated region immediately upstream of the authentic AUG initiation codon for the polyprotein. The 3′ untranslated region ends in a poly (A) tail. The ORF is divided into L, P1 (blue) encoding the four capsid proteins, P2 (yellow) three nonstructural proteins, and P3 (red) four nonstructural proteins, including the 3C cysteine protease which makes all but two of the cleavages in the polyprotein, and the 3D, the RNA-dependent RNA polymerase. Cleavage dipeptides are shown above viral protein boundaries. Finally, the location of the L* protein that is translated out-of-frame is shown near the N-terminus of the polyprotein.

## Translation: Polyprotein Processing and Final Gene Products

The 12 TMEV gene products are the result of post-translational processing of a 2303 amino acid polyprotein (mol. weight of 256 kDa) (**Figure 3**). The polyprotein of GDVII virus contains no insertions or deletions; however, two VP1 amino acids are deleted in DA, TO4, and WW viruses. The processing scheme follows a standard L-4-3-4 picornavirus polypeptide arrangement, that is, the leader protein (L), four capsid proteins in part one (P1) of the genome, three proteins in P2, and four proteins in P3 (**Figure 3**). The coding limits of individual viral proteins have been predicted by analogy with those of EMCV since the only confirmation to date of a deduced sequence is that of the N terminus of 1D. The eight amino acids flanking the putative cleavage sites are highly conserved for the two viruses. All of the cleavage sites in the polyprotein except for two, 1A/1B and 2A/2B, are processed by the viral protease 3C. The TMEV 3C protease therefore processes Q-C, as well as Q-S and Q-A, dipeptides and, in addition, the E-N dipeptide at the 1D/2A cleavage. However, only 6 of 8 Q-G, 2 of 13 Q-S, and 1 of 7 Q-A dipeptides in the polyprotein are cleaved by 3C, indicating that involvement of secondary, tertiary, or both types of structure is also important for recognition of these particular dipeptides. The tetrapeptide NP/GP at 2A/2B which is the primary cleavage site in the cardiovirus polyprotein is cleaved autocatalytically, as it is in EMCV.

Cleavage of the polyprotein gives rise to three primary products, the first of which (116 kDa) contains the leader protein (8 kDa), the P1 capsid proteins, and the first P2 protein 2A (15 kDa). Thus, the initial precursor released

from the polyprotein is like that of the other cardioviruses but differs from that of other groups of picornaviruses. The capsid proteins are arranged in the following order: 1A (VP4; 7 kDa), 1B (VP2; 29 kDa), 1C (VP3; 25 kDa), and 1D (VP1; 30 kDa). The second processing precursor (2BC) is 51 kDa and gives rise to 2B (14 kDa) and 2C (37 kDa). The third or C-terminal precursor protein is 88 kDa and is processed into the four mature proteins 3A (10 kDa), 3B (2 kDa), 3C (24 kDa), and 3D (52 kDa). The functions of the nonstructural proteins are shown in **Table 1**. Another protein, termed L*, translated out-of-frame, is initiated 22 nt downstream of the authentic AUG in the polyprotein, giving rise to an 18 kDa protein that was originally shown to be involved in the TMEV persistent infection.

## Viral RNA Replication

Cardiovirus replication is similar to that of other picornaviruses. Following entry, VPg is removed from the 5′ end of the RNA, and the RNA is directly translated using cellular factors. The viral genomic RNA (plus-sense), is then transcribed into negative-strand copies, and each one is used as template for reiterative synthesis of ~25–50 plus-sense RNAs identical to the genome of the virus. An RNA structure located within the VP2 sequence of TMEV is necessary for RNA replication, and is referred to as the *cis*-acting replicative element (CRE). The CRE functions as a template for uridylylation of viral protein 3B (VPg) forming $VPgpUpU_{OH}$ which primes positive-strand RNA synthesis. Viral protein 3D is the RNA-dependent RNA polymerase which catalyzes both of these processes.

## Viral Genomic Determinants in Pathogenesis

The existence of two naturally occurring TMEV neurovirulence groups provides a useful system for investigating molecular pathogenesis. Moreover, the difference in neurovirulence in terms of mean 50% lethal dose between high and low neurovirulence strains is of the order of $10^5$ plaque forming units. With the advent of reverse genetics the generation of full-length cDNA clones of high neurovirulence GDVII and low virulence DA and BeAn viruses was feasible. Viral RNAs transcribed from cDNAs are infectious upon transfection of mammalian cells. To identify pathogenetic determinants, for example, those of neurovirulence and persistence, recombinant viruses between parental cDNAs have been assembled and point mutations introduced into wild-type strains for analysis in cell culture and mice.

Neurovirulence and persistence have been mapped to the L-P1 regions encoding the L and L* proteins and the capsid proteins. The results suggest that the mechanism for the pathogenetic properties of neurovirulence and persistence involve several determinants, including an exclusive role for the capsid in neurovirulence and the out-of-frame L* protein and capsid (exterior surface of the virion) in persistence. The latter observation suggested that receptor-mediated events may be involved in persistence; it was demonstrated that persistence required the ability of low neurovirulence strains to bind to its sialic acid co-receptor. The L* protein was initially recognized because only the low neurovirulence strains have an out-of-frame AUG start codon. However, the ACG codon in high neurovirulence strains was then shown to initiate L* translation, and chimeric TMEVs that contain a high neurovirulence L protein in a low neurovirulence background were shown to persist in the mouse CNS as well as the low neurovirulence parental virus. The role of the L* protein in persistence will require further study.

## Transmission and Tissue Tropism

TMEVs are transmitted by the fecal–oral route and are separable into two biological groups based on neurovirulence (**Table 2**). The first group, consisting of three isolates, GDVII, FA, and ASK-I, possesses high neurovirulence,

**Table 1**    Functional activities of the TMEV nonstructural proteins

| Nonstructural protein | Activities |
| --- | --- |
| Leader (L) | Binds to Ran, inhibiting import and export of proteins to and from the nucleus, including those involved in the innate interferon response |
| L* | Out-of-frame 19-kDa protein initiated by AUG or ACG codons immediately downstream of the authentic AUG for polyprotein translation; has a putative role in TMEV persistence |
| 2A | A C-terminal tetrapeptide NP/GP responsible for autocatalytic cleavage of 2A/2B, the primary cleavage in the cardiovirus polyprotein |
| 2B | Possible role in cell membrane permeability |
| 2C | A multifunctional protein involved in viral RNA replication, including ATPase, GTPase, membrane binding, and RNA binding activities |
| 3A | Inhibition of ER-to-Golgi transport that results in reduction of host cell cytokine secretion |
| 3B | Covalently linked to the 5′-terminal uridine of the single-stranded RNA and primer for the viral RNA-dependent RNA polymerase |
| 3C | Cysteine-reactive protease responsible for all of the monomolecular and bimolecular cleavages in the polyprotein except for the assembly-dependent maturation cleavage of VP0 (1A/1B) and autocatalytic cleavage at 2A/2B |
| 3D | RNA-dependent RNA polymerase responsible for viral RNA replication |

**Table 2**    Two TMEV neurovirulence groups

| Characteristic | High neurovirulence | Low neurovirulence |
| --- | --- | --- |
| Isolates (strains) | GDVII, FA, ASK-1 | DA, BeAn 8386, Yale, WW, TO4, TO(B15), Vie415HTR |
| Disease | Encephalomyelitis | Poliomyelitis/demyelination |
| Incubation period | 1–10 days | 7–20 days/>30 days |
| CNS target cell | Cortical and motor neurons | Motor neurons/macrophages and oligodendrocytes |
| $LD_{50}$ | 1–10 PFU | $>10^5$ PFU |
| Persistent infection | No | Yes |
| Temperature sensitive | No | Yes |
| Carbohydrate co-receptor | Heparan sulfate | α2,3-linked sialic acid |
| Differences in virion structure | Only in the Cα chain of the VP2 puff B | |

causing a rapidly fatal encephalitis in mice. Some 10–15 isolates, including viruses recovered from the CNS of spontaneously paralyzed mice and feces of asymptomatic mice, form a second, low neurovirulence group. Experimentally, the low neurovirulence strains produce poliomyelitis (early disease) followed by demyelinating disease (late disease). When mice are inoculated intracerebrally with cell culture-adapted low neurovirulence strains, the poliomyelitis phase is attenuated (subclinical); whereas, brain-derived stocks of these viruses produce both disease phases.

## Pathogenesis

Very little information is available about the pathogenesis of TMEV infection following peripheral routes of infection, including the oral route. In general, isolates from either of the neurovirulence groups do not readily produce CNS disease following peripheral routes of inoculation, with the exception of TO(B15), a mutant selected for its invasiveness from the intestinal tract. When mice are inoculated intracerebrally with the high neurovirulence strains, virus replicates widely in the brain and spinal cord, causing encephalitis or encephalomyelitis. Thus, neurons as well as glial cells (astrocytes and oligodendrocytes) become infected in the cerebral cortex, hippocampus, basal ganglia, thalamus, brainstem, and spinal cord. Affected mice develop hunched posture and hind-limb paralysis. A rapid demise is the result of widespread cytolytic infection. The following sections focus on the pathogenesis of the biphasic disease produced by the low neurovirulence strains, which provides an experimental model system for human demyelinating disease, multiple sclerosis.

## Clinical Features of Infection

The intracerebral route of inoculation maximizes the incidence of neurological disease. Following intracerebral inoculation, the low neurovirulence strains produce a distinct biphasic CNS process in susceptible strains of mice, which is characterized by poliomyelitis during the first 2 weeks post infection, followed by chronic, inflammatory demyelination that begins during the second or third week post infection and becomes clinically manifest between 1 and 3 months post infection. Some investigators who inoculated lower amounts of virus observed an even later onset of demyelinating disease. Mice with poliomyelitis develop flaccid paralysis, usually of the hind limbs; only one limb may be affected or paralysis may involve both hind limbs and spread to involve the forelimbs, occasionally leading to death. In contrast to the fatal outcome of paralysis produced by the Lansing strain of human poliovirus type 2, complete recovery from TMEV-induced

poliomyelitis is usually seen. Residual limb deformities may be seen as the result of extensive anterior horn cell infection and severe paralysis (early disease).

Gait spasticity is the clinical hallmark of the demyelinating (late) disease. Late disease is first manifest by slightly unkempt fur and decreased activity, followed by an unstable, waddling gait. Subsequently, generalized tremulousness and ataxia develop, and the waddling gait evolves into overt paralysis. Incontinence of urine and priapism are seen. As the disease advances, prolonged extensor spasms of the limbs occur spontaneously followed by difficulty in righting. Extensor spasms can be induced by turning an animal over on its back by quickly rotating the tail. Weight loss occurs during late disease. The clinical manifestations of late disease are progressive and lead to an animal's demise in several to many months post infection. A functional motor assay using a rotorod apparatus has been used to quantitate motor function in this disease.

## Pathogenesis and Histopathology

Motor neurons in the brainstem and spinal cord are the main targets of infection during poliomyelitis, but sensory neurons and astrocytes are also infected. TMEVs do not replicate in endothelial and ependymal cells. A brisk microglial reaction is elicited, with the appearance of numerous microglial nodules, particularly in the anterior gray matter of the spinal cord. Examples of neuronophagia are quite frequent at this time, but little lymphocytic response is seen. The poliomyelitis phase lasts 1–4 weeks, after which time little residual gray matter involvement is inapparent other than for astrocytosis.

As early as 2 weeks post infection, inflammation of the spinal leptomeninges begins to appear, followed by involvement of the white matter. Initially, the inflammatory infiltrates are almost exclusively composed of lymphocytes, but at later times plasma cells and macrophages become numerous (**Figure 4(a)**). The influx of macrophages is in close temporal and anatomic relationship with myelin breakdown. Both light microscopic and ultrastructural studies show that myelin breakdown is related to the presence of macrophages (**Figure 4**), which either actively strip myelin lamellae from otherwise normal-appearing axons or are found in contact with myelin sheaths undergoing vesicular disruption. Foci of inflammation and myelin destruction extend from the perivascular spaces into the surrounding white matter, leading to sharply demarcated plaques of demyelination (**Figure 4(b)**). The ultrastructure studies during the initial phase of myelin breakdown have not shown alterations in oligodendroglia, which are in close apposition with naked but otherwise normal axons; however, oligodendrocytopathology has been observed later although it appears to be a minor contributor to demyelination.

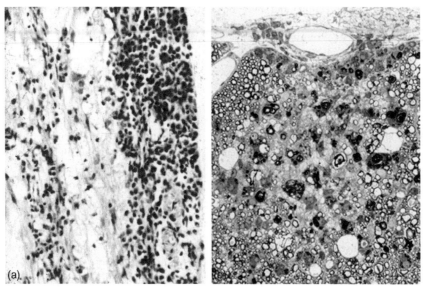

**Figure 4** Histopathology of TMEV-induced demyelinating disease (late disease) in an SJL mouse. (a) H&E-stained longitudinal section (6 μm) of the spinal cord showing intense mononuclear inflammatory cell infiltrates in the leptomeninges (right) and parenchyma where many vacuolated macrophages are observed. (b) Toluidine blue-stained, Epon-embedded coronal section (1 μm) of a spinal cord showing a discrete plaque-like area of demyelination (many naked axons present) and lipid-laden macrophages at the cord margin and surrounded by normal myelinated axons. Magnification ×400 (a); ×300 (b).

## Sites of TMEV Persistence

TMEV persistence clearly involves active virus replication, since infectious virus can be readily isolated from the CNS of infected mice and high viral genome copy numbers are present. *In situ* hybridization has revealed two populations of CNS cells differing in the number of viral genomes. Virus replication in the majority of these cells (>90%) appears to be restricted, as they contain <500 viral genomes. A small percentage of CNS cells contain >1500 genomes, possibly as many as $10^4$–$10^5$, and are probably productively infected. The absolute number of viral genomes as determined by *in situ* hybridization is probably only an approximation. Restricted virus production has been demonstrated in macrophages isolated from the CNS of diseased mice; therefore, macrophages appear to be the primary target for persisting virus. It is also possible that some of the cells with restricted infection are astrocytes. The kinetics of virus replication in the CNS cells with restricted infection remains to be elucidated – the length of the replicative cycle and whether the cells are lysed or continue to produce infectious virus for longer times is not known. TMEV infection *in vitro* only occurs in monocytes once they have differentiated into macrophages. Virus production in infected macrophage cell lines is restricted but viral translation, polyprotein processing, and assembly of virion intermediates (protomers and pentamers) as well as virions appear to be normal. Ultimately infected macrophages undergo apoptosis, which is caspase-9 and -3 dependent, consistent with activation of the mitochondrial pathway. In contrast, oligodendrocytes appear to be productively infected, since ultrastructural analysis has shown crystalline arrays of virions in oligodendrocytes in demyelinating lesions in mice. Oligodendrocytes may correspond to the CNS cells containing large numbers of viral genomes by *in situ* hybridization. These data suggest that a cytolytic infection of oligodendrocytes contributes to demyelination along with immune-mediated mechanisms of myelin damage.

## Immune Response

During the first week, TMEV-infected mice mount a virus-specific humoral immune response that reaches a peak by 1–2 months post infection and is sustained for the life of the host. Neutralizing and other virus-specific antibodies have been measured. The majority of the antiviral IgG response in persistently infected, susceptible mice is IgG2a subclass, with little antiviral IgM detected by day 14 post infection, whereas IgG1 antiviral antibodies appear to predominate in resistant as well as in immunized mice. Murine CD4+ T cells of the Th1 subset mediate delayed-type hypersensitivity (DTH) and regulate IgG2a production via interferon-γ production, whereas CD4+ Th2 cells regulate IgG1 and IgE production via interleukin 4. Thus, the predominant IgG2a antiviral response in susceptible mice may be an *in vivo* measure of preferential stimulation of a Th1-like pattern of cytokine synthesis. Virus-specific CD8+ cytolytic T-cell responses have also been shown to help in virus clearance during the acute phase of the infection, and may be responsible for the resistance of C57BL/6 mice to the demyelinating disease.

Infected, susceptible strains of mice also produce substantial levels of virus-specific CD4+ T-cell responses. T-cell proliferation and DTH appear by 2 weeks post infection and remain elevated for at least 6 months. Both DTH and T-cell proliferation have been shown to be specific for TMEV and mediated by CD4+ class II restricted T cells. A temporal correlation has also been found between the onset of demyelination and the appearance of virus-specific CD4+ T-cell responses, as well as for high levels of virus-specific DTH. High levels of the Th1 cytokines interferon-$\gamma$ and TNF-$\alpha$ also correlate temporally with the evolution of demeylination. DTH and CD4+ T-cell proliferative responses in infected and immunized susceptible SJL mice are directed toward immunodominant regions (peptides) in each of the three major coat proteins. T-cell responses to these epitopes in VP1 and VP2 are believed to participate in the immunopathology.

Although mice mount virus-specific humoral and cellular immune responses early in the infection and peak CNS virus titers fall by 100 000-fold, TMEVs somehow evade immune clearance to persist at low infectious levels indefinitely. Extraneural persistence has not been observed. Current dogma holds that humoral immunity is more important than cellular immunity in clearing infections by nonenveloped viruses, such as picornaviruses. Evidence has been presented for a role for both neutralizing antibodies and cytolytic CD8+ T cells in TMEV clearance. The precise mechanism by which TMEVs evade immune surveillance is not known but does not appear to involve antigenic variation. Although complement and virus-antibody deposition in the CNS parenchyma has detected extracellular transport of virus as infectious virus antibody complexes, viral aggregates, or as virus contained within cellular membranes, are a possible means whereby virus could be protected from TMEV-specific immune responses and continue to infect other cells. This is an area for further study to enable a better understanding of how TMEV evade immune surveillance.

## Immune-Mediated Mechanism of Demyelination

Appropriately timed immunosuppression can prevent the clinical signs and pathological changes of TMEV-induced demyelinating disease, indicating that the immune response participates in myelin breakdown. A number of different immunosuppressive modalities have proved to be effective, including cyclophosphamide, antilymphocyte serum, antitumor necrosis factor antibodies, and monoclonal anti-IA, CD4+, and CD8+ antibodies. If given too early in the course of early disease,

the infection in neurons is potentiated and results in encephalitis and a high mortality rate. Thus, immunosuppression may be most effective when administered after the first week of infection. The incidence of demyelinating disease is increased in SJL mice infected with a dose of virus that normally produces a low incidence of disease and adoptively immunized with TMEV VP2-specific T-cell line. This observation supports a role for CD4+ T cells in mediating TMEV-induced demyelinating disease.

The effector mechanism by which a nonbudding virus, such as TMEV, might lead to immune-mediated tissue injury is unknown. Because TMEV antigens have been primarily found in macrophages, it has been proposed that myelin breakdown results from an interaction between virus-specific T cells trafficking into infected areas of the CNS and the virus. Thus, myelinated axons may be nonspecifically damaged as a consequence of a virus-specific immune response, that is, an 'innocent bystander' response. In this circumstance, cytokines produced by MHC class II-restricted, TMEV-specific $T_{DTH}$ cells primed by interaction with infected macrophages lead to the recruitment and activation of additional macrophages in the CNS, resulting in nonspecific macrophage-mediated demyelination. This hypothesis is consistent with the CNS pathology observed in mice exhibiting TMEV-induced demyelinating disease and the fact that antigen-specific T cells and T-cell lines have been shown to cause bystander CNS damage via macrophage activation in other model systems. Alternatively, in the case of extensive infection of oligodendrocytes, demyelination might result from immune injury to these myelin-maintaining cells expressing TMEV antigens in conjunction with H-2 class I determinants. CD8+ T cells would then be the likely T cells to kill infected oligodendrocytes; however, widespread degeneration of oligodendrocytes has not been observed.

## Acknowledgments

The authors thank Jan-Yve Sgro for providing the GRASP image of a BeAn virion and Paul Chipman for the cryoelectron micrograph of a GDVII virion.

## Further Reading

Adami C, Pritchard AE, Knauf T, Luo M, and Lipton HL (1998) Mapping a determinant for central nervous system persistence in the capsid of Theiler's murine encephalomyelitis virus (TMEV) with recombinant viruses. *Journal of Virology* 71: 1662–1665.

Borson NO, Paul C, Lin X, *et al.* (1997) Brain-infiltrating cytolytic T lymphocytes specific for Theiler's virus recognize H2D$^b$ molecules complexed with a viral VP2 peptide lacking a consensus anchor residue. *Journal of Virology* 71: 5244–5250.

Dethlefs S, Brahic M, and Larsson-Sciard EL (1997) An early, abundant cytotoxic T-lymphocyte response against Theiler's virus is critical for preventing viral persistence. *Journal of Virology* 71: 8875–8878.

Grant RA, Filman OJ, Fujinami RS, Icenogle JP, and Hogle JM (1992) Three-dimensional structure of Theiler virus. *Proceedings of the National Academy of Sciences, USA* 89: 2061–2065.

Jelachich ML, Bramlage C, and Lipton HL (1999) Differentiation of M1 myeloid precursor cells into macrophages results in binding and infection by Theiler's murine encephalomyelitis virus (TMEV) and apoptosis. *Journal of Virology* 73: 3227–3235.

Kumar ASM, Reddi HV, Kung A, and Lipton HL (2004) Virus persistence and disease in a mouse model of multiple sclerosis requires binding to the sialic acid co-receptor. *Journal of Virology* 78: 8860–8867.

Lobert PE, Escriou N, Ruelle J, and Michiels T (1999) A coding RNA sequence acts as a replication signal in cardioviruses. *Proceedings of the National Academy of Sciences, USA* 96: 11560–11565.

Luo M, He C, Toth KS, Zhang CX, and Lipton HL (1992) Three-dimensional structure of Theiler's murine encephalomyelitis virus (BeAn strain). *Proceedings of the National Academy of Sciences, USA* 89: 2409–2413.

Paul S and Michiels T (2006) Cardiovirus leader proteins are functionally interchangeable and have evolved to adapt to virus replication fitness. *Journal of General Virology* 87: 1237–1246.

Penna-Rossi C, Delcroix M, Huitinga I, *et al.* (1997) Role of macrophages during Theiler's virus infection. *Journal of Virology* 71: 3336–3340.

Peterson JO, Waltenbaugh C, and Miller SD (1992) IgG subclass responses to Theiler's murine encephalomyelitis virus infection and immunization suggest a dominant role for Th1 cells in susceptible mouse strains. *Immunology* 75: 652–658.

Roussarie J-P, Ruffie C, and Brahic M (2007) The role of myelin in Theiler's virus persistence in the central nervous system. *PLoS Pathogens* 3(2): e23(doi:10.1371/journal.ppat.0030023).

Simas JP and Fazakerley JK (1996) The course of disease and persistence of virus in the central nervous system varies between individual CBA mice infected with the BeAn strain of Theiler's murine encephalomyelitis virus. *Journal of General Virology* 77: 2701–2711.

Trottier M, Wang W, and Lipton HL (2001) High numbers of viral RNA copies in the central nervous system during persistent infection with Theiler's virus. *Journal of Virology* 75: 7420–7428.

Yauch RL, Palma JP, Yahikozawa H, Chang-Sung K, and Kim BS (1998) Role of individual T-cell epitopes of Theiler's virus in the pathogenesis of demyelination correlates with the ability to induce a Th1 response. *Journal of Virology* 72: 6169–6174.

# Yatapoxviruses

**J W Barrett and G McFadden,** The University of Western Ontario, London, ON, Canada

## Introduction

The most recently accepted ICTV designation for the *Poxviridae* includes a new primate genus in the subfamily *Chordopoxvirinae*. The genus *Yatapoxvirus* contains two recognized members: the type species, *Yaba monkey tumor virus* (YMTV) and *Tanapox virus* (TPV).

## History

Poxvirus members of the genus *Yatapoxvirus* have been identified relatively recently following infection of monkeys at primate centers in Nigeria (1957) and in several states of the USA (1967), and infection of native African populations of equatorial Africa (late 1950s and early 1960s). YMTV infection produces benign histiocytomas in man and monkeys that rapidly proliferate, leading to large subcutaneous masses that are considered benign tumors. TPV infection causes localized, dermal lesions which are located on the extremities and which resolve slowly. The yatapoxviruses have been shown to infect humans and other primates only (**Table 1**). Based on genomic sequence data and morphology studies, the yatapoxviruses are structurally similar to other members of the *Poxviridae*.

YMTV was first observed following a spontaneous outbreak of subcutaneous tumors in a colony of captive rhesus monkeys housed in open-air pens in June 1957 at Yaba, near Lagos, Nigeria. The superficial growths were first observed in a single rhesus monkey and subsequently spread to 20 of 35 rhesus monkeys from that colony over the following several weeks. Although this primate center housed several other species in close proximity, only a single other species of primate (dog-faced baboon) was affected during this outbreak. The lesions in all cases eventually regressed.

TPV was first identified (1957) following two outbreaks among local people living in villages along the Tana River of Kenya. The illness was characterized by acute febrile reaction and associated pox-like skin lesions. A more widespread illness of 50 cases occurred in 1962 that included both genders and a spread of ages. The observation that the infection occurred during years of dramatic floods and increased mosquito activity, and the fact that the lesions appeared only on areas of exposed skin suggested that a biting insect, most likely a mosquito, was the vector of transmission. Virus isolated from infected humans could only be grown *in vitro* on various human and monkey cell lines. In addition, further transmission of infection by the inoculation virus was successful only in man and monkey. Therefore, most likely, an undefined local monkey species acts as the reservoir species for TPV.

Supporting these conclusions was the occurrence of mild poxvirus infections in three primate centers in the

**Table 1**    Members of the *Yatapoxvirus* genus

| Member | Abbreviation | Natural host | Major arthropod vector | Natural host disease | Length of infection |
|---|---|---|---|---|---|
| Yaba monkey tumor virus | YMTV | Monkeys of Africa and Malaysia | Probably mosquito | Large, multicellular masses (2–5 cm) | Spontaneously regresses 6–12 weeks |
| Tanapox | TPV | Humans | Probably mosquito | Individual, round, raised nodules | Resolution in 3–4 weeks |
| Yaba-like disease | YLDV | Captive primates/ human handlers | Probably mosquito in monkeys, possibly scratches or bites to human handlers | Individual-few raised nodules | Resolution in 3–4 weeks |

USA in 1966. The affected monkeys, mainly rhesus macaques, exhibited lesions that were similar in appearance and histology to those of the native Kenyans infected with tanapox. The lesions were hypertropic, slow in developing, with little evidence of vesiculation, and these characteristics were quite different from the lesions produced by a similarly appearing nodule that arises from monkeypox infection of man. In addition, at least two handlers at these centers contracted an infection which produced symptoms and lesions that clinically and histologically resembled tanapox infection.

## Taxonomy and Classification

The prefix 'yata' is a contraction from the names of the two recognized members of the yatapoxviruses: *ya*ba monkey tumor virus and *ta*napox virus. The members of the yatapoxviruses are closely related by sequence similarity, serology, and immunodiffusion tests. This genus is comprised of only two recognized members (YMTV and TPV) that so far have only been shown to infect primates, including humans. The members of this genus are immunologically distinct from members of the seven other *Chordopoxvirinae* genera. Vaccination by poxviruses from other genera, including vaccinia virus, will not protect from infection by the yatapoxviruses and, conversely, a previous infection with a yatapoxvirus will not block other poxvirus infections.

A third member, yaba-like disease virus (YLDV), considered a strain of TPV, has been isolated from monkeys and their human handlers at several primate centers in the USA. Although ICTV does not recognize YLDV, the complete genomic sequence has been deposited in GenBank and provides scientists with genetic information about the closely related TPV.

## Properties of the Virion

Morphologically, the yatapoxvirus viruses resemble typical oval-shaped poxvirus virions. YMTV and TPV particles contain a lipid outer membrane, inner membrane, and enclosed dumbbell-shaped core and lateral bodies. The virus measures between 250 and 300 nm on the long axis.

## DNA Replication, Transcription, and Translation

Generally, viral DNA replication and protein synthesis of the yatapoxviruses is similar to, albeit slower than, the prototypical poxvirus, vaccinia virus. Yatapoxvirus DNA synthesis occurs in the cytoplasm of infected cells in 'virus factories'. Sequencing has confirmed that the genomes of the yatapoxviruses encode the standard suite of conserved poxvirus housekeeping genes, including transcription factors and enzymes required for viral replication, transcription, and translation.

One consistent difference between YMTV and other poxviruses has been the observation that YMTV replicates more efficiently *in vitro* at 35 °C rather than 37 °C. The reason for this temperature sensitivity is undefined; however, it may be the result of a required viral-encoded enzyme that is temperature sensitive or prolonged passage in a poikilothermic, nonmammalian host. Regardless, the cycle of replication follows standard poxvirus early gene expression, DNA synthesis, late gene expression, and morphogenesis. Viral DNA synthesis is detected as early as 3 h post infection (p.i.). Progeny virus first appears at 24 h p.i. *in vitro* and plateaus at 72 h p.i. This replication cycle is six to ten times longer than for vaccinia virus. YMTV has a narrow host range in tissue culture. In addition, *in vitro* infection involves a prolonged replication cycle and generally low virus yield. Continuous cells from cercopithecus monkey kidney cells (CV-1) are susceptible to YMTV infection; however, cell lines derived from other monkeys (BGMK, OMK) and other species (e.g., HeLa, RK13, and CEFs) do not support productive infection.

In contrast, TPV replication is most efficient at 37 °C. TPV replication follows the typical cascade of poxvirus DNA synthesis and production of infectious progeny but exhibits slower kinetics when compared to vaccinia virus, although it is much faster than YMTV. The eclipse period ranges from 24 to 48 h p.i.; however, this variation is dependent on the multiplicity of infection.

Transient expression of native yatapoxvirus genes from standard mammalian expression vectors results in low-to-no protein expression. However, if the viral coding sequence is optimized to favor the use of more commonly used human codons, the result is generally much higher protein expression levels from transfected human cells.

## Properties of the Genome

The members of the yatapoxviruses encode the smallest characterized genomes within the *Poxviridae* (**Table 2**). Complete genomic sequencing information is now available for all yatapoxviruses. The genomes of the yatapoxvirus members are very A+T- rich, a characteristic shared by other members of the *Poxviridae* including members of the ortho-, sui-, capri-, and avipoxviruses. The YMTV genome is 70% A+T, 134.7 kbp long, and encodes for 140 genes. In contrast, TPV is 144.6 kbp, 73% A+T, and encodes for 155 genes (**Table 2**). Comparison between the complete YLDV sequence and the sequenced genomes of TPV indicates a high degree of sequence identity of approximately 98%, supporting the claim that TPV and YLDV are strains of the same virus. Comparison of the genomic sequences of YMTV and TPV indicates 78% identity. All of the genes identified in YMTV are also encoded by TPV; however, YMTV has lost 13 open reading frames (ORFs) found in TPV. The yatapoxviruses encode many of the same structural and housekeeping genes that are found in other poxviruses. The immunomodulatory genes of the yatapoxviruses also include a handful of novel genes predicted to be involved in regulation of immune response that are unique to the yatapoxvirus or are found in only a few other poxviruses. These include a new inhibitor of human tumor necrosis factor (TNF α (2L), virally encoded versions of chemokine receptors (7L and 145R), and TPV/YLDV (but not YMTV) encodes a viral IL-10 homolog (134R).

## Immunity

YMTV and TPV show minimal to moderate cross-reactivity in collected sera. However, YMTV infection can protect nonhuman primates from TPV challenge. Monkeys infected with TPV and then challenged with YMTV exhibit reduced tumors and delayed symptoms. Comparison between YMTV and TPV infection identified both type-common and type-specific antigens. Circulating neutralizing antibodies, although present in the sera of several species of monkeys, are ineffective in preventing growth of YMTV tumors or reinfection. Immunity to superinfection is observed as long as tumors are present or regressing; however, following total tumor regression a new infection results in new tumor formation. Complement-fixing and complement-fixing-inhibiting antibodies are present in clinical and convalescent stages, respectively, of rhesus monkeys infected with either TPV or YMTV. The persistence of complement-fixing antibodies in monkeys infected with TPV is 10–12 weeks. Complement-fixing antibody was detected up to 35 weeks p.i. in monkeys infected with YMTV.

## Tropism and Transmission – Humans

Naturally occurring YMTV infections have only been identified in nonhuman primates. However, accidental and volunteer infections have been established in humans. Infected humans develop lesions similar to those observed in monkeys although the proliferative responses are less pronounced and regression occurs earlier than in monkeys. Recovery of infectious virus from human lesions followed by serial passage and titration confirmed that YMTV was able to replicate productively in primary human tissue. Inoculation of rabbits, guinea pigs, hamsters, rats, mice, and dogs failed to produce proliferative lesions. In addition, no lesions were observed following inoculation of embryonated eggs. Testing of nonhuman primates suggests that rhesus and cynomolgus species are most susceptible as hosts.

TPV infections have only been identified in native populations of equatorial Africa or visitors to that region. The fact that infections appeared during years of extensive flooding, and that lesions are observed only on exposed areas of skin and occur on the extremities, suggests that transmission is via a biting arthropod vector (e.g., mosquitoes).

YLDV infection of monkey handlers at primate centers of the US exhibited a brief fever followed by production of a few raised, necrotic nodules that completely resolved.

**Table 2**    Features of the yatapoxvirus genomes

| Member | Genome size (bp) | Single copy genes | Duplicated genes | Terminal inverted repeat (bp) | % A+T |
|--------|------------------|-------------------|------------------|-------------------------------|-------|
| TPV | 144 565 | 155 | 1 | 1868 | 73 |
| YMTV | 134 721 | 139 | 1 | 1962 | 70.2 |
| YLDV | 144 575 | 150 | 1 | 1883 | 73 |

## Tropism – Nonhuman Primates

YMTV and YLDV have been identified from monkeys kept as research subjects at primate centers. Monkeys infected with YMTV were kept in open-air pens and infection spread from a single individual to other segregated monkeys, suggesting biting arthropods as the likely transmission vector. Research groups have screened sera collected from monkeys of various parts of the world for antibodies against either YMTV or TPV. Generally, antibodies against YMTV and TPV were identified from various monkey species from Africa, as well as cynomolgus monkeys from Malaysia, suggesting that these species suffer from infection, possibly subclinical, with TPV or YMTV. No antibodies to either virus were detected in Indian rhesus monkeys or from any of the monkey species tested from South America. Since rhesus monkeys are highly susceptible to clinical infection by both yatapoxviruses, it is surprising that none of the collected samples confirmed any previous infection. Although natural infection must be rare, the geographical location of the Indian primate species that are located between the African and Malaysian species (both of which were YMTV/TPV positive) suggests that negative serology results from primates in India may be misleading.

## Pathogenesis

Infection of susceptible primates by YMTV targets histiocytes which rapidly divide and produce tumors. Histiocytes are cells, of either macrophage or Langerhans cell lineage, that migrate to areas of cellular disturbance. Following YMTV inoculation, histiocytes migrate to the site of virus inoculation during the first 48 h. The infiltrating histiocytes begin to exhibit cellular alterations, including enlargement of the nucleus and the prominence of nucleoli, by 72 h p.i. By day 5, the altered histiocytes become spindle shaped and exhibit mitotic activity. Also by day 5, inclusion bodies begin to become visible. Actively dividing cells begin to assume spiral forms between days 7 and 9 and acquire well-defined reticular patterns. By week 2, many degenerating cells along with other actively dividing cells become apparent. This scenario continues for the next 4–6 weeks. Eventually, the number of degenerating cells starts increasing and the number of dividing cells diminishes. Host immune response to infection is generally insignificant until regression of the lesion is nearly complete. At this point, there is evidence of lesion infiltration with host mononuclear cells. Necrosis of the center of the lesion is generally not part of the regression process; however, the tumor will exhibit surface ulceration. The beginning of degeneration is characterized by eosinophilic cytoplasmic mass, cytoplasmic lipid accumulation, vacuolization, and eventual cell dissolution. Tumor regression is not correlated to serum antibody titers. It is postulated that tumor regression is due to *in vivo* cytopathic effects rather than an innate immune response. However, the cytopathogenic effect of the virus eventually kills the cells and the tumor regresses. Natural regression can take up to several months, after which the individual is susceptible to reinfection.

TPV infection begins with a short febrile illness lasting several days that may include severe headaches, general fatigue, and body aches. This is followed by the appearance of a single, or a few, pock-like lesions that initially resemble those of variola. Tanapox lesions begin as a papule and develop into a hard, raised nodule and are normally located on the extremities. Nodules normally regress after 3–4 weeks.

## Geographic and Seasonal Distribution

Naturally occurring yatapoxvirus infections have been extremely rare and geographically limited. TPV infections in human populations have only been observed in the equatorial belt of Africa between Zaire and Kenya. Recent TPV infections of humans have been limited to very few cases. Infection of human handlers with YLDV at primate centers in the US was effectively stopped by appropriate changes to biological safety conditions. YMTV infections have only been observed in nonhuman primates in Africa primate centers. Although a worldwide survey of primate sera has identified antibodies against YMTV in monkeys in both Africa and Malaysia, and TPV-neutralizing antibodies in native populations of equatorial Africa, the numbers of observed cases are rare.

The yatapoxviruses are probably transmitted by biting arthropod vectors (mosquitoes?) and therefore environmental conditions such as rainy seasons, excessive flooding, and natural occurrences that bring humans into closer contact with infected nonhuman primates will lead to increased observation of infections.

## Immune Modulation

TPV is a self-limiting infection in humans and natural infection for YMTV has not been observed in humans. Only a small amount of research has been done on the molecular aspects of a TPV infection and none has been undertaken with YMTV. It is known that TPV-infected cells secrete a 38 kDa glycoprotein that has been shown to bind human interferon-$\gamma$, human IL-2, and human IL-5. In addition, the secreted, early protein 2L of TPV represents a new class of virally encoded tumor necrosis factor (TNF)-binding proteins found in the members of the yatapoxviruses, swinepox, and the unclassified deerpox virus. This 2L protein binds human TNF$\alpha$ with high affinity but is unable to bind other members of the human TNF superfamily. In addition, TPV 2L inhibits human TNFα from binding to TNF receptors I and II, as well as blocking TNF-induced cytolysis. However, 2L protein was shown to be unable to bind IFN-γ, IL-2, or IL-5 under experimental conditions.

TPV has been isolated from humans living in (or visiting) equatorial Africa and YLDV from workers at primate centers in the USA. The complete genomic sequence is presently available from TPV, YLDV and YMTV. Based on these sequences, it is clear that the TPV and YLDV genomes are 98% identical, which is clearly on the level of genetic similarity between strains of vaccinia virus. Based on the sequencing, a large number of host-modulating viral genes were predicted but only a handful have been studied. These include a new viral homolog of CCR8, a novel TNF inhibitor, and a viral-encoded member of the IL-10 family.

## Epidemiology

YMTV is likely endemic in African monkeys. Neutralizing antibodies have been detected in monkeys from Africa and Malaysia, suggesting that YMTV possibly represents a latent infection in several monkey species. If this is true, it is surprising that monkeys from India have not yet been reported to contain the same neutralizing antibodies. Infection in man has only occurred through injection of isolated YMTV.

The reservoir host for TPV is thought to be wild monkeys in equatorial Africa, from which natives can be infected by mosquito transmission. TPV infection is more common in years of heavy flooding when high water forces monkeys and man into closer proximity, while at the same time mosquito populations are at their zenith.

## Prevention and Control

Control of YMTV and YLDV infection in man requires normal biological safety protocols to be exercised by animal handlers, including the wearing of protective clothing. TPV infection in equatorial Africa will require mosquito control measures. Separation of Asian and African monkey species at primate centers and markets and protective clothing for merchants and animal handlers may also help.

## Future Perspectives

The reservoir status of primates with the yatapoxviruses is not a major human health concern. However, the features of infection, including YMTV targeting of histiocytes and tumor formation, the lack of long-term protection following regression of the initial infection, the observation that early TPV infection is difficult to distinguish from monkeypox infection, and the observation that members of this genus of poxviruses do in fact infect humans without eliciting an effective immune response may offer some unique insights into the mechanism of human zoonotic infections. Given the current concerns for early diagnoses of any and all human poxvirus infections, research on this group of poxviruses is likely to continue.

## Further Reading

Brunetti CR, Amano H, Uedo Y, et al. (2003) Complete genomic sequence and comparative analysis of the tumorigenic poxvirus yaba monkey tumor virus. Journal of Virology 77: 13335–13347.

Brunetti CR, Paulose-Murphy M, Singh R, et al. (2003) A secreted high-affinity inhibitor of human TNF from tanapox virus. Proceedings of the National Academy of Sciences, USA 100: 4831–4836.

Downie AW and Espana C (1973) A comparative study of tanapox and yaba viruses. Journal of General Virology 19: 37–49.

Knight JC, Novembre FJ, Brown DR, Goldsmith CS, and Esposito JJ (1989) Studies on tanapox virus. Virology 172: 116–124.

Lee HJ, Essani K, and Smith GL (2001) The genome sequence of yaba-like disease virus. Virology 281: 170–192.

Nazarian SH, Barrett JW, Frace AM, et al. (2007) Comparative genetic analysis of genomic DNA sequences of two human isolates of Tanapox virus. Virus Research 129: 11–25.

## Relevant Website

http://www.poxvirus.org – Poxvirus Bioinformatics Resource Center.

# AVIAN VIRUSES

# Fowlpox Virus and Other Avipoxviruses

**M A Skinner,** Imperial College London, London, UK

## Taxonomy

*Fowlpox virus*, the prototype of the *Avipoxvirus* genus, is the best-studied species. There are currently nine other recognized species (*Canarypox virus, Juncopox virus, Mynahpox virus, Pigeonpox virus, Psittacinepox virus, Quailpox virus, Sparrowpox virus, Starlingpox virus,* and *Turkeypox virus*) and three tentative species (Crowpox virus, Peacockpox virus, and Penguinpox virus). Avipoxvirus infections have been observed in more than 230 of the known 9000 species of birds, spanning 23 orders, yet little is known about the genome diversity, host range, and host specificity of the causative agents.

## History

With its characteristic lesions, ubiquitous distribution among domesticated poultry, and large virion size, fowlpox virus (FWPV) was one of the earliest recognized viruses. It also played important roles in the development of modern virological techniques during the middle decades of the twentieth century. Fowlpox was one of the first diseases of livestock and poultry for which effective vaccines were developed, as early as the late 1920s. These vaccines led to effective control of the disease and its virtual eradication from commercial poultry production in temperate regions. Fowlpox remains enzootic in most tropical and subtropical regions where poultry is produced. It represents, after Newcastle disease, the second largest virus infection of backyard poultry in Africa and is thus of considerable socioeconomic importance.

## Virion Structure

Like other poxviruses, the brick-shaped avipoxviruses are large enough (at $330\,nm \times 280\,nm \times 200\,nm$) to be resolved by light microscopy. Indeed, the particles were originally observed following staining with basic dyes (such as basic fuchsin in Gimenez stain) and were termed 'elementary particles' or 'Borrel bodies'. Overall, the structure of the avipoxvirus virion is assumed to be similar to that of the much better studied vaccinia virus (VACV). Likewise, the replication cycle of the avipoxviruses is assumed to be essentially similar to that elucidated for the mammalian poxviruses. However, there are differences between avipoxviruses and the commonly studied mammalian poxviruses in the complement of structural genes and in morphogenesis of extracellular enveloped virions (described below), both indicative of significant structural differences at the molecular level. As a consequence, it is not clear which proteins are present in the envelope of avipoxvirus extracellular enveloped virus (EEV).

## Genome Size and Organization

The avipoxviruses appear to have some of the largest known genomes of viruses of vertebrates, more than 300 kbp for canarypox virus (CNPV), encoding about 300 proteins. By way of comparison, this is 100 times the size of the smallest animal virus genomes and half the size of the genome of the smallest free-living bacterium. Among mammalian poxviruses, the central two-thirds of the genome generally encode conserved structural proteins and enzymes. In contrast, the terminal regions are more variable and divergent, encoding genus and species-specific, nonessential proteins, which are frequently involved in virus–host interactions affecting host–range, pathogenesis, and virulence. This general distribution holds in the avipoxviruses but, relative to the mammalian poxviruses, several large genome rearrangements (translocations, inversions, and transversions), which could have occurred in either avian or mammalian lineages (or both), have resulted in transfer of likely nonessential genes into more central locations.

## Gene Complement

Although avipoxviruses appear to encode equivalents of most of the internal structural proteins of the VACV core, they lack some important proteins found on the surface of the intracellular mature virus (IMV) of VACV (such as D8 and A27), on the surface of the EEV (such as A33, A56, and B5), as well as on the surface of intracellular enveloped viruses, or IEV (such as A36).

Avipoxviruses also encode proteins not found in mammalian poxviruses, such as homologs of the host PC-1 nucleotide phosphodiesterase, DNaseII (DLAD), alpha-SNAP, and the lipid-pathway enzyme involved in Stargardt's macular dystrophy (ELOVL4). Such proteins appear to be nonessential for replication in tissue culture and are presumed to be nonstructural. Avipoxviruses also encode multiple members of several gene families, notably the 31 ankyrin-repeat proteins encoded by FWPV (51 by CNPV) and the six copies of the massive B22 ortholog

(2000 amino acid residues) found only as a single copy in some mammalian poxviruses, such as variola virus (VARV), cowpox virus (CPXV), and molluscum contagiosum virus (MOCV). The latter gene family therefore accounts for about 35 kbp of the additional sequence found in the avipoxvirus genome.

## Antigens

Three major immunodominant antigens of FWPV that are recognized by murine monoclonal antibodies have been identified. They correspond to immunodominant antigens recognized by hyperimmune serum from FWPV-infected chickens and to equivalent immunodominant antigens of mammalian poxviruses. They are the 30/35 kDa IMV surface protein fpv140 (corresponding to VACV H3), the 39 kDa virion core protein fpv168 (corresponding to VACV A4), and the 63 kDa 'virion occlusion' protein fpv191 (corresponding to the p4c protein retained in very few VACV strains). Neutralizing antisera or monoclonal antibodies have not been reported.

## Survival Factors

### A-Type Inclusion Protein

The avipoxviruses express a number of proteins that might be considered as factors to potentiate their survival in the face of various environmental stresses. These include the A-type inclusion (ATI) protein, which forms large cytoplasmic inclusions. These inclusions can contain large assemblies of embedded virions (analogous to spheroidin inclusions in the entomopoxviruses), which would probably be better protected from dessication in desquamated dermis. It is likely that entry of avipoxviruses into the ATI requires the presence of fpv191 (p4c, virion occlusion protein) on the surface of the IMV, assuming the mechanism is as elucidated for CPXV.

### Photolyase

Avipoxviruses encode photolyases (e.g., fpv158), which are capable of repairing ultraviolet (UV)-induced pyrimidine dimers in DNA in a light-dependent manner. Such lesions might be induced in viral genomic DNA when the virion is exposed to the environment in desquamated epithelium, or while the virion is near the surface of a skin lesion.

### Glutathione Peroxidase

Like MOCV, avipoxviruses encode a glutathione peroxidase. Such proteins might be able to protect the virus from environmental oxidative stress. However, the FWPV protein (fpv064) is probably not an ortholog of the MOCV protein (MC066), which is most closely related to cellular glutathione peroxidase. Instead it is probably a paralog, most closely related to cellular phospholipid hydroperoxide glutathione peroxidase. The avipoxvirus proteins might protect infected cells from the oxidative burst of immune cells or affect cell signaling pathways.

## Immunomodulators

Unlike most mammalian poxviruses, but in common with MOCV, no obvious candidates for proteins interfering with the host type I interferon response have been identified. Thus the avipoxviruses lack orthologs of the VACV double-stranded RNA-binding protein (E3) and the eIF2 mimic (K3). No soluble homologs of type I interferon receptors (equivalent to VACV B18) have yet been identified in the avipoxviruses, although a soluble binding protein (e.g., fpv016) for type II interferon has been identified biochemically. Conversely, avipoxviruses also encode proteins not generally found in mammalian poxviruses, such as homologs of transforming growth factor β (e.g., fpv080), which has also been found in deerpox virus, and IL10 (e.g., CNPV018), also found in orf parapoxvirus.

No obvious soluble chemokine-binding proteins encoded by avipoxviruses have been identified, in contrast to the mammalian poxviruses. However, proteins resembling cellular serpentine chemokine receptors of the 7-transmembrane spanning G-protein-coupled receptor family are encoded by avipoxviruses (e.g., fpv021, fpv027, and fpv208), as are single copies by some mammalian poxviruses (capripoxviruses, suipoxviruses, yatapoxviruses, and deerpox virus). Like MOCV, avipoxviruses encode putative IL18-like proteins (e.g., fpv214) and chemokine-like proteins (e.g., fpv060, fpv061, fpv116, and fpv121).

## Features of Avipoxviruses Shared with Molluscum Contagiosum Virus

The mammalian poxvirus to which the avipoxviruses are most closely related phylogenetically is MOCV. The avipoxviruses also share a number of other features with MOCV. For example, they lack orthologs of the VACV proteins E3 and K3 involved in evading the type I interferon response. Whereas avipoxviruses encode a family of proteins (e.g., fpv097, pfv098, fpv099, fpv107, fpv122, and fpv123) with homology to the large VARV protein B22, MOCV (like VARV and CPXV) encodes only a single protein (MC035). In CPXV, as in VARV, the gene encoding the B22 ortholog (CPXV219) is located in the variable region at the right terminus of the genome. The gene encoding the MOCV ortholog MC035 is, however, more central, located between orthologs of VACV E4L and E6R. This is syntenic with the location of FWPV genes encoding B22 orthologs fpv097, fpv098, and fpv099, also found between orthologs of VACV E4L and E6R.

Like the avipoxviruses, MOCV lacks orthologs of VACV IMV surface proteins A27 and D8 as well as EEV proteins A56 and B5 (though, unlike the avipoxviruses, MOCV does encode orthologs of VACV EEV protein A33 and IEV protein A36).

## Virus Replication

### Host Range Restriction

Avipoxviruses are incapable of productive replication in mammalian cell lines, including those (such as BHK-21) permissive or semipermissive for the host-range-restricted MVA variant of VACV, and those defective in the type I interferon pathway, such as Vero cells. Otherwise, the replicative cycle is largely similar to that elucidated for VACV, although considerably slower (taking about 24 h rather than 12 h). Genome transcription and replication mechanisms are essentially the same, with relatively well conserved polymerases and other enzymes. VACV promoters function well in cells infected with avipoxviruses and are frequently used to drive foreign gene expression in recombinant avipoxviruses, and the inverse appears to be true. Virus-induced shut-off of host gene expression, clearly observed with VACV, is far less dramatic with FWPV.

### Genetic Reactivation

The long-recognized phenomenon of 'genetic reactivation' illustrates that many of the essential replicative components of poxviruses are interchangeable. Thus the proteins of a UV-inactivated poxvirus can rescue the genome of a heat-inactivated poxvirus, even when the two viruses are from different genera. This is well illustrated by the modern practise of rescuing naked (and often genetically manipulated) genomic DNA of a mammalian poxvirus by infection of transfected cells with FWPV. The rescued mammalian poxvirus can be recovered and amplified by passage through mammalian cells, which eliminates the rescuing FWPV due to its host range restriction.

### Virion Morphogenesis

The most obvious difference between the replication cycles of avipoxviruses and that of VACV is in the formation of EEV. VACV EEV formation predominantly involves wrapping of IMV with a double membrane derived from the *trans*-Golgi network (to form IEV) followed by subsequent exocytosis to form cell-associated enveloped virus (CEV) and EEV. Avipoxviruses, however, form EEV by a more conventional pathway in which IMV buds through the cell membrane to acquire an envelope. This difference, observed by electron microscopy (**Figure 1**), is consistent with the absence from the avipoxvirus genome of genes involved in wrapping and exocytosis in VACV.

### Lipid Metabolism

There have been reports that FWPV has a profound effect on host cell lipid metabolism. It is tempting to speculate that this might be attributable to some of the unusual genes carried by FWPV, notably fpv048 encoding a protein with unusually high sequence similarity to the ELOVL4 host protein, a fatty acid elongation factor implicated in macular degeneration.

## Virus Propagation

Avipoxviruses replicate only in avian cells; replication in mammalian cells is abortive and no infectious progeny are produced. Some vaccine strains of FWPV, such as the Cyanamid Webster FPV-M vaccine, even display a preference for chick embryo skin cells (CESs) over chick embryo fibroblast cells (CEFs). FWPV FP9 has been effectively adapted to CEFs but it displays a distinct preference for primary as opposed to secondary CEFs. Plaques on CEFs are not lytic, but the cytopathic effects manifest as changes in cell morphology, resulting in areas of altered refractive index with the plaques best viewed by dark field illumination. FWPV fails to plaque and replicates poorly in the recently derived chicken fibroblast cell line, DF-1. Replication is similarly poor in the chemically transformed cell line OU-2. It can be plaqued and replicated quite efficiently in quail cell lines, such as QT-35, but the presence in these cells of viable endogenous Marek's disease virus (a herpesvirus) means that their use for preparation of vaccines is not advisable. Of these possible cell substrates for avipoxvirus propagation, currently only CEFs and CESs are licensed for use in the production of human vaccines.

Publications reporting the replication of uncharacterized avipoxviruses of unknown origin in embryonic bovine tracheal cells or in BHK-21 are atypical and, until corroborated, should be viewed with caution.

## Molecular Phylogenetics

The taxonomy and classification of avipoxviruses are important to the study of epidemiology and hence to the future ability to control the diseases. Recent molecular studies confirm earlier impressions that avipoxviruses can jump species to cause disease. Thus isolation of a

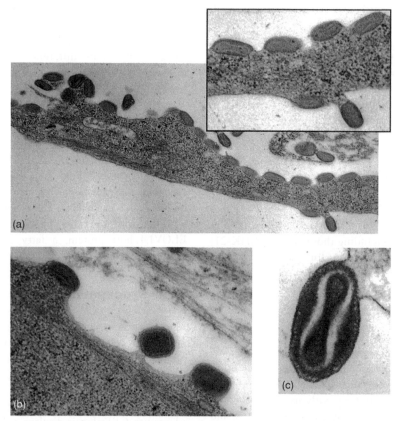

**Figure 1**  FWPV IMV particles budding through the membranes of infected chick embryo fibroblasts. Magnifications: (a) ×27 000 (inset ×51 000); (b) ×60 000; (c) ×170 000. Reproduced from Boulanger D, Smith T, and Skinner MA (2000) Morphogenesis and release of fowlpox virus. *Journal of General Virology* 81: 675–687, with permission from the Society for General Microbiology.

virus from a turkey, for instance, is not sufficient to demonstrate that turkeypox virus is the cause and, more importantly, that the outbreak can be controlled by a turkeypox virus vaccine.

Avipoxviruses can be highly diverged at the molecular level. For instance, the relatively highly conserved FWPV and CNPV P4b proteins (encoded by genes fpv167 and cnpv240, respectively) share only 64.2% amino acid sequence identity. This level of divergence is comparable to that seen between different genera of mammalian poxviruses (see **Figure 2**). In fact, recent molecular studies have demonstrated that avipoxviruses fall into three major diverged groups: (1) the FWPV-like viruses, (2) the CNPV-like viruses, and (3) the psittacinepox viruses (**Figure 2**). As their name suggests, the psittacinepox viruses have so far only been isolated from psittacines. In contrast, viruses of the FWPV-like and CNPV-like groups appear either inherently capable of infecting a wider range of birds or have evolved and adapted to be able to infect different birds. FWPV-like viruses have been isolated from turkeys, pigeons, ospreys, albatrosses, doves, and falcons. Viruses closely related to, and even barely distinguishable from, CNPV can cause disease in

great tits, sparrows, stone curlews, and houbaras. CNPV-like viruses have been isolated from pigeons and starlings. A report in 2006 from Virginia in the USA indicated that one particular CNPV-like virus caused disease in a wide range of birds (robins, crows, herons, finches, doves, hawks, gnatcatchers, mockingbirds, and cardinals). It was not known whether the virus that caused the epornitic had a wider geographic distribution throughout the USA.

It is apparent that pigeonpox can be caused by two distinct types of virus, either FWPV-like or CNPV-like. The FWPV-like virus is very closely related to viruses from turkeys and osprey, and a little less closely related to those from an albatross, a falcon, and a dove. The CNPV-like virus is closely related to one from a starling. Infection of avian species outside the normal host range of the particular avipoxvirus can result in altered pathogenesis compared to that observed in the normal host. For instance, a virus which was isolated from an Andean condor (*Vultur gryphus*), in which it had caused an aggressive, diphtheritic form of the disease, produced only mild lesions in inoculated chickens. Conversely, viruses causing mild poxvirus lesions in wild birds, such as those found in 50% of short-toed larks

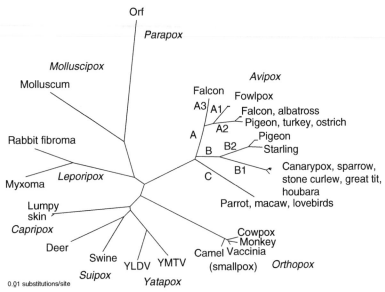

**Figure 2**   A phylogram showing phylogenetic relationships and evolutionary distances of avipoxvirus clades and mammalian poxvirus genera based on neighbor-joining analysis (supported by bootstrapping) of P4b orthologs.

(*Calandrella rufescens*) and 28% of Bertholet's pipits (*Anthus berthelotti*) in the Canary Islands, might cause more severe disease in naive populations of other avian species. It is, for instance, suspected that canaries might not be the natural reservoir for CNPV, which causes them a devastating disease.

## Epizootiology

Evidence of poxvirus infection has been observed in many avian species but little is known about the natural host range of the causative agents, due to the lack of robust techniques for the identification and differentiation of isolates. Initially, the viruses were distinguished by their ability to cause disease in a range of test species, such as chickens, pigeons, turkeys, and quail. Such infectivity studies probably overestimate the degree of similarity between the viruses, as many isolates seem able to cause disease in the test species, possibly due to the inoculation of high doses. *In vivo* analysis of antigenic cross-reactivity allowed the viruses to be grouped or distinguished by their ability or inability to induce protective immunity against each other. Thus, psittacinepox virus offered no protection against FWPV or pigeonpox virus, or vice versa, nor did quailpox virus. Similarly, mynahpox virus showed no cross-protection with fowl, pigeon, psittacine, quail, or turkey poxviruses, and a condor poxvirus induced no protection against FWPV. *In vitro* serological techniques were applied to only a small proportion of the observed isolates because initial propagation in chick embryos or chick embryo fibroblast cells often failed. Possibly as a consequence of the limited characterization of isolates, there are only the ten recognized species of avipoxviruses.

Reintroduction programs appear to be particularly susceptible to problems caused by poxvirus infection. For instance, houbara bustard reintroduced into the Middle East have proved susceptible to uncharacterized avipoxvirus infections from unknown sources. Similar programs, such as that for the closely related great bustard on Salisbury Plain, Wiltshire, in the UK may face similar threats. There are also concerns that avipoxviruses might threaten marginal species such as some species of birds in the Hawaiian Islands and especially the kakapo, the flightless, nocturnal New Zealand owl parrot.

## Transmission

Poxviruses produce two types of virion particles that are both infectious: IMV released into the environment only by desquamation of skin lesions and EEV released from the cell to spread to secondary sites of infection. In the wild, the primary route of infection is mechanical transmission of blood-borne EEV by biting insects (mosquitoes and midges). Lesions are therefore characteristically restricted to the featherless areas around the eyes and nares, on the comb, wattle, lower legs, and feet. Fowlpox remains a problem when control of biting insects is difficult but is generally not a problem for intensive production systems in the temperate areas of Northern Europe and the northern USA, even in the absence of vaccination. Problems with epizootics have emerged with free-range flocks, presumably because they are more exposed to biting insects, as well as to pecking by infected birds. In subtropical and tropical climates, fowlpox poses a significant problem requiring vaccination of commercial flocks.

FWPV can also transmit via inhalation or ingestion of dust (or dander, representing virus-infected cells shed from cutaneous lesions), or aerosols, leading to the 'diphtheritic form' of the disease, with lesions on the mucous membranes of the mouth, pharynx, larynx, and sometimes trachea. More likely to occur at high population density, this form of the disease is associated with commercial poultry flocks or collections of captive or domesticated birds (including quarantine facilities). However, such lesions may also form as a consequence of secondary viremia following primary cutaneous lesions, and viral genetic factors may play a role. Avipoxvirus infections of passerine birds (e.g., canaries and finches) can cause significantly higher rates of mortality than those of chickens or turkeys.

## Diagnosis

### Clinical Signs

FWPV and many other avipoxviruses primarily cause disease in mature birds. The cutaneous form of avipox, including fowlpox in chickens and turkeys, spread mechanically by biting insects or pecking, is normally relatively mild (**Figures 3** and **4**) but the diphtheritic form (**Figure 5**) causes higher mortality by occlusion of the oropharynx. A third form of poxvirus disease causes a pneumonia-like illness in canaries, with high mortality.

### Histology

Smears of material scraped from cutaneous lesions or postmortem sections from diphtheritic lesions (or airway epithelium in the case of pneumonia) can be stained with hematoxylin/eosin, or Gimenez stain. The presence of eosinophilic inclusions (A-type inclusions, Bollinger bodies) in the cytoplasm is diagnostic of poxviruses.

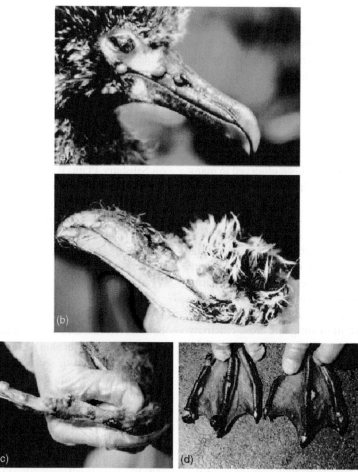

**Figure 3**  Typical avipoxvirus lesions seen on the head and feet of a Laysan albatross. Reproduced from Hansen W (1999) Avian pox. In: Friend M and Franson JC (eds.) *Field Manual of Wildlife Diseases, General Field Procedures and Diseases of Birds*, pp. 163–169, with permission from USGS.

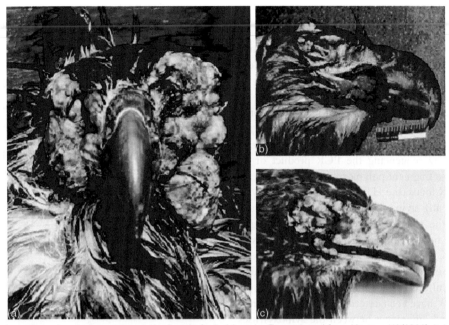

**Figure 4** Extensive avipoxvirus lesions seen on the head of a bald eagle. Reproduced from Hansen W (1999) Avian pox. In: Friend M and Franson JC (eds.) *Field Manual of Wildlife Diseases, General Field Procedures and Diseases of Birds*, pp. 163–169, with permission from USGS.

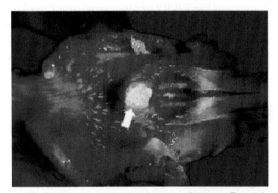

**Figure 5** Diphtheritic lesion in a Laysan albatross. Reproduced from Hansen W (1999) Avian pox. In: Friend M and Franson JC (eds.) *Field Manual of Wildlife Diseases, General Field Procedures and Diseases of Birds*, pp. 163–169, with permission from USGS.

Basophilic (or B-type) inclusion bodies may also be seen in the cytoplasm (these represent the sites of virus replication, the so-called 'viral factories'), as may Borrel bodies (the virions themselves).

## Virus Isolation and Detection

Virus may be passaged and amplified *in vivo* through specific pathogen-free chickens via wing web scarification or through embryonated eggs via chorio-allantoic membrane infection. The method of choice for virus propagation, however, is *in vitro* culture on CEFs for amplification

through liquid culture or for plaque purification under semisolid overlay. Not all avipoxvirus isolates will form plaques, or even propagate, on CEFs. Primary cultures of other poultry species (duck, turkey, or quail) may also be used.

## Serology

Serological methods such as enzyme-linked immunosorbent assays (ELISAs), available as commercial flock monitoring kits, can be used to provide evidence for ongoing or prior infection in the flock. Virus neutralization tests are more specific but are technically more demanding and the responsible antigenic epitopes have not been identified.

## Monoclonal Antibodies

Monoclonal antibodies against the three major immunodominant structural antigens of FWPV have been isolated and characterized, as described above. None appears to be neutralizing but all can be used in ELISAs and western blotting.

## Restriction Enzyme Digestion and Southern Blotting

Before extensive genome sequencing, Southern blotting was the only available molecular diagnostic method, involving examination of restriction enzyme digest profiles. Without the use of radioisotopes, the method was relatively insensitive.

## PCR-Based Analysis

With the advent of DNA sequence data for the avipoxviruses, polymerase chain reaction (PCR) amplification became the molecular diagnostic method of choice to identify avipoxvirus infections. This has been based routinely on the sequence of the gene encoding the P4b protein (the A3 ortholog encoded by gene fpv167), with primers for a 578 bp fragment. However, all avipoxviruses produce fragments of the same length, so the avipoxvirus could only be identified either by sequencing the PCR product or by restriction enzyme fragment polymorphism profiling.

A second PCR locus (the H3 locus), which works with most (but not all) avipoxviruses, has the advantage that viruses of the two major groups (CNPV-like and FWPV-like) can be discriminated purely on the basis of the size of the PCR product (**Figure 6**).

The genome sequences of two different FWPV strains, one extensively culture-passaged and attenuated, and of a pathogenic CNPV have been determined. They confirmed the divergence and differences between the avipoxviruses and the mammalian poxviruses typified by VACV. In fact, phylogenetic analysis showed that avipoxviruses are most closely related to MOCV of humans, a relationship confirmed by other specific aspects of their molecular biology (see **Figure 2**). Despite having sequence information for the prototypic members of the two major groups of avipoxviruses, it has still proved extremely difficult to identify conserved primer sequences that work in PCR

reactions for all other members of the genus, further illustrating the extent of sequence divergence and diversity within this group of viruses.

## Intraspecies and Interstrain Differentiation

Despite their large genome size, the high level of conservation within species of avipoxviruses makes it difficult to differentiate between different strains or isolates or between vaccines and pathogenic strains. Although numerous loci within FWPV have been surveyed, only one locus (the H9 locus), has been reported to allow clear differentiation. It appears to be an unstable region, with deletions of different lengths found in various FWPV strains, isolates, and vaccines. Three commercial fowlpox vaccines were found to have the same parental sequence found in two clinical isolates, while two other different commercial vaccines shared an identical deletion at the H9 locus (see **Figure 7**).

## Control and Prevention

### Vaccination

Since its introduction in the 1920s, vaccination against fowlpox using live FWPV or pigeonpox virus (now known to be closely related antigenically to FWPV) has become commonplace and extensive, such that the disease has been nearly eradicated from developed countries in

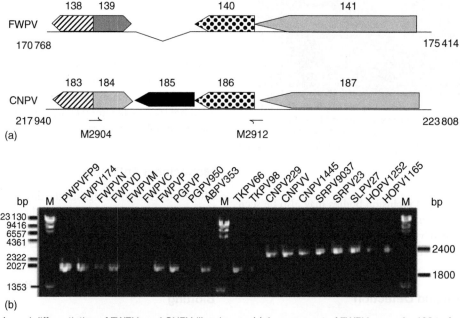

**Figure 6** PCR-based differentiation of FWPV- and CNPV-like viruses. (a) Arrangement of FWPV genes fpv138 to fpv141 at the H3 locus aligned with their CNPV orthologs. The positions of primers used for PCR analysis are indicated. (b) The PCR analysis shows the length difference in the amplified DNA fragment obtained from FWPV-like viruses (1800 bp) and from CNPV-like viruses (2400 bp). Reproduced from Jarmin S, Manvell R, Gough RE, Laidlaw SM, and Skinner MA (2006) Avipoxvirus phylogenetics: Identification of a PCR length polymorphism that discriminates between the major clades. *Journal of General Virology* 87: 2191–2201, with permission from the Society for General Microbiology.

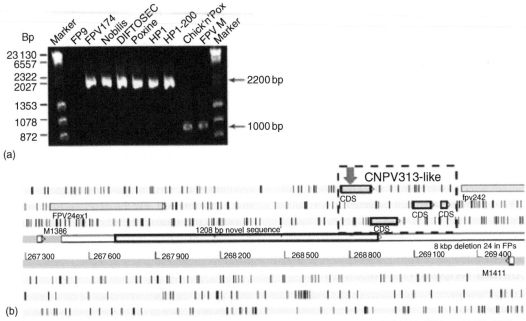

**Figure 7** PCR analysis of the H9 locus of FWPV. (a) The 2200 bp product for field viruses (FPV174, HP1, and HP1-200) and three vaccines (Nobilis, DIFTOSEC, and Poxine) and identically deleted 1000 bp products for two other vaccines (Chick'n'Pox and FPV M). No product was seen for an extensively passaged and attenuated virus FP9. (b) Organization (to scale) of the H9 locus (FWPV genes fpv241 to fpv242), including the 1200 bp product, which is deleted from the vaccines, shown for FWPV HP1. The positions of primers used for the PCR are shown. Reproduced from Jarmin SA, Manvell R, Gough RE, Laidlaw SM, and Skinner MA (2006) Retention of 1.2 kbp of 'novel' genomic sequence in two European field isolates and some vaccine strains of fowlpox virus extends open reading frame fpv241, *Journal of General Virology* 87: 3545–3549 with permission from the Society for General Microbiology.

temperate zones. Most currently available commercial vaccines originate from early isolates, though a minority were isolated in the mid-1960s.

Vaccination may be undertaken from 10 days or 4 weeks of age, depending on the residual pathogenicity of the vaccine, which is often related to whether the vaccine is propagated in cell culture or in embryonated eggs. Inoculation is into the wing web using a bifurcated needle or by scarification of the thigh. The formation of a small lesion at the site of vaccination 6–8 days later indicates a good take, with immunity developing in 8–15 days. Though desirable, alternative routes for vaccination (aerosol, intranasal, or via drinking water) have not generally proved successful.

## Treatment

There are no demonstrated effective treatments for avipoxvirus infections other than palliative treatment and to prevent or treat secondary bacterial infections.

## Variant FWPVs

### Antigenic Variants

Outbreaks of fowlpox have been reported within flocks previously vaccinated with FWPV or pigeonpox virus

vaccines. If the vaccination had been effective, which is often not the case, antigenic variation might be suspected, though serotype specificity would be novel among poxviruses. Little is known about protective epitopes for humoral or cellular immune responses in FWPV and there has only been preliminary characterization of the 'variant' isolates.

### Tumorigenic Variants

FWPV has also been associated with cases of dermal squamous cell carcinoma in poultry in Brazil. It is not clear whether FWPV is a causative agent and, if so, whether a variant is involved.

### The Role of Integrated Reticuloendotheliosis Virus Sequences

FPV-S, a commercial FWPV vaccine known to be contaminated with reticuloendotheliosis virus (REV), was found to carry a near full-length, infectious progenome of REV integrated into the poxvirus genome. The provirus has subsequently been found in most, if not all, pathogenic field isolates of FWPV, but the majority of vaccine strains of FWPV carry only noninfectious, long terminal repeat (LTR) sequences of REV. The provirus and the LTR sequences have only ever been found at the same single locus, although differences exist between the REV LTR sequences retained in different viruses. It appears likely that a single, ancestral event inserted the provirus into the FWPV genome between genes fpv201 and fpv203, in contrast to the multiple REV insertions that have been observed in Marek's disease virus. It is not known whether REV can reintegrate at the site of a retained LTR or whether this would regenerate a pathogenic virus. There are no REV sequences in the completely sequenced genome of CNPV, but they have been detected in a commercial CNPV vaccine as well as in some commercial pigeonpox virus vaccines. Full-length REV sequences have been detected in an isolate from a turkey.

## Recombinant Avipoxvirus Vaccines

### Recombinant FWPV as a Vaccine Vector in Poultry

Shortly after the development of methods for isolating recombinant VACV in the early 1980s, FWPV was developed as an equivalent recombinant vector for use in poultry. Several commercial vaccine and laboratory attenuated strains were used as vectors against a number of important poultry pathogens, especially avian influenza virus, Newcastle disease virus, infectious bronchitis virus, avian hemorrhagic enteritis virus, Marek's disease virus, turkey rhinotracheitis virus, REV, and infectious bursal disease virus, as well as *Mycoplasma gallisepticum*. Commercial recombinant FWPV vaccines against Newcastle disease virus and avian influenza virus have been licensed for commercial use in the USA. Those against avian influenza have also been licensed for use in Mexico; indeed, between 1997 and 2003, approximately 459 million doses of a recombinant fowlpox-H5 vaccine were used in Mexico as part of a program to control H5N2. The same recombinant and similar viruses developed in China are being used in Southeast Asia to counter the highly virulent avian influenza H5N1 strain.

### Recombinant Avipoxviruses as Vaccine Vectors in Mammals

It was demonstrated in the late 1980s that recombinant avipoxviruses (initially FWPV and then CNPV) carrying antigens from mammalian viral pathogens could enter mammalian cells and express the foreign antigens, even though the recombinants could not replicate and spread to neighboring cells. Moreover, vaccination of mammals with the recombinants could elicit immune responses, which could be protective against viral challenge. This discovery,

which was surprising because of the low level of antigen expressed from the single-round, abortive infections, offered the prospect of extremely safe recombinant vaccines. Several recombinant avipoxvirus vaccines, mainly based on CNPV, have been developed primarily for veterinary use. However, the more recent focus on T-cell-mediated immunity has seen more use of FWPV-based vectors. Many clinical trials have been conducted, are underway, or are planned, against viral diseases such as acquired immune deficiency syndrome (AIDS), parasitic diseases including malaria, and various cancers. In many of these trials, the recombinant avipoxviruses are used in combined (so-called 'prime-boost') regimes with the same antigens expressed by different vectors, such as DNA plasmids, the host-restricted MVA variant of VACV, or adenoviruses. These regimes allow immune responses to be boosted by multiple vaccinations without eliciting excessive responses against vector-specific proteins.

Recombinant avipoxvirus vaccines are yet to be licensed for agricultural use in Europe, though recombinant CNPV vaccines against equine influenza and feline leukemia have received European Medicines Agency (EMEA) approval. Both are licensed for use in the USA, besides similar recombinants against canine distemper and West Nile virus (for use in horses).

*See also:* Entomopoxviruses; Herpesviruses of Birds; Leporipoviruses and Suipoxviruses; Mousepox and Rabbitpox Viruses; Parapoxviruses.

## Further Reading

Boulanger D, Smith T, and Skinner MA (2000) Morphogenesis and release of fowlpox virus. *Journal of General Virology* 81: 675–687.

Hansen W (1999) Avian pox. In: Friend M and Franson JC (eds.) *Field Manual of Wildlife Diseases, General Field Procedures and Diseases of Birds*, pp. 163–169. Madison, WI: US Geological Survey.

OIE (World Organisation for Animal Health) (2004) Page on Fowlpox diagnostic tests and vaccines from Manual of Diagnostic Tests and Vaccines for Terrestrial Animals (5th edn.) http://www.oie.int/eng/normes/mmanual/A_00113.htm (updated 23 July 2004).

Jarmin S, Manvell R, Gough RE, Laidlaw SM, and Skinner MA (2006) Avipoxvirus phylogenetics: Identification of a PCR length polymorphism that discriminates between the major clades. *Journal of General Virology* 87: 2191–2201.

Jarmin SA, Manvell R, Gough RE, Laidlaw SM, and Skinner MA (2006) Retention of 1.2 kbp of 'novel' genomic sequence in two European field isolates and some vaccine strains of fowlpox virus extends open reading frame fpv241. *Journal of General Virology* 87: 3545–3549.

Skinner MA, Laidlaw SM, Eldaghayes I, Kaiser P, and Cottingham MG (2005) Fowlpox virus as a recombinant vaccine vector for use in mammals and poultry. *Expert Review of Vaccines* 4: 63–76.

Skinner MA (2007) *Poxviridae*. In: Pattison M, McMullin P, Bradbury J, and Alexander D (eds.) *Poultry Diseases*, 6th edn. New York: Elsevier.

Tripathy DK and Reed WM (2003) Pox. In: Saif YM, Barnes HJ, Fadly A, Glisson JR, McDougald LR, and Swayne DE (eds.) *Diseases of Poultry*, 11th edn., pp. 253–265. Ames, IA: Iowa State University Press.

# Hepadnaviruses of Birds

**A R Jilbert,** Institute of Medical and Veterinary Science, Adelaide, SA, Australia
**W S Mason,** Fox Chase Cancer Center, Philadelphia, PA, USA

## Introduction

The avian hepadnaviruses belong to the genus *Avihepadnavirus* in the family *Hepadnaviridae*. Within this genus, duck hepatitis B virus (DHBV) and heron hepatitis B virus (HHBV) are assigned to the species *Duck hepatitis B virus* and *Heron hepatitis B virus*, respectively. These avian viruses are related phylogenetically through similarities in genome sequence and organization of open reading frames (ORFs) to human hepatitis B virus (HBV) and other hepadnaviruses that infect mammals (genus *Orthohepadnavirus*). The major site of hepadnavirus infection and replication is the hepatocyte, the predominant cell type of the liver, constituting about 60–70% of liver cell mass. There are $\sim 5 \times 10^{10}$ hepatocytes in the liver of an adult duck.

Hepadnaviruses contain a relaxed circular double-stranded DNA (rcDNA) genome which is converted in the nucleus to covalently closed circular DNA (cccDNA). cccDNA acts as the virus transcriptional template and is used by host RNA polymerase II to produce a greater than genome length, 'pregenomic' RNA, referred to as the pregenome, and a number of other mRNA species. Hepadnaviruses have a unique method of replication that involves reverse transcription of pregenomic RNA into DNA. Virus replication and release are generally considered to be noncytopathic and disease activity is attributed to the host immune response to infected hepatocytes.

The avian hepadnaviruses are naturally transmitted *in ovo* via vertical transmission of virus from an infected female duck to the egg, with virus replication occurring in the yolk sac and liver of the developing embryo. Ducks infected *in ovo* develop widespread and persistent DHBV infection of the liver but have minimal or no liver disease as they are immune tolerant to the virus. Although experimental infection of newly hatched ducks also leads to widespread and persistent DHBV infection of the liver, DHBV-infected ducks, unlike HBV-infected humans, do not develop severe liver disease, cirrhosis, or liver cancer. However, they provide a reproducible experimental system for studying virus kinetics and immune clearance, and much of what we know of the hepadnavirus replication strategy has been discovered from studies of DHBV *in vitro* and *in vivo*. DHBV-infected ducks are also used to evaluate new antiviral therapies and vaccines with the ultimate aim of applying the same strategies to the treatment of HBV infections in humans.

## Virion and Particle Structure

Like the mammalian hepadnaviruses, avian hepadnaviruses are enveloped viruses possessing an icosahedral nucleocapsid and $\sim 3000$ nt rcDNA genome (**Figure 1**). DHBV, the prototypic avian hepadnavirus, has a diameter of 40–45 nm, and different isolates contain genomes ranging in length from 3021 to 3027 nt. In infected ducks, mature enveloped DHBV virions are released from hepatocytes directly into the bloodstream. Virus titers in chronically infected ducks are up to $1 \times 10^{10}$ virions per ml of serum.

The envelope of DHBV is composed of a lipid bilayer containing multiple copies of two transmembrane virus proteins, Pre-S/S and S (36 and 17 kDa, respectively). These two proteins are synthesized from the same virus ORF, with initiation of Pre-S/S occurring upstream of S. The two proteins share a common carboxy terminus. An additional 28 kDa protein antigenically related to Pre-S/S and S has been detected in DHBV-infected liver but it is unclear whether this is a degradation product of Pre-S/S or is translated from an AUG codon mapping between the start sites of Pre-S/S and S. As for HBV, the envelope proteins not only participate in virion formation but also self-assemble into noninfectious virus-like DHBV surface antigen particles (DHBsAg particles). This process occurs in the endoplasmic reticulum and results in the release from infected hepatocytes of a 500- to 1000-fold excess of DHBsAg particles over infectious virions. DHBsAg particles do not contain a virus nucleocapsid and lack virus nucleic acids. DHBsAg particles are pleomorphic and spherical, with a diameter of $\sim 35$–60 nm, and the larger particles are almost indistinguishable from DHBV virions by electron microscopy (EM). In contrast, during HBV infection, filamentous forms of surface antigen-containing particles (HBsAg) are produced as well as 22 nm spherical HBsAg particles, both of which are readily distinguished from those of HBV by EM.

The nucleocapsid of DHBV is icosahedral, as observed by cryoelectron microscopy, and is comprised of dimers of 30 kDa nonglycosylated DHBV core antigen (DHBcAg). In mature virions, the rcDNA genome and a virus-encoded DNA polymerase are contained in the virus nucleocapsid (**Figure 1**), which also contains cellular chaperones.

The DHBV polymerase is a 90 kDa molecule that functions as both an RNA-dependent DNA polymerase and a DNA-dependent DNA polymerase. The polymerase also has an RNase H activity that digests the RNA

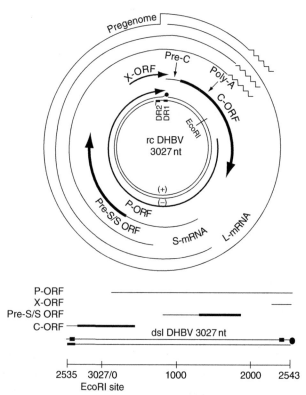

**Figure 1** Organization of the DHBV genome. The rcDNA genome is shown at the top center, with the virus polymerase covalently attached to the 5′ end of the negative strand and an 18 nt RNA bound to the 5′ end of the positive strand. The DHBV genome contains two direct repeat (DR) sequences (DR1 and DR2). The locations of the virus ORFs, DR1 and DR2 and maps of the virus mRNAs are also shown. None of the major mRNAs is spliced. Thus, each has its own promoter. However, they share a common polyadenylation (poly-A) signal in the virus C-ORF. The pregenome RNA is terminally redundant and serves as the mRNA for both the C-ORF and, less frequently, the downstream P (polymerase) ORF. The pregenome lacks the AUG of the Pre-C/C-ORF, which instead is translated from an mRNA a few nt longer at the 5′ end than the pregenome (not shown). The L and S mRNAs encode the Pre-S/S and S envelope proteins, respectively. The more rarely synthesized double-stranded linear (dsl) virus genome is shown at the bottom. The common nucleotide numbering system is also displayed, proceeding in a clockwise direction from a conserved EcoRI restriction site.

pregenome during virus replication. The protein sequence of the DHBV polymerase has four separate domains listed from the N terminal end, that include a terminal protein (TP), 'spacer', reverse transcriptase (RT), and RNase H domain. Each of these domains has one or more key roles during virus replication, as described below.

Also released from hepatocytes and circulating in the blood of infected ducks is the so called DHBV e antigen (DHBeAg), a proteolytically processed form of the 35 kDa Pre-C/C protein. Different forms of DHBeAg range in size from a nonglycosylated 27 kDa to 30–33 kDa glycosylated forms. DHBeAg is thought to play an important

role in either the initiation or maintenance of persistent infection by delaying or diverting the host immune response to DHBcAg. Both DHBsAg and DHBcAg are highly immunogenic. Anti-DHBc antibodies can be detected by ELISA in the serum of ducks during acute and persistent DHBV infections. Anti-DHBs antibodies are produced during the resolution phase of acute DHBV infection and are generally not detected in ducks with persistent infection except in complexes with circulating DHBsAg. Anti-DHBs antibodies bind virus particles and are able to block DHBV infection of cells. For this reason, ducks that have recovered from acute DHBV infection are immune to challenge with DHBV.

## Genome Organization

As noted above, all hepadnaviruses have a similar genome organization, despite the low DNA sequence identity between the mammalian and avian hepadnaviruses (40%). The negative strand of the DHBV genome contains S-ORF, C-ORF, and P-ORF encoding the surface or envelope proteins, core and e antigen proteins, and polymerase protein, respectively (**Figure 1**). The DHBV genome was originally thought to contain only these three ORFs and to lack an ORF encoding a protein analogous to the X protein of the mammalian hepadnaviruses. It was subsequently discovered that avian hepadnaviruses, including HHBV and DHBV, have a fourth ORF, the X-ORF, which directs synthesis of a candidate X protein that is translated using an unconventional start codon. The significance of this observation is still unclear. Using woodchuck hepatitis virus (WHV), a close relative of HBV, the X gene was shown to be essential for successful WHV infections *in vivo*. In contrast, knockout of the X gene of DHBV did not alter the time course of DHBV infection. As with wild-type DHBV, the X gene knockout of DHBV spread rapidly through the liver of newly hatched ducks and caused persistent DHBV infection.

The positive strand of the DHBV genome does not contain any functional ORFs. All virus mRNA species are produced from the negative strand of the virus genome.

The difference in size between the genomes of the avian (e.g., DHBV with a genome of 3027 nt) and the mammalian hepadnaviruses (e.g., HBV with a genome of 3200–3300 nt), is due in part to deletion of a 150 nt stretch in S-ORF. This region in the HBV genome encodes the so-called 'a' determinant, a highly immunodominant region to which most of the neutralizing anti-HBV antibodies are directed. This region in HBV is present on the small form of HBsAg, the S protein. The absence of this region in DHBV results in a lack of immunodominance, and both DHBV Pre-S/S and S domains have been shown to induce high titer, neutralizing, anti-DHBs antibodies.

## Replication Cycle

Hepatocytes, the major parenchymal cell of the liver, are the primary site of DHBV infection. The cell specificity of infection is determined by the presence of specific receptors required for virus binding and entry into hepatocytes. In early studies, DHBsAg particles, which appear to have the same envelope structure as DHBV virions, were shown to bind cell surface receptors on primary duck hepatocytes in a species-specific manner. Receptor binding occurs via the Pre-S/S region of DHBV and is followed by cell entry via receptor-mediated endocytosis. Recent studies have determined that the cellular protein carboxypeptidase D (180 kDa) binds DHBsAg particles and DHBV with high affinity and is found on both internal and external membranes of the cell. However, whereas DHBV has a narrow host range, carboxypeptidase D is expressed on many cell types that are not susceptible to DHBV infection. In addition, despite the observed binding of DHBsAg to carboxypeptidase D, transfection of cells with carboxypeptidase D cDNA does not confer susceptibility to DHBV, suggesting that other co-receptors or mechanisms may be operating. An additional DHBV-binding protein, glycine decarboxylase (120 kDa) has been identified. Its cellular expression is restricted to the liver, kidney, and pancreas. Interestingly, DHBV infection and replication has been detected in a few percent of cells in both the kidney and pancreas (see below and **Figure 5**). Thus, these proteins are potential components of a DHBV receptor complex and probably have a role in determining DHBV organ tropism. However, definite proof that these are the receptors that lead to DHBV binding, receptor-mediated endocytosis, and infection is still lacking.

Whatever the receptor, the immediate sequel to virus uptake is transport of the rcDNA genome to the nucleus to form cccDNA (**Figure 2**). The negative strand of the rcDNA DHBV genome is nicked, with a 9 nt terminal redundancy and with the virus polymerase molecule covalently attached to its 5′ end. Covalent attachment of the virus polymerase occurs during priming of reverse transcription through a tyrosine located in the TP domain of the polymerase. Similarly, the positive strand of the DHBV genome has an 18 nt RNA primer attached to its 5′ end (**Figure 1**). In addition, the positive strand is incomplete, with a minimum gap of 12 nt. Thus, following transport to the nucleus, the covalently linked polymerase protein, the RNA primer, and the terminal redundancy in the negative strand are removed, the positive strand is completed, and ligation of the ends of each strand takes place. As noted above and discussed in detail below, ~10% of circulating DHBV virions contain double-stranded linear (dsl) genomes that result from a defect that occurs during synthesis of positive-strand DNA. Following infection these dsl genomes can also enter the nucleus to form cccDNA, which in this case is formed

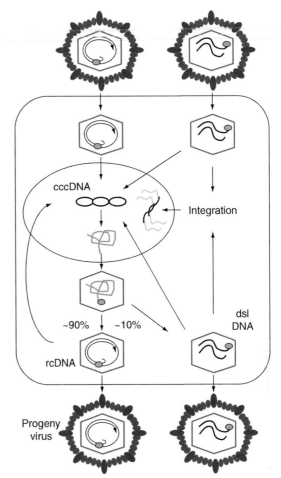

**Figure 2** DHBV infection of hepatocytes. Virions, shown at the top, may have either an rcDNA or, more rarely, a dsl DNA genome. Upon infection virus nucleocapsids are uncoated and move to the nucleus. Virus DNA is released from nucleocapsids and probably enters the nucleus at nuclear pores. Both rcDNA and dsl DNA give rise to cccDNA, the virus transcriptional template. cccDNA is used by host-cell RNA polymerase II to produce pregenomic RNA that is reverse transcribed to rcDNA or dsl DNA. dsl DNA also has a propensity to integrate into host-cell DNA (see text). Early in infection, cccDNA copy number increases by intracellular amplification from rcDNA and dsl DNA made in the cytoplasm via reverse transcription. Later, this pathway is shut down and nucleocapsids containing rcDNA and dsl DNA bud into the endoplasmic reticulum and are released as progeny virus.

by illegitimate recombination between the ends of the dsl DNA. This recombination event typically involves some loss of sequences, and cccDNA formed from dsl genomes is generally defective.

DHBV cccDNA molecules exist within the nucleus of each infected hepatocyte as a population of virus minichromosomes that bind up to 20 nucleosomes per 3000 nt molecule. cccDNA does not undergo semiconservative replication. New copies are therefore formed from rcDNA and dsl DNA synthesized in the cytoplasm of infected hepatocytes. Once formed, cccDNA is transcribed by host RNA polymerase II to produce pregenomic and other virus mRNAs (**Figures 1** and **2**), followed by protein production, assembly of nucleocapsids from the viral core protein and packaging of pregenomic RNA. Each virus mRNA is produced from its own promoter and virus RNA molecules including the pregenome have a 5′ cap and are polyadenylated at a common site (nt 2778–2783) on the DHBV genome numbered according to the sequence of the Australian strain of DHBV (Gen-Bank AJ006350) where the unique EcoRI site is nucleotide 1.

Packaging of pregenomic RNA is facilitated by the presence of an encapsidation signal, epsilon (ε), located at the 5′ end (nt 2566–2622) and at the 3′ end of the pregenome, within the terminal redundancy (**Figure 3(a)**). Pregenome packaging is dependent upon binding of the virus polymerase to the 5′ ε sequence. In fact, the pregenome is able to serve as the mRNA for both core and polymerase proteins (**Figure 1**). However, once

polymerase is translated, it may bind to its own message and block its further translation. Once packaging into nucleocapsids has occurred, virus DNA synthesis takes place via reverse transcription of the pregenomic RNA, with production of replicative intermediate DNA (RI DNA) to produce rcDNA and dsl DNA genomes in a ∼10:1 ratio (**Figures 3(f)** and **3(h)**).

DNA synthesis begins with reverse transcription of 4 nt (5′ UUAC 3′) in the bulge in the stem–loop structure of ε, leading to synthesis of 4 nt of DNA (5′ GTAA 3′) (**Figure 3(b)**). As noted above, a tyrosine residue in the TP domain of the polymerase serves as the primer of reverse transcription. Following synthesis by reverse transcription of the first 4 nt, the complex is translocated to DR1, in particular the 3′ copy of DR1, DR1* (**Figure 3(c)**).

DR1 is a 12 nt sequence located 6 nt from the 5′ end of the pregenome at nt 2541–2552. It is therefore also present in the terminal redundancy of the pregenome. The same sequence known as DR2 is located about 50 nt

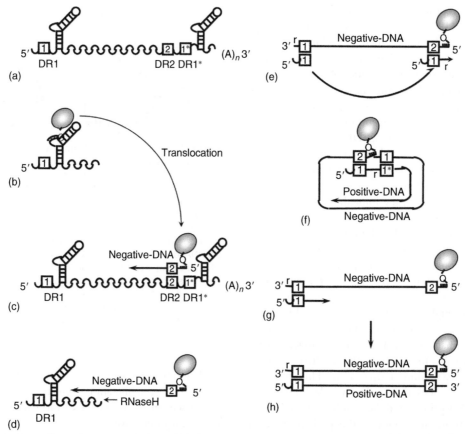

**Figure 3** Mechanism of DHBV DNA synthesis. Virus DNA synthesis begins with reverse transcription of 4 nt (5′ UUAC3′) of the bulge in the stem–loop structure, ε, and leads to synthesis of the first 4 nt (5′ GTAA3′) of negative-strand DNA, as shown in (b). Polymerase with the nascent transcript then translocates to the right-hand copy of DR1, DR1*, and reverse transcription of the negative strand and degradation of the pregenomic RNA template by RNase H proceeds as shown in (c) and (d). Following completion of the negative strand, the 5′ 18 nt of the pregenome, including the cap, are typically translocated to DR2 and positive-strand DNA synthesis then initiates from this RNA primer. In this case, rcDNA formation is of necessity an early step in positive-strand synthesis ((e) and (f)). About 10% of the time, positive-strand synthesis initiates without translocation of the primer (g), leading to the formation of dsl DNA (h). The details of DNA synthesis are described in greater detail in the text.

upstream of the terminal redundancy at nt 2483–2494. Once transferred to DR1*, where the 4 nt can base pair due to sequence homology, reverse transcription re-initiates and continues to the 5′ end of the pregenome, to produce a full-length negative strand with a 9 nt terminal redundancy (**Figures 3(d)** and **3(e)**). Most of the pregenome is degraded during negative-strand elongation by the RNase H activity of the virus polymerase. However, the 5′ ~18 nt of the pregenome, including the cap and all of the 5′ copy of DR1, escapes RNase H degradation and serves as the positive DNA strand primer. Positive-strand synthesis leading to rcDNA formation initiates near the 5′ end of the negative strand. The primer is first translocated from its original location at the 3′ end of the template to DR2 where it can hybridize due to the sequence identity of DR1 and DR2 (**Figure 3(e)**). Following positive-strand elongation to the 5′ end of the negative strand, circularization occurs to facilitate continuation of positive-strand synthesis to produce mature rcDNA (**Figure 3(f)**). Circularization is facilitated by the 9 nt terminal redundancy on the negative-strand template.

dsl DNA genomes reflect a failure of positive-strand primer translocation from DR1 to DR2, resulting in a phenomenon known as *in situ* priming to produce a DNA that is collinear with pregenomic RNA up to DR1* (**Figure 3(h)**). Interestingly, both the polymerase, the protein primer of negative-strand synthesis and the RNA primer of positive-strand synthesis remain associated with virus DNA throughout virion assembly. Biochemical evidence suggests that each nucleocapsid contains only a single copy of polymerase protein, implying that a single protein is simultaneously the primer of DNA synthesis and the polymerase for both RNA- and DNA-dependent DNA synthesis.

Newly made rcDNA and dsl DNA are enveloped by budding into the endoplasmic reticulum and exported as progeny virus via the Golgi apparatus, or are transported to the nucleus to make additional copies of cccDNA, typically found at 10–30 copies per hepatocyte. Nuclear transport is negatively regulated by the virus envelope proteins, which direct nucleocapsids into the pathway of virus assembly. This negative regulation is essential because excessive accumulation of cccDNA will kill the host cell. Strong negative regulation may also be important because of the stability of cccDNA, and new synthesis of cccDNA may only be necessary to restore cccDNA levels in the progeny following division of infected hepatocytes. Negative regulation of cccDNA synthesis also appears to occur during HBV infection, but it is still not known whether the viral envelope proteins have an essential role in this process.

dsl DNA also integrates randomly into chromosomal DNA and has been detected in ~0.01–0.1% of hepatocytes during acute infections by both DHBV and the mammalian hepadnaviruses. Higher levels of integrated virus DNA accumulate during chronic infections. This probably reflects ongoing import of rcDNA and dsl DNA into the nucleus to restore cccDNA copy number as infected hepatocytes divide to replace those killed by the host immune response, thereby providing new dsl DNA genomes for integration. Integrated forms of hepadnavirus DNA are usually unable to act as templates for transcription of pregenomic RNA since the promoter for this virus RNA is located at the 3′ end of the integrant, not the 5′ end, and integrated DNA is therefore not able to direct virus replication (see **Figure 1**). In addition, virus sequences may be lost during the integration process, particularly from the ends of the dsl molecule.

Since each integrated virus–cell DNA junction is unique, and will be present only once in the liver unless the infected hepatocyte divides, integration sites can be used to identify and track the fate of individual hepatocyte lineages. In particular, assays for integrated DNA were used to show that hepatocytes present in the liver following recovery from an acute WHV infection were derived from previously infected hepatocytes, indicating the existence of mechanisms for removal of cccDNA from infected hepatocytes.

## Phylogenetic Information

Assigned species within the genus *Avihepadnavirus* include DHBV isolated from Pekin ducks (*Anas domesticus*) and HHBV from grey herons (*Ardea cinerea*). Many DHBV isolates have been found in domesticated ducks and, in the wild, in the mallard, the species from which most domesticated ducks are derived. Viruses less closely related to DHBV have been isolated from geese and other duck species and include the Ross's goose hepatitis B virus (RGHBV) from Ross's geese (*Anser rossii*), Mandarin duck hepatitis B virus (MDHBV) from Mandarin ducks (*Aix galericulata*), and the snow goose hepatitis B virus (SGHBV) from snow geese (*Anser caerulescens*). The stork hepatitis B virus (STHBV) has been isolated from white storks (*Ciconia ciconia*), with additional viruses isolated from demoiselle (*Anthropoides virgo*) and grey crowned cranes (*Balearica regulorum*) (**Figure 4**). By genome sequencing, HHBV and STHBV are the most distant from DHBV (**Figure 4**). HHBV was assigned as a species based both on genome divergence and a host range difference from DHBV. Current information does not provide clear evidence for designation of additional new species among the isolates shown in **Figure 4**.

Thus, the avihepadnaviruses are currently classified phylogenetically into 'Chinese' and 'Western Country' isolates as well as four highly distinct lineages that include SGHBV, RGHBV, plus MDHBV, STHBV, and HHBV. Sequence divergence within the 'Chinese' and 'Western Country' DHBV strains is 5.99% and 3.35%, respectively,

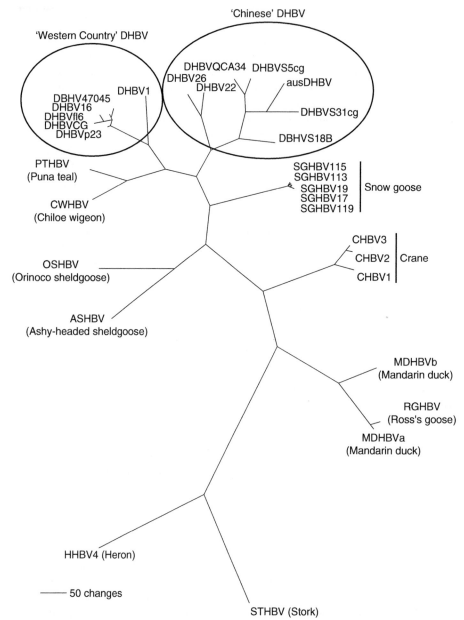

**Figure 4**  Phylogenetic relationships of avian hepadnaviruses. A dendrogram file was constructed using Clustal X and full-length virus sequences and displayed using Treeview. The following sequences were included: 'Chinese' DHBV isolates, accession numbers M32990, M32991, X60213, AJ006350, M21953, X58568, X58569; 'Western Country' DHBV isolates, K01834, M60677, X12798, X74623, AF047045, X58567; snow goose hepatitis B virus isolates: AF110996, AF110997, AF110998, AF110999, AF11000; Ross's goose hepatitis B virus: M95589; grey heron hepatitis B virus: M22056; stork hepatitis B virus: AJ251937; crane hepatitis B virus isolates: AJ441111, AJ441112, AJ441113; Mandarin duck hepatitis B virus isolates: AY494848, AY494849; Chiloe wigeon hepatitis B virus: AY494850; puna teal hepatitis B virus: AY494851; Orinoco sheldgoose hepatitis B virus: AY494852; and ashy-headed sheldgoose hepatitis B virus: AY49485.

while divergence between the strains is 9.8%. SGHBV diverges from DHBV by 11–13%, RGHBV and MDHBV by 17–19% and STHBV and HHBV by 22–24%. Additional closely related viruses have been isolated from the puna teal (*Anas puna*), ashy-headed sheldgoose (*Chloephaga poliocephala*), Orinoco sheldgoose (*Neochen jubata*), and Chiloe wigeon (*Anas sibilatrix*) (**Figure 4**).

## Pathogenesis and Control of Diseases

In persistently DHBV-infected ducks, the natural route of virus transmission is from the bloodstream to the egg. Virus replication then occurs in the yolk sac and developing liver and pancreas of the embryo (**Figures 5(a)–5(c)**) and results in congenital DHBV infection. Congenitally

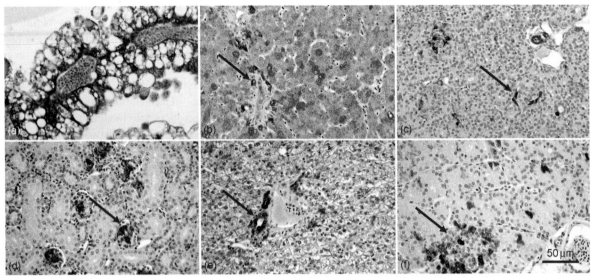

**Figure 5** Hepatic and extrahepatic infection with DHBV of a 14-day-fertilized duck embryo (a–c) and a 2-week-old congenitally infected duck (d–f). Immunoperoxidase staining of DHBV core antigen in yolk sac (a), liver (b, e), pancreas (c, f), and kidney (d). DHBV is transmitted *in ovo* from the bloodstream of the persistently DHBV-infected female duck to the egg, resulting in DHBV replication in yolk sac cells (a), hepatocytes and bile duct cells (arrow) in the liver (b), and pancreatic acinar cells (c). DHBV infection persists in congenitally DHBV-infected ducks in glomerular cells in the kidney ((d); arrow), in >95% of hepatocytes and in bile duct cells of the liver ((e); arrow shows high levels of DHBV core antigen detection in bile duct cells), and in pancreatic acinar and islets cells ((f); arrow indicates a group of DHBV core antigen-positive pancreatic beta islet cells; alpha islets also positive (not shown)). Tissues were fixed in ethanol:acetic acid, immunostained with polyclonal anti-DHBV core antibodies and counterstained with hematoxylin.

DHBV-infected ducks remain persistently infected for life, with infection in >95% of hepatocytes (**Figure 5(e)**). Bile duct cells are also infected with DHBV and express high levels of DHBcAg and DHBsAg (**Figure 5(e)**). Virus replication also occurs in acinar and islet cells in the pancreas (**Figure 5(f)**), and in glomeruli (**Figure 5(d)**) and tubular epithelial cells in the kidney. Cells located in the germinal centers of the spleen contain nonreplicating DHBV DNA, which is thought to be associated with follicular dendritic cells. In ducks with congenital infection, levels of DHBV DNA and DHBsAg in the bloodstream gradually decrease over 800 days and anticore antibodies can be detected from ~90 days post hatch, consistent with a high degree of immune tolerance.

Persistent DHBV infection also results following experimental inoculation of newly hatched ducks, and inoculation of infected serum containing the equivalent of one virion is sufficient to initiate DHBV infection. Infection of newly hatched ducks with DHBV has allowed detailed studies of the kinetics and tissue specificity of DHBV infection. Inoculation of 2- to 4-week-old ducks with DHBV results in either acute or persistent infection depending on the age of the duck at the time of inoculation and the dose of DHBV administered. Ducks from this age group that develop persistent infection have histological changes in the liver with mild mononuclear cell infiltration of portal tracts but no evidence of lobular hepatitis

or extensive liver damage. Experimental inoculation of 4-month-old ducks with high doses of DHBV leads to either persistent infections with mild to marked liver disease or to transient infections that are rapidly cleared.

Since hepadnavirus infection is noncytopathic, the liver damage seen during DHBV infection has been attributed to the immune response directed against infected hepatocytes. Although cirrhosis and primary hepatocellular carcinoma (HCC) are not reported to occur in DHBV infection, the clinical and serological events, hepatocyte specificity, and ability of the host to rapidly resolve an infection involving the entire hepatocyte population are similar for DHBV, WHV, and HBV.

Humans infected with HBV, especially when less than a year of age, often develop a healthy carrier state which can last for several decades without clinically evident liver disease. Similarly, persistent infection with avian hepadnaviruses, resulting either from *in ovo* infection or experimental inoculation after hatching, generally results in only mild hepatitis similar to the 'healthy' carrier state in humans. The failure to detect liver disease, cirrhosis and HCC in persistently DHBV-infected ducks may to be linked to the timing and mode of transmission of these viruses, since they are usually transmitted vertically by *in ovo* transmission resulting in congenital infection with immune tolerance and an absence of, or only mild, liver disease. The inability of DHBV-infected ducks to progress to HCC may also be affected by their limited life span in captivity, which is generally less than 5 years. HCC was detected in ducks in a Chinese province but in those areas aflatoxin exposure may have been common and the key contributory factor in the development of the liver cancers.

## Conclusion

Although the avian hepadnaviruses share only 40% nucleotide sequence identity with HBV and the other mammalian hepadnaviruses, they are nearly identical in genome organization and replication strategy. Indeed, the molecular details of hepadnavirus replication were initially worked out with DHBV and later extended to HBV, and the similarities were found to be striking. The biology of infection of HBV and DHBV is also strikingly similar, with hepatocytes the primary target of infection and immune-mediated cell death the primary cause of liver disease in infected hosts.

The only major difference between the two viruses is how they are able to persist in their respective host populations. DHBV appears to be maintained primarily by vertical transmission to the developing embryo, whereas the primary route for maintenance of HBV in the human population is by horizontal transmission during the first year of life from mother to child, or among young children. Both routes lead to chronic infection, but it is generally believed that the degree of immune tolerance to the virus is much greater following vertical than horizontal transmission. This probably explains the greater disease activity in chronically infected humans than ducks. This difference is also seen in the woodchuck model. Chronic WHV infection results, as in HBV in humans, primarily from horizontal transmission, leading to a much more rapid disease progression than found in ducks.

HBV was discovered in 1967, WHV in 1978, and ground squirrel hepatitis B and DHBV viruses shortly thereafter. Among these, DHBV was the easiest to work with because of the ready availability of hosts from commercial sources. Thus, in the initial absense of a cell culture system, much of the early work on hepadnavirus replication focused on DHBV. As a result, DHBV provided much of the information on how the hepadnaviruses replicate as well as detailed early information on the biology of infection and virus spread, including possible identification of the cell surface receptor for the virus. Studies of DHBV have also provided important information on how cccDNA is made and on its high degree of stability in nondividing cells. In addition, the DHBV model has been used to demonstrate the reproducible and rapid kinetics of the spread of DHBV infection *in vivo* and to determine the high specific infectivity of DHBV, where one virus particle has been shown to be infectious in neonatal ducks.

Because of the reproducible nature of the kinetics of infection and the predictable outcomes of infection using defined doses of DHBV, the model is especially useful for the evaluation of new antiviral therapies and vaccine strategies for HBV infection in humans. Similarities in the replication strategy and polymerase enzymes of the avian and human hepadnaviruses allow evaluation of new antiviral drugs in *in vivo* models of HBV infection, including the development of antiviral drug-resistant mutants and competition between wild-type and mutant DHBV strains.

## Further Reading

Foster WK, Miller DS, Scougall CA, Kotlarski I, Colonno RJ, and Jilbert AR (2005) The effect of antiviral treatment with Entecavir on age- and dose-related outcomes of duck hepatitis B virus infection. *Journal of Virology* 79: 5819–5832.

Funk A, Mhamdi M, Will H, and Sirma H (2007) Avian hepatitis B viruses: Molecular and cellular biology, phylogenesis, and host tropism. *World Journal of Gastroenterology* 13: 91–103.

Gong SS, Jensen AD, Chang CJ, and Rogler CE (1999) Double-stranded linear duck hepatitis B virus (DHBV) stably integrates at a higher frequency than wild-type DHBV in LMH chicken hepatoma cells. *Journal of Virology* 73: 1492–1502.

Guo H, Mason WS, Aldrich CE, *et al.* (2005) Identification and characterization of avihepadnaviruses isolated from exotic anseriformes maintained in captivity. *Journal of Virology* 79: 2729–2742.

Jilbert A and Locarnini S (2005) *Avihepadnaviridae*. In: Thomas H, Lemon S,, and Zuckerman A (eds.) *Viral Hepatitis,* 3rd edn., pp. 193–209. Adelaide: Blackwell Publishing.

Jilbert AR, Freiman JS, Gowans EJ, Holmes M, Cossart YE, and Burrell CJ (1987) Duck hepatitis B virus DNA in liver, spleen, and pancreas: Analysis by *in situ* and Southern blot hybridization. *Virology* 158: 330–338.

Jilbert AR and Kotlarski I (2000) Immune responses to duck hepatitis B virus infection. *Developmental and Comparative Immunology* 24: 285–302.

Jilbert AR, Miller DS, Scougall CA, Turnbull H, and Burrell CJ (1996) Kinetics of duck hepatitis B virus infection following low dose virus inoculation: One virus DNA genome is infectious in neonatal ducks. *Virology* 226: 338–345.

Jilbert AR, Wu TT, England JM, *et al.* (1992) Rapid resolution of duck hepatitis B virus infections occurs after massive hepatocellular involvement. *Journal of Virology* 66: 1377–1388.

Meier P, Scougall CA, Will H, Burrell CJ, and Jilbert AR (2003) A duck hepatitis B virus strain with a knockout mutation in the putative X ORF shows similar infectivity and *in vivo* growth characteristics to wild-type virus. *Virology* 317: 291–298.

Miller DS, Bertram EM, Scougall CA, Kotlarski I, and Jilbert AR (2004) Studying host immune responses against duck hepatitis B virus infection. *Methods in Molecular Medicine* 96: 3–25.

Summers J, Smith PM, and Horwich AL (1990) Hepadnavirus envelope proteins regulate covalently closed circular DNA amplification. *Journal of Virology* 64: 2819–2824.

Yang W and Summers J (1995) Illegitimate replication of linear hepadnavirus DNA through nonhomologous recombination. *Journal of Virology* 69: 4029–4036.

Yang W and Summers J (1999) Integration of hepadnavirus DNA in infected liver: Evidence for a linear precursor. *Journal of Virology* 73: 9710–9717.

Zhang YY, Zhang BH, Theele D, Litwin S, Toll E, and Summers J (2003) Single-cell analysis of covalently closed circular DNA copy numbers in a hepadnavirus-infected liver. *Proceedings of the National Academy of Sciences, USA* 100: 12372–12377.

# Herpesviruses of Birds

**S Trapp and N Osterrieder,** Cornell University, Ithaca, NY, USA

## Introduction

A large number of herpesviruses are found in avian host species of several different orders. Similar to their mammalian counterparts, they generally have a relatively narrow host range *in vitro* and *in vivo*. At present, only the gallid herpesviruses (GaHV-1, GaHV-2, and GaHV-3), meleagrid herpesvirus 1 (MeHV-1; also referred to as herpesvirus of turkeys, HVT), and psittacid herpesvirus 1 (PsHV-1) have been classified taxonomically by the International Committee on Taxonomy of Viruses (ICTV) as members of the *Alphaherpesvirinae* subfamily. Genomic sequences have been reported for all of these alphaherpesviruses and deposited in the GenBank sequence database. Avian beta- or gammaherpesviruses have not been identified.

Taxonomically unclassified herpesviruses have been discovered in a wide variety of avian hosts; including the bald eagle (acciptrid herpesvirus 1, AcHV-1), duck (anatid herpesvirus 1, AnHV-1), black stork (ciconiid herpesvirus 1, CiHV-1), pigeon (columbid herpesvirus 1, CoHV-1), falcon (falconid herpesvirus 1, FaHV-1), crane (gruid herpesvirus 1, GrHV-1), bobwhite quail (perdicid herpesvirus 1, PdHV-1), cormorant (phalacrocoracid herpesvirus 1, PhHV-1), black-footed penguin (sphenicid herpesvirus 1, SpHV-1), and owl (strigid herpesvirus 1, StHV-1). Of these viruses, only AnHV-1 causes a known disease, duck virus enteritis (DVE), which accounts for significant economic losses. DVE, also referred to as duck plague, is a highly contagious acute disease of ducks, geese, and swans, and is characterized by hemorrhagic lesions in the blood vessels, gastrointestinal mucosa, and lymphoid tissues. The clinical symptoms of DVE are unspecific, and often mortality is the first observation in infected waterfowl flocks. Morbidity and mortality in domestic ducks may range from 5% to 100%.

Gallid herpesvirus 1 (GaHV-1), frequently referred to as infectious laryngotracheitis virus (ILTV), belongs to the type species of the genus *Iltovirus* and is the causative agent of a highly contagious, acute respiratory tract disease of domestic fowl termed infectious laryngotracheitis (ILT). ILT causes considerable economic losses to the poultry industry worldwide owing to mortality and decreased egg production associated with the disease. Epizootic forms of ILT are characterized clinically by severe respiratory symptoms such as dyspnea and hemorrhagic expectorations, and are generally associated with high mortality (5–70%). Enzootic infections, predominantly those occurring in poultry flocks of developed countries, are associated

with mild symptoms (nasal discharge, conjunctivitis, and decreased egg production) or subclinical symptoms. Modified-live vaccines against ILTV infections are available, but their use is commonly restricted to areas where ILT is enzootic. However, most of the current modified-live virus vaccines have residual virulence, and several ILT outbreaks have been attributed to reversions of the ILTV vaccine strains to a virulent phenotype.

ILTV is the only virus allocated to the genus *Iltovirus*. However, recent genomic information indicates clearly an affiliation of PsHV-1 with this genus. PsHV-1 causes Pacheco's disease, a generally fatal disease of psittacine birds characterized by acute onset and massive necrotizing lesions of the crop, intestines, pancreas, and liver. Parrot species from multiple geographic regions are highly susceptible to Pacheco's disease. However, captive parrots such as macaws, Amazon parrots, and cockatoos account for the majority of clinical cases of Pacheco's disease; hence, the disease is of great concern to pet traders and exotic bird breeders worldwide. An association of subclinical PsHV-1 infections with mucosal papillomatosis in neotropical (Central and South American) parrots has been reported, but causality has not yet been demonstrated. Recently, genomic DNA of a novel psittacine alphaherpesvirus has been amplified from mucosal and cutaneous papillomas of African grey parrots. This virus is related to, but phylogenetically distinct from, PsHV-1, and has been designated psittacid herpesvirus 2 (PsHV-2).

Gallid herpesvirus 2 (GaHV-2) or Marek's disease virus (MDV) is the etiologic agent of Marek's disease (MD), an economically important, neoplastic, and neuropathic disease of chickens. MDV is highly infectious and routinely causes >90% morbidity and mortality in susceptible, unvaccinated animal populations. MD manifests as various clinical syndromes of varying severity. Of these, T-cell lymphoproliferative syndromes, including fowl paralysis (classic MD) and fatal MD lymphoma (acute MD), are most frequently associated with the disease. However, infections of chickens with the most recent clade of MDV strains are characterized by massive inflammatory brain lesions that are clinically manifested as transient paralysis and/or peracute death. Owing to its biological features, namely its lymphotropism and oncogenic potential, MDV was long thought to be related to Epstein–Barr virus, a lymphomagenic gammaherpesvirus. However, based on its genomic organization, MDV was reclassified as an alphaherpesvirus; thus, MDV is genetically more closely related

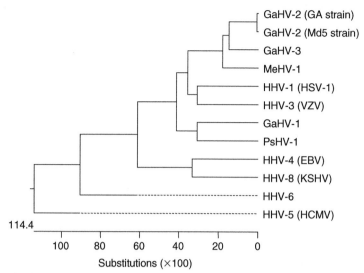

**Figure 1** Genetic relationship of avian herpesviruses. A ClustalV-based comparison of the amino acid sequences of the DNA polymerase proteins of the viruses is shown. Human herpesviruses 5 (human cytomegalovirus) and 6, representatives of the *Betaherpesvirinae*, were chosen as outgroups. It is evident that the two representatives of the *Iltovirus* genus, GaHV-1 (ILTV) and PsHV-1 are closely related, as are the three members of the genus *Mardivirus*, GaHV-2 (MDV), GaHV-3, and MeHV-1 (HVT). These results also indicate independent evolution of *Alphaherpesvirinae* (GaHV-1 and GaHV-2) within one bird species (*Gallus gallus*). EBV, Epstein–Barr virus; HCMV, human cytomegalovirus; HHV, human herpesvirus; HSV-1, herpes simplex virus type 1; KSHV, Kaposi's sarcoma-associated herpesvirus; VZV, varicella-zoster virus.

to herpes simplex virus 1 (HSV-1) and varicella-zoster virus (VZV) (**Figure 1**). MDV belongs to the type species of the genus *Mardivirus*, into which two other closely related but distinct species have been grouped, represented by gallid herpesvirus 3 (GaHV-3) and MeHV-1 (HVT). Although the three viruses are closely related, only MDV causes MD while GaHV-3 and HVT are nonpathogenic. Therefore, the old nomenclature referring to GaHV-3 and HVT as MDV (serotypes) 2 and 3 is misleading and should be avoided.

Control of MDV-caused syndromes by vaccination was started in the late 1960s using an attenuated MDV strain (HPRS-16att) or the nonpathogenic HVT. Because MDV field strains are evidently evolving toward greater virulence in the face of vaccination, combination vaccines consisting of HVT and GaHV-3 or an attenuated MDV strain (CVI988-Rispens) are currently used to immunize chickens against the latest clade of MDV strains. Based on their ability to cause breaks of vaccinal immunity, MDV strains are subdivided into four different pathotypes: mildly virulent (m), virulent (v), very virulent (vv), and very virulent plus (vv+).

## History

ILT was first described in 1925 as tracheolaryngitis, and shortly thereafter its viral etiology was demonstrated. The term infectious laryngotracheitis was adopted in 1931 by the Special Committee on Poultry Diseases of the American Veterinary Medical Association. ILT was the first major viral avian disease against which an effective vaccine was developed, being achieved in the 1930s by Hudson and Beaudette at Cornell University. Pacheco's disease was first recognized by Pacheco and Bier in the late 1920s in Brazil, but was not seen again until the 1970s, when outbreaks of the disease occurred in wild-caught neotropical parrots and a psittacine herpesvirus was identified as the etiologic agent.

The first account of MD dates from 1907, when József Marek (after whom the disease was named in 1960), a preeminent clinician and pathologist at the Royal Hungarian Veterinary School in Budapest, reported a generalized neuritis interstitialis or polyneuritis in four adult cockerels, which were affected by paralysis of the limbs and wings. Marek's detailed histological examination revealed that the sciatic nerve and areas of the spinal cord of the affected birds were infiltrated by mononuclear cells, an observation that is still made today after infection with most MDV strains. In the late 1920s, Pappenheimer and colleagues at Rockefeller University recognized the lymphoproliferative character of MD, and proposed that polyneuritis and visceral lymphoma were manifestations of the same disease. The identification of a highly cell-associated herpesvirus as the etiological agent of MD in the late 1960s by Churchill and colleagues led to the development of vaccines that achieved unparalleled success in preventing the disease, and provided the first example of immune prophylaxis against a cancer induced by an oncogenic virus.

## Host Range and Virus Propagation

Like most avian herpesviruses, ILTV exhibits a very narrow host range. The chicken is the primary natural host, but pheasants and peafowl have also been reported to be susceptible. Turkeys have been shown to be susceptible to infection under experimental conditions, but other avian species are probably refractory. Embryonated chicken eggs are also susceptible, and can be used to propagate the virus. Chorioallantoic membrane (CAM) plaques resulting from necrosis and proliferative tissue reactions can be observed as early as 2 days post inoculation (pi). The virus can also be propagated in a variety of primary avian cell cultures, including chicken embryo liver cells (CELCs), chicken embryo kidney cells (CEKCs), and chicken kidney cells (CKCs). In addition, a permanent chicken cell line (LMH) derived from a chemically induced liver tumor was shown to permit replication of cell culture-adapted ILTV. Viral cytopathology *in vitro*, characterized by the formation of syncytia and nuclear inclusion bodies, can be observed as early as 4–6 h pi.

PsHV-1 infects a broad spectrum of psittacine species. In addition, it has been isolated from a superb starling, and some evidence suggests that other passerine species, such as the common cardinal, zebra finch, and canary, are also susceptible to PsHV-1 infections. Embryonated chicken eggs and primary chicken embryo cells (CECs) derived from 10- to 12-day-old chicken embryos are used for virus propagation *in vitro*.

MDV infections and MD-like symptoms have been observed in quail, turkeys, and pheasants, but the chicken is considered the natural host of MDV. Primary chicken cells (CKCs and CECs) or duck embryo fibroblasts (DEFs) are used routinely to propagate the virus *in vitro*. However, for primary isolation and propagation of low-passage MDV isolates, the use of CKC or DEF is recommended to retain wild-type properties of the virus. Permanent avian cell lines such as OU2, DF-1, and QM7 allow only low level or abortive MDV replication. On permissive cells, MDV-induced plaques ($\leq$1 mm in diameter) develop very slowly (in 5–14 days pi) on primary isolation and 3–7 days pi after cell culture adaptation. In addition, 1-day-old chicks can be used for primary isolation and propagation of MDV *in vivo*.

## Morphology

All herpesvirus particles share a complex and characteristic multilayered structure in which the nucleocapsid containing the viral DNA is separated from the envelope by a proteinaceous layer called the tegument. While both MDV and ILTV capsids have a diameter of approximately 125 nm, the incorporation of highly variable amounts of tegument into ILTV virions results in diameters of enveloped ILTV particles that vary between 195 and 350 nm. In contrast, enveloped MDV particles have a diameter of 150–160 nm. The morphologies of GaHV-3 and HVT closely resemble that of MDV, but, in thin sections, HVT capsids commonly show a characteristic cross-shaped appearance. The morphology of PsHV-1 has not been studied in detail, but typical herpesvirus particles have been visualized.

## Genetics

The genomes of herpesviruses are linear, double-stranded DNA molecules that range in size from approximately 120 to 300 kbp. A total of six different genome organizations, referred to as classes A through F, are distinguished in the *Herpesviridae*, and only class D and E genomes are found in the *Alphaherpesvirinae*. ILTV and PsHV-1 have class D genomes and the three members of the *Mardivirus* genus (MDV, GaHV-3, and HVT) have class E genomes. Class D genomes consist of two unique sequence regions (unique-long, $U_L$; unique-short, $U_S$) with inverted repeats (internal repeat, IR; terminal repeat, TR) flanking $U_S$. Class E genomes consist of $U_L$ and $U_S$, each bracketed by inverted internal ($IR_L$, $IR_S$) and terminal repeats ($TR_L$, $TR_S$).

The ILTV genome sequence, as assembled from 14 overlapping genome fragments from different virus strains, is approximately 147 kbp in length and has a G+C content of 48.2%. The PsHV-1 genome is 163 kbp in length and has a nucleotide composition of 61% G+C. ILTV and PsHV-1 contain 76 and 73 protein-coding open reading frames (ORFs), respectively, and the majority of these ORFs exhibit significant homologies to genes of the prototypic alphaherpesvirus, HSV-1. However, ILTV and PsHV-1 exhibit several unusual structural features, for example, a large internal inversion of the region within $U_L$ containing genes UL22 to UL44 (a suffix is sometimes used in gene name, e.g., $U_L$ 22). Also, $U_L$ in both viruses contains a unique cluster of five ORFs (designated A to E) that do not share significant sequence similarity with known viral or cellular genes. The function of these ORFs is unknown, but they have been shown to be dispensable for ILTV replication *in vitro*. Another striking feature is the localization of the UL47 gene, which encodes a tegument protein and is usually localized in the $U_L$ region of alphaherpesvirus genomes. UL47 is absent from the corresponding position in the ILTV and PsHV-1 genomes, but both viruses are still predicted to encode a homolog of UL47 (ILTV: UL47; PsHV-1: sORF1) in $U_S$.

One major structural difference between the closely related viruses ILTV and PsHV-1 can be found in the inverted repeat regions of the genomes. The ILTV repeats are considerably (18.5%) shorter than those of PsHV-1, and each harbors three genes: ICP4, US10, and sORF4/3. In contrast, ICP4 is the only gene located in the PsHV-1 repeat, and the US10 and sORF4/3 genes are located in $U_S$.

Moreover, PsHV-1 $U_L$ contains a homolog of UL16, an ORF that is conserved throughout the herpesvirus subfamilies but is absent from the ILTV genome, having presumably been lost during evolution. Conversely, ILTV $U_L$ contains the UL48 gene and ILTV-specific UL0 gene, neither of which is found in the PsHV-1 genome.

The complete genomic sequences of representatives of all three species in the genus *Mardivirus* have been determined. The gene contents and linear arrangements of the genomes of MDV, GaHV-3, and HVT are similar in general, but vary considerably with regard to G+C content and size. Whereas the ~180 kbp MDV genome has a G+C content of 44.1%, the ~165 kbp GaHV-3 genome has a nucleotide composition of 53.6% G+C; the ~160 kbp HVT genome has a G+C content in between these two values (47.2%). A total of 103 (MDV), 102 (GaHV-3), and 99 (HVT) genes have been clearly identified in the mardivirus genomes. The majority of these genes are homologous to genes encoded by other alphaherpesviruses, but genus- and species-specific genes are also present.

Most of the differences between the three mardiviruses concern the $TR_L$ and $IR_L$ regions. In pathogenic MDV, they harbor a unique cluster of three species-specific genes, which are designated vTR, vIL-8, and meq. vTR, which encodes a viral homolog of telomerase RNA (vTR), exhibits 88% sequence identity to chicken telomerase RNA, and was presumably pirated from the chicken genome. The vIL-8 ORF encodes a CXC chemokine (viral interleukin-8, vIL-8) of 18–20 kDa in size, which functions as a chemoattractant for chicken mononuclear cells. The meq gene encodes the 339-residue oncoprotein Meq (<u>M</u>DV <u>E</u>co<u>R</u>I <u>Q</u>), a transcriptional regulator that is characterized by an N-terminal bZIP domain and a proline-rich C-terminal transactivation domain.

In addition, a genus-specific ORF (pp38), which is located in the junctions between the $U_L$ and the adjacent repeat regions of all three mardivirus genomes, encodes a pp38 phosphoprotein of variable size dependent on the virus and the phosphorylation status of the protein. Another mardivirus-specific ORF, vLIP, is located in $U_L$ in close proximity to pp38, and encodes a 120 kDa N-glycosylated protein, a portion of which shows significant similarity to the $\alpha/\beta$ hydrolase fold of pancreatic lipases and was thus termed viral lipase (vLIP). The HVT-specific vN-13 ORF encodes a 19 kDa protein (vN-13) that exhibits 63.7% amino acid sequence identity to cellular N-13, an anti-apoptotic member of the Bcl-2 family. While Bcl-2-like sequences have been identified in several gammaherpesviruses, HVT is the only alphaherpesvirus that encodes a Bcl-2 homolog.

One striking feature of all three mardiviruses is the presence of heterogenic telomeric repeat sequences at the genome termini. Interestingly, similar telomeric repeat sequences have been identified in the genomes of two betaherpesviruses, human herpesviruses 6 and 7 (HHV-6 and HHV-7), and one gammaherpesvirus, equid herpesvirus 2 (EHV-2). The structural or functional significance of these telomeric repeats is unknown, but they might be responsible for genome integration and maintenance of virus genomes in latently infected (tumor) cells.

## Pathobiology

### Pathogenesis, Clinical Features, and Pathology of Iltovirus Infections

ILTV is readily transmitted from infected to susceptible chickens, and virus shedding and spread mainly occur via the respiratory and ocular routes. Early cytolytic replication of ILTV in the epithelia of the upper respiratory tract results in syncytia formation and subsequent desquamation. Following the acute phase of infection, which lasts for approximately 6–8 days, ILTV establishes latency in the central nervous system (CNS), in particular in trigeminal ganglia. No clear evidence exists for a viremic phase in the course of lytic infection, latency, or reactivation. Sporadic reactivations from the latent state are usually asymptomatic, but generally lead to productive replication in the upper respiratory tract and virus shedding, which can result in infection of susceptible contact animals. The severity of clinical symptoms of ILT depends on the virulence of a particular ILTV strain or isolate, and mortality rates range from 0% to 70%. Severe epizootic forms of ILT are characterized clinically by marked dyspnea and hemorrhagic expectorations. Clinical signs of the milder, enzootic forms include nasal discharge, conjunctivitis, sinusitis, gasping, and decreased egg production. The incubation period of ILT ranges from 6 to 12 days. Pathomorphological alterations may be found in the conjunctiva and throughout the respiratory tract, but are most consistently detected in the larynx and trachea. Typical gross lesions include mucoid to hemorrhagic tracheitis, conjunctivitis, infraorbital sinusitis, and necrotizing bronchitis. However, in the case of the mild enzootic forms of ILT, conjunctivitis and sinusitis are often the only detectable gross lesions. Microscopic lesions include epithelial syncytia, desquamation, and submucosal edema. Eosinophilic intranuclear inclusion bodies in epithelial cells are detectable from day 1 to 5 pi, but disappear as desquamation of infected epithelial cells progresses.

Similar to ILTV, PsHV-1 is shed from the upper respiratory tract but also in the feces of infected parrots. Transmission of the virus occurs by direct contact between infected and susceptible animals or indirectly by contact with contaminated fomites or environmental contamination. The target sites for primary lytic viral replication and the establishment of latency are unknown. The systemic character of Pacheco's disease strongly argues for a viremic phase of infection during which the virus disseminates into multiple organ sites. Anorexia, depression, diarrhea, nasal discharge, and ataxia are among the most common clinical signs of the disease, but a variety of symptoms may be observed, largely depending on which organ system is affected. However, the majority of diseased animals die peracutely, that is, before the onset of clinical symptoms. Latently infected parrots that survive the disease play an important epidemiological role as asymptomatic virus carriers and shedders. The incubation time of Pacheco's disease ranges from 3 to 14 days. Gross pathological lesions are unspecific and may be found in a multitude of organ systems, including the respiratory and gastrointestinal tract, liver, and CNS. Microscopically, Pacheco's disease is characterized by a necrotizing hepatitis with minimal associated inflammation and the presence of intranuclear inclusion bodies (Cowdry type A).

## Pathogenesis, Clinical Features, and Pathology of MD

MDV shed from the skin and associated with feathers and dander is highly infectious and can persist for extended periods in the environment. Transmission of the virus occurs by inhalation, either through direct contact or through virus present in dust and dander. In the current model of MDV pathogenesis, phagocytic cells in the lower respiratory tract become infected either directly or after an initial round of replication in epithelial cells. Within 24 h of uptake, the virus is detectable in the primary and secondary lymphoid organs such as thymus, bursa of Fabricius, and spleen. Following primary productive replication, which takes place in B-lymphocytes, the virus infects activated $CD4^+$ lymphyocytes, and, rarely, $CD4^-CD8^-$ T-cells or $CD8^+$ T-cells. Infected $CD4^+$ T-cells serve as the target for the establishment of MDV latency and are also the means of virus dissemination within an infected animal. Besides epithelial layers in visceral organs, MDV enters the feather follicle epithelium, where cell-free infectious virus is assembled and released into the environment.

In latently infected T-cells, viral DNA is commonly integrated into the cellular genome. MDV is one of the few herpesviruses that achieve genome maintenance during the quiescent stage of infection through this mechanism, the details of which are entirely enigmatic. It is well known that latency is a prerequisite for oncogenic transformation by MDV, but only small subsets of latently infected T-cells become ultimately transformed and proliferate to generate tumors. Depending on the virulence of the virus strain and the susceptibility of the chicken population, mortality rates range from 0% to >90%. Clinical and pathological signs of MD vary according to the specific syndrome. The leading symptom of the classical form of the disease (fowl paralysis) is flaccid or spastic paralysis of the limbs and/or wings caused by lymphoproliferative peripheral nerve lesions. Chickens affected by MD lymphoma (acute MD) generally exhibit unspecific symptoms such as weight loss, anorexia, depression, and ruffled plumage, but (transient) paralysis may also be seen. Unlike the classic form of paralysis, transient paralysis is caused by inflammatory lesions of the CNS and peripheral nervous system. Most v and vv MDV strains induce MD lymphoma and/or (transient) paralysis in susceptible chicken lines. Recent outbreaks of MD caused by vv+ MDV strains are characterized clinically by transient paralysis, a massive rash affecting mainly the extremities, and/or peracute death.

Enlarged peripheral nerves and lymphomatous lesions are the most frequently observed gross pathological findings in MD. Lymphomatous lesions can develop as early as 14 days after infection and generally manifest as diffuse infiltrations and/or solid lymphomas, which affect a variety of organs, including the viscera (heart, liver, spleen, kidney, gonads, adrenal gland, etc.), skeletal muscle, and skin. Two main peripheral nerve pathologies are described: neoplastic proliferation that sometimes involves secondary demyelination (type A) and primary inflammatory cell-mediated demyelination (type B). MD lymphomas are cytologically complex and essentially comprised of lymphocytes and macrophages. MD tumors mainly consist of T-cells, but only a minority of these are transformed, the majority representing immune T-cells that try to contain the neoplasm.

Tumors induced by avian retroviruses represent a differential diagnosis for MDV-induced tumors, but onset of disease is delayed and nerve lesions are generally absent. Histologically, intranuclear inclusions are always absent from retrovirus-infected cells. A hallmark of MDV-transformed cells is expression of the viral oncoprotein Meq, and upregulation of the Hodgkin's antigen, CD30, has also been reported.

## Prevention and Control

### Control of Iltovirus Infections

ILTV-infected chickens produce peak virus-neutralizing antibody titers around 21 days post infection or vaccination. ILTV-neutralizing antibodies decline over the following months, but remain detectable for years. Although the detection of ILTV-specific antibodies by virus neutralization test is an important means of serological diagnosis, neutralizing antibody titers do not reflect the immune status of infected chickens or vaccinees, as immunity against ILT largely rests on local and cell-mediated immune response in the upper respiratory tract. Maternal antibodies to ILTV are transmitted to the chicken embryo via the egg yolk, but do not confer passive immunity against ILT or interfere with vaccination. For many years, modified-live virus (MLV) vaccines have been used to immunize chickens against ILT. They are administered via the intraocular route and for rapid mass vaccination via the drinking water or aerosolization. Immunization of chickens with attenuated ILTV vaccine strains results in latently infected carrier animals and spread of vaccine virus to nonvaccinates. However, spread to non-vaccinates results in consecutive bird-to-bird passages during which the vaccine virus may revert to a virulent phenotype. Therefore, the use of ILTV MLV vaccines has commonly been restricted to areas where infectious laryngotracheitis is enzootic. Experimental inactivated whole-virus vaccines and subunit preparations containing affinity-purified immunogenic ILTV glycoproteins were tested successfully as an immune prophylactic alternative to MLV vaccines. However, due to high costs of production and individual administration, the practical use of these vaccines in the field is debatable. Thus, the generation of MLV vaccines based on genetically engineered ILTV strains appears to be a more promising approach to the development of safe and efficacious ILTV vaccination protocols for the future.

Immune prophylaxis against Pacheco's disease is available in the form of an inactivated vaccine that is administered subcutaneously or intramuscularly. However, the vaccine is only protective against certain PsHV-1 serotypes, and its administration has been associated with adverse side effects, including granuloma formation and paralysis. Treatment with antiherpetic nucleoside analogues such as acyclovir can be used for pro- and metaphylactic measures in aviaries affected by Pacheco's disease. Strict quarantine protocols together with diagnostic screenings and isolation of birds that have been exposed to PsHV-1 are the most effective control measures for parrot breeding facilities and pet stores.

## Control of MD

MD is controlled worldwide by vaccination of 18-day-old embryos *in ovo* or 1-day-old chickens by subcutaneous/intramuscular injection into the neck. Vaccine practices, however, vary between countries and, for example, broilers usually remain unvaccinated in Europe whereas all chickens are vaccinated in the USA. These different vaccine regimens exist largely because of differences in the production practices of broilers, which live longer in the Americas to produce carcasses with higher body mass as preferred by the consumer. Prior to the introduction of vaccines against MD in the late 1960s and early 1970s, the disease had an economically devastating impact on the poultry industry, and mortality rates reached as high as 30–60%. All MD vaccines used today are MLV preparations, and some of them have been used for almost 40 years. The first vaccines were based on HVT isolate FC126 (used mainly in the USA) and on HPRS16att (Europe), a formerly virulent strain that was rendered nonpathogenic by serial passage in cultured cells. Shortly after the

introduction of vaccination in Europe, a naturally avirulent MDV strain, CVI988, was isolated, which has formed the basis of the MDV-based vaccines that are currently in use worldwide.

It became evident early on that MD vaccination is able to reduce and delay tumor development, but does not induce sterile immunity, which leads to a situation where constant evolutionary pressure is on field viruses to adapt to, and ultimately escape, vaccination. Consistent with this hypothesis, new MDV strains have been isolated that are able to break vaccine protection provided by HVT. The appearance of new, more virulent strains led to the introduction of so-called bivalent vaccines consisting of HVT and GaHV-3 strain SB-1. The latter was isolated from chickens, is completely avirulent, and is closely related genetically and antigenically to HVT and MDV. The bivalent vaccine was able to protect against more virulent (vv) viruses, but in the early 1990s even more virulent (vv+) MDV strains began to emerge. Most recently, repeated vaccinations using various combinations of vaccines (HVT + GaHV-3, HVT + MDV, MDV alone) are employed mainly in the USA to keep MD in check.

With the threat of new, even more virulent strains breaking through the current vaccination protocols, the development of novel vaccines is a huge challenge to the scientific community. Next to the efficacy of the vaccine preparations, the production process of vaccines in primary chicken embryo cultures is a major problem. The cost of producing these vaccines is high for several reasons, most notably the maintenance of pathogen-free chicken flocks, and approaches to find alternatives have been undertaken. The availability of infectious clones of various MDV strains and of HVT holds promise for a novel generation of rationally designed and efficacious vaccines.

*See also:* Herpesviruses of Horses; Retroviruses of Birds.

## Further Reading

Davison F and Nair V (eds.) (2004) *Marek's Disease: An Evolving Problem.* London: Academic Press.

Guy JS and Bagust TJ (2003) Laryngotracheitis. In: Saif YM, Barnes HJ, Fadly A, Glisson JR, McDougald LR,, and Swayne DE (eds.) *Diseases of Poultry,* 11th edn., ch. 5, pp. 121–134. Ames, IA: Iowa State.

Kaleta EF (1990) Herpesviruses of free-living and pet birds. In: Purchase HG, Arp LH, Domermuth CH,, and Pearson JE (eds.) *A Laboratory Manual for the Isolation and Identification of Avian Pathogens,* pp. 97–102. Athens, GA: American Association of Avian Pathologists.

Osterrieder N, Kamil JP, Schumacher D, Tischer BK, and Trapp S (2006) Marek's disease virus: From miasma to model. *Nature Reviews Microbiology* 4: 283–294.

Panigraphy B and Grumbles LC (1984) Pacheco's disease in psittacine birds. *Avian Diseases* 28: 808–812.

Thureen DR and Keeler CL, Jr. (2006) Psittacid herpesvirus 1 and infectious laryngotracheitis virus: Comparative genome sequence analysis of two avian alphaherpesviruses. *Journal of Virology* 80: 7863–7872.

# Retroviruses of Birds

**K L Beemon,** Johns Hopkins University, Baltimore, MD, USA

## History

Avian retroviruses have been studied for 100 years. Avian leukosis virus (ALV) was discovered in 1908 by Ellermann and Bang, and the related Rous sarcoma virus (RSV) was isolated by Peyton Rous in 1911. Numerous isolates of ALV and of transforming viruses, which cause sarcomas and a variety of hematopoietic neoplasms, were reported in the decades that followed. Progress in understanding their nature was very slow until the development of cell culture assays in the late 1950s and the use of genetic and cell biological approaches to study replication and transformation. The discovery of reverse transcriptase (RT) in 1970 and of the origin and mechanism of action of viral oncogenes in the decade following led to an explosion of research activity. In addition to the genetic information of ALV needed for replication, RSV has a transduced oncogene, *src*, that enables it to induce sarcomas rapidly *in vivo* and to transform cells in culture. Src was the first retroviral oncogene to be characterized and the first tyrosine kinase to be identified. Currently, avian retroviruses provide a robust system for studies of retroviral gene expression and of virion assembly *in vitro*, as well as for studies of oncogenesis.

## Taxonomy and Classification

The avian leukosis viruses comprise a single genus *Alpharetrovirus*, of the family *Retroviridae* and the subfamily *Orthoretrovirinae*. Although they share structural and biological characteristics with the mammalian C-type gammaretroviruses (such as murine leukemia virus), these two groups are not closely related. All ALVs are closely related to one another sharing considerable sequence and antigenic identity. Isolates are differentiated by subgroup (i.e., receptor utilization) and the presence or absence of oncogenes.

## Distribution, Host Range, and Propagation

ALVs are endemic in flocks of domestic chickens (*Gallus gallus*) worldwide, and natural infections seem limited to this species, within which they are of some economic importance. Related endogenous viruses are found in ring-necked and golden pheasant (but not other related birds, such as turkeys), but exogenous viruses have not been isolated from other species. ALV will replicate efficiently in species closely related to the chicken such as quail, turkeys, and pheasants, but less so in more distant species such as ducks. RSV of some subgroups can transform mammalian cells and induce tumors in mammals, but with greatly reduced efficiency, and virus replication in mammalian cells cannot be reproducibly observed. The restriction of the virus to avian species is due to a lack of suitable receptors for most subgroups as well as to blocks to viral gene expression. The rare transformants that arise in RSV-infected mammalian cells often display rearrangements in proviral DNA that relieve this block.

A variety of cell types from gallinaceous birds (including chickens, turkeys, and quail) can be used to propagate ALVs and their relatives. Primary and secondary fibroblast cultures or cell lines (DF-1) are most commonly used, as well as lines derived from quail tumors (QT6). To avoid problems associated with frequent recombination, it is advisable to use cells that do not contain related endogenous proviruses, such as cells from species other than chickens or from chickens bred to contain no such proviruses.

## Properties of the Virion

Like all retroviruses, ALVs are transmitted as enveloped virions of about 100 nm diameter, derived by budding from the host cell membrane. Lipids derived from the host plasma membrane are present in the viral envelope and make up 35% of the virion weight. Within the retrovirus family, they are defined as having a C-type morphology. Small, dispersed spikes project from the surface of the virion; these consist of trimers of the two *env*-encoded proteins, SU (surface) and TM (transmembrane). The internal core of the virion is of uncertain symmetry in mature virions but appears in electron micrographs as a centrally located, roughly spherical structure about 30 nm in diameter. Immature virions seen during or shortly after budding have a more open, spherical core structure, substantially larger in diameter than the processed one. The core comprises about 1500 copies each of the four gag-encoded proteins (as well as protease) and about 100 copies each of RT and integrase.

## Properties of the Genome

The ALV genome consists of a homodimer of positive-sense, single-stranded (ss) RNA about 7500 bp in length. Transforming viruses, in which an oncogene has been inserted, have genomes varying in length from about 3.2 kbp (for UR2 virus) to about 9.3 kbp (for nondefective Rous sarcoma virus). In most of these viruses, the oncogene has replaced some of the normal genome, leading to genetically defective virus, which requires co-infection with helper ALV for replication. The genome is modified and processed by cell machinery. It contains a 5′m7GpppGm capping group and a 3′ poly (A) sequence, as well as some internal m6A residues. In *in vitro* translation systems, it is capable of serving as mRNA for the *gag-pro* and *gag-pro-pol* gene products. As with all retroviruses, the order of genes is 5′-*gag-pro-pol-env*-3′.

Important noncoding regions found near the end of the genome are necessary to provide signals for virus replication. These include an 18–21 base sequence (R) repeated at each end as well as unique sequences U3 (*c.* 250 bp) near the *3*′ end and U5 (*c.* 80 bp) near the *5*′ end which are duplicated in the long terminal repeat (LTR) during reverse transcription. The LTR contains sequences controlling transcription initiation and polyadenylation. Adjacent to these are the sites for initiation of reverse transcription: the primer binding (PB) sequence next to U5. Between PB and the beginning of *gag* is an approximately 300 bp leader region, which contains signals important for the dimerization and packaging of the genome into virions. The direct repeat (DR) sequences flanking the *src* gene in RSV are necessary for cytoplasmic accumulation and packaging of full-length viral RNA. ALV has one copy of the DR sequence. Other regulatory sequences are within coding sequences. The negative regulator of splicing (NRS) within the *gag* gene suppresses splicing and also promotes polyadenylation. ALVs with mutations in the NRS can lead to rapid-onset lymphomas *in vivo*, characterized by readthrough and splicing from the viral genome into downstream oncogenes or onco-miRs.

## Properties of the Proteins

The virion contains nine proteins, the products of four coding regions. The Gag proteins constitute the major structural components and are sufficient to form recognizable virions if expressed alone. The Gag-Pro precursor is processed during release of virus into four Gag proteins: MA (matrix, about 19 kDa) which interacts with the cell membrane; p10, a 10 kDa protein of unknown function and location; CA (capsid, about 27 kDa) which forms the core shell structure; and NC (nucleocapsid, about 12 kDa), an RNA-binding protein necessary for specific encapsidation of genome RNA. The Gag-Pro precursor also contains the 15 kDa PR (protease) peptide necessary for processing all internal virion proteins. The Pol reading frame is expressed as a fusion protein with Gag and Pro, processed to yield RT (usually present as a heterodimer of 98 and 66 kDa reflecting partial processing by PR), and

integrase (IN, about 32 kDa); these are the two enzymatic activators necessary for synthesis and integration of the DNA provirus. The *env* gene encodes the Env precursor (Pr95) which is processed as a membrane protein and cleaved by host cell proteases to yield the SU glycoprotein, which has an apparent molecular weight of about 85 kDa, about half of which is due to the provision of *c.* 14 N-linked carbohydrate side chains, and the TM glycoprotein, which has an apparent molecular weight of about 37 kDa. The SU and TM products remain as a disulfide-bonded heterodimer with SU containing the activity necessary for receptor binding and TM-mediating fusion with the cellular membrane.

## Physical Properties

Virions of ALV have an equilibrium density in sucrose solutions of about 1.16–1.18 g ml$^{-1}$ and a sedimentation coefficient of about 600S. They are quite labile and are readily inactivated by extremes of pH, as well as by heat or mild detergent treatments. They are somewhat radiation resistant, perhaps reflecting the recombinational repair capability provided by the dimeric genome.

## Replication

Replication of ALV is like that of other retroviruses, and this group of viruses provided some of the important early models for studying the process. Entry of the virion follows interaction with a specific receptor on the cell surface. Genetically, at least ten subgroups (A–J) have been identified on the basis of distinct receptor recognition. The presence of receptors for specific subgroups is polymorphic among birds. Three unlinked genetic loci (*Tv-a*, *Tv-b*, and *Tv-c*) for ALV receptors have been genetically identified in chickens. The dominance of susceptibility over resistance alleles at each of these loci implies that they encode the receptor directly. The *Tv-b* locus has several alleles, controlling susceptibility to subgroups B, D, and E. Receptors for ASLV subgroups A, B, D, and E have been cloned. The Tv-a receptor resembles a portion of the receptor for low-density lipoprotein and is unrelated to other known retroviral receptors. The receptors for B, D, and E are all in the tumor necrosis factor receptor family. Chickens have two alleles that can act as receptors for these viruses. Entry of the virion core into the cell is by fusion of viral and cellular membranes, perhaps following endocytosis.

Once within the cytoplasm of the infected cell, the process of reverse transcription within the poorly defined core structure copies the ssRNA genome into a molecule of double-stranded (ds) DNA. This process – which varies little from that of other retroviruses – includes a series of 'jumps' from one end of the template to the other. The product is a dsDNA molecule, which differs from the genomic RNA by the presence at either end of the LTR. The LTR contains sequences necessary for DNA integration and for synthesis and processing of viral RNA.

Integration of viral DNA into more or less random sites in the cell genome is accomplished by the IN protein which has entered the cell with the virion and remains with the DNA in an ill-defined structure. The process of integration leads to the insertion of the viral DNA into cell DNA in the same general organization as both genome and unintegrated DNA. Integrated ALV DNA is characterized by the loss of two bases from each end of the viral sequence and the duplication of six bases of cell DNA at the integration site.

Transcription of the provirus into genomic and mRNA is mediated by cellular RNA polymerase II directed to the correct initiation site by promoter and enhancer sequences in the LTR. The strength of the enhancer elements is a major factor distinguishing pathogenic from nonpathogenic ALV isolates. Unlike some other retroviruses, there is no apparent role of virus-encoded proteins in regulating the transcription process. Processing of the viral transcripts includes addition of poly(A) following a canonical signal (AAUAAA) in the RNA derived from the 3' LTR and splicing of the fraction of the transcripts destined to become mRNA for the *env* gene. The splicing removes most of the *gag, pro,* and *pol* sequences, leaving the beginning of *gag* fused to *env.*

Translation of the full-length RNA leads to two products: The Gag-Pro precursor of about 76 kDa and the Gag-Pro-Pol precursor of about 180 kDa. Synthesis of the latter molecule is made possible by a −1 translational frameshift about 5% of the time, bypassing the termination codon at the end of Pro. Assembly of the precursors is at the cell surface, and is coincident with budding, implying a simultaneous association of the precursors with the genome, with the cell membrane, and with one another. Release of the immature particle (characterized by a hollow, symmetrical core which almost fills the virion) is rapidly followed by cleavage of the Gag-Pro and Gag-Pro-Pol precursors to yield the finished proteins. This cleavage is accompanied by condensation of the core into its mature form. Since the PR protein embedded in the Gag-Pro precursor contains only one-half of the active site, dimerization of this domain is necessary for cleavage to occur. This requirement probably helps to delay cleavage until the appropriate time.

Once infected, the host cell is usually not killed by virus replication. A strong superinfection resistance due to blockage or loss of viral receptors develops soon after infection and prevents accumulation of proviruses by reinfection. In some cases, weak or slow development of superinfection resistance is associated with a cytopathic interaction of the virus with its host cell.

## Transformation

A unique characteristic of ALV and a few other retroviruses is their ability to incorporate certain host sequences into their genome and alter the function of these proto-oncogenes to generate oncogenes. The presence of an oncogene renders the virus capable of inducing malignant transformation of cells in culture and one of a variety of malignant and rapidly fatal diseases in birds. At least 20 distinct cell sequences have been incorporated by ALV into a very large number of distinct isolates. RSV, which contains *src*, is the prototype oncogene-containing virus. Other notable oncogene-containing ALV variants include avian myeloblastosis virus (AMV; containing *myb*); avian myelocytomatosis virus-29 (MC-29; *myc*); avian erythroblastosis virus (AEV; *erb*-A and *erb*-B); Fujinami sarcoma virus (FSV; fps); and University of Rochester sarcoma virus-2 (RU-2; *ros*). Study of the genetic alterations that distinguish these oncogenes from proto-oncogenes, and the enzymatic and physiological function of the proteins they encode has been a keystone of modern cancer research. Incorporation of oncogenes into the virus genome is usually at the expense of some viral genes and co-infection of a cell with a wild-type (helper) ALV is thus necessary to provide viral proteins for replication of oncogene-containing viruses. RSV, which is a replication-competent transforming virus, is the exception.

## Endogenous Viruses

Another unique feature shared by ALV and a few other retrovirus groups is their ability to become established in the germline and inherited stably as endogenous proviruses. Naturally occurring endogenous proviruses form a distinct lineage of ALVs, showing a specific host range (subgroup E) for which many domestic chickens lack receptors (a phenomenon known as xenotropism), and a reduced replication capacity and pathogenicity relative to exogenous viruses. Endogenous viruses are usually expressed at a very low rate, due largely to methylation of CpG residues in the proviral DNA, and are often (but not always) defective in sequence.

## Genetics

Strain differences among ALV isolates are primarily in host range and are encoded by differences within the central portion of SU; other parts of the genome, with the exception of the U3 end of the LTR, are quite highly conserved. Like other retroviruses, ALVs exhibit very high rates of homologous recombination – a consequence of the diploid genome and the 'jumping' mechanism of reverse transcription. The latter also permits relatively high rates of nonhomologous recombination, leading to frequent (but not usually lethal) rearrangements of the genome as well as the occasional acquisition of foreign sequences such as oncogenes.

## Evolution

Amino acid sequence relationships reveal a common origin of all retroviruses, but the ALV group forms a divergent branch, with its closest relative being the mouse mammary tumor virus. Whereas the recent spread of viruses among chickens is probably due largely to human intervention, the virus group is of considerable antiquity, since distantly related endogenous viruses are widespread in the genomes of avian and even mammalian species. The closely related endogenous viruses seem to be recent introductions derived by germline infection with exogenous virus since they are found only in *Gallus gallus*, and not in other species of *Gallus*, although they do appear in more distantly related pheasants.

## Transmission and Tissue Tropism

Transmission of virus is principally vertical by infection of the offspring through virus secreted into the egg. Indeed, high titers of ALV are often detectable in commercial hen's eggs. Horizontal spread of virus is naturally much more rare, requiring close contact, but virus can be readily spread from infected birds via contaminated needles during vaccination or through vaccines prepared from infected eggs or cell cultures.

All isolates of ALV replicate efficiently in fibroblast cultures and in the bursa. Tropism for other tissues varies among isolates and is determined by both *env* and LTR sequences.

## Pathogenicity

ALVs induce a wide spectrum of disease in naturally or experimentally infected animals. The prototypic disease induced by ALV is a B-cell lymphoma arising in the bursa of Fabricius starting a few months after infection and spreading to the liver and other organs during its course. Other malignancies, including erythroleukemia, sarcoma, and others, are not uncommon depending on the strain of virus and bird and the time and route of inoculation. The malignant diseases induced by viruses, which do not contain oncogenes, are the consequence of insertional activation of cellular proto-oncogenes (such as *c-myc* in the case of lymphoma, *c-erb*-B in erythroleukemia, and others). In addition to malignancies, these viruses also induce hemangiomas, osteopetrosis, and wasting diseases.

In some cases, an immune response against infected cells may be important; in others, cytopathic effects of the sort noted above may play a significant role.

Acquisition of oncogenes by ALVs greatly alters the nature and course of the disease. Infection of newly hatched chicks with AMV, for example, can lead to their death from myeloblastic leukemia in as few as 5 days. Moribund animals display enormously elevated myeloblast counts and a level of viremia sufficient to render the plasma noticeably turbid. Similarly, birds inoculated with RSV develop rapidly growing, usually fatal, sarcomas at the site of injection in a few weeks. It should be noted that the oncogene-containing viruses are not efficiently transmitted from one animal to another due to their rapid pathogenicity. In most cases, they have probably arisen in the animal from which they were isolated and would have died out if not brought into the laboratory.

Not all members of this group are highly pathogenic. RAV-0 (an endogenous virus) can infect susceptible chickens and induce viremia, but disease is rare and occurs only after a long latent period. The reduced virulence is probably an important feature of viruses inherited in the germline.

## Immune Response

In infected birds, the only significant immune response is the appearance of type-specific neutralizing antibodies, which apparently recognize the regions of Env involved in receptor recognition. Group specific responses against Env or other proteins are not usually observed in infected chickens, although inoculation of virus into mammals induces antibodies capable of recognizing all virion proteins in the absence of subgroup-specific reactivity. The limited immune response observed in infected chickens has been attributed to the presence of endogenous proviruses whose expression (even at a low level) can induce tolerance to antigens in common with infecting virus. Indeed, it has been suggested that induction of tolerance might be a desirable feature for the animal, since it could prevent or limit immunopathological sequelae of infection. Postinfection immune response seems to be of little consequence in preventing subsequent malignant disease, since the cells, which will eventually form the tumor, are probably infected quite soon after infection, and the long latency reflects the necessity for subsequent rare events (such as mutations in other genes) rather than a continuing period of virus replication.

## Prevention and Control

ALV-induced disease is a cause of some economic loss to the poultry industry in the United States, and occasional more serious epizootics (such as a recent outbreak of hemangioma in Israel) due to ALV have occurred. Control of infection is generally by detection and culling of infected individuals. No useful vaccination strategy has been developed. In principle, it should be possible to virtually eliminate the disease by breeding the appropriate *Tv-a* and *Tv-b* alleles into commercial strains; in practice, this has not been done very often. A more recent strategy is to introduce defective proviruses encoding envelope protein into the germline of birds; these can block infection by inducing superinfection resistance.

## Future

Although of economic importance to the poultry industry, the value of ALV and the related oncogene-containing viruses to science has been far greater. The study of these viruses as models will continue to illuminate fundamental aspects of retrovirus biology. Continued searches for new transforming viruses and selected retroviral integration sites are likely to yield novel and important oncogenes. The goal of eradication of ALV disease from commercial chickens is attainable with present technology; its realization is largely a matter of economic considerations.

*See also:* Endogenous Retroviruses.

## Further Reading

Coffin JM, Hughes SH, and Varmus HE (1997) *Retroviruses.* Cold Spring Harbor, NY: Cold Spring Harbor Laboratory.
Flint SJ, Enquist LW, Racaniello VR, and Skalka AM (2004) *Principles of Virology, Molecular Biology, Pathogenesis, and Control of Animal Viruses,* 2nd edn. Washington, DC: ASM Press.
Goff SP (2006) *Retroviridae*: The retroviruses and their replication. In: Knipe DM, Howley PM, Griffin DE, *et al.* (eds.) *Fields Virology,* 5th edn., pp. 1871–1940. Philadelphia, PA: Lippincott Williams and Wilkins.

# VIRUES OF AQUATIC SPECIES

# Aquareoviruses

**M St. J Crane and G Carlile,** CSIRO Livestock Industries, Geelong, VIC, Australia

## Introduction

*Aquareovirus*, as the name implies, is a genus (one of 12 genera) of the family *Reoviridae*. Species in this genus infect aquatic animals – finfish, crustaceans, and mollusks – from both marine and freshwater environments. The name *Reoviridae* is derived from *r*espiratory *e*nteric *o*rphan viruses, and 'orphan' viruses are those viruses that are not associated with any known disease. Although, originally, reoviruses commonly may have been associated with subclinical or asymptomatic infections, it is now known that many are associated with disease. Reo-like viruses have been reported from aquatic animals since the 1970s and, as for other reoviruses, the majority of aquareoviruses are of low pathogenicity and have not attracted much attention. However, others have been isolated from populations with mortality rates higher than normal and some with mortality rates as high as 80%. There are at least six (A–F) recognized aquareovirus species based on RNA–RNA blot hybridization, RNA electrophoresis, antigenic properties, and nucleic acid sequence analysis (**Table 1**). More than 40 aquareoviruses have been isolated to date, with the majority classified within species groups A and B. However, some aquatic reoviruses such as the marine crab reoviruses, P and W2, do not fit this classification and these and several other aquareoviruses are yet to be classified.

## Taxonomy and Classification

The genus *Aquareovirus* forms one of 12 genera (*Orthoreovirus*; *Orbivirus*; *Rotavirus*; *Coltivirus*; *Seadornavirus*; *Aquareovirus*; *Idnoreovirus*; *Cypovirus*; *Fijivirus*; *Phytoreovirus*; *Oryzavirus*; *Mycoreovirus*) that make up the family *Reoviridae*. The *Reoviridae* is one of the six families of viruses possessing a double-stranded RNA (dsRNA) genome. Of these, the *Reoviridae* is one of only two families that infect vertebrates and the only family that infects mammals. Within the family, each genus can be placed in a subset based on whether the virion is turreted (*Orthoreovirus*; *Aquareovirus*; *Idnoreovirus*; *Cypovirus*; *Fijivirus*; *Oryzavirus*; *Mycoreovirus*) or unturreted (*Orbivirus*; *Rotavirus*; *Coltivirus*; *Seadornavirus*; *Phytoreovirus*). The reovirus genome is made up of 10–12 segments of dsRNA. Each segment encodes one to three (usually one) proteins. Aquareovirus genomes are made up of 11 segments of dsRNA. Except for segment 11, which usually encodes two proteins,

each segment encodes a single protein. Interestingly, segment 11 of chum salmon reovirus is tricistronic. Aquareoviruses have been reported from finfish, crustaceans, and mollusks and from both freshwater and marine host species.

For aquareoviruses, the primary species demarcation criteria are RNA cross-hybridization and antibody-based cross-neutralization. Currently, six genogroups or species (A–F) have been identified with several aquareoviruses remaining unclassified (**Table 1**). Ultrastructural similarity between orthoreoviruses and aquareoviruses has been noted and the relatively high level of sequence homology between some isolates of these two genera indicates a common evolutionary lineage. Despite this relatedness, other properties, such as host range, different numbers of genome segments, and absence of antigenic similarity, support classification into two genera.

## Virion Structure and Morphology

The structure and morphology of aquareovirus virions are similar to other members of the family *Reoviridae*, particularly members of the genus *Orthoreovirus*. Virions are spherical in appearance, have icosahedral symmetry, and are *c.* 80 nm in diameter (**Figure 1**). The capsid consists of two concentric shells made up of three layers of protein. The outer capsid surrounds the inner core which is approximately 60 nm in diameter. For members of the genus *Aquareovirus*, the core is turreted – turrets or spikes project from the surface of the inner core and interconnect with the outer capsid layers. The inner protein layer of the core surrounds the 11 segments of the dsRNA.

A study of the turbot aquareovirus has indicated that its replication and morphogenesis generally follow that typical of other reoviruses. Virions were observed to be internalized by direct penetration of the host cell plasma membrane. In infected cells, two sizes of virus particles were observed in the cytoplasm: particles, 30 nm in diameter, which were probably inner cores; and single-shelled particles, 45 nm in diameter, located in the endoplasmic reticulum. Viral replication was observed to occur in the cytoplasm and immature virions (45 nm in diameter) formed complete, mature, double-shelled virions (75–80 nm in diameter) by budding through the plasma membrane so that complete viral particles were only observed outside host cells.

**Table 1**    Aquareovirus species, host species, and geographical distribution

| Virus | Host species | Pathogenicity | Mortality rate | Country |
|---|---|---|---|---|
| *Aquareovirus A* | | | | |
| Geoduck clam aquareovirus (CLV) | *Panope abrupta* | NS | 0% | USA |
| Herring aquareovirus (HRV) | *Clupea harengus* | NS | 0% | USA |
| Striped bass aquareovirus (SBRV) | *Morone saxatilis* | L | NR | USA |
| American oyster reovirus (13$_{p2}$RV) | *Crassostrea virginica* | NS | 0% | USA |
| | *Lepomis macrochirus* | H | 44% | Exp |
| | *Oncorhynchus mykiss* | H | 60% | Exp |
| Angelfish aquareovirus (AFRV) | *Pomacanthus semicirculatus* | L | L | USA |
| Chum salmon aquareovirus (CSRV) | *Oncorhynchus keta* | L | 0% to L | Japan |
| Smelt aquareovirus (SRV) | *Osmerus mordax* | H | H | Canada |
| Atlantic salmon reovirus (ASRV) | *Salmo salar* | NS | NR | Canada |
| Atlantic salmon reovirus (TSRV) | *S. salar* | L | L | Australia |
| Atlantic salmon reovirus (HBRV) | *S. salar* | NS | NR | USA |
| Chinook salmon reovirus (DRCRV) | *Oncorhynchus tshawytscha* | NS | NR | USA |
| Guppy aquareovirus (GRV) | *Poecilia reticulata* | L | L | Singapore |
| *Aquareovirus B* | | | | |
| Coho salmon aquareovirus (CSRV) | *Oncorhynchus kisutch* | L | L | USA |
| Coho salmon reovirus (LBS) | *O. kisutch* | NS | NR | USA |
| Chinook salmon reovirus (YRCV) | *O. tshawytscha* | NS | NR | USA |
| Chinook salmon reovirus (ICRV) | *O. tshawytscha* | NS | NR | USA |
| Coho salmon reovirus (GRCV) | *O. kisutch* | NS | NR | USA |
| Coho salmon reovirus (CSRV) | *O. kisutch* | NS | NR | USA |
| Coho salmon reovirus (ELCV) | *O. kisutch* | NS | NR | USA |
| Coho salmon reovirus (SSRV) | *O. kisutch* | NS | NR | USA |
| *Aquareovirus C* | | | | |
| Golden shiner aquareovirus (GSRV) | *Notemignous crysoleucas* | L | L | USA |
| | *Semotilus atromaculatus* | L | NR | USA |
| | *Pimephales promelas* | M | M | USA |
| Grass carp reovirus (GCRV) (GCHV) | *Ctenapharyngodon idellus* | H | 70–95% | China |
| *Aquareovirus D* | *Mylopharyngodon piceus* | H | 70–80% | China |
| Channel catfish reovirus (CCRV) | *Ictalurus punctatus* | L | <5% | USA |
| *Aquareovirus E* | | | | |
| Turbot aquareovirus (TRV) | *Scophthalmus maximus* | L | <5% | Spain |
| *Aquareovirus F* | | | | |
| Chum salmon reovirus (PSRV) | *O. keta* | NR | NR | NR |
| Chinook salmon reovirus (SCRV) | *O. tshawytscha* | NR | NR | NR |
| *Unclassified aquareoviruses* | | | | |
| Haddock reovirus | *Melanogrammus aeglefinus* | NR | 0% | UK |
| Golden ide reovirus (GIRV) | *Leuciscus idus* | NR | 0% | Germany |
| Gilthead seabream reovirus | *Sparus aurata* | M | M | Spain |
| Red grouper reovirus | *Plectropomus maculatus* | H | 30–90% | Singapore |
| Landlocked salmon virus | *Oncorhynchus masou* (Breroort) | L | L | Taiwan |
| Tench reovirus (TNRV) | *Tinca tinca* | NS | 0% | Germany |
| Japanese eel reovirus | *Anguilla japonica* | NR | NR | Japan |
| Fancy carp reovirus | *Cyprinus carpio* | NR | NR | Japan |
| Halibut reovirus | *Hippoglossus hippoglossus* | H | H | Canada, UK |
| Chub reovirus (CHRV) | *Leuciscus cephalus* | NS | 0% | Germany |
| Marine threadfin fish reovirus | *Eleutheronema tetradactylus* | H | Up to 100% | Singapore |
| | *Lates calcarifer* | H | 60% | Exp |
| Brown trout reovirus | *Salmo trutta* | L | 0% | UK |
| | *O. mykiss* | L | 0% | Exp |
| Snakehead reovirus (SKRV) | *Channa striata* | NS | 0% | Thailand |
| Mediterranean shore crab reovirus (RC84) | *Carcinus mediterraneus* | L | 0% | France |
| Mediterranean shore crab reovirus (W2) | *C. mediterraneus* | M | NR | France |
| Mediterranean swimming crab reovirus (P) | *Macropipus depurator* | L | NR | France |
| Chinese mitten crab reovirus | *Eriocheir sinensis* | NR | NR | China |
| Tiger shrimp reovirus | *Penaeus japonicus* | M | M | France |
| Tiger prawn reovirus | *Penaeus monodon* | H | 95% | Malaysia |

Exp, Experimental infections; L, low; M, moderate; H, high; NS, no significant pathology; NR, not reported.

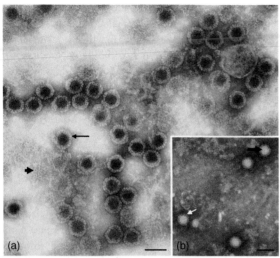

**Figure 1** Transmission electron micrographs of negative-stained preparations of Tasmanian Atlantic salmon aquareovirus (TSRV). (a) Image of a purified preparation where the stain has penetrated the inner capsid. (b) Image of similar aquareovirus particles derived from the supernatant of infected cells. Thin arrows (black and white): surface projections associated with the outer capsid. Thick arrows indicate locations of hexameric (or tetrameric) clusters of surface projections (thin arrows). Scale = 100 nm (a, b). Courtesy of Electron Microscopy Group, Australian Animal Health Laboratory, CSIRO Livestock Industries, Geelong, VIC, Australia.

## Genome Organization and Transcription Strategy

The genus *Aquareovirus* is relatively diverse, being made up of at least six species. The genomes of viruses in each species consist of 11 segments of dsRNA which migrate as three size classes in 1% agarose gels. Segments 1–3 are the large-size class, segments 4–6 medium, and segments 7–11 small. The complete genomic sequence of golden shiner reovirus (GSRV), comprising 23 696 bp, and grass carp reovirus (GCRV), comprising 23 695 bp, have been determined. The sequences of some segments of other aquareovirus isolates have also been determined. Apart from segments 7 and 11, each segment is monocistronic, containing a single open reading frame (ORF). For most aquareoviruses, segment 11 encodes two proteins (**Table 2**); segment 11 from chum salmon reovirus (CSRV) encodes three proteins. Thus, there are seven structural proteins (VP1–VP7) and five nonstructural proteins (NS1, NS2, NS4, NS15, and NS29). There is variation in the estimated molecular mass of each polypeptide for different aquareoviruses. For example, when compared by electrophoresis in a single polyacrylamide gel, the estimated molecular masses of the five major structural viral proteins for four aquareoviruses ($13_{p2}$, GSRV, CSRV, channel catfish reovirus (CCRV)) varied in the ranges 132–137 kDa (VP1), 126–130 kDa (VP2), 63–72 kDa (VP5), 43–45 kDa (VP6), and 32–36 kDa (VP7). **Table 2** shows the data reported for

**Table 2** *Aquareovirus A* genome segments and encoded polypeptides with the estimated mass and location

| Genome segment | Protein | Estimated Mass (kDa) | Protein location |
|---|---|---|---|
| 1 | VP1 | 130 | Core turret |
| 2 | VP2 | 127 | Inner capsid |
| 3 | VP3 | 126 | Inner capsid |
| 4 | NS1 | 97 | NS |
| 5 | VP5 | 71 | Inner capsid |
| 6 | VP4 | 73 | Outer capsid |
| 7[a] | NS4 | 28 | NS |
| 8 | VP6 | 46 | Inner capsid |
| 9 | NS2 | 39 | NS |
| 10 | VP7 | 34 | Major outer capsid protein |
| 11[b] | NS29 | 29 | NS |
| | NS15 | 15 | |

[a]Segment 7 of GCRV and GSRV has been reported as bicistronic encoding two nonstructural proteins with estimated masses of 16 (NS5) and 31 kDa (NS4).
[b]Segment 11 of CSRV is tricistronic encoding three nonstructural proteins with estimated masses of 13, 15, and 16 kDa.

*Aquareovirus A.* As stated above, segment 11 of CSRV has been reported to be tricistronic encoding three polypeptides with estimated masses of 16.9, 15.1, and 13.0 kDa, and segment 7 of GCRV/GSRV appears to be bicistronic encoding two nonstructural proteins.

Putative functions of the aquareovirus proteins have been predicted based on the functions established for the equivalent mammalian orthoreovirus proteins. Accordingly, VP1 is the homologue of λ2 protein, pentamers of which form the turrets. This protein has important functions in particle assembly, as well as guanylyltransferase and methyltransferase activities in mRNA capping. VP2, equivalent to λ3, is located in the inner capsid or core and has RNA-dependent RNA polymerase activity associated with transcription and replication. VP3 (λ1) is the main component of the inner capsid and possesses NTPase, RTPase, and helicase activities. VP4 (μ1) is located in the outer capsid and is believed to function in penetration of the cellular membrane to allow virus entry into the cell. The function of VP5 (μ2) is not fully understood but it is known to bind RNA and possess NTPase activity, indicating that VP5 may be an RNA polymerase cofactor. VP6 (σ2), together with VP3, forms the core shell. VP6 functions are poorly understood; it binds to RNA and is thought to be involved in replicase-particle assembly. VP7 (σ3) is the major outer capsid protein and is thought to play important roles in outer capsid assembly and in stabilizing virions in extracellular environments. VP7 also binds dsRNA and functions in translational control in infected cells. The nonstructural proteins NS1 and NS2 are likely to be involved in RNA replication and packaging during virus particle assembly and the function of NS4 is unclear thought to be the cell attachment protein. The functions of the nonstructural proteins encoded by RNA segment 11 are also unknown.

## Geographic Distribution and Host Range

Most aquareoviruses have been isolated from healthy aquatic animals and are likely to be of low pathogenicity. Thus, the presence of aquareoviruses is likely to be under-reported. Moreover, it is unlikely that routine surveillance for aquareoviruses has been undertaken in any systematic manner. Many isolations of aquareoviruses have occurred incidentally during surveillance activities for other, more significant, pathogens. It is during these surveillance activities that several aquareoviruses have been isolated from apparently healthy aquatic animals. **Table 1** lists most of the known aquareoviruses, their hosts, and country of isolation, cited in the readily accessible scientific literature. Some of the reoviruses listed have not been fully characterized and it may eventuate that some of the viruses will be classified outside of the currently recognized taxa.

Clearly, both the host range and the geographical distribution of aquareoviruses are broad and it is probable that, with ongoing surveillance, the known host range and geographical distribution will be extended. As aquaculture expands and the interaction between wild and farmed aquatic animal species increases, it can be expected that the number of known viruses, including reoviruses, will increase. A good example is virus $13_{p2}$, originally isolated from healthy American oysters has been shown to infect and cause disease in more than one finfish species, indicating that the primary host and wild reservoir of this virus are unclear.

While *Aquareovirus A* appears to be the most diverse species with virus isolates obtained from several host species from very different parts of the world, it appears that *Aquareovirus B* has very limited host and geographical ranges, based on the several available isolates. The isolates of *Aquareovirus B* listed in **Table 1** may be the same virus merely isolated on different occasions. However, such a conclusion may be premature since many of the aquareoviruses have not been fully characterized and a large number of aquareoviruses remain unclassified with respect to species assignment.

## Pathology

As stated above, the majority of known aquareoviruses are of low pathogenicity and have been isolated from apparently healthy animals. Nevertheless, some of the known aquareoviruses are highly pathogenic. For example, GCRV

and others that have been isolated from normal animals may, under certain environmental conditions, be pathogenic. There are several examples in which stocking density and water temperature influence the pathogenicity of the virus. A good example is GSRV. Mortality rates associated with GSRV are normally around 5% but, under crowded conditions and high temperatures, acute epizootics with mortality rates of 50–75% have been reported.

It is also of note that isolation of aquareoviruses often occurs during investigations of conditions with apparently mixed etiology, involving either other viruses or a concomitant bacterial infection. In mixed infections with bacteria, treatment with antibiotics does not always resolve the condition, suggesting that the reovirus may play some role in the disease, if not as the primary pathogen. In other cases of mixed infections, the respective roles of each agent are not at all clear and it is difficult to ascribe disease signs to either agent.

Several reoviruses isolated from apparently healthy finfish with no gross external signs have been shown to cause low-level pathology in experimental infections. While these viruses have been shown to replicate in experimental fish, mortality is rare. The pathology is characterized by a diffuse multifocal necrosis of the liver which, in some cases, subsequently resolves.

For those aquareoviruses that have been isolated from disease outbreaks in finfish hosts, external signs are those typically found for systemic infections and include lethargy, inappetance, anorexia, abnormal swimming behavior, petechial hemorrhages on the body surface, lateral recumbency, distended abdomen, and high mortality rates. Internal signs included discoloration of the liver. Histological examination may reveal hepatic lesions with varying degrees of severity. Syncytial giant cell formations of hepatocytes have been reported.

GCRV is one of two highly pathogenic aquareoviruses isolated to date. The virus, first reported in 1984, is responsible for an acute hemorrhagic disease affecting grass carp (*Ctenopharyngodon idella*) and black carp (*Mylopharyngodon piceus*) in China. Disease outbreaks occur in the summer with mortality rates in the range of 70–95%. As with most viral diseases of finfish, younger age classes are more susceptible than older fish. External signs include exophthalmia and hemorrhages at the fin bases and gill covers. Internally, hemorrhages have been reported to occur in all the major organs – intestinal tract, liver, spleen, kidneys, and throughout the musculature. Recent studies indicate that GCRV and GSRV are variants of the same virus.

The other highly pathogenic reovirus was isolated in 1998 from cultured threadfin (*Eleutheronema tetradactylus*) fingerlings undergoing a mass mortality at a farm in Singapore. Following isolation, the virus was used in experimental infections of threadfin fingerlings and sea bass (*Lates calcarifer*). Clinical signs (dark pigmentation, lethargy, recumbency with sudden bursts of swimming) developed within 1 day post infection (d.p.i.), resulting in 100% cumulative mortality in the infected threadfin within 4 d.p.i. and 60% cumulative mortality in the sea bass within 7 d.p.i.

Several reoviruses or reo-like viruses have been isolated from crustaceans such as shrimp and crabs, some of which harbored mixed infections with other agents. As commonly reported for other viral diseases, external signs have included discoloration and abnormal behavior such as lethargy and inappetance. While virus particles have been observed in different tissues/organs (hepatopancreas, gills, digestive tract, lymphoid organ), a common feature appears to be involvement of the hepatopancreas where the most obvious lesions occur.

## Host Response to Infection

There are no detailed studies of the immune response of finfish to infection by aquareoviruses but, from observations that have been reported, it is clear that cellular and humoral immune reactions are stimulated. While not consistent, local infiltration of host inflammatory cells, particularly in the liver of infected fish, has been observed during aquareovirus infections. Moreover, in studies in which sera have been collected from infected fish, specific neutralization titers of >1:4000 have been obtained in neutralization tests. Further evidence of an immune response comes from studies with a vaccine produced in China for use against GCRV. A crude inactivated GCRV vaccine was produced in the late 1970s and was reported to provide good protection (70% survival of fingerlings).

Of further interest is a study reporting aquareovirus interference-mediated resistance of rainbow trout to infectious hematopoietic necrosis. Pre-exposure of rainbow trout to coho salmon reovirus (CSRV) induced a protective response to subsequent challenge with the rhabdovirus infectious hematopoietic necrosis virus. Protection appeared to be mediated by innate immune factors.

## Transmission

The natural transmission cycle has not been studied in detail for any of the aquareoviruses. Experimentally, infection and disease can be transmitted horizontally by injection and by immersion in diluted tissue culture supernatants from reovirus-infected fish cell lines. It is not known whether vertical transmission occurs.

## Genetic Diversity

Within the family *Reoviridae*, viruses in only three genera, *Mycoreovirus*, *Rotavirus*, and *Aquareovirus*, possess an 11-segmented dsRNA genome. Other properties such as host range, RNA sequence, and serological differences justify the classification of the aquatic reoviruses into a separate genus. Interestingly, there are some relatively high sequence identities in some proteins of aquareoviruses and orthoreoviruses, indicating these two genera share a common ancestral lineage. It is also noteworthy that some reoviruses, or reo-like viruses, that infect aquatic animals, such as viruses P and W2, isolated from marine crabs, possess 12 segments of dsRNA and may represent a new reovirus genus.

Currently, there are six genogroups/species (A–F) within the genus *Aquareovirus*. This classification is based on RNA–RNA blot hybridization, RNA electrophoresis, antigenic properties, and nucleotide sequence analysis (**Table 1**). While reciprocal RNA–RNA hybridization and cross-neutralization assays provide useful data for the classification of aquareoviruses, genomic sequence provides more precise data. For example, based on RNA–RNA hybridization, it had been suggested that GCRV may represent a seventh species group (G) but subsequent nucleotide sequence analysis has clearly indicated that it should be placed within genogroup C.

In a study that analyzed the relative electrophoretic mobility of the 11 RNA segments of 19 aquareoviruses, distinct electropherotypes were observed. Whilst there was no correlation with the host species from which the viruses were isolated, there was a correlation with geographical location. Further studies are required to determine whether, as for other members of the *Reoviridae*, electrophoretic mobility will be useful for strain identification within the aquareoviruses.

A comparison of deduced amino acid sequences of segment 10 (encoding major outer capsid protein VP7) of viral isolates representing the species *Aquareovirus A*, *Aquareovirus B*, and *Aquareovirus C*, has indicated sequence identities in the range 19–100%. Within a species, sequence identities were >80% and, for some, >99%. Between viruses in different species, identities were in the range 19–22%. Similar results have been obtained in other studies.

With the current level of knowledge, it is difficult to determine any correlation between *Aquareovirus* species, host and geographical ranges, and pathogenicity.

## Diagnosis and Disease Management

External signs of disease associated with infection by highly pathogenic aquareoviruses, including lethargy, inappetance, anorexia, abnormal swimming behavior, petechial hemorrhages, lateral recumbency, distended abdomen, high mortality rates, are not pathognomonic and laboratory investigation is required for definitive diagnosis. Several of the known aquareoviruses have been detected by virus isolation on any of a number of fish cell lines in common use in diagnostic laboratories. Depending on the aquareovirus isolate and local conditions, cell lines used for viral isolation and replication have included bluegill fry cell line (BF-2), chinook salmon embryo cell line (CHSE-214), fathead minnow cell line (FHM), *Epithelioma papillosum cyprini* cell line (EPC), channel catfish ovary cell line (CCO), brown bullhead cell line (BB), grass carp kidney cell line (CIK), Asian seabass cell line (SB), rainbow trout mesothelioma cell line (RTM), striped snakehead cell line (SSN-1), and rainbow trout gonad cell line (RTG-2). The appearance of the cytopathic effect (CPE) caused by aquareoviruses in fish cell lines is quite variable, depending on the aquareovirus isolate and the cell line

used for isolation. Examples of CPE caused by Tasmanian Atlantic salmon reovirus (TSRV) in two cell lines are shown in **Figure 2**. Where pathogenic aquareoviruses are endemic, more rapid, sensitive, and specific diagnostic tests are highly desirable. Species-specific antisera are currently not available but would provide useful diagnostic reagents in a variety of immunoassays. A rapid test, based on a reverse-transcription polymerase chain reaction (RT-PCR), has recently been developed for local pathogenic strains of threadfin aquareovirus and grass carp reovirus that are endemic in China and Singapore. Tentative assignment of species/genogroup can be achieved by comparing isolates with known aquareovirus species by reciprocal RNA–RNA hybridizations and cross-neutralization assays. Precise genogroup assignment can only be achieved by RT-PCR, subsequent sequence analysis, and comparison with sequences of other known genogroup isolates.

Apart from the GCRV vaccine, no vaccines or therapeutics are currently available for the control of diseases

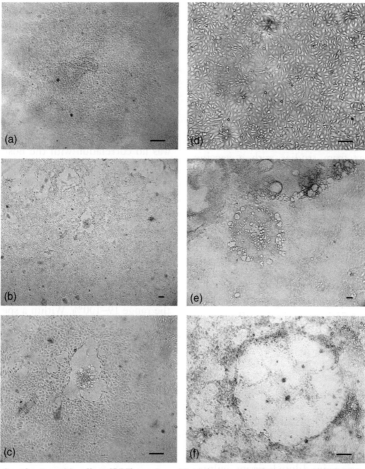

**Figure 2** Photomicrographs of cytopathic effect (CPE) produced by infection by TSRV. (a–c) CHSE-214 and (d–f) EPC cell cultures. (a, d) Uninfected cultures; (b, e) low magnification image; (c, f) high magnification image. Scale = 100 μm (a–f). Courtesy of Nette Williams, Australian Animal Health Laboratory, CSIRO Livestock Industries, Geelong, VIC, Australia.

associated with aquareovirus infections. As for other viral diseases of aquatic animals, avoidance is the preferred strategy. Thus, when available, pathogen exclusion can be attempted using good biosecurity and sanitary protocols in hatcheries and on farms. These can include the selection of specific pathogen-free (SPF) broodstock using virus isolation on cell lines and RT-PCR as screening tools, disinfection of fertilized eggs, and rearing water with, for example, ozone. In addition, stress reduction by maintaining high water quality and low stocking density is important. As aquareoviruses appear to have broad host and geographical ranges, the farming of aquatic animals where they are exposed to wild host species could present risks. Vaccines, when available, are likely to provide an additional level of protection.

## Current Status

The classification of aquareoviruses is not fully resolved, with many viral isolates remaining unclassified, and this is an important area for further research. For many of the species/genogroups, there are insufficient numbers of available isolates to allow determination of the key biological properties within each species. Thus, there does not appear to be correlation between host species, geographical range, pathogenicity, and species group. Many of the aquareoviruses, including the pathogenic threadfin aquareovirus, remain unclassified. As sequence data are available for only a few of the aquareoviruses, phylogenetic analysis has been limited. Further research is required not only to clarify the phylogenetic relationships within the genus *Aquareovirus* but also to assist in a better understanding of the role each segment plays in viral pathogenesis. Furthermore, the classification of the crustacean reo-like viruses and their relationship to other reoviruses, including aquareoviruses, requires clarification.

The isolation of different *Aquareovirus* species from both healthy and diseased fish indicates that, as for many other viruses of fish, pathogenicity is influenced by host (e.g., species, concomitant infections, immunocompetency) and environmental factors (e.g., water temperature, water quality, stocking density). In addition to elucidation of virulence factors (virus factors), further investigation on the respective roles of host and environmental factors on the pathogenicity of aquareoviruses is required. Based on knowledge to date, it seems likely that, for some *Aquareovirus* species at least, disease outbreaks will occur under adverse conditions of water quality/stocking density/temperature, and possibly in new host species. Thus, as the aquaculture industry expands globally, the interactions between farmed species and wild aquatic animal species will become more numerous, increasing the chance of virus transfer between wild and farmed animals. With this situation, taken together with their broad geographic range, it appears inevitable that aquareoviruses will produce disease in an increasing number of aquatic animal species in the future.

*See also:* Fish Viruses.

## Further Reading

Attoui H, Billoir F, Cantaloube JF, Biagini P, de Micco P, and de Lamballerie X (2000) Strategies for the sequence determination of viral dsRNA genomes. *Journal of Virological Methods* 89: 147–158.

Attoui H, Fang Q, Mohd Jaafar F, *et al.* (2002) Common evolutionary origin of aquareoviruses and orthoreoviruses revealed by genomic characterization of golden shiner reovirus, grass carp reovirus, striped bass reovirus and golden ide reovirus (genus *Aquareovirus*, family *Reoviridae*). *Journal of General Virology* 83: 1941–1951.

Dopazo CP, Bandin I, Rivas C, Cepeda C, and Barja JL (1996) Antigenic differences among aquareoviruses correlate with previously established genogroups. *Diseases of Aquatic Organisms* 26: 159–162.

Goodwin AE, Nayak DK, and Bakal RS (2006) Natural infections of wild creek chubs and cultured fathead minnow by Chinese grass carp reovirus (golden shiner virus). *Journal of Aquatic Animal Health* 18: 35–38.

Kim J, Tao Y, Reinisch KM, Harrison SC, and Nibert ML (2004) Orthoreovirus and aquareovirus core proteins: Conserved enzymatic surfaces, but not protein–protein interfaces. *Virus Research* 101: 15–28.

Lupiani B, Hetrick FM, and Samal SK (1993) Genetic analysis of aquareoviruses using RNA–RNA blot hybridization. *Virology* 197: 475–479.

Lupiani B, Subramanian K, and Samal SK (1995) Aquareoviruses. *Annual Review of Fish Diseases* 5: 175–208.

McEntire ME, Iwanowicz LR, and Goodwin AE (2003) Molecular, physical and clinical evidence that golden shiner virus and grass carp reovirus are variants of the same virus. *Journal of Aquatic Animal Health* 15: 257–263.

Meyers TR (1980) Experimental pathogenicity of reovirus 13$_{p2}$ for juvenile American oysters *Crassostrea virginica* (Gmelin) and bluegill fingerlings *Lepomis macrochirus* (Rafinesque). *Journal of Fish Diseases* 3: 187–201.

Rivas C, Noya M, Cepeda C, Bandin I, Barja JL, and Dopazo CP (1998) Replication and morphogenesis of the turbot aquareovirus (TRV) in cell culture. *Aquaculture* 160: 47–62.

Samal SK, Attoui H, Mohd Jaafar F, and Mertens PPC (2005) *Reoviridae – Aquareovirus*. In: Fauquet CM, Mayo MA, Maniloff J, Desselberger U, and Ball LA (eds.) *Virus Taxonomy: Eighth Report of the International Committee on Taxonomy of Viruses*, pp. 511–516. San Diego, CA: Elsevier Academic Press.

Seng EK, Fang Q, Chang SF, *et al.* (2002) Characterisation of a pathogenic virus isolated from marine threadfin fish (*Eleutheronema tetradactylus*) during a disease outbreak. *Aquaculture* 214: 1–18.

Seng EK, Fang Q, Lam TJ, and Sin YM (2004) Development of a rapid, sensitive and specific diagnostic assay for fish *Aquareovirus* based on RT-PCR. *Journal of Virological Methods* 118: 111–122.

Subramanian K, Hetrick FM, and Samal SK (1997) Identification of a new genogroup of aquareovirus by RNA–RNA hybridization. *Journal of General Virology* 78: 1385–1388.

Subramanian K, McPhillips TH, and Samal SK (1994) Characterization of the polypeptides and determination of genome coding assignments of an aquareovirus. *Virology* 205: 75–81.

# Fish and Amphibian Herpesviruses

**A J Davison,** MRC Virology Unit, Glasgow, UK

This article is a revision of the previous edition articles by Andrew J Davison, volume 1, pp 553–557, and Allan Granoff, volume 1, pp 51–53, © 1999, Elsevier Ltd.

## Glossary

**Fingerling** Young fish between the fry and adult stages.
**Fry** Newly hatched or very young fish.
**Tegument** The layer of proteins situated between the capsid and the envelope in herpesvirus particles; equivalent to the matrix in other viruses.

## Classification and History

Most currently recognized fish herpesviruses infect species that are farmed or harvested from the wild for human consumption. The conditions used in aquaculture may enhance the disease potential of these pathogens and increase their likelihood of detection. It is probable, therefore, that many more fish herpesviruses await discovery. A similar prospect applies to amphibian herpesviruses, since the two known examples originated from a single host species. Herpesviruses of fish and amphibians, like those of higher vertebrates, are usually highly species specific in the natural setting. This indicates that they have evolved in close association with their hosts over long periods of time. Many of these viruses cause mortality only in young fish, and some are also agents of epidermal hyperplasia or neoplasia. Some have been studied to such a limited extent that causal links with the disease whose occurrence led to their identification have not yet been established adequately.

Several fish and amphibian herpesviruses have been classified as members of the family *Herpesviridae*. These include viruses that infect white sturgeon, *Acipenser transmontanus* (acipenserid herpesviruses 1 and 2), Japanese eel, *Anguilla japonica* (anguillid herpesvirus 1), carp, *Cyprinus carpio* (cyprinid herpesvirus 1), goldfish, *Carassius auratus* (cyprinid herpesvirus 2), northern pike, *Esox lucius* (esocid herpesvirus 1), rainbow trout, *Oncorhynchus mykiss* (salmonid herpesvirus 1), channel catfish, *Ictalurus punctatus* (ictalurid herpesvirus 1), Pacific salmon, *Oncorhynchus* species (salmonid herpesvirus 2), walleye, *Stizostedion vitreum* (percid herpesvirus 1), and turbot, *Psetta maxima* (pleuronectid herpesvirus 1). Only one of these viruses (ictalurid herpesvirus 1) has been classified further into a species (*Ictalurid herpesvirus 1*) and a genus (*Ictalurivirus*). Candidate herpesviruses have also been reported in black bullhead (*Ictalurus*

*melas*), Japanese flounder (*Paralichthys olivaceus*), pilchard (*Sardinops sagax*), and redstriped rockfish (*Sebastes proriger*). The viruses representing the classified amphibian herpesviruses (ranid herpesviruses 1 and 2) originated from the leopard frog, *Rana pipiens*. The tenuous genetic relationships between herpesviruses of fish and amphibians and those of higher vertebrates have prompted the proposal that the former group be separated into a new family (*Alloherpesviridae*) and grouped with other herpesviruses into an order (*Herpesvirales*). Elucidation of the genetic relationships among these viruses, upon which detailed subclassification will depend, is at an early stage.

This article focuses on three principal viruses, one infecting an amphibian and two infecting fish. These are Lucké tumor herpesvirus (LTHV; ranid herpesvirus 1), channel catfish virus (CCV; ictalurid herpesvirus 1), and koi herpesvirus (KHV; proposed cyprinid herpesvirus 3). Comments are made on other viruses where appropriate.

In 1934, Lucké reported that intranuclear acidophilic inclusion bodies typical of certain virus infections were present in renal adenocarcinomas of the leopard frog. He concluded 4 years later that the tumor was caused by a virus. Almost two decades elapsed before herpesvirus particles were observed in frog kidney tumor cells by electron microscopy (**Figure 1**), and another decade followed before a causative relationship was established between LTHV and the tumor. The complete genome sequence of the McKinnell strain of LTHV was published in 2006 along with that of the other amphibian herpesvirus, the Rafferty strain of frog virus 4 (FV4; ranid herpesvirus 2).

In 1968, Fijan reported the first isolation of CCV from young channel catfish, in which it causes an acute disease of high mortality. The first detailed characterization of the virus was published 3 years later, and showed that capsids with the typical herpesvirus morphology are assembled in infected cell nuclei. Three-dimensional reconstructions derived by cryoelectron microscopy have shown that, apart from minor dimensional differences, the CCV capsid is strikingly similar to that of herpes simplex virus type 1 (HSV-1) (**Figure 2**). The complete genome sequence of the Auburn strain of CCV was published in 1992.

In 1998, a herpesvirus-like agent was identified as the cause of high mortality among carp, including expensive ornamental fish known as koi. The first outbreaks of this new disease may have occurred as early as 1996. In initial

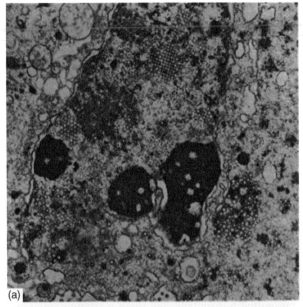

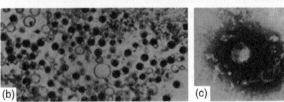

**Figure 1**   (a) Thin section of an inclusion-bearing Lucké tumor cell with typical herpesvirus particles in various stages of development in the nucleus. Magnification ×19 400. (b) Enveloped extracellular virions. Magnification ×24 000. (c) Negatively stained nonenveloped particles showing typical herpesvirus morphology. Magnification ×110 000. Reproduced from Granoff A (1972) Lucké tumor-associated viruses – a review. In: Biggs PM, de-The G, and Payne LN (eds.) *Oncogenesis and Herpesviruses*, pp. 171–182. Lyons: International Agency for Research on Cancer, with permission from WHO.

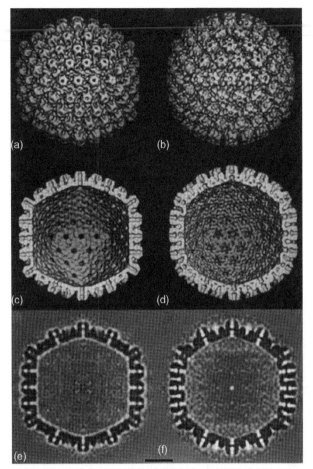

**Figure 2**   Comparison of the three-dimensional capsid structures of CCV (a, c, e) and HSV-1 (b, d, f). The capsids are viewed along a twofold symmetry axis. Outer surfaces (a and b); inner surfaces (c and d); central thin sections (e and f). The distribution of capsomers (a and b) is distinctive for the triangulation number, $T = 16$, with lines of three hexons connecting pentons along each edge of the icosahedral surface lattice. Scale = 25 nm. Reproduced from Booy FP, Trus BL, Davison AJ, and Steven AC (1996) The capsid architecture of channel catfish virus, an evolutionarily distant herpesvirus, is largely conserved in the absence of discernible sequence homology with herpes simplex virus. *Virology* 215: 134–141, with permission from Elsevier.

studies, this agent (KHV) was also known as carp interstitial nephritis and gill necrosis virus. Consideration of developmental, morphological, and, most recently, genetic attributes have led to the virus being proposed formally as a member of the proposed family *Alloherpesviridae*. The complete genome sequences of three strains of KHV (from Japan, USA, and Israel) were published in 2007.

## Geographic and Seasonal Distribution

The Lucké tumor occurs in north-central and northeastern parts of the USA and southern Canada. In the 1960s, the frequency of affected frogs reached 9% in some collections. However, leopard frog populations have since declined drastically, and the tumor has also become very rare. Production of LTHV within tumors is temperature dependent and therefore seasonal. Tumor cells contain

acidophilic intranuclear inclusions and virus particles at temperatures below 11.5 °C but not at higher temperatures, and transition between these states can be induced by temperature shift. The mechanisms by which temperature regulates virus growth have not been elucidated, and their operation *in vivo* and *in vitro* (explanted tumors) indicates that the immune system is not a primary factor. Despite the absence of virus particles at higher temperatures, there is some evidence that tumors express virus-specific proteins.

The occurrence of CCV disease has paralleled the intensification of channel catfish farming in the southern

USA and other warmer temperate regions. The lack of reported CCV isolations from wild channel catfish indicates that factors such as dense stocking and poor environmental conditions may predispose farmed fish stocks to outbreaks of disease. A key factor is water temperature, since epizootics occur in the summer months and the incubation period has been shown to be considerably shorter at higher temperatures up to 30 °C.

KHV has spread to many countries worldwide, presumably as a result of intensive aquaculture and unregulated transport of live fish in the absence of diagnostic assessment. Water temperature is an important seasonal factor influencing disease, with losses tending to occur during periods at 18–25 °C (spring and autumn). In one study, experimental infections of koi resulted in a cumulative mortality of 95% at 23 °C, with marginally fewer deaths occurring more rapidly at 28 °C and more slowly at 18 °C. Mortalities did not occur at 13 °C, but shifting virus-exposed fish from 13 to 23 °C resulted in rapid onset of mortality.

## Pathology, Clinical Features, and Pathogenesis

Little information is available on the natural transmission of LTHV and the factors that influence the occurrence of tumors. It is possible that virus is transmitted by contact with urine or by infection of oocytes in tumor-bearing frogs. Although FV4 infects the embryos and larvae of *R. pipiens*, surviving animals do not develop tumors. Examinations of the gene complements of the two viruses have not provided a ready explanation of this biological difference.

CCV causes an acute hemorrhagic disease in juvenile channel catfish. It is readily transmitted from fish to fish, probably entering through the gills. In artificial settings, it can also be transmitted by injection or orally by ingestion of contaminated food. After experimental infection, CCV can be isolated from the kidneys and then from other organs, in some of which impressively high titers of virus may be attained. The primary route for virus shedding is probably via the urine.

CCV can be remarkably virulent in susceptible populations of channel catfish. Under optimal conditions the incubation period can be as short as 3 days, and mortality can rise rapidly to 100%. Signs of distress may be accompanied by convulsive swimming, including a 'head-up' posture, and lethargy and death follow. Externally, affected fish may display protruding eyes, a distended abdomen and hemorrhages, largely on the ventral surface. Internally, viscera may be enlarged and hemorrhagic, but certain organs, such as kidneys, liver, and spleen, may be pale. The digestive tract is empty of food, instead containing a mucoid secretion, and a fluid accumulation

is present in the peritoneal cavity. Histopathological examination reveals widespread and profound changes. Initially, the kidneys show edema, hemorrhage, and necrosis, and then these features develop in the liver and digestive tract. Electron microscopic studies reveal virus particles in affected organs.

Given the virulence of CCV in young catfish, it is reasonable to suppose that the virus might persist in an inapparent or latent form in adult fish, as do higher vertebrate herpesviruses in their hosts. There is evidence in support of this. Viral mRNA and antigens have been detected in adult fish and, in more recent studies, virus was recovered by co-cultivation of tissues from wintering adult fish and virus DNA was detected by polymerase chain reaction (PCR) in various tissues of surviving fish many months after infection. There is evidence that the CCV genome may exist in circular or concatemeric form in surviving fish. However, the site of latency has not been identified. Reactivated CCV from adult fish could be transmitted horizontally, and there is circumstantial evidence that vertical transmission may also occur.

KHV is highly contagious, has an incubation period of 2–3 days, and exhibits mortality rates of 80–100%. Clinical signs include increased mucus production, pale patches on the skin and gills, labored breathing, and swelling and then necrosis of the gill filaments. Pathological lesions are evident primarily in the gills but may be present in the kidney, skin, liver, spleen, brain, and gastrointestinal tract. Gill disease is characterized by hyperplasia and then fusion of secondary lamellae, inflammation of the gill rakers, and subsequent necrosis. Kidney disease, if present, is characterized by a peritubular and interstitial nephritis. Virus particles are present in affected organs. The routes of infection and shedding are not known, though the gills and skin are obvious candidates, and cohabitation is an effective means of transmitting the disease. Depending on water temperature, virus may survive for periods of days to weeks. Immunohistochemistry and PCR analyses have demonstrated large amounts of the virus in the gills, skin, kidneys, and spleen with smaller amounts in liver, brain, and intestinal tract, mirroring the pathological involvement of these organs. Given its identity as a herpesvirus, it is likely that KHV has a latent aspect to its life cycle. There is some evidence for this, in that temperature-dependent reactivation of KHV has been shown to occur experimentally in surviving carp several months after initial exposure.

Two other carp herpesviruses have been characterized. From limited DNA sequence data, both appear to be closely related to, though distinct from, KHV. Carp pox herpesvirus (cyprinid herpesvirus 1) has been implicated as the cause of a localized epithelial hyperplasia, which manifests itself as benign smooth nodules on the skin and may be transferred by applying material from the lesions to the abraded skin of other fish or following bath exposures of young carp or koi to virus from cell culture. The agent is difficult to grow successfully in cell culture, and thus is isolated infrequently from clinical cases. Hematopoietic necrosis herpesvirus of goldfish (cyprinid herpesvirus 2) was first observed in Japan in 1992, and since then severe outbreaks of the associated disease have occurred in several countries. The virus affects goldfish and not carp, and the disease shares some pathological manifestations similar to that caused in carp by KHV, although the hematopoietic tissue in the kidney rather than the gills is the principal virus target. Similar to cyprinid herpesvirus 1, the goldfish virus is difficult to isolate, although it has been successfully cultured on occasion, with the experimental demonstration that upon bath exposure goldfish will succumb to typical signs of the disease and death.

Two salmonid herpesviruses have been shown to cause virulent disease either naturally or experimentally. Herpesvirus salmonis (salmonid herpesvirus 1; SalHV-1) was isolated on several occasions from a rainbow trout hatchery in the state of Washington. Oncorhynchus masou virus (salmonid herpesvirus 2; SalHV-2) was isolated from Japanese land-locked salmon, and has the property of causing epithelial tumors in survivors of experimental infection. Two additional herpesviruses, the NeVTA and Yamame tumor viruses, have been isolated from *Oncorhynchus* species. They appear to be related to each other, but it is not known whether they represent distinct salmonid herpesviruses or whether they are isolates of SalHV-2 or, as seems less likely, SalHV-1.

Diseases ostensibly due to several other fish herpesviruses have been described. Walleye herpesvirus is associated with epidermal hyperplasia, but causality has not been demonstrated. Similarly, the role of turbot herpesvirus has not been proven in episodes of substantial mortality among farmed fry.

## Growth Properties

The Lucké tumor occurs naturally in *R. pipiens*. Tumors can be induced readily in *R. pipiens* embryos or larvae inoculated with LTHV-containing extracts of Lucké tumors or virus purified by density gradient centrifugation. The ascites frequently produced by tumor-bearing frogs contains virus that can induce tumors when inoculated into embryos. Tumors have also been induced experimentally in other species of the host genus. Despite attempts employing cell lines from a wide range of hosts, it has not proved possible to culture LTHV *in vitro* from homogenates of Lucké tumors or the urine of

tumor-bearing frogs. Therefore, it has not been possible to investigate the replication cycle. In contrast, FV4 can be grown in cell culture, and produces cytopathic effects typical of herpesviruses within 10–21 days after infection of *R. pipiens* embryo or adult kidney cells at 25 °C. These include cell rounding and vacuolization, enlargement of nuclei and development of intranuclear inclusions, and formation of syncytia.

CCV causes acute infection only in young channel catfish up to about 6 months old, the degree of mortality depending on the strain of fish. Certain other closely related species, such as the blue catfish (*Ictalurus furcatus*), may be infected experimentally by injection, but other species are refractory even by this route. Host cell requirements are a little less stringent in cell culture, but virus growth still only occurs in ictalurid and clariid fish cell lines. Among commonly used cell lines BB (*Ictalurus nebulosus* or brown bullhead) and CCO (channel catfish ovary), the latter is more susceptible. Optimal virus yield is obtained at 25–30 °C, and about 50% of progeny virus is released into the culture medium. Virus infection causes the formation of syncytia, particularly at lower multiplicities of infection, followed eventually by disaggregation and lysis. Under optimal conditions, peak virus yield may be attained only 12 h after infection. Thus, CCV is one of the fastest growing herpesviruses *in vitro*.

Experimental determinations have shown that about 50 CCV proteins are expressed or induced in infected cell culture. As with other herpesviruses, expression appears to be coordinately regulated. The major immediate early protein, which is likely to regulate the expression of other virus genes, has an apparent molecular mass of 117 000 Da. The capsid contains an abundant constituent (the major capsid protein) with a molecular mass of 128 000 Da and at least two smaller proteins. The major capsid protein of higher vertebrate herpesviruses is invariably larger, having a molecular mass of about 150 000 Da. Different isolates of CCV may be differentiated by restriction endonuclease digestion of their DNAs, but are recognizably similar. CCV DNA replicates in the nuclei of infected cells via head-to-tail concatemers made up of a unit comprising the unique region linked to a single copy of the direct repeat.

KHV disease is restricted to koi and common carp, and other fish tested have been shown to be resistant even after extensive exposure to infected carp at permissive temperatures. A cell line derived from koi fin has been used to culture KHV, with optimal growth occurring at 15–25 °C and no growth at 10 or 30 °C. The highest virus yields are generated 7 days after infection at 20 °C, with most infectivity released into the culture medium. KHV strains are highly similar to each other as assessed by restriction endonuclease and sequence analyses. A total of 31 virion proteins have been detected. Studies of KHV gene expression are in their infancy.

SalHV-1 causes disease when injected into young rainbow trout maintained at 6–9 °C, but not in other salmonid species. A similar temperature optimum is characteristic of growth in the rainbow trout cell line RTG-2. SalHV-2 has a slightly wider host range, causing virulent disease in the young of several members of the genus *Oncorhynchus* and the rainbow trout. It has a higher temperature optimum for growth in RTG-2 cells than SalHV-1 (15 °C).

## Genetics and Evolution

The complete genome sequences of two fish and two amphibian herpesviruses have been determined: those of CCV, KHV, LTHV, and FV4. Partial data are available for other viruses in this group. **Table 1** shows some of the basic characteristics of the sequenced genomes. All have a type A genome structure, consisting of a unique region (U) flanked by a direct repeat at the termini (TR). However, this structure is not universal among fish and amphibian herpesviruses, as the SalHV-1 genome has a type D structure. All of the sequenced genomes contain a number of families of genes that are related (usually distantly) to each other and have presumably arisen by gene duplication. KHV has the largest genome thus far reported for any herpesvirus.

**Figure 3** shows the predicted gene layout in CCV, which has the smallest sequenced genome among the fish and amphibian herpesviruses. Analysis of the sequence indicates the presence of 62 genes in U (two spliced) and 14 genes in TR. Several gene functions have been predicted from computer-aided comparisons of predicted CCV proteins with proteins from other organisms. Ten genes belong to four gene families: two encoding related sets of protein kinases (PK1 with ORF14, ORF15, and ORF16; PK2 with ORF73 and ORF74), one encoding proteins similar to a bacteriophage deoxynucleoside monophosphate kinase (dNMPK; ORF76 and ORF77), and one encoding proteins containing a potential zinc-binding domain (RING; ORF9, ORF11, and ORF12). Other genes encode a potential zinc-binding protein (ORF78), a protein containing a

myosin-like domain (ORF22), a helicase (ORF25), a DNA polymerase (ORF57, composed of two exons), a deoxyuridine triphosphatase (ORF49), a thymidine kinase (ORF5), a subtilisin-like proprotein convertase (ORF47), the ATPase subunit of the putative terminase (ORF62, composed of three exons), a putative primase (ORF63), a protein containing an ovarian tumor (OTU)-like cysteine protease domain (ORF65), an envelope glycoprotein (ORF46), and seven other membrane-associated proteins (ORF6, ORF7, ORF8, ORF10, ORF19, ORF51, and ORF59). The principal constituent proteins of CCV virions have been identified by proteomic analysis. The capsid includes the major capsid protein (ORF39), a potential scaffold protein (ORF28), and two other proteins that possibly constitute the intercapsomeric triplex (ORF27 and ORF53). Several virus proteins in the tegument have been identified, in addition to actin. The major envelope protein is specified by ORF59.

LTHV, FV4, and KHV have substantially more genes than CCV, and many of these are members of gene families or genes apparently captured from the cell or other viruses. For example, the frog herpesviruses, unlike the fish herpesviruses, encode a DNA (cytosine-5-)-methyltransferase and, presumably as a result, have extensively methylated genomes. Overall, the two frog herpesvirus genomes are the most closely related of the four, sharing 40 genes (when genes with marginal similarity are excluded). CCV shares 19 genes with the frog herpesviruses and only 15 with KHV. The modest number of conserved genes indicates that the evolutionary distance among lower vertebrate herpesviruses is substantially greater than that among higher vertebrate herpesviruses.

Where functions may be predicted for the conserved genes, they are central to herpesvirus replication, being involved in capsid morphogenesis, nucleotide metabolism, DNA replication, and DNA packaging. The arrangement of homologous genes in LTHV and FV4 is collinear, except for one block of genes that is in a different position and orientation in the two genomes. In contrast, homologous genes in the frog herpesviruses are situated in several rearranged blocks in the more distantly related fish herpesviruses. This parallels the situation among members of different subfamilies of higher vertebrate herpesviruses.

**Table 1**    Characteristics of sequenced fish and amphibian herpesvirus genomes

| Virus | Genome size[a] (bp) | G + C composition (mol.%) | Genes[b] | Gene families |
|---|---|---|---|---|
| CCV | 134 226 [18 556] | 56.2 | 76 | 4 |
| KHV | 295 146 [22 469] | 59.2 | 156 | 5 |
| LTHV | 220 859 [636] | 54.6 | 132 | 15 |
| FV4 | 231 801 [912] | 52.8 | 147 | 15 |

[a]The total size of the DNA sequence is given, with the size of TR in square brackets.
[b]Genes that are duplicated by virtue of their presence in the terminal repeat are counted only once.

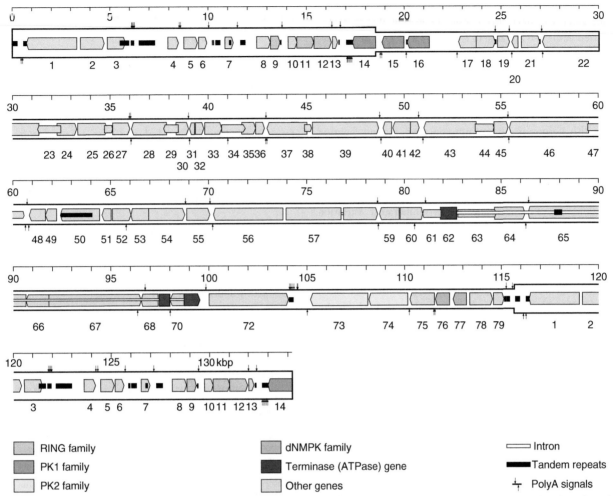

**Figure 3** Arrangement of predicted protein-coding open reading frames (ORFs) in the CCV genome. ORFs are colored and numbered with the 'ORF' prefix omitted. The thinner portion of the genome denotes the unique region (U) and the thicker portions the terminal repeats (TR).

As with higher vertebrate herpesviruses, homologous genes tend to be located centrally in the genomes.

The salmonid viruses SalHV-1 and SalHV-2 have been shown to be distinct viruses on the base of serological comparisons, DNA hybridization studies, and limited DNA sequencing. The SalHV-1 genome is approximately 174 kbp in size and has homologues of at least 18 CCV genes in several rearranged blocks. Sequence data indicate that these two viruses are related to each other and, more distantly, to CCV.

No proteins encoded by fish and amphibian herpesviruses are detectably related in their primary sequences to proteins that are specific to higher vertebrate herpesviruses (e.g., those that make up the capsid, of which the structure is conserved). This observation suggests that the two groups diverged from their common ancestor a long time ago. The best (and perhaps only) sequence-based evidence for a common evolutionary origin of the two groups depends on conservation of the putative ATPase subunit of the terminase, which is encoded by a spliced gene containing three exons (**Figure 3**). This protein is thought to be involved in packaging replicated DNA into the capsid and is also distantly conserved in T4-like bacteriophages, thus contributing to the notion that herpesviruses may share an ancient origin with bacteriophages.

## Immune Response

Understanding of the immune responses to amphibian and fish herpesviruses is not well developed, and data obtained under relatively normal conditions of infection are limited largely to CCV. Adult channel catfish produce peak neutralization titers on average 8 or 9 weeks after primary immunization with CCV, and a further moderate increase in titer of short duration is apparent after boosting. The importance of virus growth in eliciting the immune response is indicated by the observation that heat-inactivated virus is poorly immunogenic. Serum neutralization indexes have been used to document a link between outbreaks of CCV disease and potential carriers of the virus. These studies, though not extensive, have given some indication that seroconverted adult fish are able to transmit CCV.

## Control and Prevention

The devastating economic losses occasioned by certain of the fish herpesviruses prompt the need for intervention protocols. Avoidance and containment of outbreaks presently involve the use of ostensibly virus-free or partially resistant breeding stock, as clean environmental conditions as practicable, destruction of affected populations, and disinfection of ponds. The use of temperature variation regimes to aid the survival of infected fish has also been mooted. It is clear from the KHV situation, where individual fish may be very valuable, that effective diagnosis and monitoring of stock movements should be considered in order to avoid the spread of highly virulent diseases.

CCV is sensitive to nucleoside analogs that inhibit the growth of higher vertebrate herpesviruses. In general, these compounds are phosphorylated by the virus, but not the cellular, thymidine kinase. Further steps in phosphorylation probably involve cellular enzymes. The triphosphate form then inhibits DNA replication by direct interaction with the DNA polymerase or by incorporation into nascent DNA. These compounds include the widely used antiherpetic drug acyclovir. Phosphonoacetate, which inhibits the DNA polymerase by mimicking pyrophosphate, is also inhibitory. Against considerations of cost and administration, however, it is doubtful whether antiviral therapy will ever be generally practicable for the treatment of fish herpesvirus diseases.

The poor immunogenicity of inactivated CCV and KHV preparations suggests that the use of live, attenuated viruses is likely to be more effective in vaccination strategies. However, given the potential for latent vaccine virus to revert to wild type, thorough characterization of vaccine candidates and development of assays to differentiate vaccine from wild-type virus are essential (for a precedent in higher vertebrate herpesviruses, consider pseudorabies virus). The use of avirulent strains of virus in which virulence genes are replaced by detection markers may lead in the long term to safe, efficacious vaccines.

CCV attenuated by passage in a clariid fish cell line was able to provide substantial protection against the lethal effect of infection by virulent virus, particularly when the initial immunization was boosted. This virus exhibits several genomic differences from wild type, most notably a substantial deletion in ORF50, which potentially encodes a secreted glycoprotein. In this context, deletion of ORF5, which encodes thymidine kinase, has been shown to cause attenuation of virulence in channel catfish fingerlings. Attenuated versions of KHV produced by serial passage in koi fin cell culture and subjecting clones to further

mutation *in vitro* did not induce lethal disease and protected immunized fish against challenge. This protection correlated with antibody production.

DNA vaccines also hold promise in combating fish herpesvirus diseases, particularly in their avoidance of utilizing intact virus. From seven CCV genes tested, ORF59 (encoding the major envelope glycoprotein) and ORF6 (encoding a predicted membrane protein) produced significant resistance to challenge, with combined vaccination even more effective.

## Acknowledgments

The author is grateful to Ronald Hedrick for comments on the pathological features of KHV in light of his unpublished data.

*See also:* Pseudorabies Virus.

## Further Reading

Aoki T, Hirono I, Kurokawa K, *et al.* (2007) Genome sequences of three koi herpesvirus isolates representing the expanding distribution of an emerging disease threatening koi and common carp worldwide. *Journal of Virology* 81: 5058–5065.

Booy FP, Trus BL, Davison AJ, and Steven AC (1996) The capsid architecture of channel catfish virus, an evolutionarily distant herpesvirus, is largely conserved in the absence of discernible sequence homology with herpes simplex virus. *Virology* 215: 134–141.

Davison AJ (1992) Channel catfish virus: A new type of herpesvirus. *Virology* 186: 9–14.

Davison AJ, Cunningham C, Sauerbier W, and McKinnell RG (2006) Genome sequences of two frog herpesviruses. *Journal of General Virology* 87: 3509–3514.

Gilad O, Yun S, Adkison MA, *et al.* (2003) Molecular comparison of isolates of an emerging fish pathogen, koi herpesvirus, and the effect of water temperature on mortality of experimentally infected koi. *Journal of General Virology* 84: 2661–2667.

Granoff A (1972) Lucké tumor-associated viruses – a review. In: Biggs PM, de-The G, and Payne LN (eds.) *Oncogenesis and Herpesviruses*, pp. 171–182. Lyons: International Agency for Research on Cancer.

Granoff A (1983) Amphibian herpesviruses. In: Roizman B (ed.) *The Herpesviruses*, vol. 2, pp. 367–384. New York: Plenum.

Ilouze M, Dishon A, and Kotler M (2006) Characterization of a novel virus causing a lethal disease in carp and koi. *Microbiology and Molecular Biology Reviews* 70: 147–156.

McKinnell RG, Lust JM, Sauerbier W, *et al.* (1993) Genomic plasticity of the Lucké renal carcinoma: A review. *International Journal of Developmental Biology* 37: 213–219.

Naegele RF, Granoff A, and Darlington RW (1974) The presence of Lucké herpesvirus genome in induced tadpole tumors and its oncogenicity: Koch–Henle postulates fulfilled. *Proceedings of the National Academy of Sciences, USA* 71: 830–834.

Pikarsky E, Ronen A, Abramowitz J, *et al.* (2004) Pathogenesis of acute viral disease induced in fish by carp interstitial nephritis and gill necrosis virus. *Journal of Virology* 78: 9544–9551.

Plumb JA (1989) Channel catfish virus. In: Ahne W and Kurstak E (eds.) *Viruses of Lower Vertebrates*, pp. 198–216. Berlin: Springer.

Wolf K (1983) Biology and properties of fish and reptilian herpesviruses. In: Roizman B (ed.) *The Herpesviruses*, vol. 2, pp. 319–366. New York: Plenum.

# Fish Retroviruses

**T A Paul, R N Casey, P R Bowser,** and **J W Casey,** Cornell University, Ithaca, NY, USA
**J Rovnak** and **S L Quackenbush,** Colorado State University, Fort Collins, CO, USA

## Glossary

**Cytopathic effect** Morphologic changes in cells resulting from virus replication.
**Dysplasia** An abnormality in the appearance of cells and indicative of a preneoplastic change.
**Hyperplasia** An increase in the number of cells of an organ or tissue.
**Leiomyosarcoma** Neoplasia of smooth muscle cells.
**Malpighian cells** Cells of the deepest layer of the epidermis.
**Neoplasia** An abnormal growth of cells.
**Oncogene** Cellular or viral gene whose products are capable of inducing a neoplastic phenotype.
**Proto-oncogene** A normal cellular gene which when inappropriately expressed or mutated becomes an oncogene.

## Introduction

Retroviruses have been documented in a wide range of vertebrate species including lower vertebrates such as frogs, snakes, sharks, fish, birds, and turtles. To date, however, the majority of these reported sequences represent only partial fragments of the retrovirus. In recent years, the complete genomic sequence of exogenous fish retroviruses from Atlantic salmon (*Salmo salar*), walleye (*Sander vitreus*), and snakehead (*Ophicephalus striatus*), and an endogenous retrovirus of zebrafish (*Danio rerio*) have been determined. Analysis of these viral genomes indicates a high degree of diversity among the fish retroviruses as well as several unique features compared to mammalian and avian retroviruses.

The etiological relationship between retroviruses and cancer is well established in mammalian and avian systems. Simple retroviruses can promote cell proliferation by inducing the ectopic expression of captured cellular oncogenes (viral transduction for acutely transforming viruses) in which an oncogene recombines into the viral genome, or by integration near or within the coding sequence of cellular proto-oncogenes (nonacute transforming viruses). Transcription factors encoded by some complex retroviruses, like human T-cell leukemia virus-1 (HTLV-1), also have nonacute oncogenic potential by deregulating cellular pathways controlling cell proliferation.

Like their mammalian and avian counterparts, many fish neoplastic/proliferative diseases are suspected of having a retroviral etiology. Retroviruses are reported to be associated with 13 spontaneous proliferative diseases of fish based on the observation of retrovirus-like particles and, in some cases, reverse transcriptase activity in neoplastic lesions. Seven of these diseases with putative viral etiologies display a seasonal cycle, that is, they develop and regress annually. Retrovirus-associated tumors of the skin have received the most attention, since they are most visible and easily sampled. Skin tumors with suspected viral etiologies have been found in white sucker (*Castostomus commersoni*), walleye, yellow perch (*Perca flavescens*), and European smelt (*Osmerus eperlanus*). Retroviruses have also been linked to lymphoma in northern pike (*Esox lucius*), leukemia in chinook salmon (*Oncorhynchus tshawytscha*), and leiomyosarcoma of the swimbladder in Atlantic salmon. One noteworthy piscine retrovirus, the snakehead fish retrovirus (SnRV), has not been associated with tumor induction. In most of these systems, the etiologic relationship of retroviral infections and neoplasms rests on circumstantial evidence such as observations of viral particles by electron microscopy and the presence of reverse transcriptase activity. However, sequencing of fish retroviruses has facilitated use of molecular-based diagnostic reagents and, in some cases, shed light on potential modes of pathogenesis. In particular, the walleye retroviruses, walleye dermal sarcoma virus (WDSV) and walleye epidermal hyperplasia virus type 1 (WEHV-1) and type 2 (WEHV-2), express a subset of accessory genes exclusively during oncogenesis, specifically implicating the encoded proteins in the process of tumorigenesis.

## Retroviruses and their Life Cycle

Retrovirus particles are composed of viral structural and enzymatic proteins and two copies of the positive-sense single-stranded RNA genome. The proteins are surrounded by a lipid bilayer, acquired from the host cell, in which viral envelope glycoproteins are embedded. Retroviral infection is initiated when the surface glycoprotein binds to its cognate receptor on the surface of a susceptible cell. Upon fusion of the viral and cellular membranes, the viral core enters the cytoplasm where the virally encoded enzyme, reverse transcriptase, copies the RNA genome into DNA. The viral integrase protein binds reverse transcribed DNA and mediates its integration into the genomic DNA of the host. In rare cases, retroviral infection of host germ-line cells and subsequent integration into the chromosomes can establish retroviral sequences as heritable genetic elements, known as endogenous retroviruses.

Based on the complexity of the viral genome, retroviruses can be divided into two broad categories: simple and complex. Simple retroviruses, including members of the *Gammaretroviruses* and *Alpharetroviruses*, contain three genes: *gag, pol,* and *env.* Expression of a full-length unspliced messenger RNA (mRNA) and a spliced mRNA serve as the templates for translation of the retroviral structural and enzymatic proteins. These proteins are first translated as polyproteins from *gag* and *pol,* respectively, and are processed by a virally encoded protease. The viral envelope glycoprotein is encoded from a singly spliced viral transcript containing the *env* gene.

Complex retroviruses are distinguished from simple retroviruses on the basis of their additional coding capacity and pattern of viral gene expression. This category of retroviruses includes *Lentiviruses* such as human immunodeficiency virus type 1 (HIV-1), *Spumaviruses,* and the *Deltaretroviruses,* human T-cell leukemia virus (HTLV-1), and bovine leukemia virus (BLV). Complex retroviruses produce multiply spliced transcripts that encode two classes of accessory/regulatory proteins. One class includes transcriptional regulatory proteins such as HTLV-1 Tax and HIV-1 Tat, which act *in trans* to directly regulate the activity of the viral promoter. A second class, including HTLV-1 Rex and HIV-1 Rev, act post transcriptionally, to facilitate transport of unspliced and singly spliced viral transcripts to the cytoplasm. The combined action of these proteins divides the replication cycle into two temporal phases: an early, regulatory phase, and a later, structural phase. During the regulatory phase, low levels of fully spliced transcripts encoding *trans*-activators increase levels of transcription leading to the accumulation

of post-transcriptional regulatory proteins. These proteins allow production of unspliced and singly spliced mRNAs that encode the viral structural proteins.

Both simple and complex retroviruses have been identified in fish species. Retroviruses isolated from walleye and snakehead fish resemble complex retroviruses based upon their genome structure and transcriptional profile, while simple retroviruses have been identified in Atlantic salmon and zebrafish.

## Skin Tumors in Walleye and Their Associated Retroviruses

Walleye dermal sarcoma (WDS) and walleye discrete epidermal hyperplasia (WEH) are neoplastic and hyperplastic skin lesions in walleye that have been etiologically associated with infection by three distinct retroviruses (**Figure 1**). WDS and WEH were first reported in 1969 on fish from Oneida Lake in New York. Since then, WDS and WEH have been reported on walleyes throughout North America. These diseases have a seasonal cycle; tumor incidence is highest in the late fall and early spring months at frequencies of 27% and 5% for WDS and WEH, respectively. Lower tumor prevalence in summer months is associated with regression on individual adult fish.

WDS appears as a cutaneous mesenchymal neoplasm arising multicentrically within the superficial dermis and overlaid with epidermis. Fall tumors appear highly vascularized due to a network of capillaries, while spring tumors are frequently white with ulcerated surfaces. Invasive tumors are rarely observed in feral fish. WEH lesions are benign mucoid-like plaques with distinct boundaries. They can range from 2 to 3 mm in diameter to large lesions with irregular borders that may be as large as

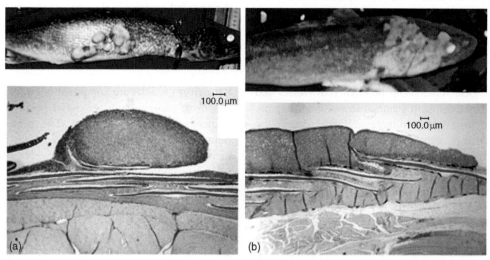

**Figure 1**    (a) Gross and histological images of walleye dermal sarcoma and (b) walleye epidermal hyperplasia.

50 mm across. Histologically, this disease appears as an epidermal proliferation consisting primarily of Malpighian cells.

Experimental transmission of WDS and WEH has been achieved with cell-free filtrates. Interestingly, only cell-free filtrates prepared from the spring, regressing WDS, not fall, developing WDS, are able to transmit disease. Infection of walleye fingerlings less than 9 weeks of age results in the frequent development of invasive tumors.

Electron microscopic observation of retrovirus particles and cell-free transmission of both diseases suggest a retroviral etiology for WDS and WEH. WDSV was isolated from WDS tissue, and two independent retroviruses, WEHV1, WEHV2, were isolated from WEH lesions. Similar hyperplastic lesions on yellow perch in Oneida Lake are associated with two new retroviruses, perch epidermal hyperplasia virus types 1 and 2 (PEHV1, PEHV2).

## Isolation and Sequencing of Retroviruses from WDS and WEH Lesions

WDSV, WEHV1, and WEHV2 have been molecularly cloned and sequenced (**Figure 2**). The genome structures of WDSV, WEHV1, and WEHV2 indicate large and complex viral genomes (12.7, 12.9, and 13.1 kbp, respectively). All three viruses have intact open reading frames (ORFs) capable of encoding the structural and enzymatic genes *gag*, *pol*, and *env*. *gag* (viral capsid) and *pol* (reverse transcriptase) are in the same reading frame and synthesized as a polyprotein through a termination suppression mechanism. *pro* (viral protease), responsible for cleaving the polyprotein, is located in the same reading frame as *pol*. A unique feature of all three viruses is the presence of additional orfs that have tentatively been called *orfa*, *orfb*, and *orfc*. The *orfa* and *orfb* genes are located between *env* and the 3′ long terminal repeat (LTR), while *orfc* is located between the 5′ LTR and the start of *gag*.

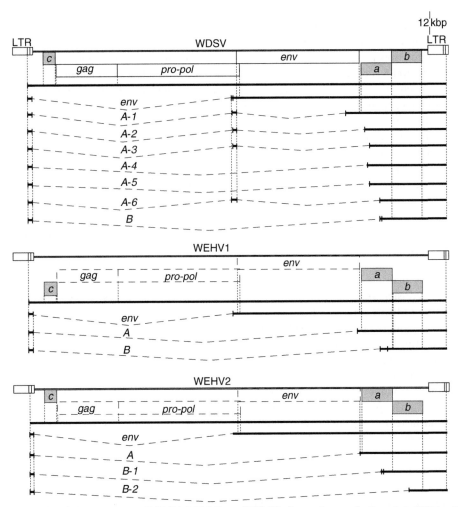

**Figure 2** Genomic and transcriptional maps of WDSV, WEHV1, and WEHV2. Genomic organization of viral DNA with retroviral genes and accessory genes *orfa*, *orfb*, and *orfc* is depicted under each virus heading. The envelope-spliced transcript (*env*) and additional spliced transcripts (*A* and *B*), which are capable of expressing accessory genes, are illustrated. The vertical dashed lines indicate the boundaries of the exons, introns, and open reading frames.

Database searches with OrfA protein amino acid sequences suggest limited homology with D-type cellular cyclins within the cyclin-box motif, and are referred to as rv-cyclins. WEHV1 rv-cyclin has a 20% amino acid identity and 35% similarity with human cyclin D-3, whereas WEHV2 and WDSV rv-cyclin are most similar to human cyclin D-1 (22%/35% and 19%/29% amino acid identity/similarity). Similarities with known walleye and other piscine cyclins are not significantly greater. The WEHV cyclin homologs are 37% identical within the cyclin box motif and 21–28% identical with the WDSV cyclin. Sequence homologies between rv-cyclin and OrfB in the walleye retroviruses suggest they arose by a gene duplication event.

## Roles of the WDSV Accessory Proteins in Pathogenesis

Transcriptional mapping by RT-PCR and Northern blot analyses of developing and regressing WDS and WEH have demonstrated temporal gene expression profiles and complex splicing patterns analogous to those seen in the complex retroviruses of mammals. In developing WDS tumors, only low levels of multiply spliced subgenomic transcripts are detected. These transcripts predominantly contain the coding sequences for rv-cyclin and OrfB. Regressing spring tumors contain high levels of full-length and subgenomic transcripts as well as unintegrated viral DNA and transmissible virus. OrfC is likely encoded by the full-length transcript coincident with tumor regression.

A detailed transcriptional analysis of WDSV showed an alternative splicing pattern of the *orfa* transcript (**Figure 2**). In developing tumors, the *orfa* transcript contains the coding sequence for a full-length rv-cyclin protein that localizes to the nucleus of mammalian and walleye cells. Alternatively spliced forms of this transcript encode amino-terminal truncated forms of the rv-cyclin protein, which localize in the cytoplasm of cells. The different forms of rv-cyclin may play functionally different roles in developing and regressing tumors. A single, spliced transcript encodes the OrfB protein, which is predominantly localized in the cytoplasm in tumor explant cells, but is capable of shuttling into and out of the nucleus when expressed in piscine and mammalian cells.

The OrfC protein from WDSV has been shown to localize to mitochondria and to disrupt mitochondrial function, which results in apoptosis. Only the full-length viral transcript found in regressing tumors is capable of encoding OrfC. Apoptotic cells are present in regressing, but not developing, WDS tumor sections. Therefore, the OrfC protein may be responsible for a direct viral mechanism of tumor regression.

WDSV *orfa* and *orfb* are the only virus transcripts found in developing tumors, suggesting direct roles for rv-cyclin and OrfB in the process of tumorigenesis, and their oncogenic potential has been demonstrated by several experimental approaches. WDSV *orfa* supported growth of a yeast (*Saccharomyces cerevisiae*) strain conditionally deficient for the synthesis of the G1 to S cyclins that are necessary for cell cycle progression. WEHV *orfa* did not support yeast growth in this model. Transgenic expression of WDSV *orfa* in mice from a skin-specific promoter caused a moderate to severe squamous epithelial hyperplasia and dysplasia dependant on skin injury. This suggests that rv-cyclin is not oncogenic as a result of a 'single-hit' mechanism, but rather, that secondary genetic or epigenetic events (possibly wound repair) are necessary for tumor development and progression. A similar phenotype has been described in transgenic mice expressing *v-jun* oncogene from the H-2K$^k$ major histocompatibility complex (MHC) class I antigen gene promoter. When expressed in mammalian or piscine cell culture, WDSV rv-cyclin localized in the nucleus and was found by co-immunoprecipitation to be associated with cyclin dependent kinase 8 and cyclin C, general transcription initiation factors, and RNA polymerase II transcription complexes. In piscine cells, rv-cyclin inhibited transcription from the WDSV promoter independent of *cis*-acting DNA sequences. However, rv-cyclin can activate other viral promoters in fish cells, and can activate the WDSV promoter in select mammalian cells; thus rv-cyclin activation and inhibition of transcription are dependent on both the promoter and the cell type. WDSV rv-cyclin contains a defined transcription activation domain in the carboxy end of the protein, and the isolated activation domain is capable of interacting with co-activators of transcription. WEHV rv-cyclins do not have a corresponding carboxy-region activation domain. WDSV rv-cyclin may exhibit oncogenic potential by differential regulation of host gene expression such as proto-oncogenes or tumor suppressors.

Less is known about the capabilities of the OrfB protein, but initial studies indicate its direct association with the regulation of signal transduction pathways. It is concentrated, in tumor explant cells, at focal adhesions, and along actin stress fibers. Established OrfB-expressing lines are resistant to the chemical induction of apoptosis, suggesting a role in oncogenesis.

The origins of the accessory genes of complex retroviruses are unclear. This includes the origins of the WDSV accessory genes encoding rv-cyclin, OrfB, and OrfC. In the case of rv-cyclin and OrfB, their extreme divergence from host cyclin sequences indicates that any transduction event was ancient and led, ultimately, to an exclusive, complex viral species. The OrfC protein, like the accessory proteins of other complex retroviruses, has no clear homology to host proteins.

## Control of the Seasonal Cycle of Disease

An interesting aspect of WDS is the control of the seasonal switch in viral gene expression and associated tumor regression. Potential modulators of viral gene expression include host immunity and endocrine activity (accompanying spawning) and environmental factors such as water temperature, physical trauma, and sunlight. A number of *cis*-acting elements important for transcription activation have been identified in the WDSV promoter. There is differential binding of proteins from developing and regressing tumor nuclear extracts to a 15 bp repeat region in the WDSV promoter. This element may be critical to the induction of high levels of virus expression. The WDSV rv-cyclin protein negatively regulates the WDSV promoter in tissue culture cells. Presumably, it is advantageous for the virus to have lower levels of gene expression during tumor development to avoid immune surveillance as well as the cytopathic effects associated with virus production. While rv-cyclin may function in the repression of virus expression during tumor growth, the host, environmental, or viral signals that switch on full virus expression are yet to be determined.

## Snakehead Retrovirus

The SnRV was isolated from a productively infected cell line derived from a Southeast Asian striped snakehead fish. Cell culture supernatant from these infected cells demonstrated high levels of RT activity and the presence of type C-like retrovirus particles. Additionally, supernatant from the infected cell line induced cytopathic effects in cultures of a bluegill cell line (BF-2).

Molecular approaches were utilized to identify and sequence the SnRV from infected cells. The large 11.2 kbp genome of SnRV contains intact coding regions for *gag*, *pol*, and *env* (**Figure 3**). An arginine tRNA primer binding site used for reverse transcription initiation distinguishes SnRV from other retroviruses. The structure and transcriptional profile of SnRV suggests a complex expression pattern capable of encoding an ORF located between *env* and the 3′ LTR and two very small ORFs termed ORF1

and ORF2. Within the leader sequence of SnRV resides a start codon located just upstream of the major splice donor site that could potentially encode a 14 amino acid peptide (LP). Expression of Env from a singly spliced transcript is predicted to utilize the LP initiation codon and fuses this 14 amino acid peptide in frame to downstream *env* sequences. A transcript with four exons and two initiator codons would encode ORF1 and ORF2 proteins. The 3′ ORF would be expressed from a transcript containing three exons and would encode a protein of 24 kDa. Finally, the fourth spliced transcript may encode 3′ ORF or possibly a LP-Env cytoplasmic domain (CD) fusion protein. The 3′ ORF contains an N terminal acidic domain, cysteine residues, and a basic region, motifs commonly found in transcriptional activators. These small ORFs have no significant homology to any known proteins in the databases, and their role in the viral life cycle is unknown. No endogenous copies of SnRV have been identified in the snakehead genome and an uninfected cell line has been established.

Although the presence of SnRV in wild populations has not been thoroughly examined, the virus has been independently isolated from two separate snakehead cell lines derived from whole fry tissue and from caudal peduncle tissue from juvenile fish. In all cases, fish from which these cell lines were derived appeared healthy.

## Salmon Swimbladder Sarcoma-Associated Retrovirus

An outbreak of neoplastic disease of the swimbladder of Atlantic salmon was first reported at a Scottish commercial marine fish farm in 1975. Affected salmon were sluggish and in poor condition. A viral etiology was suspected, and electron microscopic evaluation of tumors revealed the presence of budding viral particles with retroviral morphology. A second outbreak occurred between 1995 and 1997 in brood stock salmon held at the North

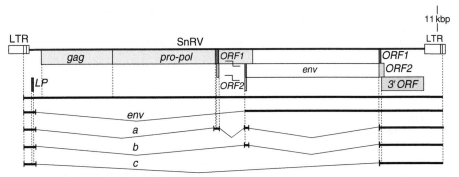

**Figure 3** Genomic and transcriptional map of SnRV. Predicted coding regions are shown as open or shaded boxes. The envelope-spliced transcript (*env*) and additional spliced transcripts (*a*, *b*, *c*), which are capable of expressing accessory genes, are illustrated. LP indicates the location of a predicted leader peptide. The vertical dashed lines indicate the boundaries of the exons, introns, and open reading frames.

Attleboro National Fish Hatchery in Massachusetts. The fish exhibited skin discoloration and hemorrhages on the fins and body and showed a general debilitation and lack of vigor. In May of 1997, significant mortality was noted at the facility such that 35% of the population was affected by late spring of 1998. All of the affected fish displayed swollen abdomens due to multinodular masses on internal and external surfaces of the swimbladder. In several cases, these multinodular masses occupied the entire swimbladder (**Figure 4**). Histologic examination revealed that the tumors were composed of well-differentiated fibroblastic cells that were arranged in interlacing bundles, which were classified as leiomyosarcomas.

## Isolation of a Retrovirus from Salmon Swimbladder Sarcoma

An exogenous retrovirus, termed Atlantic salmon swimbladder sarcoma virus (SSSV), was initially identified in tumors by degenerate RT-PCR of tumor RNA, and the entire viral sequence completed by DNA sequencing of proviral DNA. In contrast to the complex walleye

retroviruses, SSSV is a simple retrovirus. The viral genome contains ORFs capable of expressing *gag, pol,* and *env* (**Figure 5**). Additionally, a short 25 amino acid leader peptide of unknown function is located upstream of the Gag-Pol polyprotein ORF. SSSV differs from other simple retroviruses by not having related endogenous sequences in the host genome, and SSSV is the only retrovirus to use a methionine-tRNA as a plus-strand primer. Additionally, sequences in *pol* display homology to central polypurine tract regions identified in complex retroviruses. Central polypurine tracts facilitate the formation of a single-stranded DNA region called a central DNA flap as a result of reverse transcription priming from this internal site. In HIV-1, this feature plays a major role in complex retroviral replication and allows efficient infection of nondividing cells. It is intriguing that SSSV displays a high proviral copy number (greater than 30 copies per cell) with a polyclonal integration pattern in swimbladder tumors. SSSV must be capable of initiating multiple rounds of infection within the same cell. The specific mechanisms leading to the high copy number and its implications in the pathogenesis of disease are of significant interest for future research.

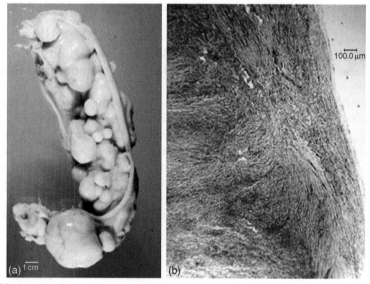

**Figure 4**    (a) Gross and (b) histological images of Atlantic salmon swimbladder sarcoma.

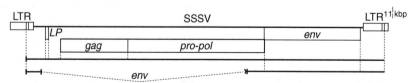

**Figure 5**    Genomic and transcriptional map of SSSV. Predicted coding regions are shown as open boxes. The envelope-spliced transcript (*env*) is illustrated. LP indicates the location of a predicted leader peptide. The vertical dashed lines indicate the boundaries of the exons, introns, and open reading frame.

## Sequence Comparisons of SSSV with Other Retroviruses

A comparison of the sequence of SSSV viral proteins with other retroviruses indicates large regions of homology with mammalian type C and type D viruses in Pol and Env. Additionally, a 179 amino acid region in the C terminus of Gag and a 1064 amino acid region of Pro–Pol displays 23% and 33% identity to the related WDSV proteins, respectively. SSSV has striking homology to the sequence of the zebrafish endogenous retrovirus (ZFERV). BLAST analysis of the Gag, Pol, and Env ORFs of SSSV reveals a 25% identity with ZFERV over 533 amino acids within Gag, a 40% identity over 533 amino acids of Pol, and a 39% identity over 429 amino acids of Env.

## Prevalence, Seasonality, and Transmission of SSSV

A PCR diagnostic assay was developed using sequences within the *pol* gene of SSSV. Prevalence at the North Attleboro fish facility has been found to be 52% and 5% of a natural stock of Pleasant River salmon were found to harbor SSSV.

Like other retroviral diseases of fish, observations suggest that salmon swimbladder sarcoma is seasonal. First, of the 34% fish mortality at the North Attleboro facility between 1997 and 1998, 57% occurred in June. Second, in the following year, the surviving salmon had an SSSV incidence (measured by PCR) that cycled with a peak in late summer to early winter and then diminished in late winter to early spring. The period of highest SSSV incidence correlated with salmon spawning runs in late fall. Interestingly, WDSV prevalence, which peaks during late spring, also correlates with the time of spawning. This suggests that endocrine changes during spawning runs may be a critical factor in the observed seasonal variation in disease incidence.

## Pathogenesis of SSSV

The existence of SSSV sequences in association with an outbreak of the swimbladder sarcoma suggests a role for the retrovirus in pathogenesis of the disease. As a simple retrovirus with no transduced cellular oncogenes, one possible mechanism of tumorigenesis is the insertional activation of a cellular proto-oncogene. The high copy number of proviruses in tumors has made the analysis of insertional activation events difficult, but multiple insertions increase the likelihood of such a mechanism. It is also feasible that SSSV may express an oncogenic viral gene product. This mechanism of oncogenesis has been proposed for the Jaagsiekte sheep retrovirus (JSRV) in the induction of ovine pulmonary adenocarcinoma and in Friend spleen focus-forming virus (SFFV)-associated

erythroid hyperplasia in mice. Additionally, the presence of common integration sites within JSRV associated tumors suggests that insertional mutagenesis may act in concert with the envelope in tumor development. Thus, a multifactorial mechanism for the development of salmon swimbladder sarcoma must also be considered.

In addition to sarcoma, a number of other distinct pathologies are associated with SSSV infection. These diseases are frequently debilitating and are, therefore, of significance to the aquaculture industry. Atlantic salmon at the North Attleboro hatchery, during the SSSV outbreak, presented with multifocal hemorrhages, sloughing of the epidermis, lethargy, wasting, and failure to mature sexually in addition to swimbladder tumors.

## Zebrafish Endogenous Retrovirus

Endogenous retroviruses have been identified in almost all vertebrate genomes, and most are defective due to mutations and deletions. An endogenous retrovirus, ZFERY with a genome of 11.2 kbp has been identified in the Tubingen stock of zebrafish, and contains intact coding regions for *gag*, *pol*, and *env*. The *gag* and *pol* genes are in the same reading frame. While the majority of endogenous retroviruses are transcriptionally silent because of mutation or methylation, ZFERV remains transcriptionally active. In addition to genomic transcripts that encode Gag and Pol proteins, an unusual multiply spliced *env* transcript is produced. Expression appears highest in the larval and adult zebrafish thymus, and no expression was detected in 2-day old embryos, suggesting that ZFERV expression may be tied to thymic development.

## Phylogeny of Fish Retroviruses

Retroviruses have been classified into seven genera based largely on highly conserved amino acid sequences in the retroviral reverse transcriptase gene. While the majority of the viral sequences employed in this classification represent mammalian and avian retroviruses, a new genus termed *Epsilonretroviruses*, representing the fish retroviruses WDSV, WEHV-1, WEHV-2, has been added to the most recent classification. As more retroviral sequences from lower vertebrates have been identified, it has become apparent that this classification scheme may be inadequate to represent the apparent diversity.

Based on the unique characteristics of SnRV, including its genomic organization, tRNA primer, and complex transcriptional profile, the virus is yet to be definitively placed in the current classification. The large size of the genome, genetic organization, and presence of additional ORFs suggest that SnRV is closest to the spumaviruses and walleye retroviruses, but its limited sequence homology suggests SnRV is divergent from these groups.

Phylogenetic analysis indicates that, while the walleye retroviruses cluster in a group representing the *Epsilonretroviruses*, SSSV and ZFERV appear to represent a new branch of piscine retroviruses between the walleye retroviruses and the *Gammaretroviruses*, a genera that includes the murine leukemia virus (MLV)-related retroviruses (**Figure 6**). The SnRV appears quite divergent from the other fish retroviruses by its placement in a distinct branch near the *Spumaviruses*. This would suggest that SnRV is quite divergent from the genus *Epsilonretrovirus* and may represent yet another group of retroviruses. Interestingly, a more encompassing phylogenetic analysis using all known retroviral sequences from lower vertebrates, including partial endogenous retroviral *pol* fragments from Stickleback (*Gasterosteus aculeatus*), brook trout (*Salvelinus fontinalis*), Brown trout (*Salmo trutta*), freshwater whiting

(*Corogonus lavaretus*), and puffer fish (*Fugu rubripes*), indicates that the majority of the fish viruses, excluding SnRV, cluster together with MLV-related viruses in a group separate from most non-MLV related mammalian retroviruses. This raises the possibility that some retroviral groups maybe restricted to particular vertebrate classes. However, it is evident from the diversity among the fish retroviruses, that there is a high degree of heterogeneity within this group.

## Acknowledgments

This research was supported in part by USDA grants 99-35204-7485 and 02-35204-12777 to J.W.C., National Oceanic and Atmospheric Administration award no. NA86RG0056 to the Research Foundation of State University of New York for New York Sea Grant to P.R.B., American Cancer Society grant RPG-00313–01-MBC to S.L.Q., and National Institutes of Health grant CA095056 to S.L.Q. T.A.P. was supported by National Institutes of Health training grant 5T32CA09682.

*See also:* Equine Infectious Anemia Virus; Feline Leukemia and Sarcoma Viruses; Foamy Viruses; Mouse Mammary Tumor Virus; Retroviruses of Birds; Simian Retrovirus D; Visna-Maedi Viruses.

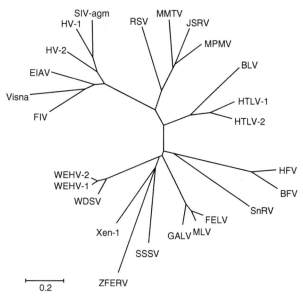

**Figure 6** Unrooted phylogenetic tree of representative retroviruses based on an amino acid alignment of seven conserved domains in reverse transcriptase.
Retroviruses are designated as follows: MPMV (Mason–Pfizer monkey virus), JSRV (Jaagsiekte sheep retrovirus), MMTV (mouse mammary tumor virus), RSV (Rous sarcoma virus), EIAV (equine infectious anemia virus), FIV (feline immunodeficiency virus), Visna (visna virus), HIV-2 (human immunodeficiency virus-2), HIV-1 (human immunodeficiency virus-1), SIV-agm (simian immunodeficiency virus-agm), HTLV-1 (human T-cell leukemia virus type 1), HTLV-2 (human T-cell leukemia virus 2), BLV (bovine leukemia virus), SSSV (salmon swimbladder sarcoma virus), SnRV (snakehead retrovirus), BFV (bovine foamy virus), HFV (human foamy virus), FeLV (feline leukemia virus), MLV (murine leukemia virus), GALV (gibbon ape leukemia virus), WDSV (walleye dermal sarcoma virus), WEHV-1 (walleye epidermal hyperplasia virus type 1), WEHV-2 (walleye epidermal hyperplasia virus type 2), ZFERV (zebrafish endogenous retrovirus), Xen-1 (Xenopus endogenous retrovirus-1).

## Further Reading

Bowser PR, Wolfe MJ, Forney JL, and Wooster GA (1988) Seasonal prevalence of skin tumors from walleye (*Stizostedion vitreum*) from Oneida Lake, New York. *Journal of Wildlife Diseases* 24: 292–298.

Coffin JM, Hughes SH,, and Varmus HE (eds.) (1997) *Retroviruses,* Cold Spring Harbor, NY: Cold Spring Harbor Laboratory Press.

Hart D, Frerichs GN, Rambaut A, and Onions DE (1996) Complete nucleotide sequence and transcriptional analysis of the snakehead fish retrovirus. *Journal of Virology* 70(6): 3606–3616.

Hernious E, Martin J, Miller K, Cook J, Wilkinson M, and Tristem M (1998) Retroviral diversity and distribution in vertebrates. *Journal of Virology* 72(7): 5955–5966.

Holzschu DL, Fodor SK, Quackenbush SL, *et al.* (1995) Nucleotide sequence and protein analysis of a complex piscine retrovirus, walleye dermal sarcoma virus. *Journal of Virology* 69(9): 5320–5331.

Lairmore MD, Stanley JR, Weber SA, and Holzschu DL (2000) Squamous epithelial proliferation induced by walleye dermal sarcoma retrovirus cyclin in transgenic mice. *Proceedings of the National Academy of Sciences, USA* 97(11): 6114–6119.

LaPierre LA, Casey JW, and Holzschu DL (1998) Walleye retroviruses associated with skin tumors and hyperplasias encode cyclin D homologs. *Journal of Virology* 72: 8765–8771.

LaPierre LA, Holzschu DL, Bowser PR, and Casey JW (1999) Sequence and transcriptional analyses of the fish retroviruses walleye epidermal hyperplasia virus types 1 and 2: Evidence for a gene duplication. *Journal of Virology* 73(11): 9393–9403.

Paul TA, Quackenbush SL, Sutton C, Casey RN, Bowser PR, and Casey JW (2006) Identification and characterization of an exogenous retrovirus from Atlantic salmon swimbladder sarcomas. *Journal of Virology* 80(6): 2941–2948.

Poulet FM, Bowser PR, and Casey JW (1994) Retroviruses of fish, reptiles, and molluscs. In: Levy JA (ed.) *The Retroviridae*, vol. 3, pp. 1–38. New York: Plenum.

Quackenbush SL, Holzschu DL, Bowser PR, and Casey JW (1997) Transcriptional analysis of walleye dermal sarcoma virus (WDSV). *Virology* 237: 107–112.

Rovnak J, Hronek BW, Ryan SO, Cai S, and Quackenbush SL (2005) An activation domain within the walleye dermal sarcoma virus retroviral

cyclin protein is essential for inhibition of the viral promoter. *Virology* 342(2): 240–251.

Rovnak J and Quackenbush SL (2002) Walleye dermal sarcoma virus cyclin interacts with components of the mediator complex and the RNA polymerase II holoenzyme. *Journal of Virology* 76: 8031–8039.

Shen CH and Steiner LA (2004) Genome structure and thymic expression of an endogenous retrovirus in zebrafish. *Journal of Virology* 78(2): 899–911.

# Fish Rhabdoviruses

**G Kurath and J Winton,** Western Fisheries Research Center, Seattle, WA, USA

Published by Elsevier Ltd.

## Glossary

**Cytopathic effect (CPE)** Damage caused in cultured cells due to insult such as infection with virus.

**Genogroup** Grouping of virus isolates within a species based on genetic data, such as nucleotide sequences and phylogenetic analyses.

**Novirhabdovirus** A member of the taxonomic genus *Novirhabdovirus*, within the family *Rhabdoviridae*. This genus contains many important fish rhabdoviruses.

**Nucleocapsid** For a rhabdovirus, the inner structure of the virion comprised of the viral genomic RNA wrapped in nucleocapsid (N) protein with associated phosphoprotein (P) and polymerase (L) proteins.

**Spill-over and spill-back events** Transmission of pathogens, and consequently disease, between wild and cultured populations of animals (in this case, fish).

**Vesiculovirus** A member of the taxonomic genus *Vesiculovirus*, within the family *Rhabdoviridae*. This genus currently contains only mammalian rhabdoviruses but several fish rhabdoviruses are very closely related to this genus.

## Introduction

Some of the most significant viral pathogens of fish are members of the family *Rhabdoviridae*. The viruses in this large and important group cause losses in populations of wild fish as well as among fish reared in aquaculture. While many of the best known fish rhabdoviruses produce acute disease and high mortality, others have been isolated from chronic or asymptomatic infections. Fish rhabdoviruses

often have a wide host and geographic range, and infect aquatic animals in both freshwater and seawater.

The diseases caused by fish rhabdoviruses are generally characterized as acute, hemorrhagic septicemias affecting multiple organs. Death is usually due to organ failure and subsequent loss of osmoregulation. In addition to petechial hemorrhages, gross signs include accumulation of ascites, darkening, and exopthalmia. Internally, necrosis of multiple organs is evident upon histological examination. Mortality is frequently highest in younger fish and can be explosive in aquaculture settings, resulting in losses approaching 100% in some cases. Fish that survive infection typically develop protective immunity. Transmission of fish rhabdoviruses occurs both horizontally between fish, and vertically through egg-associated transmission from an infected adult to its progeny. The role of long-term carriers and reservoirs is an area requiring further research.

Understanding of fish rhabdovirus infections improved significantly following the establishment of a variety of fish cell lines, beginning in the 1960s. Infection of cultured cell lines produces typical cytopathic effects (CPEs) consisting of cell rounding and necrosis following the release of mature virions by budding. The rate of the appearance of CPE is related to the incubation temperature, which is typically set to mirror the temperature optimum for the fish host (e.g., 10–25 °C). Highly reproducible laboratory challenge models have been developed for several important fish rhabdoviruses and their principal hosts. These tools have been used extensively to further our understanding of host–pathogen relationships and the role of environmental factors such as temperature on the virus replication cycle and the disease process.

The rhabdoviruses recovered from fish and described in the literature comprise a diverse collection of isolates (**Table 1**). Those studied in detail have been assigned to one of two quite different groups: isolates that are members, or likely members, of the established genus,

**Table 1** Fish rhabdoviruses from the published literature and their status in the *Eighth Report of the International Committee on Taxonomy of Viruses* (ICTV). Virus names shown as indented are isolates described in the literature that are either now considered to be indistinguishable from a recognized species (indicated in parentheses), or those that appear to be similar to the virus directly above but require further characterization

| Named virus | Abbreviation | Status in 8th ICTV |
| --- | --- | --- |
| **I. Species and tentative species in the genus *Novirhabdovirus*** | | |
| *Infectious hematopoietic necrosis virus* | IHNV | Type species of the genus |
|    Oregon sockeye virus (IHNV) | OSV | |
|    Sacramento River Chinook virus (IHNV) | SRCV | |
| *Viral hemorrhagic septicemia virus* | VHSV | Formal species in genus |
|    Egtved virus (VHSV) | | |
|    Brown trout rhabdovirus (VHSV) | | |
|    Cod ulcus syndrome rhabdovirus (VHSV) | | |
|    Carpione brown trout rhabdovirus (VHSV) | 583 | |
| *Hirame rhabdovirus* | HIRRV | Formal species in genus |
| *Snakehead virus* | SHRV | Formal species in genus |
| Eel virus B12 | EEV-B12 | Tentative species in genus |
| Eel virus C26 | EEV-C26 | Tentative species in genus |
| **II. Vesiculovirus-like viruses from fishes** | | |
| Spring viremia of carp virus | SVCV | Tentative species in genus |
|    Swim bladder inflammation virus (SVCV) | SBI | |
| Pike fry rhabdovirus | PFRV | Tentative species in genus |
|    Grass carp rhabdovirus | GCV | None |
|    Tench rhabdovirus | | None |
| Eel virus American | EVA | Tentative species in genus |
|    Eel virus European X | EVEX | None |
|    Eel virus C30, B44 and D13 | C30, B44, D13 | None |
|    *Rhabdovirus anguilla* | None | |
| Ulcerative disease rhabdovirus | UDRV | Tentative species in genus |
| Perch rhabdovirus | | None |
|    Pike perch rhabdovirus | | None |
|    Pike rhabdovirus | DK5533 | None |
|    Grayling rhabdovirus | | None |
| European lake trout rhabdovirus | 903/87 | None |
|    Swedish sea trout rhabdovirus | SSTV | None |
| Starry flounder virus | SFRV | None |
| **III. Incompletely characterized fish rhabdoviruses** | | |
| Rio Grande cichlid virus | | Unassigned animal rhabdovirus |
| *Siniperca chuatsi* rhabdovirus | SCRV | None |
| *Scophthalmus maximus* rhabdovirus | SMRV | None |

*Novirhabdovirus*, and those fish rhabdovirus isolates that are most similar to members of the genus *Vesiculovirus* (**Figure 1**). Formal species names have been assigned to only four fish rhabdoviruses, all within the genus *Novirhabdovirus*, while several others are recognized as tentative members of a genus. There are also several partially characterized or unusual isolates that have been reported as rhabdoviruses based largely on their characteristic bullet-shaped morphology in electron micrographs. Upon further study, some of the fish rhabdo-viruses listed in **Table 1** may be shown to be the same virus species.

## Novirhabdoviruses of Fish

The genus *Novirhabdovirus* was established in 1998, and includes four official species as shown in **Table 1**.

Infectious hematopoietic necrosis virus (IHNV) and viral hemorrhagic septicemia virus (VHSV) are economically significant viruses that cause epidemics in salmonid fish. IHNV is endemic in salmonids of northwestern North America and has become established in Europe and Asia through historical aquaculture-related activities. VHSV was originally known as a major pathogen of trout in Western Europe, but in recent years it has also been revealed as a relatively ubiquitous pathogen of numerous species of marine fish in both the Pacific and Atlantic Oceans. Hirame rhabdovirus (HIRRV) and snakehead rhabdovirus (SHRV) are important pathogens of cultured fish in Asia. Hirame rhabdovirus has been isolated from several species of wild and cultured marine fish suffering from a hemorrhagic septicemia. In Japan and Korea, HIRRV causes economically significant disease, especially in cultured Japanese flounder (hirame). Snakehead rhabdovirus has been isolated from both wild and

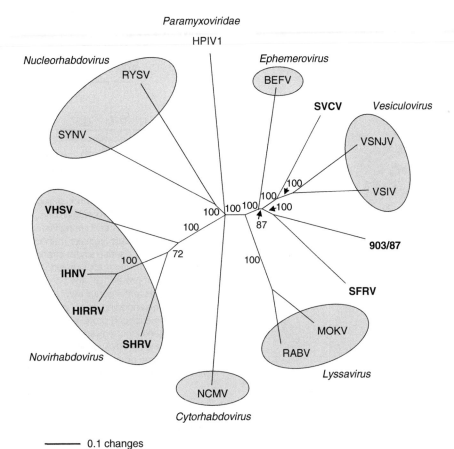

——— 0.1 changes

**Figure 1** Phylogenetic tree showing the relationship of fish rhabdoviruses (in bold) with other representative members of the family *Rhabdoviridae*. Partial polymerase protein sequences comprising ∼460 amino acids at the N-terminus of the L protein were used in a neighbor-joining distance program. Two groups of fish rhabdoviruses are shown either as members of the genus *Novirhabdovirus* or as vesiculovirus-like isolates. Abbreviations used are: BEFV, bovine ephemeral fever virus; SVCV, spring viremia of carp virus; VSNJV, vesicular stomatitis New Jersey virus; VSIV, vesicular stomatitis Indiana virus; 903/87, European lake trout rhabdovirus; SFRV, starry flounder rhabdovirus; MOKV, Mokola virus; RABV, rabies virus; NCMV, northern cereal mosaic virus; SHRV, snakehead virus; HIRRV, hirame rhabdovirus; IHNV, infectious hematopoietic necrosis virus; VHSV, viral hemorrhagic septicemia virus; SYNV, sonchus yellow net virus; RYSV, rice yellow stunt virus. The paramyxovirus human parainfluenza virus 1 (HPIV-1) was used as the outgroup. Phylogenetic analysis used 1000 bootstrapped data sets, and nodes with bootstrap values less than 70% were collapsed to polytomies.

cultured snakehead in Southeast Asia where it causes a severe ulcerative disease. These four viruses have all been well studied, and each one has been developed as an important research model for studies of various aspects of fish rhabdovirus molecular biology. In addition to these formal species in the genus, there are two tentative members that have been isolated from eel, but these and several other fish rhabdoviruses reported in the literature are less well characterized.

The virions of novirhabdoviruses have the typical bullet-shaped morphology of rhabdoviruses and are *c.* 150–190 nm in length and 65–75 nm in diameter (**Figure 2(a)**). Virions are comprised of five viral proteins. The single glycoprotein (G) on the surface of enveloped virus particles has been shown to be a major antigenic protein that is, by itself, capable of eliciting a protective immune response. The matrix protein (M) is an inner

component of the virions that binds both the cytoplasmic domain of the G protein and the viral nucleocapsid and, for IHNV, has been shown to downregulate host transcription. The major structural component of the nucleocapsid is the viral nucleocapsid (N) protein that associates with full-length viral genomic RNA and facilitates its interaction with the viral polymerase. The large polymerase protein (L) is a complex protein that carries out most of the enzymatic functions of genome replication and transcription. The phosphoprotein (P) is an essential cofactor that is required for polymerase function. These five virion proteins are found in all known rhabdoviruses and, to date, it appears that their roles are conserved across genera. In addition to these familiar rhabdovirus proteins, the hallmark of the novirhabdoviruses is the presence of a sixth protein, the nonvirion (NV) protein, which has not yet been identified in any rhabdovirus of another genus. The

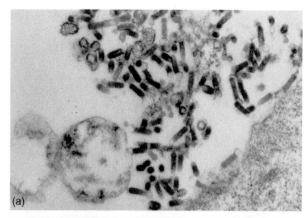

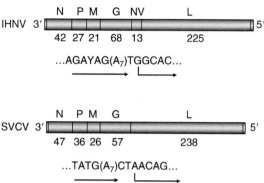

**Figure 3**　Genome organization of representatives of the two major subgroups of fish rhabdoviruses. IHNV represents the genus *Novirhabdovirus* and spring viremia of carp virus (SVCV) represents the vesiculovirus-like rhabdoviruses of fish. Both have negative-sense single-stranded RNA genomes of c. 11 000 nt containing nucleocapsid (N), phosphoprotein (P), matrix (M), glycoprotein (G), and polymerase (L) genes as shown. Species in the genus *Novirhabdovirus* have an additional gene encoding an NV protein. Approximate sizes (in kDa) of the encoded proteins are shown below each gene. Conserved gene junction sequences for each virus are shown in positive-sense (mRNA) orientation below the genome with arrows indicating putative transcription stop (ending with seven A's) and start signals.

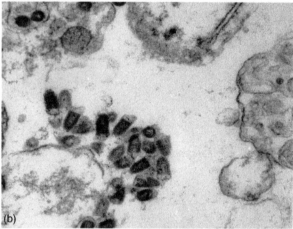

**Figure 2**　Electron micrograph showing a representative member of each of the two groups of fish rhabdoviruses. (a) *Viral hemorrhagic septicemia virus*, a species in the genus, *Novirhabdovirus*. (b) Starry flounder rhabdovirus, a vesiculovirus-like rhabdovirus of fish. Scale = 200 nm (a, b).

NV protein is not found in virus particles, but it is synthesized, often in only trace amounts, within infected cells. The presence of an apparently functional NV gene is conserved in all novirhabdovirus isolates examined to date, but the role of this protein is not well defined. Through the use of reverse genetics, it has been shown that the NV gene and its encoded protein product are not essential for replication in cultured cells or in fish, but in some cases it enhances replication and pathogenicity.

Fish rhabdovirus replication occurs in the cytoplasm of infected cells by processes common to all rhabdoviruses. During the replication cycle the viral RNA-dependent RNA polymerase (L) transcribes individual mRNAs for each viral gene, and also copies the RNA genome to produce progeny genomes. Viral mRNAs are translated into viral proteins that traffic to the outer cell membrane where assembly with viral genomic RNA occurs and budding through the cell membrane releases new enveloped virus particles. All novirhabdovirus genomes are single-stranded minus-sense RNA molecules *c.* 11 000 nt in length. The genome organization is conserved across the genus, and is

shown for the type species *Infections hematopoietic necrosis virus* in **Figure 3**. The six viral genes occur in the order 3′-N-P-M-G-NV-L-5′. This is identical to the genome organization of members of the genera *Vesiculovirus* and *Lyssavirus*, with the exception of the additional NV gene at the G-L junction. The genome termini have complementary leader and trailer regions of approximately 50–60 and 40–115 nt, respectively. The untranscribed, intergenic regions are single nucleotides, typically A or T, at all gene junctions except for the G-NV junction, which is slightly more variable. Putative transcription start and stop signals for each gene, shown in **Figure 3**, are highly conserved among individual genes. They are also conserved among novirhabdovirus species and differ from the conserved regulatory sequences of rhabdoviruses in other genera.

Genetic diversity within novirhabdovirus species has been well characterized for IHNV and VHSV. Genetic typing of hundreds of IHNV field isolates from North America, as well as from Europe, Russia, and Asia, has shown surprisingly low diversity, with a maximum of 9% nucleotide sequence diversity in a relatively variable region of the G gene. Despite this overall low diversity, genetic typing clearly resolves IHNV isolates into three major genogroups that correlate with their geographic origin in North America. Similar typing of extensive global collections of VHSV isolates has revealed much greater diversity, with up to 16% nucleotide diversity in full-length G gene sequences, and four phylogenetic subgroups that also correlate with geographic range.

For both the IHNV and VHSV subphylogenies, additional studies with partial nucleocapsid (N) gene sequences have confirmed the genogroups defined by partial G gene analyses. Diversity between species of novirhabdoviruses can be illustrated with full G protein amino acid sequences. Within the genus, IHNV and HIRRV are most closely related with 74% identity (83% similarity) in their G proteins. Within the entire genus, the G proteins of the four member species are more divergent, with as little as 37% identity (54% similarity). Comparisons outside the genus reveal 13–23% identity (27–48% similarity) between the G proteins of novirhabdoviruses and the fish vesiculovirus-like isolates or members of other rhabdovirus genera.

## Vesiculovirus-Like Viruses of Fish

At present, no fish rhabdoviruses are accepted as formal species within the genus *Vesiculovirus*, but many rhabdoviruses isolated from fish are clearly closely related to members of this genus, and distinct from the members of the genus *Novirhabdovirus*. Some vesiculovirus-like fish rhabdoviruses are considered tentative species in the genus *Vesiculovirus* (**Table 1**). The best studied vesiculo-like fish rhabdovirus is spring viremia of carp virus (SVCV), which has a long history of causing severe epidemics among cultured carp in Europe. SVCV is well characterized at both the biological and molecular levels, and it is considered the representative of the vesiculovirus-like fish rhabdoviruses. Full-length genome sequences are available for several strains of SVCV, and numerous other isolates are partially sequenced, facilitating phylogenetic analyses that confirm its close relationship to the mammalian vesiculoviruses. Many isolates of a similar virus, pike fry rhabdovirus, have also been described, and several other fish rhabdoviruses have been isolated from various cold- and warm-water hosts including various species of eel, snakehead, trout, and perch. By serological assays and phylogenetic analyses, at least some of these isolates appear to be distinct vesiculo-like viral species. Phylogenetic trees of partial G or L gene sequences indicate that these isolates form an emerging cluster of tentative species around the mammalian genus *Vesiculovirus*, as illustrated in **Figure 1**. Future work by the ICTV will likely establish some formal species among the vesiculo-like fish rhabdoviruses and clarify whether they should be accepted as members of the genus *Vesiculovirus*.

Virions of the fish vesiculo-like rhabdoviruses are typically shorter and wider than novirhabdoviruses, with bullet-shaped particles measuring *c.* 80–150 nm in length and 60–90 nm in diameter (**Figure 2(b)**). Particles are composed of five viral proteins that correspond to the five major virion proteins found in all rhabdoviruses. The virus replication cycle roles of the N, P, M, G, and L proteins are as described above for novirhabdoviruses. Among fish rhabdoviruses, the distinguishing feature of the fish vesiculo-like viruses is the absence of an NV gene at the G–L junction, indicating that, whatever the role of the NV protein in novirhabdoviruses, it is not essential for rhabdovirus replication in fish *per se*.

The negative-sense RNA genome of SVCV is just over 11 000 nt in length, and it has genes encoding the five major viral proteins in the same order found in all rhabdovirus genomes (**Figure 3**). The upstream untranslated region of each gene is a conserved 10 nt sequence and the downstream untranslated regions are more variable. The 3′ and 5′ termini of the genome have complementary leader and trailer regions of *c.* 20–60 and 12–20 nt, respectively. The untranscribed, intergenic regions between genes are dinucleotides, which, for SVCV, are all CT with the exception of the G–L junction that has the tetranucleotide CTAT. Putative transcriptional start and stop signals, shown in **Figure 3**, are highly conserved among individual genes and among SVCV isolates. These regulatory signals at the SVCV gene junctions are nearly identical to those of mammalian virus members of the genus *Vesiculovirus*, and they differ from the regulatory sequences conserved among members of other rhabdovirus genera, including novirhabdoviruses. As an example of the levels of sequence similarity, the SVCV G protein has 31–33% amino acid sequence identity (52–53% similarity) with the G proteins of members of the genus *Vesiculovirus*, but only 19–24% identity (40–47% similarity) with G proteins of 11 rhabdoviruses from all other genera including *Novirhabdovirus*. Among several viruses reported as isolates of SVCV, partial G gene nucleotide sequences have 83–100% identity, and phylogenetic analyses resolved four genogroups that correlated with geographic origin in Eurasia. Among SVCV and other tentative species of fish vesiculo-like rhabdoviruses, partial G or L gene nucleotide sequences typically have 70–80% identity.

## Fish Rhabdovirus Detection and Control

Because the diseases caused by fish rhabdoviruses are important to aquaculture, diagnostic methods for the detection and identification of the most significant pathogens are well established. Many cultured cell lines derived from finfish support the replication of a broad range of fish rhabdoviruses and are used routinely in cell culture-based assays to detect the presence of infections or to quantify infectious virus. Serological methods using polyclonal or monoclonal antibodies are used for both diagnostics and research, and molecular techniques such as DNA probes, polymerase chain reaction (PCR) assays, and quantitative polymerase chain reaction (qPCR) assays have been developed for confirmatory diagnosis, identification, and quantification of the most significant rhabdoviruses affecting fish. In many regions of North America, Europe, and Asia, the majority of all cultured fish stocks are surveyed on a regular basis for viral pathogens by fish health professionals.

Understanding the potential impacts of fish rhabdovirus infections on the health of native species and fish reared in aquaculture has led to increased attention to biosecurity and in measures to prevent the spread of aquatic animal diseases. During the mid-1900s, the inadvertent spread of several fish rhabdoviruses by movement of infected eggs or juvenile fish was responsible for several intercontinental introductions of pathogens with serious economic impacts. National and international standards now require health inspections for certain fish species prior to international or interstate transport. Several fish rhabdoviruses are on the list of pathogens for which inspections are required. The global trade in aquaculture species is reasonably well regulated. However, the huge global trade in ornamental fish is essentially unregulated and is a documented source of transboundary virus movement.

Considerable attention has also been given to improving methods for the control or prevention of aquatic animal diseases. These include sound management practices such as improved sanitation, the use of pathogen-free well water sources for early life-stage rearing, the installation of water treatment technologies for facilities using large volumes of water from open sources, and more frequent fish health inspections that make use of improved technologies. In aquaculture settings, the ability to break the cycle of vertical transmission between generations by the disinfection of eggs with an iodine solution has been an important control approach for fish rhabdoviruses.

Research on vaccines to protect fish from rhabdovirus infections has been conducted for more than 30 years. Initially, this work focused on traditional approaches including inactivated viruses or live-modified vaccines. Later, recombinant DNA technology produced experimental vaccines using bacterial or baculovirus expression systems as well as peptide immunogens. While some of these traditional and molecular vaccines were reported to be highly efficacious in both laboratory and field trials, prohibitive development and licensing costs, inconsistent efficacy, or safety concerns have prevented their use on a commercial scale. More recently, DNA vaccines have been engineered for protecting fish against the novirhabdoviruses, IHNV, VHSV, and HIRRV. These vaccines have been studied extensively and show exceptionally high efficacy against severe viral challenges under a wide range of conditions. An IHNV DNA vaccine was licensed for use in Canada in 2005. With regulatory concerns and vaccine delivery methods currently being addressed, it is possible that these will be among the first DNA vaccines to be used commercially for preventative veterinary care.

## Current Aspects

The number of reported fish rhabdoviruses continues to grow as a result of the growth of aquaculture, the increase in global trade, the development of improved diagnostic methods, and the expansion of surveillance activities. The increase in nucleotide sequence information available for many fish rhabdoviruses has not only improved our understanding of the genetic diversity among members of the group, but also complicated our ability to form neat taxonomic categories. Upon further analysis, the creation of several new virus species and, possibly, genera may be needed to accommodate the range of fish rhabdoviruses, particularly the unassigned or less well characterized members of the family.

Due to their economic importance, the rhabdoviruses of finfish are among the best studied of all aquatic animal viruses, providing models for their function, movement, and persistence in the environment. There is an increasing understanding that rhabdoviruses are important pathogens of wild or free-ranging fish in both freshwater and marine ecosystems. Extensive oceanographic surveys have revealed marine fish as important reservoirs for virus infections of fish in freshwater and marine aquaculture. In addition to causing natural mortality that may limit population size, anthropogenic stressors can act synergistically to amplify the effects of disease on the overall health and survival of aquatic species. Field studies of the relatively unique disease interface between cultured and wild aquatic host populations are providing insight into virus spill-over and spill-back events, and anthropogenic impacts on fish health in altered environments.

Fish rhabdoviruses are also serving as useful components of model systems to study vertebrate virus disease, epidemiology, and immunology. The availability of a variety of established fish cell lines, the creation of new-generation reagents and tools, and the well-established laboratory challenge models that can use statistically robust numbers of trout, catfish, or zebrafish make these model systems particularly attractive and powerful. Recent work includes the use of DNA vaccines against fish rhabdoviruses in mechanistic studies to determine how DNA vaccines elicit strong innate and adaptive immune responses in vertebrate hosts. Reverse genetics systems for both IHNV and SHRV have been developed and used to investigate the roles of individual viral genes and proteins. These studies have already shown that the G genes of different fish rhabdovirus species can be interchanged, and that the NV gene is not essential for virus replication. In the area of immunology, quantitative real-time PCR assays and microarray analyses have been used to profile the fish immune gene response following either viral infection or DNA vaccination. Future work will include the use of these models to address questions such as the genetics of host disease resistance, viral host specificity and virulence, viral fitness and competition, and host immune selection as a driver of virus evolution.

*See also:* Fish Viruses; Vesicular Stomatitis Virus.

## Further Reading

Ahne W, Bjorklund HV, Essbauer S, Fijan N, Kurath G, and Winton JR (2002) Spring viremia of carp (SVC). *Diseases of Aquatic Organisms* 52: 261–272.

Betts AM, Stone DM, Way K, *et al.* (2003) Emerging vesiculo-type virus infections of freshwater fish in Europe. *Diseases of Aquatic Organisms* 57: 201–212.

Bjorklund HV, Higman KH, and Kurath G (1996) The glycoprotein genes and gene junctions of the fish rhabdoviruses spring viremia of carp virus and hirame rhabdovirus: Analysis of relationships with other rhabdoviruses. *Virus Research* 42: 65–80.

Bootland LM and Leong JC (1999) Infectious hematopoietic necrosis virus. In: Woo PTK and Bruno DW (eds.) *Fish Diseases and Disorders, Vol. 3: Viral, Bacterial and Fungal Infections*, pp 57–121. New York: CABI.

Bremont M (2005) Reverse genetics on fish rhabdoviruses: Tools to study the pathogenesis of fish rhabdoviruses. *Current Topics in Microbiology and Immunology* 292: 119–141.

Einer-Jensen K, Ahrens P, Forsberg R, and Lorenzen N (2004) Evolution of the fish rhabdovirus viral haemorrhagic septicaemia virus. *Journal of General Virology* 85: 1167–1179.

Hoffmann B, Beer M, Schutze H, and Mettenleiter TC (2005) Fish rhabdoviruses: Molecular epidemiology and evolution. *Current Topics in Microbiology and Immunology* 292: 81–117.

Kim D-H, Oh H-K, Eou J-I, *et al.* (2005) Complete nucleotide sequence of the hirame rhabdovirus, a pathogen of marine fish. *Virus Research* 107: 1–9.

Kurath G (2005) Overview of recent DNA vaccine development for fish. In: Midtlyng PJ (ed.) *Fish Vaccinology, Developments in Biologicals*, vol. 121, pp. 201–213. Basel: Karger.

Kurath G, Garver KA, Troyer RM, Emmenegger EJ, Einer-Jensen K, and Anderson ED (2003) Phylogeography of infectious haematopoietic necrosis virus in North America. *Journal of General Virology* 84: 803–814.

Smail DA (1999) Viral haemorrhagic septicaemia. In: Woo PTK and Bruno DW (eds.) *Fish Diseases and Disorders, Vol. 3: Viral, Bacterial and Fungal Infections*, pp 123–147. New York: CABI.

Snow M, Bain N, Black J, *et al.* (2004) Genetic population structure of marine viral haemorrhagic septicaemia virus (VHSV). *Diseases of Aquatic Organisms* 61: 11–21.

Stone DM, Ahne W, Sheppard AM, *et al.* (2002) Nucleotide sequence analysis of the glycoprotein gene of putative spring viraemia of carp viruses and pike fry rhabdovirus isolates reveals four distinct piscine vesiculovirus genogroups. *Diseases of Aquatic Organisms* 53: 203–210.

Tordo N, Benmansour A, Calisher C, *et al.* (2004) Family *Rhabdoviridae*. In: Fauquet CM, Mayo MA, Maniloff J, Desselberger U, and Ball LA (eds.) *Virus Taxonomy: Eighth Report of the International Committee on Taxonomy of Viruses*, pp. 623–644. San Diego, CA: Elsevier Academic Press.

Wolf K (1988) *Fish Viruses and Fish Viral Diseases*. Ithaca, NY: Cornell University Press.

# Fish Viruses

**J C Leong,** University of Hawaii at Manoa, Honolulu, HI, USA

## Glossary

**Anadromous** Migrating from the sea to freshwater to spawn.

**Cardiomyopathy** A weakening of the heart muscle or a change in heart muscle structure.

**Salmonid** Belonging to, or characteristic of the family Salmonidae which includes the salmon trout and whitefish.

**Swimbladder** An air-filled sac near the spinal cord in many fishes that helps maintain buoyancy.

## Introduction

Viruses that infect fish and cause disease are represented in 14 of the families listed for vertebrate viruses by the International Committee on the Taxonomy of Viruses (27 May 2005). The fish viruses containing DNA genomes are listed in the families *Iridoviridae*, *Adenoviridae*, and *Herpesvirdae* and those with RNA genomes are listed in the families *Picornaviridae*, *Birnaviridae*, *Reoviridae*, *Rhabdoviridae*, *Orthomyxoviridae*, *Paramyxoviridae*, *Caliciviridae*, *Togaviridae*, *Nodaviridae*, *Retroviridae*, and *Coronaviridae*. As more fish species are brought under culture, there will be additions to this list, and possibly new viruses will be assigned to families not previously characterized in vertebrates.

Viral diseases have had a tremendous economic impact on both wild and farm-reared fish. A herpesvirus outbreak in 1998 and early 1999 reduced the pilchard (*Sardinops sagax neophilchardus*) fishery in southern Australia by two-thirds. In 2001, infectious salmon anemia virus (ISAV) was discovered in cultured Atlantic salmon in Cobscook Bay, Maine. The discovery of this orthomyxovirus virus forced farmers to destroy about 2.6 million fish in an effort to contain the spread of the disease. The cost to the Maine salmon industry (valued at more than $100 million) was about $24 million (USDA Animal and Plant Health Inspections Service (APHIS) estimates).

**Table 1**    Diseases of fish listed by the OIE, 2006

| | |
|---|---|
| Epizootic hematopoietic necrosis | Iridovirus |
| Infectious hematopoietic necrosis | Novirhabdovirus |
| Spring viremia of carp | Vesiculovirus |
| Viral hemorrhagic septicemia | Novirhabdovirus |
| Infectious salmon anemia | Orthomyxovirus |
| Epizootic ulcerative syndrome | Fungal infection |
| Gyrodactyloses | Flat worm fluke |
| Red sea bream iridovirus diseases | Iridovirus |
| Koi herpesvirus disease | Herpesvirus |

More recently, the rhabdovirus viral hemorrhagic septicemia virus (VHSV), a very serious pathogen of marine and freshwater fish in Europe, was detected in the Great Lakes of North America in 2005. On 24 October 2006, APHIS issued an emergency order that blocked the live export of 37 fish species from any of the eight Great Lakes states. The order caused strong protests from fish farmers who make their living with live bait shipments and fish-stocking programs that sustain the Great Lakes' $4.5 billion fishing industry. Since vaccines and/or therapeutics for fish viruses are not readily available, containing the spread of these viruses by restricting movement and destruction of the affected population has been the only effective control strategy. Thus, the World Animal Health Organization (OIE) lists nine reportable diseases of fish (**Table 1**), seven of which are viral diseases.

Known and characterized fish viruses numbered only 16 in 1981, with an additional 11 observed by electron microscopy. Now, there are over 125 described viruses of fish and countless reports of electron microscopic observations of viruses in wild-caught and cultured fish. The dramatic increase in reports of new fish viruses correlates with growth of the aquaculture industry that has increased production more than fivefold since 1985 to now represent more than 30% of global fishery production.

## RNA Viruses of Fish

### Rhabdoviridae

Fish rhabdoviruses are considered among the most serious viral pathogens of aquacultured fish, affecting predominantly salmon and trout. The first fish rhabdovirus was described in 1938 by Schaperclaus in European rainbow trout and, 6 years later, the Sacramento River Chinook virus was reported by Rucker. Since then, these viruses have been isolated, grown in tissue culture cells, and the genomes have been cloned and sequenced. The salmon virus is now called *Infectious hematopoietic necrosis virus* (IHNV) which is the type species for a new genus *Novirhabdovirus* in the *Rhabdoviridae*. Other fish rhabdovirus species assigned to this genus include *Viral hemorrhagic septicemia virus* (VHSV), *Hirame rhabdovirus* (HIRRV), and *Snakehead rhabdovirus* (SHRV). All of these viruses have

negative-sense ssRNA genomes with a physical map ordered from the 3'-end as follows: leader-N-P-M-G-NV-L, where N is the nucleoprotein gene, P is the phosphoprotein gene, M is the matrix protein gene, G is the glycoprotein gene, NV is the nonvirion protein gene, and L is the virion RNA polymerase gene. The presence of the NV gene distinguishes the rhabdoviruses in the genus *Novirhabdovirus*, 'novi' standing for nonvirion.

Reverse genetic analysis of the IHNV, SHRV, and VHSV NV genes has, to date, provided mixed results. For IHNV and VHSV, deletion of the NV gene ameliorated virus-induced cytopathic effect (CPE) in tissue culture cells and reduced pathogenicity in fish. However, deletion of the NV gene for SHRV did not affect virus production or virus-induced CPE in tissue culture cells, or reduce pathogenicity in live fish challenges.

IHNV is a virus of salmonid fish and outbreaks of this virus in rainbow trout (*Oncorhynchus mykiss*), sockeye salmon (*O. nerka*), Chinook salmon (*O. tshawytscha*), Atlantic salmon (*Salmo salar*), and masou salmon (*O. masou*) have been economically devastating to the fish farmers. This virus prefers colder temperatures with optimal growth at 8–15 °C. VHSV is also a serious pathogen of salmonid fish, but its host range is broader and it has been shown to kill Pacific herring (*Clupea pallasi*), Pacific cod (*Gadus macrocephalus*), whitefish (*Coregonus* sp.), European sea bass (*Dicentrarchus labrax*), and turbot (*Scophthalmus maximus*). This broad host range has caused a great deal of concern to authorities in the USA since VHSV was first reported there in 2006 and found to affect freshwater drum (*Aplodinotus grunniens*), round goby (*Neogobius melanostomus*), smallmouth bass (*Micropterus dolomieu*), bluegill (*Lepomis machrochirus mystacalis*), crappie (*Pomoxis nigromaculatus*), gizzard shard (*Dorosoma cepadianum*), and other species occurring in the Great Lakes. HIRRV affects hirame, the Japanese flounder (*Paralychthys olivaceus*), which is a highly prized food fish in Japan. Its host range includes ayu (*Pleuroglossus altivelis*) as well as salmonid fish. SHRV was isolated from snakehead fish (*Channa striatus*) suffering from epizootic ulcerative syndrome (EUS) in Thailand. It is not considered the etiologic agent of EUS which is caused by a fungal pathogen. However, zebrafish (*Brachydanio rerio*), exposed to tissue culture grown SHRV develop, will develop petechial hemorrhages and die.

Spring viremia of carp virus (SVCV), unlike the fish rhabdoviruses described above, does not contain an intervening gene between its glycoprotein and L genes. Analysis of the SVCV genome sequence indicates that it clusters with the members of the genus *Vesiculovirus* that includes vesicular stomatitis virus. SVCV was first identified as the etiologic agent of an acute hemorrhagic disease in common carp (*Cyprinus carpio*) in Europe in 1972. The disease has since been found in Asia, the Middle East, and most recently in South and North America. Outbreaks in the USA have raised concerns that indigenous fish species in the minnow family (*Cyprinidae*), some of which are endangered species, may be susceptible to SVCV. Other virus isolates that are closely related in nucleotide sequence to SVCV are the pike fry rhabdoviruses (PFRV) from a variety of freshwater fish in Europe including pike (*Esox lucius*), common bream (*Abramis brama*), roach (*Rutilus rutilus*), eel virus Europe X (EVEX), eel virus American (EVA); ulcerative disease rhabdovirus (UDRV); the grass carp rhabdovirus isolated from grass carp (*Ctenopharyngdon idella*); trout rhabdovirus 903/87 (TRV 903/87); and sea trout rhabdovirus 28/97 (STRV-28/97).

Phylogenetic analyses comparing aligned data for the N and G genes of members of the family *Rhabdoviridae* have confirmed the classification of the six genera: *Lyssavirus*, *Vesiculovirus*, *Ephemerovirus*, *Cytorhabdovirus*, *Nucleorhabdovirus*, and *Novirhabdovirus*. To date, fish rhabdoviruses are restricted to the genera *Novirhabdovirus* and *Vesiculovirus*. Analyses using the viral P gene sequences indicate that the aquatic vesiculoviruses form a separate cluster from the arthropod-borne vertebrate vesiculoviruses.

### Paramyxoviridae

The first description of a paramyxovirus-like virus in fish was reported in 1985. During a routine health assessment of Chinook salmon juveniles in Oregon, tissue culture cells inoculated with a cell-free homogenate of organ tissue exhibited syncytia formation. Electron micrographs of the infected cell line showed enveloped, pleomorphic virus particles with a diameter of approximately 125–250 nm and a single helical nucleocapsid with a diameter of 18 nm and a length of 100 nm. No disease syndrome was observed in trout and salmon fingerlings in subsequent infectivity trials with the tissue cultured virus. A second fish paramyxovirus that caused epidermal necrosis in juvenile black sea bream (*Acanthopargrus schlegeli*) was identified in Japan by electron microscopy. This virus was never cultured *in vitro*. The most recent description of a fish paramyxovirus was from Atlantic salmon post-smolts suffering from inflammatory gill disease in Norway. The genome of this virus has been cloned and partial sequences from the viral L protein have been used to determine the phylogenetic placement of this virus among the *Paramyxoviridae*. The Atlantic salmon paramyxovirus (ASPV) clustered with the subfamily *Paramyxovirinae*, in the genus *Respirovirus* that includes human parainfluenza virus and Sendai virus.

### Orthomyxoviridae

Infectious salmon anemia virus (ISAV) is the only fish orthomyxovirus that has been fully described to date. There are eight RNA segments in the ISAV genome. Segment 1 encodes PB2, a component of the virion RNA polymerase; segment 2 encodes PB1; segment 3, the nucleocapsid protein NP; segment 4, the RNA polymerase PA; segment 5, acetylcholinesterase P3 or fusion protein; segment 6, hemagglutinin; segment 7, protein P4 and P5; and segment 8, proteins P6 and P7. The proteins P4 and P5 may be the ISAV counterparts to the membrane proteins M1 and M2 of influenza A virus; proteins P6 and P7 may be related to the nonstructural proteins NS1 and NEP of influenza A virus. The ISAV hemagglutinin does agglutinate fish red blood cells or mammalian red blood cells.

A comparative sequence analysis of the PB1 gene of ISAV and other members of the *Orthomyxoviridae* led to its assignment as the type species of a new genus *Isavirus*. More recent comparative analyses of the fusion protein gene (segment 5) and the hemagglutinin gene (segment 7) indicate that ISAV isolates can be divided into two subtypes, a North American subtype and a European subtype.

ISAV causes a highly lethal disease with affected farmed Atlantic salmon displaying severe anemia, leucopenia, ascetic fluids, hemorrhagic liver necrosis, and petecchiae of the viscera. The virus also causes disease in sea trout (*Salmo trutta*), rainbow trout, and Atlantic herring.

### Picornaviridae

The first reported observation of picorna-like viruses in fish was made in 1988 from rainbow smelt (*Osmerus mordax*) in New Brunswick, Canada. Since then, picornaviruses have been isolated from barramundi, turbot, sea bass, grass carp, blue gill, grouper (*Epinephelus tauvina*), Japanese parrotfish (*Oplegnathus fasciatus*), and salmonid fish. In most of these descriptions, the presumptive characterization of the etiologic agent as a picornavirus was based on growth in tissue culture cells and the observation of crystalline arrays in the cytoplasm of small virus particles with a size and morphology consistent with picornaviruses. Analysis of RNA extracted from purified blue gill virus has indicated that it is single-stranded RNA virus. Sequence characterization of the viral genomes has not been carried out and there is some suggestion that at least some of these viruses might actually be betanodaviruses. In many cases, diseased fish infected with these viruses contain picorna-like virus particles in the brain and medulla and the victims display corkscrew-like swimming and eventually die.

### Nodaviridae

Members of the *Nodaviridae* that infect fish belong to the genus *Betanodavirus* for which the type species is *Striped jack nervous necrosis virus* (SJNNV). These viruses are nonenveloped with icosahedral symmetry and virion diameters of approximately 30 nm. The viral genome consists of two molecules of positive-sense ssRNA. RNA1, the largest RNA genome segment encodes the viral polymerase. RNA2 encodes the virion capsid protein. A third RNA, transcribed from the 3′ terminal region of

RNA1, encodes a 75 amino acid protein that bears little similarity with the B2 and B1 proteins encoded by a similar RNA3 in the alphanodaviruses. Despite this, the SJNNV B2 protein RNA has RNA silencing-suppression activity, as does the B2 protein of insect-infecting alphanodaviruses.

The betanodaviruses are the causative agents of viral nervous necrosis or viral encephalopathy and retinopathy in a variety of cultured marine fish. The disease affects young fish and produces a necrosis and vaculoation in the brain, spinal cord, and retina in most cases. It has been reported in striped jack (*Pseudocaranx dentex*), grouper (*Epinephelus* spp.), red drum (*Sciaenops ocellatus*), guppy (*Poicelia reticulate*), barfin flounder (*Verasper moseri*), red sea bream, tiger puffer (*Takifugu rubripes*), Japanese flounder, Atlantic halibut (*Hippoglossus hippoglossus*), amberjack (*Seriola dumerili*), sea bass, and barramundi. The recent detection of betanodaviruses in apparently healthy aquarium fish and invertebrates has raised concerns that the disease could be spread by trade in aquarium fish, particularly from Southeast Asia. Comparative sequence analyses of the coat protein genes for 25 isolates suggest that there are four genotypic variants: tiger puffer nervous necrosis virus (TPNNV), striped jack nervous necrosis virus (SJNNV), barfin flounder nervous necrosis virus (BFNNV), and red-spotted grouper nervous necrosis virus (RGNNV).

### Nidovirales

The family *Coronaviridae* comprises two genera, *Coronavirus* and *Torovirus*, and is classified with the families *Arteriviridae* and *Roniviridae* in the order *Nidovirales*. Members of the *Coronaviridae* share the common feature of pleomorphic, enveloped virions with diameters of 126–160 nm and prominent surface projections. The nucleocapsid is helical and contains a single molecule of linear, positive-sense ssRNA. Coronavirus-like particles have been isolated from a common carp from Japan showing petecchial hemorrhages on the skin and abdomen. A similar virus has also been isolated from moribund colored carp (*Cyprinus carpio*) with ulcerative dermal lesions. The investigators were able to grow the virus in epithelioma papulosum cyprini (EPC) cells and produce the same disease in carp injected with the tissue culture grown virus. Further characterization of these virus isolates was never carried out and there was no confirmation that they are, indeed, coronaviruses.

Recently, a novel virus with morphological features resembling those found in rhabdo-, corona-, and baculoviruses has been detected during the routine diagnostic screening of white bream (*Blicca bjoerkna*) in Germany. Ultrastructural studies indicated that the cell-free virions contain of a rod-shaped nucleocapsid similar to that seen in baculoviruses. Virions are bacilliform-shaped structures somewhat reminiscent of plant rhabdoviruses with an envelope containing coronavirus-like spikes. Sequence analysis has indicated that the 26.6 kbp white bream virus (WBV) contains five open reading frames, ORF1a, -1b, -2, -3, and -4, which are produced from a 'nested' set of 3'-coterminal mRNAs. The largest mRNA is of genome length. ORF1a and ORF1b form the viral replicase gene. ORF1a encodes several membrane domains, a putative ADP-ribose 1'-phospatase, and a chymotrypsin-like serine protease. ORF1b encodes the putative polymerase, helicase, ribose methyltransferase, exoribonuclease, and endoribonuclease activities. These characteristics are consistent with classification of WBV in the order *Nidovirales*. Phylogenetic analyses of the helicase and polymerase core domains indicate that WBV is more closely related to toroviruses than to coronaviruses and it has been suggested that a new nidovirus genus *Bafinivirus* be established (from bacilliform fish nidoviruses).

### Togaviridae

The family *Togaviridae* comprises the genera *Alphavirus* and *Rubivirus* among the vertebrate viruses. These viruses have spherical virions, 70 nm in diameter, with a lipid envelope containing glycoprotein peplomers and a ssRNA genome which is capped at the 5'-end and polyadenylated at the 3'-end. Salmonid alphaviruses (SAVs) cause mortality in salmon and trout in Europe (Norway, France, UK, and Ireland). At least three subtypes of SAV exist: Salmon pancreas disease virus (SPDV/SAV-1) in Atlantic salmon; sleeping disease virus (SDV/SAV-2) in rainbow trout; and Norwegian salmonid alphavirus (NSAV/SAV-3). An early study on the evolutionary relationships of the alphaviruses has indicated that SAVs represent a separate and distant group in the genus *Alphavirus*.

Pancreas disease, due to SPDV (SAV-1) infection, was first described in Scotland in Atlantic salmon. It occurs during the first year at sea following transfer of young fish from freshwater tanks. The fish become anorexic and exhibit sluggish swimming activity with mortality rates reaching 10–50%. Histological examination of the affected fish has shown pancreatic acinar necrosis, and cardiac and skeletal myopathy. In rainbow trout, SDV (SAV-2) infection is characterized by the unusual behavior that fish lie on their side at the bottom on the tank. The lesion responsible for this behavior is red and white muscle degeneration. The histological lesions are similar to those observed in SPDV infection with progressive pancreatic necrosis and atrophy, mulifocal cardiomyopathy and muscle degeneration.

### Caliciviridae

San Miguel sea lion virus (SMSV) is classified in the species *Vesicular exanthema of swine virus* in the genus *Vesivirus* in the family *Caliciviridae*. Investigators have found that the serotype 7 strain of the virus (SMSV-7), isolated from the opaleye fish (*Girella nigrigans*), can produce vesicular exanthema in swine. Thus, it is a virus that can jump from fish to mammals. The same serotype has also been reported in elephant seals and a sea lion trematode. Tissue culture grown serotype 5 SMSV injected into opaleye replicated to high titer 15 °C, producing $10^{7.6}$ TCID$_{50}$ per gram of spleen. There is no apparent disease in opaleye caused by this virus.

SMSV virions are nonenveloped with icosahedral symmetry and are 27–40 nm in diameter. The genome consists of a 7.5–8.0 kbp linear, positive-sense ssRNA that contains a covalently linked protein (VPg) attached to its 5′-end. The 3′-end of the genome is polyadenylated. The nonstructural polypeptides are encoded as a polyprotein in the 5′-end of the genomic RNA, while the single structural protein is encoded in the 3′-end. The identity of nonstructural polypeptides 2C (RNA helicase), 3C (cysteine protease), and 3D (RNA-dependent RNA polymerase) has been suggested by similarity to highly conserved amino acid motifs in the nonstructural proteins of the picornavirus superfamily. Phylogenetic analysis of the capsid protein region of caliciviruses including the Sapporo-like human caliciviruses indicate that the genus *Vesivirus* includes SMVL-1, SMSV-4, SMSV-13, SMSV-15, SMSV-17, three feline caliciviruses, and the primate calicivirus Pan-1. These viruses are distant from the human caliciviruses and the rabbit caliciviruses.

### Retroviridae

The family *Retroviridae* consists of two subfamilies, the *Orthoretrovirinae*, containing six genera, and the *Spumaretrovirinae*, containing only one genus. The piscine retroviruses constitute the genus *Epsilonretrovirus*, a genus established within the *Orthoretrovirinae* to include the piscine retroviruses: walleye dermal sarcoma virus (WDSV), walleye epidermal hyperplasia virus type 1 (WEHV-1), walleye epidermal hyperplasia virus type 2 (WEHV-2), and snakehead retrovirus (SnRV). The genomes of all of these viruses have been sequenced. There are also numerous reports of C-type (retrovirus-like) particles of about 110–150 nm in epidermal papillomas of European smelt (*Osmerus eperlanus*) and in cells cultured from neurofibromas of damselfish (*Pomacentrus partitus*). A retrovirus has also been suggested as the etiological agent of plasmacytoid leukemia in Chinook salmon.

The first report of a retrovirus-like agent in fish was made in 1976 in lymphosarcoma of northern pike and muskellunge (*Esox masquinongy*). The lymphosarcoma lesions contained a reverse transcriptase-like DNA polymerase with a temperature optimum of 20 °C. The first molecular evidence for a piscine retrovirus was reported in 1992 for a type C retrovirus from dermal sarcomas that form on the surface of adult walleye. These tumors are formed on the surface of adult walleye (*Stizostedion*

*vitreum*) in the fall and regress in the spring. The genome of the virus (13.2 kbp) was larger than all other known retroviruses at the time. Sequence analysis indicated that WDSV contained three additional open reading frames: ORF C at the 5′ terminal end; and ORF A and ORF B at the 3′ terminal end. ORF A encodes a D-cyclin homolog (retroviral cyclin) that locates in the nucleus of tumor cells in interchromatic granule clusters. ORF C encodes a cytoplasmic protein that targets the mitochondria and is associated with apoptosis. It is expressed in regressing tumors when full-length viral RNA is synthesized. The function of the protein encoded in ORF B, which is distantly related to ORF A, remains unknown. The WDSV protease cleavage sites have been identified to contain glutamine in the P2 position. The WDSV reverse transcriptase is rapidly inactivated at temperatures greater than 15 °C; a finding that is consistent with adaptation to growth in a coldwater fish species.

Two additional retroviruses have been cloned from epidermal hyperplasias on walleye. The genome sequences indicate that they are distinctly different from each other (77% identity) and from WDSV (64% identity). Walleye epidermal hyperplasia viruses 1 and 2 (WEHV-1 and -2) have genome organizations similar to WDSV. Each of the walleye retroviruses produces lesions when a cell-free filtrate from homogenized tumors is injected in naïve walleye juveniles.

Complete nucleotide sequence and transcriptional analyses of snakehead fish retrovirus have also been reported. The proviral genome is arranged in a typical 5′-LTR-gag-pol-env-LTR-3′ retrovirus organization. There are three additional ORFs: ORF1 encoding a 52 aa protein (5.7 kDa); ORF2 encoding a 94 aa protein (11 kDa); and ORF3 encoding a 205 aa protein (24 kDa). BLAST searches for possible homologs of these proteins have not produced any meaningful matches and their functions remain unknown. The SnRV genome differs from the retroviruses of walleye in that it has no ORF between the Unique region in the 5′ LTR (U5) and the gag region. The pathogenicity of SnRV has also not been determined.

In 2006, a novel piscine retrovirus was identified in association with an outbreak of leiomyosarcoma in the swimbladders of Atlantic salmon. The swimbladder sarcoma virus (SSSV) provirus is 10.9 kbp in length with a simple *gag, pro-pol, env* gene arrangement similar to that of murine leukemia viruses. Phylogenetic analysis of pol sequences suggests that SSV is most closely related to the sequenced zebrafish endogenous retrovirus (ZFERV) and that these viruses represent a new group of piscine retroviruses.

### Reoviridae

Reoviruses that infect aquatic animals are grouped in the genus *Aquareovirus* in the family *Reoviridae* and are characterized by a nonenveloped double capsid shell, 11 segments of double-stranded RNA and seven structural proteins. John Plumb isolated the first finfish reovirus, golden shiner virus, GSRV, from golden shiner (*Notemigonus crysoleucas*) in 1979. Since then, several reovirus-like agents have been reported in piscine, molluscan, and crustacean hosts. Each has 11 segments of dsRNA and grow at temperatures that reflect their host range. The aquareoviruses have been divided by RNA–RNA hybridization kinetics into six groups (A–F) and several tentative species (**Table 2**). The type species of the genus *Aquareovirus* is *Aquareovirus A* which includes striped bass (*Morone saxatilis*) reovirus (SBRV). Like other reoviruses, the aquareoviruses are ether resistant and resistant to acid to pH3.

Most aquareovirus isolates are nonpathogenic or of low virulence in their host species. Grass carp virus (GCV; species *Aquareovirus C*) is the exception and appears to be the most pathogenic aquareovirus. GCV was isolated from grass carp in the People's Republic of China, causing

**Table 2**    Species and tentative species of aquareoviruses

*Aquareovirus A*
  Angelfish reovirus AFRV
  Atlantic salmon reovirus HBR
  Atlantic salmon reovirus ASV
  Atlantic salmon reovirus TSV
  Chinook salmon reovirus DRC
  Chum salmon reovirus CSV
  Threadfin reovirus
  Herring reovirus HRV
  Masou salmon reovirus MSV
  Smelt reovirus
  Striped bass reovirus
*Aquareovirus B*
  Chinook salmon reovirus B
  Chinook salmon reovirus LBS
  Chinook salmon reovirus YRC
  Chinook salmon reovirus ICR
  Coho salmon reovirus CSR
  Coho salmon reovirus ELC
  Coho salmon reovirus SCS
*Aquareovirus C*
  Golden shiner reovirus[a]
  Grass carp reovirus
*Aquareovirus D*
  Channel catfish reovirus
*Aquareovirus E*
  Turbot reovirus
*Aquareovirus F*
  Chum salmon reovirus PSR
  Coho salmon reovirus SSR
Tentative species of Aquareoviruses
  Chub reovirus
  Landlocked salmon reovirus
  Tench reovirus

[a]Grass carp reovirus and Golden shiner reovirus are variants of the same virus. Table 2 taken from *ICTVdB-The Universal Virus Database*, version 4. http://www.ncbi.nlm.nih.gov/ICTVdb/ICTVdB.

severe hemorrhagic disease and affecting about 85% of infected fingerling and yearling populations.

Full-length and partial genome sequences for several members of the genus *Aquareovirus* have been reported. The complete sequence is available for several isolates of GCV, golden shiner reovirus (species *Aquareovirus C*), chum salmon (*O. keta*) reovirus (species *Aquareovirus A*), golden ide (*Leuciscus idus melanotus*) reovirus (tentative species), and striped bass reovirus (species *Aquareovirus A*). Segment 6 of the guppy reovirus has been determined and threadfin (*Eleutheronema tetradactylus*) reovirus (untyped) segments 10, 6, and 11 are available. Segment 1 encodes a putative guanylyl/methyl transferase; segment 2 encodes the RNA-dependent RNA polymerase; segment 3 encodes a dsRNA binding protein with NTPase and helicase activity; segment 4, a nonstructural protein; segment 5, a NTPase core protein; segment 6, the outer capsid protein; segment 7, a nonstructural protein; segment 8, a core protein; segment 9, a nonstructural protein; segment 10, the external capsid protein; and segment 11, a nonstructural protein. Phylogenetic comparisons of the available sequences support the current taxonomic classification of the aquareoviruses and orthoreoviruses in two different genera, a distinction that was made originally on their genome segment number and specific econiches.

## *Birnaviridae*

Members of the *Birnaviridae* have single-shelled nonenveloped capsids and genomes comprising two segments of double-stranded RNA. There are three genera in this family: *Aquabirnavirus*, *Avibirnavirus*, and *Entomobirnavirus*. The names of each genus denote the host specificity. The larger genome segment A encodes a polyprotein containing the virion capsid protein VP2, an autocatalytic protease NS, and an internal capsid protein VP3 in the physical order 5′-VP2-NS-VP3–3′ in the positive sense. There is an additional 17 kDa protein encoded in a second reading frame at the 5′-end of RNA segment A and it has been shown to be a novel anti-apoptosis gene of the Bcl-2 family. Segment B encodes the virus RNA-dependent RNA polymerase. There is no evidence of 5′-capping of any of the viral mRNAs.

The type species of the genus *Aquabirnavirus* is *Infectious pancreatic necrosis virus* (IPNV). Infectious pancreatic necrosis is a highly contagious viral disease of salmonid fish. The disease most characteristically occurs in fry of rainbow trout, brook trout (*Salvelinus fontinalis*), brown trout (*S. trutta*), Atlantic salmon, and several species of Pacific salmon. In salmonid fish, the virus causes an acute gastroenteritis and destruction of the pancreas. The signs of the disease are typically darkening, a pronounced distended abdomen, and a spiral swimming motion. The virus has also been associated with disease in Japanese eels (*Anguilla japonica*) in which it causes nephritis, menhaden (*Brevoortia tryrranus*) in which it causes a 'spinning disease', and in yellowtail fingerlings (*Seriola quinqueradiata*). A birnavirus has been associated with hematopoietic necrosis, causing high mortalities in turbot with renal necrosis, and birnaviruses have been isolated from clams exhibiting darkened gills and gill necrosis. A nontypical apoptosis has been observed in cultured cells infected by IPNV.

Transmission of the virus can occur via the feces of piscivorous birds. Fish that survive an IPNV outbreak become IPNV carriers and continue to shed the virus for life. Most IPNV isolates are antigenically related and belong to one large serogroup A. There is only one virus in serogroup B, a clam Tellina virus. More recent studies using comparisons of the deduced VP2 amino acid sequence have identified six genogroups. Genogroup 1 (equivalent to serotype A1) comprises four subgroups: genotypes 1, 2, 3, and 4. With increased culture of marine species of fish, there have been increasing reports of mortalities in yellow tail and amberjack in Japan from marine aquabirnaviruses.

Several vaccines have been developed for IPNV, including bacterially produced capsid protein and a DNA vaccine. The protein vaccine has been moderately effective in reducing the lethal effects of IPNV infection in Atlantic salmon in Norway. However, control methods still reply on quarantine and certification of eggs/fry as disease free.

## DNA Viruses of Fish

### Iridoviridae

In the family *Iridoviridae*, the genera *Iridovirus*, *Lymphocystivirus*, *Ranavirus*, and *Megalocystivirus* contain all of the known iridoviruses that infect fish. Their common features are icosahedral virions, 120–350 nm in diameter, that may acquire an envelope, and a viral genome consisting of one molecule of linear dsDNA of 100–303 kbp. Lymphocystis disease was one of the first fish diseases to be described due, in large part, to the characteristic giant cells observed in the connective tissue and benign nodules in the skin of plaice (*Pleuronectes platessa*) and flounder (*Platichthys flesus*). The causative agent, lymphocystis disease virus (LCDV), has been detected in more than 140 species of freshwater, estuarine, and marine fishes.

Six iridoviruses genomes have been completely sequenced, including those of the *Lymphocystis disease virus 1* (LCDV-1, genus *Lymphocystivirus*), Chilo iridescent virus (CIV, species *Invertebrate iridescent virus 6*, genus *Iridovirus*), Tiger frog virus (TFV, species *Frog 3 virus*, genus *Ranavirus*), *Infectious spleen and kidney necrosis virus* (ISKNV, genus *Megalocystivirus*), *Abystoma tigrinum virus* (ATV, genus *Ranavirus*), and Singapore grouper iridovirus (SGIV, tentative species, genus *Ranavirus*). Comparisons of the different iridovirus genomes have revealed that many genes have been conserved during evolution and, among closely related species, the gene order is well preserved. The number of genes (ORFs) in viruses of this family range from 93 (ATV) to 468 (CIV). There are 195 ORFs in LCDV-1 and 120 ORFs in GIV.

Other iridovirus diseases of fish include epizootic hematopoietic necrosis which is caused by viruses in the species *Epizootic hematopoietic necrosis virus* (EHNV, genus *Ranavirus*) in perch and rainbow trout, European sheatfish virus (ESV, genus *Ranavirus*) in sheatfish (*Silurus glanis*), and European catfish virus (ECV, genus *Ranavirus*) in catfish. ESV and ECV are classified as the same species, *European catfish virus*. Santee–Cooper ranavirus (SCRV) is the species name given to three iridoviruses: largemouth bass iridovirus (LMBV), doctor fish virus (DFV-16), and guppy virus (GV-6). The white sturgeon iridovirus group (WSIV) is comprised of a group of unassigned viruses that infect sturgeon in North America and Russian sturgeon (*Acipenser guldenstadi*) in Europe. Red seabream iridoviruses (RSIV) (genus *Megalocystivirus*) causes mortality in cultured juvenile red sea bream in Japan. It has also been observed in grouper in Thailand. Two goldfish iridovirus-like viruses (goldfish virus 1 and 2, GFV-1 and -2) have been isolated from swimbladder tissue culture of healthy goldfish. Electron microscopic observations of iridoviruses in the cytoplasm of erythrocytes (viral erythrocytic necrosis, VEN) have been observed in many marine and anadromous bony fish.

### Herpesviridae

Herpesviruses have been isolated from channel catfish (*Ictalurus punctatus*), common and koi carp (*C. carpio*), common goldfish (*Carassius auratus*), eel (*Anguilla* spp.), rainbow trout, masou salmon, lake trout (*S. namaycush*), sturgeon, walleye, and Japanese flounder. Channel catfish virus is the only fish herpesvirus assigned to the genus, *Ictalurivirus*, and this genus is not assigned to any of the three subfamilies (*Alphaherpesvirinae*, *Betaherpesvirinae*, and *Gammaherpesvirinae*) of the family *Herpesviridae*. The other fish herpesviruses, cyprinid herpesviruses 1 and 2 (CyHV-1 and CyHV-2), koi herpesvirus (CyHV-3), salmonid herpesvirus 1 and 2 (SalHV-1 and -2), eel herpesvirus (Anguilla herpesvirus, AngHV-1), and the acipenserid or white sturgeon herpesviruses remain as unassigned members of the family *Herpesviridae*. Electron micrographic evidence of herpesviruses has been found in sharks, eels, pike, flounder, perch, angelfish, grouper, and other fish.

The genomes of fish herpesviruses range in size from 134 to 295 kbp and the physical organization of the genome varies sufficiently to suggest that they have evolved separately from the herpesviruses of birds and mammals. The genome of *Ictalurid herpesvirus 1* (IcHV-1) or Channel catfish virus has a unique long (UL) region flanked by a substantial direct repeat that is similar to the betaherpesviruses of the genus *Roseolovirus*. The SalHV-1 genome is more similar in organization to the alphaherpesviruses of the genus *Varicellovirus* with a unique short (US) region flanked by a unique long (UL) region which is not flanked by a repeat. Phylogenetic comparisons of the individual genes including the DNA polymerase gene, the major capsid protein gene, the intercapsomeric triplex protein gene, and the DNA helicase gene indicate that the three cyprinid viruses are closely related and are distinct from IcHV-1.

These viruses are serious pathogens in their respective hosts. IcHV-1 outbreaks among juvenile catfish result in mortality and fish that survive the infection become carriers. The cyprinid herpes viruses produce a systemic disease with lesions in hematopoietic tissue in goldfish and papillomas on the caudal regions in koi carp. SalHV-2 was isolated from the ovarian fluid of masou salmon and it induces syncytia formation and lysis of infected cells. Epithelial papillomas are induced in young masou salmon injected with tissue culture-grown virus. The acipenserid herpesviruses cause serious losses in hatchery-reared young of white sturgeon (*Acipenser transmontanus*).

### Adenoviridae

Adenovirus particles have been observed in lesions in a number of fish species and have been isolated from white sturgeon, dabs (*Limanda limanda*), cod, and Japanese red sea bream. The white sturgeon adenovirus has been isolated in tissue culture and its hexon protein and protease gene sequences are available. Based on an alignment of partial DNA polymerase gene sequences of the sturgeon adenovirus and 24 other adenovirus types, it is clear that the fish adenovirus is distantly related to the other adenoviruses, and might constitute a fifth genus of the *Adenoviridae*.

Adenovirus infection in cod produces an epidermal hyperplasia. In California, white sturgeon adenovirus affects young fish in hatcheries. Infection is characterized by epithelial hyperplasia and enlarged cell nuclei. A lympholeukemia has been observed in red sea bream and papillomas have been observed in dabs infected with adenoviruses.

*See also:* Fish and Amphibian Herpesviruses; Fish Rhabdoviruses; Fish Retroviruses; Aquareoviruses; Infectious Salmon Anemia Virus.

## Further Reading

Attoui H, Fang Q, Jaafar FM, *et al.* (2002) Common evolutionary origin of aquareoviruses and orthoreoviruses revealed by genome characterization of Golden shiner reovirus, Grass carp reovirus, Striped bass reovirus, and Golden ide reovirus (genus *Aquareovirus*, family *Reoviridae*). *Journal of General Virology* 83: 1941–1951.

Essbauer S and Ahne W (2001) Viruses of lower vertebrates. *Journal of Veterinary Medicine, Series B* 48: 403–475.

Hoffmann B, Beer M, Schutz H, and Mettenleiter TC (2005) Fish rhabdoviruses: Molecular epidemiology and evolution. *Current Topics in Microbiology and Immunology* 292: 81–117.

Lewis TD and Leong JC (2004) Viruses of fish. In: Leung KY (ed.) *Current Trends in the Study of Bacterial and Viral Fish and Shrimp Diseases. Molecular Aspects of Fish & Marine Biology,* vol. 3, 39–81.

Paul TA, Quackenbush SL, Sutton C, Casey R, Bowser P, and Casey JW (2006) Identification and characterization of an exogenous retrovirus from Atlantic salmon swimbladder sarcomas. *Journal of Virology* 80: 2941–2948.

Phelan PE, Pressley ME, Witten PE, Mellon MT, Blake S, and Kim CH (2005) Characterization of Snakehead rhabdovirus infection in zebrafish (*Danio rerio*). *Journal of Virology* 79: 1842–1852.

Schutze H, Ulferts R, Schelle B, *et al.* (2006) Characterization of White bream virus reveals a novel genetic cluster of Nidoviruses. *Journal of Virology* 80: 11598–11609.

Skall HF, Olesen NJ, and Mellergaard S (2005) Viral haemorrhagic septicaemia virus in marine fish and its implications for fish farming – A review. *Journal of Fish Diseases* 58: 509–529.

Troyer RM and Kurath G (2003) Molecular epidemiology of infectious hematopoietic necrosis virus reveals complex virus traffic and evolution within southern Idaho aquaculture. *Diseases of Aquatic Organisms* 55: 175–185.

Wolf K (1988) *Fish Viruses and Fish Viral Diseases.* Ithaca, NY: Cornell University Press.

# Infectious Salmon Anemia Virus

**B H Dannevig,** National Veterinary Institute, Oslo, Norway
**S Mjaaland and E Rimstad,** Norwegian School of Veterinary Science, Oslo, Norway

### Glossary

**Ascites** Accumulation of serous fluid in the peritoneal cavity.
**Coprophagy** Eating of feces.
**Exophthalmia** Protrusion of the eyeballs.
**Fry** Young offsprings, presmolt stage.

**Hemagglutinin-esterase** A surface glycoprotein responsible for both receptor-binding (hemagglutinin) and receptor-destroying (esterase) activities.
**Pathognomonic** Pathological changes typical for a specific disease.

**Smolt** The stage in the life cycle of young anadromous salmonids when the fish is physiologically adapted to seawater, that is, farmed salmonids can be moved from freshwater to seawater.
**Well boats** Boats that are used for transportation of live fish.

## Introduction

Infectious salmon anemia virus (ISAV) is the causative agent of infectious salmon anemia (ISA), a disease of farmed Atlantic salmon (*Salmo salar*). ISA primarily affects fish held in or exposed to seawater. The disease appears as a systemic condition characterized by severe anemia and hemorrhages in several organs. Mortality during an outbreak of ISA varies significantly. Daily mortality in affected net pens ranges from 0.2% to 1%, but may increase during an outbreak and the cumulative mortality may exceed 90% in severe cases.

ISA was recognized in 1984 in Norway, and was soon identified as a contagious viral disease. The disease increased in prevalence and showed a peak in 1990. In the following years, the incidence of ISA was greatly reduced by the implementation of legislatory measures or husbandry practices based on general hygiene. These included mandatory health control in hatcheries and health certification for fish, restrictions on transportation of live fish, regulations of disinfection of wastewater from fish slaughterhouses and of water supplies to hatcheries. Approximately 10 years after the first recognition of ISA, the causative virus, ISAV, was isolated in cell culture using the SHK-1 cell line established from Atlantic salmon head kidney. The subsequent investigations showed that the morphological, physiochemical, and genetic properties of ISAV are consistent with classification in the *Orthomyxoviridae*.

## Virus Properties and Classification

ISAV is a pleiomorphic, enveloped virus, 100–130 nm in diameter, with 10–12 nm surface projections (**Figure 1**). The virus hemagglutinates erythrocytes of several fish species and it has receptor-destroying and membrane fusion activities. Endothelial and leukocytic cells are the main target cells and the virus replicates by budding from the cell membrane. ISAV has two main surface glycoproteins: the hemagglutinin-esterase (HE) responsible for the receptor-binding and receptor-destroying activities, and a fusion protein (F).

The buoyant density of virus particles in sucrose or cesium chloride is $1.18 \, \mathrm{g \, ml^{-1}}$. The virus is stable at

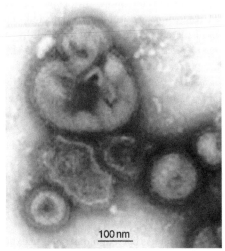

**Figure 1** Electron micrograph of negative-stained ISAV particles purified from infected cell culture medium. Photo by Ellen Namork, The Norwegian Institute of Public Health, Oslo, Norway.

pH 5.7–9.0. The virus replicates in the salmon cell lines SHK-1, TO, and ASK, with a replication optimum of 10–15 °C. Some strains also replicate in the CHSE-214 cell line. There is no replication in SHK-1 cells at 25 °C or higher and, even at 20 °C, the yield of virus in SHK-1 cells is only 1% of the yield at 15 °C.

The 14.3 kb genome consists of eight single-stranded RNA segments of negative polarity in the size range of 1.0–2.4 kb. The amino acid identity between the ISAV proteins and those of other orthomyxoviruses is low (13–25%), and the organization of ISAV genes is unique. ISAV is therefore classified as the type species of the genus *Isavirus* within the family *Orthomyxoviridae*.

## Geographic Distribution and Host Range

After the first recorded outbreak in 1984, ISA was considered to be a uniquely Norwegian disease. In 1996, a disease in Canada (New Brunswick) designated as hemorrhagic kidney syndrome was verified as ISA. The disease has thereafter been reported in Scotland (1998), the Faroe Islands (2000), and in the USA (Maine, 2001).

While natural outbreaks of ISA have only been described in Atlantic salmon, the virus may survive and replicate in other salmonid fish under experimental conditions. ISAV has been detected in wild Atlantic salmon and brown trout (*Salmo trutta*). Outbreaks of ISA in farmed Atlantic salmon have occurred mainly during the seawater stage, but indications of disease outbreaks in the freshwater stage have been reported. Disease and transmission are readily induced experimentally in Atlantic salmon kept in either freshwater or seawater. Wild Atlantic salmon are susceptible to ISA and show the same clinical signs as farmed fish when experimentally infected. The virus has been isolated from apparently healthy rainbow trout (*Oncorhynchus mykiss*) in Ireland (2002). ISAV has also been reported to have been isolated from Coho salmon (*Oncorhynchus kitsutch*) in Chile, but this observation needs to be confirmed. Subclinically infected feral salmonids (Atlantic salmon, brown trout, and sea brown trout) have been identified in Scotland and Norway by reverse transcriptase-polymerase chain reaction (RT-PCR). However, reports of RT-PCR-positive samples from marine, nonsalmonid fish (Atlantic cod (*Gadus morhua*) and pollock (*Pollachius virens*)) need to be corroborated as samples were collected from the vicinity of cages holding ISA-diseased Atlantic salmon.

ISAV replication has been demonstrated in experimentally infected brown trout and in rainbow trout, but disease and mortality have only been produced in rainbow trout by experimental infection. ISAV has also been detected by RT-PCR in experimentally infected Arctic charr (*Salvelinus alpinus*) but neither virus replication nor clinical signs of disease have been demonstrated. ISAV could be reisolated from Pacific salmon species (*O. mykiss, Oncorhynchus keta, O. kitsutch, Oncorhynchus tshawytscha*) injected intraperitoneally with various Canadian and Norwegian virus isolates but no mortality was observed. Pacific salmon are therefore considered more resistant to ISA than Atlantic salmon but should not be ignored as potential virus carriers. Among marine fish, ISAV is able to propagate in herring (*Clupea harengus*) after bath challenge, but attempts to induce infection in pollock have failed. There are no indications that ISAV can infect mussel (*Mytilus edulis*) or scallops (*Pecten maximus*).

## Transmission, Vectors and Reservoir Hosts

Epidemiological and experimental studies have shown that ISA may spread by water-borne transmission. The risk of ISA is closely linked to geographical proximity to farms with ISA outbreaks or to slaughterhouses and processing plants. The spread of the disease over long distances may be caused by transportation of infected fish by well boats.

The virus may be shed into the water by various routes such as skin, mucus, feces, and urine. The most likely route of virus entry is through the gills and skin lesions but transmission by coprophagy has also been proposed. ISAV may retain infectivity for long periods outside the host. No significant loss in virus titer was observed after incubation of virus supernatants for 14 days at 4 °C and 10 days at 15 °C, and infectivity of tissue preparations is retained for at least 48 h at 0 °C, 24 h at 10 °C, and 12 h at 15 °C. A 3-$\log_{10}$ reduction in virus titer after 4 months

storage in sterile seawater at 4 °C has been observed, but ISAV survival time in natural seawater may be shorter.

There are indications that ISAV may be transmitted vertically. ISAV has been detected by real-time RT-PCR in fertilized eggs from ISA-diseased brood fish. However, it is not known if this represents infective virus as recovery of virus by isolation in cell culture was not performed. Eggs, fry, and juveniles from ISAV-infected parents have been demonstrated ISAV-positive by real-time RT-PCR. On the other hand, ISAV could not be detected in progeny from healthy but virus-positive brood fish. Furthermore, ISAV has been detected by real-time RT-PCR in Atlantic salmon parr and smolt sampled from hatcheries, that is, from the freshwater stage. However, there are no verified field observations that can confirm vertical transmission of ISA disease. Nevertheless, the detection of virus in progeny from infected brood fish and the few reported outbreaks in the freshwater stage indicate that this route of transmission cannot be excluded.

The sea louse (*Lepeophtheirus salmonis*) has been suggested as a possible vector for ISAV, but it is not clear if this is by passive transfer or active virus replication. Reservoir hosts of ISAV have not been identified, but the virus replicates in sea trout, which are abundant in Norway in fiords and coastal areas in the vicinity of the fish farms. However, the possible role of sea trout as a reservoir host for ISAV can only be speculated at this time.

## Genetics

Nucleotide sequences of all eight ISAV genome segments have been described. The genome encodes at least 10 proteins (**Table 1**). Segments 1, 2, and 4 encode the viral polymerase subunits PB1, PB2, and PA, respectively. Segment 3 encodes the 68 kDa nucleoprotein (NP). Segments 5 and 6 encode the two major surface glycoproteins: the 50 kDa fusion (F) protein, and the 42 kDa HE responsible for receptor-binding and receptor-destroying activities. The two smallest ISAV genomic segments each contain two overlapping reading frames (ORFs). Two mRNAs are transcribed from genome segment 7 – one is collinear with the viral RNA (vRNA) and the other is spliced in an arrangement similar to the two smallest gene segments of influenza A virus. The unspliced mRNA of segment 7 encodes a nonstructural protein that has been suggested to interfere with the interferon type 1 response of the cell. The protein encoded by the spliced mRNA has not yet been characterized. No splicing of transcripts from segment 8 ORFs has been detected, indicating that ISAV uses a bicistronic coding strategy for this genomic segment. The smaller ORF1 encodes a 22 kDa matrix protein, while the collinear mRNA transcript from the larger ORF2 encodes an RNA binding structural protein of about 26 kDa with putative interferon antagonistic properties. ISAV gene segments and the respective encoded proteins are summarized in **Figure 2**.

The 3'- and 5'-terminal structure of vRNAs, and the ISAV transcription strategy, resemble those of influenza viruses.

As for all members of the *Orthomyxoviridae*, each ISAV genome segment contains partially self-complementary termini that are essential for the replication process. However, compared to the 12–13 nucleotides conserved in the

**Table 1** Genome segments and encoded proteins of ISA virus

| Segment (kb) | Encoded protein | ORF (bp) | Protein (kDa) |
|---|---|---|---|
| 1 (2.3) | Polymerase, PB2 | 2127 | 80.5[a] |
| 2 (2.3) | Polymerase, PB1 | 2169 | 79.5[a] |
| 3 (2.2) | Nucleoprotein, NP | 1851 | 66–74[b] |
| 4 (2.0) | Polymerase, PA | 1840 | 65.3 |
| 5 (1.7) | Fusion, F | 1332 | 53 |
| 6 (1.5) | Hemagglutinin-esterase, HE | 1176[c] | 38–46[b] |
| 7 (1.3) | Two open reading frames | | |
| | • ORF1 = nonstructural (NS) | 903 | 34 |
| | • ORF2 = spliced protein | 369 | 17.5 |
| 8 (1.0) | Two open reading frames | | |
| | • Matrix, M | 588 | 22–24 |
| | • as RNA-binding protein | 726 | 26 |

[a]Estimations based on amino acid sequence.
[b]The estimated molecular masses of some of the proteins differ slightly in the literature, probably due to differences in experimental conditions. For HE, this could also be due to differences in glycosylation as well as in the highly polymorphic region (HPR).
[c]Length of ORF for the reference ISAV isolate Glesvaer/2/90. The length varies between isolates due to the HPR characterized by deletions/gaps. The proposed ancestral ORF sequence is estimated to 1236 bp.

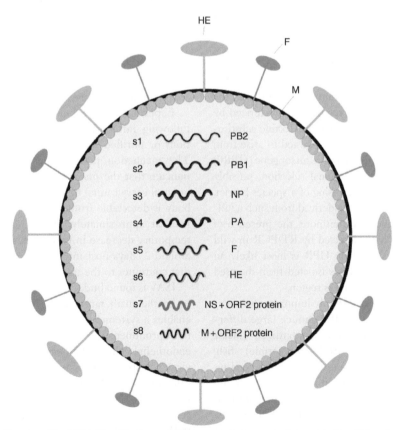

**Figure 2** Schematic diagram of the ISAV virion. The two smallest genomic segments (segments 7 and 8) each contain two open reading frames (ORFs). The proteins encoded by each ORF is yet to be characterized. s, Genomic segment; PB2/PB1/PA, polymerase subunits; NP, nucleoprotein; F, fusion protein; HE, hemagglutinin-esterase; NS, nonstructural protein; M, matrix protein. Adapted from Ida Skaar.

influenza A virus, only 8–9 nucleotides are conserved in ISAV, most likely reflecting the lower replication temperature optimum for this virus. As for the influenza viruses, the terminal 21–24 nucleotides are predicted to form self-complementary panhandle structures important for transcriptional regulation of viral RNA. ISAV also exerts cap-stealing in the host cell's nucleus, transferring 8–18 nucleotide 5′-cap structures from host mRNAs to the viral mRNAs and affecting the normal transcription and protein synthesis in the cell. ISAV mRNAs are polyadenylated, a process that is regulated from a signal 13–14 nucleotides downstream the 5′-terminus of the vRNAs. Altogether, the ISAV replication strategy is similar to those of the other orthomyxoviruses.

ISAV isolates vary in virulence, as observed by differences in disease development and clinical signs in field outbreaks and in experimental trials using genetically standardized fish. However, analysis of important virulence factors is still in its infancy. The ISAV genome is highly conserved, both over time and geographical distance, with 98–99% overall nucleotide similarity between Norwegian isolates. However, small, but relevant, differences between isolates both within and between defined geographical areas do exist, and analysis of the 5′-terminal end of the HE gene has demonstrated the presence of two major groups of isolates, one European and one North American. The European group may be further divided into three major subgroups.

The surface glycoprotein HE gene displays the highest sequence variation (94–97%) which is mainly concentrated in a small highly polymorphic region (HPR) of the HE protein that is predicted to lie immediately outside the viral envelope. Variation in this region is characterized by the presence of gaps rather than single-nucleotide substitutions. The polymorphism has been suggested to arise from differential deletions of a full-length precursor gene (HPR0) as a consequence of strong functional selection, possibly related to a recent or ongoing crossing of a species barrier. All HPRs described to date can be derived from such a full-length precursor sequence. Furthermore, the presence of a long HPR0 gene has been detected by RT-PCR in wild Atlantic salmon. The variation in HPR is most likely an important virulence factor as virus isolated from diseased fish always contains a deletion in this region.

Other genes are also most certainly important for virulence as isolates with identical HPR induce large differences in mortality in genetically standardized (major histocompatibility complex (MHC)-compatible) fish. Candidate genes include genome segment 5 encoding the surface glycoprotein with fusion activity and genome segment 7 and 8 encoding the putative IFN I antagonists in alternative reading frames. The synthetic IFN I inducer poly I:C induces no or only minor protection against ISAV infection in Atlantic salmon or cell culture, demonstrating the efficiency of the ISAV IFN I antagonistic

properties. In orthomyxoviruses, reassortment of gene segments occurs frequently and is a major contributor to the evolution of these viruses and the emergence of new virulent strains. Alignments and phylogenetic studies of full-length sequenced ISAV isolates provide evidence for both genome segment reassortment and recombination. A 30 bp insert found in close proximity to the putative cleavage site of the fusion protein in several unrelated isolates combined with extensive sequence internal homology in this region suggests the presence of a recombinational hot-spot in this gene.

## Pathogenesis

The mortality rate during an ISA outbreak may vary significantly. Variation in the seriousness in disease outbreaks may be influenced by the environmental and management parameters, genetics of the fish, and the virus strain.

In affected populations of farmed fish, individuals may harbor the virus for weeks or months before the development of disease. Prior to an outbreak, a slightly increased mortality over a period of 1–3 weeks is often seen. Outbreaks are often restricted initially to one or two net pens and up to 12 months can pass before clinical ISA spreads to neighboring pens in a farm. The signs exhibited by infected fish range from none to severe. The disease may appear throughout the year. The course of the disease may vary from an acute form with rapid development and high mortality, to a chronic form in which a slow increase in mortality is observed over several months, but several immediate forms may exist.

Experimentally, ISA can be induced in Atlantic salmon following intraperitoneal injection with tissue preparations or purified virus, or through infected cohabitants. The incubation period is usually 10–20 days. Studies indicate that the major portal of ISAV entry is the gills but oral entry cannot be excluded. Viral spread within the body is detectable from 5 days post-infection and cumulates at approximately 15 days. This is followed by a temporary decrease in viral load, reaching a minimum at around 25 days post-infection, followed by a second rise that continues to the terminal stage of ISA.

ISAV is found budding from endothelial cells that seem to be the main target cells. Their ubiquitous presence enables a systemic infection. By *in situ* hybridization, the most prominent ISAV-specific signals are detected in the endothelial cells of the heart. The presence of infectious virus has also been reported in leukocytes. ISAV specifically binds to glycoproteins containing 4-O-acetylated sialic acids. The viral esterase is specific for this sialic acid, indicating that it may be a receptor determinant for ISAV. ISAV infects cells via the endocytic pathway and fusion between virus and cell membrane takes place in the acidic environment of endosomes.

## Clinical Features and Pathology

Fish infected with ISAV show a range of pathological changes, from none to severe. None of the described lesions is considered pathognomonic. Diseased fish appear lethargic and, in terminal stages, often sink to the bottom of the cage. The disease appears as a systemic condition characterized by severe anemia (hematocrit values below 10) and hemorrhages in several organs. The most prominent external signs are pale gills, exophthalmia, distended abdomen, and petechia in the eye chamber; skin hemorrhages in the abdomen, and scale edema. The major gross postmortem findings are circulatory disturbances in several organs caused by endothelial injury in peripheral blood vessels. These pathological manifestations of ISA are mainly recognized in the liver, kidney, gut, and gills, but not all of these organs are affected to the same extent during a disease outbreak. In some cases, the pathological manifestations are more clearly seen in one single organ than in others.

Abundant ascitic fluid is often present. A fibrinous layer may cover the liver capsule and the liver may be partly or diffusely dark red. The spleen and kidney may appear dark and swollen and the intestinal wall congested and dark. Petechial hemorrhages are seen on the surface of several organs as well as the adipose tissue and skeletal muscle. The major histopathological findings have been observed in the liver, kidneys, and intestine. The lesions result in extensive congestion of the liver with dilated sinusoids and, in later stages, the appearance of blood-filled spaces. Multifocal to confluent hemorrhages and/or necrosis of hepatocytes at some distance from large vessels in the liver are often seen. In the kidney, interstitial hemorrhage with tubular necrosis in the hemorrhagic areas, and accumulation of erythrocytes in the glomeruli may occur. Accumulation of erythrocytes in blood vessels of the intestinal lamina propria and hemorrhage into the lamina propria may be observed. In the spleen, accumulation of erythrocytes and distention of stroma may be found, and numerous erythrocytes may be present in central venous sinus and lamellar capillaries of the gills.

In ISA outbreaks on the American East Coast in the 1990s, histopathological changes were prominent in the kidneys. The major pathological findings included renal interstitial hemorrhage with tubular necrosis and casts, branchial lamellar and filamental congestion, and congestion of the intestine and pyloric cecae. The disease therefore initially became known as hemorrhagic kidney syndrome (HKS). The gross appearance of the fish was somewhat similar to that reported for ISA in Norway. However, liver congestion was a rare finding in fish from outbreaks in New Brunswick. HKS was later confirmed to be ISA by RT-PCR and cell culture isolation of the virus. Similar kidney and intestinal manifestations of the disease has now also been reported in Norway.

## Diagnosis

Diagnosis of ISA was initially based on macroscopic, histological, and hematological findings. A dark liver was considered as a typical finding and the presence of multifocal, hemorrhagic liver necrosis with a 'zonal' appearance and hematocrit values below 10 confirmed the diagnosis. However, following the isolation of ISAV in SHK-1 cells, a number of methods for detection of virus in tissue samples were established.

Detection of ISAV antigens in kidney imprints from Atlantic salmon exhibiting clinical signs with the use of an indirect fluorescent antibody technique (IFAT) has been an important method for verification of ISA. The production of an anti-ISAV HE monoclonal antibody to be used as the primary antibody in the IFAT was an important step in the development of specific diagnostic tools. Polyclonal antibodies suitable for immunohistochemistry have also been developed, and this method has recently been implemented in the routine diagnostics of ISA.

ISAV was first isolated in the salmonid cell line SHK-1, but other salmonid cell lines such as CHSE-214, ASK, and TO also support viral propagation. Development of cytopathic effect (CPE) may be observed in infected cell cultures, but the extent of CPE may vary dependent on cell type and virus strain. The isolated virus may be identified using IFAT on infected cell cultures. Strain variations with respect to cell susceptibility have been observed. The Atlantic salmon cell lines SHK-1, TO, and ASK do not support growth of all ISAV variants as virus cannot be recovered from some RT-PCR-positive samples. The CHSE-214 cell line supports growth of some ISAV isolates, but others, such as the European variants of ISAV, do not replicate in this cell line at all. This limits the utility of the CHSE-14 cell line for virus isolation. Currently available fish cell lines appear to be either not sensitive enough or not permissive for all ISAV strains.

RT-PCR techniques have been widely in use since the RT-PCR for ISAV was described in 1997, and several different primer sets have been found to be suitable for detection of ISAV. Real-time RT-PCR has also been established for ISAV, allowing a further increase in specificity and sensitivity.

## Immune Response, Prevention and Control

Due to lack of standardized molecular and experimental tools in fish, detailed knowledge of immune responses to viral agents is limited. This represents a major problem for the development of effective vaccines against fish viral diseases. For ISA, the ability to induce a strong lymphocyte proliferative response correlates with survival and virus clearance, while induction of a humoral response is less protective, as shown in experimental trials using MHC-compatible fish.

Currently available vaccines against ISA contain inactivated whole virus grown in cell culture added to mineral oil adjuvants. Vaccines are approved by the United States Department of Agriculture (USDA) and the Canadian Food Inspection Agency (CFIA) and are commercially available in Canada and the USA. Vaccination has also been used in the Faroe Islands. The use of vaccines against ISA in the rest of Europe is subject to EU/European Fair Trade Association approval. The present policy is that control of ISA should normally be based on a nonvaccination strategy. However, due to the severe disease problems in the Faroe Islands, exceptions to these rules have been made. The efficacy of ISAV vaccines has been evaluated using a vaccination-challenge model in the laboratory. Data on the evaluation of vaccines in field situations have so far not been presented. Currently available vaccines do not result in total clearance of virus in immunized fish.

The incidence of ISA may be greatly reduced by geneal husbandry practices and control of the movement of fish, mandatory health controls, and transport and slaughterhouse regulations. Specific measures including health restrictions on affected, suspected, and neighboring farms, enforced sanitary slaughtering, segregation of different generations of fish, as well as disinfection of offal and wastewater from fish slaughterhouses and fish-processing plants, also contribute to reduction in the incidence of the disease.

## Further Reading

Falk K, Aspehaug V, Vlasak R, and Endresen C (2004) Identification and characterization of viral structural proteins of infectious salmon anemia virus. *Journal of Virology* 78: 3063–3071.

Falk K, Namork E, Rimstad E, Mjaaland S, and Dannevig BH (1997) Characterization of infectious salmon anaemia virus, an orthomyxo-like virus isolated from Atlantic salmon (*Salmo salar* L.). *Journal of Virology* 71: 9016–9023.

Koren CWR and Nylund A (1997) Morphology and morphogenesis of infectious salmon anaemia virus replicating in the endothelium of Atlantic salmon *Salmo salar*. *Diseases of Aquatic Organisms* 29: 99–109.

Krossoy B, Devold M, Sanders L, *et al.* (2001) Cloning and identification of the infectious salmon anaemia virus haemagglutinin. *Journal of General Virology* 82: 1757–1765.

Mjaaland S, Hungnes O, Teig A, *et al.* (2002) Polymorphism in the infectious salmon anemia virus hemagglutinin gene: Importance and possible implications for evolution and ecology of infectious salmon anemia disease. *Virology* 302: 379–391.

Mjaaland S, Rimstad E, and Cunningham C (2002) Molecular diagnosis of infectious salmon anaemia. In: Cunningham CO (ed.) *Molecular Diagnosis of Salmonid Diseases*, pp. 1–22. Boston: Kluwer Academic.

Mjaaland S, Rimstad E, Falk K, and Dannevig BH (1997) Genomic characterization of the virus causing infectious salmon anaemia in Atlantic salmon (*Salmo salar* L.): An orthomyxo-like virus in a teleost. *Journal of Virology* 71: 7681–7686.

Rimstad E and Mjaaland S (2002) Infectious salmon anaemia virus. An orthomyxovirus causing an emerging infection in Atlantic salmon. *Acta Pathologica Microbiologica et Immunologica Scandinavica* 110: 273–282.

# Shellfish Viruses

**T Renault,** IFREMER, La Tremblade, France

## Glossary

**Aquaculture** Cultivation of aquatic animals or plants.
**Bivalve** Marine or freshwater mollusks having a soft body with plate-like gills enclosed within two shells hinged together.
**Gills** Respiratory organ of aquatic animals that breathe oxygen dissolved in water.
**Hatchery** A place where eggs are hatched under artificial conditions.
**Hemocyte** Any blood cell especially in invertebrates.
**Larva** The immature free-living form of most invertebrates which on hatching from the egg is fundamentally unlike its parent and must metamorphose.
**Mantle** A protective layer of epidermis in mollusks that secretes a substance forming the shell.

**Mollusk** Invertebrates having a soft unsegmented body usually enclosed in a shell.
**Nursery** A place for the cultivation of juveniles under controlled conditions.
**Shellfish** Aquatic invertebrates belonging to the crustacean or mollusk families.
**Velum** Membrane of mollusk larvae that allows swimming activity.

## Introduction

A natural abundance of shellfish was common in many areas of the world until the early twentieth century. However, industrial and urban development and population growth in coastal areas, coupled with extreme harvest pressure, appear to have contributed to a stready decline in natural shellfish populations. This decline in wild harvests, together with a greater demand for seafood from an increasing world population, have driven the development of technology for the intensive management and cultivation of shellfish. As a result, global shellfish production, the greatest proportion of which is bivalves, was estimated to be 10 732 000 metric tons in the year 2000. However, as husbandry practices have developed, the significant impact of infectious diseases on productivity and product quality has been increasingly recognized. Numerous examples worldwide have demonstrated that entire shellfish industries in coastal areas are susceptible to diseases and that the production of healthy shellfish is a key to the economic viability of mollusk farming.

The study of shellfish diseases is a relatively young science and the discovery of viruses in marine mollusks is a fairly recent event. Viral diseases have seriously affected the aquaculture industry during the last decades. Viral pathogens are often highly infectious and easily transmissible, and are commonly associated with mass mortalities. Viruses interpreted as members of the families *Iridoviridae*, *Herpesviridae*, *Papovaviridae*, *Reoviridae*, *Birnaviridae*, and *Picornaviridae* have been reported as associated with disease outbreaks and causing mortality in various mollusks. However, there is currently a lack of information concerning the occurrence of mollusk viruses worldwide, and the basic method for identification and examination of suspect samples is still predominantly histopathology. This technique enables the identification of cellular changes associated with infection but does not provide conclusive identification of mollusk viruses unless completed by other methods such as transmission electron microscopy. Moreover, as there is a lack of marine mollusk cell lines and, since invertebrates lack antibody-producing cells, the direct detection of viral agents remains the only possible approach to diagnosis.

As filter feeders, bivalves may also bioaccumulate viruses from humans and other vertebrates, acting as a transient reservoir. The consumption of raw or undercooked shellfish can result in human disease and contamination of shellfish cultivated in coastal marine waters by microorganisms that are pathogenic to humans is a public health concern worldwide. The association of shellfish-transmitted infectious diseases with sewage pollution has been well documented since the late nineteenth and early twentieth centuries. Human enteric viruses, including rotaviruses, enteroviruses, and hepatitis A virus, are the most common etiological agents transmitted by shellfish. These enteric viruses are associated with several human diseases ranging from ocular and respiratory infections to gastroenteritis, hepatitis, myocarditis, and aseptic meningitis. Many of these viruses are transmitted by the fecal–oral route and are highly prevalent in locations with poor sanitation. There is considerable literature on the implications for human health. However, this is not the subject of the present article.

## Irido-Like Viruses

### Hosts and Locations

Infections by irido-like viruses have been reported in oysters in France and in the USA. Two distinctive conditions have been associated with mass mortalities in adult Portuguese oyster, *Crassostrea angulata*, along French coasts: gill necrosis virus disease and hemocytic infection virus disease. A viral infection similar to the latter was reported in the Pacific oyster *Crassostrea gigas* during summer mortalities in the Bay of Arcachon (Atlantic coast, France) long after the disappearance of the Portuguese oyster. A third type of irido-like virus, the oyster velar virus (OVV), has been reported from hatchery-reared larval Pacific oysters on the west coast of North America (Washington State, USA).

### Disease Manifestations and Epizootiology

Gill necrosis virus disease is regarded as the primary cause of disease outbreaks and mortalities that occurred in the late 1960s among Portuguese oysters on the Atlantic coast of France. The disease appears to have affected up to 70% of oyster populations with maximum losses reported in 1967. Losses subsequently declined and survivors recovered from the disease. The first gross signs were small perforations in the center of yellowish discolored zones of tissue on gills and labial palps. Further development and extension of the lesions resulted in larger and deeper ulcerations. In advanced stages, total destruction of affected gill filaments was observed. Yellow or green pustules also developed on the adductor muscle and mantle.

In 1970, high mortality rates were again reported in *C. angulata* oysters in France. Mortality was first observed in the basin of Marennes Oleron (Altantic coast) and in Brittany. The high mortality rates that occurred during this epizootic led to almost total extinction of French *C. angulata* by 1973. The disease affected adult oysters. No distinctive clinical signs were noted (e.g., no gill lesions). Histological observations included an acute cellular infiltration consisting of atypical virus-infected hemocytes. Pacific oysters seemed to be resistant to the vius and subsequently replaced *C. angulata* in France. However, a morphologically similar virus was reported from Pacific oysters during an outbreak of summer mortality in the Bay of Arcachon (Atlantic coast, France) in 1977. Although affected Pacific oysters exhibited virtually no gross signs, the presence of atypical cells interpreted as infected hemocytes and degeneration of connective tissues were reported in infected animals.

Oyster velar virus disease (OVVD) of the Pacific oyster occurred in the USA from mid-March through mid-June each year from 1976 to 1984, suggesting that the expression of the disease may be related to particular environmental conditions. When cultured at 25–30 °C, mortalities in oyster larvae greater than 170 μm in shell length typically begin at about 10 days of age. The infection results in the sloughing of ciliated velar epithelial cells and detachment of infected cells from the velum. Other cells lose cilia and infected larvae become unable to move normally.

## Descriptive Histopathology

Histologically, gill necrosis virus disease is characterized by tissue necrosis with massive hemocytic infiltration around the lesions. The most distinctive lesion is the occurrence of giant polymorphic cells which may be up to 30 μm in size and contain large fuchsinophilic granules in the cytoplasm. In some giant cells, a voluminous basophilic inclusion (5–15 μm) occupies the greatest part of the cytoplasm in which finer basophilic granules (0.4–0.5 μm) are also present. Electron microscopy indicates that the inclusions are the viroplasm, and the fine granules are large viral particles. The most characteristic histological lesion of hemocytic infection virus disease is an acute cellular infiltration with the presence of atypical hemocytes in the connective tissues. Basophilic intracytoplasmic inclusion bodies are found in atypical blood cells in which irido-like virus particles can be observed in ultrathin sections. OVVD disease manifests histologically by the presence of intracytoplasmic inclusion bodies, 1.2–4 μm in diameter, located most commonly in the ciliated velar epithelium. The presence of DNA in the inclusion bodies is suggested by a positive Feulgen and Rosenbeck reaction.

## Viruses

Mature icosahedral virions (380 nm diameter) are scattered throughout the cytoplasm of infected cells (**Figure 1(a)**). The outer shells of virions appear to consist of two trilaminar layers. The electron-opaque core (250 nm diameter) is limited by a three-layered fringe of definite width and surrounded by a layer of dense material (**Figure 1(b)**). Morphogenesis takes place in the cytoplasm. Oyster irido-like viruses have not been isolated from infected tissue and have not been characterized biochemically. However, the presence of viral DNA was demonstrated by histochemical techniques including acridine orange staining and the Feulgen and Rosenbeck reaction. The characteristic morphology and cytoplasmic localization of these large DNA viruses suggest that they may eventually be classified as members of the family *Iridoviridae*. However, no molecular characterization has yet been conducted and there remains a need for definitive demonstration of viral etiology for the reported diseases.

## Herpesviruses

### Hosts and Locations

Herpes-like virus infections have been identified in various marine mollusk species throughout the world, including the USA, Mexico, France, Spain, the UK, New Zealand, Australia, and Taiwan. The first description of a virus

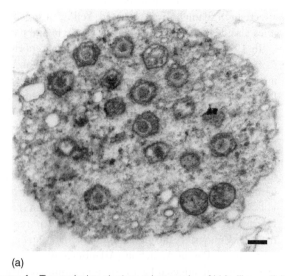
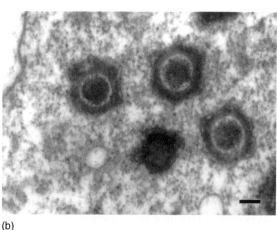

(a)                                    (b)

**Figure 1**  Transmission electron micrographs of irido-like particles infecting *Crassostrea angulata* oysters. (a) Intracytoplasmic irido-like virus particles in an infected *C. angulata* cell (gill necrosis virus disease). Scale = 200 nm. (b) Irido-like virus particles from *C. angulata*. Virions are icosahedral in shape with a central electron-dense core, surrounded by an electron-lucent zone followed by another dense layer. Two unit membranes separated by a clear zone enclose the particle. Scale = 100 nm.

morphologically similar to members of the family *Herpesviridae* in a bivalve mollusk was reported in 1972 in the eastern oyster, *Crassostrea virginica*. Since then, a wide host range has been reported for herpes and herpes-like viruses infecting bivalve species, including the Pacific oyster *C. gigas*, the European oyster *Ostrea edulis*, the Antipodean flat oyster *Ostrea angasi*, the Chilean oyster *Tiostrea chilensis*, the Manila clam *Ruditapes philippinarum*, the carpet shell clam *Ruditapes decussatus*, the Portuguese oyster *C. angulata*, the Suminoe oyster *C. ariakensis*, and the French scallop *Pecten maximus*. It is noteworthy that recently a herpes-like virus has also been observed by transmission electron microscopy in the gastropod mollusk *Haliotis diversicolor supertexta* in Taiwan associated with high mortality rates.

## Disease Manifestations and Epizootiology

Herpesvirus and herpes-like virus infections have been associated with high mortalities of hatchery-reared larvae and juveniles stages of several bivalve mollusk species. Observations by transmission electron microscopy indicate that larvae exhibit generalized infections, whereas focal infections usually occur in juveniles. Although viral infections have also been observed in adult bivalves, they are apparently less sensitive than younger stages. Infected larvae exhibit velar and mantle lesions. They swim weakly in circles and shortly before death settle at the bottom of the tanks. Infected juveniles exhibit sudden high mortalities in a short period of time (less than 1 week) often during the summer. Histologically, lesions are confined to connective tissues. Fibroblast-like cells exhibit abnormal cytoplasmic basophilia and enlarged nuclei with marginated chromatin. Other cell types including hemocytes and myocytes show extensive chromatin condensation. Peculiar patterns of chromatin, ring-shaped or crescent-shaped, are also observed suggesting that apoptosis may occur. Viral DNA and proteins have been detected in asymptomatic adult oysters. Like other herpesviruses, the *C. gigas* herpesvirus seems to be capable of long-term persistence in the infected host. The pathogenicity of the virus for the larval stages of *C. gigas* has been demonstrated by experimental transmission to axenic larvae. Attempts to reproduce symptoms experimentally in juveniles and adult oysters have so far been inconclusive.

## Virus Ultrastructure

Based primarily on virion morphology and aspects of morphogenesis and genome organization, Ostreid herpesvirus 1 (OsHV-1) is currently classified as an unassigned member of the family *Herpesviridae*. Particles present in the nucleus are circular or polygonal in shape. Empty particles are presumed to be capsids; others containing an electron-dense toroidal or brick-shaped core are interpreted as nucleocapsids (**Figure 2(a)**). Capsids and nucleocapsids are scattered throughout the nucleus in infected cells (**Figure 2(b)**). An electron–lucent gap of approximately 5 nm with fine fibrils is observed between core and capsid. Digital reconstruction of the OsHV-1 capsid based on cryoelectron microscopic images indicates an icosahedral structure with a triangulation number of $T = 16$, which is an architecture unique to herpesviruses. Prominent external protrusions at the hexon sites, and a relatively flat and featureless appearance of the inner surface, reported for OsHV-1 capsids, are also characteristic features of herpesviruses. Extracellular particles are usually enveloped with a trilaminar unit-membrane and measure 100–180 nm in diameter (**Figure 2(c)**). Tegument between the outer membrane and the capsid shell of enveloped particles is either absent or minimal (**Figure 2(c)**).

## Genome Structure and Organization

Virus particles have been purified from fresh infected *C. gigas* larvae and the entire OsHV-1 genome has been cloned and sequenced (GenBank accession number AY509253). The total genome size is 207 439 bp. The overall genome organization is $TR_L$-$U_L$-$IR_L$-X-$IR_S$-$U_S$-$TR_S$ (**Figure 3**) in which $TR_L$ and $IR_L$ (7584 bp) are inverted repeats flanking a unique region ($U_L$, 167 843 bp), $TR_S$ and $IR_S$ (9774 bp) are inverted repeats flanking a unique region ($U_S$, 3370 bp), and X (1510 bp) is located between $IR_L$ and $IR_S$. A somewhat similar genome structure has been reported for certain vertebrate herpesviruses (e.g., herpes simplex virus and human cytomegalovirus). A small proportion of OsHV-1 genomes either lacks the X-sequence or contains an additional X-sequence at the left terminus. Since herpesvirus genomes are packaged into capsids from head-to-tail concatemers, this minor genome form may result from rare cleavage of concatemers at X–$TR_S$ rather than at $IR_L$–$IR_S$. Moreover, approximately 20–25% of genomes contain a 4.8 kbp region of $U_L$ in inverse orientation. The two orientations of $U_L$ and $U_S$ are present in approximately equimolar amounts in viral DNA, giving rise to four genomic isomers. This is also a feature of the vertebrate herpesvirus genomes with similar structures and results from recombination between inverted repeats during DNA replication. The genome termini are not unique but a predominant form is apparent for each. The $IR_L$–$IR_S$ junction is also not unique, but the predominant form corresponds to a fusion of the two termini if each possesses two unpaired nucleotides at the 3′-end. Unpaired nucleotides are characteristic of herpesvirus genome termini.

Detailed analysis of the OsHV-1 genome sequence indicates that there are 124 unique open reading frames (ORFs). Owing to the presence of inverted repeats, 12 ORFs are duplicated resulting in a total of 136 genes in the viral genome. These numbers include several fragmented genes, each of which is counted as a single ORF. It is not yet known if splicing contributes to further

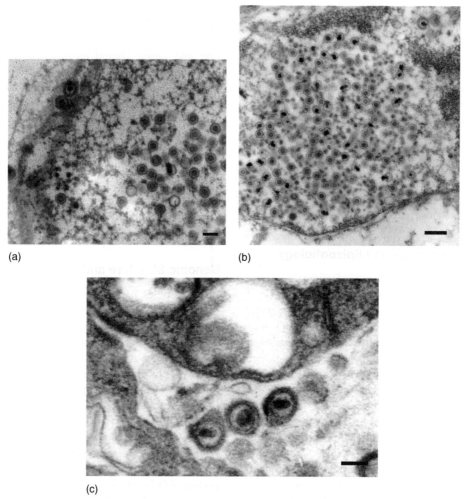

(a)

(b)

(c)

**Figure 2** Transmission electron micrographs of ostreid herpesvirus 1 (OsHV-1) infecting Pacific oyster larvae. (a) Intranuclear spherical or polygonal virus particles; some particles appear empty and other contain an electron-dense core. Scale = 100 nm. (b) Nucleus of an infected interstial cell containing empty capsids and nucleocapsids. Scale = 200 nm. (c) High magnification of extracellular enveloped particles. Scale = 100 nm.

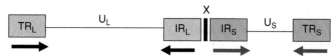

**Figure 3** General genome organization of ostreid herpesvirus 1 (OsHV-1). $TR_L$ and $IR_L$ are inverted repeats flanking the unique region $U_L$. $TR_S$ and $IR_S$ are inverted repeats flanking the unique region $U_S$.

elaboration of gene expression. A total of 38 genes shares sequence similarities with other genes of the virus, defining 12 families of related genes. These include one gene family encoding proteins containing helicase motifs, one family encoding product related to inhibitors of apoptosis (IAPs), one family derived from a deoxyuridine triphosphatase gene, three families predicted to encode membrane-associated proteins, two families encoding RING-finger proteins, two families whose products are predicted to be secreted, and two other families. Gene families are also present in all other sequenced herpes-

viruses. The observation that IAPs are also encoded by baculoviruses and entomopoxviruses (both of which have insect hosts) underscores the importance of the apoptotic responses of invertebrates against viral infections. Vertebrate herpesviruses and poxviruses do not encode IAPs, and subvert the battery of host defenses by other pathways. Amino acid sequence comparisons have provided functional information on 25 genes that are not members of families. Seven genes encode enzymes. These include the catalytic subunit of DNA polymerase, two subunits of ribonucleotide reductase, a helicase, a putative primase, and the ATPase subunit of terminase. Two additional genes encode RING-like proteins. One protein is related to a eukaryotic protein of unknown function which is brain-specific in vertebrates. The ORF30 protein is related in an N-terminal cysteine-rich domain to a protein of unknown function in mammalian herpesviruses. A total of 15 genes encodes proteins which have predicted signal or transmembrane sequences and therefore may be associated with membranes, one specifying a putative ion channel protein.

## Evolution and Taxonomy

Even though OsHV-1 shares a similar capsid architecture, amino acid sequence comparisons have failed to identify a single protein that has homologs in proteins unique to herpesviruses, with the exception of ORF30 which contains a domain found to date only in a subset of mammalian herpesviruses. Several OsHV-1 proteins have homologs that are distributed widely in nature (e.g., DNA polymerase), but these are no more closely related to homologs in other herpesviruses or to homologs in other organisms. This finding is also characteristic of comparisons between herpesviruses that infect fish or amphibians and those that infect mammals or birds. The strongest genetic indication of a common origin resides with the ATPase subunit of the terminase, which is involved in packaging DNA into the capsid. Homologs of this gene are present in all herpesviruses, and T4 and related bacteriophages. The T4 and OsHV-1 genes are unspliced, whereas those in herpesviruses of mammals and birds contain one intron and those in herpesviruses of fish and amphibians contain two introns. The available data support the view that herpesviruses of mammals and birds, of fish and amphibians, and of invertebrates form three major lineages of the herpesviruses. The invertebrate herperviruses would have evolved as a separate lineage about a billion years ago, and the fish viruses about 400 million years ago. OsHV-1 is currently the single representative of what may be a large number of invertebrate herpesviruses. Recent data show that OsHV-1 can infect several bivalve species. This contrasts with vertebrate herpesviruses which are generally confined to a single species in nature. Consequently, the true host of OsHV-1 is unknown. The apparent loss of several gene functions in OsHV-1 prompts the speculation that this may have promoted interspecies transmission in the context of introduction of non-native bivalve species and use of modern aquaculture techniques.

## Diagnosis and Epidemiological Surveys

Light microscopy remains the preferred method for diagnosis of herpes-like virus infections in suspect samples. However, this method is poorly suited to diagnosis of viral diseases and should be supported by other techniques such as transmission electron microscopy. Even so, microscopic techniques are time consuming and unsuitable for epidemiological surveys. The lack of bivalve cell lines precludes *in vitro* culture and the observation of virus cytopathic effects. The purification of OsHV-1 from fresh infected larval *C. gigas* has served as a platform for the generation of molecular biological reagents for diagnosis. Procedures to detect herpesviruses in oysters using polymerase chain reaction (PCR) and *in situ* hybridization (ISH) have been developed and are suitable for epidemiological surveys of field samples, such as are currently being performed on oyster spat and larvae from commercial hatcheries and shellfish farms in France.

## Picorna-Like Viruses and Other Small Virus-Like Particles

Virus-like particles of 27 nm in diameter have been reported in *Mytilus edulis* mussels from Denmark. These particles were enclosed in vesicles and arranged singly or in paracrystaline arrays. Acute cellular infiltrations were associated with virion detection and were interpreted as granulocytomas. Electron-dense, unenveloped virus-like particles (25–45 nm) have also been detected in farmed *Perna canaliculus* and *Mytilus galloprovincialis* mussels suffering mortalities in New Zeland. Extensive hemocytosis and necrosis of interstitial cells, basal cells, and digestive tubule epithelial cells were observed. Small DNA-negative virus-like particles (22–30 nm) were also reported in digestive and secretory cells of scallops, *Pecten novaezelandiae*, and toheroa, *Paphies ventricosum*, from New Zealand. Mass mortalities in Japanese pearl oysters, *Pinctada fucata martensii*, which have occurred in Japan since 1994, have been associated with a nonenveloped virus (25–33 nm) called Akoya virus. The disease was characterized by necosis and degeneration of muscle fibers. A morphologically similar virus was detected in the pearl oyster, *Pinctada margaritifera*, from French Polynesia associated with granulomas and focal necrosis within the adductor muscle. These lesions were similar to those reported in the mussel *M. edulis* suffering from granulocytomas. Paraspherical or polygonal-shaped virus-like particles (40 nm) consisted of a membrane-like envelope coating a central 35 nm electron-dense core. Icosahedral–spherical (27–35 nm), nonenveloped virus particles have also been detected in the cytoplasm of connective tissue cells from cultured carpet shell clams, *R. decussatus*, suffering mortalities in Galicia (Spain). More recently, nonenveloped, icosahedral (19–21 nm) virus-like particles have been associated with large foci of massive hemocytic infiltration in cockles, *Cerastoderma edule*, from the same area (Galicia, Spain). The detection of red deposits on histological sections after methyl green pyronin staining suggested that this is an RNA virus.

All these virus-like particles are similar to those described first in mussels from Denmark. Due to their size, morphology, and the formation of paracrystalline arrays, they have been assumed to belong to the family *Picornaviridae*. However, no molecular information is available on these viruses to date.

## Papova-Like Viruses

Intranuclear, nonenveloped virus-like particles (50–55 nm) with icosahedral symmetry were first reported from the gonadal epithelia of eastern oysters, *C. virginica*, in the USA in 1976 and in Canada in 1994. The virions were interpreted as papova-like viruses. A papova-like virus has also been detected in gonadal tissues during a health survey of cultured Pacific oyster, *C. gigas*, from the southern coast of Korea. More recently, histological examination of *C. gigas* oysters in France has revealed several cases of abnormally large basophilic cells in gonadal tissues. Electron microscopy examination has revealed nonenveloped icosahedral particles 50 nm in diameter.

## Reo-Like Viruses and Birnaviruses

A virus tentatively assigned the family *Reoviridae* has been isolated from juvenile eastern oysters, *C. virginica*, using a fish cell line. Virions have been described as slightly oval particles (79 nm in diameter) containing a distinct inner core and clear spike-like projections on the outer capsid. Birnaviruses have been isolated from different bivalve species in Europe and Taiwan. A virus tentatively named 'marine birnavirus' (MABV) has also been isolated during a high mortality episode from oysters cultured in the Uma Sea (Japan). MABVs have been defined as a group within the genus *Aquabirnavirus*. Although the pathogenicity of certain MABV strains appears to be weak in shellfish, it has been observed in some mollusk species (the clam *Meretrix lusoria*, the Agemaki or jack knife clam *Sinovacura constricta*, and the Japanese pearl oyster, *P. fucata*) that stressors such as changes in temperature, spawning, and exposure to heavy metals can result in mortality by increasing host suceptibility. MABVs may thus be opportunistic pathogens that persistently infect marine organisms and become pathogenic under stressful conditions. Birnavirus-like particles were also isolated from the thin telling, *Tellina tenuis*, and the flat oyster, *Ostrea edulis*, from the coast of Britain and east coast of Canada. MABVs isolated from shellfish appear to be pathogenic to fish. Moreover, based on serological and genomic properties, strains isolated from shellfish and fish seem similar. This may indicate that the host range of MABV may be broad. Assays to reproduce experimentally the infection using the reovirus-like and birnavirus-like particles isolated on

a fish cell line have shown inconsistent results, and a firm conclusion on the significance of these viruses for shellfish is still unknown.

## Conclusion

In some cases, mollusk viruses have been detected only as inconsequential infections in animals that are suffering from another known disease or from an environmental stress such as pollution. However, several mass mortality outbreaks in mollusks have been attributed to viral infections. The almost total extermination of the Portuguese oyster, *C. angulata*, in French and European Atlantic waters in 1973 has been associated with irido-like virus infections. Viruses morphologically similar to members of the *Herpesviridae* have also been associated with high mortality rates in various marine mollusk species around the world.

The production of healthy shellfish from hatcheries and nurseries is a critical aspect of the conservation and management of natural populations and extensive farming areas. Selective breeding of hatchery stock will also be important for aquaculture development. This may lead to a substantial international trade in bivalve gametes and larvae to allow distribution of genetically improved seed stock. However, significant production problems including the elimination of viral diseases must be solved before hatcheries can become a major supplier for the industry. High-density production systems including commercial hatcheries and nurseries are an important source of viral diseases in aquaculture and the movement of stock must be considered as one of the major risks of disease spread. The risk of viral disease in invertebrate aquaculture species is accentuated by the lack of specific chemotherapies and vaccines. Improved knowledge and understanding of shellfish viruses is needed to develop new tools for disease control.

## Further Reading

Arzul I, Renault T, Lipart C, and Davison AJ (2001) Evidence for inter species transmission of oyster herpesvirus in marine bivalves. *Journal of General Virology* 82: 865–870.

Barbosa-Solomieu V, Dégremont L, Vazquez-Juarez R, *et al.* (2005) Ostreid herpesvirus 1 detection among three successive generations of Pacific oysters (*Crassostrea gigas*). *Virus Research* 107: 47–56.

Chang PH, Kuo ST, Lai SH, *et al.* (2005) Herpes-like virus infection causing mortality of cultured abalone *Haliotis diversicolor supertexta* in Taiwan. *Diseases of Aquatic Organisms* 65: 23–27.

Chou HY, Chang SJ, Lee HY, and Chiou YC (1998) Preliminary evidence for the effect of heavy metal cations on the susceptibility of hard clam (*Meretrix lusoria*) to clam birnavirus infection. *Fish Pathology* 33: 213–219.

Comps M and Duthoit JL (1979) Infections virales chez les huîtres *Crassostrea angulata* (Lmk) et *C. gigas* (Th.). *Haliotis* 8: 301–308.

Davison AJ, Trus BL, Cheng N, *et al.* (2005) A novel class of herpesvirus with bivalve hosts. *Journal of General Virology* 86: 41–43.

Farley CA, Banfield WG, Kasnic JRG, and Foster WS (1972) Oyster herpes-type virus. *Science* 178: 759–760.

Le Deuff R-M and Renault T (1999) Purification and partial genome characterization of a herpes-like virus infecting the Japanese oyster, *Crassostrea gigas. Journal of General Virology* 80: 1317–1322.

Lees D (2000) Viruses and bivalve shellfish. *International Journal of Food Microbiology* 59: 81–116.

Lipart C and Renault T (2002) Herpes-like virus detection in *Crassostrea gigas* spat using DIG-labelled probes. *Journal of Virological Methods* 101: 1–10.

McGeoch DJ, Rixon FJ, and Davison AJ (2006) Topics in herpesvirus genomics and evolution. *Virus Research* 117: 90–104.

Meyers TR and Hirai K (1980) Morphology of a reo-like virus isolated from juvenile American oysters (*Crassostrea virginica*). *Journal of General Virology* 46: 249–253.

Rasmussen LPD (1986) Virus-associated granulocytomas in the marine mussel, *Mytilus edulis*, from three sites in Denmark. *Journal of Invertebrate Pathology* 48: 117–123.

Renault T and Novoa B (2004) Viruses infecting bivalve molluscs. *Aquatic Living Resources* 17: 397–409.

Renault T, Le Deuff R-M, Lipart C, and Delsert C (2000) Development of a PCR procedure for the detection of a herpes-like virus infecting oysters in France. *Journal of Virological Methods* 88: 41–50.

# Shrimp Viruses

**J-R Bonami,** CNRS, Montpellier, France

## Glossary

**Cephalothorax** The shrimp head, containing the main organs, hepatopancreas, stomach, foregut and midgut, gonads, heart, gills.

**Epizootic** An epidemic in animal populations. Rapid spreading of a disease.

**Hepatopancreas** Organ of the digestive tract with secretion–absorption functions and located in the cephalothorax (head) of shrimp. Also called the digestive gland.

**Postlarvae** Stage of shrimp development, after the larval stages.

## Introduction

To date, more than 20 viral diseases have been reported in shrimp and prawns. Most of the described viruses are related, but often only on the basis of morphological characteristics to known virus families. Two of the most important pathogens of shrimp have been sufficiently characterized to be accepted by the International Committee on Taxonomy of Viruses (ICTV) as members of new virus families within the classification and nomenclature of viruses. Yellow head virus (YHV), together with closely related gill-associated virus (GAV), have been classified as members of the new genus *Okavirus* in the new family *Roniviridae*. White spot syndrome virus (WSSV) has been classified as the only known member of the new genus *Whispovirus* in the new family *Nimaviridae*. A third major pathogen, Taura syndrome virus (TSV), has been accepted for classification in the family *Dicistroviridae*. Although not yet officially accepted by the ICTV, six other shrimp viruses have been sufficiently well characterized to be considered as possible members of four existing virus families: *Totiviridae* (infectious myonecrosis virus, IMNV), *Nodaviridae* (macrobrachium rosenbergeii nodavirus, MrNV), *Parvoviridae* (infectious hypodermal and hematopoietic necrosis virus, IHHNV, and hepatopancreatic parvovirus, HPV) and *Baculoviridae* (BP-type and MBV-type viruses).

## History

Three periods can be defined in the recent history of shrimp virus discovery: the first was during the 1970s, in which observations of viral agents were made by 'chance'; the second period commenced in the 1980s, in which evidence of viral pathogenic agents was obtained as a result of disease observations or mortalities occurring in shrimp farms; and finally, since the early 1990s with the development of molecular biology, more structured and intensive approaches to the descriptions of the pathogens and the associated diseases were undertaken.

The first virus of Crustacea was reported in 1966 by Vago in the Mediterranean crab *Portunus depurator*. The virus appeared to be related to members of the *Reoviridae*. In shrimp, occluded bacilliform particles were reported in 1973 by Couch during investigations on the effect of pollutants in pink shrimp (*Penaeus duorarum*). The agent was reported to be closely related to members of the *Baculoviridae*.

In 1981, Sano and colleagues reported the detection of a 'nonoccluded baculovirus' in kuruma shrimp (*Penaeus japonicus*) during mortalities in hatchery-reared shrimp in two prefectures in Japan. Two years later (1983), Lightner reported a transmissible disease named infectious hypodermal and hematopoietic necrosis (IHHN) as the Pacific blue shrimp (*Penaeus stylirostris*) as the source of mortalities in ponds. While at first thought to be related to members of the *Picornaviridae*, IHHNV was later assigned to the *Parvoviridae* after investigations on the structure of the genome. Since that time, reports of new viruses have increased in parallel with the rapid development of shrimp farming globally and, to date, more than 20 viruses have been reported in shrimp (**Table 1**).

The major developments in shrimp virus research commenced in the early 1990s following the development and application of molecular tools. Cloning and sequencing of genome fragments allowed construction of specific and sensitive tools for detection and diagnosis. These DNA-based methods, such as the polymerase chain reaction (PCR) and dot-blot hybridization, have led to the use of commercial diagnostic kits for selection of healthy shrimp and the production of specific pathogen-free (SPF) breeding stock. SPF shrimp have proven to be particularly useful, not only in limiting or preventing production losses due to disease on farms, but also as experimental animals for studies on shrimp viruses.

## Impact of Viral Diseases on Farmed Shrimp Production

The rapid progress in shrimp virology during the past two decades is clearly related to the high commercial value of

**Table 1**    Known shrimp viruses

| Genome | Virus family[a] | Acronym | Virus name | Host | Genomic data |
|---|---|---|---|---|---|
| ssRNA | *Dicistroviridae* | TSV | Taura syndrome virus | *P. vannamei* | Complete |
| | *Roniviridae* | YHV | Yellow head virus | *P. monodon* | Complete |
| | | GAV | Gill-associated virus | | Complete |
| | *Bunyaviridae* | MoV | Mourilyan virus | *P. monodon* | Partial |
| | | | | *P. japonicus* | |
| | *Totiviridae* | IMNV | Infectious myonecrosis virus | *P. vannamei* | Complete |
| | *Rhabdoviridae* | RPS | | *P. stylirostris* | n.d. |
| | | | | *P. vannamei* | |
| | *Togaviridae* | LOVV | Lymphoid organ vacuolisation virus | *P. vannamei* | n.d. |
| | *Nodaviridae* | MrNV/XSV | Macrobrachium rosenbergii nodavirus/extra small virus | *M. rosenbergii* | Complete |
| | | LSNV | | *P. monodon* | n.d. |
| dsRNA | *Birnaviridae* | IPN-like virus | Infectious pancreatic necrosis-like virus | *P. japonicus* | n.d. |
| | *Reoviridae* | Reo-Pj | | *P. japonicus* | n.d. |
| | | Reo-Pm | | *P. monodon* | n.d. |
| | | Reo-Pv | | P. vannamei | n.d. |
| | | PBRV | | *Palaemon* sp. | n.d. |
| ssDNA | *Parvoviridae* | IHHNV | Infectious hemocytic and hematopoietic virus | *P. stylirostris* | Complete |
| | | HPV | Hepatopancreatic parvovirus | *P. semisulcatus* | Complete |
| | | HPV-like | | *P. merguiensis* | n.d. |
| | | | | *M. rosenbergii* | n.d. |
| | | | | | n.d. |
| | | SMV | | *P. monodon* | n.d. |
| | | LPV | | *P. monodon* | n.d. |
| | | | | *F. merguiensis* | n.d. |
| | | | | *P. esculentus* | n.d. |
| dsDNA | *Iridoviridae* | | | *Protrachypene precipua* | n.d. |
| | Nonoccluded bacilliform virus | BMNV or (PjNOB) | Baculoviral midgut gland necrosis virus | *P. japonicus* | Partial |
| | | PHRV | | | n.d. |
| | | CcBV | | *Crangon crangon* | n.d. |
| | *Baculoviridae* | PvNPV or (BP-type) | Single-nucleocapsid polyedrosis virus | *P. duorarum* | n.d. |
| | | PmNPV or (MBV-type) | Single-nucleocapsid polyedrosis virus | *P. vannamei* | Partial |
| | | MbNPV | Single-nucleocapsid polyedrosis virus | *P. monodon* | Partial |
| | | | | *Metapenaeus bennettae* | n.d. |
| | *Nimaviridae* | WSSV | White spot syndrome virus | Penaeids and numerous other crustaceans | Complete |

[a]Only TSV, GAV, YHV, IHHNV, and WSSV have been formally classified to date.

these farmed crustaceans. This has significantly increased our understanding of viruses infecting only invertebrates which previously had been confined primarily to insect viruses. However, in contrast to most insect viruses in which investigations were oriented primarily toward biological control of insect pests and their potential use as gene expression vectors, shrimp virus research has focused on disease prevention.

It is difficult to know the impact of viral diseases on shrimp populations in the natural environment. Diseased shrimp are rarely found, essentially due to predation and cannibalism when animals appear weakened. However, under farming conditions, where the density of the shrimp population can easily exceed 300 000 postlarvae per hectare, the consequence of a disease outbreak and associated mass mortalities can be disastrous. In 2003, total world production from shrimp farming was more than 1.6 million metric tons, representing a value of almost US$ 9000 million and accounting for about 25% of marketable shrimp production (capture and farming). Viral disease has been a major problem for this large and expanding industry and the economic and socioeconomic impacts have been severe. For example, a report commissioned by the World Bank in 1996 estimated the annual global cost of disease (primarily viral) to shrimp farming was US$ 3000 million or 40% of production capacity at that time. In China and Thailand alone, annual production losses due to WSSV have reached US$ 500–1000 million. In Ecuador, the emergence of WSSV in 1999 resulted in a 75% drop in annual production and 130 000 industry workers were reported to have lost their jobs. The production records of these major shrimp-producing countries exhibit depressions coinciding with the sequential emergence of major viral pathogens. In contrast, in Brazil, which was free of the major diseases until 2003, shrimp production constantly increased. Nevertheless, Brazil has also experienced significant production losses since that time with the emergence of infectious myonecrosis caused by a new toti-like virus.

# Factors Responsible for Viral Disease Emergence in Shrimp

Disease emergence in shrimp aquaculture can be attributed to three primary factors: (1) the common practice in the shrimp farming industry of introducing each season fresh wild broodstock collected from the natural environment as the source of seed (postlarval shrimp) for farms; (2) national and international trade in broodstock and commercial seed (postlarvae) to be transferred to ponds until they reach the marketable size; and (3) the culture of shrimp in earthern ponds in high densities.

The use of wild brooders in hatcheries commonly occurs without adequate knowledge of their health status or adequate quarantine. This often results in the introduction

of pathogens into the farming system and it is a practice that persists even though SPF shrimp, bred in biosecure facilities, are now readily available in many countries.

Trade in broodstock and seed also commonly occurs without checking for at least the known pathogens. This practice was responsible for the rapid worldwide spread of the IHHNV, the introduction of TSV to the Eastern Hemisphere, and the rapid spread of WSSV from the Eastern to the Western Hemisphere. The practice of farming in brackish water earthern ponds creates an environment in which new pathogens may be encountered and disease spread rapidly once outbreaks occur. As a result, short explosive epizootics may, in few days, wipe out the whole shrimp population of a farm.

Environmental and host factors also play an important role in the emergence of shrimp disease. Poor-quality pond conditions (e.g., high salinity, pH, or nitrogen) can cause physiological stress in shrimp leading to increased susceptibility to disease. The shrimp culture medium (brackish water) allows very efficient transfer of free viruses, either as free infectious agents or in pathogen vectors. As ectotherms, shrimps are susceptible to water temperature shifts that can stimulate the replication of viruses that commonly persist in shrimp as unapparent infections. Shrimp also lack the sophisticated adaptive immune mechanisms (antibodies, cytokines, T-cells) deployed by vertebrates to combat viral infections and so have less capacity to survive disease.

# Characteristics of Some Shrimp Viruses

## Shrimp Baculoviruses

Two distinct groups of viruses, sharing numerous characters with members of the family *Baculoviridae*, have been described in shrimp. They have been improperly called BP-type viruses (BP, baculovirus penaei) and MBV-type viruses (MBV, monodon baculovirus) on the basis of the morphology of their occlusion bodies (OBs). The BP-type group exhibits tetrahedral OBs; the MBV group exhibits rounded OBs. It is classified as a tentative species (*Penaeus monodon* NPV, PemoNPV) in the genus *Nucleopolyhedrovirus* of the family *Baculoviridae*.

### General characteristics

All baculoviruses detected in shrimp develop in the nuclei of digestive epithelial cells (hepatopancreas and mid-gut) with the release of OBs within feces. They are bacilliform in shape and comprise a trilaminar envelope surrounding a rod-shaped nucleocapsid. Virions may be occluded in paracrystalline occlusion bodies. Only small fragments of the double-stranded DNA (dsDNA) genome have been cloned and sequenced for a few shrimp baculoviruses. For the BP-type virus, Penaeus duorarum single nuclear polyhedrosis virus (PdSNPV), the genome has been shown by electron microscopy to be a circular structure with an estimated size of $75 \times 10^6$ kDa (113–115 kbp). There appear to be different morphotypes of BP-type baculoviruses which were distinguished based on differences in particle size; two different BP genotypes have been reported in the same shrimp tissue section by *in situ* hybridization.

### Polyhedra

In contrast to insect baculoviruses, shrimp baculovirus OBs are unenveloped and comprise large subunits (SuOBs) of polyhedrin which are icosahedral in shape (**Figure 1**). The SuOBs are always associated in triplets. They are organized in two different crystalline forms: the BP-type viruses form

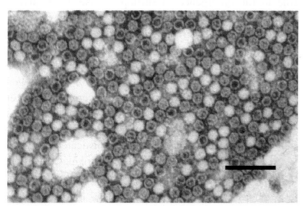

**Figure 1** Purified SuOBs (polyhedrin) from PmSNPV (MBV-type virus). Note the full and empty virus-like particles. The particles were negatively stained with 2% phosphotungstic acid (PTA). Scale = 100 nm. Reproduced from Bonami: JB, Aubert H, Mari J, Poulos BT, and Lightner DV (1997) The polyhedra of the occluded baculoviruses of marine decapod crustacea: A unique structure, crystal organization, and proposed model. *Journal of Structural Biology* 120: 134–145, with permission from Elsevier.

parallel rows in all three dimensions (**Figure 2(a)**); the MBV-type viruses assemble four triplets to form a 'rosette' (hollow sphere) as the building block of the OB (**Figure 2(b)**). MBV-type OBs are more sensitive to thaw–freezing but each OB type disaggregates spontaneously in CsCl gradients. Compared to insect baculovirus polyhedrin subunits, both BP- and MBV-type SuOBs are larger in dimensions (15–22 nm compared to 6.5–9 nm diameter) and molecular mass (52–58 kDa compared to ~30 kDa ).

There is evidence of antigenic cross-reactivity between PdSNPV and MBV SuOBs, but this requires confirmation as, unexpectedly, PdSNPV SuOBs were also found to cross-react with both polyhedrin and granulin from the insect baculoviruses Autographa californica nuclear polyhedrosis virus and and Trichoplusia ni granulosis virus, respectively.

### Viral infection cycle

All life stages of the pink shrimp (*P. duorarum*), white shrimp (*Penaeus setiferus*), and the brown shrimp (*Penaeus aztecus*) are susceptible to BP-type baculovirus, while only larval and postlarval stages of the Pacific white shrimp (*Penaeus vannamei*) and Pacific blue shrimp (*P. stylirostris*) have been observed to be infected. In the black tiger shrimp (*Penaeus monodon*), postlarvae, juveniles, and adults have been observed to be infected with MBV.

For PdSNPV in *P. duorarum*, the major steps in the infection cycle have been described including the appearance of naked nucleocapsids in the cytoplasm of epithelial digestive cells, nucleoprotein release at nuclear pores, followed by all morphogenesis steps in infected nuclei and the development of tetrahedral OBs. Cellular pathological changes include nuclear hypertrophy and perinuclear membranous proliferation. Nuclear hypertrophy associated with increasing size of OBs leads to the release of the nuclear contents into the digestive lumen of

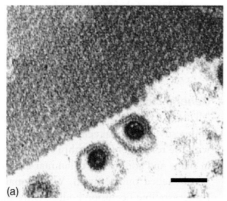
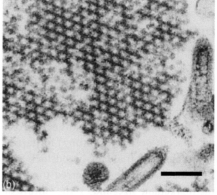

**Figure 2** Ultrathin sections in occlusion bodies of shrimp baculoviruses; (a) PvSNPV (BP-type virus) and (b) PmSNPV (MBV-type virus). The two types of crystal (bullet-like arrangement and rosette formation) are evident. Scale = 100 nm (a, b). Reproduced from Bonami JB, Aubert H, Mari J, Poulos BT, and Lightner DV (1997) The polyhedra of the occluded baculoviruses of marine decapod crustacea: A unique structure, crystal organization, and proposed model. *Journal of Structural Biology* 120: 134–145, with permission from Elsevier.

hepatopancreatic tubules and gut, and the excretion of OBs in the feces. The infection cycle is completed by oral ingestion and OB dissolution in the digestive tract of the new host. A similar infection cycle is hypothesized for MBV-type baculoviruses. In addition to horizontal transmission, vertical transmission is suspected, based on the presence of OBs in very young postlarvae a few days after hatching.

### Geographic distribution and host range

BP-type virus infection is widespread in farmed and wild penaeid shrimp in the Americas. The known distribution is from the Gulf of Mexico in the north through the Caribbean, the east coast of South America as far south as the State of Bahia in Central Brazil. On the Pacific coast, the distribution ranges from Mexico to Peru. BP-type virus has also been observed in wild shrimp from Hawaii. Several penaeid shrimp species have been reported to be infected, both in aquaculture facilities and in the wild environment. These include *P. duorarum, P. aztecus, P. vannamei, P. setiferus, P. stylirostris, P. penicillatus, P. schmitti, P. paulensis, P. subtilis, Trachypenaeus similis,* and *Protrachypene precipua.*

MBV-type virus infections are widely distributed in penaeid shrimp of the Eastern Hemisphere, particularly in the Indo-Pacific countries of China, India, Indonesia, Philippines, Malaysia, Thailand, Sri Lanka, and Australia where the virus is enzootic in wild stocks. The virus has also been reported in Kuwait, Oman, Israel, Italy, and West Africa (Kenya and Gambia). It has been observed in imported penaeid shrimp in Tahiti and Hawaii, Mexico, Ecuador, Brazil, Puerto Rico, and some states of the USA. The known host range includes *P. monodon, P. merguiensis, P. semisulcatus, P. indicus, P. penicillatus, P. esculentus,* and *P. vannamei.*

## Shrimp Parvoviruses

Two viruses sharing the primary characteristics of members of the family *Parvoviridae* have been reported in penaeid shrimp. IHHNV causes a systemic infection of multiple organs of ectodermal and mesodermal origin as and is described in the Pacific blue shrimp (*P. stylirostris*). It is associated with runt and deformity syndrome (RDS) in Pacific white shrimp (*P. vannamei*) and occurs commonly as a low-level persistent infection in apparently healthy black tiger shrimp (*P. monodon*). HPV causes an infection of the digestive system (epithelial cells of hepatopancreas and mid-gut) in black tiger shrimp *P. monodon* and in the fleshy prawn (*P. chinensis*). HPV isolates from *P. monodon* (HPVmon) and *P. chinensis* (HPVchin) represent two distinct genetic lineages. A third parvo-like virus, spawner-isolated mortality virus (SMV) infects *P. monodon* but is less well characterized.

IHHNV and HPV are each nonenveloped icosahedral viruses, 22 nm in diameter and containing a linear single-stranded DNA (ssDNA) genome. IHHNV virions have been reported to contain four polypeptides as detected by sodium dodecyl sulfate polyacrylamide gel electrophoresis (SDS-PAGE) and silver staining (74, 47, 39, and 37.5 kDa). For HPVchin, only one virion structural protein has been observed (54 kDa) but analysis of HPVmon has revealed a doublet protein band (57 kDa major band and 54 kDa minor band). In addition to differences in tissue tropism, the viruses display differences in cytopathology. During HPV infection, cellular lesions correspond to typical densonucleosis in insects with the formation of enlarged, densely stained, and Feulgen-positive nuclei. In IHHNV infections, lesions are discrete, often difficult to detect, and display characteristic eosinophilic intranuclear Cowdry type A inclusion bodies.

### Genomic organization

The IHHNV genome comprises 4075 nucleotides (according to a recent GenBank submission) and contains three long open reading frames (ORFs) on the complementary (positive) strand (**Figure 3**). The three ORFs are referred to as left, mid, and right. The left ORF is in a different reading frame (+1) to mid- and right ORFs. As for other parvoviruses, noncoding termini at each end of the genome contain palindromic sequences. The left ORF encodes a 666 amino acid protein with high homology with putative major nonstructural protein (NS-1) of mosquito brevidensoviruses. The mid-ORF overlaps the left ORF and encodes a 363 aa protein of unknown function (possibly an NS-2 protein). The right ORF overlaps the left ORF by 62 nt and encode a 329 aa protein. By analogy to other parvoviruses, it has been speculated that the right ORF encodes the capsid proteins but this is not consistent with the four structural proteins reported in purified virions. The negative strand also contains an ORF with a coding capacity of 134 amino acids. Further work is required to define the IHHNV expression strategy.

The HPV genome comprises 6321 nucleotides containing three long ORFs in the complementary (positive) strand and palindromic noncoding termini that form hairpin-like structures, as found in other parvoviruses (**Figure 3**). ORF1 (left ORF) encodes a 428 amino acid putative nonstructural protein-2 (NS-2) of unknown function. ORF2 (mid-ORF), in −1 frame relative to ORF1 encodes a 579-amino-acid polypeptide that contains conserved replication initiator motifs, NTP-binding, and helicase domains similar to NS-1 of other parvoviruses. The right ORF (ORF3), which is in the same frame as ORF1, encodes the 818-amino-acid capsid protein (VP protein).

### Taxonomic position

In terms of morphology and genome structure and organization, both IHHNV and HPV share similarities with

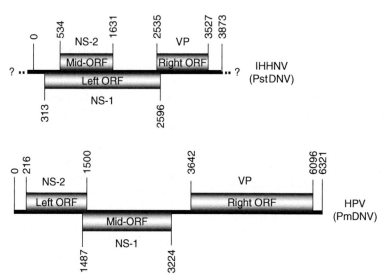

**Figure 3** Genome organization of IHHNV and HPV. IHHNV (PstDNV) is according to Shike H, Dhar AK, Burns JC, *et al.* (2000) Infections hypodermal and haematopoietic necrosis virus of shrimp is related to mosquito brevidensoviruses. *Virology* 277: 167–177.

members of the family *Parvoviridae*. Genomic analysis has clearly indicated that IHHNV is closely related to mosquito densoviruses and it has recently been classified as a tentative species (*Penaeus stylirostris densovirus*), in the genus *Brevidensovirus*. Similarly, HPV was recently proposed as new member of subfamily *Densovirinae* to be designated as the species *Penaeus monodon densovirus*.

### Geographic distribution and host range

HPV was first observed in wild and farmed penaeid shrimp in Australia, China, Korea, Philippines, Indonesia, Malaysia, Kenya, Kuwait, and Israel. It has also been reported subsequently from several locations in North and South America (Pacific coast of Mexico and El Salvador). Natural infections have been reported in *P. merguiensis*, *P. semisulcatus*, *P. chinensis*, *P. esculentus*, *P. monodon*, *P. japonicus*, *P. penicillatus*, *P. indicus*, *P. vannamei*, and *P. stylirostris*.

IHHNV is widely distributed in the Americas (Brazil, Ecuador, Central America, Mexico, Peru, southeast USA), the Central Pacific (Guam, Hawaii, Tahiti, and New Caledonia), and Asia and the Indo-Pacific area (Indonesia, Malaysia, Philippines, Thailand, and Australia). Natural infections have been reported in *P. stylirostris*, *P. vannamei*, *P. occidentalis*, *P. californiensis*, *P. monodon*, *P. semisulcatus*, and *P. japonicus*. It is likely that infection with IHHNV or a similar virus also occurs in other penaeid shrimp species.

Recent investigations have revealed evidence of the integration of IHHNV-related sequences within the genomes of *P. monodon* populations from Africa (Madagascar, Tanzania, Mozambique) and Australia. The integrated sequences vary by up to 14% from epidemic IHHNV and do not appear to be associated with the formation of complete or infections virions.

## Infectious Myonecrosis Virus

In 2002, a new disease associated with low mortalities was reported in the Pacific white shrimp *Penaeus vannamei* from northeastern Brazil. Clinical signs included necrotic areas in muscles, resulting sometimes in a whitish and opaque appearance to the tail. The causative agent was named infectious myonecrosis virus (IMNV) on the basis of the clinical signs.

### General properties

In infected animals, virions accumulate in the cytoplasm of target cells (muscular cells, hemocytes, and connective tissue cells) forming basophilic inclusions. IMNV has a density of $1.366 \, \text{g ml}^{-1}$ in cesium chloride. It is a nonenveloped icosahedral virus, 40 nm in diameter (**Figure 4**) with a genome consisting of a single segment of double-stranded RNA (dsRNA), 7560 bp in length. The capsid contains a single major polypeptide of 106 kDa.

### Genomic organization

The IMNV genome organization is illustrated in **Figure 5**. Two large nonoverlapping ORFs in different reading frames (ORF1 and ORF2) are flanked by 3′ untranslated region (UTR) and 5′ UTR of 109 and 135 nt, respectively, and are separated by a noncoding region of 287 nt. ORF1 contains a dsRNA-binding motif (DSRM) of 60 amino acids in the N-terminal region. The translated sequence of 901 amino acids corresponds approximately to the size determined in SDS-PAGE for the major capsid protein (106 kDa). ORF2 encodes an RNA-dependent RNA polymerase (RdRp) with significant sequence similarity to members of the family *Totiviridae*.

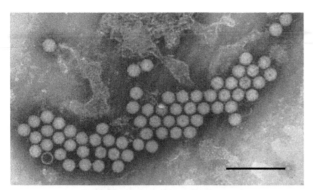

**Figure 4** Purified IMNV virions. The particles were negatively stained with 2% phosphotungstic acid (PTA). Scale = 200 nm. From Poulos BT, Tang KFJ, Pantoja CR, Bonami JR, and Lightner DV (2006) Purification and characterization of infectious myonecrosis virus of penaeid shrimp. *Journal of General Virology* 87: 987–996.

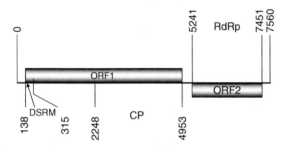

**Figure 5** Genome organization of IMNV.

## Taxonomic position

Phylogenetic analysis of IMNV RdRp clusters this virus within members of the genus *Giardiavirus* in the family *Totiviridae*. The genome structure and organization are also consistent with classification in the *Totiviridae*. However, as known giardiviruses infect only flagellated protozoan parasites (*Giardia lamblia* and *Trichomonas vaginalis*), further consideration of the properties of IMNV will be required before formal classification can be obtained.

## Geographic distribution and host range

The disease was, until recently, restricted to farmed *P. vannamei* in northeastern Brazil. However, recently the virus and the disease have been reported at several sites in Indonesia where infected *P. vannamei* postlarvae have been introduced from Brazil. *Penaeus stylirostris* and *P. monodon* shrimps are susceptible to experimental infection with IMNV.

## MrNV/XSV Complex

White tail disease occurs in farmed giant freshwater prawns (*Macrobrachium rosenbergii*) and is named after the obvious clinical signs in diseased postlarvae. Two viruses, Macrobrachium rosenbergii nodavirus (MrNV) and a

very small virus-like particle named XSV (extra small virus), are each found in diseased prawns. The disease was first observed in a hatchery in Guadeloupe Island in French West Indies where abnormal and sudden mortalities had been recorded since 1994. Losses were variable in intensity (5–90% cumulative mortality), depending on the broodstock used to generate the postlarvae. The first gross sign of the disease is the presence of whitish postlarvae 2–3 days after emergence. The prevalence of opaque and milky postlarvae increases dramatically 1–2 days later and changes are particularly obvious in abdomen (tail). The mortality rate reaches a maximum 5 days after the first observation of gross signs.

In diseased prawns, the most affected tissues are the striated muscles in the abdomen and cephalothorax and the connective tissues of all organs. The cytoplasm of infected cells contains discrete, pale to darkly basophilic inclusions, ranging from <1 to 40 μm in diameter. Muscles exhibit multifocal areas of hyaline necrosis of the fibers, with moderate edema.

### General properties of isolated particles

Two types of particles are observed in the cytoplasm of infected cells (**Figure 6**). The larger particles are nonenveloped, icosahedral in shape, and 26–27 nm in diameter, with a density in CsCl of 1.27–1.28 g ml$^{-1}$. The genome consists of two segments of linear single-stranded RNA (ssRNA) of 3202 (RNA1) and 1250 nt (RNA2). The capsid contains a single major protein of 43 kDa (CP43). The properties of this virus are similar to those of nodaviruses and it has been named Machrobrachium rosenbergii nodavirus (MrNV).

The smaller particles are nonenveloped, icosahedral, and 15 nm in diameter, and have a density in CsCl of 1.325 g ml$^{-1}$. The genome is composed of a single segment of linear ssRNA 796 nt in length. The capsid comprises coat proteins of 16 kDa (CP16) and 17 kDa (CP17). Because the particles are very small, this agent has been called extra small virus (XSV).

### Genomic organization

The organization of the MrNV genome is shown in **Figure 7**. RNA1 and RNA2 each encodes a long ORF flanked by terminal noncoding regions, and lacks a 3' poly(A) tail. The coding capacity is 1046 and 371 amino acids, equivalent to 122 and 43.5 kDa, for ORF1 and ORF2, respectively. Similar to other nodaviruses, RNA1 contains two long ORFs encoding nonstructural proteins: ORF1 encodes the 1046-amino-acid (~122 kDa) A protein which contains motifs characteristic of the RdRp; and ORF1b, located at the 3' end of the segment, encodes the 134-amino-acid (~13 kDa) B protein. ORF2 encodes the 371-amino-acid (~43.5 kDa) capsid protein (CP43). The coding assignment of RNA2 has been demonstrated by N-terminal amino acid sequencing of CP43. As for all

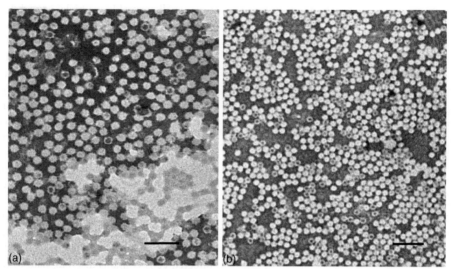

**Figure 6** Purified MrNV and XSV particles. The particles were negatively stained with 2% phosphotungstic acid (PTA). Scale = 50 nm. (a, b) Reproduced from Bonami JR, Shi Z, Qian D, and Sri Widada J (2005) White tail disease (WTD) associated virions and characterization of MrNV as a new type on nodavirus. *Journal of Fish Diseases* 28: 23–31, with permission from Blackwell Publishing.

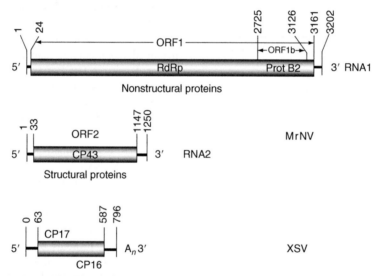

**Figure 7** Genome organizations of MrNV and XSV.

other nodaviruses, a nonencapsidated RNA3 of 453 nucleotides has also been detected. The MrNV RNA3 is longer than that of any other nodavirus RNA3 (~380–400 nt) and is likely to be a subgenomic mRNA encoding ORF1b.

The 796 nt XSV genome contains a single ORF located between nucleotides 63 and 587, and a short poly(A) tail. A potential polyadenylation signal (AAUAAA) is located 6 nt upstream of the poly(A). The ORF encodes both capsid proteins (CP16 and CP17). Amino acid sequence analysis indicates that CP16 is synthesized by internal initiation at a second methionine residue 11 amino acids downstream of the first initiation codon. The two forms of the capsid protein are synthesized in an equimolar ratio.

**Taxonomic position**

No formal taxonomic classification of MrNV has yet been assigned. The particle morphology and genome organization are similar to those of members of the family *Nodaviridae*. Amino acid sequence alignments of the RdRp indicate highest homology with members of the genera *Alphanodavirus* (insect nodaviruses) and *Betanodavirus* (fish nodaviruses). Sequence similarities are higher with alphanodaviruses than with betanodaviruses. However, coat protein sequence alignments indicate that the distance between MrNV and alphanodaviruses is similar to those separating alphanodaviruses and betanodaviruses. This suggests that MrNV may represent a possible third genus within the family.

The appropriate taxonomic classification of XSV is currently unclear. Sequence similarity searches have not indicated any significant homology with known virus genomes. As the monocistronic genome encodes only the capsid proteins, it is possible that the RdRp required for replication and transcription may be provided by MrNV. This agent meets the primary criteria of satellite viruses and appears more similar to the known satellite viruses infecting plants (e.g., tobacco necrosis satellite virus-like) than those infecting insects (e.g., chronic bee paralysis-associated satellite virus).

### MrNV/XSV relationships

MrNV and XSV are each always found associated in white tail disease infections in *M. rosenbergii* in all hatcheries and farms where disease is reported. Analysis by quantitative (real-time) polymerase chain reaction (PCR) has indicated variable proportions of MrNV RNA and XSV RNA in different isolates. However, nothing is known to date about their respective roles in the disease or its severity.

### Geographic distribution and host range

White tail disease was first recognized in a hatchery in Guadeloupe Island and was then reported in Martinique Island and in the Dominican Republic. It is suspected that infected postlarvae were introduced to Puerto Rico.

In China, the disease was recorded in Zhejiang, Jiangsu, Shanghai, Guangxi, and Guangdong Provinces and, more recently, it has been reported in Taiwan. In India, the disease has been reported in Andhra Pradesh and Tamil Nadu on the east coast and in Kerala on the west coast where *M. rosenbergii* farming was developed to replace marine (*P. monodon*) culture following the dramatic effects of the WSSV epidemic.

To date, white tail disease has only been reported in the giant freshwater prawn *M. rosenbergii*. However, marine shrimp (*P. monodon*, *P. indicus*, and *P. japonicus*) are susceptible to experimental infection, suggesting a possible role as reservoir. No disease has been reported in marine shrimp species.

## Control of Viral Diseases in Shrimp

As invertebrates, marine shrimp and freshwater prawns lack the acquired immune systems that exist in vertebrates. Consequently, a disease control based on vaccination cannot be used. Some antiviral defense reactions (innate immunity) have been reported in Crustacea but the mechanisms by which these occur are largely unknown and prevention appears as the most useful method for control. For this reason, specific and sensitive DNA-based tools for early detection are now available for most of the viral diseases. These tools allow selection of healthy broodstock and a good knowledge of the health status of postlarval seed introduced into ponds. The availability of these tools has also led to the estab-lishment of biosecure breeding programs for commercial production of specific pathogen-free (SPF) broodstock. The more widespread use of SPF stock will significantly reduce the risk of future emergence of devastating viral diseases in shrimp aquaculture.

*See also:* White Spot Syndrome Virus; Yellow Head Virus.

## Further Reading

Bonami JR, Aubert H, Mari J, Poulos BT, and Lightner DV (1997) The polyhedra of the occluded baculoviruses of marine decapod crustacea: A unique structure, crystal organization, and proposed model. *Journal of Structural Biology* 120: 134–145.

Bonami JR, Mari J, Poulos BT, and Lightner DV (1995) Characterization of the HPV, a second unusual parvovirus pathogenic for penaeid shrimp. *Journal of General Virology* 76: 813–817.

Bonami JR, Shi Z, Qian D, and Sri Widada J (2005) White tail disease of the giant freshwater prawn, *Macrobrachium rosenbergii*: Separation of the associated virions and charaterization of MrNV as a new type of nodavirus. *Journal of Fish Diseases* 28: 23–31.

Bonami JR, Trumper B, Mari J, Brehelin M, and Lightner DV (1990) Purification and characterization of the infectious hypodermal and haematopoietic necrosis virus penaeid shrimps. *Journal of General Virology* 71: 2657–2664.

Couch JA (1991) *Baculoviridae*. Nuclear polyhedrosis viruses. Part 2: Nuclear polyhedrosis viruses of invertebrates other than insects. In: Adam JR and Bonami JR (eds.) *Atlas of Invertebrate Viruses*, pp. 205–226. Boca Raton, FL: CRC Press.

Lightner DV (1988) Diseases of cultured penaeid shrimp and prawns. In: Sindermann CJ and Lightner DV (eds.) *Diseases Diagnosis and Control in North American Marine Aquaculture*, pp. 8–127. Amsterdam: Elsevier.

Lightner DV (ed.) (1996) *A Handbook of Shrimp Pathology and Diagnostic Procedures for Diseases of Cultured Penaeid Shrimp*, 304pp. Baton Rouge, LA: World Aquaculture Society.

Mari J, Bonami JR, and Lightner DV (1993) Partial cloning of the genome of the IHHNV, an unusual parvovirus pathogenic from penaeid shrimp. Diagnosis of the disease using a specific probe. *Journal of General Virology* 74: 2637–2643.

Pillai D, Bonami JR, and Sri Widada J (2006) Rapid detection of macrobrachium rosenbergii nodavirus (MrNV) and extra small virus (XSV), the pathogenic agents of white tail disease of *Macrobrachium rosenbergii* (De Man), by loop-mediated isothermal amplification. *Journal of Fish Diseases* 29: 275–283.

Poulos BT, Tang KFJ, Pantoja CR, Bonami JR, and Lightner DV (2006) Purification and characterization of infectious myonecrosis virus of penaeid shrimp. *Journal of General Virology* 87: 987–996.

Sahul Hameed AS, Yoganandhan K, Sri Widada J, and Bonami JR (2004) Studies on the occurrence of macrobrachium rosenbergii nodavirus and extra small virus-like particles associated with white tail disease of *M. rosenbergii* in India by RT-PCR detection. *Aquaculture* 238: 127–133.

Shike H, Dhar AK, Burns JC, *et al.* (2000) Infectious hypodermal and haematopoietic necrosis virus of shrimp is related to mosquito brevidensoviruses. *Virology* 277: 167–177.

Sri Widada J, Richard V, and Bonami JR (2004) Characteristics of the monocistronic genome of extra small virus (XSV), a virus-like particle associated with macrobrachium rosenbergii nodavirus (MrNV): Possible candidate for a new species of satellite virus. *Journal of General Virology* 85: 643–646.

Sukhumsirichart W, Attasart P, Boonsaeng V, and Panyim S (2006) Complete nucleotide sequence and genomic organization of hepatopancreatic parvovirus (HPV) of *Penaeus monodon*. *Virology* 346: 266–277.

Zhang H, Wang J, Yuan J, *et al.* (2006) Quantitative relationship of two viruses (MrNV and XSV) in white tail disease of *Macrobrachium rosenbergii* de Man. *Diseases of Aquatic Organisms* 71: 11–17.

# White Spot Syndrome Virus

**J-H Leu, J-M Tsai, and C-F Lo,** National Taiwan University, Taipei, Republic of China

## Glossary

***In situ* hybridization (ISH)** A technique that uses a labeled complementary DNA or RNA probe to hybridize and detect a specific DNA or RNA sequence in a section of tissue (*in situ*).

**Microarray** A DNA microarray is a collection of microscopic dsDNA or oligonucleotide spots that are deposited on a solid glass slide at high density. Each spot commonly represents a single gene. DNA microarrays use DNA–DNA or DNA–RNA hybridization to perform simultaneous large-scale analyses of the expression levels of the corresponding genes.

**RNAi (RNA interference)** RNAi refers to the introduction of homologous double-stranded RNA to specifically interfere with the target gene's expression in the cells/organisms. It was originally discovered in *C. elegans*, and is now widely used in many organisms for null mutation. Recent studies suggest that RNAi can be applied in shrimp as well through intramuscular injection of dsRNA.

## Introduction

White spot disease (WSD) is a highly contagious viral disease of penaeid shrimp. Its onset is rapid, and high levels of mortality can result within just a few days. Following the first outbreak of WSD in China and Taiwan in 1992–93, this viral disease spread quickly to other shrimp-farming areas, including Japan (1993), Thailand (1993), the United States (1995), Central and South America (1999), France (2002), and Iran (2002). Nowadays, WSD is considered endemic in almost all shrimp-producing countries in Asia and the Americas, causing serious economic damage to the shrimp culture industry. The causative agent of WSD is white spot syndrome virus (WSSV), which is a large ($80–120 \times 250–380$ nm), non-occluded, rod-shaped to elliptical, double-stranded (ds) DNA virus. The virus has a remarkably broad host range among crustaceans, including many species of shrimp, crayfish, crab, and lobster. WSSV replication and virion assembly occur in the hypertrophied nuclei of infected cells without the production of occlusion bodies. The WSSV virion consists of a rod-shaped nucleocapsid surrounded by a trilaminar envelope and a unique, tail-like extension at one end. The virions contain a circular, supercoiled, dsDNA genome of about 300 kilobase pairs (kbp). Complete genome sequence analyses have shown that most of the WSSV open reading frames (ORFs) encode proteins bearing no homology to known proteins, while some identifiable genes are more homologous to eukaryotic genes than to viral genes. Based on these genetic analyses and on its unique morphological features, WSSV has been classified as the sole member of a new virus family.

## Taxonomy

After its initial discovery, WSSV was classified as the genus *nonoccluded Baculovirus* (*NOB*) of the subfamily *Nudibaculovirinae* of family *Baculoviridae*. However, based on its unique morphological features, on its genomic structure and composition, and on phylogenetic analyses, *White spot syndrome virus 1* was reassigned by the International Committee on Taxonomy of Viruses in 2004 as the type species of the genus *Whispovirus* and the sole member within the new virus family *Nimaviridae*. The family name refers to the thread-like, polar extension on the virus particle (*nima* is Latin for 'thread'). Today, there is still only a single species within the genus *Whispovirus*. However, various geographical isolates with genotypic variability (variants) have been identified within this species. Other names that have been used in the literature for WSSV include: hypodermal and hematopoietic necrosis baculovirus (HHNBV), rod-shaped nuclear virus of *Penaeus japonicus* (RV-PJ), systemic ectodermal and mesodermal baculovirus (SEMBV), and white spot baculovirus (WSBV).

## Transmission, Host Range, and Epidemiology Studies of WSSV

WSSV is contagious and highly virulent in penaeid shrimp. In cultured shrimp, WSSV infection can cause a cumulative mortality of up to 100% within 3–10 days of the first signs of disease. WSSV can be transmitted horizontally, either *per os* when the shrimp feed on diseased individuals, contaminated food or infected carcasses, or else through exposure to virus particles in the water, in which case the route of infection is primarily through the gills or other body surfaces. The virus is also transmitted vertically from brooder to offspring. However, transmission is not transovarial because the virus appears to attack only young developing oocytes, which die before reaching maturation. It is therefore more likely that vertical transmission is caused by contamination of the egg mass. Penaeid shrimp are highly susceptible to WSSV. Although there is evidence of resistance during the larval and early (younger than PL6) postlarval stages, WSSV can cause disease in shrimp at any growth stage.

WSSV has a remarkably broad host range. Almost every species of penaeid shrimp is susceptible to WSSV infection. Moreover, the virus can infect other marine, brackish, and freshwater crustaceans, including crayfish, crabs, and spiny lobsters. However, in contrast to penaeid shrimp, infection is often not lethal in these species, and consequently they may serve as reservoirs and carriers of the virus. Furthermore, at least one insect, the shore fly (a member of the family Ephyridae), as well as copepods collected from WSSV-affected farms, have been diagnosed as WSSV-positive by PCR, suggesting that they are also possible reservoir hosts.

In epidemiological studies of WSSV, variations in the number of the 54 bp tandem repeat located between the *rr1* and *rr2* genes (see the section titled 'Identification through homology comparison') have been used as a strain-specific, genetic marker. The number of repeats varies greatly when infected shrimps are collected from different ponds or from the same ponds at different times, but in almost every outbreak of WSD, shrimps from the same pond usually have the same number of repeats. This suggests that in each pond, a single WSSV isolate is the causative agent. High variations in the number of 54 bp repeats have been reported in strains of WSSV from Thailand, India, and Vietnam. In Vietnam, a particular repeat pattern was observed in shrimps from outbreak ponds, but no repeat pattern was found to be useful as a prediction of pathogenicity or geographical origin in any of these different strains. On the other hand, cultured shrimps and wild crustaceans from the same WSD outbreak pond had different 54 bp repeat patterns, suggesting that the wild crustaceans may not have been responsible for infecting the cultured shrimp. However, this interpretation has been questioned by a recent study showing that the number of the 54 bp repeats as well as the pathogenicity changed when a given WSSV isolate was passaged through different crustacean hosts. This study further implies that the variations in repeat number could result from host selection rather than geographical isolation.

## Clinical Features and Pathology

The most commonly observed clinical sign of WSD in shrimp is white spots in the exoskeleton and epidermis. These may range in size from minute spots to disks several millimeters in diameter which may coalesce into larger plates. The spots may result from abnormal deposits of calcium salts by the cuticular epidermis or result from disruption to the transfer of exudates from the epithelial

cells to the cuticle. Infected animals are lethargic, reduce their food consumption, and display a reddish to pink body discoloration due to expansion of cuticular chromatophores. Moribund shrimp exhibit systemic destruction of target tissues with many infected cells showing homogeneous hypertrophied nuclei. At advanced stages of infection, numerous virus particles are released into the hemolymph from the lesions, causing a general viremia.

It should be noted that although the white spots are a typical and characteristic clinical sign of WSD, white spots on the carapace of shrimp can also be caused by other environmental stress factors, such as high alkalinity or a bacterial shell disease. Conversely, moribund shrimp with WSD may have few, if any, white spots.

To date, no species of penaeid shrimp is known to show significant resistance to WSD.

## Histopathology

The prime targets for WSSV replication are tissues of ectodermal (cuticular epidermis, fore- and hindgut, gills, and nervous tissue) and mesodermal (lymphoid organ, antennal gland, connective tissue, and hematopoietic tissue) origin. Tissues of endodermal origin (hepatopancreas and midgut) are not affected by the virus. Histopathological observation reveals similar cellular changes upon WSSV infection in all target tissues. In the early stage of infection, affected cells display nuclear hypertrophy (**Figure 1**), nucleoli dissolution, and chromatin margination, and the central area changes into a homogeneous eosinophilic region. The infected cells then proceed to develop an intranuclear eosinophilic Cowdry A-type

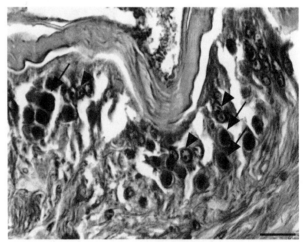

**Figure 1** Hematoxylin and eosin (HE) staining of tissue section from *Penaeus monodon* cuticular epithelium of eyestalk infected with WSSV. Degenerated cells characterized by hypertrophied nuclei (black arrows) are readily seen. The cells with normal nuclei are also indicated with arrowheads. Scale = 20 μm.

inclusion, which subsequently becomes a light basophilic, denser inclusion separated by a transparent zone from the marginated chromatin. During this time, the cytoplasm becomes less dense and more lucent. In the late stage of infection, the nuclear membrane is disrupted, causing the intranuclear transparent zone to fuse with the lucent cytoplasm. At the end of cellular degeneration, the nucleus or whole cell disintegrates, leading to loss of cellular architecture. In moribund shrimp, most tissues and organs are heavily infected with the virus, and they exhibit severe multifocal necrosis.

Temporal studies coupled with *in situ* hybridization (**Figure 2**) have shown that the first WSSV-positive signals are detected in the stomach, gills, cuticular epidermis, and connective tissue of the hepatopancreas. At later stages of infection, the lymphoid organ, antennal gland, muscle tissue, hematopoietic tissue, heart, midgut, and hindgut also become positive. As infection proceeds, the stomach, gill, hematopoietic tissue, lymphoid organ, antennal gland, and cuticular epidermis become heavily infected with WSSV, which leads to serious damage and necrosis (and/or apoptotsis; see the section titled 'Viral–host relationships').

## Viral Morphology and Morphogenesis

The WSSV virion is a nonoccluded particle with a trilaminar envelope. It is elliptical to bacilliform (olive-like) in shape and measures about $270 \times 120$ nm. A long, tail-like projection is often seen extending from the narrow end of the purified virion (**Figure 3(a)**). The cylindrical, rod-shaped nucleocapsid is about $300 \times 65$ nm, which is longer than the intact virion. The nucleocapsid displays a very distinctive pattern consisting of a stacked series of rings (about 16 in total) that run perpendicular to the longitudinal axis of the capsid. The thickness of these rings is quite constant, at about 20 nm. Each ring consists of two rows of 12–14 globular subunits, each approximately 10 nm in diameter (**Figure 3(b)**).

The entire WSSV replication cycle takes place in the nucleus and, in an acutely infected shrimp, can be completed within 24 h post infection. Initial signs of WSSV replication in the nucleus include nuclear hypertrophy and chromatin margination. Viral morphogenesis begins with *de novo* formation of the viral envelope, which can be seen at first as fibrillar fragments in the nucleoplasm. As infection progresses, these fragments form into the

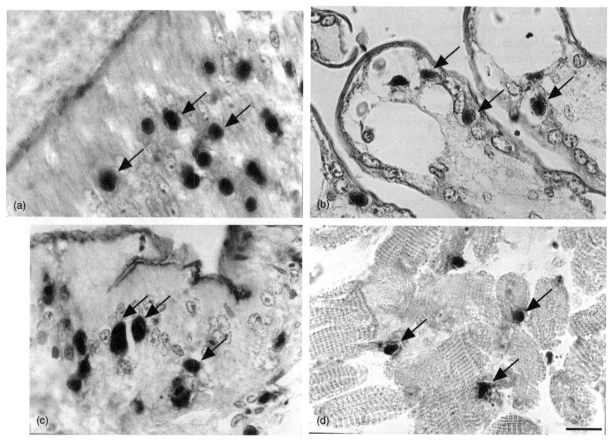

**Figure 2** *In situ* hybridization analysis of WSSV positive cells (arrows) in (a) the integument, (b) the gill, (c) the stomach, and (d) the heart from experimentally infected *Penaeus monodon* at 60 hpi. The infected cells shown here in the heart are connective tissue cell; muscle cells are not usually targeted by WSSV. Scale = 20 μm.

membranous and/or vesicular precursors of the viral envelope. The development of nucleocapsids begins with the formation of long empty tubules (**Figure 4(a)**) which have a diameter similar to that of empty

nucleocapsids and a segmentation similar to that of nucleocapsids. They can exist individually or may be laterally aligned in groups of two or three to form a larger structure. The assembled tubules break into fragments of 12–14 rings to form empty naked capsids (**Figure 4(b)**) which are then surrounded by envelopes, leaving an opening at one end. Nucleoproteins, which have a filamentous appearance, enter the capsid through this open end, while simultaneously increasing the diameter of the virion. Finally, the open end of the nucleocapsid is closed, and the envelope narrows at the open end to form the apical tail of the mature virion, which has now obtained its characteristic olive-like shape.

## Virion Structure and Composition

WSSV virions have a complex SDS-PAGE protein profile (**Figure 5(a)**). Early structural protein studies used SDS-PAGE coupled with Western blot analyses and/or N-terminal sequencing of proteins to identify at least six structural proteins, including VP35, VP28, VP26, VP24, VP19, and VP15. More recent studies have used mass spectrometry to analyze the protein profiles of purified WSSV virions separated by SDS-PAGE and 2-D electrophoresis, and more than 40 structural proteins have now been identified. The major structural proteins are VP664, VP28, VP26, VP24, VP19, and VP15 (**Figures 5** and **6**). A biochemical fractionation study using differential concentrations of salt and detergent has tentatively classified

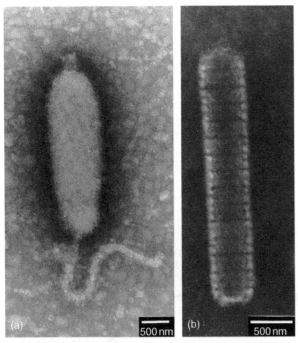

**Figure 3** Morphology of the WSSV virions. (a) Intact WSSV virion showing the tail-like extension on one end.
(b) A WSSV nucleocapsid showing the stacked ring structures, which are made up of two rows of globular subunits.

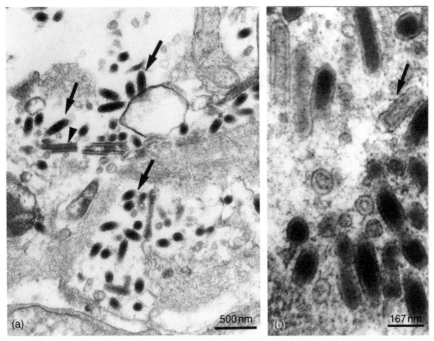

**Figure 4** Transmission electron micrograph of WSSV-infected tissues from beneath the cephalothoracic exoskeletoal cuticle. (a) The viral particles spread among the necrotic area. The complete viral particles are indicated with arrows and the long empty tubules with an arrowhead. (b) High magnification of virus particles with rod-shaped morphology. A viral particle with an empty nucleocapsid is indicated with an arrow.

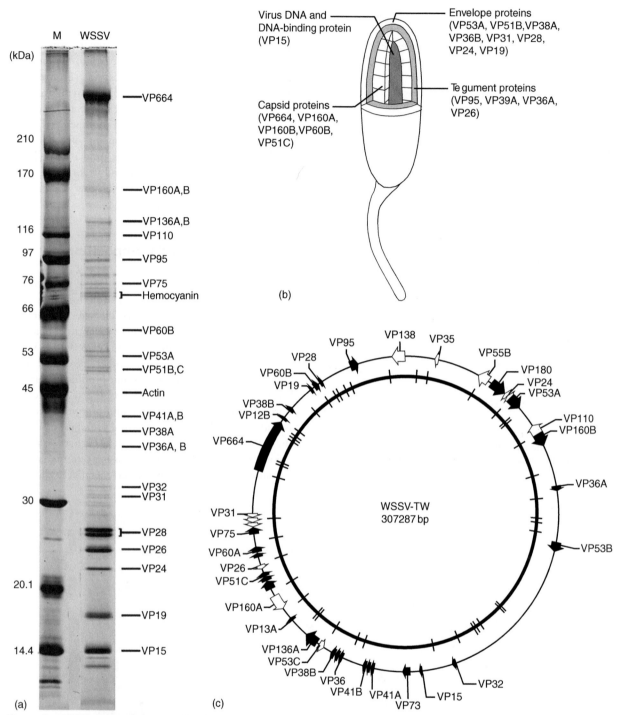

**Figure 5**  WSSV structural proteins. (a) SDS-PAGE profile of purified WSSV virions. The six major and some minor structural protein bands are indicated. The bands corresponding to two host proteins co-purified with the virion are also indicated. (b) A proposed schematic diagram to show the WSSV virion structure and the possible location of WSSV structural proteins and its DNA. (c) Distribution of 41 WSSV structural protein genes in the WSSV-TW genome. The inner circle shows predicted HindIII restriction enzyme cutting sites.

the WSSV structural proteins into envelope, tegument, and capsid proteins. VP15 is a basic capsid protein with *in vitro* DNA-binding activity, and it has high homology to the lysine- and arginine-rich DNA-binding proteins of the insect baculoviruses. This protein is therefore thought

to be responsible for packing the WSSV DNA into the nucleocapsid. VP26, a tegument protein, can interact with actin, but the importance of this interaction remains unknown. VP19, VP24, and VP28 are envelope proteins, and an *in vitro* physical interaction between VP24 and

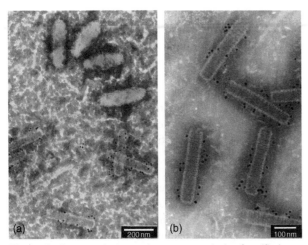

**Figure 6** Immunoelectron microscopy analysis of purified WSSV virions detected with VP664 antibody followed by gold-labeled secondary antibody. (a) The VP664 antibody specifically binds to the nucleocapsid and not to the viral envelope. (b) Most of the gold particles are localized at the perimeter of the nucleocapsid.

VP28 has been reported. VP664, the major capsid protein, takes its name from its calculated molecular weight of 664 kDa, and it is not only the largest protein encoded by the WSSV genome, but also the largest viral structural protein ever found. This protein is encoded by the intron-less giant ORF (*wssv419*) of 18 234 nt. Immunoelectron microscopy of purified virions has shown that VP664 forms the globular subunits that are visible in the nucleocapsid ring structures (**Figure 6**). In addition to VP15 and VP664, the capsid contains at least four other minor proteins: VP160A (WSSV344), VP160B (WSSV94), VP60B (WSSV474), and VP51C (WSSV364) (**Figure 5**).

A number of viruses use the Arg-Gly-Asp (RGD) motif to bind to cellular integrins during infection and this cell attachment site signature can be identified in at least six WSSV structural proteins. It has been shown that one of these six structural proteins, VP110 (WSV035), can attach to shrimp host cells, and that this adhesion can be blocked by synthetic RGDT peptides, suggesting that the RGD motif in VP110 may play a role in WSSV infection. VP28 may also bind to host cells even though it lacks the RGD motif, and virus neutralization tests originally suggested that VP28 was critical for systemic WSSV infection. However, recent studies have shown that the observed phenomenon was, in fact, a nonspecific inhibitory effect of rabbit serum. Thus, to date, although SDS-PAGE indicates that VP28 is the most abundant virion protein, its role remains elusive. In addition to VP28, virus neutralization tests have been used to identify other structural proteins in the envelope and determine their role in WSSV infection. However, considering what is now known for VP28, the results of neutralization tests should be interpreted with care.

None of the five small major WSSV structural proteins (VP28, VP26, VP24, VP19, and VP15) appears to be glycosylated. However, increased migration in SDS-PAGE after N-linked glycosidase F treatment of structural protein VP180 (encoded by *wsv001*) suggests that this large collagen-like protein is N-glycosylated. This is the first reported evidence of an intact collagen gene in a virus genome.

## WSSV Genome Structure

The WSSV genome is a large ds circular DNA of about 300 kbp. The complete genome sequences of three isolates originating from China (WSSV-CN), Taiwan (WSSV-TW), and Thailand (WSSV-TH) indicated sizes of 305, 307, and 297 kbp, respectively. Genetic variations among these isolates include two major polymorphic loci (a 13 kbp deletion in WSSV-TH and a variable region prone to recombination), a transposase sequence that was only present in WSSV-TW, and variation in the number of repeats and single nucleotide mutations. Not including the two major polymorphic loci and the transposase sequence, these three isolates share an overall nucleotide sequence identity of 99.32%. It has been shown that differences in the major polymorphic 13 kbp deletion locus are related to differences in virulence of WSSV isolates.

The WSSV genome has a total G + C content of 41% uniformly distributed over the genome. Although most WSSV genome sequences are unique, 3% of the genome consists of highly repetitive sequences, which are organized into nine homologous regions (hrs). These are distributed throughout the genome, and are located largely in intergenic regions. The presence of hrs is a feature of many baculovirus genomes. Baculovirus hrs function as enhancers of early gene transcription and as initiation sites for DNA replication. They have also been implicated as sites of DNA recombination. It is likely that WSSV hrs will be shown to have similar functions.

A total of 532 putative ORFs consisting of a minimum of 60 codons have been identified by sequence analysis of the WSSV-TW isolate. Of these, 140 ORFs have a potential downstream polyadenylation site (AATAAA). The size of proteins encoded by these predicted ORFs ranges from 60 to 6077 amino acids. Only 30% of the predicted ORFs encode proteins homologous to any other known proteins or motifs. As about 40 structural proteins have been identified, approximately 8% of the ORFs encode structural proteins. Some of the predicted ORFs encode proteins that share significant similarities (40% or even higher) to each other and can therefore be classified into the same gene family. There are ten putative gene families in the WSSV genome, and it is possible that these families arose from gene duplication.

## WSSV Genes

### Identification through Homology Comparison

The WSSV genome contains several genes that can be identified unambiguously through homology searches. These genes are involved in nucleotide metabolism and DNA replication, and encode *thymidylate synthase, dUTPase, ribonucleotide reductases* (*rr1* and *rr2*; two separate ORFs encoding the two subunits), chimeric *thymidylate/thymidine kinase* (*TK-TMK*), and *DNA polymerase*. The chimeric *thymidylate/thymidine kinase* gene is a unique feature of WSSV, as these genes in other large DNA viruses are encoded in separate ORFs. The enzymatic activities of dUTPase, ribonucleotide reductase, and TK/TMK have been demonstrated by using purified recombinant proteins.

Some proteins from predicted ORFs show weak similarity to known proteins, including nonspecific nuclease (WSV191), TATA-box binding protein (TBP; WSV303), CREB-binding protein (CBP; WSV100), and helicase (WSV447). The activity of the nonspecific nuclease has been demonstrated using a purified recombinant protein produced in *Escherichia coli*.

Some proteins contain well-defined domains or motifs, and therefore their possible functions can be inferred. Two protein kinases, PK1 (WSSV482) and PK2 (ORF61), have been identified because they each contain the catalytic domain of serine/threonine protein kinase. Two proteins containing the EF-hand, calcium-binding motif have also been identified (WSV079 and WSV427; WSV427 is a latency-related gene), suggesting that WSSV might modulate calcium levels in infected cells. Four proteins with RING-H2 finger motifs have been annotated (WSV199, WSV222, WSV249, and WSV403). This motif has been implicated in ubiquitin-conjugating enzyme (E2)-dependent ubiquitination; many proteins containing a RING finger play a key role in the ubiquitination pathway. Ubiquitination activity has been demonstrated for WSV222 and WSV249, and their interacting host proteins have been identified using yeast-two hybrid screening. Some proteins contain conserved zinc finger or leucine zipper motifs. These motifs have been shown to be involved in DNA-protein interactions and in regulation of transcriptional activation. Of these, *wssv126* is one of three immediate early genes that have been identified to date.

### Identification through Functional Studies

As most WSSV gene products show no significant homology to known proteins, *ab initio* research is required to identify their functions. For large dsDNA viruses, gene expression is usually categorized sequentially as immediate early, early, and late. Immediate early genes are expressed in the absence of *de novo* viral protein synthesis, early genes are involved in DNA synthesis, and late genes are expressed following viral DNA replication and encode the viral structural proteins and proteins required for assembly, maturation, and release of viral particles. Three immediate early genes, *ie1* (*wssv126*), *ie2* (*wssv418*), and *ie3* (*wssv242*), have been identified in WSSV-infected shrimp by showing that their transcription is not inhibited by cycloheximide. IE1 contains the Cys2/His2-type zinc finger motif, which is implicated in DNA-binding activity, suggesting that IE1 might function as a transcription factor. The gene products of *ie2* and *ie3* contain no recognizable functional motifs, and their functions remain unknown. Three latency–related genes have been identified: *wsv151, wsv427*, and *wsv 366*. These genes have been shown to be relatively highly expressed in asymptomatic carrier shrimp that tested negative for WSSV using a commercial PCR detection kit. When expressed as recombinant proteins in Sf9 insect cells, WSV151 is a nuclear protein of approximately 165 kDa, while WSV427 interacts *in vitro* with a novel shrimp serine/threonine protein phosphatase. A novel anti-apoptosis protein (ORF390) has also been identified. WSSV infection induces bystander, noninfected cells to undergo apoptosis, whereas WSSV-infected cells are not apoptotic. ORF390 has been shown to inhibit apoptosis induced either by infection with a mutant baculovirus or by treatment with actinomycin D. The protein has two putative caspase9 cleavage sites and a caspase3 cleavage site, and therefore might function like the AcMNPV P35 protein by directly binding to and inhibiting the activity of caspase9 and/or caspase3.

## WSSV Gene Expression and Regulation

Since no suitable shrimp cell line is available, studies of WSSV gene expression have long been carried out *in vivo* in penaeid shrimp or crayfish by using RT-PCR. In the black tiger shrimp, *P. monodon*, WSSV immediate early and early genes (e.g., *rr1, rr2, pk1, tk-tmk, dnapol, ie1, ie2*, and *ie3*) are detected as early as 2–4 hpi (hours post infection) and their transcription levels either steadily and slowly increase till the end of the study (48 or 60 hpi) or else reach a plateau phase at 12–18 hpi. For late genes (the major viral structural protein genes), although very low levels could be detected as early as 2–4 hpi, transcription levels surged at 12–18 hpi and steadily increased thereafter. In crayfish, expression of the late genes was not observed until at least 18–24 hpi.

WSSV gene expression has been globally analyzed using microarrays. In one study, the results revealed that about 23.5% of WSSV genes began to express at 2 hpi, 4.2% at 6 hpi, 17.7% at 12 hpi, and 47.9% at 24 hpi. Most of the WSSV structural protein genes were expressed either at 12 hpi (9 WSSV structural protein genes) or at 24 hpi (14 WSSV structural protein genes). However, several structural protein genes were expressed at 2 hpi, suggesting that these proteins might also have important roles in the early infection stage. In another microarray study, clustering of the transcription profiles of the individual WSSV genes during infection showed two major classes of genes; the first class reached maximal expression at 20 hpi and the second class at 2 days post infection. Since most of the known WSSV early genes were found in the first class, the other genes in this class were also thought to be early genes. Conversely, the genes that clustered with the structural protein genes in the second class were likewise thought to be late genes. Therefore, RT-PCR and microarray studies suggest that, as for other large dsDNA viruses, the expression of WSSV genes is regulated in a coordinated series of cascades.

The promoter regions of WSSV early and late genes have been analyzed. The upstream region of WSSV early genes contains a TATA box and an initiator. This is similar to the *Drosophila* RNA polymerase II core promoter sequences, suggesting that the WSSV early genes are under the control of cellular transcription machinery. Alignment of the regions upstream of all the major structural protein genes has identified a degenerate motif (ATNAC) that could be involved in WSSV late gene transcription, while only one of these genes was found to contain a functional TATA box. These differences between the promoter regions of the early and late genes are sufficient to account for the differential transcription patterns between early and late genes, and they also suggest that WSSV uses at least two different classes of transcription machinery for gene expression. Since the WSSV genome contains no homologs of RNA polymerase subunits, at least one novel transcription factor (e.g., IE1, IE2, or IE3) would need to be induced at the early infection stage. These factors, which are presumably able to recognize a late gene-specific motif (such as the 'ATNAC' motif), could then recruit the host cellular transcription machinery to transcribe the late genes.

## Viral–Host Relationships

### Apoptosis

Apoptosis is a cell suicide program that enables multicellular organisms to direct and control cell numbers in tissues and to eliminate cells, including virus-infected cells that may be harmful to the survival of the organism. If apoptosis occurs during the early stage of infection, virus production is severely limited; because it inhibits the spread of progeny virus in the host, apoptosis is recognized as an antiviral defense. In consequence, most animal viruses have evolved strategies to evade or delay an early apoptosis response. The classical signs of apoptosis can be identified in WSSV-infected shrimp, including nuclear disassembly,

fragmentation of DNA into a ladder, and increased caspase3 activity. Furthermore, there is a positive correlation between the severity of WSSV infection and the number of apoptotic cells. Among the WSSV target tissues, the subcuticlar and abdominal epithelia are the most seriously damaged, and these epithelial tissues exhibit the highest incidence of apoptotic cells. However, it is significant that cells displaying apoptotic characteristics do not contain virions, whereas those containing WSSV virions are not apoptotic. It is therefore reasonable to suppose that apoptosis is employed by shrimp as a protective response to prevent the spread of WSSV, while in the infected cells, the anti-apoptosis protein ORF390 blocks apoptosis and thus facilitates multiplication of the virus.

## Hemocyte Responses to WSSV Infection

In crustaceans, the hemocytes (blood cells) mediate many defense-related activities that are essential for the nonspecific immunity, including phagocytosis, melanization, encapsulation, cytotoxicity, and clotting. They also produce a vast array of antimicrobial proteins, such as agglutinins, antimicrobial peptides, and lysozymes. Hemocyte responses to WSSV have been investigated thoroughly in penaeid shrimp and crayfish. WSSV infection decreases the total hemocyte count (THC) in shrimp but not in crayfish. The reduced THC in shrimp is probably due to lysis by the virus of infected hemocytes as well as due to virus-induced apoptosis in both circulating hemocytes and hematopoietic tissue. In addition, circulating hemocytes migrate to tissues that have a high number of virus-infected cells, although this is probably a general defensive response rather than a specific antiviral response. WSSV infection also induces apoptosis in crayfish hemocytes but the percentage of apoptotic hemocytes is much lower in crayfish (1.5%) than in shrimp (20%).

WSSV infection differentially affects the three morphologically and functionally distinct hemocyte types that have been identified in crustacean hemolymph, commonly referred to as semigranular cells (SGCs), granular cells (GCs), and hyaline cells (HCs). In shrimp and crayfish, both SGCs and GCs can be infected with WSSV but SGCs are the preferential target. This suggests that SGCs are more susceptible to WSSV and that the virus replicates more rapidly in SGCs than in GCs. However, the melanization activity of GCs in WSSV-infected crayfish is reduced. The third type of hemocyte (HC) is refractory to WSSV infection in shrimp but their role in antiviral defense is still not clear. On the other hand, GCs and SGCs each play a major defensive role and WSSV infection of these cell types is likely to weaken shrimp defenses and reduce shrimp health. Since hemocytes are also necessary for clotting, the low THC also accounts for the phenomenon that hemolymph withdrawn from

WSSV-infected shrimp and crayfish always has a delayed (or sometimes completely absent) clotting reaction.

## Protection of Shrimp Against WSSV Infection Using Vaccination and RNAi Strategies

Since the earliest outbreaks of WSD, several advances have been made in our understanding of how shrimp might be protected against WSSV infection. For example, although it is generally thought that shrimps lack the immunoglobulin-based adaptive immune system, recent studies have shown that when *Penaeus japonicus* shrimps survive either natural or experimental WSSV infections, they sometimes show resistance to subsequent challenge with WSSV. This 'quasi-immune response' suggests that shrimps may have an innate immune system that includes specific memory. Further research into this phenomenon has shown that intramuscular injection or oral adminis-tration of either inactivated WSSV virions or recombinant structural protein VP28 similarly provide shrimps and crayfish with some degree of protection against WSSV infection. Another potential means of limiting WSSV infec-tion is to take advantage of the *in vivo* roles of RNA interference induced by dsRNA. In *Litopenaeus vannamei* shrimp, whereas long dsRNA was shown to induce both sequence-dependent and sequence–independent antiviral responses, WSSV gene-specific dsRNAs produce strong anti-WSSV activity. Similar results have also been reported for the gene-specific dsRNAs of another shrimp virus, yel-low head virus. However, the anti-WSSV activity of WSSV gene-specific dsRNAs varies greatly from one WSSV gene to another, and the effectiveness of each candidate needs to be tested empirically. Further, the antiviral activity of WSSV gene-specific small interfering RNA (21–23 bp dsRNA) has not yet been conclusively demonstrated.

*See also:* Shrimp Viruses.

## Further Reading

Leu JH, Tsai JM, Wang HC, *et al.* (2005) The unique stacked rings in the nucleocapsid of the white spot syndrome virus virion are formed by the major structural protein VP664, the largest viral structural protein ever found. *Journal of Virology* 79: 140–149.

Lo CF, Wu JL, Chang YS, *et al.* (2004) Molecular characterization and pathogenicity of white spot syndrome virus. In: Leung KY (ed.) *Molecular Aspects of Fish and Marine Biology, Vol. 3: Current Trends in the Study of Bacterial and Viral Fish and Shrimp Diseases*, pp. 155–188. Singapore: World Scientific.

Marks H, Ren XY, Sandbrink H, *et al.* (2006) *In silico* identification of putative promoter motifs of white spot syndrome virus. *BMC Bioinformatics* 7: 309–322.

Robalino J, Bartlett T, Shepard E, *et al.* (2005) Double-stranded RNA induces sequence-specific antiviral silencing in addition to nonspecific immunity in a marine shrimp: Convergence of RNA interference and innate immunity in the invertebrate antiviral response? *Journal of Virology* 79: 13561–13571.

Tsai JM, Wang HC, Leu JH, *et al.* (2004) Genomic and proteomic analysis of thirty-nine structural proteins of shrimp white spot syndrome virus. *Journal of Virology* 78: 11360–11370.

Tsai JM, Wang HC, Leu JH, *et al.* (2006) Identification of the nucleocapsid, tegument, and envelope proteins of the shrimp white spot syndrome virus virion. *Journal of Virology* 80: 3021–3029.

van Hulten MCW, Witteveldt J, Peters S, *et al.* (2001) The white spot syndrome virus DNA genome sequence. *Virology* 286: 7–22.

Witteveldt J, Cifuentes CC, Vlak JM, *et al.* (2004) Protection of *Penaeus monodon* against white spot syndrome virus by oral vaccination. *Journal of Virology* 78: 2057–2061.

Wongteerasupaya C, Pungchai P, Withyachumnarnkul B, *et al.* (2003) High variation in repetitive DNA fragment length for white spot syndrome virus (WSSV) isolates in Thailand. *Diseases of Aquatic Organisms* 54: 253–257.

Yang F, He J, Lin X, *et al.* (2001) Complete genome sequence of the shrimp white spot bacilliform virus. *Journal of Virology* 75: 11811–11820.

Zhang X, Huang C, and Hew CL (2004) Use of genomics and proteomics to study white spot syndrome virus. In: Leung KY (ed.) *Molecular Aspects of Fish and Marine Biology, Vol. 3: Current Trends in the Study of Bacterial and Viral Fish and Shrimp Diseases*, pp. 204–236. Singapore: World Scientific.

Zuidema D, van Hulte MCW, Marks H, *et al.* (2004) Virus–host interaction of white spot syndrome virus. In: Leung KY (ed.) *Molecular Aspects of Fish and Marine Biology, Vol. 3: Current Trends in the Study of Bacterial and Viral Fish and Shrimp Diseases*, pp. 237–255. Singapore: World Scientific.

# Yellow Head Virus

**P J Walker,** CSIRO Australian Animal Health Laboratory, Geelong, VIC, Australia
**N Sittidilokratna,** Centex Shrimp and Center for Genetic Engineering and Biotechnology, Bangkok, Thailand

## Glossary

**Antennal gland** Complex excretory glands located behind the eyes on antenna on the head of decapods.

**Hepatopancreas** An organ of the digestive tract of arthropods and fish that provides the functions which are performed separately by the liver and pancreas in mammals.

**Lymphoid organ** Also known as the Oka organ, a component of the hematopoeitic system of penaeid shrimp consisting of lymphoid cells around the two subgastric arteries.

**Pseudoknot** A complex folded structure in an RNA molecule.

**Slippery sequence** A nucleotide sequence at which ribosomal slippage can occur during translation to cause a change in the reading frame.

## Introduction

Yellow head virus (YHV) is a pathogen of the black tiger shrimp (prawn), *Penaeus monodon*, which is one of the world's major aquaculture species. Yellow head disease was first reported in central Thailand in 1990 from which it spread rapidly along the eastern and western coasts of the Gulf of Thailand to southern farming regions. Outbreaks of yellow head disease have since been reported from most of the major shrimp farming countries in Asia. It is suspected that the YHV (rather than monodon baculovirus, which is not usually pathogenic for juvenile shrimp) may have previously caused the crash of the shrimp farming industry in Taiwan during the late 1980s. Mortalities usually occur during the mid-late stages of grow-out in ponds with complete crop loss commonly occurring within 3 days of the first signs of disease. YHV is one genotype in a complex of closely related viruses infecting black tiger shrimp. Other genotypes include gill-associated virus (GAV) which has been associated with relatively less severe forms of disease in farmed shrimp in Australia, and at least four other genotypes for which no disease association has yet been established. YHV and the other genotypes are endemic throughout the Indo-Pacific region, occurring commonly as low-level chronic infections in healthy shrimp.

## Taxonomy and Classification

YHV is a positive-sense single-stranded RNA (ssRNA) virus that shares aspects of genome organization, replication, and transcription with coronaviruses, toroviruses, and arteriviruses with which it is classified in the order *Nidovirales*. In 2002, the International Committee on Taxonomy of Viruses (ICTV) established the genus *Okavirus* in the new family *Roniviridae* to accommodate YHV and closely related GAV. *Okavirus* is derived from the Oka or lymphoid organ of penaeid shrimp in which the virus is commonly detected; *Roniviridae* is derived from the sigla rod-shaped nidovirus. *Gill-associated virus* was assigned as the type species of the genus because its biological

and molecular characterization were more complete. YHV is currently classified as a member of the species *Gill-associated virus*. No virus other than those described in the yellow head complex is currently assigned to the *Roniviridae* but several viruses with similar morphology have been reported in crabs and fish. Roniviruses are the only members of the order *Nidovirales* that are currently known to infect invertebrates.

## Virion Structure and Morphology

YHV virions are rod-shaped, enveloped particles ($\sim$50 nm $\times$ $\sim$175 nm) with prominent diffuse spikes ($\sim$8 nm $\times$ $\sim$11 nm) projecting from the surface (**Figure 1(a)**). Internal helical nucleocapsids are approximately 25 nm in diameter and have a periodicity of 5–7 nm. Filamentous nucleocapsid precursors, approximately 15 nm in diameter and of variable length ($\sim$80–450 nm), are observed in the cytoplasm, sometimes densely packed in paracrystalline arrays (**Figure 1(b)**). Nucleocapsids acquire trilamellar lipid envelopes by budding through membranes into intracytoplasmic vesicles or at the cell surface (**Figure 1(c)**). It has been reported that long nucleocapsid precursors generate elongated, enveloped structures that subsequently fragment into mature virions. The morphology of GAV virions is indistinguishable from that of YHV.

YHV virions contain a polyadenylated 26.6 kDa ($+$) ssRNA genome and three structural proteins. The nucleoprotein (p20) is a highly hydrophilic, basic protein that complexes with the genomic RNA in nucleocapsids. Transmembrane glycoproteins gp64 and gp116 are components of the envelope that form the visible projections on the virion surface. YHV infectivity can be at least partially neutralized by antibody to gp116 but not by antibody to gp64. It is reported that gp116 docks with a 65 kDa cell membrane protein (pmYRP65) that mediates YHV entry into susceptible shrimp cells. Knockdown of pmYRP65 expression has been reported to totally abrogate susceptibility of shrimp cells to YHV infection.

## Genome Organization and Transcription Strategy

The 26 662 nt YHV genome comprises four long open reading frames (ORFs) designated ORF1a, ORF1b, ORF2, and ORF3 (**Figure 2**). ORF1a (12 216 nt) and ORF1b (7887 nt) encode all of the elements of a large replicase complex. ORF1a encodes a 4072 aa polyprotein (pp1a) that contains a 3C-like cysteine protease catalytic domain flanked by putative transmembrane domains. The pp1a protease has autolytic activity and appears to be involved in processing the replicase polyproteins. ORF1b overlaps ORF1a by 37 nt. Expression of ORF1b requires

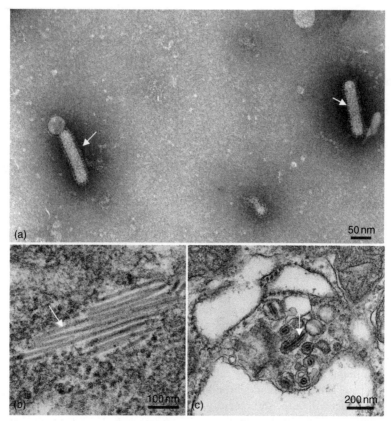

**Figure 1** Transmission electron micrographs of YHV. (a) Image of virions stained with heavy metal salts showing the external appearance of the enveloped particles (arrows). (b) Image of an ultrathin section of helical nucleocapsids (arrow) within the gill of an infected shrimp. (c) Image of an ultrathin section of virions (arrow) within the gill of an infected shrimp. Kindly provided by Dr. Alex Hyatt, CSIRO, Australian Animal Health Laboratory, Geelong, Australia.

a −1 ribosomal frameshift at a slippery sequence (AAAUUUU) near a complex pseudoknot structure in the mRNA. The extended 6688 aa polyprotein (pp1ab) contains RNA-dependent RNA polymerase (RdRp), multinuclear zinc-binding (ZBD), helicase (HEL), 3′-5′ exoribonuclease (ExoN), uridylate-specific endoribonuclease (NendoU), ribose-2′-O-methyltransferase (O-MT) catalytic domains, and other cysteine/histidine-rich domains that are conserved in pp1ab of other nidoviruses. ORF2 encodes the 146 aa nucleocapsid protein (p20). Roniviruses are unique among known nidoviruses in that the nucleocapsid protein gene is located upstream rather than downstream of the glycoprotein genes. ORF3 encodes a 1666 aa polyglycoprotein that is processed to generate virion envelope glycoproteins gp64 and gp116. Proteolytic cleavage of ORF3 occurs at two [Ala-X-Ala] motifs immediately following predicted transmembrane domains that appear to function as signal peptides. The cleavage also generates a 228 aa (∼22 kDa) protein that contains triple membrane-spanning domains and resembles M-proteins in coronaviruses. The YHV M-like protein appears to be present in infected cells at relatively low levels. The YHV genome also features significant noncoding regions, including a 71 nt untranslated region (UTR) at the

5′-terminus, a 352 nt UTR between ORF1b and ORF2, and a 54 nt UTR between ORF2 and ORF3. The 677 nt region between ORF3 and the 3′-poly[A] tail contains no long ORFs (>65 nt) and so also appears to be a long UTR (**Figure 2**).

Much of our understanding of YHV molecular biology has been obtained by comparison with closely related GAV. The 26 235 nt GAV genome is similar in structural organization to YHV, varying principally in the size and structure of the UTRs. In GAV, the ORF1b–ORF2 UTR comprises only 93 nt. The 638 nt region downstream of GAV ORF3 encodes a 252 nt ORF (ORF4) that has potential to express an unidentified 83 aa polypeptide with a deduced molecular weight ∼9.2 kDa. A short ORF in the corresponding region of the YHV genome is truncated with a termination codon after only 20 aa and is unlikely to be expressed. Like other nidoviruses, the GAV genome is transcribed as a nested set of 3′-co-terminal mRNAs comprising the full-length genome and two subgenomic messenger RNAs (sg mRNAs) that initiate at conserved transcription-regulating sequences (TRSs) in noncoding regions immediately upstream of ORF2 and ORF3. However, unlike coronaviruses and arteriviruses, conserved GAV (and YHV) TRSs are not present in the 5′-UTR of

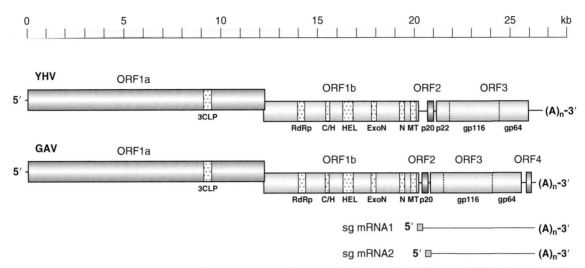

**Figure 2** Genome organization of YHV and GAV indicating the locations of subgenomic mRNAs (sg mRNA1 and sg mRNA2) and functional domains in ORF1a (3CLP) and ORF1b (RdRp, C/H, HEL, ExoN, N, and MT). Also indicated are proteolytic cleavage sites in the ORF3 polyprotein that is processed post-translation to generate triple-membrane-spanning protein (p22) and transmembrane glycoproteins (gp116 and gp64).

genomic RNA and so do not mediate splicing of common 5′-leader sequences on to the sg mRNAs. Sequences with partial identity to the conserved ORF2 and ORF3 TRSs occur upstream of GAV ORF4 (and the truncated YHV ORF4) but these do not appear to be functional.

## Geographic Distribution and Host Range

Surveys for the presence of viral genomic RNA have indicated that YHV and other genotypes in the complex are endemic in black tiger shrimp populations across its natural geographic range throughout the Indo-Pacific. Yellow head disease has been reported in farmed tiger shrimp from Thailand, Taiwan, China, the Philippines, Vietnam, Malaysia, Indonesia, India, Sri Lanka, and Madagascar. Although natural infection and disease have been reported only in black tiger shrimp and kuruma shrimp (*Marsupenaeus japonicus*), YHV can cause high rates of mortality following experimental infection of most other farmed marine shrimp species, including Pacific white shrimp (*Litopenaeus vannamei*), Pacific blue shrimp (*Litopenaeus stylirostris*), brown tiger shrimp (*Penaeus esculentus*), white banana shrimp (*Fenneropenaeus merguiensis*), white shrimp (*Litopenaeus setiferus*), brown shrimp (*Farfantepenaeus aztecus*), hopper and brown-spotted shrimp (*Farfantepenaeus duorarum*), red endeavour prawn (*Metapenaeus ensis*), and Jungas shrimp (*Metapenaeus affinis*). Some species of palemonid shrimp and krill are also susceptible to experimental infection. Crabs appear to be refractory to YHV infection and disease.

GAV has been associated with a less-aggressive disease of juvenile black tiger shrimp in Australia called mid-crop mortality syndrome. However, several other viruses have also been detected in shrimp with this condition and the etiology remains uncertain. GAV does cause disease and mortalities following experimental infection of several farmed shrimp species, including black tiger, brown tiger, and kuruma shrimp. GAV and other genotypes in the YHV complex have also been detected in healthy black tiger shrimp from Taiwan, the Philippines, Malaysia, Brunei, Indonesia, Vietnam, Thailand, India, Mozambique, and Fiji. A very high prevalence of GAV infection has been reported in healthy black tiger shrimp from eastern Australia. Evidence of GAV infection has also been detected in mud crab (*Scylla serrata*) in an experimental aquaculture facility.

## Pathology

Shrimp are susceptible to YHV infection from late post-larval stages but mass mortality in ponds usually occurs in early-to-late juvenile stages. Disease and mortalities usually occur within 2–4 days of a period of exceptionally high feeding activity followed by an abrupt cessation of feeding. Moribund shrimp congregate at pond edges near the surface and may exhibit a bleached overall appearance and discoloration of the cephalothorax caused by yellowing of the underlying hepatopancreas.

YHV infects tissues of ectodermal and mesodermal origin, including lymphoid organ, hemocytes, hematopoietic tissue, gill lamellae, and spongy connective tissue of the subcutis, gut, antennal gland, gonads, nerve tracts, and ganglia. In severe infections, there is a generalized cell degeneration with prominent nuclear condensation, pyknosis and karyorrhexis, and basophilic, perinuclear cytoplasmic inclusions in affected tissues.

There is evidence of apoptosis, including chromatin condensation and DNA fragmentation, in hemocytes, lymphoid organ, and gill tissues and it has been suggested that widespread apoptosis rather than necrosis is the cause of disease and mortalities.

YHV, GAV, and other viruses in the yellow head complex can also occur as low-level chronic infections in apparently healthy shrimp. Chronic infections have been observed in shrimp of all life stages collected from hatcheries and farms, and in the survivors of experimental infection. For GAV, the progression of infection following experimental challenge has been shown to be dose related. Shrimp infected with a high dose of GAV progress rapidly to disease with high viral loads and typical pathology leading to mortalities. Shrimp infected with a low dose do not develop disease and the virus persists as a low-level infection for at least 60 days. There is also evidence that stress can lead to rapid increases in viral load. For YHV, the onset of disease has been associated with the stress of molting. During chronic infections, there is little histopathology other than the accumulation of partitioned foci of cells with hypertrophic nuclei (spheroid bodies) in the lymphoid organ. Spheroid bodies appear to form in shrimp as part of a nonspecific defense mechanism for clearance of infectious agents and other foreign bodies.

## Host Response to Infection

As invertebrates, shrimp lack antibodies, cytokines, T-lymphocytes, and other powerful components of the vertebrate immune system that allow a specific adaptive response to viral infection, clearance of virus and infected cells, and long-term immunological memory. There is also no evidence in shrimp of interferon, natural killer (NK) cells, or other key components of the vertebrate natural immune system that allow an immediate nonspecific defense against viruses. Nevertheless, shrimp do appear to have a capacity to respond to viral infection and highly pathogenic viruses are commonly present as low-level chronic infections in apparently healthy shrimp. For YHV, there is no evidence of an inflammatory response at the primary sites of infection. However, YHV accumulates in spheroid bodies in the lymphoid organ during chronic persistent infections, and it is thought that the lymphoid organ has an important role in filtering granulated hemocytes and the clearance of viruses from infected shrimp. It has been reported that cells within lymphoid organ spheroids become apoptotic during infection and may be cleared during molting. Apoptotic cells have been observed in lymphoid organs, hemocytes, and gills during acute YHV infections in what appears to be a fundamental host defensive reaction. It has also been reported that double-stranded RNA (dsRNA) corresponding to sequences in viral replicase and glycoprotein genes specifically inhibits YHV infection *in vitro* and *in vivo*, suggesting that RNA interference may play a role in the host response to infection.

## Transmission

The natural transmission cycle of YHV has not been studied in detail. Experimentally, YHV infection and disease can be transmitted horizontally by injection, ingestion of infected tissue, immersion in membrane-filtered tissue extracts, or by cohabitation with infected shrimp. Transmission of disease by ingestion has been demonstrated from the late postlarval stages onward. Transmission has also been demonstrated by injection of black tiger shrimp with extracts of paste shrimp (*Acetes* sp.) and mysid shrimp (*Palaemon styliferus*) collected from infected ponds. For GAV, there is evidence that horizontal transmission can occur from chronically infected shrimp in the absence of disease.

There is no direct evidence of vertical transmission of YHV but it can be detected as a chronic infection in broodstock prior to spawning, and polymerase chain reaction (PCR) screening to eliminate infected broodstock and seed is increasingly being used to reduce risks of yellow head disease in ponds. GAV has been detected in spermatophores and mature ovarian tissue of broodstock, and in fertilized eggs and nauplii spawned from infected females. Examination by electron microscopy has revealed virions in seminal fluid but not in sperm cells. Artificial insemination of infected broodstock has shown that vertical transmission occurs efficiently from both male and female parents. Transmission is probably by surface contamination or infection of tissue surrounding the fertilized egg. The high prevalence of yellow head complex viruses in postlarvae collected from hatcheries in Australia and several Asian countries supports the view that vertical transmission has an important role in the infection cycle of all genotypes, particularly during propagation for aquaculture.

## Genetic Diversity

YHV is one of several closely related genotypes that have been detected in black tiger shrimp in the Indo-Pacific region. Analysis of nucleotide and deduced amino acid sequences in a relatively conserved region of the ORF1b gene has identified at least six distinct genetic lineages in the complex (**Figure 3**). In pairwise alignments, nucleotide sequence identity between consensus sequences representing each genotype ranges from 80.3% to 96.5%. Variation within genotypes is generally low,

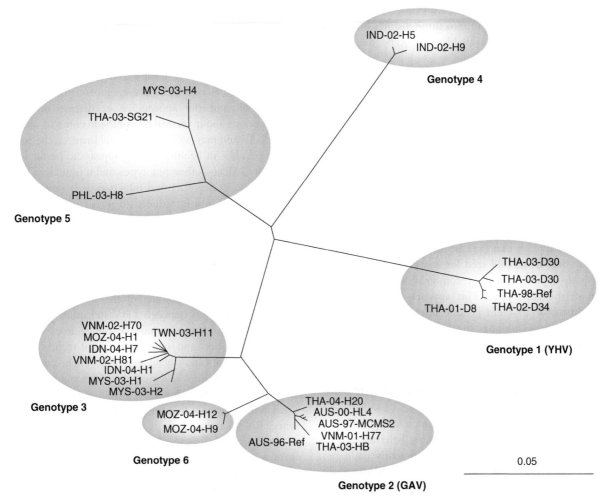

**Figure 3** Phylogenetic tree constructed from an alignment of nucleotide sequences obtained from 26 viruses detected in *Penaeus monodon* shrimp from the Indo-Pacific region. The sequences correspond to a 671 nucleotide region of the ORF1b gene encompassing elements of the HEL domain. The alignment illustrates the six known genotypes in the yellow head complex including YHV (genotype 1), GAV (genotype 2), and four other genotypes (genotypes 3, 4, 5, and 6) that have been detected only in healthy shrimp. The viruses were obtained from shrimp collected in India (IND), Malaysia (MYS), Thailand (THA), the Philippines (PHL), Australia (AUS), Vietnam (VNM), Mozambique (MOZ), Indonesia (IDN), and Taiwan (TWN) between 1997 and 2004. Sequences kindly provided by Mrs Priyanjalie Wijegoonawardane, CSIRO Livestock Industries, St. Lucia, Australia.

with nucleotide sequence identities between isolates in the range 97.1–100%, except genotype 5 for which three available isolates have been reported to share 93.0–97.1% identity.

YHV (genotype 1) is the only genotype that has been detected in shrimp with typical signs of yellow head disease. Although the disease has been reported from many sites in Asia, isolates are currently available only from Thailand and Taiwan. Genotype 1 is the most distantly related to other lineages and appears to occur less commonly than other genotypes in healthy shrimp. GAV (genotype 2) is the only other lineage known to be associated with disease of any form. Analysis of complete genome sequences of prototype strains of YHV and GAV indicates similar nucleotide sequence identities for ORF1a (79.7%), ORF1b (82.3%), ORF2 (81.0%),

and a slightly lower level of identity for ORF3 (73.2%). Amino-acid-sequence identities between YHV and GAV proteins are similar for the replicase pp1ab (84.9%), nucleoprotein p20 (84.4%), and glycoprotein gp64 (83.9%), and lower for the M-like protein p22 (74.8%) and glycoprotein gp116 (71.7%).

GAV has been detected in black tiger shrimp from Australia, Vietnam, and Thailand. Phylogenetic analysis of sequences analyzed to date suggests that all isolates may have originated from translocated Australian shrimp. Genotype 3 has been detected to date in Taiwan, Vietnam, Indonesia, Malaysia, Thailand, and Mozambique. It appears to be the most widely distributed and most frequently detected genotype. Genotype 4 has been detected only in India. Genotype 5 has been detected in the Philippines, Malaysia, and Thailand. As indicated above, genotype 5 is genetically the most diverse genotype and may be split into three distinct lineages as more isolates become available. Genotype 6 has been detected only in Mozambique.

Assignment of these genotypes has been based primarily on comparisons of sequences in a conserved region of the ORF1b gene. Analysis of nucleotide sequences in the 5′-terminal region of the ORF3 polyglycoprotein gene indicates more genetic variability and suggests that genetic recombination is contributing to diversity in the complex. Of 24 isolates examined recently, almost one-third were assigned to different genotypes in comparative phylogenetic analyses of nucleotide sequences in the ORF1b and ORF3 regions. Genetic recombination is a phenomenon known to occur commonly in other nidoviruses. It appears that the vast international trade in live shrimp broodstock and seed for aquaculture is providing adequate opportunities for recombination and diversification of the gene pool. This appears to confound the assignment of coherent genetic lineages and may have significant consequences for both the emergence and definitive diagnosis of disease.

## Diagnosis and Disease Management

Gross clinical signs of YHV infection including yellowing of the carapace and erratic swimming behavior are not observed consistently and are not sufficiently pathognomonic to be useful for disease diagnosis. Histologically, moderate to large numbers of basophilic, spherical, cytoplasmic inclusions in tissues of ectodermal and mesodermal origin are indications of YHV infection and can be used for presumptive diagnosis. Confirmatory diagnosis of yellow head disease requires the use of electron microscopy or molecular methods such as the reverse transcriptase-polymerase chain reaction (RT-PCR) or *in situ* hybridization assays. Antibody-based tests such as western blotting and dot-blot nitrocellulose enzyme immunoassay (NC-EIA) are also available. Low-level chronic infections with YHV and other genotypes can be detected by nested RT-PCR or other highly sensitive molecular genetic tests such as real-time PCR or loop-mediated isothermal amplification (LAMP). Accurate genotype assignment can only be achieved by PCR, sequence analysis, and comparison with sequences of other known genotypes.

No effective vaccines or therapeutics are currently available for the control of YHV and no genetically resistant shrimp stocks have been reported yet. Disease management is primarily through pathogen exclusion by PCR screening of broodstock and/or seed, the application of on-farm biosecurity and sanitary measures, and stress reduction by careful management of water quality during grow-out.

## Current Status

Key aspects of the biology of YHV infection are yet to be resolved and yellow head continues to be a disease of concern to aquaculture farmers. No direct link has been demonstrated between the presence of virus in infected broodstock and the appearance of disease on farms. Assumptions about vertical transmission come by analogy with GAV and may well be accurate. However, the prevalence of YHV in healthy shrimp appears to be far lower than for GAV and other genotypes, and it is unclear how it maintains a cycle of natural infection. It is possible that YHV is commonly introduced to ponds in healthy wild shrimp or other carrier crustaceans but surveys to date have not revealed a likely source. The host–viral interaction during the chronic phase of infection, the transition from chronic to acute phases, and the role of stress in disease emergence are also poorly understood, and there is little understanding of the molecular basis of virulence variations between YHV and other genotypes. A more comprehensive study of the sources of YHV infection and host and/or environmental factors leading to emergence of yellow head disease should be conducted. Emerging capabilities in shrimp genomics and proteomics will greatly facilitate this work.

There is an emerging understanding of RNA interference (RNAi) as a potentially powerful mechanism for the control of viral diseases. Inhibition of YHV infection in primary lymphoid organ cell culture has been demonstrated by treatment with dsRNA corresponding to YHV protease, polymerase, and helicase domains. Injection of shrimp with protease domain dsRNA has also been shown to inhibit YHV replication and mortalities. Knockdown of the shrimp dicer-1 endoribonuclease gene expression has demonstrated that the antiviral effects of dsRNA are caused by RNAi. RNAi technology has useful applications in studies of the molecular biology of YHV infection and, if delivered cost-effectively, could potentially find commercial application in the management of yellow head disease.

Roniviruses are also seen as important links in understanding the evolutionary biology of (+) ssRNA viruses. Considerations of virion structure and the size, complexity and structural organization of the genome suggest that roniviruses form a genetic lineage ancestral to coronaviruses and toroviruses. Studies of the ronivirus 3C-like cysteine protease encoded in ORF1a have also revealed structural similarities to coronaviruses in the catalytic site but substrate specificity and binding sites are more similar to those of potyviruses, suggesting that they bridge the gap between these distantly related proteases. A pseudoknot structure and slippery sequence at the ribosomal frameshift site is also distinct from the H-type structures characteristic of many vertebrate nidoviruses. Further molecular studies of ronivirus structure and function should provide insights into the evolution of these unusual viruses.

## Further Reading

Assavalapsakul W, Smith DR, and Panyim S (2006) Identification and characterization of a *Penaeus monodon* lymphoid cell-expressed receptor for yellow head virus. *Journal of Virology* 80: 262–269.

Chantanachookin C, Boonyaratpalin S, Kasornchandra J, *et al.* (1993) Histology and ultrastructure reveal a new granulosis-like virus in *Penaeus monodon* affected by 'yellow-head' disease. *Diseases of Aquatic Organisms* 17: 145–157.

Cowley JA, Cadogan LC, Spann KM, Sittidilokratna N, and Walker PJ (2004) The gene encoding the nucleocapsid protein of gill-associated nidovirus of *Penaeus monodon* prawns is located upstream of the glycoprotein gene. *Journal of Virology* 78: 8935–8941.

Cowley JA, Dimmock CM, Spann KM, and Walker PJ (2000) Gill-associated virus of *Penaeus monodon* shrimp: An invertebrate virus with ORF1a and ORF1b genes related to arteri- and coronaviruses. *Journal of General Virology* 81: 1473–1484.

Cowley JA, Dimmock CM, and Walker PJ (2001) Gill-associated nidovirus of *Penaeus monodon* prawns transcribes 3′-coterminal subgenomic RNAs that do not possess 5′-leader sequences. *Journal of General Virology* 83: 927–935.

Cowley JA, Hall MR, Cadogan LC, Spann KM, and Walker PJ (2002) Vertical transmission of covert gill-associated virus (GAV) infections in *Penaeus monodon*. *Diseases of Aquatic Organisms* 50: 95–104.

Cowley JA and Walker PJ (2002) The complete genome sequence of gill-associated virus of *Penaeus monodon* prawns indicates a gene organisation unique among nidoviruses. *Archives of Virology* 147: 1977–1987.

Dhar AK, Cowley JA, Hasson KW, and Walker PJ (2004) Genomic organization, biology and diagnosis of Taura syndrome virus (TSV) and yellowhead virus (YHV) of penaeid shrimp. *Advances in Virus Research* 63: 353–421.

Gorbalenya A, Enjuanes L, Ziebuhr J, and Snijder EJ (2006) *Nidovirales*: Evolving the largest RNA virus genome. *Virus Research* 117: 17–37.

Jitrapakdee S, Unajak S, Sittidilokratna N, *et al.* (2003) Identification and analysis of gp116 and gp64 structural glycoproteins of yellow head nidovirus of *Penaeus monodon* shrimp. *Journal of General Virology* 84: 863–873.

Sittidilokratna N, Hodgson RAJ, Cowley JA, *et al.* (2002) Complete ORF1b-gene sequence indicates yellow head virus is an invertebrate nidovirus. *Diseases of Aquatic Organisms* 50: 87–93.

Sittidilokratna N, Phetchampai N, Boonsaeng V, and Walker PJ (2006) Structural and antigenic analysis of the yellow head virus nucleocapsid protein p20. *Virus Research* 116: 21–29.

Walker PJ, Bonami JR, Boonsaeng V, *et al.* (2005) *Roniviridae*. In: Fauquet CM, Mayo MA, Maniloff J, Desselberger U,, and Ball LA (eds.) *Virus Taxonomy: Eighth Report of the International Committee on Taxonomy of Viruses*, pp. 973–977. San Diego, CA: Elsevier Academic Press.

Walker PJ, Cowley JA, Spann KM, *et al.* (2001) Yellow head complex viruses: Transmission cycles and topographical distribution in the Asia-Pacific region. In: Browdy CL and Jory DE (eds.) *The New Wave: Proceedings of the Special Session on Sustainable Shrimp Culture, Aquaculture*, pp. 292–302. Baton Rouge: World Aquaculture Society.

Ziebuhr J, Bayer S, Cowley JA, and Gorbalenya AE (2003) The 3C-like proteinase of an invertebrate nidovirus links coronavirus and potyvirus homologs. *Journal of Virology* 77: 1415–1426.

# VIRUSES WHICH INFECT BACTERIA

# Filamentous ssDNA Bacterial Viruses

**S A Overman and G J Thomas Jr.,** University of Missouri – Kansas City, Kansas City, MO, USA

## Glossary

**Cloning vector** The DNA molecule of a virus, plasmid, or cell into which a foreign DNA fragment can be integrated without loss of self-replicating activity. The vector introduces the foreign DNA fragment into an appropriate host cell for autonomous replication, usually in large quantity.

**Phage library** An ensemble of up to about $10^{10}$ phage clones, each harboring a different foreign coding sequence in-frame with either the N- or C-terminal region of a capsid protein gene. The clone thus allows display of a different 'guest' peptide on the virion surface.

**Raman spectroscopy** The branch of optical spectroscopy (named after its 1928 founder, C. V. Raman) concerned with measurements of the intensities of light scattered inelastically by molecules that have been excited by monochromatic radiation. The resulting spectrum, usually a plot of scattering intensity (in arbitrary units) versus energy (in wave number or $cm^{-1}$ units), reflects the transfer of discrete energy quanta from the impingent photons to vibrational energy states of the molecules. The Raman spectrum, which is determined by both intramolecular bonding arrangements (covalency and conformation) and intermolecular interactions, provides a sensitive signature of molecular structure and local environment.

**Trans-envelope network** A multiprotein complex that is located in the envelope of a bacterial cell and brings the inner and outer membranes in close proximity to one another.

**Ultraviolet resonance Raman spectroscopy (UVRR)** A type of Raman spectroscopy (see above) in which the wavelength of the exciting monochromatic radiation is in the ultraviolet region (i.e., wavelength $\lambda < 400$ nm, or wave number $\sigma > 25\,000$ $cm^{-1}$), so as to achieve resonance with electronic absorption processes of the molecules. In UVRR spectra, only the vibrational states of the chromophore are represented.

## Introduction

The filamentous ssDNA viruses (genus *Inovirus*) are members of a genus of morphologically similar virions that infect different bacteria via molecular recognition of a host-specific pilin. The most well studied of these phages are the closely related M13, fd, and f1 virions, which infect *Escherichia coli* displaying a conjugative F-pilus. The genome sequences of these F-specific phages are sufficiently similar that they are collectively called Ff phage. Other filamentous phages that have been studied include IKe, which infects *E. coli* displaying a conjugative N-pilus, Pf1, which infects *Pseudomonas aeruginosa* strain PAK by binding to the bacterial type IV pilus, Pf3, which infects *P. aeruginosa* strain PAO by binding not to the inherent type IV pilus but to the conjugative RP4 pilus, and PH75, which infects *Thermus thermophilus*. These filamentous phages are nonlytic and nonlysogenic. On the other hand, the filamentous ssDNA bacteriophage CTXφ, which infects *Vibrio cholera* by recognition of a toxin-co-regulated pilus (TCP), is lysogenic.

Genetic, biochemical, and biophysical methods have been used to study the Ff bacteriophage life cycle, which is unique in its use of the bacterial cell envelope for virus assembly. Features of the nonlytic Ff assembly pathway are (1) the prolific production of phage particles, (2) the extrusion of progeny virions through the cell envelope, and (3) the requirement of stable transmembrane (TM) domains in virally encoded proteins that participate in the assembly process. Also noteworthy in Ff morphogenesis is that genomes of variable size can be packaged without deleterious consequences. For example, although the single-stranded DNA (ssDNA) genome of wild-type Ff ($\sim$6400 nt) is sheathed by 2750 copies of the major capsid protein, viable variants have been isolated containing as many as 12 000 nt and corresponding modifications in the filament length and number of subunits in the sheath. Biophysical studies have shown that the Ff phage particles are highly thermostable and highly flexible. Polymorphism of the viral capsid is also revealed by electron cryomicroscopy.

The life cycle of the filamentous ssDNA bacteriophage enables its use as a model for membrane-associated nucleoprotein assembly and as a valuable tool for molecular cloning, phage display, and pharmacotherapy. The filamentous ssDNA bacteriophage also serves as a vehicle for orientation of small molecules in solution spectroscopic (nuclear magnetic resonance, NMR) applications and as a model for nanowire self-assembly. Details of the molecular structure and life cycle of the filamentous ssDNA bacteriophage are considered in this article.

## Taxonomy and Classification

The filamentous ssDNA bacterial viruses, which are visualized in electron micrographs as thin cylindrical filaments about 7 nm in diameter and ranging from 700 to 2000 nm in length, belong to the genus *Inovirus* of the family *Inoviridae*. They are distinguished from rod-shaped members of the genus *Plectrovirus* of the same family (typically $85–280 \times 10–15$ nm dimensions) by their greater contour length, smaller diameter, and lower flexural rigidity. The many species of the genus *Inovirus* so far identified have been categorized into four broad groups on the basis of the types of bacteria infected. The species encompassed by these four groups are listed in **Table 1**, in accordance with the classification of the International Committee on Taxonomy of Viruses (ICTV). The best characterized of the filamentous viruses with respect to both biological and structural properties is the coliphage M13, which serves as the prototype of the species *Enterobacteria phage M13*. This species also includes the closely related phages f1, fd, AE2, dA, Ec9, HR, and ZJ/2.

## Physical Properties

**Table 2** lists selected physical properties of several well-studied filamentous ssDNA bacterial viruses. Although each of the viruses included in **Table 2** exhibits a characteristic filamentous shape, significant differences occur in their contour lengths and in the mass ratio of capsid protein to DNA. Accordingly, differences are also anticipated in the packing arrangement of capsid subunits with respect to the encapsidated genome. The overall length of the viral filament is dictated by both the genome size and the number of subunits required to electrostatically balance the negatively charged DNA phosphates, which is accomplished by the distribution of basic side chains (Lys and Arg) near the subunit C-terminus. On the basis of fiber X-ray diffraction

results, two distinct symmetry classes (I and II) have been defined to categorize subunit/DNA packing arrangements: subunits of the class I phages (e.g., M13, f1, and fd) are arranged with approximate $C_5S_2$ symmetry, while class II phages (e.g., Pf1, Pf3, and PH75) exhibit $C_1S_{5.4}$ symmetry. Further details of virion structure are discussed in the section titled 'Composition and structure'.

## Genome Organization

The genomes of many filamentous viruses, including M13, f1, fd, IKe, Pf1, Pf3, PH75, and CTX, have been sequenced. Comparative analyses indicate that at least those of M13, f1, fd, IKe, and PH75 are similarly organized, as shown in **Figure 1** for fd.

Of the 11 virally encoded Ff genes, two (X and XI) overlap and are in-frame with larger genes (II and I, respectively). The Ff genome contains only one significant noncoding region (intergenic region, IG) consisting of about 500 nt. The IG contains the origin of replication, as well as a functionally and structurally distinct region called the packaging signal (PS), which is capable of forming a hairpin of 78 nt. During the phage life cycle, recognition of the genomic PS by virally encoded proteins initiates assembly of the viral particle. The viral genes are expressed from the origin of replication in a counterclockwise direction and are organized on the genome in functional groups, such that genes II, V, and X are grouped together and express proteins that facilitate DNA replication; genes III, VI, VII, VIII, and IX are grouped together and express structural proteins found in the mature infectious virion; and genes I, IV, and XI are grouped together and express proteins that direct virus assembly. The CTX genome lacks gene IV but contains genes that encode proteins specific to the CTX life cycle.

## Composition and Structure

The typical filamentous virion consists of a covalently closed, ssDNA genome (5–10 kbp) sheathed by several thousand copies of the major capsid protein (pVIII, ~5 kDa) plus a few copies of minor proteins at the filament ends (**Figure 2**). The numbers of pVIII subunits and DNA

**Table 1** Species of the genus *Inovirus*[a]

| Host type | Species |
| --- | --- |
| Enterobacteriaceae | *Enterobacteria phage M13,*[b] *C-2, If1, IKe, I2–2, PR64FS, SF, tf-1, X,* and *X-2* |
| Spirillaceae | *Vibrio phage 493, fs1, fs2, CTX, v6, Vf1, Vf33,* and *VSK* |
| Pseudomonadaceae | *Pseudomonas phage Pf1, Pf2,* and *Pf3* |
| Xanthomonadaceae | *Xanthomonas phage Cf16, Cf1c, Cf1t, Cf1tv, Lf, Xf, Xfo,* and *Xfv* |

[a]The species are categorized by host type.
[b]Enterobacteria phages fd, f1, and several others have been classified as a type of *Enterobacteria phage M13*.

**Table 2** Physical properties of filamentous ssDNA bacteriophages

| Property | M13 | Pf1 | Pf3 | Xf | PH75[a] |
|---|---|---|---|---|---|
| Virion length (nm) | 880 | 1900 | 680 | 980 | 910 |
| Percent mass protein | 87 | 93 | 85 | 85 | 84 |
| Capsid subunits per virion | 2750 | 7370 | 2500 | 3500 | 2700 |
| Residues per subunit | 50 | 46 | 44 | 44 | 46 |
| Nucleotides per genome | 6407 | 7390 | 5830 | 7420 | 6760 |
| Nucleotides per subunit | 2.3 | 1.0 | 2.3 | 2.1 | 2.5 |
| $\lambda_{max}$ (nm) | 269 | 270 | 264 | 263 | 267 |
| Extinction coefficient ($cm^2\,mg^{-1}$) | 3.84 | 2.07 | 4.53 | 3.52 | 3.77 |
| Symmetry class[b] | I | II | II | II | II |

[a]The thermophilic filamentous ssDNA bacteriophage, PH75, which infects *Thermus thermophilus*, has not yet been assigned to a species, genus, or family by the International Committee on Taxonomy of Viruses.

[b]Class I phages have capsid subunits arranged with $C_5S_2$ symmetry (fivefold rotational symmetry and approximately twofold screw axes) and class II phages have capsid subunits arranged with $C_1S_{5.4}$ symmetry (no rotational symmetry and a single-start superhelical array of approximately 5.4 subunits per turn).

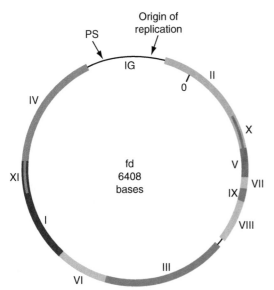

**Figure 1** The genome organization of the Ff (fd) bacteriophage. All genes (I–XI) are labeled and color-coded by function of the gene product (blue, DNA synthesis; green, capsid; red, virus assembly). The single-stranded DNA genome of fd contains 6408 nt, which are numbered clockwise from the unique *Hind*II site located in gene II. The intergenic region (IG) is located between genes II and IV and includes the packaging signal (PS) and the origin of replication. Adapted from Petrenko VA and Smith GP (2005) Vectors and modes of display. In: Sidhu S (ed.) *Phage Display in Biotechnology and Drug Discovery*, pp. 63–110. Boca Raton, FL: CRC Press.

nucleotides in several well-studied filamentous phages are given in **Table 2**. The pVIII subunits of the *Enterobacteria phage M13* species members (including phages M13, f1, and fd) have been studied extensively and can be discussed collectively. (Note that the amino acid sequence of the pVIII subunits in fd and f1 are identical and differ from that of M13 by a single amino acid change, namely Asp12 of fd (and f1) is replaced by Asn12 in M13; see **Table 3**.) It is evident from **Table 3** that the pVIII sequence in many filamentous viruses comprises three distinct components, an acidic N-terminal region, a hydrophobic central region, and a basic C-terminal region, suggesting that these fulfill distinct functions in phage morphogenesis.

Here, we consider in further detail the composition and structure of phage fd, which has served as the focus of many detailed and comprehensive biochemical and biophysical studies. The pVIII subunit is generally modeled as a gently curved α-helix that is tilted at a small average angle ($16 \pm 4°$) relative to the filament axis. The N-terminus of pVIII is exposed on the exterior of the capsid and the C-terminus lines the core, where it is presumed capable of contacting phosphates of the packaged ssDNA. Fiber X-ray diffraction studies indicate that pVIII subunits of the capsid lattice are arranged in a right-handed slew with near-fivefold rotational symmetry and twofold screw symmetry (**Figure 2**). Five copies of each of four minor proteins form the ends of the fd filament. The initially assembled end ('head') contains minor proteins pVII (3.6 kDa) and pIX (3.6 kDa), while the ultimately assembled end ('tail') contains minor proteins pIII (42.6 kDa) and pVI (12.3 kDa). The packaged genome is oriented with its IG region (PS hairpin) at the head, gene III region near the tail, and the intervening non-base-paired antiparallel strands of the DNA loop spanning the length of the filament core (**Figure 2**). Phage display and genetic studies suggest further that the minor proteins pVII and pVI at the head and tail, respectively, form contacts with the neighboring pVIII subunits, while pIX and pIII decorate the surfaces of the filament tips. Each pIII subunit is known to contain a globular N-terminal domain that is visible in electron micrographs (**Figure 2**).

In the mature fd virion, pVIII is predominantly α-helical and the C-terminal end of the α-helix (residues 40–50) consists of 'basic' and nonpolar side chains along opposite faces. Although direct experimental evidence is lacking, model-building exercises have revealed that it is possible to position the positively charged side chains of this amphipathic helix proximal to the surface of the capsid core, where interaction with packaged DNA would be facilitated. The net positive charge of the C-terminal region apparently functions to neutralize the negatively charged DNA phosphates. This is supported by the fact that mutating Lys 48 of pVIII to an uncharged side chain results in the assembly of an appropriately elongated (~35%) fd virion;

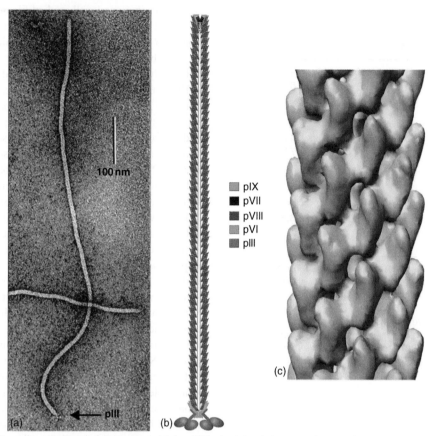

□ pIX
■ pVII
■ pVIII
□ pVI
□ pIII

**Figure 2** The fd filamentous ssDNA bacteriophage. (a) A negatively stained electron micrograph showing one complete virion (top to bottom) oriented with the pIII tail (arrow) at the bottom. The flexibility of the virion, which is apparent, is consistent with the experimentally determined equilibrium persistence length of 1.0 µm. (b) Cartoon of fd (not to scale) showing locations of the minor coat proteins. (c) Reconstruction of a 24 nm segment of fd at ~8 Å resolution from images obtained by electron cryomicroscopy. (a) Courtesy of Carla W. Gray, University of Texas, Dallas. (c) Courtesy of E. H. Egelman, University of Virginia.

**Table 3**    pVIII sequences for filamentous ssDNA bacteriophages

| Phage | pVIII sequence[a] |
|---|---|
| M13 | [1]AEGDDPAKAAFNSLQASATEYIGYAWAMVVVIVGATIGIKLFKKFTSKAS[50] |
| Pf1 | [1]GVIDTSAVESAITDGQGDMKAIGGYIVGALVILAVAGLIYSMLRKA[46] |
| Pf3 | [1]MQSVITDVTGQLTAVQADITTIGGAIIVLAAVVLGIRWIKAQFF[44] |
| Xf | [1]SGVGDGVDVVSAIEGAAGPIAAIGGAVLTVMVGIKVYKWVRRAM[44] |
| PH75 | [1]MDFNPSEVASQVTNYIQAIAAAGVGVLALAIGLSAAWKYAKRFLKG[46] |

[a]The hydrophobic segment of each pVIII sequence is underlined.

that is, additional pVIII subunits are required to package the genomic complement. The opposite nonpolar (hydrophobic) face of the C-terminal helix provides a suitable surface for intersubunit contacts.

The N-terminal region of pVIII (residues 1–20) also forms an amphipathic helix, in this case with 'acidic' and nonpolar faces. The former is exposed on the capsid surface, while the latter is presumably engaged in inter-subunit contacts. In aqueous environments of low or moderate ionic strength, electron micrographs reveal extensive intervirion

clustering, which may be mediated by the acidic (and/or polar) residues of the capsid surface. In some micrographs, liquid-crystalline phase formation is evident. Although high ionic strength conditions tend to disfavor such inter-virion clustering, the bundles once formed are not readily dissociated.

The highly hydrophobic central region of the pVIII α-helix (residues 21–39) appears to serve as the pillar of capsid stability. This α-helical segment also appears to function as a distinct domain in the assembly process, as is discussed in the next section. Studies based upon site-directed and random mutations of residues throughout the central α-helix region have contributed significantly to an understanding of inter-subunit contacts in both the mature virion and its assembly precursors. As implied above, hydrophobic contacts between subunits involve not only the central region of the α-helix but also the nonpolar faces of the N- and C-terminal segments. The periodicity of small nonpolar side chains (Gly, Ala) along specific faces of the α-helix facilitates close packing of subunits. For example, small side chains appear to be required at pVIII positions 25, 34, 35, and 38 for fd capsid stability. A similar requirement applies to the capsid subunits of other filamentous bacteriophages.

Genetic and biophysical studies of proteins show that the pentapeptide motif Gly/Ala-X-X-X-Gly/Ala (where X is any residue) increases the thermostability of packed α-helices. Of the sequences listed in **Table 3**, all contain at least one Gly/Ala-X-X-X-Gly/Ala motif within the central hydrophobic region (residues 21–39). Interestingly, the corresponding segment of the pVIII subunit of the thermophilic *T. thermophilus* phage PH75 contains four Gly/Ala-X-X-X-Gly/Ala motifs among 11 small side chains (residues Ala and Gly). Conversely, the mesophile infecting fd phage contains two Gly/Ala-X-X-X-Gly/Ala motifs among six small side chains of the 19-peptide region. In summary, hydrophobic interactions lead to close packing of pVIII helices, which is likely the principal source of capsid stability.

The multifunctional minor capsid protein pIII, which directs host infection, progeny virus assembly termination, and virion tail stabilization, has been the subject of several structural studies. The 406-amino-acid protein comprises three domains, namely two closely associated and globular N-terminal domains (N1 and N2, consisting of residues 1–67 and 88–218, respectively) that protrude from the capsid, and a stalk-like C-terminal domain (residues 253–406) that is anchored to the capsid. The domains are linked by flexible, glycine-rich sequences. The crystal structure of the N1–N2 fragment indicates a largely β-stranded structure.

The conformation of the packaged genome is not known for fd or any other filamentous phage. Because DNA typically represents a very small percentage of the virion mass (6–16%, **Table 2**), most biophysical probes do not yield definitive structural information regarding the packaged genome. Methods that selectively probe the ssDNA bases, such as ultraviolet resonance Raman (UVRR) spectroscopy, reveal strong hypochromic effects in the fd genome, which implies close contact between the purine and pyrimidine bases. Conversely, UVRR studies of Pf1 suggest unstacked bases in its packaged genome. Raman spectroscopy also indicates very different local deoxynucleoside conformations in the packaged ssDNA molecules of phages fd and Pf1.

## Life Cycle

### Infection

The mechanism of host cell infection by a filamentous bacteriophage has been studied in detail only for the bacteriophage Ff, which recognizes the conjugative F pilus of *E. coli* cells harboring the F plasmid. The process involves a trans-envelope network of host proteins – the Tol–Pal system – that is located in the *E. coli* cell envelope and serves to maintain the stability of the outer membrane. The Tol–Pal system includes the cytoplasmic membrane proteins TolA, TolR, and TolQ, which are anchored to the inner membrane, and the proteins TolB and Pal, which are associated with the outer membrane. TolA consists of an N-terminal TM domain, a periplasmic spanning α-helix, and a C-terminal globular domain also located in the periplasmic space. These domains are linked by glycine-rich segments. Like TolA, TolR has TM and periplasmic domains, whereas TolQ lacks a periplasmic domain and is located predominantly in the cytoplasm. TolA, TolR, and TolQ are associated with one another via their TM domains and all are necessary for viral infectivity. TolB is a periplasmic protein and Pal is a lipoprotein that is anchored to the outer membrane. Interaction of TolA with both TolB and Pal connects the outer and inner membranes of the *E. coli* cell. In the initial step of infection (**Figure 3**), the N2 domain of pIII binds the F-pilus, inducing a conformational change in N1–N2 that exposes a site of the N1 domain specific for TolA binding. The conformational change in N1–N2 allows a fast *cis–trans*-isomerization of the peptide bond between Gln212 and Pro213. When the peptide bond is in the more stable *trans*-form, the TolA binding site is exposed. Isomerization to the initial *cis*-form is a slow reaction, the rate of which is determined by the sequence of amino acids flanking Pro213. The rapid isomerization of the Gln212–Pro213 bond to the *trans*-form is a molecular switch controlled by the slower reverse reaction, which acts as a molecular timer. During the time that the N1 TolA binding site is exposed, the F-pilus is believed to retract through a secretin channel in the outer membrane of the host cell, by depolymerization of pilin, thus translocating pIII into the periplasm. The N1 domain of pIII binds the periplasmic C-terminal domain of TolA, the second phage receptor, forming a bridge between the adsorbed phage particle and the bacterial inner membrane. Subsequently, the C-terminal domain of pIII directs continuation of the infection process. Genetic studies suggest that the TolA–N1 interaction causes a conformational change in the pIII C-terminal domain, which 'unlocks' the capsid. Once unlocked, a TM region of the pIII C-terminal domain likely interacts with the inner membrane to initiate dissociation of the capsid proteins, pVIII, pVII, and pIX, into the inner membrane with concomitant

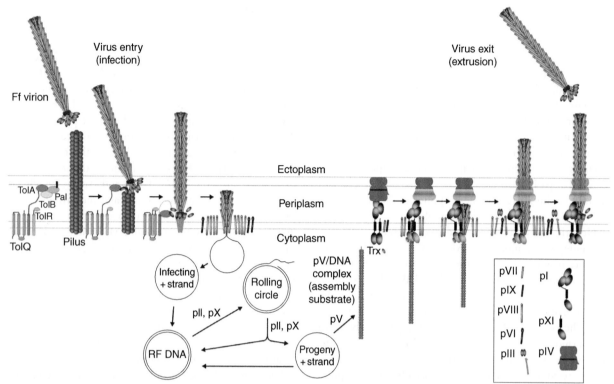

**Figure 3** Schematic representation of the Ff life cycle. In the periplasmic space, the arrows show progressive stages of disassembly (left) and assembly (right) as discussed in the text. Viral and bacterial components are not drawn to scale (e.g., the actual dimensions of the Ff virion are 6.5 × 880 nm). Pilin biogenesis proteins are not shown.

release of the viral genome into the cytoplasm. The capsid proteins of the infecting virion are retained in the membrane for use in the assembly of progeny virions.

## DNA and Protein Synthesis

Upon entry into the cytoplasm, the ssDNA viral genome is converted into a replicative double-stranded form (RF) by the activity of host-encoded polymerases (RNA Pol and DNA Pol III) and a host-encoded single-stranded DNA-binding protein (SSB). To initiate this event, Pol synthesizes a short RNA primer beginning at nucleotide 5753. Pol III extends this primer the length of the viral strand, and Pol I and ligase close the complementary strand to produce a circular, dsDNA molecule. Gyrase supercoils the circle, thus resulting in the RF DNA, which serves as the template for transcription of viral genes.

Synthesis of ssDNA viral molecules requires the virally encoded protein pII, which specifically nicks the viral strand ((+)-strand) of RF DNA. The resultant 3′ hydroxyl group is used by the host DNA synthesizing apparatus (Pol III, SSB, and Rep helicase) to generate a new (+)-strand by the rolling-circle mode of replication, thus displacing the parent (+)-strand, which is subsequently circularized by pII. The newly synthesized RF DNA is closed and supercoiled for additional rounds of replication. The displaced and circularized (+)-strand can serve as

either a substrate for additional RF DNA formation (template for (−)-strand synthesis) or a virus genome (encapsidation). At early stages of infection, the former path is more likely; at later stages, as the concentrations of virally encoded proteins become large, encapsidation is favored.

The (−)-strand serves as the template for transcription of viral genes, beginning at gene II. The presence of two strong terminators, one of which is rho-independent between genes VIII and III and the other rho-dependent in the IG, divides the genome into regions that are relatively frequently (genes II–VIII) and infrequently (gene III–IG) transcribed. The former has three strong promoters that lead to three primary transcripts. Post-transcriptional modification of these primary transcripts results in a set of six smaller and more stable mRNA molecules, all of which encode pVIII and a subset (four) of which encode pV. Multiple transcripts facilitate synthesis of the large amounts of pV and pVIII required to coat the prolifically produced (+)-strands (up to 200–300 progenies per cell). The frequently transcribed region also includes genes for the minor capsid proteins pVII and pIX. However, the translational initiation sites for synthesis of these proteins are weak. Accordingly, pVII and pIX are not produced in abundance. Proteins pII and pX, which likewise are encoded in the frequently transcribed region but not required in abundance, are regulated at the translational level via pV binding to the mRNA transcripts.

This inhibition is evident at high cellular concentrations of pV, when amounts of the protein exceed the threshold required to sequester (+)-strands targeted for viral assembly.

Transcription of the genome and translation of the mRNA transcripts produces 11 viral proteins, of which pII, pX, and pV are required for (+)-strand synthesis, pIII, pVI, pVII, pVIII, and pIX are incorporated into the capsid, and pI, pIV, and pXI facilitate membrane-associated assembly. pII (409 residues) is a strand-specific endonuclease required for (+)-strand and RF syntheses; pX (111 residues) is synthesized from an AUG site within and in-frame with the C-terminal coding region of pII; pV (87 residues) forms a stable homodimer, the crystal structure of which has been solved to 1.8 Å and gives insight into the mechanism of binding of antiparallel ssDNA strands.

Each of the five capsid proteins of Ff exhibits a sequence consistent with an α-helical TM domain. All reside in the cytoplasmic membrane prior to assembly into the virion. Nascent pVIII contains a 23-residue signal sequence, which is removed from the N-terminus by a periplasmic signal peptidase, yielding the 50-residue subunit of the mature capsid. The N-terminal segment (1–19) of the mature subunit resides on the periplasmic face of the inner membrane, the middle 20 or so residues span the membrane, and the C-terminal segment (40–50) is situated in the cytoplasm. Although Sec proteins of *E. coli* ordinarily facilitate membrane insertion and translocation, these processes for pVIII are Sec-independent and mediated instead by the host-encoded protein YidC. Maturation of the pIII precursor, which contains an 18-residue N-terminal signal, is also accomplished following membrane translocation. A C-terminal sequence of 23 hydrophobic residues anchors pIII to the inner membrane, while most of the protein is located in the periplasmic space. The three remaining minor capsid proteins, pVI (112 residues), pVII (33 residues), and pIX (32 residues), are membrane-inserted without the aid of a signal sequence.

The three morphogenetic proteins of Ff are also located in the bacterial cell envelope. pI (348 residues) contains an internal TM region and spans the inner membrane with residues 1–253 in the cytoplasm and 273–348 in the periplasm. pXI (108 residues), which is synthesized from within the pI coding region, shares the sequence of the pI C-terminal segment. Accordingly, pXI is anchored to the membrane by a short N-terminal TM region, while most of the protein resides in the periplasm. The only viral protein located in the outer membrane is pIV. The 426-residue precursor is translocated into the periplasm where a 21-residue signal sequence is removed. The resulting 405-residue protein is integrated into the outer membrane as an oligomer of 14 subunits, each with its N-terminus in the periplasm. A cryoelectron microscopy-based image reconstruction of detergent solubilized pIV at 22 Å resolution reveals a barrel-like cylindrical complex of three domains – an N-terminal ring (N-ring) of inner diameter 6.0 nm, a middle ring (M-ring) blocked by protein density, and a C-terminal ring (C-ring) of inner diameter 8.8 nm. In a recent model of the pIV multimer, it has been proposed that the C-ring is embedded in the outer membrane and the M- and N-rings are located in the periplasmic space, where a virus assembly-induced conformational change would allow opening of the gated M-ring and widening of the narrow N-ring.

## Virus Assembly

Virus assembly occurs in the bacterial envelope at sites where the inner and outer membranes are associated by a trans-envelope network of proteins comprising the virally encoded pI, pIV, and pXI. This network is not transient and exists even in the absence of virus assembly. In addition to pI, pIV, and pXI, virus assembly is also dependent on host-encoded thioredoxin, ATP hydrolysis and the proton motive force across the cytoplasmic membrane. Thioredoxin must be in the reduced state; however, redox capability of the protein is unnecessary. pI likely catalyzes ATP hydrolysis, since its cytoplasmic domain contains an ATP-binding Walker motif, which is necessary for phage assembly.

The substrate for assembly is the pV-coated viral genome, in which the PS is exposed at one end. The PS likely forms an initiation complex with the cytoplasmic domains of pI, pVII, and pIX. pV is stripped from the genome concurrent with association of the positively charged C-terminal pVIII domain to the ssDNA molecule. The viral genome is translocated across the inner membrane as pVIII subunits assemble to it. A proposed hinge region between the TM and N-terminal amphipathic domains of pVIII may facilitate the transition of the capsid subunit from the inner membrane to the viral coat, although direct experimental evidence is lacking. Concurrent with assembly of the capsid, the progeny virion exits the bacterial cell through the pIV channel. The periplasmic N-terminal and middle domains of the pIV channel must undergo large conformational changes to allow passage of the 7 nm virus particle. The narrow N-terminal ring of the channel (6 nm i.d.) must expand and the gated middle ring must open. Since pI binds to both the initiation complex and the pIV channel, the initiation of virus assembly may be coupled to pIV conformational change by way of pI, which would avoid unintended channel opening. Additionally, if energy is necessary to widen the pIV channel or open its gate, pI may provide this energy via ATP hydrolysis.

Elongation of the progeny phage continues until the end of the viral genome is reached, at which time pVI and pIII associate with the tip of the viral capsid to terminate assembly and release the virion into the extracellular milieu. Without pVI and pIII, virus assembly continues by packaging additional genomes, one after the other, until the resultant polyphage is removed from the cell by mechanical shearing. Genetic studies have shown that separate regions of the C-terminal domain of pIII are important for termination of virus assembly, release of the viral filament from the host cell, and stabilization of the virion particle. An 83-residue C-terminal segment (residues 324–406) allows incorporation of pVI, but not release of the progeny phage. Ten additional residues (313–322) within the 313–406 segment confer the ability to release progeny phage from the bacterial cell envelope. A pIII C-terminal fragment of at least 121 residues is needed to release stable filamentous ssDNA bacteriophage progeny from an *E. coli* cell.

## Biotechnology

Several aspects of the unique life cycle and morphology of the Ff bacteriophage have been exploited for biotechnological applications. (1) The size of the packaged genome is variable, such that it can easily tolerate an insertion of up to 6 kbp, which is compensated by the additional assembly of the proportionate number of pVIII subunits, as noted earlier. (2) The orientations of pVIII within the capsid lattice and pIII at the virion tail allow fusion of non-native peptides and proteins to exposed sites of the viral particle without significant disruption of phage viability or capsid stability. (3) The mature virion is very stable to changes in pH, temperature, and ionic strength. (4) Phage preparations yield high titers resulting in efficient and inexpensive large-scale phage production. (5) The phages are distinct from animal and plant viruses, and are generally not toxic to mammalian cells.

The filamentous ssDNA bacteriophage M13 has been used as a cloning vector for decades. The foreign gene to be cloned is usually inserted between functional sequences of the IG region of the genome. The virus assembly process allows up to 12 kbp of DNA to be packaged without adverse effects on phage viability. Inserts greater than 6 kbp, which result in a genome larger than 12 kbp, are possible with compensatory mutations elsewhere in the genome. One advantage of cloning with M13 is that both single-stranded and double-stranded products can be isolated from progeny phage and intracellular RF DNA, respectively.

Most biotechnological applications of M13 are byproducts of the revolutionary exploitation of the phage as a platform from which peptides (or proteins) can be displayed. To produce a phage that displays a foreign peptide, the coding sequence is inserted in-frame with that of a capsid protein, usually pVIII or pIII, so that the fused peptide is exposed on the surface of the virion. Minor capsid proteins pVI, pVII, and pIX have also been successfully used for phage display, although to a lesser extent than pIII and pVIII. The display of the peptide must not interfere with capsid protein function. In the case of pVIII tethering, the peptide must be compatible with translocation of the capsid subunit across the inner membrane and with capsid assembly. Accordingly, peptides are usually fused to the pVIII N-terminus. For pIII, the peptide must not occlude the pilin binding site. Interference of the displayed peptide with the life cycle and/or stability of the phage can often be overcome by using a helper phage to facilitate production of hybrid virions containing both wild-type and fused capsid proteins, thus minimizing the adverse effect of the display. When sequences from a DNA library are inserted into the genome for display, a phage library containing up to $10^{10}$ different displayed peptides is produced.

The applications of phage display for biotechnological progress range from identification of molecular recognition elements between interacting proteins and ligands to targeted drug delivery for treatment of diseased mammalian cells. Biomedical applications include (1) antibody selection using a phage-displayed epitope library to facilitate the design of vaccines with optimal binding affinity for target epitopes; (2) immunopharmacotherapy for cocaine addiction, in which cocaine-sequestering antibodies displayed on a filamentous ssDNA bacteriophage are delivered to the central nervous system intranasally; (3) *in vivo* visualization of β-amyloid plaques by delivery of phage-displayed anti-β-amyloid antibodies to the brain with subsequent staining with fluorescent-labeled anti-phage antibody; and (4) cell-targeted gene and drug delivery, in which the phage is essentially a therapeutic nanocourier. Filamentous ssDNA bacteriophage display systems have also been successfully applied for nonmedical biotechnological purposes, for example, in the synthesis and assembly of nanowires for lithium ion battery electrodes. In this case, the tetrapeptide Glu-Glu-Glu-Glu is fused to the N-terminus of pVIII and treated to bind cobalt oxide forming a $Co_3O_4$ nanowire. These $Co_3O_4$ viral nanowires electrostatically self-assemble to form a nanostructured monolayer, which is used as the negative electrode in the construction of a Li-ion battery.

*See also:* Icosahedral Tailed dsDNA Bacterial Viruses.

## Further Reading

Bennett NJ and Rakonjac J (2006) Unlocking of the filamentous bacteriophage virion during infection is mediated by the C domain of pIII. *Journal of Molecular Biology* 356: 266–273.

Davis BM and Waldor MK (2005) Filamentous phages linked to virulence of *Vibrio cholera*. *Current Opinion in Microbiology* 6: 35–42.

Eckert B, Martin A, Balbach J, and Schmid FX (2005) Prolyl isomerization as a molecular timer in phage infection. *Nature Structural and Molecular Biology* 12: 619–623.

Frenkel D and Solomon B (2002) Filamentous phage as vector-mediated antibody delivery to the brain. *Proceedings of the National Academy of Sciences, USA* 99: 5675–5679.

Nam KT, Kim D-W, Yoo PJ, *et al.* (2006) Virus-enabled synthesis and assembly of nanowires for lithium ion battery electrodes. *Science* 312: 885–888.

Opalka N, Beckmann R, Boisset N, *et al.* (2003) Structure of the filamentous phage pIV multimer by cryo-electron microscopy. *Journal of Molecular Biology* 325: 461–470.

Petrenko VA and Smith GP (2005) Vectors and modes of display. In: Sidhu S (ed.) *Phage Display in Biotechnology and Drug Discovery.* pp. 63–110. Boca Raton, FL: CRC Press.

Samuelson JC, Chen M, Jiang F, *et al.* (2000) YidC mediates membrane protein insertion in bacteria. *Nature* 406: 637–641.

Tsuboi M and Thomas GJ, Jr. (2007) Polarized Raman and polarized infrared spectroscopy of proteins and protein assemblies. In: Uversky VN and Permyakov EA (eds.) *Protein Structures: Methods in Protein Structure and Stability Analysis*, ch. 3.4. Hauppage, NY: Nova Science Publishers.

Wang YA, Yu X, Overman SA, *et al.* (2006) The structure of the filamentous bacteriophage. *Journal of Molecular Biology* 361: 209–215.

Webster RE (1999) Filamentous phages. In: Granoff A and Webster RG (eds.) *Encyclopedia of Virology,* 2nd edn., pp. 547–552. London: Academic Press.

# Fuselloviruses of Archaea

**K M Stedman,** Portland State University, Portland, OR, USA

## Glossary

**Acidophile** An organism whose optimal growth is at acidic pH, often 2 or below.

**Archaea** One of the three domains of life as defined by Carl Woese, completely microbial and separate from bacteria.

**Archaeon** Singular of Archaea or Archaebacteria.

**Cryptic plasmid** Plasmid with no known function.

**Cryptic protein** Protein with no known function.

**Extreme thermophile** An organism whose optimal growth temperature is above 80 °C.

**Fusiform** Having a spindle shape.

**Thermoacidophile** An organism that is thermophilic and acidophilic.

**Thermophile** An organism whose optimal growth temperature is above 50 °C.

**Tyrosine recombinase** One of a family of DNA recombining enzymes with an active site tyrosine.

## Introduction

Fuselloviruses are unique spindle-shaped viruses with a short tail at one end that have so far only been observed in archaeal viruses or extreme environments dominated by Archaea (**Figure 1**). The first fusellovirus to be found and characterized was SSV1, a virus-like particle of *Sulfolobus shibatae,* an extremely thermoacidophilic archaeon (optimal growth at 80 °C and pH 3). Fusellovirus genomes are relatively small double-stranded circular DNA molecules from 15 to 17 kbp. Only one gene, the viral integrase, shows clear similarity to genes outside the fuselloviruses.

Their genomes persist in host cells both as episomes and integrated into the host genome. The genome is positively supercoiled when packaged in virus particles. Virus production can be induced by UV-irradiation. Virion production is usually constitutive at a low level and does not impede host growth or lyse the host cells. Viruses appear to be produced by budding at the cellular membrane.

Fuselloviruses have been found throughout the world and five complete genomes have been reported (**Table 1**). Fusellovirus-like DNA sequences have been found in many more locations by culture-independent techniques. Intriguing virus-plasmid hybrids have been discovered along with the SSV1-like viruses. SSV1, or portions thereof, has been used to make the first widely used vectors for genetic manipulation in thermophilic Archaea. Biochemical characterization has focused on the viral integrase with recent results showing that the integrase is similar to eukaryotic recombinases. Interestingly, the integrase gene and integration do not appear to be absolutely necessary for virus function. Nonetheless, the presence of the integrase gene appears to give such viruses a competitive advantage. Two structures of SSV1 encoded proteins have been solved to high resolution, but elucidation of the structure of the entire virion and many of the proteins remains elusive.

A number of archaeal viruses have been described as having a similar morphology to the SSV viruses. However, the spindle-shaped viruses of methanogens that were originally grouped with the fuselloviruses are very pleiomorphic and probably do not belong in this family. Additionally, the haloviruses His1 and His2 have very different genomes and replication and have been placed in the new genus *Salterprovirus.* Other spindle-shaped viruses of Archaea are much larger than the fuselloviruses.

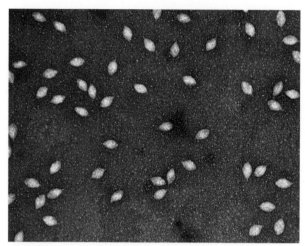

**Figure 1**    SSV1 image. Typical transmission electron micrograph of negatively stained SSV1 virions. Virus particles are 60 nm across and 90 nm long.

**Table 1**    Sequenced fuselloviruses

| Virus | Genome size (bp) | Location of isolation |
| --- | --- | --- |
| SSV1 | 15 495 | Kyushu, Japan |
| SSV2 | 14 794 | Reykjanes, Iceland |
| SSV3 | 15 230 | Krisovik, Iceland |
| SSV-RH | 16 473 | Yellowstone, USA |
| SSV-K1 | 17 385 | Kamchatka, Russia |
| pSSVx[a] | 5 705 | Reykjanes, Iceland |

[a]Satellite.

## History

The virus SSV1 was originally detected as a UV-inducible plasmid in a *Sulfolobus* isolate from Beppu Onsen in Kyushu, Japan by Wolfram Zillig and his co-workers in the early 1980s. Production of a $60 \times 90$ nm spindle-shaped virus-like particle was shown soon thereafter. The term 'virus-like particle' was used because infection of an otherwise uninfected strain could not initially be shown. It appears to be very difficult, if not impossible, to cure a *Sulfolobus* strain of a fusellovirus once infected. This may be due to the integration of the virus genome into a tRNA gene in the host genome by the virus integrase gene. SSV1 integrates into the CCG arginyl tRNA gene, whereas other fuselloviruses integrate into other tRNA genes. SSV1 became a model for the understanding of transcription in Archaeaa. It was in the study of SSV1 genes and their promoters that Wolf-Dieter Reiter noticed that they resembled eukaryotic promoters with their canonical TATA-boxes. Together with previous work from the Zillig laboratory that had shown that the DNA-dependent RNA polymerases in Archaea were similar to eukaryotic DNA-dependent RNA polymerases, there was a strong evidence that the archaeal transcription machinery was eukaryote-like. The complete 15 495 bp

genome sequence of SSV1 was determined in 1990. Genome analysis showed that other than the previously characterized virus coat protein genes, VP1 and VP3, an apparent DNA-binding protein, VP2, and the viral integrase (see below), none of the other 34 open reading frames (ORFs) showed any similarity to proteins in the known databases (**Figure 2**).

A major breakthrough in the study of SSV1 was made when Christa Schleper showed that SSV1 could infect *Sulfolobus solfataricus*, an uninfected *Sulfolobus* isolated from Pisciarelli, Italy, showing conclusively that SSV1 was a virus. She was also able to transform *Sulfolobus* for the first time using this DNA. With this technique, plaque tests were established, the virus could be characterized, and large quantities could be purified. *Sulfolobus solfataricus* is one of the best studied of the thermophilic Archaea and a complete genome sequence and many other data are available. The development of the plaque test also allowed screening for fuselloviruses (and other viruses) in samples from throughout the world.

## Fuselloviruses

### Isolates

Using a plaque test and related spot-on-lawn halo techniques, first Wolfram Zillig's group and then others isolated fuselloviruses from Iceland, the USA, and Russia, in addition to SSV1 from Japan. The Zillig group found that approximately 8% of isolates from habitats with $T > 70\,°C$ and $pH^+ < 4$ contained SSVs that could be detected by their ability to infect *S. solfataricus*. First characterized was SSV2, from Iceland, followed by SSV-RH from Yellowstone National Park in the USA and SSV-K1 from the Kamchatka peninsula in Russia. All of these viruses had the typical spindle-shape and size of fuselloviruses and all contained *c.* 15 kbp genomes (**Table 1**). Those tested appeared to integrate into the host genome and were also inducible with UV-irradiation. However, the level of induction varied greatly between isolates as did the tRNA gene used as the site of virus integration into the host genome.

The complete genome sequences of all of these new fuselloviruses were determined and it was found that only about 50% of the genome is conserved (**Figure 2**). In some cases there is no sequence similarity whatsoever between parts of the virus genomes. The overall nucleotide identity is only about 55%, but the level of amino acid identity varies from undetectable to about 80%. The genomes have similar organization, with the exception of a large insertion and inversion in the SSV-K1 genome. Strangely, the putative DNA-binding protein, VP2, is missing in all genomes other than SSV1. The question then arose whether these genomic differences were due to geographical isolation of the viruses or to large

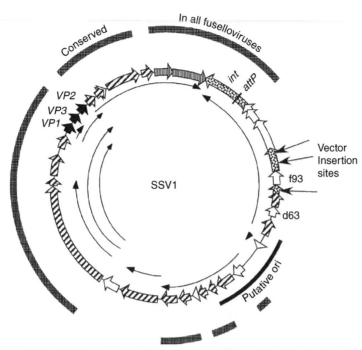

**Figure 2** The SSV1 genome with its ORFs is shown, together with mapped transcripts. The attachment site in the viral integrase gene is shown as 'attP'. Known viral genes are labeled. VP1, VP3, and VP2 are virus structural genes. The location of the ORFs whose products have been crystallized, f93 and d63, are labeled. The putative origin of replication is labeled as 'Putative ori'. Insertion points for full-length shuttle vectors are shown with arrows outside the viral genome. Dotted ORFs have been shown to be not essential for virus function. Diagonally striped ORFs appear to be important for virus function. Vertically striped ORFs are conserved in pSSVx. ORFs conserved in all fusellovirus genomes are indicated by a stippled curve, outside of the ORF map.

amounts of local heterogeneity. To address this question the complete genome of a new SSV from Iceland, SSV3, was determined and compared to SSV2. It was found to have about 70% overall nucleotide identity to SSV2 and most of the ORFs were well conserved between the two viruses. However, there were a number of ORFs that were not conserved in SSV2, the other Icelandic virus, but were found in fuselloviruses from other parts of the world.

## Culture-Independent Studies

The availability of multiple genome sequences for the fuselloviruses allowed the design of oligonucleotide probes that could be used to amplify conserved parts of fusellovirus genomes using the polymerase chain reaction. This technique was used on DNA samples collected directly from the environment, pioneered by Mark Young and his group. They showed that in a single spring that was known to harbor both *Sulfolobus* and fuselloviruses, the composition and relative abundance of fusellovirus sequences changed on at least a monthly basis. They also showed that a great deal of diversity was present in a single spring, much more diversity than seen in their hosts. Analysis of the sequence data over time indicated that there was a great deal of migration between

springs and possibly a very large reservoir of fuselloviruses worldwide. Similar data from Lassen Volcanic National Park in the USA indicate this to be the case. These data contrast with the conservation seen between the whole SSV2 and SSV3 genomes from Iceland mentioned above. This conundrum remains to be resolved.

## Plasmid Virus Hybrids

During the investigation of SSV2 from Iceland, a small virus-like particle was observed. This virus-like particle corresponded to a small plasmid, then named pSSVx, that was present in the same culture as SSV2 and appeared to be dependent on it or another complete fusellovirus for propagation. The genome sequence of pSSVx indicated that it was a fusion of a plasmid from the pRN family of cryptic *Sulfolobus* plasmids and two ORFs from a fusellovirus. It is not clear if activity of these ORFs is required for the plasmid to be packaged or if a *cis*-acting DNA sequence is required. At least one more of these virus-plasmid pairs has been reported in viruses from Iceland. This plasmid not only provides insight into virus and plasmid function but also is the basis for new genetic tools for *Sulfolobus*.

## Fusellovirus-Based Vectors

One of the major reasons for sequencing the *S. solfataricus* genome and for isolation of viruses and plasmids of thermophilic Archaea was to be able to establish a genetic system for the analysis of these organisms. Many of the first and most successful steps have been taken using SSV1 or other fuselloviruses as the basis for plasmids that replicate in *Sulfolobus* and allow recombinant DNA to be transformed into *Sulfolobus*. A number of repeated sequences near the UV-inducible promoter, Tind, together with divergent promoters, led to the proposition that this region was the origin of replication (**Figure 2**). Pieces of the SSV1 genome containing this region have been incorporated into vectors that appear to replicate in *S. solfataricus* after transformation. However, these vectors have not been widely used. More successful vectors use the whole SSV1 genome with an insertion of an *Escherichia coli* plasmid in a region that was shown not to be critical for virus function to create infectious clones (**Figure 2**). Vectors based on this technique are now in their third generation. They have been successful in complementing mutants, overexpressing homologous and heterologous genes, and for preliminary gene-expression studies.

## Fusellovirus Integrases

The only gene in fusellovirus genomes to show clear similarity to other genes is the virus integrase gene. It shows distant but clear similarity to the large family of site-specific tyrosine recombinases. Fusellovirus integrases are, however, unlike most other integrases in that the viral attachment site is within the integrase gene. Thus, integration disrupts the viral integrase gene. The attachment site in all fusellovirus integrases is in the N-terminal domain of the protein, and it is assumed, but not proved, that the remainder of the protein is not active, even though it contains all of the conserved catalytic amino acids responsible for recombination. The host attachment sites are in tRNA genes and proviral insertion preserves most of the tRNA gene so that it should remain functional. Intriguingly, all of the fuselloviruses sequenced to date integrate or are predicted to integrate into different tRNA genes. No additional host or virus genes appear to be required for either integration or excision. No excision of a provirus has been observed to date. Extensive *in vitro* studies with the SSV1 integrase indicate that the integrase itself is necessary and sufficient for both integrative or deletion reactions. Elegant molecular genetic studies have shown that the active site of the integrase is shared between two monomers and performs 'trans-cleavage', similar to eukaryotic recombinases, but not bacterial ones.

Very recently, it was shown that the virus integrase and integration are not necessary for virus function.

This was somewhat surprising due to the conservation of the integrase gene in all fusellovirus genomes sequenced to date. Additionally, a number of partial integrase genes, apparently made by past virus integration events, are present in not only the *S. solfataricus* genome but also in many other extremely thermophilic Archaea where they are thought to be highly involved in horizontal gene transfer.

Viruses lacking the integrase gene appeared not to integrate, but were stably maintained in laboratory cultures and under a number of stress conditions. However in head-to-head competition experiments between viruses containing and lacking the virus integrase gene respectively, the construct without the integrase was rapidly out-competed.

## Structures

A structural genomics program to elucidate all of the structures of the products of all of the ORFs in the SSV1 genome has produced two high-resolution structures to date. The first, the product of ORF f93, is clearly a winged helix-domain containing protein, almost undoubtedly involved in DNA binding. However, its role in virus function is not clear. This ORF is also not conserved in most of the other SSV genomes. A high-resolution structure for the ORF product d63 has been solved. It is a very simple four-helix bundle which may be involved in protein–protein interactions but again its function is not clear. Recently developed genetic tools may help in the elucidation of these functions.

## Other 'Fusiform' Viruses

The viruses of extremely halophilic Archaea, His1 and His2, have strikingly similar morphology to the *Sulfolobus* fuselloviruses, but their genomes are linear and their replication is protein primed. Therefore, they have been recently assigned to the new floating genus *Salterprovirus*. The virus-like particle reported from *Methanococcus voltae* strain A3 at first glance appears to be very similar to the *Sulfolobus* fuselloviruses, but it has a much larger genome and many different shapes in transmission electron microscopy. A virus-like particle with a similar shape to the *Sulfolobus* fuselloviruses, PAV1, has been isolated from a deep-sea *Pyrococcus abysii* strain. This virus has not yet been fully characterized and its infectivity has not yet been shown. Its genome has no sequence similarity to the *Sulfolobus* SSVs.

A number of other viruses with a spindle shape with or without projections at one or both ends have been isolated from a number of thermoacidophilic Archaea. Most of them, however, have either been assigned to other virus families or have not yet been classified. Generally, their genomes are very different both in size and sequence from the known fuselloviruses and often their virions have very different sizes.

*See also:* Viruses Infecting Euryarchaea.

## Further Reading

Albers SV, Jonuscheit M, Dinkelaker S, *et al.* (2006) Production of recombinant and tagged proteins in the hyperthermophilic archaeon *Sulfolobus solfataricus. Applied and Environmental Microbiology* 72(1): 102–111.

Arnold HP, She Q, Phan H, *et al.* (1999) The genetic element pSSVx of the extremely thermophilic crenarchaeon *Sulfolobus* is a hybrid between a plasmid and a virus. *Molecular Microbiology* 34(2): 217–226.

Prangishvili D, Forterre P, and Garrett RA (2006) Viruses of the Archaea: A unifying view. *Nature Reviews Microbiology* 4(11): 837–848.

Schleper C, Kubo K, and Zillig W (1992) The particle SSV1 from the extremely thermophilic archaeon *Sulfolobus* is a virus:

Demonstration of infectivity and of transfection with viral DNA. *Proceedings of the National Academy of Sciences, USA* 89(16): 7645–7649.

Stedman KM (2005) Fuselloviridae. In: Fauquet CM, Mayo MA, Maniloff J, Desselberger U,, and Ball LA (eds.) *Virus Taxonomy Eighth Report of the International Committee on Taxonomy of Viruses,* pp 107–110. San Diego, CA: Elsevier Academic Press.

Stedman KM, Clore A, and Combet-Blanc Y (2006) Biogeographical diversity of archaeal viruses. In: Logan NA, Pappin-Scott HM,, and Oynston PCF (eds.) *SGM Symposium 66: Prokaryotic Diversity: Mechanisms and Significance,* pp. 131–144. Cambridge: Cambridge University Press.

Stedman KM, Prangishvili D, and Zillig W (2005) Viruses of Archaea. In: Calendar R (ed.) *The Bacteriophages,* 2nd edn., pp. 499–516. New York: Oxford University Press.

Stedman KM, She Q, Phan H, *et al.* (2003) Relationships between fuselloviruses infecting the extremely thermophilic archaeon *Sulfolobus:* SSV1 and SSV2. *Research in Microbiology* 154(4): 295–302.

Wiedenheft B, Stedman KM, Roberto F, *et al.* (2004) Comparative genomic analysis of hyperthermophilic archaeal *Fuselloviridae* viruses. *Journal of Virology* 78(4): 1954–1961.

# Icosahedral dsDNA Bacterial Viruses with an Internal Membrane

**J K H Bamford,** University of Jyväskylä, Jyväskylä, Finland
**S J Butcher,** University of Helsinki, Helsinki, Finland

## Glossary

**DNA packaging** Energy-requiring process where the empty virus capsid is filled by the virus genome.
**Protein-primed DNA replication** Duplication of a linear DNA genome utilizing a protein covalently linked to the DNA terminus to initiate the reaction.
**Triangulation number** T number ($T$), a parameter for icosahedral capsids that describes the geometrical arrangement of the protein subunits.

## Introduction

Bacterial viruses with an internal membrane all have double-stranded DNA (dsDNA) genomes. They are classified into two families, the *Tectiviridae* and the *Corticoviridae.* The former family consists of several viruses, whereas the latter has only one representative. The type species of the *Tectiviridae* is PRD1, which infects a wide variety of Gram-negative bacteria. Its host range is limited to bacteria that contain a conjugative antibiotic resistance plasmid, since it utilizes the plasmid-encoded cell surface

DNA-transfer complex as a receptor. The type species of the family *Corticoviridae* is PM2.

The family *Tectiviridae* can be divided into two groups: viruses infecting Gram-negative bacteria and viruses infecting Gram-positive bacteria. The group infecting Gram-negative bacteria contains six extremely similar phages (PRD1, PR3, PR4, PR5, PR772, and L17) with a linear dsDNA genome. Their sequence similarity is between 91.9% and 99.8%, which is surprising since they have been isolated from different parts of the world. The other group infects Gram-positive bacteria (different *Bacillus* species). The length of the genomes (about 15 kbp) and the order of the genes is conserved in all the tectiviruses, but there is no sequence similarity between the two groups. The genomes of the tectiviruses encode about 35 proteins (**Table 1**).

The corticovirus PM2 was isolated in 1968 from seawater off the coast of Chile. The host is a marine bacterium, *Pseudoalteromonas espejiana.* PM2 has a negatively supercoiled circular dsDNA of about 10 kbp. It encodes about 17 proteins (**Table 2**). The combination of a membrane and a supercoiled DNA genome makes PM2 a unique virus. The entry and the DNA-packaging mechanisms are likely to differ from those of other viruses.

**Table 1**    PRD1 genes, corresponding proteins, and protein functions

| Gene | Protein | Mass (kDa) | Description[a] |
|------|---------|-----------|------------|
| I | P1 | 63.3 | DNA polymerase (N) |
| II | P2 | 63.7 | Receptor binding (S) |
| III | P3 | 43.1 | Major capsid protein (C) |
| V | P5 | 34.2 | Trimeric spike protein (S) |
| VI | P6 | 17.6 | Minor capsid protein, DNA packaging (C, P) |
| VII | P7 | 27.1 | DNA delivery, transglycosylase (L, M) |
| VIII | P8 | 29.5 | Genome terminal protein (N) |
| IX | P9 | 25.8 | Minor capsid protein, DNA packaging ATPase (C, P) |
| X | P10 | 20.6 | Assembly (A, N) |
| XI | P11 | 22.2 | DNA delivery (M) |
| XII | P12 | 16.6 | ssDNA binding protein (N) |
| XIV | P14 | 15.0 | DNA delivery (M) |
| XV | P15 | 17.3 | Muramidase (L) |
| XVI | P16 | 12.6 | Infectivity (M) |
| XVII | P17 | 9.5 | Assembly (A, N) |
| XVIII | P18 | 9.8 | DNA delivery(M) |
| XIX | P19 | 10.5 | ssDNA binding protein (N) |
| XX | P20 | 4.7 | DNA packaging (M, P) |
| XXII | P22 | 5.5 | DNA packaging (M,P) |
| XXX | P30 | 9.0 | Minor capsid protein (C) |
| XXXI | P31 | 13.7 | Pentameric base of spike (S) |
| XXXII | P32 | 5.4 | DNA delivery (M) |
| XXXIII | P33 | 7.5 | Assembly (A, N) |
| XXXIV | P34 | 6.7 | (M) |
| XXXV | P35 | 12.8 | Holin (L) |

[a](N) nonstructural early protein; (M) integral membrane protein; (S) spike complex protein; (A) assembly protein; (P) packaging protein; (C) capsid protein; (L) lysis protein.

**Table 2**    PM2 genes, corresponding proteins, and protein functions

| Gene | Protein | Mass (kDa) | Description |
|------|---------|-----------|-------------|
| I | P1 | 37.5 | Spike protein |
| II | P2 | 30.2 | Major capsid protein |
| III | P3 | 10.8 | Membrane protein |
| IV | P4 | 4.4 | Membrane protein |
| V | P5 | 17.9 | Membrane protein |
| VI | P6 | 14.3 | Membrane protein |
| VII | P7 | 3.6 | Membrane protein |
| VIII | P8 | 7.3 | Membrane protein |
| IX | P9 | 24.7 | Potential ATPase |
| X | P10 | 29.0 | Membrane protein |
| XII | P12 | 73.4 | Replication initiation protein |
| XIII | P13 | 7.2 | Transcription factor |
| XIV | P14 | 11.0 | Transcription factor |
| XV | P15 | 18.1 | Transcription factor |
| XVI | P16 | 10.3 | Transcription factor |
| XVII | P17 | 6.0 | Lysis |
| XVIII | P18 | 5.7 | Lysis |

## Virion Structure and Properties

### Overall Structure

The virion of PRD1 is an icosahedrally symmetric particle approximately 65 nm in diameter (**Figure 1**). It is composed of about 70% protein, 15% lipid, and 15% DNA and has a mass of about 66 MDa. The structure of the virion has been studied extensively using electron microscopy and X-ray crystallography (**Figure 2**). X-ray crystallography results have indicated the roles of four proteins in controlling virus assembly. There are 240 hexagonally shaped trimers of the major capsid protein, P3 (**Figure 2(b)**), occupying the surface of the capsid on a pseudo $T = 25$ lattice, an arrangement that is also found in the human adenovirus capsid. In PRD1, a dimer of the linear glue protein P30 extends from one vertex to the next, cementing the P3 facets together (**Figure 2(c)**). At the vertex, pentamers of P31 interlock with P3 and the transmembrane protein P16.

The majority of the PRD1 vertices have two proteins attached to them: one is a trimer of P5 (**Figure 3(a)**) attached by the N-terminus, the other is a monomer of P2 (**Figure 3(b)**), the receptor-binding protein. Both P5 and P2 are elongated molecules (P5 is 17 nm long, P2 is 15.5 nm long). P2 is a club-shaped molecule with a pseudo β-propeller head and a long tail formed from extended β-sheet. The head is proposed to be the site of receptor binding, lying distal to the virus. A specific vertex is used for packaging the phage DNA.

The overall size and structure of the phage Bam35 is very similar to that of PRD1. However, the exact counterparts of many of the PRD1 structural proteins have not yet been clearly identified. One of the major differences between PRD1 and Bam35 is the presence of a large transmembrane protein complex in Bam35 that modulates the curvature of the membrane under the capsid facets. Also, the host cell recognizing spike complex is likely to be different.

The corticovirus PM2 particle is icosahedral and measures 77 nm in diameter from spike to spike. The capsid is approximately 60 nm in diameter. Like the tectiviruses, it does not have a tail. The mass of the virion is $\sim4.5 \times 10^7$ Da and it is composed of protein (72%), lipid (14%), and DNA (14%). The capsid is composed of 200 trimers of the major capsid protein arranged on a pseudo $T = 21$ lattice. Pentameric receptor-binding spikes protrude from the vertices.

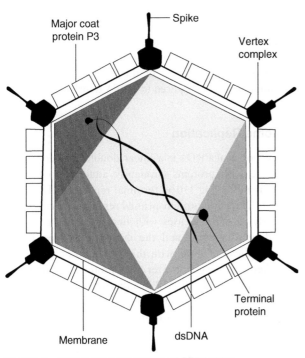

**Figure 1** Schematic presentation of PRD1 virion.

## Membrane and DNA

In PRD1, about half of the virion proteins are associated with the membrane (**Table 1**). The lipid headgroups are predominantly phosphatidylethanolamine (53%) and phosphatidylglycerol (43%) with 4% of cardiolipin. The membrane is well ordered, following the icosahedral outline of the capsid. Many interactions occur between the membrane and both the capsid and the underlying DNA. The average separation of the concentric layers of DNA is approximately 2.5 nm, similar to that found in other bacteriophages and animal viruses. Removal of the capsid and spike proteins by heat or guanidinium hydrochloride treatment results in aggregation of the membrane vesicle.

In PM2, the membrane, lying underneath the capsid, follows the shape of the capsid as in PRD1, and there are many interactions mediated by additional minor proteins. The lipid composition is approximately 64% phosphatidylglycerol, 27% phosphatidylethanolamine, and 8% neutral lipids and a small amount of acyl phosphatidylglycerol. Release of the capsid and spike proteins from the virion by freeze–thawing or by chelation of calcium ions with ethylene glycol tetraacetic acid (EGTA) results in a soluble vesicle called the lipid core.

## Life Cycle

PRD1 is a lytic phage that exploits the transcription functions of its host. The host cell is selected by specific recognition of a plasmid-encoded receptor on the cell surface. PRD1 belongs to the class of broad-host-range, donor-specific phages, which infect cells only when an IncP-, IncN-, or IncW-type multiple-drug resistance conjugative plasmid is present. The primary function of the receptor is in bacterial conjugation. Among the hosts are several opportunistic human pathogens such as *Escherichia coli*, *Salmonella enterica*, and *Pseudomonas aeruginosa*. After

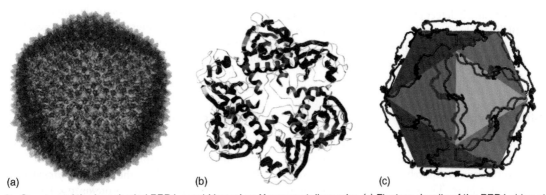

**Figure 2** Structure of the icosahedral PRD1 capsid based on X-ray crystallography. (a) Electron density of the PRD1 virion at 4 Å resolution. (b) The major coat protein P3, top view. P3 has a double β-barrel fold, resulting in a hexameric shape of the trimer. (c) The structure of the virion revealed the location of the cementing protein P30 at the twofold positions. The icosahedron is representing the viral membrane. Dimers of P30 are lying underneath the capsid stabilizing the virion structure.

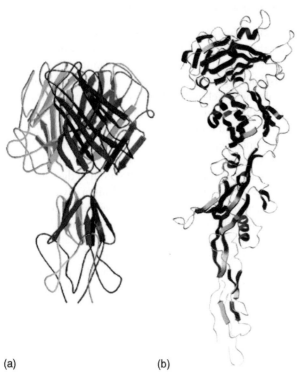

(a)                              (b)

**Figure 3**  Structure of the vertex proteins of PRD1 based on X-ray crystallography. (a) The trimeric spike protein P5. (b) The monomeric receptor-binding protein P2. (a) Reproduced from Merckel MC, Huiskonen JT, Bamford DH, Goldman A, and Tuma R (2005) The structure of the bacteriophage PRD1 spike sheds light on the evolution of viral capsid architecture. *Molecular Cell* 18: 161–170, with permission from Elsevier.

adsorption, the phage genome is injected into the cell cytosol, leaving the capsid outside. After the production of the phage components, both virus- and host-encoded factors assist in particle assembly. Host cell lysis releases some 500 progeny viruses. Bam35 is a temperate phage, either growing lytically like PRD1, or existing in a dormant state within the host. In contrast to PRD1, the host range of Bam35, and its relatives GIL01 and GIL16, is limited to one species, *Bacillus thuringiensis*. AP50 infects *Bacillus anthracis*, and a defect phage replicating as a linear plasmid (pBClin15) has been described for *Bacillus cereus*. The corticovirus PM2 is lytic. Of all the dsDNA phages with an internal membrane, the life cycle of PRD1 is best understood and is described below.

### Receptor Recognition

A single phage structural protein, P2, is responsible for PRD1 attachment to its host. Each of the PRD1 receptor recognition vertices is a metastable structure and possibly capable of DNA release. The injection vertex is likely to be determined by P2 binding to the receptor. The association of P2 with the receptor activates, possibly by P2 removal, the injection process. This leads to irreversible

binding. Both empty and DNA-containing particles are bound equally tightly to cells, indicating that DNA injection is not a prerequisite for this tight interaction.

### DNA Entry

Isolation and analysis of PRD1 mutants have resulted in the identification of eight, phage-specific, structural proteins essential for infectivity. In addition to the spike-complex proteins (P2, P5, and P31) needed for adsorption, protein P11 starts the DNA delivery process and membrane proteins P14, P18, and P32 are involved in later stages of the DNA delivery. Mutant particles missing protein P7 (a lytic transglycosylase) are infectious but the DNA entry process is delayed.

The PRD1 membrane can undergo a structural transformation from a spherical vesicle to a tubular form. A similar process has been described for Bam35 and AP50, thus occurring in all members of the *Tectiviridae*. This tube formation might be required for DNA translocation.

### Genome Replication

The genome of PRD1 is a linear double-stranded DNA molecule with proteins covalently attached to both 5′ termini and having 110 bp terminal repeats. PRD1 replicates its DNA by a protein-primed replication mechanism similarly to other viruses with linear dsDNA genomes, including adenovirus and the φ29-type phages. PRD1 DNA replication starts with the formation of a covalent bond between the genome terminal protein, P8, and the 5′ terminal nucleotide, dGMP, in a reaction catalyzed by the phage DNA polymerase, P1. The minimal origin of replication resides in the 20 first-terminal base pairs of both genome ends, and the fourth base from the 3′ end of the template directs, by base complementation, the linking of deoxyribonucleoside monophosphate (dNMP) to the terminal protein. The 3′ end DNA sequence is maintained by sliding back of the polymerase complex.

After initiation, elongation of the initiation complex by the same DNA polymerase takes place resulting in the formation of full-length daughter DNA molecules. Two phage-encoded single-stranded DNA binding proteins, P12 and P19, are involved in replication *in vivo*.

### Particle Assembly

Approximately 15 min post infection, the major capsid protein P3 and the spike-complex proteins P2, P5, and P31 are found soluble in the host cell cytosol, whereas the phage-encoded membrane proteins (e.g., P7, P11, P14, and P18) are addressed to the host cell cytoplasmic membrane (CM). Correct folding of the soluble proteins and assembly of a number of viral membrane proteins are dependent on the host GroEL/ES chaperonins. Upon assembly, a virus-specific patch from the host CM is translocated into the forming procapsid using the membrane-bound scaffolding protein P10. In addition, two small phage-encoded proteins are implicated in the assembly process: P17 and P33.

Correct assembly results in an empty capsid enclosing a membrane rich in phage-specific proteins. The linear double-stranded DNA genome is packaged into the prohead by the packaging ATPase P9. Unlike packaging ATPases of most other icosahedral dsDNA bacteriophages, P9 is part of the mature virus structure. It resides at a single vertex that also contains proteins P6, P20, and P22. P6 is a soluble protein needed for efficient DNA packaging and the latter two are integral membrane proteins connecting the portal structure to the viral membrane.

## Cell Lysis

At the end of the infection cycle, the newly synthesized progeny virions are released via host cell lysis. Two genes, *XV* and *XXXV*, are involved in this step, which means that a two-component, holin–endolysin system operates in phage PRD1. The product of gene *XV*, protein P15, is a soluble β-1,4-*N*-acetylmuramidase that degrades the peptidoglycan of the Gram-negative cell causing host cell lysis. The PRD1 particle carries another muramidase, protein P7, which has a lytic transglycosylase activity assisting in genome entry. The presence of two lytic activities probably reflects the broad host range of PRD1.

In addition to lytic enzymes, bacteriophages quite often encode helper protein factors (holins) that facilitate the access of lytic enzymes to the susceptible bond in the cell wall and control the timing of lysis. The PRD1 holin is protein P35.

## Genomes and Genomics

The length of the PRD1 genome is 14 927 bp and the guanine–cytosine (GC) content is 48.1%. It has 110 bp long inverted repeat sequences at the ends, which are 100% identical. The genomes of the other Gram-negative bacteria-infecting tectiviruses are very close to that of PRD1, varying between 14 935 and 14 954 bp. They are remarkably similar in nucleotide sequence, the overall identity being 91.9–99.8%. The Bam35 genome is 14 935 bp long with a GC content of 39.7%. The inverted repeat for Bam35 is 74 bp long. These Bam35 inverted terminal repeats (ITRs) have 81% identity. PRD1 and Bam35 do not share much sequence similarity. The discovery of the almost invariant genomes for the two *Tectiviridae* groups contrasts sharply with the situation in the tailed bacteriophages. The nucleotide identity is 100% between Bam35 and GIL01 and 83% between GIL01 and GIL16.

PRD1 genome is organized into two early and three late operons (**Figure 4**). Bam35 operons have not been mapped, but the gene order and the length of the genes are similar to those of PRD1 (**Figure 4**). Although there is no overall sequence similarity between PRD1 and Bam35 genomes, Bam35 genes for DNA polymerase, packaging ATPase, and lytic enzyme can be recognized by corresponding conserved amino acid sequence motifs in the databases. The coat protein gene can be identified by comparing the N-terminal amino acid sequence of the major virion protein to the DNA sequence. The only genes of Bam35, which seem to be in different positions in the genome compared to PRD1, are those responsible for the host cell recognition (the spike protein).

The circular PM2 genome is 10 079 bp long with a GC content of 42.2%. It contains 21 putative genes, of which 17

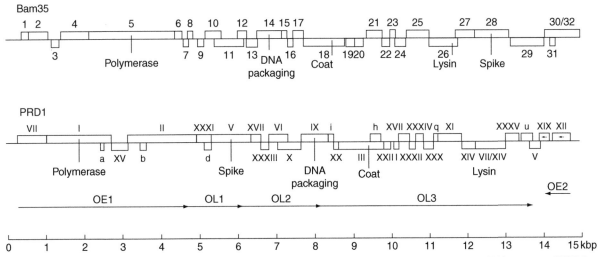

**Figure 4** Alignment of the genomes of Bam35 (top) and PRD1 (middle). The two early (OE) and three late (OL) operons of PRD1 are shown at the bottom. In Bam35, the open reading frames (ORFs) are marked by Arabic numerals from left to right. PRD1 ORFs have a Roman numeral if they have been shown to encode protein, otherwise they are marked with a lowercase letter.

have so far been shown to be functional. Promoter mapping by primer extension has revealed three operons, which are expressed in a timely fashion during infection. The first early operon is highly similar to the maintenance region of the *Pseudoalteromonas* plasmid pAS28. The second early operon contains genes for DNA replication and regulation of late phage functions. The PM2 genome replicates via a rolling-circle mechanism. Protein P12 has conserved sequence motifs common to superfamily I replication initiation proteins. This superfamily consists of the A proteins of certain bacteriophages, such as $\phi$X174 and G4, and the initiation proteins of cyanobacterial and archaeal plasmids. The function of the late operon is activated by two phage-encoded transcription factors, P13 and P14. P14 has sequence similarity to the TFIIS-type general eukaryotic transcription factors most closely resembling those of the archaeal organisms *Thermococcus celer* and *Sulfolobus acidocaldaricus*.

The structural proteins encoded by the late genes are, similar to the corresponding proteins of tectiviruses, either membrane associated or soluble. Based on the conserved amino acid sequence motifs deduced from the nucleotide sequence, one of the structural virion proteins is a putative packaging ATPase. The packaging process of the circular supercoiled PM2 DNA is not understood at the moment.

*See also:* Replication of Bacterial Viruses; Transcriptional Regulation in Bacteriophage; Virus Evolution: Bacterial Viruses.

## Further Reading

Abrescia NGA, Cockburn JJB, Grimes JM, *et al.* (2004) Insights into assembly from structural analysis of bacteriophage PRD1. *Nature* 432: 68–74.

Bamford DH (2005) Family *Tectiviridae*. In: Fauquet CM, Mayo MA, Maniloff J, Desselberger U, and Ball LA (eds.) *Virus Taxonomy. Eighth Report of the International Committee on Taxonomy of Viruses*, pp. 81–85. San Diego, CA: Elsevier Academic Press.

Bamford DH and Bamford JKH (2006) Lipid-containing bacteriophage PM2, the type-organism of *Corticoviridae*. In: Calendar R (ed.) *The Bacteriophages*, pp. 171–174. New York: Oxford University Press.

Bamford JKH (2005) Family *Corticoviridae*. In: Fauquet CM, Mayo MA, Maniloff J, Desselberger U, and Ball LA (eds.) *Virus Taxonomy: Eighth Report of the International Committee on Taxonomy of Viruses*, pp. 87–90. San Diego, CA: Elsevier Academic Press.

Benson SD, Bamford JKH, Bamford DH, and Burnett RM (1999) Viral evolution revealed by bacteriophage PRD1 and human adenovirus coat protein structures. *Cell* 98: 825–833.

Benson SD, Bamford JKH, Bamford DH, and Burnett RM (2004) Does common architecture reveal a viral lineage spanning all three domains of life? *Molecular Cell* 16: 673–685.

Cockburn JJB, Abrescia NGA, Grimes JM, *et al.* (2004) Membrane structure and interactions with protein and DNA in bacteriophage PRD1. *Nature* 432: 122–125.

Grahn AM, Butcher SJ, Bamford JKH, and Bamford DH (2006) PRD1-dissecting the genome, structure and entry. In: Calendar R (ed.) *The Bacteriophages*, pp. 161–170. New York: Oxford University Press.

Grahn AM, Daugelavicius R, and Bamford DH (2002) Sequential model of phage PRD1 DNA delivery: Active involvement of the viral membrane. *Molecular Microbiology* 46: 1199–1209.

Merckel MC, Huiskonen JT, Bamford DH, Goldman A, and Tuma R (2005) The structure of the bacteriophage PRD1 spike sheds light on the evolution of viral capsid architecture. *Molecular Cell* 18: 161–170.

Ravantti JJ, Gaidelyte A, Bamford DH, and Bamford JKH (2003) Comparative analysis of bacterial viruses Bam35, infecting a Gram-positive host, and PRD1, infecting Gram-negative hosts, demonstrates a viral lineage. *Virology* 313: 401–414.

Salas M (1991) Protein-priming of DNA replication. *Annual Review of Biochemistry* 60: 39–71.

# Icosahedral Enveloped dsRNA Bacterial Viruses

**R Tuma,** University of Helsinki, Helsinki, Finland

## Glossary

**Carrier state** A partial or complete viral genome is maintained inside the host cell as a stable episome without lysis or infection.

**Genomic precursor** ssRNA destined for packaging.

**Genomic segment** A piece of genomic dsRNA.

**Packaging** A process of genomic precursor acquisition.

***Pac site*** A specific signal at 5' end of a genomic precursor which targets it for selective packaging.

**Polymerase complex** Viral assembly which contains the polymerase and is able to replicate and transcribe the viral genome. Usually it also contains the viral genomic dsRNA.

**Procapsid** Empty capsid assembly which is capable of acquiring the genomic precursors.

**Reverse genetics** RNA virus genome manipulation and rescue from cDNA clones.

**Viral core** dsRNA containing inner part of the virus which is capable of transcription.

## Introduction – The *Cystoviridae* Family

Members of the family *Cystoviridae* are lipid-containing bacteriophages with segmented dsRNA genomes. The first recognized member, the bacteriophage φ6, was isolated in 1973. Several other members were discovered in the late 1990s. All known cystoviruses were isolated from the leaves of various plants and consequently infect primarily plant-pathogenic bacteria (pseudomonads). All share a similar architecture with a proteinaceous viral core hosting the three genomic segments (L, M, and S, approx. 6.5, 4, and 3 kbp in size, respectively). The core is enclosed in a lipid envelope which contains the host cell attachment proteins. The viral core contains an RNA-dependent RNA polymerase (RdRP) which plays a central role in RNA metabolism. Despite infecting prokaryotic hosts these phages exhibit structural and functional features that parallel those of the family *Reoviridae*. Because reverse genetics had been developed early on for φ6, the system has been a model for studying the assembly and replication of other dsRNA viruses.

An *in vitro* assembly of infectious nucleocapsids from purified constituents has been achieved for bacteriophages φ6 and φ8. Similarly, RNA packaging and replication have been extensively studied *in vitro*. Together with the reverse genetics system the *in vitro* methods have been instrumental in delineating the virus replication mechanisms. The host entry mechanism mimics that of viruses infecting eukaryotic cells and involves both membrane fusion and an endocytotic-like event. Structural and extensive biochemical characterization of individual proteins and subviral assemblies made the cystoviral system a paradigm for studying mechanisms of molecular machines in atomic details. The self-assembly and replication system shows promise in biotechnology and nanotechnology applications.

## Classification and Host Range

Based on their sequences and host range five out of the recently discovered cystoviruses (φ7, φ9, φ10, φ11, φ14) are close relatives of φ6 while the remaining three (φ8, φ12, and φ13) are only distantly related to the φ6 group

and among themselves. φ6 and the related phages attach to the host cell via a specific type IV pilus while the members of the second group utilize rough lipopolysaccharides (LPSs). This limits the host range to *Pseudomonas syringae* (*Pseudomonas pseudoalcaligenis* for certain mutants) for the former group while phages belonging to the latter can also infect rough LPS of other Gram-negative bacteria without forming plaques. Only φ8 form plaques on a heptose-less strain of *Salmonella typhimurium*. A common laboratory host of φ6 is *P. syringae* strain HB10Y. The φ8 phage is usually propagated on *P. syringae* strain LM2509.

## Virion Structure and Properties

### Physico-Chemical Properties

Virion molecular weight (MW, in dalton units, Da) $\sim 9.9 \times 10^7$ Da, sedimentation coefficient $S_{20w}$ $\sim 405$S, density $1.24\,\mathrm{g\,cm^{-3}}$ (sucrose), nucleocapsid MW $\sim 4.0 \times 10^7$ Da. Composition: 70% (w/w) protein, 14% dsRNA, 16% phospholipids. RNA packaging density $350\,\mathrm{g\,cm^{-3}}$.

### Architecture of the Polymerase Complex and the Nucleocapsid

**Figure 1** depicts schematically the architecture and localization of the proteins for the φ6 virion. The innermost structure is the polymerase complex (PC) which is composed of 120 copies of major structural protein P1 (MW 85 kDa), 12 copies of RdRP P2 (75 kDa), 12 hexamers of packaging motor P4 (subunit MW 35 kD), and 60 copies of assembly factor P7 (17 kDa). Structural details of the dodecahedral P1 skeleton are depicted in **Figure 2**. The $T = 1$ lattice is composed of 60 asymmetric P1 dimers as seen for other dsRNA viruses. However, the arrangement of dimers within the asymmetric unit is different from that seen in the reovirus or bluetongue virus cores. P2 monomers are attached to the inner surface of the PC shell, possibly at the fivefold vertices. P4 hexamers form turret-like protrusions on the outer surface of the fivefold vertices. Location of the P7 within the PC is not known.

PC undergoes a series of large conformational changes (expansions) during RNA packaging and genome replication. The empty dodecahedral PC (procapsid) expands into a more round, icosahedral dsRNA-filled PC, which is sometimes called the viral core. The expansion consists of motions of whole P1 subunits around hinges that run roughly parallel with the twofold edges of the dodecahedral skeleton (**Figure 2**). The expansion increases the inner volume by a factor of 2.4 and makes room for the dsRNA genome. The mature PC is subsequently enclosed in an icosahedral shell ($T = 13$) made of 200 P8 (subunit MW 16 kDa) trimers (**Figure 2**). The resulting structure is called the nucleocapsid (NC). The packaged dsRNA genome is arranged in concentric shells (layers) with

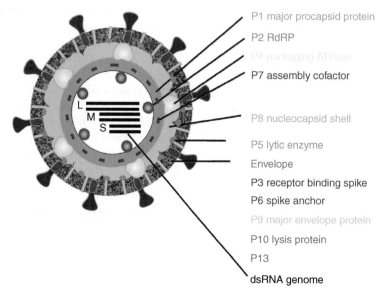

P1 major procapsid protein

P2 RdRP

P4 packaging ATPase

P7 assembly cofactor

P8 nucleocapsid shell

P5 lytic enzyme

Envelope

P3 receptor binding spike

P6 spike anchor

P9 major envelope protein

P10 lysis protein

P13

dsRNA genome

**Figure 1**   Schematics of φ6 virion architecture. Function of individual proteins: P1-major structural protein of PC, forms the dodecahedral skeleton of the procapsid; P2-RdRP; P3-spike protein, host cell attachment; P4-packaging ATPase, ssRNA translocation; P5-lytic enzyme (lysozyme); P6-integral membrane protein, P3 anchoring and membrane fusion; P7-assembly, packaging and replication cofactor, PC stabilization; P8-nucleocapsid coat protein; P9-membrane protein; P10-host cell lysis, perhaps holin; P11-membrane protein (most likely nonessential).

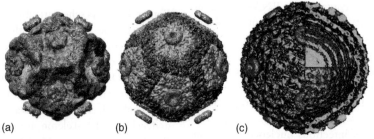

(a)                    (b)                    (c)

**Figure 2**   Structure of the polymerase complex and the nucleocapsid of φ6 as revealed by electron cryo-microscopy. (a) Modeled empty PC (void of RNA, precursor for packaging) which is also called the procapsid. (b) The $T = 1$ (triangulation number) shell of the expanded, mature, PC which contains dsRNA genome and is transcription competent. (c) The $T = 13$ P8 shell which makes the outer surface of NC together with the protruding P4 hexamers. P4 is gray, the two P1 monomers in the asymmetric dimer are colored red and blue, respectively. P8 shell is rendered purple. Reproduced from Huiskonen JT, de Haas F, Bubeck D, Bamford DH, Fuller SD, and Butcher SJ (2006) Structure of the bacteriophage φ6 nucleocapsid suggests a mechanism for sequential RNA packaging. *Structure* 14: 1039–1048, with permission from Elsevier.

average spacing 31 Å. This is larger than the 24–26 Å spacing which has been observed for other dsDNA and dsRNA viruses and reflects the lower packaging density.

The structures of P1 (PC) and P8 (NC) shells are related to the structure of dsRNA containing cores isolated from viruses belonging to the family *Reoviridae*. However, the empty packaging competent precursors have not been detected nor has a conformational change akin to the PC expansion been observed for the latter viruses.

## Structure of Individual Proteins

### P1

Current structural model of φ6 P1 monomer is based on high-resolution (7.5 Å) electron cryo-microscopy (**Figure 3**).

The structure is composed of α-helices that are packed together to form a flat sheet. The few remaining densities have been tentatively assigned to β-sheets. The exact tracing of the polypeptide chain was not possible at this resolution; however, the two conformers in the asymmetric unit were clearly resolved.

### P2

Several structures of φ6 P2 alone and in complex with various substrates were solved by X-ray diffraction. P2 is a compact, globular, monomer with α/β fold (**Figure 3**) with a domain arrangement resembling a hand (i.e., palm, fingers, and thumb domains). The fold is similar to those of other viral polymerases, for example, hepatitis C virus and HIV reverse transcriptase. RNA substrate

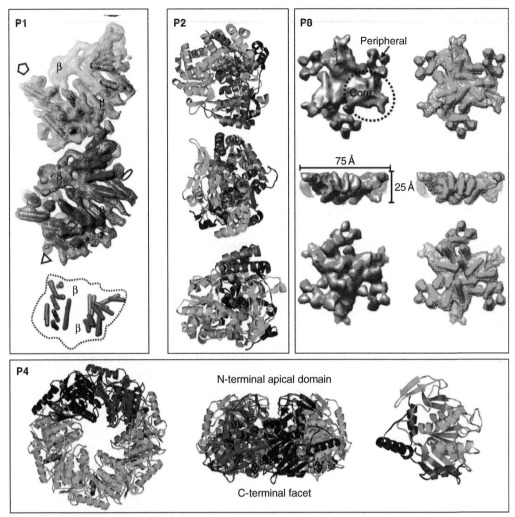

**Figure 3** Structure of individual cystoviral proteins. (P1) φ6 P1 structure was derived from cryo-EM. The electron densities of the two conformers found in the asymmetric unit (see **Figure 2**) are shown in blue and red, respectively. Bottom panel shows the tentative secondary structure assignment to the electron density. Reproduced (P2) Ribbon diagram of P2 polymerase structure from phage φ6 in complex with RNA (spacefill representation). Based on PDB id 1UVI, Salgado *et al.* (2004) *Structure* 12: 307–316. Top view shows the C-terminal domain (red) blocking the RNA exit site. Middle panel displays view down the RNA template channel. Bottom panel exhibits view of the template RNA through the substrate channel. Ribbon coloring from N-terminus (blue) to C-terminus (red). (P4) P4 hexamer, the packaging motor (ATPase) structure solved by X-ray diffraction. Based on PDB id 1W44, Mancini EJ, Kainov DE, Grimes JM, Tuma R, Bamford DH, and Stuart DI (2004) Atomic snapshots on an RNA packaging motor reveal conformational changes linking ATP hydrolysis to RNA translocation. *Cell* 118: 743–755. Left panel: top view down the central channel, subunits in different colors. Middle: Side view. Right: One subunit colored from N-terminus (blue) to C-terminus (red). (P8) P8 structure derived from cryo-EM. Reproduced from Huiskonen JT, de Haas F, Bubeck D, Bamford DH, Fuller SD, and Butcher SJ (2006) Structure of the bacteriophage φ6 nucleocapsid suggests a mechanism for sequential RNA packaging. *Structure* 14: 1039–1048, with permission from Elsevier.

binds in a template channel and the putative dsRNA exit site is partially occluded by the C-terminal domain in the crystal structure (**Figure 3**).

## P4

The structures of φ12 P4 hexamer in apo and nucleotide-bound forms have been solved by X-ray diffraction (**Figure 3**). The hexamer has a dome-like structure with a central channel through which RNA passes during packaging. Six equivalent ATP binding sites are located between the subunits at the hexamer periphery. The subunit structure encompasses a catalytic core which is conserved among many ATPases, including Rec-A and hexameric helicases. P4 hexamer interacts with the procapsid dodecahedral framework predominantly via its C-terminal facet.

## P8

The structure of the φ6 P8 trimer was derived by fragmentation of the cryo-EM density map at 7.5 Å resolution. The P8 subunit is highly α-helical. The trimer is flat (only 25 Å thick, 75 Å effective diameter) and each sub-unit is composed of the central, four-helix bundle core and a peripheral four helix bundle (**Figure 3**).

## Membrane Envelope

Lipids are derived from the host cytoplasmic membrane but the viral envelope is enriched in phosphatidylglycerol and contains less phosphatidylethanolamine presumably due to high viral membrane curvature and charge repulsion. Lipids constitute about 40% of membrane mass while the remaining 60% are membrane proteins. The membrane is loosely associated with the nucleocapsid and the membrane-associated proteins lack icosahedral symmetry.

## Genome Organization and Sequence Similarity

The φ6 genome (13385 bp) is organized into three segments (**Figure 4**): L (6374 bp in φ6) codes for the procapsid structural proteins, M (4063 bp in φ6) codes for the spike and membrane proteins, and S (2948 bp in φ6) codes for nucleocapsid and membrane proteins. The (coding) plus strand of each segment contains a short conserved sequence at the 5′-end. This sequence is followed by a packaging signal that is unique to each segment (*pac* site, about 200 nt). The dsRNA genome remains sequestered inside the PC throughout the viral life cycle and only the plus strands are extruded into the cytoplasm where they serve as messenger RNAs or packaging precursors.

Two genes, 12 and 14, code for the two nonstructural proteins identified thus far. While the former is essential for membrane morphogenesis, the latter is dispensable under laboratory conditions.

Genomic maps of the other cystoviruses are similar to φ6 with several exceptions. The viruses which attach directly to rough LPS (φ8, 12, 13) possess several separate genes for the receptor binding spike structure (3a, 3b, and 3c in φ12 and φ13). In addition, gene 7 is positioned after gene 1 in the φ8 L-segment and its expected place is occupied by ORF H. The functions of the nonessential ORFs F, G, and H are not known.

Identity at the amino acid sequence level is high among φ6, 7, 9, and 10, while φ8, 12, and 13 exhibit only limited sequence similarity to φ6 and among themselves. The limited similarity is restricted to the conserved motifs of the polymerase and the packaging ATPase. Sequence similarities for the structural proteins P1 and P7 are generally statistically insignificant for the latter group of phages despite conservation of the procapsid structure. However, high sequence identity detected in restricted regions (e.g., lysis proteins of φ12 and φ6, identical 3′-end of M segments in φ6 and φ13) indicate significant genetic interaction (e.g., recombination) among cystoviruses.

## Replication Cycle

The virus life cycle is schematically illustrated in **Figure 5**. The steps were elucidated for φ6 but many features are likely to be similar for the other cystoviruses.

## Host Cell Attachment and Outer Membrane Fusion

The φ6 and related phages attach to the pilus using the P3 spike protein. The pilus contracts and brings the virion into contact with the outer cell membrane (OM). The φ8, 12, 13 phages utilize a spike composed of proteins P3a, P3b, and P3c (missing in φ8) to attach directly to the rough LPS. The viral envelope then fuses with the OM using the virion fusogenic protein P6. Then the virion-associated lysozyme (P5) degrades the peptidoglycan layer to allow direct contact of the nucleocapsid with the plasma membrane (PM).

## Plasma Membrane Penetration

The φ6 nucleocapsid is first enclosed in an endocytic-like vesicle which is brought into the cytoplasm. The NC coat protein P8 disassembles and disrupts the membrane vesicle in order to release the PC into the cytoplasm. The mechanism of the P8-assisted release is still elusive.

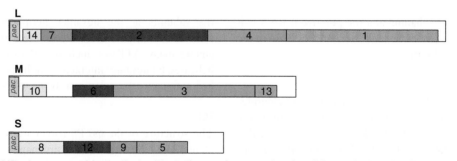

**Figure 4**   The phi6 genome map showing the locations of genes (gene numbers) and the packaging signal sequences (*pac*).

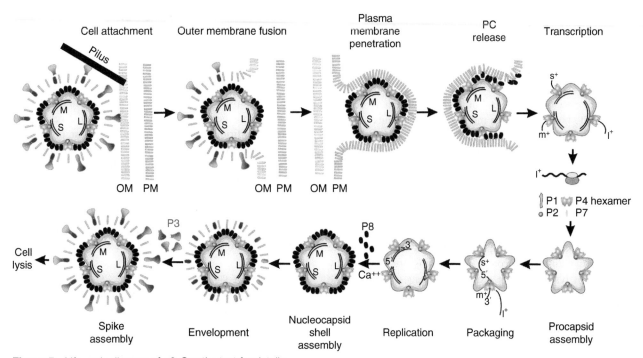

**Figure 5** Life cycle diagram of φ6. See the text for details.

## Transcription

The depolymerization of the P8 layer activates the PC to perform transcription of the dsRNA genome which produces the plus-strand copies of the three segments ($s^+$, $m^+$, $l^+$). These copies are made inside the PC by the P2 polymerase using a semiconservative mechanism. Several polymerase molecules may engage each segment simultaneously. The resulting RNAs are extruded via P4 hexamers into the cytoplasm where they serve as mRNA for the synthesis of phage proteins and as ssRNA precursors for packaging. Transcription of the three segments is regulated, $s^+$ and $m^+$ being produced in a several-fold excess over $l^+$. The regulation is due to specific interactions between the 3'-end of the minus strand and the polymerase.

## PC assembly

The major structural protein P1 co-assembles with P2, P4, and P7 into empty PC (procapsid). The assembly is nucleated by a P1–P4 (P1–P2 in φ8 phage) interaction and intermediates are further stabilized by protein P7 (a 'glue' protein).

## Packaging

The unique *pac* sites at the 5'-end of RNA plus strands are specifically recognized in a sequential fashion by the assembled P1 framework. This initial and selective binding brings the 5'-end to the vicinity of the packaging ATPase

(P4) hexamer. The P4 ring opens and topologically encloses the RNA inside the central channel. The presence of RNA stimulates the ATPase activity. P4 translocates the ssRNA in the 5'–3' direction into the procapsid at the expense of ATP hydrolysis. The sequential packaging order is accomplished by increasing the PC affinity for $m^+$ ($l^+$) *pac* sequence after packaging of $s^+$ ($m^+$). This switching is mediated by the expansion which is in turn driven by the increased amount of the packaged RNA (cf. the headfull packaging of dsDNA bacteriophages). The *in vivo* packaging fidelity is high. However, specific *in vitro* packaging conditions may result in acquisition of multiple $s^+$ segments or of $m^+$ segment in the absence of prior packaging of $s^+$. A heterologous RNA can be packaged by φ8 PCs and the sequential dependence of *in vitro* packaging is weak for this phage.

## Replication and NC Maturation

During φ8 or after φ6 packaging, the polymerase performs replication (minus-strand synthesis) of ssRNA into the genomic dsRNA. P2 polymerase interacts with a specific sequence at the 3'-end of each plus strand to initiate the self-primed reaction and makes a full copy of each packaged template. This reaction doubles the amount of RNA inside the PC and yields the mature icosahedral PC. The mature PC can be coated with a layer of P8 trimers in a calcium-dependent reaction. This yields the nucleocapsid. Alternatively, PC may remain in the transcription mode and produce more plus-strand RNA. In φ8 virus the P8 protein is directly associated with the membrane and consequently the PC becomes directly enveloped. The mature φ8 PC is also infectious to host cell spheroplasts.

## Membrane Acquisition and Host Cell Lysis

NC is enveloped with a lipid bilayer, which is derived from the host cell plasma membrane. It contains only the viral membrane proteins. The virion-associated lytic enzyme P5 is also incorporated at this stage. Structural protein P9 and the nonstructural protein P12 are essential and sufficient for membrane envelopment in φ6. These two proteins alone can produce lipid vesicles inside the host cell suggesting that envelopment takes place within the cytoplasm. The envelope is subsequently decorated with P3 receptor binding spike which is anchored by the integral membrane protein P6. Virions are released by host cell lysis which is assisted by phage-encoded lytic proteins P5 and P10.

## Recombination

Recombination in the *Cystoviridae* is mostly heterologous requiring only about three identical nucleotides. The mechanism of recombination is template switching. The frequency of recombination is increased by truncating the 3′-end of one of the packaged plus strands. Such truncation may be a result of cellular nuclease cleavage and yields a poor substrate for replication. Hence, recombination may serve as an effective way of correcting the nuclease damage. In addition, homologous recombination, requiring an identical sequence of about 600 nucleotides, has been demonstrated for the φ8 phage. Another mode of recombination is the exchange of whole genomic segments as also seen for other segmented genome viruses.

## Genetic Tools and Applications

### Reverse Genetics

A reverse genetics system allows systematic testing of the effects of engineered mutations on specific steps in the phage life cycle. Thus, it greatly facilitates delineation of the viral packaging and replication mechanisms. There are two ways to introduce a foreign gene into the dsRNA genome. (1) By constructing a recombinant ssRNA transcript containing the foreign sequences and a 5′-end *pac* site. This substrate is then packaged into procapsids, replicated and matured into NC *in vitro*. The NCs infect host cell spheroplasts to produce the engineered virus progeny. (2) A more efficient method for reverse genetics is based on electroporation of cDNA plasmids, containing the three genomic segments, into cells expressing either SP6 or T7 RNA polymerase. The foreign sequence may be introduced between the 5′-end *pac* sites and the conserved 3′-end replication sequences of each segment.

## *In Vitro* Assembly, Packaging, and Replication System

φ6 procapsid can be efficiently produced in *Escherichia coli* by simultaneously expressing proteins P1, P2, P4, and P7 from a plasmid containing a cDNA copy of the L segment. These procapsids are capable of packaging and replicating the three genomic precursors *in vitro*. Even under optimal conditions only about 5–10% of these procapsids are successfully packaged *in vitro*. Despite the low efficiency the *in vitro* packaging system has been instrumental in delineating the sequential packaging rules and the replication specificity. Incomplete procapsids (containing proteins P1P4, P1P2P4, P1P4P7, P1P2P7) can be produced in *E. coli* and tested for packaging and polymerase activity or used for assembly of specifically labeled procapsids.

Procapsids can be assembled *in vitro* from purified proteins. The *in vitro* assembly system allowed the identification of the minimum assembly requirements and the nucleation mechanism. The *in vitro* system also allows incorporation of chemically labeled or modified subunits to facilitate biophysical and structural studies.

## Carrier State

Bacteriophages φ6 and φ8 can establish a carrier state during which the viral genome (or portion of it) replicates as a stable episome inside the host cell cytoplasm. The stable episome constitutes the phage dsRNA inside polymerase complexes that assemble in the cytoplasm. Consequently, the L segment cDNA coding for the PC protein is required to establish the state. The carrier state is maintained by a selective resistance marker engineered into one of the phage genomic segments (usually M or S).

The carrier state is established by electroporating ColE1 suicide plasmids containing the cDNAs of the phage segments into a pseudomonas host that expresses T7 RNA polymerase. These plasmids cannot replicate in pseudomonads and are used to introduce the phage ssRNA into the cytoplasm.

A carrier state may be used to probe RNA packaging or to select new phage mutants. Given the high number of mutations introduced during the phage RNA replication cycle, the carrier state constitutes a good vehicle for targeted evolution of proteins or RNA with novel functions or a way to produce large quantities of siRNA.

## Polymerase Applications

φ6 RdRP has the unique capacity to perform self-primed, primer-independent, replication and transcription of RNA substrates. This feature can be used, for example, to obtain complete copies of viral RNA genomes (amplification), or for primer-independent RNA sequencing. An engineered version of RdRP is commercially available.

*See also:* Replication of Bacterial Viruses.

## Further Reading

Bamford DH, Ojala PM, Frilander M, Walin L, and Bamford JKH (1995) Isolation, purification, and function of assembly intermediates and subviral particles of bacteriophages PRD1 and φ6. In: Adolph KW (ed.) *Methods in Molecular Genetics, Vol. 6: Microbial Gene Techniques*, pp. 455–474. San Diego: Academic Press.

Butcher SJ, Grimes JM, Makeyev EV, Bamford DH, and Stuart DI (2001) A mechanism for initiating RNA-dependent RNA polymerization. *Nature* 410: 235–240.

Huiskonen JT, de Haas F, Bubeck D, Bamford DH, Fuller SD, and Butcher SJ (2006) Structure of the bacteriophage φ6 nucleocapsid suggests a mechanism for sequential RNA packaging. *Structure* 14: 1039–1048.

Kainov DE, Tuma R, and Mancini EJ (2006) Hexameric molecular motors: P4 packaging ATPase unravels the mechanism. *Cellular and Molecular Life Sciences* 63: 1095–1105.

Makeyev EV and Bamford DH (2000) The polymerase subunit of a dsRNA virus plays a central role in the regulation of viral RNA metabolism. *EMBO Journal* 19: 6275–6284.

Makeyev EV and Bamford DH (2004) Evolutionary potential of an RNA virus. *Journal of Virology* 78: 2114–2120.

Mancini EJ, Kainov DE, Grimes JM, Tuma R, Bamford DH, and Stuart DI (2004) Atomic snapshots on an RNA packaging motor reveal conformational changes linking ATP hydrolysis to RNA translocation. *Cell* 118: 743–755.

Mindich L (1999) Precise packaging of the three genomic segments of the double-stranded-RNA bacteriophage φ6. *Microbiology and Molecular Biology Reviews* 63: 149–160.

Mindich L (1999) Reverse genetics of the dsRNA bacteriophage φ6. *Advances in Virus Research* 53: 341–353.

Mindich L (2005) Phages with segmented double-stranded RNA genomes. In: Calendar R (ed.) *The Bacteriophages,* 2nd edn., pp. 197–207. New York: Oxford University Press.

Poranen MM, Paatero AO, Tuma R, and Bamford DH (2001) Self-assembly of a viral molecular machine from purified protein and RNA constituents. *Moleculer Cell* 7: 845–854.

Poranen MM, Tuma R, and Bamford DH (2005) Assembly of double-stranded RNA bacteriophages. *Advances in Virus Research* 64: 15–43.

Sun Y, Qiao X, and Mindich L (2004) Construction of carrier state viruses with partial genomes of the segmented dsRNA bacteriophages. *Virology* 319: 274–279.

# Icosahedral ssDNA Bacterial Viruses

**B A Fane, M Chen, and J E Cherwa,** University of Arizona, Tucson, AZ, USA
**A Uchiyama,** Cornell University, Ithaca, NY, USA

## Glossary

**Procapsid** A viral assembly intermediate containing a full complement of scaffolding proteins but devoid of genome.

**Scaffolding protein** A protein that directs the assembly of the virus, found in the procapsid assembly intermediate but not in the mature virion.

**S** Sedimentation constant in Svedberg units, measured by analytical ultracentrifugation.

**T = 1 icosahedron** A geometric shape consisting of 20 faces and 12 vertices. A T = 1 virion is composed of 60 viral coat proteins.

## History

Bacteriophage øX174, the most well known virus of the family *Microviridae* (micro: Greek for small) was isolated in the 1920s by Sertic and Bulgakov. From the onset, this phage appeared very different from the other bacteriophages isolated during this extensive period of discovery. It was unusually tiny, readily passing through the smallest of ultrafilters. This biophysical characteristic defined its 'race': race X (Roman numeral ten) and the isolate was placed in a vial labeled #174, from which the phage derived its name, race X phage in test tube #174. And there it sat, relatively unperturbed, for decades. The first electron micrographs revealed small, vague isometric particles, vastly different from the tailed morphologies, which came to represent bacteriophages in general. Robert Sinsheimer unraveled the odd nature of the genome in 1959 and øX174 became the first recognized single-stranded (ss) DNA phage. While genetic maps of other phages consisted of orderly linear gene progressions, the øX174 map was most peculiar with genes located within genes. When Sanger and colleagues sequenced the genome, the first one ever sequenced, the complex arrangement of overlapping reading frames was confirmed, so beguiling that many suspected an extraterrestrial origin. As the *New York Times* reported the theory, an advanced race engineered øX174 and disseminated it into the cosmos where it would "persist until the evolution of intelligent life and finally of investigators interested in the genetics of phage." Although attempts were actually made to decipher the hypothesized hidden message, they all failed. However, rumors persist that the code has been broken, it reads, "Behold this marvelous little thing."

This small virus would continue to have a large impact on molecular biology. Arthur Kornberg and colleagues used it to elucidate the molecular mechanism of prokaryotic DNA replication. Masaki Hayashi and colleagues defined the øX174 assembly pathway and were the first to demonstrate that viral DNA packaging could be achieved *in vitro*. As the genome sequence initially defied imagination in 1978, the atomic structure of the viral procapsid, the first such structure solved, beguiled structural virologists, with its unusual external scaffolding protein lattice. And when events were at their most bizarre, the skeletons in the family *Microviridae* closet emerged, the gokushoviruses (Japanese for very small). These viruses escaped detection for decades, hiding out in their obligate intracellular parasitic bacterial hosts.

## Virion Morphology and Genome Content

All members of the family *Microviridae* have ssDNA circular genomes of positive polarity and a T = 1 icosahedral capsid. The bulk of the capsid is composed of 60 copies of a major capsid protein (**Figure 1** and **Table 1**), which exhibits the common β-barrel motif found in most icosahedral virion capsid proteins. In addition to the major capsid protein, microviruses also contain 60 copies each of the major spike protein G and DNA binding protein J. The fourth structural protein, the DNA pilot protein, is buried within vertex channels running through the fivefold axes of symmetry. Particles lacking this protein extrude DNA from these locations. Protein H stoichiometry varies among the microviruses, in which there are three major clades represented by bacteriophages G4, α3, and øX174. In øX174, there are 10–12 H proteins per virion, while in bacteriophage α3 only 4–6 copies are required for viability.

Bacteriophage øX174 typifies the microvirus morphology (**Figure 1**), in which 70 Å-diameter G protein pentamers adorn the fivefold axes of symmetry, rising 30 Å from the surface of the 250 Å-diameter capsid. The gokushoviruses lack major spike proteins: hence, the fivefold axes of symmetry are not decorated. The cryoelectron microscopy image reconstruction of gokushovirus SpV4 reveals mushroom-shaped protrusions at the threefold axes of symmetry, which rise 54 Å above the surface of the 270 Å-diameter capsids (**Figure 1**). These threefold related structures appear to be composed of amino acid sequences of three interacting coat proteins. The gokushovirus VP2 is also a structural protein. Although its function has not been experimentally defined, bioinformatic approaches suggest it is analogous to the microvirus DNA pilot protein H. These proteins share a predicted N-terminal transmembrane and a central coiled-coil domain. VP8

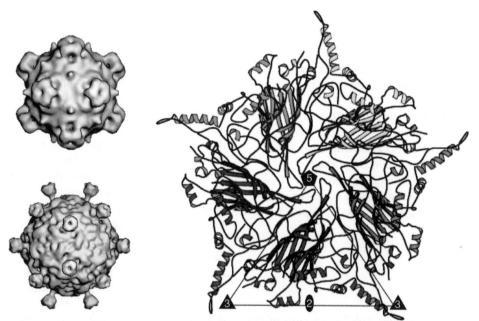

**Figure 1**   Virion structures. Top left, cryoelectron microscopy (cryoEM) image reconstruction of microvirus øX174. Bottom left, cryoEM of gokushovirus SpV4. Right, the arrangement of five øX174 coat proteins around a fivefold axis of symmetry. Numbers indicate axis of symmetry and the number of coat proteins that would be interacting at that axis.

may be analogous to the DNA binding protein J, both highly basic short peptides. However, it has not yet been detected in a gokushovirus virion. This may be due to the small size and the difficulties associated with propagating large quantities of gokushoviruses for biochemical characterization.

The genetic maps of microvirus øX174 and gokushovirus Chp2 are depicted in **Figure 2**. Gokushoviral genomes encode neither external scaffolding D nor major spike G proteins. The absence of these genes accounts for the smaller genomes. The external scaffolding protein has at least three known functions in øX174 morphogenesis. It mediates procapsid assembly, stabilizes the assembled procapsid at the two- and threefold axes of symmetry, and directs the placement of the major spike protein G pentamers into the fivefold related capsid craters. These functions are either not required or performed by different proteins in the gokushoviruses. In the gokushoviruses, procapsid assembly is most likely mediated by the internal scaffolding protein VP3, as is seen with the øX174 internal scaffolding protein B. Despite the small compact nature of microvirus genomes, two proteins A*

**Table 1**    Microviridae gene products

| Microvirus protein | Gokushovirus protein | Function |
|---|---|---|
| A | VP4 | Stage II and stage III DNA replication. |
| A* | UD[a] | An unessential protein for viral propagation. It may play a role in the inhibition of host cell DNA replication and superinfection exclusion. |
| B | VP3 | Internal scaffolding protein, required for procapsid morphogenesis and the assembly of early morphogenetic intermediates. Sixty copies present in the procapsid. |
| C | VP5?[b] | Facilitates the switch from stage II to stage III DNA replication. Required for stage III DNA synthesis. |
| D | NP[c] | External scaffolding protein, required for procapsid morphogenesis. 240 copies present in the procapsid. |
| E | UD | Host cell lysis. |
| F | VP1 | Major coat protein. Sixty copies present in the virion and procapsid. |
| G | NP | Major spike protein. Sixty copies present in the virion and procapsid. |
| H | VP2? | DNA pilot protein needed for DNA injection, also called the minor spike protein. Twelve copies present in the procapsid and virion. |
| J | VP8? | DNA binding protein, needed for DNA packaging, 60 copies present in the virion. |
| K | UD | An unessential protein for viral propagation. It may play a role optimizing burst sizes in various hosts. |

[a]UD, undetermined.
[b]indicates a hypothesized function based on bioinformatic data.
[c]NP, not present in gokushoviruses.

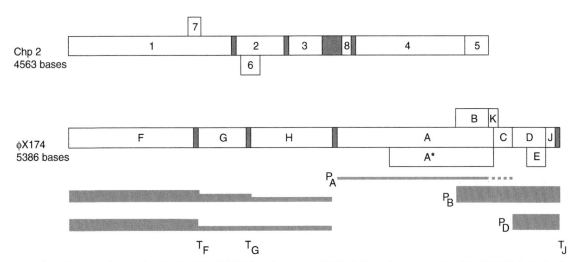

**Figure 2**    Genetic maps. Top, gokushovirus Chp2. Middle, microvirus øX174. Bottom, transcripts found in øX174 infected cells. The promoters and transcription terminators are indicated on the linear map of øX174. Line thickness indicates the relative abundance of the transcripts. The gene A transcript is very unstable; the terminator for this transcript is unknown. For protein functions, see **Table 1**.

and K with obscure or unknown functions are very strongly conserved. Three additional small ORFs are found in the H-A intercistronic region of the bacteriophage α3-like proteins. Other proteins are involved in DNA replication and lysis. These will be discussed in the context of their functions during viral replication.

## Host Cell Recognition, Attachment, and Penetration

Bacteriophage øX174 attachment requires lipopolysaccharides (LPSs) containing specific terminal glucose and galactose moieties. Most microvirus research has been conducted with øX174. Six coat protein residues constitute this $Ca^{2+}$-dependent glucose binding site. Due to the icosahedral symmetry of the capsids, each virion has 60 glucose binding sites. Attachment is a reversible reaction. Although the molecular basis of the following irreversible penetration step remains obscure, it most likely involves the spike proteins G and H. Host range mutations map to these two proteins and to coat protein residues directly surrounding the fivefold related spike complexes. Both spike proteins bind LPS of øX174 sensitive cells, but the specific details of these interactions are unknown. The location of the host range mutations argues for the existence of a second host cell penetration receptor. An analogy can be made to the large tailed bacteriophages that 'walk' along the surface of the cell, via tailspike interactions, until they find a receptor for penetration. But instead of walking, øX174 would merrily roll along.

In electron micrographs, the majority of eclipsed øX174 particles are imbedded at points of adhesion between the cell wall and inner membrane, suggesting the location of the hypothesized second receptor and indicating that the genome may be ejected directly into the cytoplasm. Penetration requires the DNA pilot protein H, which enters the cell along with the genome. Both genetic and preliminary structural data indicate that conformational changes in the capsid accompany or facilitate DNA ejection. Second-site suppressors of cold-sensitive DNA pilot proteins map to two places in the major spike protein. One set of suppressing residues lines the channel that passes through each fivefold vertex. The second set alters the interface between β-strands B and I of the G protein β-barrel, suggesting that conformational switches within this interface may mediate the channel opening.

Due to their recent discovery, the details of gokushovirus attachment and penetration have yet to be defined. The results of bioinformatic approaches combined with host range studies with the chlamydiaphages suggest that the threefold related protrusion may govern host cell specific attachment. However, there is no direct experimental evidence to support this hypothesis. Unlike microviruses, gokushoviruses appear to utilize a host cell protein, as opposed to LPS, as a receptor molecule. The exact location of the hypothesized DNA pilot protein, VP2, at the three- or fivefold axes of symmetry, is unknown as is the conduit through with the genome is ejected.

## DNA Replication

The studies of øX174 DNA replication are of historical significance. Positive polarity ssDNA replication strategies are complex, occurring in three separate stages, which are described below (**Figure 3**). Kornberg and colleagues reconstituted the first two stages *in vitro* while Hayashi and colleagues reconstituted the third stage of DNA replication, which includes concurrent packaging of the single-stranded genome. Collectively, these studies established the first defined viral genome replication process on the biochemical level.

Single-stranded viral DNA is delivered into the infected cell. Stage I DNA replication involves the conversion of the ss genome into a covalently closed, double-stranded (ds), circular molecule, called replicative form one (RFI) DNA. Since purified single-stranded microvirus DNA produces progeny when transfected, host cell proteins are both necessary and sufficient for stage I replication *in vivo*. A stem–loop structure in the FG intercistronic region serves as the host cell and protein recognition site, which initiates the assembly of the primosome. After primosome assembly, the complex migrates along the ssDNA in a $5' \rightarrow 3'$ direction synthesizing the requisite RNA primers for DNA replication. Addition of the holoenzyme leads to chain elongation. The 13 host cell proteins required for this stage of synthesis are the same proteins involved in replicating the host cell chromosome.

During stage II DNA synthesis, RF1 DNA is amplified. In addition to the host cell proteins required for stage I replication, stage II replication is dependent on the viral A protein and the host cell *rep* protein, which functions as a helicase. The viral A protein binds to the origin of replication and nicks it to initiate (+) strand synthesis, which will occur via a rolling circle mechanism. After nicking, protein A forms a covalent ester bond with the DNA, forming a relaxed circular molecule called RFII. The host cell *rep* protein unwinds the helix and the host ssDNA binding protein (ssb) stabilizes the separated strands. After one round of rolling circle synthesis, protein A cuts the newly generated origin and acts as a ligase, generating a covalently closed circular molecule. Minus strand synthesis is mechanistically similar to stage I DNA synthesis.

Stage III DNA synthesis involves the concurrent synthesis and packaging of the ssDNA genome. Procapsids and viral protein C are required for this reaction along with all the proteins involved in the previous stages of replication with the exception of the ssb. Thus, a single-stranded genome is not synthesized unless there is a

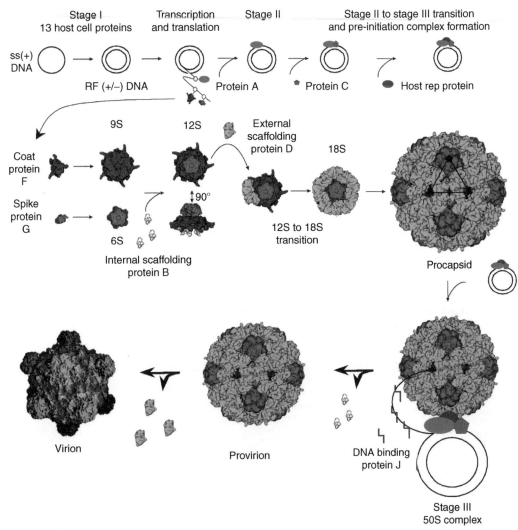

**Figure 3** Morphogenesis and DNA replication of øX174.

procapsid in which to package it. The competition between ssb and protein C for binding ssDNA most likely signals the commencement of stage III synthesis. Proteins A, C, and *rep* form a complex on the dsDNA that docks to procapsids, presumably in a groove that spans one of the twofold axes of symmetry. Procapsid binding does not occur in the absence of protein C. Mechanistically, stage III DNA synthesis is similar to the stage II (+) rolling circle synthesis. As the new (+) strand is synthesized, it is translocated into the procapsid. After one round of synthesis, protein A, which is covalently attached to the origin of replication, cuts the newly synthesized origin and acts as a ligase to generate a covalently closed circular molecule.

## Gene Expression

Since microviruses contain single-stranded genomes of positive polarity, stage I DNA synthesis, which generates the negative strand, must occur before transcription. Unlike large bacteriophages, gene expression in the members of the family *Microviridae* is neither temporal nor mediated by *trans*-acting mechanisms. Thus, the timing and relative production of viral proteins is entirely dependent on *cis*-acting regulation signals: promoters, transcription terminators, mRNA stability sequences, and ribosome binding sites. Promoters are found upstream of genes A, B, and D and terminators are found after genes J, F, G, and H (**Figure 2**). Since terminators are not 100% efficient, a wide variety of transcripts are produced. Yet there is a rough correlation between the abundance of a gene transcript and the amount of the encoded protein required for the viral life cycle. For example, gene D transcripts, which encode the external scaffolding protein, are the most abundant in the cell and the requirement of protein D is the greatest for progeny production. Similarly, there are more gene F, J, and G transcripts than transcripts of gene H. The relative stoichiometry of these structural proteins are

5:5:5:1, respectively. Protein expression is also affected by mRNA stability. Each mRNA species decays with a characteristic rate. Transcripts of gene A decay very rapidly, ensuring that this nonstructural protein is not overexpressed. Finally, regulation can also be achieved on the translational level. Despite gene E's location within gene D, the most abundant transcript, few E proteins, which mediate cell lysis, are translated due to an extremely ineffective ribosome binding site.

## Morphogenesis

Despite extensive searches, a dependence on host molecular chaperones, such as groEL, and groES, has never been documented. Thus, chaperone independence is another factor that distinguishes the microviruses from dsDNA bacteriophages. The first virally encoded microvirus assembly intermediates are the 9S and 6S particles, respective pentamers of the major coat F and spike G proteins

(**Figure 3**). After 9S pentamer formation, five internal scaffolding proteins bind to the 9S underside, which will become the capsid's internal surface, forming the 9S* intermediate. 9S* particles then associate with spike protein pentamers to produce 12S assembly intermediates. The internal scaffolding protein also facilitates the incorporation of the DNA pilot protein H. However, the exact time protein H enters the assembly pathways remains somewhat obscure. The addition of 20 external scaffolding proteins results in the construction of the 18S particle.

The external scaffolding protein has been the focus of many research endeavors due to its inherent ability to achieve different structures. The four D subunits (D1, D2, D3, and D4) per coat protein (**Figure 4**), are arranged as two similar, but not identical, asymmetric dimers (D1D2 and D3D4). Each subunit makes a unique set of contacts with the underlying coat protein, the spike protein, and neighboring D protein subunits. Accordingly, the structure of each subunit is unique. The atomic structure of the assembly naive D protein dimer has also been determined.

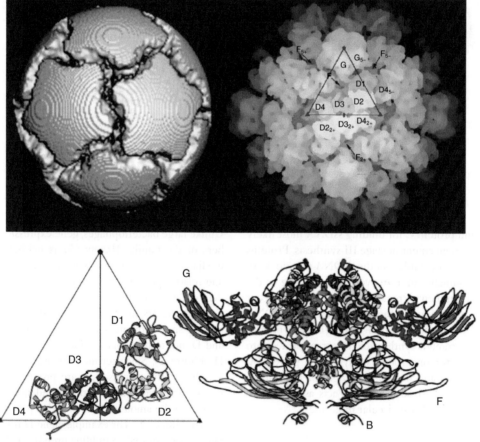

**Figure 4**   CryoEM and atomic renderings of the ⌀X174 procapsid. Top left, rendering of the procapsid with the removal of the external scaffolding protein. Note that the coat protein pentamers do not contact each other. Top right, isosurface tracing of the ⌀X174 procapsid, the four structurally unique external scaffolding proteins are depicted as D1–D4. Bottom left, the Cα backbones of the four external scaffolding protein subunits. Bottom right, cross-section of the procapsid along a twofold axis of symmetry, showing the positions of the internal B and external D scaffolding proteins relative to the coat F and spike G proteins.

The subunits within that dimer, DA and DB, appear poised to achieve the four structures found in the procapsid. DA has a structure somewhat between D1 and D3, while DB has a structure midway between D2 and D4.

External scaffolding proteins are rare, only observed in parasitic satellite virus systems such as bacteriophage P4, in which the satellite virus encodes an external scaffolding protein that forces the helper's virus capsid to form a smaller capsid. Thus, microviruses are the only nonsatellite viruses known to encode an external scaffolding protein. This protein performs many of the functions typically associated with internal scaffolding proteins in one-scaffolding-protein systems, the organization of assembly precursors into a procapsid, and the stabilization of that structure. However, its function is physically and temporally dependent on the internal scaffolding protein, which can be eliminated from the pathway (see the section titled 'Evolution and evolutionary studies' below). Procapsid morphogenesis is completed with the association of the 12 18S particles. The structure is almost exclusively held together via external scaffolding protein contacts across twofold axes of symmetry. Remarkably, there appear to be no associations between coat protein pentamers (**Figure 4**).

Gokushovirus genomes do not encode an external scaffolding protein. The details of the early assembly pathway remain to be elucidated. A gokushovirus particle containing VP3 in addition to the structural coat and DNA pilot proteins has been isolated. Unlike virions, these particles are devoid of DNA. This particle most likely represents a procapsid and indicates that VP3 functions as an internal scaffolding protein.

## DNA Packaging and the DNA Binding Protein

Genome biosynthesis and packaging are concurrent processes in øX174. The pre-initiation complex, consisting of the host cell *rep*, viral A and C proteins, associates with the procapsid forming the 50S complex. As described above, the viral A protein binds the origin of replication in replicative form DNA. The results of genetic studies indicate that the pre-initiation docking site resides along a twofold axis of symmetry. The DNA binding protein J enters the procapsid during packaging and is absolutely required for genome encapsidation. Once in the procapsid, the C-terminus of the protein, which is very hydrophobic and aromatic, competes with the internal scaffolding protein for binding to a cleft in the viral coat protein. This competition results in the extrusion of the internal scaffolding protein during the packaging reaction.

Microvirus J proteins are extremely basic proteins that bind the genome via electrostatic interactions. The genome also interacts with a small cluster of basic amino acid residues in the capsid. Unlike large dsDNA bacteriophages, the øX174 genome does not exist as a dense core in the capsid. Instead, the DNA is tethered to the capsid's inner surface. In the atomic model, the protein forms an S-shaped polypeptide chain devoid of secondary structure. The C-terminus is tightly associated with the cleft located near the center of the coat protein. Each of the 60 proteins traces a path toward the fivefold axis of symmetry, crosses over to the adjacent capsid protein, and veers toward the C-terminus of the adjacent J protein. Thus, the DNA binding protein guides the incoming genome into a somewhat ordered conformation and a portion of the genome is ordered in the X-ray structure. The biophysical characterization of fully packaged particles with foreign genome-length DNA or øX174 genomes with mutant DNA binding proteins suggest that protein–DNA interactions influence the final stages of morphogenesis. Morphogenesis terminates with the provirion to virion transition: the dissociation of the external scaffolding protein and an 8.5 Å radial collapse of capsid pentamers around the genome. The tethered genome constrains the spatial orientation and secondary structure of the remaining nucleotides. Therefore, altering the tether or the base composition of the packaged nucleic acid may affect the magnitude or the integrity of the collapse. However, the role of DNA–capsid interactions in øX174 is not as dramatic as those seen in other viral systems in which abrogating genome–capsid interactions lead to severely aberrant particles.

## Lysis

Unlike large double-stranded bacteriophages, microviruses do not have the genetic capacity to encode two-component endolysin and holin lysis systems. Instead, they have evolved a small protein, lysis protein E that inhibits peptidoglycan biosynthesis. Thus, lysis is dependent on host cell division, during which the cell becomes sensitive to osmotic pressure. The results of several elegant genetic studies elucidated protein E function. By selecting for lysis resistant cells, Ryland Young and colleagues first uncovered the *slyD* (*s*ensitivity to *l*ysis) gene, which encodes a peptidly-prolyl cis-transferase-isomerase, or PPIase. However, it is unlikely that the *slyD* gene product is the E protein target. Considering the function of PPIase's in protein folding and the E protein's five prolyl bonds, it seemed more likely that the E protein was a substrate for the host cell enzyme. In fact, gene E mutants, *Epos*-plates on *slyD*, can be readily isolated. The *Epos* proteins were used in a second round of selection with *slyD* cells, surviving colonies containing mutations in the *mraY* gene, which encodes tanslocase I. This enzyme catalyzes the formation of the first lipid-linked intermediate in cell wall biosynthesis and most likely the target of protein E.

## Evolution and Evolutionary Studies

Due to the small genomes and the ability to interpret amino acid substitutions within the context of the virion and procapsid atomic structures, the microviruses have become one of the leading systems for molecular evolution analyses. In studies pioneered by Jim Bull, Holly Wichman, and colleagues, viruses are placed under selective conditions, and grown for numerous generations in a chemostat. At various time intervals, individual genomes are sequenced, allowing the appearance and disappearance of beneficial mutations to be monitored. Of course, the mutations obtained differ according to the selection conditions. While these studies identify beneficial changes in both structural and nonstructural proteins, many mutations are in genetic regulatory sequences, which most likely optimize the relative level of viral proteins synthesized under the experimental conditions.

The results of an exhaustive search for new *Escherichia coli* microviruses reveal that the 47 known species can be divided into three separate clades, typified by bacteriophages øX174, G4, and α3. Although there is evidence for some horizontal gene transfer between the species, the extent is considerably lower than that observed for dsDNA viruses. The one gene that seems to be the most recent acquisition, at least in its present form, is the external scaffolding protein gene, which appears to have originated in the øX174 clade and spread to the other two.

The evolutionary relationship between the gokusho and microviruses remains somewhat obscure. There is a deep evolutionary rift between the two groups, with no known intermediate species. The rift appears to be a function of the biology of their hosts, not the hosts' evolutionary relationship. The gokushoviruses have been isolated from obligated intracellular parasitic bacteria or mollicutes. For example, the *Bdellovibrio* host for the gokushovirus øMH2K is a proteobacterium, like other microvirus hosts, but øMH2K is closely related to the phages of chlamidia. One of the primary differences between the two groups is the external scaffolding protein.

While the existence of two scaffolding proteins is unique in any system, it is particularly peculiar for the T = 1 microviruses. No other T = 1 virus requires a scaffolding protein, let alone two. An accumulation of both genetic and structural data suggests that the external scaffolding protein may be more essential for morphogenesis. The internal scaffolding protein, on the other hand, may be better viewed as en efficiency protein, facilitating several morphogenetic reactions, but not absolutely essential for any one in particular. This hypothesis has recently been tested by the isolation of a sextuple mutant strain of øX174 that no longer requires the internal scaffolding protein. Although mutations in structural and external scaffolding proteins did arise, two mutations reside in the external scaffolding gene promoters, leading to the over-expression of the mutant external scaffolding protein. These three mutations appear to have a kinetic effect on virion assembly, indicating that one function of the internal scaffolding is to lower the critical concentration of the external scaffolding protein needed to nucleate the assembly. The morphogenesis of wild-type øX174 is extremely rapid, progeny virions can be detected as quickly as 5 min post-infection, which may be critical for a small phage without the genome content to encode superinfection exclusion functions. At 5 min postinfection, most other phages are just concluding early gene expression. Rapid morphogenesis may be a consequence of having two scaffolding proteins, allowing microviruses to compete with the larger and vastly more prevalent dsDNA phages. In this evolutionary model, the external scaffolding protein is a recent acquisition. Those phages that did not acquire the gene, the gokushoviruses, persisted by finding a niche free of competition, obligate intracellular parasitic hosts like chlamidia.

## Acknowledgments

The authors thank Drs. M. G. Rossmann and Timothy Baker and colleagues for assistance with figures and the support of the National Science Foundation.

*See also:* Transcriptional Regulation in Bacteriophage.

## Further Reading

Bernhardt TG, Struck DK, and Young R (2001) The lysis protein E of phi X174 is a specific inhibitor of the MraY-catalyzed step in peptidoglycan synthesis. *Journal of Biological Chemistry* 276(9): 6093–6097.

Brentlinger KL, Hafenstein S, Novak CR, *et al.* (2002) *Microviridae*, a family divided: Isolation, characterization, and genome sequence of phiMH2K, a bacteriophage of the obligate intracellular parasitic bacterium Bdellovibrio bacteriovorus. *Journal of Bacteriology* 184(4): 1089–1094.

Bull JJ, Badgett MR, Wichman HA, *et al.* (1997) Exceptional convergent evolution in a virus. *Genetics* 147(4): 1497–507.

Chipman PR, Agbandje-McKenna M, Renaudin J, Baker TS, and McKenna R (1998) Structural analysis of the Spiroplasma virus, SpV4: Implications for evolutionary variation to obtain host diversity among the Microviridae. *Structure* 6(2): 135–145.

Dokland T, McKenna R, Ilag LL, *et al.* (1997) Structure of a viral procapsid with molecular scaffolding. *Nature* 389(6648): 308–313.

Fane BA, Brentlinger KL, Burch AD, *et al.* (2006) øX174 *et al.* In: Calendar (ed.) *The Bacteriophages*, pp. 129–146. London: Oxford University Press.

Fane BA and Prevelige PE, Jr. (2003) Mechanism of scaffolding-assisted viral assembly. *Advances in Protein Chemistry* 64: 259–299.

Hafenstein S and Fane BA (2002) phi X174 genome-capsid interactions influence the biophysical properties of the virion: Evidence for a scaffolding-like function for the genome during the final stages of morphogenesis. *Journal of Virology* 76(11): 5350–5356.

Hayashi M, Aoyama A, Richardson DL, and Hayashi NM (1988) Biology of the bacteriophage øX174. In: Calendar R (ed.) *The Bacteriophages*, vol. 2, pp. 1–71. New York: Plenum.

Liu BL, Everson JS, Fane B, *et al.* (2000) Molecular characterization of a bacteriophage (Chp2) from Chlamydia psittaci. *Journal of Virology* 74(8): 3464–3469.

McKenna R, Xia D, Willingmann P, *et al.* (1992) Atomic structure of single-stranded DNA bacteriophage phiX174 and its functional implications. *Nature* 355(6356): 137–143.

Morais MC, Fisher M, Kanamaru S, *et al.* (2004) Conformational switching by the scaffolding protein D directs the assembly of bacteriophage phiX174. *Molecular Cell* 15(6): 991–997.

Novak CR and Fane BA (2004) The functions of the N terminus of the phiX174 internal scaffolding protein, a protein encoded in an overlapping reading frame in a two scaffolding protein system. *Journal of Molecular Biology* 335(1): 383–390.

Rokyta DR, Burch CL, Caudle SB, and Wichman HA (2006) Horizontal gene transfer and the evolution of microvirid coliphage genomes. *Journal of Bacteriology* 188(3): 1134–1142.

Uchiyama A and Fane BA (2005) Identification of an interacting coat-external scaffolding protein domain required for both the initiation of phiX174 procapsid morphogenesis and the completion of DNA packaging. *Journal of Virology* 79(11): 6751–6756.

# Icosahedral ssRNA Bacterial Viruses

**P G Stockley,** University of Leeds, Leeds, UK

## Glossary

**Pfu** Plaque-forming unit; that is, the number of phage particles per host cell required to generate productive infections. Theoretically, this value could be 1, but in reality only very few of the phages that attach to the edge of a pilus will get access to the inside of a cell, so values in the 100s are not uncommon.

**Polycistronic RNA** The term cistron was coined a long time ago to mean any section of an mRNA that gets translated. The RNA phage genomes are 'polycistronic', because they encode multiple protein products.

**Quasi-equivalent conformers** These are different conformations of the identical polypeptide sequences that form at the differing symmetry-related positions of viral capsids.

**Translational repression** Refers to the process whereby a protein product interacts with an mRNA molecule, thus preventing its translation.

**Triangulation number, *T*** Defined mathematically as $T = (h^2 + hk + k^2)$, where $h$ and $k$ are any pair of positive integers, including zero. For instance, giving rise to triangulation numbers of 1 for $h,k = 1,0$, and 3 for $h,k = 1,1$. These $h$ and $k$ values can be determined by analysis of real capsids viruses by analyzing them in terms of networks of equilateral triangles that cover the surface of a sphere.

## Background

Not all *Escherichia coli* cells are the same. Some of them produce a protein tube at the surface known as a pilus. It turns out that the information to build this structure is encoded by a separate genetic element, the F factor not carried by all cells. The RNA phages were initially identified because of their ability to infect *E. coli* carrying this factor. The pili encoded by F are used by the cells to swap DNA with other bacteria that lack the factor, resulting in a primitive form of sexual genetic transfer known as conjugation and the use of the term 'male' for bacteria that carry the F factor. Thus bacteria are able to swap useful genes, for example, for antibiotic resistance, rapidly within their populations. All processes in biology can be seen as opportunities ripe for exploitation, and the F pilus system, so useful to the bacteria in sharing useful genetic characteristics, presents an opening for a group of bacterial viruses to gain entry into $F^+$ cells. Tim Loeb working in Norton Zinder's laboratory at the Rockefeller University in New York was the first to realize that there might be male-specific bacterial viruses, bacteriophages. Together they isolated and began to characterize such phages from an initial sample of raw sewage. One intensively studied version known as MS2 is believed to have been named because it was male-specific factor 2, although there are unconfirmed stories that the MS also stands for metropolitan sewer.

Large numbers of similar phages were rapidly isolated worldwide after the initial discovery, and we now know that such phages are extremely common in the environment with up to $10^7$ Pfu ml$^{-1}$ in sewage. Both human and animal hosts appear to harbor *E. coli* populations able to support such phages, which are hence termed coliphage. In addition, virtually identical phages have been found that are specific to *Acinetobacter* (AP205) and other Gram-negative bacteria. In such phages, the infection process still occurs via pili but these are not the same as the sex pili of *E. coli*. For instance, phage PRR1 infects hosts via pili encoded by incompatibility type P plasmids which are widely dispersed, allowing the phage to infect a range of different bacterial cells.

All these bacteriophages turn out to have very closely related structural and genetic features. They form spherical capsids of $\sim$250 Å diameter that enclose a single-stranded RNA (ssRNA) genome of $\sim$3500–4300 nt in length. The ssRNA is the positive-sense version of the genome and acts as a messenger RNA (mRNA) while in infected cells. On the basis of immunological cross-reactivity and genome organization, the phages have been classified into two genera and these have been subdivided in turn into two groups. All these phages are members of the *Leviviridae* or the *Alloleviridae*, the latter being distinguished by having slightly longer genomes and because of the presence of read-through products from the coat protein gene. Subgroups I and II belong to the former genus and typical members are MS2 and GA, respectively, whereas group III and IV phages belong to the latter genus with typical members being Q β and SP, respectively.

These very simple pathogens have been used since their discovery to understand many basic processes of molecular biology. They have been used to probe the structure of the bacterial pilus, to dissect the function of the protein synthesis pathway, to understand RNA replication, and to identify the initiation and termination signals on prokaryotic mRNAs. These studies led to the discovery of novel forms of genetic regulation along a polycistronic RNA, including translational repression. Phage RNA was the first nucleic acid to be replicated in a test tube and was used as a model for the development of nucleic acid sequencing technology. Detailed insights into viral assembly processes and the molecular basis of sequence-specific RNA–protein recognition have also emerged. Research applications of these phages and their biology are still very active (see below).

## Capsid Structure and Life Cycle

At the time of their discovery, the three-dimensional structures of viruses were not known but it was realized that the limited coding capacity of viral nucleic acids was likely to place a constraint on the number and size of gene products that could be dedicated to building a protective container, or capsid. This in turn implied that capsids are likely to be composed of multiple copies of one or very few 'coat' protein subunits necessarily resulting in highly symmetric structures. The two most 'efficient' designs for such structures, in terms of allowing multiple copies of the smallest protein units to enclose the maximum volume, and hence encompass the largest genome, are the helix and the icosahedron. Simple spherical virus capsids are therefore based on an icosahedral surface lattice (**Figure 1**).

A mathematically perfect icosahedron would have 60 facets in it so the stoichiometry for such viruses would be 60 coat proteins per shell. However, from many early studies, it was clear that viruses often had many more than 60 subunits in their capsids, although in cases where detailed biochemistry was possible it appeared that such viruses contained simple multiples of the expected value, for example, 180, 240, etc. Don Caspar and Aaron Klug offered an explanation for such protein stoichiometries via a theory they called quasi-equivalence. They argued that viral coat proteins are three-dimensional objects that are partially flexible due to the chemical properties of their constituent polypeptide backbones and amino acid side chains. It would therefore be possible to conserve inter-subunit bonding if the precise molecular interactions at any position in the capsid were flexible enough to accommodate small changes from ideality. This theory leads immediately to predictions of 'allowed' stoichiometries for capsids with subunit numbers of 180, 240, etc., derived from what is called a subtriangulation of the sphere and defined by the triangulation number, $T$. This value is allowed to vary from 1, 3, 4, etc., yielding the observed stoichiometries of 60, 180, 240, etc. subunits. The implication of this idea is that the coat proteins within the capsids with more than 60 subunits must be able to adopt slightly different conformations depending on their relative locations in the shell. These are known as quasi-equivalent conformers and this idea has subsequently been confirmed by X-ray structure determination of many viruses. The RNA phages have 180 coat protein subunits per capsid and are therefore examples of $T = 3$ shells.

As well as the major coat protein, it is known that the capsids of RNA phages contain a minor protein that is essential for infectivity known as the maturation (or A) protein. In some of the RNA phages, another minor protein is associated with the capsids due to the production of a small percentage of read-through versions of the coat protein. The function of these minor components is largely unknown. Mature infectious capsids must contain at least one copy of the maturation protein as well as the icosahedral shell composed of the major coat protein. Infection is initiated by the interaction of the A protein with the edge of a bacterial pilus, confirming that part of this protein must project on the outer surface of the virion. This interaction triggers a release of the phage RNA from inside the phage shell and proteolytic cleavage of the A protein into two major fragments. The RNA and the A protein domains then enter the cell leaving the remainder of the capsid, that is, the major coat protein, on the outside. This implies that at least one fragment of the A protein must form a tight interaction with the phage RNA. Indeed, careful measurement of the kinetics of uptake of both phage RNA and the two fragments of the A protein suggest that they enter the cell as a single complex. Two RNA-binding sites for the A protein along the genome, one toward the 5' end and the other close to the 3' end, have been identified. It is tempting to speculate that pilin attachment leads to conformational change in the A protein, that is made irreversible by the proteolytic cleavage, and this in turn results in expulsion of the phage genomic RNA from its capsid. The precise mechanism of how the A protein–RNA complex is taken up into the cell has not been worked out in any detail. It is assumed that these complexes can transit into the cell like DNA but this does not seem to have been firmly established.

Whatever the mechanism of cell entry, once inside the cell the phage RNA then serves as an mRNA (see below). Expression of phage proteins results in replication of the phage RNA via the formation of an RNA-dependent RNA polymerase consisting of one phage-encoded replicase subunit, the host proteins S1, and elongation factors Tu and Ts, and an additional host factor. This polymerase creates negative strand versions of the genome that in turn serve as templates for the production of progeny positive-sense genomes. In an exquisite example of timing controlled by macromolecular interactions, this replication phase of infection is reined in by a translational repression event. Translation of the replicase subunit becomes blocked by interaction of a coat protein dimer with a stem–loop operator site of just 19 nt in length that includes the start codon for that cistron.

The resultant coat protein–genomic RNA complexes then serve as the assembly initiation complexes for formation of progeny phage particles. At some point, the A protein must become a part of this complex. The final

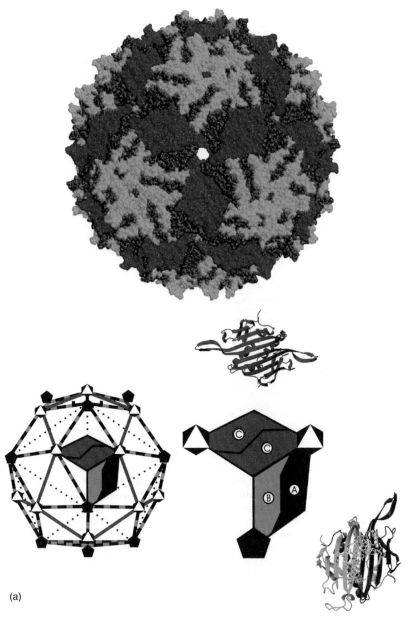

(a)

**Figure 1** Continued

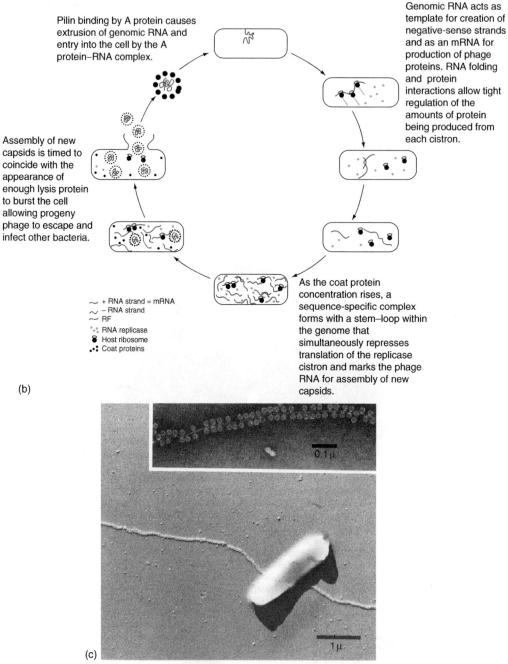

Pilin binding by A protein causes extrusion of genomic RNA and entry into the cell by the A protein–RNA complex.

Genomic RNA acts as template for creation of negative-sense strands and as an mRNA for production of phage proteins. RNA folding and protein interactions allow tight regulation of the amounts of protein being produced from each cistron.

Assembly of new capsids is timed to coincide with the appearance of enough lysis protein to burst the cell allowing progeny phage to escape and infect other bacteria.

As the coat protein concentration rises, a sequence-specific complex forms with a stem–loop within the genome that simultaneously represses translation of the replicase cistron and marks the phage RNA for assembly of new capsids.

~ + RNA strand = mRNA
~ – RNA strand
~ RF
°.°. RNA replicase
🍥 Host ribosome
.•: Coat proteins

(b)

0.1 μ

1 μ

(c)

**Figure 1** Capsid structure and life cycle. (a) Shows a space-filling representation of one face of the MS2 bacteriophage particle as determined using X-ray crystallography viewed along the icosahedral threefold axis. The differing quasi-equivalent protein conformers are colored red, green, and blue. There are 60 of each type accounting for the 180 coat protein copies per $T = 3$ shell. Note, the position of the A protein in the shell is not observed from the X-ray structure for technical reasons. Below is a cartoon of an icosahedron with the threefold (open triangles) and fivefold (solid pentagons) symmetry axes highlighted. The MS2 coat protein subunits form noncovalent dimers in solution and in the final capsid, and the way in which they pack around the axes is illustrated on the right both as a cartoon and as detailed three-dimensional representations of the differing quasi-equivalent conformers. Proteins are shown as ribbon diagrams representing their polypeptide backbones. The A/B dimer is shown bound to the translational repression RNA stem–loop (yellow); see also **Figure 3**. (b) Shows a schematic of the phage life cycle, including the attachment process, entry of the genomic RNA, replication, self-assembly of progeny phage particles, and subsequent lysis of the host. (c) Shows the process of infection with phage particles adhered along the length of a bacterial pilus. The magnification is ~16000× and reveals the relative sizes of the host and its virus particles. (b) Reproduced from Watson JD, Hapkins NH, Roberts JW, Steltz JA, and Winer AM (1993) *Molecular Biology of the Gene, Vol. I: General Principle*, 5th edn. New Delhi: Pearson Education, Inc., with permission. (c) Reproduced from Paranchych W (1975) Attachment, ejection and penetration stages of the RNA phage infectious process. In: Zinder ND (ed.) *RNA Phages*, p. 89. New York: Cold Spring Harbor Laboratory Press, with permission from Cold Spring Harbor Laboratory Press (NY).

act of infection is lysis of the host cell by the action of a lysis protein leading to release of up to 10 000 progeny particles. During this process, the phage has dramatically differing needs for each of its gene products: replicase, coat protein, maturation protein, and lysis protein. Each protein also needs to act at different times. Remarkably, both the amounts and timing of the appearance of each of these products is very tightly regulated, even though each cistron is present once on every copy of the genomic RNA. The details of that regulation are described in the following sections.

## Control of Phage Gene Expression

When the phage-encoded protein expression is analyzed (**Figure 2**), it can be seen that the first protein to be produced after the RNA gains entry to the cell is the coat protein, and its expression remains high throughout an infection cycle. There seems little regulation of this expression other than the sequence and stability of the initiator hairpin structure that binds the ribosome. There are also some data that suggest that upstream flanking sequences can act positively to promote translation, perhaps by forming structures that favor binding of the ribosome to this site.

The maturation protein is obviously needed in much smaller amounts and its appearance is slower and it is produced in much lower amounts than coat protein. It is believed that a number of regulatory features lead to this poor expression level. The start codon for the maturation gene is GUG instead of the more usual and more efficient AUG. In addition, it has been proposed that the ribosome-binding site in this cistron can be sequestered in internal base pairing with another section of the maturation protein message and, as a result, maturation protein is only expressed on nascent replicating genomic RNAs, that is, at a point when the downstream base pairing partners are yet to be replicated.

The replicase subunit is initially produced with similar kinetics and in similar amounts to the maturation protein but by 20 min after infection its levels are reduced. In fact, the phage makes more maturation protein than is strictly necessary, but the replicase is made at a level of ~5 copies/genome and its levels are always tightly controlled. This regulation is achieved in two distinct ways. Initially, the ribosome start site on the replicase subunit is sequestered in another long-range base-pairing interaction, this time with a section of the coat protein gene. Translation of the coat protein gene sequesters this complementary sequence, known as the Min Jou sequence after its discoverer, and thus frees the region around the start of the replicase gene so that it can fold to form a ribosome-binding site.

However, replication is further controlled via a translational repression complex that forms with the phage

coat protein. A stem–loop operator hairpin (**Figure 3**) can form that is bound sequence-specifically by a dimer of the coat protein in a concentration-dependent fashion. This operator encompasses the start codon for replicase and formation of this repression complex effectively switches off replicase translation. The complex also acts to trigger self-assembly of the phage coat protein shell around the phage RNA. Regulated expression is obviously tightly controlled because of the importance of timing the switch in the viral life cycle from replication to assembly of progeny phage. There may also be an additional reason to ensure that large quantities of replicase are not produced because of its role(s) in creating the active replication complex.

The phage-encoded replicase subunit is the RNA-dependent RNA polymerase responsible for copying the phage genome. However, it does not function as a separate subunit. Instead, it forms complexes with at least three cellular proteins normally involved in other functions; these are the ribosomal protein S1, which functions during the loading and initiation of mRNAs on the ribosome, and translational elongation factors EF-Tu and EF-Ts. These species form a heterotypic tetramer that appears to be the active replication enzyme for positive-sense strands of the genome, that is, in the production of the negative-sense strand. The opposite reaction, that is, the generation of the positive-sense strand from the negative strand appears not to need the S1 subunit. An explanation for this altered stoichiometry in the replication machinery has been proposed based on the fact that the positive-strand must also serve as a template for peptide synthesis. This would lead to situations in which ribosomes and replication complexes, which would be moving in opposite directions on the RNA, would collide. It is believed that S1 functions in these cases by competing with the ribosome for loading onto the RNA, thus preventing replication on actively translating RNAs. The replication complexes also appear to interact with another host protein, which appears to be hexameric, but its role(s) is unclear.

A final reason for tight regulation of the expression of replicase is that the subunit or its complexes with cellular proteins are toxic to the cell. This would interrupt the phage life cycle before progeny phages are assembled. Cell death is however the ultimate goal of the infection, thus releasing progeny phage particles, but this is actively controlled by a phage-encoded lysis protein. This cistron is read from the +1 reading frame initiating within the coat protein gene. As can be seen from **Figure 2**, the lysis protein is the last to be produced, consistent with its final function in the phage life cycle. The reason for the delayed production of this gene product appears again to be a consequence of translational control. In this case, the ribosome binding site allowing initiation of the lysis protein translation appears inaccessible until the ribosome translating the coat protein completes the translation in

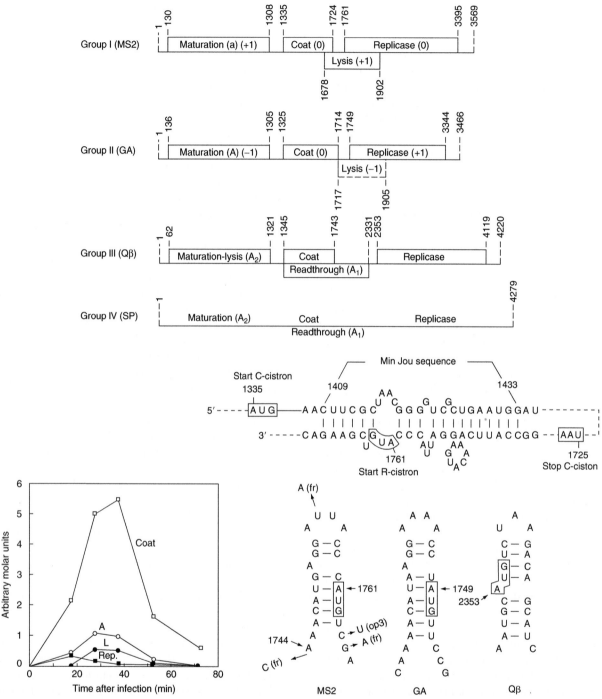

**Figure 2** Genome organization and expression. The top panel shows cartoon representations of the genomes of representative members of each of the four subgroups of the RNA bacteriophages. The locations of the encoded proteins are also shown. The middle panel left shows the amounts of each of the encoded proteins produced during an infection cycle. Although each gene is present in equal amounts along each copy of every genome, there is a dramatic difference in the amounts of each protein in the cell, reflecting the requirements for different numbers of these protein products for replication, self-assembly of progeny phage, and lysis of the host. The implication is that the expression of these protein products is tightly controlled. The middle panel right shows one type of regulation that allows control of the amount of each protein product produced. At various times in the phage life cycle, the stem–loop structures shown at the bottom of the figure are sequestered by long range Watson–Crick base-pairing interactions to a segment of the coat protein gene (illustrated here for MS2). This section of the genome contains the start codon for the phage-encoded replicase subunit, so that the tertiary interaction prevents expression of replicase until the coat protein gene begins to be translated. As a ribosome transits this base-paired region, it frees up the downstream section allowing the ribosome-binding site and replicase translation to occur. At a later stage, the re-folded stem–loop is recognized by the coat protein – a coat protein dimer binds to the site and prevents further translational initiation, an example of translational repression (**Figure 3**). (a–c) Reproduced from Van Duin J (1988) Single-stranded RNA bacteriophages. In: Calendar R (ed.) *The Bacteriophages*, vol. 1, pp. 117–167. New York: Plenum, with permission.

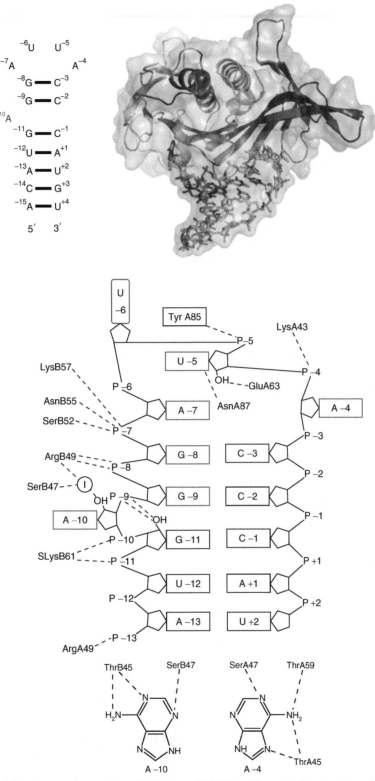

**Figure 3** The MS2 translational repression complex. The top panel left shows the secondary structure of the translational operator stem–loop and the number of the bases relative to the replicase start codon. To the right is a detailed view of the X-ray structure of the interaction of the operator stem–loop with a coat protein dimer (shown as the A/B quasi-equivalent conformers). The polypeptide (blue and green) and RNA (gold) are shown as ribbon and stick models, respectively, within a transparent representation of the molecular surfaces. The bottom panel shows the intermolecular contacts that occur within the complex. The detailed contacts at A-4 and A-10 are shown below for clearity. The dotted lines indicate hydrogen bond interactions.

its defined termination site. Experiments where the coat protein gene stop codons are moved further 3′ prevent lysis expression, implying that correctly regulated expression must be due to a defined RNA folding event similar to those controlling replicase translational repression. In principle, variations of the details of this mechanism may partially account for the frequency of read-through products in some of the coat proteins in some phages.

## The Translational Repression/Assembly Initiation Complex

As discussed above, the expression of the phage-encoded replicase subunit is controlled by a translational repression event that occurs when a coat protein dimer binds to a 19 nt stem–loop structure (**Figure 3**), thus sequestering the AUG start codon from replicase. In a set of seminal experiments, Janette Carey and Olke Ulhenbeck were able to show that all the sequence information for the specific RNA–coat protein interaction was contained within this short fragment. Furthermore, they established rapid assays for the interaction *in vitro*, allowing extensive investigation of the effects of changes to nucleotide base sequence and the chemical functional groups on the RNA that contribute to this interaction. In addition, it has proved possible to determine X-ray crystal structures for the RNA stem–loop and over 30 of its variants in complex with the coat protein shell (**Figures 3** and **1**).

The detailed intermolecular contacts revealed and confirmed by these techniques have made this complex one of the most intensively studied examples of an RNA–protein complex. It has also been possible to determine structures for variants of the coat protein mutant at the RNA-binding site. The results of these studies suggest that the interaction is remarkably robust to simple changes outside a few key residues, principally the loop adenine at position −4 (the bases are numbered with respect to the first nucleotide of the replicase start codon). The half-life of the RNA–coat protein complex *in vitro* and presumably *in vivo* is very short (<1 min), implying that translational repression is short-lived. However, this is a simplification because the RNA–protein complex created then serves as a site of assembly initiation for formation of the intact capsid (see below). The repressive function of the coat protein reconfirms the mechanism of infection described above. If significant numbers of coat protein subunits were to enter the cell with the genomic RNA, the replicase gene would never be expressed. RNA variants that have higher affinity for coat protein can be identified *in vitro* but these would be lethal *in vivo*.

When cells are co-infected with MS2 and Q β phages, the progeny phages that result consist of MS2 and Q β RNAs inside their respective coat protein shells, that is,

there is no evidence that the proteins can mispackage the competing genome. In part, this is because of the significant structural differences between the translational operator sites (**Figure 2**), but it also implies that there is direct coupling in the RNA–protein interaction leading to translational repression and assembly of progeny phage particles. It is believed that the RNA–coat protein complex that forms initially with a single coat protein dimer marks the phage RNA for assembly by addition of further coat protein subunits. All that is required to avoid misincorporation is that the coat proteins from different phages are unable to co-assemble and that seems to be the case even though there is a great deal of structural similarity between them.

The precise mechanism by which the phage capsid is generated is still unclear. When and how is the maturation protein incorporated into the structure, for instance? What we do know is that the stem–loop interaction appears to cause a conformational change in the coat protein subunits that bind, possibly between differing quasi-equivalent conformers, and provides a binding site for the stepwise addition of other coat protein dimers. These must somehow adjust their precise conformations in a structural context in order to produce a capsid of the correct size and symmetry. Recent evidence suggests that the folded genomic RNA may play a role in this process.

The major structural difference between quasi-equivalent conformers in a capsid occurs in a short loop of polypeptide connecting the F and G β-strands in each subunit. These FG loops have identical amino acid sequences in all subunits, but around the icosahedral fivefold symmetry axes they fold back toward the body of the subunit helping to create space to pack the subunits at this position. In contrast, at the icosahedral threefold axes, FG loops from two distinct quasi-equivalent subunits alternate in extended conformations, allowing six such loops to be packaged at these points. We now know that binding of the RNA translational operator causes a conformation change to occur at the FG loop, and it is tempting to assume that this interaction sets up the initial asymmetry to define a capsid structure via self-assembly. Precisely how the RNA is folded to fit into this structure and whether it folds during or before the assembly reaction is still a matter of debate.

## Applications of RNA Phages – Three-Hybrid Assay

RNA phages have become model viruses for the development of a large number of novel scientific techniques. These are remarkably varied and include the controlled release of these phages into the wider environment as markers for the passage of viruses and of the ability of water treatment systems to remove viral particulates from drinking water. One such test was even performed on the International Space Station.

A more medically orientated set of applications has also been developed. For instance, it is known that viruses present defined epitopes to the immune system of their hosts. If those epitopes are common and unchanging, the immune response that occurs after an initial infection will render the host immune to further infection by that particular virus. Many viruses however constantly alter their outer protein surfaces presenting differing epitopes to the immune system, thus escaping immune neutralization. However, modern structural immunology techniques can identify conserved functional domains/sequences within these viral proteins that cannot be altered without also causing the virus to lose the ability to replicate or assemble. Raising immune responses against such refined constant epitopes leads to potent vaccines against a range of human and animal pathogens. In fact, work in this area has shown that the immune system is particularly well evolved to recognize repeated copies of particular epitopes, such as those that appear on the surfaces of pathogenic viruses. Therefore, researchers are busy trying to turn the tables on viruses by presenting conserved epitopes from pathogenic viruses as repeated arrays on the surfaces of harmless virus particles, such as the RNA phages. Not all such applications are directed at preventing viral infections. One artificial construct based on the phage Q β presents nicotine as an artificially linked epitope and it is hoped that this virus-like particle will allow 'vaccination' of smokers who otherwise have failed to break their addictions to tobacco.

Our detailed knowledge about the coat protein–RNA operator interaction that regulates replicase translation and triggers self-assembly of progeny phage particles has also been adapted to allow encapsidation of non-phage molecules ranging from large protein toxins, to peptides and DNA oligonucleotides. These potentially therapeutic species can then be directed to specific cells by decoration of the external phage capsid surface with ligands for cell-surface receptor molecules. Once complexed at the cell surface, receptor-mediated endocytosis results in internalization of the encapsidated drug into endosomes where the pH is slightly acidic, conditions that favor disassembly of phage shells, and hence release of the 'drug' entities into the cell. Encapsidation of the plant toxin ricin A chain, that normally needs an additional B chain to cross into cells, allows this highly toxic protein to be delivered into the interior of cells carrying defined external signals resulting in reagents with effective lethal doses in the picomolar range. Controls lacking the targeting ligand are essentially nontoxic, suggesting that encapsidation reduces the nonspecific uptake of ricin A chain known from other studies to create side effects. Such artificially created virus systems have additional advantages, since they can be produced carrying a range of different therapeutic cargoes that can all be targeted to

the same cell via attachment of the identical targeting signals. The result is the possibility of refined multidrug therapy without the problems associated with each component having differing pharmacokinetic properties.

An important and very intensively used additional application of the translational repression complex is in the three-hybrid assay system. Macromolecular interactions *in vivo* are central to understanding the integrated functions of all gene products. However, there are relatively few techniques that can easily be used to detect such interactions. One screen, known as the two-hybrid assay, was developed to detect protein–protein interactions using a simple genetic phenotypic screen. It works by creating two fusion proteins. The first carries the information to encode a DNA-binding protein domain fused to a 'bait' protein whose cellular partners are sought. The second fusion protein carries a series of potential partners for the bait domain translationally fused to a transcriptional activation domain. Both fusion constructs are expressed in yeast that carries a binding site for the DNA-binding domain in close proximity to a reporter gene inferring resistance to some chemical challenge, for example, an antibiotic or essential metabolite. Only in those yeast cells where bait and target interact will the transcriptional activation domain drive production of the essential reporter gene. All other cells will not grow. Recovery of the live cells and sequencing of the constructs they carry thus reveals potential partners of the protein–protein interaction *in vivo*, although there is known to be a rate of false positives.

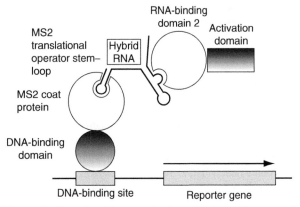

**Figure 4** Three-hybrid assay. A schematic view of the components of the three-hybrid assay for detecting RNA–protein interaction *in vivo*. A DNA-binding domain is fused to the MS2 coat protein (RNA-binding domain 1). A second potential RNA-binding domain (#2) is fused to a transcriptional activation domain. Hybrid RNAs carrying the MS2 translational operator stem–loop are also expressed in yeast cells carrying the DNA-binding target adjacent to a reporter gene. Reproduced from SenGupta DJ, Zhang B, Kraemer B, Pochart P, Fields S, and Wickens M (1996) A three-hybrid system to detect RNA-protein interactions *in vivo*. *Proceedings of the National Academy of Sciences, USA* 93(16): 8496–8501, Copyright (1996) National Academy of Sciences, USA.

In the three-hybrid variant of this approach, the protein–protein interaction is replaced by a protein–RNA interaction. This is achieved by fusing the DNA-binding domain to the MS2 coat protein, thus producing a tethered protein that will bind to RNAs carrying the translational operator site. The translational operator sequence is then embedded in transcripts that include other potential RNA-binding domains. The transcriptional activation domain is then expressed as fusions with potential binding partners for specific RNA sites (**Figure 4**). The end result is the same as for a two-hybrid assay. Only those yeast cells in which the hybrid RNA is bound by a fusion partner will survive and the RNA sequences and or binding partners can then be identified by sequencing.

*See also:* Replication of Bacterial Viruses.

## Further Reading

Caspar DLD and Klug A (1962) Physical principles in the construction of regular viruses. *Cold Spring Harbor Symposia on Quantitative Biology* 24: 1–24.

Paranchych W (1975) Attachment, ejection and penetration stages of the RNA phage infectious process. In: Zinder ND (ed.) *RNA Phages*, pp. 85–112. New York: Cold Spring Harbor Laboratory Press.

SenGupta DJ, Zhang B, Kraemer B, Pochart P, Fields S, and Wickens M (1996) A three-hybrid system to detect RNA–protein interactions *in vivo*. *Proceedings of the National Academy of Sciences, USA* 93: 8496–8501.

Stockley PG and Stonehouse NJ (1999) Virus assembly and morphogenesis. In: Russo VEA, Cove DJ, Edgar LG, Jaenisch R, and Salamini F (eds.) *Development: Genetics, Epigenetics, and Environmental Regulation*, pp. 3–20. Berlin: Springer.

Stockley PG, Stonehouse NJ, and Valegård K (1994) Molecular mechanism of RNA phage morphogenesis. *International Journal of Biochemistry* 26: 1249–1260.

Valegård K, Murray JB, Stockley PG, Stonehouse NJ, and Liljas L (1994) Crystal structure of a bacteriophage–RNA coat protein-operator complex. *Nature* 371: 623–626.

Valegård K, Murray JB, Stonehouse NJ, van den Worm S, Stockley PG, and Liljas L (1997) The three dimensional structures of two complexes between recombinant MS2 capsids and RNA operator fragments reveal sequence specific protein–RNA interactions. *Journal of Molecular Biology* 270: 724–738.

Van Duin J (1988) Single-stranded RNA bacteriophages. In: Calendar R (ed.) *The Bacteriophages*, pp. 117–167. New York: Plenum.

Watson JD, Hapkins NH, Roberts JW, Steltz JA, and Winer AM (1993) *Molecular Biology of the Gene, Vol. I: General Principle*, 5th edn. New Delhi: Pearson Education, Inc.

Witherell GW, Gott JM, and Uhlenbeck OC (1991) Specific interaction between RNA phage coat proteins and RNA. *Progress in Nucleic Acid Research and Molecular Biology* 40: 185–220.

Wu M, Sherwin T, Brown WL, and Stockley PG (2005) Delivery of antisense oligonucleotides to leukaemia cells by RNA bacteriophage capsids. Nanomedicine: Nanotechnology. *Biology and Medicine* 1: 67–76.

# Icosahedral Tailed dsDNA Bacterial Viruses

**R L Duda,** University of Pittsburgh, Pittsburgh, PA, USA

## Glossary

**Contractile tail** The tail type that defines the *Myoviridae*, composed of a baseplate that contacts the host surface, an outer protein cylinder or sheath, and an inner tail tube or core. When a host is bound the sheath contracts, driving the tube into the cell to deliver the genome to the host.

**DNA packaging** The energy-driven process by which a procapsid is filled by a phage chromosome to become a mature capsid.

**Head or capsid** The protein container for the *Caudovirales* phage genome, usually icosahedral in shape, that protects it from the environment until it is delivered to a new host.

**Horizontal gene exchange** Transfer of genetic material between different species.

**Portal** A grommet-like ring, composed of 12 copies of the portal protein, through which DNA is packaged and to which the tail is attached.

**Prohead or procapsid** An immature capsid that has a spherical shape and contains no DNA.

*T*-number The triangulation number ($T$) is a formal descriptor for complex icosahedral structures which describes the geometric arrangement of subunits for a viral capsid. The number of capsid protein subunits is $\sim 60 \times T$.

**Tail** The part of the virion responsible for attachment to the host and genome injection. This is attached to one vertex of the capsid, at the portal.

**Tail fiber** An elongated protein fiber attached to a phage tail that helps recognize a host by binding to the host by the tip of the fiber.

**Virion** The entire viral particle composed of a capsid containing the viral genome, tail, tail fibers, and other appendages.

## Introduction

The icosahedral, tailed double-stranded DNA (dsDNA) bacterial viruses or bacteriophages of the order *Caudovirales* are among the most widely recognized icons of modern molecular biology. Anyone who has participated in an advanced biology, genetics, or molecular biology class is likely to have been exposed to images of the familiar lunar-lander-shaped bacteriophage T4 virion (family *Myoviridae*) with its elongated icosahedral capsid and machine-like contractile tail (**Figure 1(a)**) or the plain icosahedral capsid and elegant, gently curving tail of bacteriophage λ (family *Siphoviridae*; **Figure 1(b)**). Both T4 and λ are bacteriophages that infect the enteric bacterial host *Escherichia coli* and have been studied extensively. Bacteriophages were originally discovered in the early twentieth century (1915–17) by English microbiologist Frederick W. Twort and French-Canadian microbiologist Felix d'Herelle. Although there was much early interest in bacteriophages because of their potential for use in treating bacterial diseases (phage therapy), research on bacteriophages for disease therapy was largely abandoned after the discovery of antibiotics. Bacteriophage research was revived in the 1940s by Max Delbrück and colleagues (the well-known Phage Group that often met at the Cold Spring Harbor Laboratories on Long Island, NY), and the focused phage research started by this group of scientists led to many fundamental biological discoveries during the birth of molecular biology. The modern-day emergence of multiply antibiotic-resistant strains of human pathogens has rekindled an interest in developing phage therapy as a means of treating human diseases.

## The Structure of Tailed dsDNA Bacteriophages

The invention and commercialization of the electron microscope led to the first images of phages as sperm-like particles with a head and tail using a technique called metal shadowing, in which images were formed by heavy metal atoms such as uranium that were evaporated in a vacuum and allowed to strike a dried specimen at an angle. The later introduction of negative stains (salts of heavy metals that dry as a thin layer without forming crystals and in which small particles such as phages could be embedded) for electron microscopy resulted in images that were far richer in detail than earlier methods and revealed the complexity and variety of phage morphology. **Figure 1** shows electron micrographs of phages T4 and λ made using the negative stain technique. Electron microscopy has remained a major tool in the study of bacteriophages and, in fact, the current taxonomic system for phages relies heavily on phage morphology as determined by electron microscopy as a major discriminating factor. **Table 1** shows a taxonomic table for the order *Caudovirales* and some of their characteristics. Members of the *Myoviridae* have contractile tails and include bacteriophages T4 (**Figures 1(a)** and **2**) and P1. Members of the *Siphoviridae* have long noncontractile tails and include phages λ

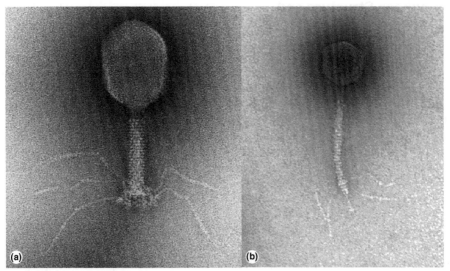

**Figure 1** Electron micrographs of bacteriophage T4 and bacteriophage λ (variant Ur-λ). (a) Negatively stained electron micrograph of bacteriophage T4, the prototypical member of the *Myoviridae*. The T4 tail is 100 nm long and the T4 head has a width of 85 nm. Many of the features labeled in **Figure 2** are visible in the micrograph, including the baseplate, tail sheath, whiskers, collar, and long tail fibers. (b) Negatively stained electron micrograph of bacteriophage λ. The micrograph is of an original isolate of λ, called Ur-λ, that has long side tail fibers. Most common laboratory strains of λ carry a mutation in the side tail fiber gene that eliminates the fibers from the particle. The length of the lambda tail is ∼150 nm (not including the protruding central fiber) and the lambda head is ∼63 nm in diameter.

**Table 1**     Tailed dsDNA bacteriophages: Order *Caudovirales*

| Family | Genus | Defining example | Capsid *T*-number | Genome size (bp) |
|---|---|---|---|---|
| *Myoviridae* (phages with contractile tails) | T4-like viruses | Enterobacteria phage T4 | $T = 13$; $Q = 20$ | 168 903 |
| | P1-like viruses | Enterobacteria phage P1 | $T = 13$? | 93 601 |
| | P2-like viruses | Enterobacteria phage P2 | $T = 7$ | 33 593 |
| | Mu-like viruses | Enterobacteria phage Mu | $T = 7$ | 36 717 |
| | SP01-like viruses | Bacillus phage SP01 | $T = 16$ | ~132 500 |
| | φ-H-like viruses | Halobacterium virus φH | $T = 7$? | ~57 000 |
| *Siphoviridae* (phages with thin noncontractile tails) | λ-like viruses | Enterobacteria phage λ | $T = 7$ | 48 502 |
| | T1-like viruses | Enterobacteria phage T1 | $T = 7$? | 48 836 |
| | T5-like viruses | Enterobacteria phage T5 | $T = 13$ | 121 750 |
| | c2-like viruses | Lactococcus phage c2 | $T = 4$?; $Q = 7$? | 22 172 |
| | L5-like viruses | Mycobacterium phage L5 | $T = 7$ | 52 297 |
| | ψM1-like viruses | Methanobacterium ψM1 | Unknown | ~23 246 |
| *Podoviridae* (phages with short stubby tails) | T7-like viruses | Enterobacteria phage T7 | $T = 7$ | 39 937 |
| | φ-29-like viruses | Bacillus phage φ29 | $T = 3$; $Q = 5$ | 19 366 |
| | P22-like viruses | Enterobacteria phage P22 | $T = 7$ | 41 724 |

A ? denotes unknown or unconfirmed values.

(**Figure 1(b)**) and T5. Members of the *Podoviridae* have shorter stubby or stumpy tails and include phages P22 and T7. The utility of morphological classification as a basis for phage taxonomy has more recently come into question as new insights into phage evolution have revealed that horizontal exchange of genes is widespread among phages, and further that some structural genes of bacteriophages and viruses that infect organisms from other domains of life appear to share common ancestors.

## Tailed Bacteriophage Structure and Function

### Capsids

In the tailed dsDNA bacteriophages, the capsid is the container for the phage genome that protects it from the environment until it is delivered to a new host by the phage tail, the organelle of attachment and genome injection. In many other types of viruses, the capsid is taken up by cells with the genome still inside and the virus particle uncoats or disassembles within the new host to initiate viral replication. The dsDNA bacteriophages' capsids do not have to disassemble in this manner to initiate infection, so they can be constructed to be highly stable – resistant to a wide variety of chemical and physical assaults from the environment – as they travel from one host to another. The dsDNA genome in bacteriophage capsids is packed to a very high density ($\sim 0.5\,\mathrm{g\,ml}^{-1}$) which results in high pressure, so the capsid shell has to be strong enough to withstand the high internal pressure from DNA. Most members of the *Caudovirales* have symmetric icosahedral capsids, but some have capsids with an elongated icosahedral shape, like T4 (**Figures 1(a)** and **2**) that have icosahedral ends and an elongated tubular middle section.

## Tails and Tail Fibers

Phage tails function to identify and bind to the correct host and to deliver the phage genome into the new host to initiate replication. Phage tails have a large variety of morphological forms with many parts and appendages, such as those labeled on the diagram of T4 in **Figure 2** and visible in the electron micrograph in **Figure 1**. We know little about the functions of some tail parts, but others are understood in considerable detail. For example, in bacteriophage T4, both the long tail fibers and the short tail fibers (which are folded under the baseplate until after the long tail fibers are bound to the host; see **Figure 2**) recognize specific host receptors. The long tail fibers of phage T4 are the primary determinants of host range, and mutations that change the T4 host range cause alterations in the fibers near their distal tips. The whiskers that are attached to the top of the T4 tail have multiple functions. The whiskers act as assembly jigs for adding the long tail fibers to the virion, and they also act as environmental sensors that sequester the long tail fibers under unfavorable conditions and thus prevent attachment to a host.

The long tail fibers of T4 have an analog in bacteriophage λ, but in the ordinary laboratory strains of λ these fibers are not made because of a mutation in the side tail fiber gene. The electron micrograph in **Figure 1(b)** shows the long side tail fibers present on Ur-λ, a primordial λ that lacks this mutation. These long side tail fibers of Ur-λ speed up the adsorption of this phage to its host, but are not required for infection, because the primary interaction of λ with its host is mediated by the central tail fiber (a trimer of the tail protein gp*J*) protruding from the end of the lambda tail. The central tail fiber of λ binds to a host maltose transport protein (called *lam*B or *mal*B) in the outer membrane of the host. Binding of phage λ to its receptor under suitable conditions acts as a signal that

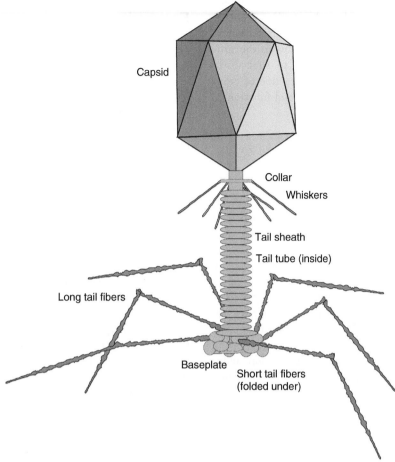

Capsid

Collar

Whiskers

Tail sheath

Tail tube (inside)

Long tail fibers

Baseplate

Short tail fibers
(folded under)

**Figure 2**  Schematic drawing of bacteriophage T4, with some of the structural components identified.

triggers the injection of the phage DNA genome into the host to initiate replication.

The structure and functions of many parts of the contractile tails of *Myoviridae* have been revealed in depth, especially for the phage T4 tail. After the T4 long tail fibers attach to the host, the short tail fibers unfold from the baseplate and bind to a second receptor on the host surface. The baseplate remains attached to the cell and undergoes a dramatic reorganization in which it changes from a hexagon to a star shape, causing the sheath to contract and drive the internal tail tube into the cell. As the nail-shaped tip of the inner tail tube passes through the outer membrane, tail lysozyme molecules are released to create a small hole in the cell wall peptidoglycan layer. These combined actions allow the tip of the tail tube to reach the inner membrane, where a channel is created that allows the dsDNA genome to enter the cell and initiate replication.

## Temperate versus Virulent Bacteriophages

Virulent bacteriophages, once they have infected a host, are committed to go through their entire growth cycle

including replication of the bacteriophage chromosome, production of progeny viral particles, and the lysis of the host cell. Temperate phages, on the other hand, are able to grow lytically like their virulent counterparts, but they are also capable of going into a dormant state within the host. This dormant state is called lysogeny, and often involves integration of the phage chromosome into the host chromosome, as occurs with phage λ, or conversion of the phage chromosome into an autonomously replicating plasmid. The seemingly normal host containing a dormant phage chromosome is called a lysogen. The dormant phage chromosome is maintained in a mostly silent state, until some change in the condition of the host (often related to stress, such as damage to the host DNA) acts as a signal to induce the phage to begin a lytic growth cycle, all the way through progeny release. The temperate phage in the lysogenic state makes a protein factor or repressor protein that can repress (nearly) all phage functions, except for the synthesis of the repressor. If the repressor is subsequently destroyed, as it may be after DNA damage occurs within the cell, the phage initiates a normal growth cycle, usually excising the phage chromosome from the host chromosome as an early step. How a temperate phage decides between a virulent and lysogenic mode of infection is a complex process that appears to depend on the conditions within the host cell at the time of infection. In a simplified version of the process, it is a balance between the production of sufficient repressor protein to shut down phage development and the antagonistic action of other factors that prevents repressor synthesis and function.

## Injection

### DNA Injection

As described above, all *Caudovirales* bacteriophage particles have tails consisting of highly specialized parts with specific roles to mediate attachment and infection. The fundamental goal of attachment is the introduction of the viral DNA into the host to begin production of progeny virions. The detailed mechanism of DNA entry varies widely from phage to phage. Although this process is called DNA injection, the phage particles do not act like syringes, as the name implies. In some cases it appears that chromosome entry is largely passive, a result of the DNA being very densely packed into the virion under very high DNA pressure. The energy stored by packaging the chromosome under pressure is used to drive the DNA out of the capsid into the host; this appears to be true for many phages, including phage T4 and phage λ. Other viruses such as phage T7 (family *Podoviridae*) and phage T5 (family *Siphoviridae*), have more elaborate mechanisms of DNA injection with an initial stage that appears to be largely passive, followed by a pause after only a fraction of the chromosome has been injected. Such paused DNA injection resumes only after proteins (encoded by the genes injected in the initial stage) act to restart chromosome entry or to pull the rest of the chromosome into the host in a controlled manner.

### Protein Injection

Many of these viruses inject both DNA and proteins into their hosts. The function of a few of these injected proteins is known, but in many cases remains mysterious. For example, phage T4 injects multiple copies of several proteins into the host. These include a protein that modifies the host RNA polymerase and other proteins of unknown function. Surprisingly, most of phage T4's injected proteins are not absolutely required for infection, and mutants that lack them are able to grow on many ordinary laboratory hosts. Phage T7 injects several large proteins that possibly play important roles in the injection process, for example, by forming channels for the passage of DNA and other proteins into the host. The injected proteins of phage T7 are essential for phage growth.

## Host Interactions and Regulation of Gene Expression

### Classes of Genes

A regulated program of gene expression begins soon after the virus has injected its DNA. The expression of phage genes can be divided by function, such as host takeover, replication, virion assembly, or lysis, but more often they are sorted by their temporal order of expression. In most cases gene expression is divided into early genes and late genes, although for some phages there may be a cascade of gene expression modes that occur sequentially. In a cascading series, early phage gene products control the expression of a set of middle gene products, which in turn control the expression of late genes.

### Early Genes

Phage early genes are usually transcribed by the normal host RNA polymerase, while the expression of late genes is dependent on the expression of the early genes. The earliest genes expressed might be ones that produce proteins to counteract the host's antibacteriophage defensive systems, as occurs in phage T7. Early genes of temperate phages are those required to make the decision to become dormant or to grow normally and carry out the first steps of these processes, including, for example, the repressor gene and integration genes, or DNA replication and recombination genes. Early genes of virulent bacteriophages, such as phage T4, include genes for genome replication and genes that shut down unneeded host functions, such as host transcription and host protein synthesis, and may include other genes required to recycle host resources, for example, by specifically degrading the host chromosome to intermediates that can be reused during the replication of the phage genome.

### Late Genes

The proteins encoded by the late genes include the structural proteins required for the assembly of the bacteriophage virion, as well as those needed for packaging the genome into the virion and for cell lysis. Late gene expression is often dependent on early (or middle) gene expression because the late genes have transcriptional promoters that are not recognized by the normal host polymerase. The early genes may direct the synthesis of transcription factors that either (1) change the specificity of the host RNA polymerase or (2) modify the polymerase in other ways, in order to express the whole set of late genes at the appropriate time with high efficiency. Alternatively, one of the early genes may encode for an entirely new RNA polymerase with a new specificity that recognizes late gene promoters. Expression of the structural proteins to high levels allows the production of a large number of progeny phages.

## Virion Assembly

### Assembly Pathways

The assembly of *Caudovirales* virions is a highly ordered process in which separate subassemblies of the virion are built and then joined to form the mature virion. The assembly of capsids, tails, and tail fibers each follows an independent assembly pathway in which individual protein components are added, usually sequentially, to a growing structure until it is complete.

### Tail Assembly

The major components of a *Caudovirales* tail are a baseplate or tail tip, major tail proteins (one for a noncontractile tail, and two for contractile tails (an inner tube protein and an outer sheath protein)), and termination or capping proteins to stabilize the completed tail and connect it to the head. Tail assembly begins with the formation of an initiator complex, which may be either a complete tail tip or a complete baseplate that is assembled via a separate pathway. The initiator complex includes a template that specifies the length of the tail, the tape measure protein complex in a compact form. The major tail proteins bind to the initiator complex and assemble into a tube around the tape measure protein until the full length of the tape measure protein is enclosed and the termination proteins can bind and stabilize the tail.

### Capsid Assembly

The capsids of these viruses are built as precursor procapsids, into which the phage genome is later packed. Procapsids are initially assembled from several types of components: a portal complex (which will connect the capsid to the tail), a major capsid protein, a scaffolding protein (which may be a separate protein or may be a disposable part of the major capsid protein), and decoration or stabilization proteins (which add to and stabilize the capsid only after the genome is packed inside). The number of capsid protein subunits needed for assembly is equal to $\sim 60 \times T$ subunits, where $T$ is the triangulation number listed in **Table 1** (or, for phages with elongated capsids, $\sim 30 \times (T + Q)$ subunits, where $T$ and $Q$ are specified in **Table 1**). So for a $T = 7$ virus, such as $\lambda$, $\sim 420$ copies are needed and more copies are needed for larger phages. Capsid assembly begins with the completion of the assembly initiator complex, usually the portal. The major capsid protein together with hundreds of copies of the scaffolding protein co-assembles onto the initiator to produce a complete shell with the scaffolding protein on the inside. After assembly is complete, the scaffolding protein is expelled intact or digested by a special protease that is also incorporated into the procapsid. Procapsids appear spherical and usually have a smaller diameter than mature capsids. When DNA is packaged into the procapsid, the capsid usually expands and changes shape, transforming into the typical angular, icosahedral shape of mature capsids. The decoration proteins add to the outside of the capsid after it expands and help to stabilize the structure. Once DNA is packaged, the capsid is made ready to join to a tail by the addition of proteins that bind to the portal.

## Lysis

Lysis of an infected host requires two phage-encoded protein factors, an endolysin or lysozyme, and a second protein called a holin. The endolysin is a soluble enzyme with the capacity to break the bonds holding the host cell wall together. The endolysin molecules accumulate within the host cytoplasm during the late stages of infection, but are unable to attack the cell wall because they are sequestered within the cytoplasmic membrane. Holin proteins allow the endolysin to get across the cytoplasmic membrane by forming holes in the inner membrane. Holins are synthesized and inserted into the membrane in a form that does not form holes at first. As the bacteriophage infection proceeds, the holins accumulate in the membrane until a predetermined time at which they suddenly and catastrophically induce membrane breakdown. The membrane holes produced by holins allow the endolysin molecules to attack the bacterial cell wall, causing rapid cell lysis and releasing the progeny virus from the cell.

## Genomes and Genomics

### Chromosome Diversity and Replication

The chromosomes that are packaged into the capsids of the *Caudovirales* are linear dsDNA. *Caudovirales* virions always contain an entire genome or slightly more than an entire genome to ensure that a complete genome is packaged into each and that every particle can initiate an infection. To achieve this, a site-specific mechanism may be used, in which DNA packaging begins and ends at defined sites that are recognized by the packaging machinery to create exactly unit-genome-length DNA chromosomes. Alternatively, the amount of virion DNA may be regulated by a head-full packaging mechanism which fills a capsid that has the capacity to hold slightly more than one genome's worth of DNA. The head-full-packaged chromosomes have the same sequence at each end and are said to be terminally redundant.

After injection, the phage genomes often rearrange to form a circular chromosome that is the primary replicative form of the genome of many dsDNA phages; however, many other phages replicate without forming such DNA circles. Chromosome replication often takes place bidirectionally from a single origin, but more complex replication schemes and multiple replication origins have also been observed. Late in infection, most phages switch to a mode of replication that produces DNA concatamers, or long strings of genome copies joined end to end, either by a rolling circle mode of replication from circular chromosomes, or by recombination between multiple overlapping genome copies. Such DNA concatamers, whether linear or branched, are the forms of the genome that are the usual substrate for DNA packaging for both head-full and site-specific mechanisms. When it does occur, circularization of the phage chromosome takes place via one of the two mechanisms. The first is by the annealing of complementary single-stranded DNA sticky ends left by the packaging enzymes (in the cases where the packaged chromosomes have defined endpoints). The second is by a recombination-like mechanism that joins the complementary regions of the overlapping, terminally redundant chromosome ends to form circular DNA molecules. Circular chromosomes are the most common form for bacterial chromosomes, but some bacteria also have linear chromosomes, and a small subset of members of this order also forms linear chromosomes that replicate as linear plasmids when in their lysogenic form.

## Diversity in Genome Size and Organization

The genomes of these viruses range in size from ~20 000 bp in phage $\phi$29, to ~170 000 bp in phage T4, and up to ~500 000 bp in other known examples. The smaller phages have proportionally fewer genes than the large phages, but are nonetheless functional and successful phages. Given this wide range of sizes and diversity of these viruses, it is not surprising that there is not a common conserved genome structure in the members of the order *Caudovirales*. Within a genus of phages there is often a common genetic structure, but within and across families there is often little resemblance in genome organization. There are notable exceptions to these generalizations; for example, the genus 'P22-like viruses' and the genus 'λ-like viruses' have rather closely related genomes.

## Common Themes in Genome Structure

Despite the differences mentioned, there are many common general features in *Caudovirales* genomes. The genes for the structural proteins, such as those for capsids, tails, or tail fibers, tend to be found clustered together, and within these clusters, the genes that encode proteins that physically interact with each other also tend to be grouped together. For example, the capsid protein genes for the portal, the scaffolding protein, and the major capsid protein usually occur together and in the order listed. Sets of late genes are often grouped together in clusters and, in some cases, the entire set of structural genes are grouped together in clusters and transcribed together from a single promoter, as is the case for phage λ.

## Horizontal Exchange of Genes Is Widespread

A large number of complete bacteriophage genomes have been fully sequenced, and hundreds of these have been deposited in GenBank and other databases. In addition, there are also many temperate phages residing in the genomes of bacterial chromosomes – some defective (or cryptic), and some complete and able to form a viable phage. Analyses of the sequences of these genomes have shown that many of the genes have highly similar counterparts in other genomes and in many cases the similarity can be inferred to be truly homologous. An important conclusion of these analyses is that there is extensive horizontal exchange of genes between phages that are not within the same species or genus or order. It appears that genetic exchange between phages by both homologous and nonhomologous recombination mechanisms is widespread and that many phages are mosaic combinations of genes found elsewhere. Many of the homologous arise genes within the *Caudovirales*, but some are from outside this order. In some cases, large modules of genes in a pair of phages are closely related (e.g., the head genes of phage HK97 (*Siphoviridae*) and phage SfV (*Myoviridae*)) despite belonging to different taxonomic groups. In other cases, a single phage tail fiber encoding gene in one phage may contain several distinct regions of homology with several other different phages.

## Common Ancestry

The exact nature of the evolutionary relationships among phages and how it relates to phage taxonomy is a controversial subject, but at the level of individual protein-coding genes, it is fairly certain that proteins with a high degree of sequence similarity in analogous proteins almost certainly share a common evolutionary ancestor. The power and utility of bioinformatics to tease out weak (sequence) similarities between distantly related proteins provides the evolutionary scientist powerful tools to detect relationships that escape casual examination. However, the reliance on sequence similarity matches to detect homologous relationships breaks down when homologous proteins have diverged so far that sequence similarity is undetectable. A notable case is that of the major capsid proteins of bacteriophages and other viruses. The three-dimensional structure and protein fold of the major capsid protein of phage HK97 was determined to high resolution by X-ray crystallography. Sensitive bioinformatic techniques were able to detect weak sequence similarities between the HK97 capsid protein sequence and the capsid proteins of a large number of other members of the *Caudovirales*, suggesting that the HK97 capsid protein fold is quite common. Subsequently, the determination of the protein folds of phages T4 (*Myoviridae*), P22, ϕ29, and ε15 (*Podoviridae*) by structural methods has shown that all of these phages also have the same protein fold as HK97, despite the lack of any detectable sequence similarity.

*See also:* Replication of Bacterial Viruses; Virus Evolution: Bacterial Viruses.

## Further Reading

Cairns J, Stent GS, and Watson JD (eds.) (1992) *Phage and the Origins of Molecular Biology*, expanded edition. Cold Spring Harbor, New York: Cold Spring Harbor Laboratory Press.

Calendar R (ed.) (2006) *The Bacteriophages*, 2nd edn. Oxford: Oxford University Press.

Caspar DL and Klug A (1962) Physical principles in the construction of regular viruses. *Cold Spring Harbor Symposium on Quantitative Biology* 27: 1–24.

Hendrix RW (2003) Bacteriophage genomics. *Current Opinion in Microbiology* 6: 506–511.

Hendrix RW and Casjens S (1988) Control mechanisms in dsDNA bacteriophage assembly. In: Calendar R (ed.) *The Bacteriophages*. New York: Plenum.

Hendrix RW and Duda RL (1998) Bacteriophage HK97 head assembly: A protein ballet. *Advances in Virus Research* 50: 235–288.

Hendrix RW, Roberts JW, Stahl FW, and Weisberg RA (1983) *Lambda II*. Cold Spring Harbor, New York: Cold Spring Harbor Laboratory Press.

Karam JD, Drake JW, Kreuzer KN, *et al.* (eds.) (1994) *Molecular Biology of Bacteriophage T4*. Washington, DC: ASM Press.

Katsura I (1990) Mechanism of length determination in bacteriophage lambda tails. *Advances in Biophysics* 26: 1–18.

Leiman PG, Kanamaru S, Mesyanzhinov VV, Arisaka F, and Rossmann MG (2003) Structure and morphogenesis of bacteriophage T4. *Cellular and Molecular Life Sciences* 60: 2356–2370.

# Replication of Bacterial Viruses

**M Salas and M de Vega,** Universidad Autónoma, Madrid, Spain

## Glossary

**Lagging strand** DNA strand synthesized as a series of 5′–3′ DNA fragments that are finally joined together to create an intact DNA strand.

**Leading strand** DNA strand whose synthesis proceeds continuously in the 5′–3′ direction as the parental duplex is unwound.

**Sliding-back mechanism** For linear chromosomes containing a terminal protein at their 5′-ends; initiation of DNA replication by which the DNA polymerase uses as template an internal 3′-end nucleotide, with the subsequent sliding of the initiation complex formed to recover the 3′-end terminal nucleotide information.

**Okazaki fragment** Short fragment of newly replicated DNA (with an RNA primer at the 5′-terminus) produced during discontinuous replication of the lagging strand.

**O-some** A first-stage initiation complex formed by the binding of lambda protein O to 100 bp of DNA close to the AT rich region of the DNA replication origin.

**Processive polymerization** Polymerization that takes place without dissociation of the DNA polymerase from the DNA.

**Procesivity factor** An accessory subunit of DNA polymerases that act to increase the processivity of polymerization.

**Replisome** The DNA-replicating structure at the replication fork consisting of two replicative DNA polymerases and a primosome.

**Primosome** A protein complex formed by a primase and a helicase that initiates synthesis of RNA primers on the lagging DNA strand during DNA replication.

**Preprimosome** For several replication systems, a protein complex assembled at the replication origin before the binding of the primase.

**Transpososome** The Mu transpososome refers to the Mu transposase protein complex and the three DNA segments bound by this protein complex.

**σ replication mode** For circular DNA, it refers to replication performed by a rolling circle mechanism.

**θ (theta) replication mode** For circular DNA, it occurs when two replication forks move in opposite directions from the replication origin, leading to a bidirectional replication mode.

## Introduction

The requirement of a DNA/RNA molecule to prime DNA synthesis imposes replication strategies that avoid the loss of genetic information contained at the 5′-end of the lagging strand. Double-stranded (ds) DNA phages have developed different mechanisms to overcome such a problem by yielding head–tail concatemers, dependent on the presence of terminal redundancies, as in phages T4, T7, and SPP1, or on the circularization and further rolling circle replication, as occurs in phage λ. Several phages, such as φ29, have evolved to use a protein to prime DNA synthesis from each genome end, the priming protein becoming covalently linked to the 5′-ends of the genome. In other cases, as in phage Mu, replication of dsDNA depends on its capacity to be integrated into the host genome, replicating as a transposable element. The 5′-replication quandary does not exist in circular single-stranded (ss) DNA phages, such as φX174, which is replicated by a looped rolling circle to produce circular unit length genomes. In the case of ss- and dsRNA phages no such a problem exists since there is specific recognition by the RNA polymerase of the 3′-end of the template RNA. In addition, in phages λ, SPP1, or φX174, the replication of their genomes requires the presence of the host replication machinery, while others such as T4, T7, and φ29 use their own replication machinery.

In this article, we summarize the different replication strategies used by some of the well-studied phages.

## Replication of dsDNA Phages

### DNA Replication of Lamboid Phages

Bacteriophage λ has served as an important model system to elucidate part of the molecular mechanisms underlying eukaryotic and viral DNA replication. The virion particle contains a 48 502 bp linear dsDNA with a single-stranded protruding region, 12 bases long at each 5′-end, complementary to each other. Early after infection of its host *Escherichia coli*, the genome is circularized by means of the complementarity of the above-mentioned 5′-ends, and ligated by a host DNA ligase. Initiation of λ DNA replication requires the products of the early transcribed genes *O* and *P*, in addition to several functions from the host. Four homodimers of protein O bind to four 18 bp long binding sites at the λ replication origin. Through protein–protein interactions, the O dimers are brought together to form the O-some complex, promoting the further melting of an adjacent AT-rich region. The O-some prepares the λ replication origin for binding the host helicase DnaB. DnaB forms a heterodimer with λ protein P, which inhibits DnaB activity bringing it to the replication origin. Host proteins DnaJ, DnaK, and GrpE lead to disassembly of the preprimosome complex, releasing protein P and triggering replication fork movement. At early stages after infection, two DnaB copies unwind the DNA in opposite directions leading to a bidirectional θ (theta) replication mode. Such bidirectionality depends

on the transcription activation from promoter $P_R$ (transcriptional activation of *ori*λ), positively controlled by DnaA. At later stages, several DNA molecules start replicating following a σ mode (rolling circle replication) producing long concatemers of λ DNA containing more than 10 genome copies, which are cut at specific sites (*cos* sites) to yield unit length genomes with protruding (cohesive) 5′-ends that will be packaged into the virions. There is uncertainty about the process that governs the switch from θ to σ replication mode, the establishment of the σ replication mode being preceded by a round of unidirectional θ replication. Recent investigations point to the positive control of $P_R$ promoter activity by bacterial DnaA in triggering such a switch. Thus, as the number of genome copies increases, free DnaA is titrated out due to its interaction with the DnaA-binding sites in λ DNA. It has been proposed that this may lead to inefficient *ori*λ transcriptional activation, leading to unidirectional θ replication followed by σ replication mode.

## DNA Replication of Phage SPP1

SPP1 bacteriophage which infects *Bacillus subtilis* is one of the best-studied phages infecting Gram-positive bacteria. Its genome is dsDNA 44 007 bp long, partially circularly permuted with a terminal redundancy of 4%. SPP1 DNA replication depends partly on several replicative proteins from its host, such as the replicative DNA polymerase III and DnaG primase. As in the case of λ phage, SPP1 starts replication following a θ replication mode followed by a σ pathway. SPP1 protein gp38 binds to *ori*L inducing a local unwinding of an adjacent AT-rich sequence. The ssDNA generated is protected by gp36, the SPP1 ssDNA binding protein (SSB). As occurs with λ DNA replication, the helicase gp40 is loaded at the replication bubble by the helicase loader gp39 that inhibits the helicase activity of gp40. gp39 interacts with gp38 forming a heterodimer that is released from the replication origin, ceasing the inactivation of gp40 that now can exert its helicase activity. Later, the primase activity of the host DnaG is required to prime DNA synthesis by the host DNA polymerase III, the replication proceeding in only one direction. The formation of concatemeric molecules requires a switch from the θ mode to σ replication mode. Such a switch is mediated by gp38 which, after one or few rounds of θ-type replication, binds to *ori*L blocking progression of DNA replication. A subsequent nick either in the lagging or the leading strand will provide a 3′ ssDNA tail. In the latter case, a previous processing by gp34 5′–3′ exonuclease is needed. The 3′-OH end can pair with the open *ori*L of other DNA molecule and prime σ replication to generate concatemeric DNA molecules. Further encapsidation is started by cleavage at the *pac* sequence by the terminase small subunit gp1, followed by translocation of the concatemer to the interior of the procapsid.

## DNA Replication of T4-Like Phages

The serologically related *E. coli* infecting bacteriophages T2, T4, and T6 are commonly called T-even phages. They have a dsDNA genome 170 kbp long whose termini contain repetitions of 3% of the genome. In addition, the genome of T-even phages contains glucosylated hydroxy-methylcytosines that protect DNA from endonucleases and confer double-strand stability. The T-even phages encode for their own replication machinery, which makes them good candidates to study the general mechanism of DNA replication.

At early stages after infection, T4 DNA replication starts from only one replication origin. The T4 helicase/primase complex (gp41/gp61), loaded on to DNA by T4 gp59, moves processively in the 5′–3′ direction in lagging strand synthesis at the same time as the primase activity periodically synthesizes the RNA primers to initiate Okazaki fragment synthesis. Leading strand synthesis is initiated by an RNA molecule synthesized by a host RNA polymerase from early or middle promoters. DNA polymerase (gp43) catalyzes DNA synthesis of both strands assisted by gp45, a trimer that acts as a sliding clamp, holding the DNA polymerase tightly to the DNA. gp44/gp62 complex uses the hydrolysis of ATP to drive the binding of gp45 to DNA. Although T4 DNA replication onset depends on the replication origin, most of T4 DNA replication forks are initiated by using intermediates of recombination as DNA primers at random positions throughout the genome. Once the replication fork reaches the 3′-end, the single-stranded portion of the chain that is templating lagging strand synthesis invades an homology region in other DNA molecules because of the terminal redundancy of its ends, accomplishing a recombination-dependent DNA replication pathway called 'join-copy replication', that depends on genes expressed from early or middle promoters, and that is initiated from the invading 3′ DNA ends. This promotes the appearance of replicating DNA intermediates containing multiple covalently linked copies of the genome. When an endonuclease cuts at either of the invaded DNA strands, 'join-cut-copy recombination' is initiated from the 3′-ends to allow copying of single-stranded segments of an invading DNA. This pathway requires the action of either endo VII or terminase proteins, predominantely synthesized at late infection times, making the join-cut-copy the late pathway for DNA replication, since origin initiation of replication ceases during T4 development (**Figure 1**).

## DNA Replication of T7-Like Phages

T7-like phages belong to the family *Podoviridae*. These phages code for a specific RNA polymerase resistant to rifampicine and specific for phage promoters. Phage T7 is the model member of this group of lytic phages.

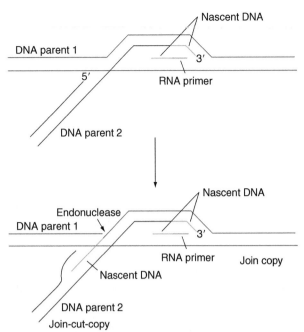

**Figure 1** Initiation of DNA replication from intermediates of homologous recombination. Figure shows how ssDNA end of parent 2 invades the homologous dsDNA of parent 1. Reproduced from Mosig G, Gewing J, Luder A, Colowick N, and Vo D (2001) Two recombination-dependent DNA replication pathways of bacteriophage T4, and their roles in mutagenesis and horizontal gene transfer. *Proceedings of the National Academy of Sciences, USA* 98: 8306–8311, copyright (2001) National Academy of Sciences, USA, with permission from National Academy of Sciences.

T7 contains a linear dsDNA 39 937 bp long with a terminal direct repetition 160 bp long, used to form concatemers during replication. This terminal repeat is different in both length and sequence in the different T7-like phages. T7 encodes for its own replication machinery and this fact has been used to study protein–protein interactions at the replication fork. Bacteriophage T7 genome is replicated as a linear monomer from replication origins in a bidirectional way at early stages after infection. The primary origin of replication is an AT-rich region (78% A+T) located downstream of φ1.1A and φ1.1B promoters. These promoters are used by T7 RNA polymerase to initiate synthesis of RNA to prime leading strand synthesis. However, alternative replication origins may exist since in the absence of T7 primase, more than 20 RNA–DNA transition sites have been detected, scattered widely downstream from the φ1.1 promoter and mostly downstream from the φ1.3 promoter. In addition, secondary replication origins have been mapped close to the left genome end by using deletion mutants lacking T7 *ori*. To accomplish T7 genome replication, the phage synthesizes four replication proteins: (1) T7 RNA polymerase (gp1), which synthesizes the RNA primer to the leading strand; (2) T7 helicase/primase (gp4) which performs two activities. On the one hand, its C-terminal half contains a helicase activity that uses the hydrolysis of dTTP to unwind duplex DNA in a 5′–3′ direction with respect to the bound strand. This part of the protein physically interacts with T7 DNA polymerase. On the other hand, the N-terminal half contains a primase activity that catalyzes the synthesis of tetraribonucleotides to function as primers for Okazaki fragments synthesis; (3) T7 DNA polymerase (gp5) that contains both a 5′–3′ synthetic activity and a 3′–5′ exonuclease activity to proofread replication errors. T7 DNA polymerase is a distributive enzyme *per se*; however, *in vivo* it forms a complex with *E. coli* thioredoxin, a protein used by the polymerase as a processivity factor; (4) T7 ssDNA binding protein (gp2.5) that interacts physically with T7 DNA polymerase and primase/helicase. This protein is required for the coordinated synthesis of both leading and lagging strands of the replication fork. This SSB protein coats the ssDNA template of the lagging strand participating in mowing the polymerase from the end of one Okazaki fragment to the initiation site for the next.

Once the replication fork has reached the end of the linear molecule, the 3′-end of the strand used as template for lagging strand synthesis remains uncopied. By means of the terminal repeat sequences, several linear DNA molecules can anneal forming long concatemers containing from 10 to >100 genome equivalents. The concatemer will have a single copy of the terminal repeat between two genomes. Before the encapsidation of unit-length genomes, the terminal repeat sequence has to be duplicated. Many efforts have been done to elucidate the duplication mechanism. Two models have been proposed.

One involves the transcription through the terminal repeat of the concatemer, promoting a displaced strand suitable to be cut by an endonuclease and generating a 3′-OH end that can be used to prime DNA synthesis and replicate the terminal repeat. A dsDNA break performed by the T7 terminase complex at the right part of the terminal repeat will provide another 3′-end that will complete duplication of the terminal repeat, allowing the genome to be packaged (**Figure 2(a)**). The presence of a palindromic sequence at the left part of the terminal repeat led to the proposal of an alternative model, invoking the formation of a cruciform structure followed by nicking by an unknown nuclease at a palindromic sequence, creating a hairpin primer for DNA polymerase, that once extended through the terminal repeat and into the genome will provide dsDNA that could be converted into mature left end. Primase initiated synthesis on the displaced strand will proceed through the terminal repeat, generating a mature right end of the next genome to be packaged (**Figure 2(b)**). Probably, both (or more) pathways could coexist to promote T7 DNA encapsidation and the yield of mature viral particles.

## Bacteriophages with Terminal Protein at the 5′ DNA Ends

Bacteriophage φ29 which is a member of the family *Podoviridae* has a linear dsDNA 19 285 bp long, with a specific protein (product of the viral gene 3) covalently linked to the two 5′-ends called terminal protein (TP). The protein contains 266 amino acids and is linked to the

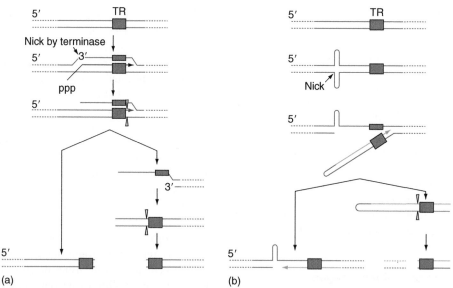

(a)                                         (b)

**Figure 2** Mechanism for TR duplication. (a) Model involving the transcription through the terminal repeat of the concatemer. (b) The palindromic model. See text for details. (a) Adapted from Fujisawa H and Morita M (1997) Phage DNA packaging. *Genes to Cells 2*: 537–547, with permission from Blackwell Publishing. (b) Reproduced from Chung YB, Nardone C, and Hinkle DC (1990) Bacteriophage T7 DNA packaging III. A "hairpin" end formed on T7 concatemers may be an intermediate in the processing reaction. *Journal of Molecular Biology* 216: 939–948, with permission from Elsevier.

DNA through a phosphoester bond between the OH group of serine 232 in the TP and 5'-dAMP.

Other *B. subtilis* phages related to φ29 that also contain linear dsDNA and TP of similar size are classified in three groups: (1) φ15, PZA, and PZE that belong to the φ29 group; (2) Nf, M2, and B103; and (3) GA-1. The DNA of all these phages have a short inverted terminal repeat (ITR), six nucleotides long (AAAGTA) for φ29, φ15, PZA, and B103, eight nucleotides long (AAAGTAAG) for Nf and M2, and seven nucleotides long (AAATAGA) for GA-1, all of them showing a reiteration AAA at their 5' DNA ends. PRD1, a member of the family *Tectiviridae* of lipid-containing phages infecting *E. coli* and other Gram-negative bacteria, contains a linear dsDNA 14 925 bp long, whose 5'-termini are linked to a 28 kDa TP by a phosphoester bond between tyrosine 190 and 5'-dGMP. The DNA of PRD1 and related phages have a 110 bp long ITR with the reiteration 5' GGGG at the ends. The *Streptococcus pneumoniae* phage Cp-1 contains a 19 345 bp linear dsDNA with a TP of 28 kDa covalently linked to the 5' DNA ends by a phosphoester bond between the OH group of threonine and 5'-dAMP. Cp-1 has an ITR of 236 bp with the reiteration 5' AAA.

In all of the above-mentioned phages, the origins of replication are located at both ends of the linear genome and are specifically recognized by their cognate replication machinery, encoded by the phage, to initiate DNA replication.

Much work has been performed to elucidate the replication mechanism of these phages, the most studied case being bacteriophage φ29. DNA polymerase from phage φ29 forms, with a free TP, a heterodimer (**Figure 3(a)**) that specifically recognizes both replication origins. The DNA polymerase catalyzes the template-directed formation of a covalent linkage between dAMP and the OH group of serine 232 of the primer TP, giving rise to the TP–dAMP initiation complex, a reaction directed by the penultimate nucleotide of the 3' reiteration (3'TTT...5') and stimulated by the φ29-encoded protein p6. The TP–dAMP complex slides-back one position to recover the terminal nucleotide, the second 3'-terminal nucleotide acting again as template to direct the incorporation of the second dAMP residue. It has also been shown that phage GA-1 DNA initiates replication at the second nucleotide from the 3' DNA end. Since the TP–dAMP covalent complex is not a substrate of the 3'–5' exonuclease proofreading activity of the φ29 DNA polymerase, the sliding-back mechanism could provide a way to ensure the fidelity of the initiation reaction. Terminal reiteration also exists in PRD1 and Cp-1 DNAs. Indeed, it was shown that initiation of PRD1 and Cp-1 DNA replication occurs at the fourth and third 3'-terminal nucleotide of the

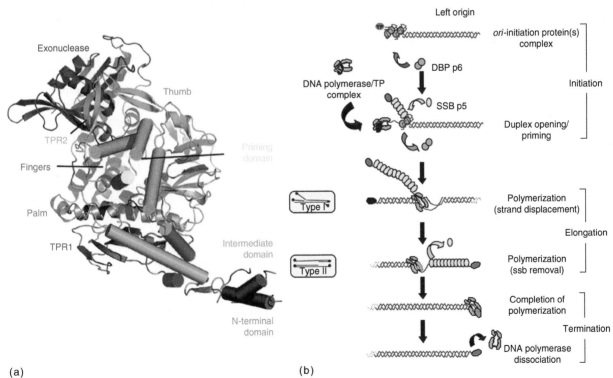

(a)                                    (b)

**Figure 3** (a) Structure of the φ29 DNA polymerase-terminal protein heterodimer. Ribbon representation of DNA polymerase colored by subdomains and terminal protein shown with cylindrical helices. (b) Schematic representation of bacteriophage φ29 TP-DNA replication. (a) Adapted from Kamtekar S, Berman AJ, Wang J, *et al.* (2006) The φ29 DNA polymerase: protein-primer structure suggests a model for the initiation to elongation transition. *EMBO Journal* 25: 1335–1343, with permission from Nature Publishing Group. (b) With permission, from the Annual Review of Biochemistry, Volume 60 © 1991 by Annual Reviews.

template, respectively. In these cases, a stepwise sliding-back mechanism has been proposed. It is likely that internal initiation and a sliding-back mechanism is a feature of the genomes that initiate replication by protein priming.

The φ29 DNA polymerase/primer TP heterodimer does not dissociate after initiation or after sliding back. There is a transition stage in which the DNA polymerase synthesizes a five nucleotide-long DNA molecule while complexed with the primer TP, undergoes some structural changes during incorporation of nucleotides 6–9 (transition), and finally dissociates from the primer TP when nucleotide 10 is incorporated into the nascent DNA chain (elongation mode).

Once dissociated from the heterodimer, the same DNA polymerase molecule starts normal DNA elongation, catalyzing highly processive polymerization coupled to strand displacement, and, therefore, complete replication of both strands proceeds continuously from each terminal-priming event. As the two replication forks move, DNA synthesis is initially coupled to strand displacement of long stretches of single-stranded φ29 DNA, producing type I replication intermediates (**Figure 3(b)**). When the two replication forks, moving in opposite directions, meet, a new type of replication intermediate (type II) is found. Electron microscopy analysis of φ29 replication intermediates *in vitro* showed that the viral protein p5 binds to the single-stranded portion of both type I and II molecules, thus acting as a SSB during φ29 DNA replication. Once replication of both strands is fulfilled, the two DNA polymerase molecules fall off the DNA to start initiation and replication of a new φ29 DNA molecule.

φ29 DNA replication takes place in close association with the bacterial membrane. Recent studies have identified p1 and p16.7 as membrane-localized, phage-encoded proteins likely to be involved in the membrane association of φ29 DNA replication. A multimeric p1 structure would provide an anchoring site for viral replisome through interaction with the primer TP, while p16.7 would recruit the φ29 DNA replication intermediates to the membrane by binding both the parental TP and the displaced ssDNA.

## Bacteriophage Mu

*E. coli* phage Mu, a member of the family *Myoviridae*, is of great interest because it is both a bacteriophage and a transposon. The size of its linear dsDNA ranges between 37 and 42 kbp with a mean value of 36.7 kbp. The variability of its length is due to the presence of 50–150 bp and 0.5–3 kbp of host genome flanking the left and right ends of the viral genome, respectively. Once Mu has infected the host cell, the linear DNA is converted into a circular form, induced by the phage protein N that is noncovalently bound to Mu DNA. The early phage protein A (transposase) specifically inserts the viral genome in a random fashion into the host chromosome, through the

genomic sequences *att*L and *att*R located at both ends of the viral DNA, following a 'nick-join-process' pathway by which the host sequences, still attached to Mu upon integration, are degraded shortly after, probably by gap repair mechanisms. Bacteriophage Mu replicates as a transposable element. Mu A protein remains bound to the Mu genome once inserted into the host genome, forming an oligomeric transpososome which promotes the transfer of the viral ends to other location of the host DNA, creating replication forks at each end. Host ClpX chaperonin reduces transpososome interaction with the DNA to promote the assembly of prereplisome. Later, primosome assembly protein PriA binds to the forked DNA structures and recruits PriB, DnaT, DnaB, and DnaC. PriA opens the dsDNA for DnaB binding that leads to the recruitment of DNA polymerase III holoenzyme to complete replisome assembly. In addition, DnaB attracts primase to catalyze lagging strand synthesis. The repetition of this integration process produces more than 100 copies of Mu DNA. Finally, these copies are cut at the *pac* sequence, located at the left end. The DNA is cut in a way that 50–150 bp of bacterial DNA at the left end are encapsidated in the phage particle. The total length of the encapsidated DNA depends on the size of the phage head, in a way that 0.5–3 kbp of host genome will flank the right end.

## φX174 and Related Phages

φX174 and related a3, St1, and G4 bacteriophages are members of the viral family *Microviridae*. All of them grow on various strains and species of *Enterobacteriaceae*, typically *E. coli*, *Salmonella*, and *Shigella* species. They contain a circular (+) ssDNA genome whose replication has been widely studied in phage φX174. The replication cycle can be divided into three stages.

*Stage I.* Once inside the host cell, the circular ssDNA is covered by the SSB protein, before starting the complementary (−)-strand synthesis. Different members of this group of phages exploit different host enzyme systems for complementary strand synthesis when ssDNA is complexed with SSB. Once covered by SSB, the assembly of preprimosome is carried out. The preprimosome is constituted by proteins PriA, PriB, PriC, DnaT, and DnaB. PriA recognizes the unique sequence *pas*, also called *n′*, that forms a stem–loop structure. PriB and PriC act as stability and specificity factors. DnaT and DnaC load the host helicase DnaB. The preprimosome associates with the host primase DnaG to produce the primosome. Such a complex travels on ssDNA following a 5′- to 3′-direction, with the concomitant synthesis of short RNA molecules by DnaG to prime DNA synthesis by host DNA polymerase III holoenzyme. Host DNA polymerase I removes RNA primers and a DNA ligase ligates the different DNA fragments to produce a circular and supercoiled dsDNA (replicative form I; RFI). The stem loops of other phages such as G4, a3, and St-1 are directly recognized by DnaG primase without the need for auxiliary proteins.

*Stage II.* Phage protein A nicks between (+)-strand nucleotides 4305 and 4306 at the replication origin (30 bp long), releasing the superhelicity of the DNA molecule to give replicative form II (RFII) DNA molecules. Protein A creates a covalent ester linkage between a tyrosine residue and the 5′-phosphate group of adenylic acid at position 4306 of viral (+)-strand. Host rep protein (helicase) forms a complex with protein A, unwinding the two strands of the duplex. In a coordinated way, DNA polymerase III holoenzyme uses the newly generated (+)-strand 3′-OH to prime the synthesis of a new (+)-strand. The 5′-end of the displaced strand travels with the replication fork in a 'looped rolling circle' way. Once the preprimosome assembly site on the displaced SSB-coated (+)-strand is available, synthesis of a new (−)-strand takes place as in stage I to give more RFI molecules that will be used as templates in further replication cycles. After one round of rolling circle synthesis, protein A cuts the newly generated replication origin, acting as a ligase to give circular (+) ssDNA molecules, protein A being transferred to the newly created 5′-end setting the stage for a new round of replication.

*Stage III.* GpC protein binds to gpA/rep/ RFII complex, enabling them to serve as template in further RF replication rounds, forcing them to be used as template for the unique generation of (+) ssDNA molecules, that will be encapsidated later.

## ss- and dsRNA Phages

The ssRNA coliphages form the family *Leviviridae*, of which the Qβ and MS2 bacteriophages are the best-studied members. Their infection depends on *E. coli* F-pili, normally used for bacterial conjugation. The genome of these phages is an ssRNA molecule with a length ranging from 3500 to 4200 nucleotides, depending on the genera. The viral (+) RNA molecule, once inside the cell, functions as messenger RNA for synthesis of phage proteins, and as template for viral replicase to multiply the viral genome. The high degree of secondary structure shown by the RNA plays a pivotal role in the fine-tuned coordination between translation (which proceeds in the 5′–3′ direction of RNA) and replication (which advances in the opposite direction), which is required to prevent a head to head collision of ribosomes and phage replicase.

To replicate their genome, ssRNA phages make use of a replicase that is composed of four proteins, only one of which coded by the phage (the replicase or β-subunit). The other three are encoded by the host: ribosomal S1 (α-subunit), and translation elongation factors EF-Tu and EF-Ts (γ- and δ-subunits, respectively). The copy of (+) ssRNA into (−) ssRNA requires also the product of the host *hfq* gene, the host factor HF. The 3′-end of (+) RNA is protected against host RNase E and other exonucleases by base pairing. This implies that the terminal nucleotides are also inaccessible to the ribosome and replicase, and suggests that S1 and HF are required. S1 is proposed to anchor the template on the polymerase in a standby complex, waiting for the occasional thermal breathing of the 3′-region, such an opening being assisted by HF. The translation elongation factors bind the RNA to the polymerase. Under such conditions, replicase initiates (−) RNA synthesis at the penultimate 3′-terminal C nucleotide, initially losing the ultimate A. Once replicase reaches the 5′-end of the (+) RNA, the terminal A nucleotide is recovered by an untemplated addition of an A at the 3′-end of the (−)-RNA. Although both (+)- and (−)-RNA chains are complementary, they do not anneal to form dsRNA. Such annealing is inhibited by the high degree of internal secondary structure formed in each ssRNA molecule. The (−)-ssRNA is used as a template to produce more (+)-ssRNA.

Members of the family *Cystoviridae* contain genomes composed of three dsRNA segments called S, L, and M. From this family, phages ø6, and more recently ø8, have been studied in great detail. Once the host cell is infected by these viruses, a transcriptionally active polymerase complex is released into the bacterial cytoplasm, where transcription of the dsRNA segments takes place. The L segment messenger RNA codes for proteins P1 (main component of the inner shell), P2 (RNA-dependent RNA polymerase), P4 (NTPase), P7 (involved in packaging and replication), and P14. The first four proteins form a polymerase complex which packages the three ssRNA(+)-strands. Such strands have an 18-base consensus sequence at their 5′-ends, and a *pac* sequence 200 bases long. Both the consensus and *pac* sequences are required and sufficient to package plus strands. The ssRNA(+) strands are packaged in a S, M, and L fashion. Once packaged within the viral particle, the polymerase complex synthesizes the minus RNA strand to convert the ssRNA into dsRNA.

*See also:* Icosahedral dsDNA Bacterial Viruses with an Internal Membrane; Icosahedral Enveloped dsRNA Bacterial Viruses; Icosahedral ssDNA Bacterial Viruses; Icosahedral ssRNA Bacterial Viruses; Icosahedral Tailed dsDNA Bacterial Viruses.

## Further Reading

Au TK, Agrawal P, and Harshey RM (2006) Chromosomal integration mechanism of infecting Mu virion DNA. *Journal of Bacteriology* 188: 1829–1834.

Bamford DH (1999) Phage ø6. In: Granoff A and Webster RG (eds.) *Encyclopedia of Virology,* 2nd edn., pp. 1205–1208. San Diego, CA: Academic Press.

Barariska S, Gabig M, Wegrzyn A, *et al.* (2001) Regulation of the switch from early to late bacteriophage λ DNA replication. *Microbiology* 147: 535–547.

Chung YB, Nardone C, and Hinkle DC (1990) Bacteriophage T7 DNA packaging III. A ''hairpin'' end formed on T7 concatemers may be an intermediate in the processing reaction. *Journal of Molecular Biology* 216: 939–948.

Fujisawa H and Morita M (1997) Phage DNA packaging. *Genes to cells* 2: 537–547.

Jiang H, Yang J-Y, and Harshey RM (1999) Criss-crossed interactions between the enhancer and the *att* sites of phage Mu during DNA transposition. *EMBO Journal* 18: 3845–3855.

Kamtekar S, Berman AJ, Wang J, *et al.* (2006) The φ29 DNA polymerase: Protein-primer stucture suggests a model for the initiation to elongation transition. *EMBO Journal* 25: 1335–1343.

Martínez-Jiménez MI, Alonso JC, and Ayora S (2005) *Bacillus subtilis* bacteriophage SPP1-encoded gene 34.1 product is a recombination-dependent DNA replication protein. *Journal of Molecular Biology* 351: 1007–1019.

Miller ES, Kutter E, Mossig G, Arisaka F, Kunisawa T, and Rüger W (2003) Bacteriophage T4 genome. *Microbiology and Molecular Biology Reviews* 67: 86–156.

Molineux IJ (2006) The T7 goup. In: Calendar R (ed.) *The Bacteriophages,* 2nd edn., pp. 277–301. Oxford: Oxford University Press.

Mosig G, Gewing J, Luder A, Colowick N, and Vo D (2001) Two recombination-dependent DNA replication pathways of bacteriophage T4, and their roles in mutagenesis and horizontal gene transfer. *Proceedings of the National Academy of Sciences, USA* 98: 8306–8311.

Nakai H, Doseeva V, and Jones JM (2001) Handoff from recombinase to replisome: Insights from transposition. *Proceedings of the National Academy of Sciences, USA* 98: 8247–8254.

Ng JY and Marians KJ (1996) The ordered assembly of the φX174-type primosome. I. Isolation and identification of intermediate protein-DNA complexes. *Journal of Biological Chemistry* 271: 15642–15648.

Ng JY and Marians KJ (1996) The ordered assembly of the φX174-type primosome. II. Preservation of primosome composition from assembly through replication. *Journal of Biological Chemistry* 271: 15649–15655.

Salas M (1991) Protein priming of DNA replication. *Annual Review of Biochemistry* 60: 39–71.

Salas M (1999) Mechanisms of initiation of linear DNA replication in prokaryotes. *Genetic Engineering (New York)* 21: 159–171.

Taylor K and Wegrzyn G (1999) Regulation of bacteriophage λ replication. In: Busby SJW, Thomas CM,, and Brown NL (eds.) *Molecular Microbiology*, pp. 81–97. Berlin: Springer.

Van Duin J and Tsareva N (2006) Single-stranded RNA phages. In: Calendar R (ed.) *The Bacteriophages,* 2nd edn., pp. 175–196. Oxford: Oxford University Press.

# Transcriptional Regulation in Bacteriophage

**R A Weisberg, D M Hinton, and S Adhya,** National Institutes of Health, Bethesda, MD, USA

Published by Elsevier Ltd.

## Introduction

Most bacteriophages regulate their own gene expression, many regulate host gene expression, and a few even regulate genes of other phages. Regulation enables temperate phages to establish and maintain lysogeny; it allows both temperate and virulent phages to carry out developmental programs in which groups of genes are expressed in an ordered, temporal sequence as their products are needed during the lytic growth cycle, and it helps phages to commandeer the transcriptional resources of their hosts. In this article we describe the biological roles and mechanisms of regulation employed by several extensively studied model phages of *Escherichia coli*: temperate phage λ and virulent phages T4, T7, and N4. We emphasize transcriptional regulation, although we present examples of regulated RNA and protein stability as well. Investigations of these regulatory strategies have not only elucidated much about phage biology, but have also yielded many insights into regulatory mechanisms that are used by the host. We also describe several other strategies found in some less extensively studied phages.

## Transcript Initiation and Elongation by Host RNA Polymerase

When a phage chromosome enters a cell, it encounters a host RNA polymerase (RNAP) that has specific requirements for promoter recognition. Prokaryotic cellular RNAPs consist of a large, multisubunit core, consisting of two copies of the α subunit, and one each of the β, β′, and ω subunits. Core has the ability to synthesize RNA, while a sixth subunit, σ-factor, is needed to identify and bind to promoters, and to initiate RNA synthesis at specific start sites. Primary σ-factors are used during exponential growth for the expression of housekeeping genes while alternate σ factors are needed to transcribe bacterial genes required under certain growth conditions or at times of stress. Many phages direct the synthesis of transcription factors that interact with, modify, or replace host σ. Another class of phage-encoded factors targets core subunits, and these factors can regulate either transcript initiation or transcript elongation.

Hundreds of prokaryotic σ factors have been identified, and they share up to four regions of similar sequence and function. Primary σ factors, like $\sigma^{70}$ of *E. coli*, have three well-characterized regions with the potential to recognize and bind promoters. Residues in region 2 interact with a $-10$ DNA element (positions $-12$ to $-7$), residues in region 3 contact an extended $-10$ (TGn) motif (positions $-15$ to $-13$), and residues in region 4 contact a $-35$ element (positions $-35$ to $-29$) (**Figure 1**; the negative numbers indicate the number of base pairs upstream of the transcription start point). Only two of these three contacts are necessary for good promoter activity, and the majority of host promoters are $-10/-35$ promoters

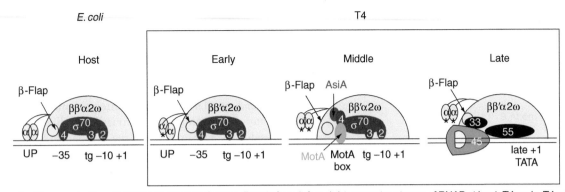

**Figure 1** Changes to (*E. coli*) RNAP during T4 infection. Panels from left to right present cartoons of RNAP at host, T4 early, T4 middle, and T4 late promoters. Core polymerase ( β, β′, α₂, and ω) is in tan. CTDs of α-subunits, which can interact with upstream promoter DNA (UP), and the β-flap are indicated. Region 2, 3, and 4 of σ⁷⁰, which recognize a −10 element, TGn, and a −35 element, respectively, are in dark blue. T4-catalyzed ADP-ribosylation of an α-CTD, which prevents the interaction of α-CTD with DNA, is denoted with a star. Recognition of a T4 middle promoter, which contains a σ⁷⁰ −10 element and a MotA box element, requires σ⁷⁰-containing RNAP, the T4 activator, MotA, and the T4 coactivator, AsiA. Recognition of a T4 late promoter, which has a TATA element at −10, requires core polymerase, a T4 σ-factor composed of gp33 and gp55, and the T4 activator gp45. See text for details.

that use the DNA binding of regions 2 and 4. The −10/−35 promoters also require an interaction between residues in region 4 and a structure in core, called the β-flap, which is required to position region 4 correctly for its contact with the DNA.

RNAP also contacts host promoters through interactions between the C-terminal domain (CTD) of the α-subunits of polymerase core and A–T-rich sequences located between −40 and −60 (UP elements). Although RNAP contains two α subunits, they are not equivalent; one is bound to β and the other is bound to β′. Each α-CTD can interact specifically with a promoter proximal UP element, centered at position −41, or a promoter distal UP element, centered at position −52. In addition, the α-CTD domains can interact nonspecifically with DNA located in the −40 to −60 region.

Initiation of transcription from a −10/−35 promoter by host RNAP is a multistep process. After binding to the promoter through the interactions of σ⁷⁰ with the −10 and −35 elements, the enzyme distorts a region around the −10 element, a step called isomerization, and becomes competent to initiate synthesis of an RNA chain that is complementary to the template strand of the DNA and that grows in a 5′ to 3′ direction. As the chain grows, its association with the template and enzyme is stabilized, principally through the formation of 8–9 bp of RNA:DNA hybrid adjacent to the 3′-end. Upstream of this point, the nascent transcript dissociates from the template strand of the DNA, and an additional 5–6 nt fill an exit channel before the chain emerges from the enzyme. During this process, the newborn elongation complex (EC) releases its grip on the promoter and begins translocating along the template at a rate of about 50 bp⁻¹s. Occupancy of the exit channel by RNA weakens binding of σ⁷⁰ to the core and facilitates σ⁷⁰ release from the EC. However, the kinetics of

σ⁷⁰ release are controversial, and there is evidence that it can remain associated with the EC even after considerable translocation.

Transcript elongation stops when the EC reaches a sequence that encodes a transcription terminator, at which point RNAP dissociates from the template and the RNA. Two classes of terminators are known in *E. coli*: intrinsic and Rho-dependent. Intrinsic terminators are nascent transcripts that can form a stable, base-paired stem–loop or hairpin that is followed by a U-rich stretch. Termination occurs within the U-rich stretch, typically 6–7 nt from the base of the hairpin. Although the nascent terminator transcript is sufficient for termination, the efficiency can be altered by proteins. Rho protein, which is necessary for termination at the second class of terminator, binds to nascent RNA upstream of the termination point. Once bound, it can use ATP to translocate in a 5′ to 3′ direction toward the EC. It is believed that termination occurs when Rho catches up to a paused EC.

## Phage T4

T4 is the best-characterized member of the T4-type phages of the family *Myoviridae*, consisting of phages distinguished by a contractile tail. T4 has a 169 kbp linear chromosome, which is terminally redundant and circularly permuted. Consequently, the T4 genome is shown as a circle (**Figure 2**). Injection of the DNA into the host initiates a pattern of T4 gene expression that results in a burst of phage about 20 min after infection. The production of phage proteins is regulated primarily at the level of temporally controlled transcription through the synthesis of early, middle, and late RNAs.

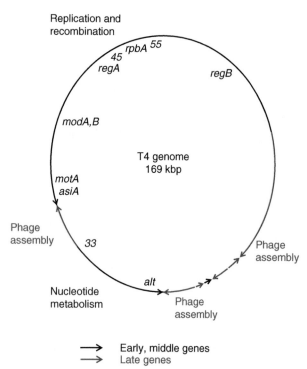

Replication and
recombination

T4 genome
169 kbp

→  Early, middle genes
→  Late genes

**Figure 2** Map of bacteriophage T4. The 169 kbp linear T4 DNA is represented as a circle because it is circularly permuted and terminally redundant. Black regions contain early/middle genes, which include genes whose products are needed for DNA replication and recombination and nucleotide metabolism. Red regions contain late genes, whose products are primarily involved in phage assembly. The positions of specific genes referred to in the text are also shown.

## T4 Early Transcription

Productive T4 infection requires exponentially growing cells. Consequently, polymerase containing $\sigma^{70}$ is the major species present when T4 infects. A top priority for T4 is to rapidly commit the host polymerase to its agenda. It accomplishes this task through multiple strategies. Immediately after infection, T4 programs strong transcription from its early promoters, which are recognized by $\sigma^{70}$ containing host RNAP. These promoters are needed for expressing early genes, many of which encode proteins that are involved in quickly moving the host resources to the phage, such as nucleases that degrade the host DNA and proteins that will be needed for middle gene expression. T4 early promoters have the recognition features of the $\sigma^{70}$-dependent $-10/-35$ promoters, but these promoters also have the extended $-10$ sequence for $\sigma^{70}$ region 3 and UP elements for $\alpha$-CTD contact. Consequently, the 40 or so early promoters are extremely strong, and they compete very efficiently with the more than 600 host promoters for productive transcription initiation by the available polymerase.

To increase further the advantage of early promoters over host promoters, T4 encodes a protein, Alt, that chemically modifies host RNAP by ADP-ribosylation. This modification specifically increases the activity of T4 early promoters relative to those of the host. Alt is actually present within the phage head, and it is injected into the host along with phage DNA. Thus, the Alt modification begins immediately after infection. Although Alt-dependent ADP-ribosylation affects a minor fraction of many *E. coli* proteins, it primarily modifies a specific residue (Arg265) on one of the $\alpha$-subunits. It is thought that this modification occurs on the same $\alpha$ on every polymerase, but which $\alpha$-subunit is unknown. Arg265 is located within the CTD of the $\alpha$-protein, and normally this residue directly contacts UP element DNA. However, ADP-ribosylation of Arg265 eliminates this DNA interaction. Sequence differences between T4 early promoters and host promoters in the $-40$ to $-60$ region (the $\alpha$-CTD binding sites) may explain how this asymmetric ADP-ribosylation favors T4 early promoters.

T4 transcription gains another advantage over the host early after infection because T4 DNA itself is modified, containing glucosylated, hydroxymethyl cytosines. This modification protects the phage genome from multiple nucleases that are encoded by T4 early genes and digest unmodified host DNA within the first few minutes of infection. In addition, T4 encodes an early protein (Alc) that specifically terminates transcription on unmodified host DNA.

## T4 Middle Transcription

T4 middle gene expression begins about 1 min after infection. Middle genes include genes that encode T4 replication proteins, transfer RNAs, and proteins that will be needed later to switch from middle to late promoter recognition. At the start of middle transcription, two early gene products, the ADP-ribosylating enzymes ModA and ModB, complete the ADP-ribosylation of Arg 265, resulting in the modification of both $\alpha$-subunits. This prevents any contact between the $\alpha$-CTD domains and the $-40$ to $-60$ sequences, thereby further decreasing initiation from host promoters. In addition, ADP-ribosylation of the second $\alpha$-subunit now lessens the activity of T4 early promoters. Thus, the action of ModA/ModB should contribute to the switch from T4 early to T4 middle transcription. Early gene expression is also decreased by the action of another early gene product, RegB endoribonuclease, which cleaves within the sequence GGAG present in the ribosome binding site of many early transcripts. Although RegB is present even after late gene expression has begun, and some middle and late T4 transcripts contain the RegB recognition sequence, only cleavage of early RNA is observed. In particular, the mRNA of the T4 MotA protein, which is required for middle promoter activation (see below), is an RegB substrate. Evidence suggests that the secondary structure of the mRNA is important for RegB recognition, but the exact nature of RegB specificity is not yet understood.

T4 middle RNA is synthesized using two separate strategies. First, early and middle genes are located together with almost all middle genes downstream of early genes (**Figure 2**). Consequently, transcription from T4 early promoters produces middle RNA as these early transcripts extend into middle genes. Although there has been speculation that this extension involves an active T4 antitermination process, perhaps like that of λ (below), definitive evidence for such a mechanism has not been found and the control of this extension is not yet understood.

Second, T4 activates the initiation of transcription at more than 30 middle promoters. These promoters contain the $\sigma^{70}$ −10 element and are dependent on RNAP containing $\sigma^{70}$ for transcription. However, they lack the $\sigma^{70}$ −35 element and have instead a different consensus sequence, the 'MotA box', centered at −30 (**Figure 1**). Activation of middle promoters occurs by a process called σ appropriation and requires two T4-encoded proteins, MotA and AsiA. MotA is a transcription activator that interacts both with the MotA box and with the far C-terminus of $\sigma^{70}$, a region that contains some of the residues that normally interact with the β-flap. AsiA is a small protein that binds tightly to $\sigma^{70}$ region 4. When MotA is present, AsiA coactivates transcription from T4 middle promoters. By itself AsiA also inhibits transcription from $\sigma^{70}$-dependent promoters that require an interaction with the −35 element.

AsiA binds to multiple residues in $\sigma^{70}$ region 4 and dramatically changes its conformation. Some of these residues normally interact with the −35 element, and some with the β-flap, but the structure that results from AsiA binding no longer interacts with either. Thus, AsiA binding inhibits transcription from $\sigma^{70}$-dependent promoters that require these interactions. Furthermore, by removing the interaction of $\sigma^{70}$ with the −35 sequences, AsiA helps MotA interact with the MotA box, centered at −30. This is because the 9 bp MotA box includes sequences that would normally interact at least indirectly with $\sigma^{70}$ region 4. In addition, AsiA frees the far C-terminus of $\sigma^{70}$ to interact with MotA, since the structural changes prevent this portion of $\sigma^{70}$ from interacting with the β-flap.

Interestingly, AsiA binds rapidly to free $\sigma^{70}$, but poorly, if at all, to $\sigma^{70}$ that is present in polymerase. Because there is an excess of core relative to $\sigma^{70}$ in *E. coli*, very little free $\sigma^{70}$ is available at any given time. Consequently, the binding of AsiA to $\sigma^{70}$ must occur when $\sigma^{70}$ is released from core, which occurs in this case after initiation at early promoters. Thus, transcription from early promoters directly promotes the switch to middle transcription, helping to coordinate the start of middle transcription with the vitality of early transcription.

## T4 Late Transcription

Late genes primarily encode proteins needed to form virions and to process replicated T4 DNA. The switch from middle to late transcription begins about 6 min after infection. The synthesis of some early and middle proteins decreases because translation of their mRNA is repressed by the T4-encoded middle protein, RegA, which competes with ribosomes for binding to the translational initiation sites of some middle mRNAs. RegA binds to an AU-rich motif but the precise requirements for binding are unknown. In addition, middle RNA synthesis decreases because the previous ADP-ribosylation of α-CTD and the binding of a T4 middle protein, RpbA, to core polymerase favor transcription from late promoters, described below, over transcription from middle promoters.

Transcription from T4 late promoters is accomplished by host core polymerase in combination with three phage-encoded middle proteins: gp33, gp55, and gp45 (**Figure 1**). Gp55 shares sequence similarity with σ region 2, and like region 2, gp55 recognizes and contacts a specific DNA element, in this case TATAAATA, centered at position −10 (**Figure 1**). Gp55 interacts with gp45 and the β'-subunit of RNAP. Gp33 interacts with gp45 and the β-flap of RNAP. Gp45 forms a ring that encircles T4 DNA and can move along it in either direction. Interaction of RNAP-bound gp33 with DNA-bound gp45 connects RNAP to DNA upstream of the gp55 DNA contact. Thus, gp33 and gp55 together can be considered a T4 σ-factor for late promoters. Interestingly, gp45 is also the DNA polymerase clamp protein, a processivity factor that is needed to keep T4 DNA polymerase from dissociating from DNA during replication. As a consequence, transcription from late promoters requires active DNA replication, because gp45 is loaded onto the DNA through its role as the DNA polymerase clamp. This connection of late transcription to the replication of phage DNA serves to coordinate the expression of late genes, whose functions are primarily DNA packaging and capsid assembly, with the amount of phage DNA. T4 late transcription continues until 20 min after infection, when the fully formed phage with the packaged phage genomic DNA are released through lysis of the cell.

## Phages T7 and T3

T7 and T3 belong to the family *Podoviridae*, comprising phages with short tails. Their virions respectively contain about 39.9 and 38.7 kbp of double-stranded nonpermuted DNA. A short segment is directly repeated at each end ('terminal redundancy'). The chromosomal arrangement of genes with identical functions is similar in the two phages, and to several other sequenced phages of the family, in accord with the modular evolution of phages. We will describe the transcriptional regulation of T7, because it is the best-studied member of the entire group, mentioning T3 when appropriate. The genetic map and the transcription pattern of T7 are shown in **Figure 3**. T7 encodes 56 open reading frames (ORFs) most of whose functions are known. The ORFs include three cases of programmed translational frameshifting.

## Temporal Expression of Genes

Studies of T7 protein synthesis after infection of the host show three temporal stages of gene expression. Early or class I genes (genes *0.3* to *1.3*), middle or class II genes (*1.4* to *6.3*) and late or class III genes (*6.5* to *19.5*) with some overlap, as described later. All T7 genes are transcribed from the same strand, from left to right. The genes in each class are physically contiguous, and the three groups, I, II and III, are also positioned from left to right in the phage chromosome in that order.

Early genes are transcribed by host $\sigma^{70}$-RNAP, and their products modify the intracellular environment so as to facilitate phage development. Only gene *1.0* in this group is essential for phage growth; it encodes a single polypeptide RNA polymerase (T7 RNAP) that specifically transcribes the class II and III genes. The class II gene products are involved in phage-specific DNA metabolic reactions, whereas the class III genes encode DNA packaging, virion assembly, and host cell lysis proteins.

## DNA Entry and Coupled Transcription

Transcription of T7 and T3 phage DNA, unlike that of some other phages, starts before the complete genome is injected into the host. After adsorption of the phage, the products of phage genes *14*, *15*, and *16* are released from the virion and form a tunnel from the tail tip across the outer and inner membranes of the host for DNA entry into the cytosol. However, only 850 bp from the left end of the phage chromosome (**Figure 3**), which include the major early promoters $P_{A1}$, $P_{A2}$, and $P_{A3}$, enter the host. Transcription from these promoters by host RNAP must begin before additional DNA can enter. The reason for the barrier to further DNA entry is not known, but it is DNA sequence independent. Mutations that allow DNA entry in the absence of transcription map in the middle of gene *16*, suggest that the middle segment of Gp16 is at least partly responsible for the blockade. Although transcription from the three early promoters in the 850 bp region is sufficient, T7 RNAP-mediated transcription takes over in completing the DNA-entry process in normal infection.

## Early Transcription

As mentioned earlier, T7 transcription begins immediately after infection at the strong adjacent $P_{A1}$, $P_{A2}$, and $P_{A3}$ promoters, although several weak promoters, as well as some RNAP binding sites, which do not initiate transcription, are distributed in the class I region (not shown in **Figure 3**). The importance, if any, of these other promoters and the RNAP binding sites is not known.

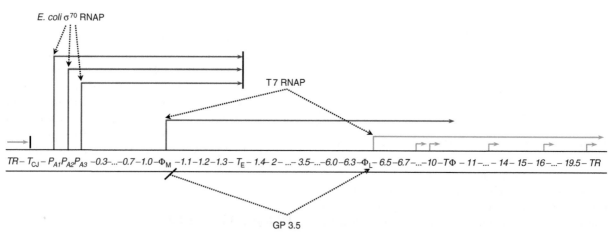

**Figure 3** Phage T7 promoters, transcripts, repressors, and activators. Only genes and sites mentioned in the text are shown, and the diagram shows the gene order as it appears in packaged DNA. *Escherichia coli* RNAP transcribes the early promoters, $P_{A1}$, $P_{A2}$, and $P_{A3}$ (blue arrows), and T7 RNAP transcribes the middle and late promoters, $\Phi_M$ and $\Phi_L$ (red and green arrows, respectively). Five other T7 RNAP-dependent promoters located downstream of $\Phi_L$ are also shown. $T_E$, $T_\Phi$, and $T_{CJ}$ are the terminators discussed in the text. TR means terminal repeat. The transcript from $\Phi_L$ (green arrow) continues through the left terminal repeat and ends at $T_{CJ}$ because T7 chromosome ends are joined by a single copy of the terminal repeat during DNA replication (see text). Activation and repression of $\Phi_L$ and $\Phi_M$ by Gp3.5 are indicated by dotted lines ending in an arrow and bar, respectively. A bar across the transcript arrow heads signify terminated transcripts.

Transcription from the early promoters continues after complete genome entry and terminates at different sites with incomplete efficiency within the ~8000 bp long polycistronic transcription unit or at a Rho-independent terminator ($T_E$) located at the end of the transcription unit encompassing genes *0.3–1.3*. T7 early transcription terminates at $T_E$ both *in vivo* and *in vitro*, but T3 early transcription terminates at $T_E$ only *in vivo*, suggesting the involvement of a termination factor in the latter phage.

## Middle Transcription

Transcription of the class II genes (from *1.4* to *6.3*) by T7 RNAP begins about 4–6 min and continues until about 15 min after infection. These genes are transcribed from several T7 RNAP specific promoters, of which the major one, $\Phi_M$, is shown in **Figure 3**. Note that three class I genes – *1.1*, *1.2*, and *1.3* – are also transcribed by T7 RNAP because they are located downstream of the middle promoter $\Phi_M$ but upstream of the early terminator $T_E$ (**Figure 3**). T7 but not host RNAP ignores the $T_E$ terminator when transcribing genes *1.1* to *1.3*. Transcription from $\Phi_M$ terminates weakly at the T7 RNAP terminator, $T_\Phi$, which is located between genes *10* and *11*. Specific transcription from $\Phi_M$ can be demonstrated *in vitro*, but only on templates that lack the class III promoters, indicating that a mechanism exists for high level transcription from $\Phi_M$ *in vivo*. It has been suggested that $\Phi_M$ has much-reduced affinity for T7 RNAP compared to that of class III promoters, but the middle promoter is stimulated *in vivo* by an unusually high local concentration of T7 RNAP, which is encoded by an adjacent gene.

## Late Transcription

There are several T7 RNAP promoters that direct expression of late genes (**Figure 3**). The first late promoter, $\Phi_L$, directs transcription of all genes located to the right of gene *6.3*, from gene *6.5* to the last gene, *19.5*. The late genes are transcribed from 8 min after infection until cell lysis occurs. Compared to the strength of $\Phi_M$, $\Phi_L$ is intrinsically strong. Note that class III genes *6.5* through *10* are transcribed from both $\Phi_M$ and $\Phi_L$, presumably because these gene products are needed in larger amounts. Although T7 RNAP initiating at $\Phi_L$ also terminates at $T_\Phi$ with reduced efficiency, all late transcription terminates at site $T_{CJ}$. $T_{CJ}$ is downstream of $\Phi_L$ in phage DNA that is actively replicating and transcribed within infected cells, but the two sites are separated by the ends of the packaged T7 chromosome (**Figure 3**). This is because replication produces concatemers – repeating units of nonredundant T7 sequence that are separated by the terminal repeat – and packaging produces the chromosome ends from the concatemers. $T_{CJ}$ has the sequence 5'-ATCTGTT with no secondary structure potential. It acts as a transcription pause site *in vitro*.

## T7 RNA Polymerase

T7 RNAP is a single subunit enzyme of 98 000 Da. It recognizes a 19 bp sequence (consensus: TAATACGACTCACTATAGG) centered on position −8 from the start point of transcription (+1), which is the first G of the final GG sequence. There are 17 identified middle and late promoters that are used exclusively by T7 and not by host RNAP. T7 RNAP does not recognize host promoters and many of the host terminators, whether the latter are Rho-dependent or Rho-independent. T7 RNAP can utilize both T7 and T3 promoters but T3 RNAP is somewhat specific. The open complexes made by T7 RNAP distort at least 10 bp of double-stranded promoter DNA and are unstable until short RNA oligomers are made. Both T3 and T7 RNAP initiate transcription with 5'-GG. Significantly, the T7 enzyme catalyzes RNA synthesis 5–10 times faster than the host RNAP. As mentioned, besides $\Phi_M$ and $\Phi_L$, there are several other promoters distributed among class II and III genes that are transcribed by T7 RNAP, and transcription from these promoters increases the products of certain genes. The 3'-ends of the RNA made by the phage enzyme without the aid of any other factors at $T_\Phi$ are also different from that by the host enzyme, $G(U)_6G$-3' for T7 versus $G/C(U)_{6-7}$-3' for the host. As mentioned below, the termination efficiency is modulated by the phage protein Gp3.5. T3, but not T7, RNAP needs the *E. coli* protein DnaB helicase for initiation, elongation, and termination of replication *in vivo*. DnaB is essential for both phage DNA replication and RNA synthesis in high salt *in vitro*. The significance of the sharing of a protein between transcription and replication is not known.

## Regulation of Transcription

T3 and T7 regulate gene expression mainly at the level of transcription. We mentioned that the gene products made from early transcripts create a favorable environment for phage growth and produce T7 RNAP. At this point, transcription of class II genes begins. As soon as the synthesis of middle proteins reaches an optimal level, both early and middle transcription are turned off, and the transcription machinery is directed exclusively to expression of late genes. The temporal control and relative amounts of transcription of different genes are achieved in several ways. First, temporal control is facilitated by positioning of the three groups of genes, I, II, and III, in the order from left to right; and second, mechanisms exist to switch from early to middle and from middle to late transcription (below). In addition, some gene products are needed in large amounts for a sustained period. The corresponding genes are located in areas of overlapping transcription and possess additional, strategically located promoters in the phage chromosome. For example, as noted earlier, genes *1.1* through *1.3* are transcribed as part of both early and middle transcription units. Next, differential levels of transcription of some class I genes are achieved by 'polarity', that is, expression of promoter proximal genes in higher amounts than promoter distal ones. Polarity is caused by Rho-dependent transcription termination signals in the early transcription unit. Finally, the mode of entry of T7 DNA into the host is also an important element in temporal control of transcription.

There are three components of the early to middle switch, and all are due to the products of early transcription. First, gene *0.7* product inactivates host RNAP. Gp0.7 is a seryl–threonyl protein kinase that phosphorylates the $\beta$- and/or $\beta'$-subunits of host RNAP. Phosphorylation decreases early transcription to about 25%. The kinase inactivates itself in a timely fashion after it is no longer needed. Second, T7 RNAP, the gene *1.0* product, accumulates. This enzyme recognizes the middle and late promoters. The host RNAP activity is also inhibited by the third factor, the middle gene *2.0* product. Gp2.0 binds to the host RNAP in a 1:1 stoichiometry. Although Gp2.0 is essential for phage growth, Gp0.7 is not. Much needs to be learned about Gp2.0 action.

The switch from middle to late transcription requires the product of middle gene *3.5*. This protein binds to T7 RNAP, forming a complex that inhibits transcription strongly from $\Phi_M$ but weakly from the late promoter, $\Phi_L$. Biochemical experiments have shown that Gp3.5 inhibits the transition from the initiating to the elongating complex. The $\Phi_M$–T7 RNAP complexes are much weaker than the corresponding late promoter complexes. Gp3.5 destabilizes the former complexes more readily than the latter ones. Interestingly, Gp3.5 has three additional functions. It is a lysozyme, which is required for release of progeny phage after infection, it stimulates DNA replication, and, indirectly, it enhances termination at $T_{CJ}$. Ordinarily, $T_{CJ}$ is a pause site for T7 RNAP, and Gp3.5 increases pausing at this site.

### RNA Processing

The long polycistronic RNA molecules made at early, middle, and late times after phage infection are cut at specific sites by the host enzyme, RNase III, to yield discrete, relatively stable mRNAs. The processing sites in early T7 RNA have been studied in more detail. RNase III cleaves at specific sites within hairpin structures that are located between coding sequences. Although some of the RNA molecules that result from RNase III cleavage are translated more efficiently than the uncut RNA, RNase III cleavage is not essential for phage growth.

### Phage N4

The virulent phage N4 uses transcription strategies that differ significantly from those of T7 or T4. Early genes are located at the left end of the N4 chromosome, in the first 10 kbp of the ~70 kbp, linear, double-stranded DNA. Transcription of the early genes requires a phage-coded, virion-encapsulated polymerase, vRNAP, which is injected into the host along with the phage DNA. This polymerase is distantly related to the T7 family of RNA polymerases (above). N4 early promoter sequences have a conserved motif and a sequence that can form a hairpin with a stem of 5–7 nt and a loop of 3 nt in single-stranded DNA. *In vivo* transcription by vRNAP requires the activity *E. coli* gyrase and *E. coli* SSB (*Eco*SSB), the host single-stranded DNA binding protein that is normally a member of the host DNA replication machinery. It is thought that gyrase-catalyzed, negative supercoiling of the DNA leads to local melting and extrusion of the hairpin, which then provides the features needed for polymerase promoter recognition. *Eco*SSB melts the complementary strand hairpin while the template strand hairpin, which is resistant to SSB melting, remains available for vRNAP recognition. In addition, SSB prevents annealing of the RNA product to the template DNA. Thus, *Eco*SSB acts as an architectural transcription factor as well as a recycling factor that makes the template DNA available for multiple rounds of early transcription.

Middle N4 genes encode the N4 replication proteins and are located within the left half of the N4 genome. Middle genes are transcribed by a second phage-encoded RNA polymerase, N4 RNAPII, composed of the N4 early products p4 and p7. This polymerase is also a member of the T7 polymerase family. N4 middle promoters contain an AT-rich sequence at the transcription start site. By itself, N4 RNAPII is inactive on double-stranded DNA and has very limited activity on single-stranded DNA. Active transcription requires another N4 protein, gp2, which interacts specifically with single-stranded DNA and with N4 RNAP II. It is thought that an as yet unidentified protein binds to the promoter element while gp2 stabilizes a single-stranded region at the promoter start and brings N4 RNAPII to the transcription start site. This system differs significantly from the other well-characterized phage transcription systems and may provide a good model system for investigating mitochondrial transcription, which is also carried out by a member of the T7 polymerase family.

Transcription of N4 late genes, which are located in the right half of the phage genome, requires *E. coli* RNA polymerase. Late promoters have regions of limited similarity to $\sigma^{70}$ DNA elements and when present in linear DNA, they are weak promoters for $\sigma^{70}$ polymerase. Transcription *in vivo* and with linear templates *in vitro* requires the N4 SSB protein. Surprisingly, the single-stranded DNA-binding function of SSB is not needed for this activation. Rather a transactivating domain of SSB that interacts with the β′-subunit of *E. coli* RNA polymerase core is required. The mechanism of this activation is not known, but is thought to occur at a step after initial binding of RNA polymerase to the promoter. Thus, this late N4 system should also provide insight into a mode of transcriptional activation that has not been previously characterized.

## Phage λ and the Regulation of Lysogeny and Lysis

Lambda is the founding member of a large family of temperate bacteriophages that are related by common gene organization and limited sequence similarity. Although λ belongs to the *family Siphoviridae* by virtue of its long, noncontractile tail, several close relatives are not members of this group. Lambda chromosomes isolated from virions consist of about 49 kbp of linear, nonpermuted, mostly double-stranded DNA. Complementary single-stranded extensions of 12 bases at each end enable the chromosome to circularize by end-joining after it is transferred from the virion into an infected cell. Transcription of all phage genes, both early and late, is catalyzed by host RNAP. Infection with λ, unlike infection with virulent phages, does not always lead to cell lysis and liberation of progeny phage. Instead, infected cells frequently survive and give rise to lysogens – cells that contain a quiescent, heritable copy of the λ chromosome

called prophage (**Figure 4**). The prophage expresses few genes and replicates in synchrony with the host, so that each daughter cell also contains a prophage. The 'decision' between lytic growth and lysogen formation after infection is controlled at many levels (below). Indeed, λ, like other temperate species, has evolved sophisticated mechanisms to ensure that a substantial fraction but not all infected cells survive and become lysogenic, and that intermediate responses, for example, survival without inheritance of a prophage (abortive lysogeny), are rare.

Once a lysogen has formed, loss of the prophage, or 'curing', is infrequent. Lambda and its relatives insert their chromosomes into specific sites in the bacterial chromosome during the establishment of lysogeny and remain there during subsequent cell division. Although site-specific prophage insertion is widespread, it is not a general feature of lysogeny; some temperate phages that are not closely related to λ use other strategies that also ensure prophage retention. For example, phage Mu, inserts its chromosome nonspecifically, while phage P1 does not insert at all, but instead exists in lysogens as a single-copy plasmid whose replication is coupled to that of the host chromosome. Lysogeny is not a dead end; the prophage can switch into an active state in which many virus genes are expressed, the prophage is excised from the bacterial chromosome, and normal lytic growth ensues (**Figure 4**). This transition, known as the genetic (or, more correctly, epigenetic) switch, is normally infrequent but can be induced experimentally by treatment of cells with DNA damaging agents. Such treatment causes a signal cascade that leads to autoproteolytic cleavage of repressor, a phage protein that prevents most

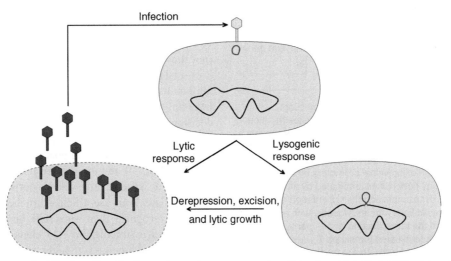

**Figure 4** The λ life cycle. After infection, the linear phage chromosome enters the cell and the single-stranded ends cohere to form a ring (in red, top panel). When the infected cell enters the lytic cycle, early and late phage genes are fully expressed, phage DNA replication ensues, the resulting replicas are packaged into phage heads, and the cell lyses, releasing infectious particles into the environment (left bottom panel). When the infected cell enters the lysogenic cycle, the phage expresses mainly early genes to a limited extent. Among these genes are *cI* and *int*. CI prevents further phage gene expression, and Int catalyzes insertion of the phage into the bacterial chromosome (lower right panel). The resulting lysogen passes a copy of the inserted, repressed prophage to its descendents. When repression fails, the prophage excises and enters the lytic cycle.

phage gene expression (below). Experimental induction of lysogens by DNA damage is not universal; lysogens of some temperate phages, such as P2, are not inducible.

## The Establishment and Maintenance of Lysogeny

Immediately after infection, host RNAP initiates transcription at the $\lambda$ early promoters, $P_L$ and $P_R$ (**Figure 5**). $P_R$ directs the transcription of the *cII* gene, whose product is the central effector of the lysogenic response. CII protein promotes lysogeny by activating the coordinate initiation of transcription at three $\lambda$ promoters: $P_{RE}$, $P_{Int}$, and $P_{aQ}$ (**Figure 5**). $P_{RE}$, the promoter for repressor establishment, directs the transcription of the *cI* gene, and $P_{RE}$ activation thus provides a burst of CI protein synthesis shortly after infection. CI, or repressor, prevents transcription of nearly all $\lambda$ genes in an established lysogen, and, indeed, is required for the maintenance of lysogeny. CI blocks the initiation of early transcripts by binding to operator sites that overlap $P_L$ and $P_R$ (below). It blocks late gene transcription indirectly, by preventing the synthesis of Q, an early protein that activates transcription of late genes (**Figure 5**). CI is not only a repressor, it is also an activator. It activates the initiation of transcription at $P_{RM}$, the promoter for repressor maintenance, a second promoter for *cI* transcription. Thus, once *cI* transcription has initiated from $P_{RE}$, it is self-sustaining.

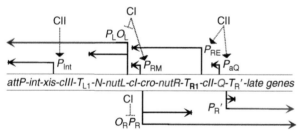

**Figure 5** Phage $\lambda$ promoters, transcripts, repressors, activators, and antiterminators. Only genes and sites mentioned in the text are shown. The top, light, horizontal line represents a DNA strand written with 5' to 3' chemical polarity, and the parallel bottom line represents the complementary strand written 3' to 5'. Activation or repression of individual promoters by CI and CII proteins is indicated by dotted lines terminated by an arrowhead or bar, respectively. Transcripts and their orientation are indicated by heavy solid lines with arrowheads, with each transcript adjacent to the transcribed strand. A bar across an arrowhead indicates a terminated transcript. $T_{L1}$ and $T_{R1}$ are the first of several transcription terminators in the $P_L$ and $P_R$ operons, respectively, and $T_R'$ is the first terminator in the $P_R'$, or late operon. N suppresses terminators by binding to ECs after they transcribe the *nutL* and *nutR* sites (see text). This is indicated by a color change from black to blue in the transcript. Q suppresses termination at $T_R'$ and downstream terminators by binding to the EC shortly after initiation at $P_R'$ (see text). This is indicated by a color change from black to red in the transcript.

This is essential to maintain lysogeny because CI prevents continued transcription of *cII*.

$P_{Int}$, the second CII-activated promoter, directs the transcription of the *int* gene. Int protein or integrase is a topoisomerase that binds to specific sequences within the phage and host 'attachment sites'. These two sites differ from each other in the number, type, and disposition of Int binding sites. The phage attachment site also contains sequences that specifically bind several molecules of IHF, a host-encoded DNA bending protein that promotes the formation of a recombinogenic structure that can capture the bacterial attachment site. Int then uses its topoisomerase activity to catalyze breakage, exchange, and rejoining of the four DNA strands at specific positions within the two sites. This inserts the prophage into the bacterial chromosome and ensures its inheritance by the progeny of the infected cell. Reversal of insertion, or excision, is rare as long as CI continues to repress transcription (below).

Finally, $P_{aQ}$, the third CII-activated promoter, directs the synthesis of an antisense RNA that inhibits the production of Q, a phage protein that promotes transcription of late genes. Inhibition of Q synthesis increases the frequency of lysogeny after infection by delaying the production of late phage proteins that would kill the cell. Once lysogeny is established, repressor prevents further transcription of Q, as noted earlier.

The rate of CII accumulation after infection is controlled by the action of several phage and host gene products, a few of which are described in more detail below. Initially, $\lambda$ Cro protein and, eventually, CI inhibit initiation of the *cII* transcript at $P_R$. Lambda N protein promotes transcript elongation through *cII* by suppressing $T_{R1}$, a rho-dependent transcription terminator (**Figure 5**). Host RNase III in concert with the antisense OOP RNA (not shown in **Figure 5**) cleaves the *cII* transcript. Finally, host FtsH protease degrades CII, but $\lambda$ CIII protein inhibits its degradation. The net effect of these multiple layers of control is probably to make the lysis–lysogeny decision responsive to internal and environmental cues. A complete quantitative description of the kinetic details of the response is cherished goal of systems biologists.

Dimers of CII and dimers, tetramers, and octamers of CI bind to specific sites that overlap the promoters they regulate. Both use a helix–turn–helix DNA binding motif to recognize their sites. CII binds specifically to sequences that straddle the $-35$ element of the relevant promoters, and binding is thought to activate transcription initiation through contacts between the tetramer and $\sigma^{70}$ RNAP. These contacts enhance binding of RNAP to the promoter and isomerization of the bound complex. CI dimers bind to repeated tandem operator sites that flank and interpenetrate each promoter: $O_{L1}$, $O_{L2}$, and $O_{L3}$ for $P_L$, and $O_{R1}$, $O_{R2}$, and $O_{R3}$ for $P_R$. One dimer binds to each operator, and neighboring dimers can interact cooperatively with each other as well as with dimers bound near the other promoter as shown in **Figure 6**. Cooperative interactions strengthen operator binding and make it more sensitive to changes in CI concentration, thus sharpening the transition between full repression and full derepression and decreasing the probability of biologically unproductive intermediate states. Repressor dimers bound to $O_{L1}$ and $O_{L2}$ occlude binding of RNAP to $P_L$, and, similarly, binding to $O_{R1}$ and $O_{R2}$ occludes $P_R$. Repressor bound at $O_{R2}$ has an additional function; it contacts the σ-subunit of RNAP bound to $P_{RM}$, promoting isomerization of the bound enzyme and subsequent *cI* transcription. $O_{R3}$ binds repressor relatively weakly and is not required for repression of $P_R$. This operator is occupied only at relatively high repressor concentration, and occupancy prevents a further

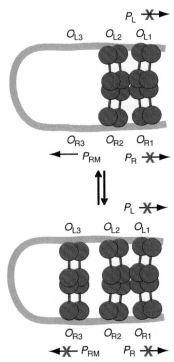

**Figure 6** Binding of repressor. The pairs of purple dumbbells represent repressor dimers bound to subsites of $O_L$ and $O_R$. One end of each dumbbell represents the N-terminal portion of the protein, which contains a DNA-binding domain. The other end represents the C-terminal portion of the protein, which contains regions that can participate in cooperative interactions with similar regions in neighboring bound dimers to form tetramers, and with a tetramer bound to a distant operator to form an octamer. At low concentrations of repressor, the cooperative interactions and the intrinsic affinities of the binding sites lead to occupancy of subsites 1 and 2 of each operator. In this configuration, promoters $P_L$ and $P_R$ are repressed and promoter $P_{RM}$ is activated (top of figure). At higher concentrations of repressor, all six subsites are occupied and all three promoters are repressed (bottom of figure). Repression is indicated by a red 'X' over the arrows representing transcripts.

increase in concentration by repressing $P_{RM}$. Thus, *cI* transcription from $P_{RM}$ is both positively and negatively autoregulated.

## Prophage Excision

If the level of repressor in a lysogen drops below the level needed to inhibit transcription, the prophage expresses genes needed for excision and lytic growth. Two λ proteins, Int and Xis, are needed for prophage excision. Int, as noted earlier, catalyzes breakage and rejoining of DNA strands. Xis is a directionality factor; it is required for excision and inhibits insertion. Analogous directionality factors are produced by many other temperate phages. Xis molecules bind specifically and cooperatively to sequences within the attachment sites and help to recruit Int to an adjacent binding sequence. This favors recombination between the two attachment sites that flank the prophage and inhibits recombination between the phage and host attachment sites. Interestingly, when Xis concentration is limiting, the host-encoded Fis protein can alleviate the deficiency. It is likely that Fis and IHF, the other host-encoded protein needed for recombination, help to couple the efficiencies of insertion and excision to the physiological state of the host.

Although Int and Xis are encoded by adjacent genes, the protein levels are differentially controlled so that the efficiency and direction of recombination are coupled to the appropriate stages of the phage life cycle. In infected cells destined for lysogeny, *int* but not *xis* is transcribed from CII-activated $P_{Int}$ (**Figure 5**). Xis, which is made from the $P_L$ transcript, is unstable, so it inhibits insertion only briefly when transcription from $P_L$ is repressed after infection. After prophage induction, both *int* and *xis* are transcribed from $P_L$, and their products promote rapid prophage excision. Excision is usually followed by phage DNA replication and the expression of late genes. Although excision is not a prerequisite for the subsequent events, it is necessary for synthesis of concatemers of λ DNA, a substrate for packaging phage chromosomes into virions.

## Lytic Growth

Lambda lytic growth is broadly similar to that of virulent phages, although the regulatory strategies differ considerably. The Cro, N, and Q proteins regulate transcription mainly during lytic growth. None of them is produced in lysogens because CI directly represses their syntheses. Cro is a transcriptional repressor, similar to CI in binding specificity and structure. However, subtle differences in binding specificity and the absence of cooperative interactions weaken Cro repression of $P_L$ and $P_R$, and adapt it to serve as a negative regulator of early gene transcription during lytic growth. Cro is essential for lytic growth because it represses transcription of *cII*, thus enabling a fraction of infected cells to enter the lytic pathway. Both N and Q are 'antiterminators'; they act during transcript elongation to suppress termination. N enhances expression of early, and Q of late genes (**Figure 5**). Nearly all λ genes are located downstream of terminators and therefore require antitermination for full expression. *Cro* and *N* are exceptions, and, indeed, they are normally expressed before any other λ proteins are produced.

What is the role of terminators in λ biology? Their role in the expression of early genes is unclear, since termination is rapidly and efficiently suppressed as N accumulates after infection. Possibly the delay in early gene expression until the concentration of N reaches an effective level influences the lysis–lysogeny decision. Indeed, it has been shown that the efficiency of translation of the N message is increased by RNase III cleavage, and that the intracellular concentration of RNase III varies with the growth phase of the culture. Alternatively, or in addition, termination adds to the effect of repressor in silencing early gene expression in lysogens. In any event, early gene terminators are likely to confer some evolutionary advantage because several are conserved in phages related to λ. By contrast, the role of termination in controlling late gene expression is clear because $P_R'$, the promoter for these genes, is constitutive. Thus, termination prevents transcription of late genes in lysogens and premature transcription of late genes during lytic growth.

Antitermination by N and Q is limited to λ transcription because both proteins bind specifically to phage nucleic acid before they act. N binds nascent transcripts of the *nutL* and *nutR* sites, which are located downstream of $P_L$ and $P_R$, respectively (**Figure 5**). RNA binding alters N structure and facilitates its transfer to the nearby elongation complex, where it acts to suppress termination. Several host proteins enhance N-dependent antitermination: NusA, NusB, NusE/RpsL, and NusG. Some of these proteins bind *nut* RNA, some bind the elongation complex, and one, NusA, binds N. All of these proteins have roles in host biology that are independent of N, and their abundance and activity might link the efficiency of antitermination to as yet unknown aspects of host physiology. Nevertheless, N is clearly the central actor since some level of antitermination has been observed *in vitro* in the absence of all of the Nus factors and the *nut* site when N is present in excess. Despite considerable effort, the location of the N binding site on the EC and the nature of the antiterminating modification are still unknown. The modification is stable *in vitro* in the presence of NusA and persists *in vivo* for considerable time and distance after it has been established. Persistence is important for λ physiology since important terminators, notably those preceding the Q and *xis* genes, are located more than 5 kbp from the *nut* sites.

Q binds to a site in the nontranscribed region of the λ late promoter, $P_R'$ (**Figure 5**). It is transferred from this site to the EC after synthesis of a 16 or 17 nt transcript. At these points the EC pauses because the $\sigma^{70}$-subunit, which has not yet been released, binds to a transcribed DNA sequence that resembles the extended −10 regions of certain genuine *E. coli* promoters. Sigma-70 interacts with Q after its transfer to the EC, but the locations of any additional contacts are unknown. Q modification of the EC decreases the duration of the 16/17 pause and suppresses downstream terminators.

Q and N suppress nearly all terminators that have been tested, both intrinsic and rho-dependent, and also increase the average rate of elongation. The mechanisms of suppression and, indeed, of termination are controversial. It is widely accepted that formation of the hairpin stem of intrinsic terminators disrupts the upstream (5′) segment of the RNA:DNA hybrid, which consists mainly of relatively weak rU:dA base pairs. It is not clear how hairpin formation is linked to hybrid disruption, and what the subsequent steps in termination consist of. Among the mechanisms that have been considered to explain N and Q action are inhibition of hairpin formation, strengthening of the weak RNA:DNA hybrid, and increase of elongation rate so that the EC escapes from the termination zone.

It is interesting that the termination/antitermination mode of gene control is not general among temperate phage. For example, it has not been found in phages Mu or P2, which regulate transcription exclusively through activators and repressors of initiation. However, several interesting variants of the termination/antitermination strategy have been discovered in other phages. In lysogens of the mycobacterial phages L5 and Bxb1, the repressor arrests the progress of the EC by binding to numerous 'stoperator' sites in the phage chromosome and physically blocking further translocation. The repressor of coliphage P4 also prevents transcript elongation, but by a quite different mechanism. P4 repressor is an RNA that activates termination by pairing with phage transcripts upstream of terminators. It has been suggested that the resulting RNA:RNA duplexes alter the secondary structure of the transcripts in such a way as to favor termination. Finally, HK022, an *E. coli* phage related to λ, uses antitermination to express its early genes but lacks a protein analogous to N. Instead, the HK022 $P_L$ and $P_R$ operons encode short, structured RNA segments that bind to the EC and suppress downstream terminator sites as efficiently as N does for λ. These RNAs act exclusively *in cis*, thus limiting antitermination to phage transcripts.

## Conclusions

Both temperate and virulent phages alter the transcriptional and translational machinery of their hosts to suit their own ends. We have described phage-encoded mechanisms that change promoter utilization, transcript elongation rate, and transcript termination efficiency. These changes can be modest or drastic, ranging from chemical modification of a host RNAP subunit to synthesis of a new and structurally dissimilar polymerase. The selective advantage conferred by some of these changes is poorly understood and may be an adaptation to evolutionary pressures that are not apparent in laboratory conditions. An example that we have not previously described is the existence of phage-encoded transfer RNAs that duplicate or augment existing host activities. Among the differences between the regulatory strategies used by temperate and by virulent phages is the lethal character of some mechanisms used by the latter group. Most striking among these is degradation of host DNA, which can be seen soon after infection by T4 and T7. Another is inactivation of host RNAP. Temperate phages can also kill their hosts, but this typically occurs after the phage enters the lytic growth pathway. The essence of the temperate lifestyle is peaceful coexistence of the prophage and the host. A prophage that conferred a selective disadvantage on its lysogenic host would probably not last long in nature. If there is a consistent difference between the regulatory strategies of the two phage types, it is the ability of temperate species to prevent the expression of genes that harm the host. In contrast, the essence of being a lytic phage is to invade, take over, and destroy as efficiently as possible. Nevertheless, the extent of this difference should not be exaggerated. Some virulent phages have close relatives that are known only as prophage-like components of bacterial chromosomes, and some temperate phages have close relatives that have lost elements required for

repressing gene expression and are, at first view, indistinguishable from virulent species. In any event, the tactics of both the temperate and virulent phages have taught researchers many elegant mechanisms for gene expression and control.

## Acknowledgment

The authors are grateful to R. Bonocora for designing Figure 1 and to Rodney King and Bill Studier for comments. This work was supported by the Intramural Research Program of the NIH, National Institute of Child Health and Human Development, National Institute of Diabetes and Digestive and Kidney Diseases, and the National Cancer Institute.

*See also:* Icosahedral ssDNA Bacterial Viruses.

## Further Reading

Calendar R (2006) *The Bacteriophages.* New York: Oxford University Press.

Greive SJ and von Hippel PH (2005) Thinking quantitatively about transcriptional regulation. *Nature Reviews Molecular Cell Biology* 6(3): 221–232.

Miller ES, Kutter E, Mosig G, Arisaka F, Kunisawa T, and Ruger W (2003) Bacteriophage T4 genome. *Microbiology and Molecular Biology Reviews* 67(1): 86–156.

Oppenheim AB, Kobiler O, Stavans J, Court DL, and Adhya S (2005) Switches in bacteriophage lambda development. *Annual Review of Genetics* 39: 409–429.

Ptashne M (2004) *A Genetic Switch. Phage Lambda Revisited.* Cold Spring Harbor, NY: Cold Spring Harbor Press.

# Virus Evolution: Bacterial Viruses

**R W Hendrix,** University of Pittsburgh, Pittsburgh, PA, USA

## Glossary

**Chromosome** The physical DNA or RNA molecule present in the virion and containing the information of the genome. The chromosome can differ from the genome by, for example, having a terminal repetition of part of the genomic sequence or being circularly permuted relative to other chromosomes in the population.

**Genome** The totality of the genetic complement of a virus. The genome is a conceptual object usually expressed as a sequence of nucleotides.

**Homologous** Having common ancestry. Homology of two sequences is often inferred on the basis of a high percentage of identity between the sequences, but homology itself is either present or not and is not expressed as a percentage.

**Novel joint** A novel juxtaposition of sequences in a genome resulting from a nonhomologous recombination event.

# Bacteriophage Evolution

Bacterial viruses ('bacteriophages' or 'phages' for short) have probably been evolving for 4 billion years or more, but it is only in recent years that we have come to a relatively detailed view of the genetic mechanisms that underlie phage evolution. Phages do not leave fossils in the conventional sense, but the sequences of phage genomes contain more detailed information about how the phages have evolved than any conventional fossil has. Because of the importance of sequence, our understanding of phage evolution has increased dramatically as more phage sequences have become available over the past few years. Even more important than the individual sequences, however, is the fact that we have multiple genome sequences that we can compare to each other. It is in such comparisons of different genomes that we see the unmistakable signatures of past evolutionary events, which would be completely invisible in an examination of a single genome alone.

Most of the work on phage evolution has addressed evolution of the double-stranded DNA (dsDNA) tailed phages, the members of the order *Caudovirales*, and most of the discussion here deals with that group. Toward the end of the article, we will consider evolution of other groups of phages as well as recent evidence suggesting deep evolutionary connections between some of the bacteriophage groups and viruses that infect members of the Eukarya and Archaea.

# The Tailed Phage Population

Nothing in phage evolution makes sense except in the light of what we have learned about the nature of the global population of tailed phages. The most remarkable fact is that the size of the population is almost incomprehensibly large – a current estimate is that there are about $10^{31}$ individual phage particles on the planet. To give a feeling for the magnitude of this number, if these phages were laid end to end, they would reach into space a distance of $\sim$200 million light years. This is apparently a very dynamic population; ecological studies of marine viruses suggest that the entire population turns over every few days. To replenish the population would then require about $10^{24}$ productive infections per second on a global scale. Each such infection is an opportunity for evolutionary change, either by mutation during replication or by recombination with the DNA in the cell, which will almost always include DNA of other phages in the form of resident prophages. At a lower frequency, cells may be co-infected by two different phages, affording a different opportunity for genetic exchange. As described below, the evolutionary events that are inferred from genome sequence comparisons include extremely large numbers of improbable events, and the only way these events could have given rise to the existing phage

population is if they have had an extremely large number of opportunities to occur.

# Evolutionary Mechanisms in the dsDNA Tailed Phages

## The Nature of the Genomes

The genomes of the dsDNA tailed phages use DNA very efficiently, with typically about 95% of the sequence devoted to encoding proteins. Spaces between genes can often be identified as containing expression signals such as transcription promoters or terminators. Genes are typically arranged in groups that are transcribed together. The specific types of genes in a genome, their numbers, and how they are arranged along the DNA are all highly variable among phages. Genome size is also variable, with the smallest known phages in this group having genomes of about 19 kbp and about 30 genes and the largest consisting genomes of 500 kbp and nearly 700 genes.

## Types of Evolutionary Changes

Comparisons of genome sequences between phages reveal the sorts of changes in the genome sequence that in aggregate constitute phage evolution. The first of these is point mutation, in which one base pair is substituted for another. The number of point mutational differences seen between two homologous sequences varies from none to so many that our ability to detect any residual similarity of the sequence, often measured at the more sensitive level of the encoded amino acid sequence, has vanished. The amount of difference between two sequences due to point mutation is a function of how long it has been since they diverged from a common ancestral sequence, because such differences accumulate progressively over time. In practice, however, it is an unreliable measure of time for a number of reasons: we do not know the mutational rates for phages in a natural setting, we do not know that those rates have been constant over evolutionary time, and different genes accumulate changes at different rates because any mutations that are detrimental to the function of the encoded protein will be lost from the population by natural selection, and different proteins have different tolerances for mutational changes in their amino acid sequences.

The other major type of evolutionary change to a genome is DNA recombination. Particularly important is 'illegitimate' or 'nonhomologous' recombination, in which two different DNA sequences are joined together to form an association of sequences that did not exist before, known as a 'novel joint'. Nonhomologous recombination can join parts of two or more genomes into one new genome; it can also cause deletion or inversion of a sequence within a genome by mediating recombination between two sequences in the genome. Nonhomologous recombination can in principle – and, it appears, also in practice – produce virtually any novel joint that can be imagined. The results of laboratory experiments have shown that homologous recombination happens many orders of magnitude more frequently than nonhomologous recombination. Unlike nonhomologous recombination, homologous recombination does not leave a novel joint that can be detected in analysis of the sequence, but it has the potential to reassort any flanking novel joints, bringing them and their associated sequences together in new combinations and providing a mechanism for them to move rapidly through the population.

## Genome Comparisons

There is typically nothing in a single phage genome sequence, viewed in isolation, that reveals the presence of changes in the phage's evolutionary past, of either mutational or recombinational origin. When multiple genomes are compared, a wealth of differences corresponding to such changes is revealed. **Figure 1** illustrates a comparison for a group of four rather similar genomes of phages infecting enteric bacterial hosts. The physical gene map shown is that of *Escherichia coli* phage HK97, and the histograms indicate the locations of sequences in the other phages that match HK97. It is apparent that the genome sequences match each other in a patchwork fashion, and the parts of the sequence that match the HK97 sequence are different for the three phages. In other words, the genomes are genetic mosaics with respect to each other. In a pairwise comparison of genomes, the transitions between where sequences match and where they do not are abrupt, even when they are examined at the level of the nucleotide sequence. This implies that there have been nonhomologous recombination events in the ancestry of the phages, creating novel joints in the resulting recombinant phages. These novel joints are detected when they are compared with a sequence that did not suffer that particular recombination event. In the comparisons shown in **Figure 1**, there is evidence for about 75 ancestral nonhomologous recombination events, occurring in either the ancestry of HK97 or in that of one of the three phages being compared. It is worth noting that this probably underestimates the number of such events, because any novel joints that lie in the common ancestry of all these phages would not have been detected.

A striking feature of the novel joints in the sequence revealed by such genome sequence comparisons is that they fall predominantly at gene boundaries. While some are precisely at the gene boundaries, some also fall in the middle of spaces between genes or even a few codons into the upstream or downstream gene's coding region. More rarely, we can see novel joints in the interior of a gene's coding region. In the case of some such genes for which the encoded proteins are well characterized, the novel

joints in the DNA sequence fall at a position corresponding to a domain boundary of the protein. Another feature of the genome comparisons that extends across all the groups of phages examined to date is that there are clusters of genes that are never, or rarely, separated by nonhomologous recombination. These are typically genes whose protein products are known to function together, such as the genes encoding the structural proteins of the head.

A frequent consequence of nonhomologous recombination among viruses is the transfer of genetic material from the genomes of one viral lineage into the genomes of a different viral lineage, a process known as 'horizontal transfer' or 'lateral transfer' of genes. This is the process that gives rise to the mosaicism in the genomes discussed above. It also means that different parts of a genome may, and most often do, have different evolutionary histories. This last fact leads to an interesting and still unresolved difficulty for viral taxonomists. That is, attempts to represent the relationships among viruses by a hierarchical taxonomy, as is conventionally done, necessarily fail to capture the multiple different sets of hierarchical relationships displayed by the individual exchanging genetic modules, deriving from their different evolutionary histories. The viruses, of course, are unaware of human attempts to classify them and so are unaffected by the resulting controversies.

## Evolutionary Mechanisms

When the mosaicism of phage genomes was first seen in DNA heteroduplex mapping experiments in the late 1960s, it was proposed that there might be special sites in the DNA, possibly at gene boundaries, that served as points of high-frequency nonhomologous recombination, either through short stretches of homology or through a site-specific recombination mechanism. This view was formulated as the 'modular evolution' model of phage evolution, in which it was proposed that exchange between genomes took place repeatedly at these special sites, leading to the observed mosaic relationship between genomes.

With the current availability of many more genomes and data at the level of nucleotide sequence, it has become clear that, while the mosaic results of phage evolution are much as described nearly 40 years ago, the mechanisms by which that state is achieved are fundamentally different than what had been proposed. That is, the observations are best explained by a model of rampant nonhomologous recombination among phage genomic sequences, with the sites of recombination being distributed, to a first approximation, randomly across the sequence with no regard for gene boundaries or other features of the sequence. Most recombinants produced this way will be nonfunctional because, for example, they have glued together parts of two encoded functional proteins into a nonfunctional chimera. The tiny fraction of such recombinants that are fully functional and competitive in the natural

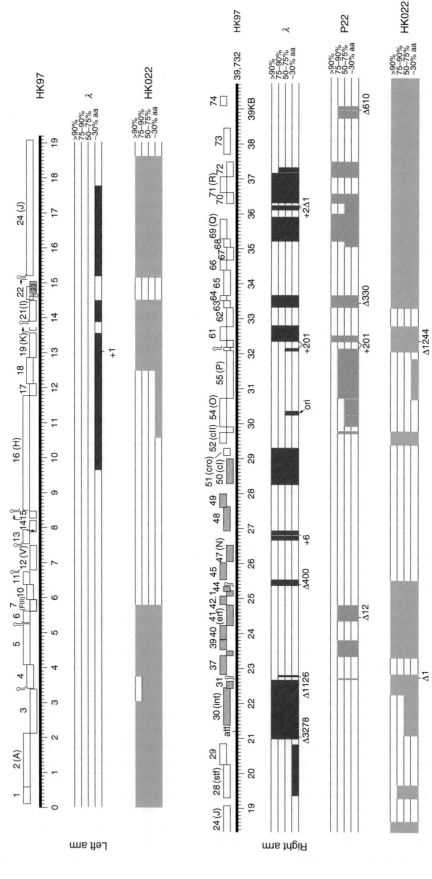

**Figure 1** The horizontal black line, scaled in kilobase pairs, represents the genome sequence of *Escherichia coli* phage HK97. The genes are indicated above the line by rectangles, with open rectangles indicating genes transcribed rightward and shaded rectangles genes transcribed leftward. The colored histograms indicate the areas of sequence similarity between HK97 and the three phages indicated to the right of each histogram: *E. coli* phages lambda and HK022 and *Salmonella enterica* phage P22. Adapted from Juhala RJ, Ford ME, Duda RL, Youlton A, Hatfull GF, and Hendrix RW (2000) Genomic sequences of bacteriophages HK97 and HK022: Pervasive genetic mosaicism in the lambdoid bacteriophages. *Jounal of Molecular Biology* 299: 27–52.

environment will be those that have recombination joints where they do no harm, like at gene boundaries; the rest will be rapidly eliminated from the population by natural selection. We would also expect that two recombining genomes would not typically be lined up in register, and this would most often lead to nonfunctional recombinants. There are a few examples of genomes with short quasi-duplications that can be explained by a slightly out of register recombination event, supporting this supposition.

Nonhomologous recombination also has the potential to bring novel genes into a genome and to mediate large-scale reorganizations of genomes, as seen for example in *E. coli* phage N15 which has head and tail structural genes homologous to those of phage lambda and, in the other half of the genome, genes from a very different, apparently plasmid-like, source. Another example is the *Shigella* phage SfV, which has head genes in the phage HK97 sequence family and tail genes like those of phage Mu.

The entire process described above can be viewed as a classical Darwinian scenario in which tremendous diversity is generated in the population by a combination of point mutations and homologous and nonhomologous recombination, and the stringent sieve of natural selection acts to eliminate all but the fittest recombinants. The survivors have largely, though not entirely, lost the appearance of having been generated by what is essentially a random mutational process.

## Evolution of Other Phage Types

Although most of the genome comparisons that have led to our current understanding of phage evolution have been carried out with the tailed phages, there has been some work done with other groups. The most extensive has been done with members of the families *Microviridae* and the *Inoviridae*, phages with small, circular single-stranded DNA (ssDNA) chromosomes, typified by the well-studied *E. coli* phages φX174 and M13. For both of these groups there is evidence for horizontal exchange of sequences, as in the tailed phages, but it is quantitatively much less prominent than what is seen in the tailed phages. There are several differences between the tailed phages and these two groups of smaller phages, some or all of which may contribute to the differences in evolutionary outcomes seen between them. These include 10- to 100-fold differences in the sizes of the genomes and the fact that the members of the *Microviridae* and *Inoviridae* do not encode recombination functions, among others.

Another study looked at evidence for evolutionary change among members of the family *Cystoviridae*, a group of phages with a double-stranded RNA (dsRNA) genome, divided into three physical segments. Comparisons among environmentally derived genome sequences showed no evidence for recombinational exchange within the segments but clear indications of reassortment of the segments. Thus it appears that evolution in this group of viruses achieves the same general outcome as evolution of the tailed phages, namely horizontal exchange of genetic modules, but by a very different mechanism. Analogous horizontal exchange by reassortment of the segments of a segmented genome has been extensively characterized in the influenza viruses, a group of animal viruses with a single-stranded RNA (ssRNA) genome of eight segments.

## Deep Evolutionary Connections

Although there are some genes that are found in all tailed phages – for example, genes encoding the major capsid protein – these are very diverse in sequence. This diversity is sufficiently great that it is not possible, on the basis of their sequences, to group them into a single sequence family, at either the DNA or the protein sequence levels. Thus the subsets of capsid protein sequences that share demonstrable sequence similarity may represent independent nonhomologous lineages of capsid proteins, or alternatively they may all be part of the same lineage but have diverged in sequence to the point that in many cases no surviving sequence similarity can be demonstrated. However, recent structural work on the polypeptide folds of capsid proteins appears to be extending our analytical reach farther back in evolutionary time and giving a resolution to this question. High-resolution X-ray structures of the capsid proteins of phages HK97 and T4 demonstrate that they have a common fold which might indicate common ancestry despite the absence of any surviving sequence similarity. Cryoelectron microscopic structures of phages representing two more capsid protein sequence groups, P22 and φ29, make a less rigorous but still convincing case that these capsid proteins also share in a common polypeptide fold and so are most likely part of the same lineage. Remarkably, a similar experiment on (the animal virus) herpes simplex virus argues that the shell-forming domain of its major capsid protein also shares the tailed phage capsid protein fold and so may be part of the same lineage.

A similar and more completely documented case for a virus lineage extending across the cellular domains of the hosts they infect can be made for a group that includes bacteriophage PRD1 (a member of the family *Tectiviridae*), archaeal virus STIV, and eukaryotic viruses adenovirus, PBCV1 (*Phycodnaviridae*), and mimivirus. This is again based on shared capsid protein folds, in this case an unusual double 'jellyroll' fold. Finally, there is compelling structural similarity between the cystoviruses, the group of phages with segmented dsRNA chromosomes, and a characteristic double protein shell discussed above, and the reoviruses of plant and animal hosts.

The simplest interpretation of these observations, though not the only possible interpretation, is that there were already viruses resembling these different types of contemporary viruses prior to the divergence of cellular life into the three current domains. The different types of viruses in this view would have co-evolved with their hosts as the hosts divided into domains and descended to the present time, with in the end nothing to indicate their common origins except the shared structure of their capsid proteins. Whatever the truth of this matter, an important caveat to such an interpretation is that the evidence for common viral ancestries across host domains is at present based primarily on conserved properties of capsid proteins, and so any conclusions about common lineages, strictly speaking, only apply to capsid protein lineages. However, despite such reservations, the data make an intriguing though still tentative case that viruses resembling at least three groups of contemporary viruses had already evolved into forms something like those of contemporary viruses before the three domains of cellular life had begun to separate, $\sim$3.5 billion years ago.

## Further Reading

Brüssow H and Hendrix RW (2002) Phage genomics: Small is beautiful. *Cell* 108: 13–16.

Casjens SR (2005) Comparative genomics and evolution of the tailed-bacteriophages. *Current Opinion in Microbiology* 8: 451–458.

Fuhrman JA (1999) Marine viruses and their biogeochemical and ecological effects. *Nature* 399: 541–548.

Hatfull GF, Pedulla ML, Jacobs-Sera D, et al. (2006) Exploring the mycobacteriophage metaproteome: Phage genomics as an educational platform. *PLoS Genetics* 2: e92. http://genetics.plosjournals.org/perlserv/?request=get-document&doi=10.1371%2Fjournal.pgen.0020092 (accessed June 2007).

Juhala RJ, Ford ME, Duda RL, Youlton A, Hatfull GF, and Hendrix RW (2000) Genomic sequences of bacteriophages HK97 and HK022: Pervasive genetic mosaicism in the lambdoid bacteriophages. *Journal of Molecular Biology* 299: 27–52.

Nolan JM, Petrov V, Bertrand C, Krisch HM, and Karam JD (2006) Genetic diversity among five T4-like bacteriophages. *Virology Journal* 3: 30–44.

Suttle CA (2005) Viruses in the sea. *Nature* 437: 356–361.

# Viruses Infecting Euryarchaea

**K Porter, B E Russ, A N Thorburn, and M L Dyall-Smith,** The University of Melbourne, Parkville, VIC, Australia

## Glossary

**Alkaliphilic** Having a requirement for an environment with a high pH.

**Burst size** The number of infectious virus particles released per cell.

**Carrier state** Persistent infection of a host cell by a virus, with the surviving host persistently carrying and continually producing virus without entering a lysogenic state.

**Circular permutation** A change in the sequence of the linear DNA termini that does not alter the relative sequence (e.g., circular permutation of ABCDEFGH could generate BCDEFGHA, CDEFGHAB, etc).

**Concatamer** Two or more DNA molecules that are linked together to form a long, linear DNA molecule.

**Cured** A host cell that was once a lysogen, but no longer carries viral DNA in any form.

**Halophilic** Having a requirement for an environment with a high salt concentration.

**Headful packaging** The mechanism of packaging viral DNA based on the size of the virus head, rather than the length of the viral genome.

**Hyperthermophile** Having a requirement for an environment with a high temperature ($>80\,°C$).

**Insertion sequences** Repetitive sequences of DNA that can move from one site to another within the viral DNA.

**Integrase/recombinase** An enzyme which can integrate viral DNA into the genome of its host cell.

**Lysogen** A host cell that has been infected by a virus that remains dormant, despite the presence of viral DNA.

**Lytic virus** A virus that is able to infect a host, replicate, and subsequently leave the host cell by rupturing (lysing) the host cell.

**Methanogenic** Having the ability to produce methane.

**Monovalent** A virus that has a host range limited to one species.

**Prophage** A virus that is dormant within the host cell.

**Protein-primed replication** Replication of DNA via the interaction of the DNA polymerase with specific proteins, rather than DNA or RNA primers.

**Temperate virus** A virus that is able to infect a host, but remain dormant within the host cell.

**Terminal redundancy** Linear DNA with the same sequence at each end.

**Transduction** The transfer of host DNA from one host cell to another by a virus.

**Transfection** The introduction of pure viral genomic DNA into a host cell, producing viable virus.

## Introduction

In comparison with the viruses infecting Bacteria and Eukarya, our understanding of viruses that infect the third domain of life, the Archaea, is still in the early stages. The first archaeal virus was accidentally discovered in 1974, 3 years before the recognition of Archaea as a separate domain. Twenty-two years later, a total of only ~35 archaeal viruses and virus-like particles (VLPs) had been reported, the vast majority of which displayed head-and-tail morphologies and possessed linear double-stranded DNA (dsDNA) genomes. By 2006, at least 63 viruses and VLPs had been described, which infect members of the two major archaeal kingdoms, Crenarchaeota, including the extremely thermophilic sulfur-metabolizers, and Euryarchaeota, including the anaerobic methanogens, the extreme halophiles, and some hyperthermophiles. All have dsDNA genomes and while the total number of archaeal viruses is still miniscule compared with the >5100 published bacteriophages, they display a wide diversity of morphologies and characteristics. This article focuses on virus representatives infecting the members of the kingdom Euryarchaeota, a group for which the diversity of known representatives has blossomed in recent years.

## Early Euryarchaeal Viruses and VLPs

In the early days of euryarchaeal virus research (1974–93), the range of virus and VLP representatives of the Euryarchaeota was limited. Attempts to isolate these particles were rare and many of the published representatives were discovered accidentally, for example, as contaminants in 'pure' preparations of archaeal flagella. In hindsight, the inability to culture the environmentally dominant Archaea restricted the isolation of viruses to those that infected easily grown laboratory strains, for example, *Halobacterium* for the haloarchaea and *Methanothermobacter* and *Methanobrevibacter* for the methanogens. Except for one oblate VLP with a circular dsDNA genome observed in cultures of *Methanococcus voltae* strain A3, all representatives possessed head-and-tail morphologies with complex protein profiles and genomes of linear dsDNA, similar to the 'classical' bacteriophages of the families *Myoviridae* (head-and-tail viruses with contractile tails) and *Siphoviridae* (head-and-tail viruses with noncontractile tails).

Like their hosts, the viruses of the extremely halophilic Archaea generally required high levels of NaCl or $MgSO_4$

for stability, although halobacterium salinarum viruses Hh-1 and ΦN were relatively stable in low salt, with the latter virus retaining infectivity even after prolonged incubation in distilled water. Many of the extremely halophilic viruses (or haloviruses) were lytic, with latent periods ranging from 6 to 17 h and burst sizes between 60 and 1300 PFU/cell. These latent periods and burst sizes appeared to be regulated by external salt concentrations, a phenomenon proposed to be significant for virus replication during changing salinity conditions in the environment. Some haloviruses such as halobacterium salinarum virus ΦH were truly temperate, while others such as halobacterium salinarum virus S45 persistently infected their host cells.

The viruses of the methanogens were lytic (by definition, no infectivity could be shown for VLP A3), with latent periods ranging from 4 to 9 h and burst sizes between 6 and 20 PFU/cell. However, some controversy still exists regarding the virus–host relationship for ψM1 and relatives (see below).

In general, the characterization of the early euryarchaeal virus and VLP isolates did not progress to the molecular level and it is likely that most of the early isolates are now lost. The exceptions were ΦH, which is one of the most thoroughly studied archaeal viruses, and methanothermobacter marburgensis virus ψM1, and relatives ψM2 and ψM100 (see below). ΦH was isolated after spontaneous lysis of its host culture and was able to infect a range of *Hbt. salinarum* strains. The virion morphologically resembled members of the family *Myoviridae* and contained a linear dsDNA genome of *c.* 59 kbp, which was packaged by a headful mechanism. The genome was partially sequenced and was shown to be transcribed in early, middle, and late phases. Although the virus particles contained linear DNA, ΦH was temperate and circular viral genomes (plasmids) could be isolated from infected cells. Genomic DNA was able to be transfected into *Hbt. salinarium* and *Haloferax volcanii* cells, producing viable virus particles. This was the first demonstration of transfection in Archaea, and allowed the optimization of plasmid transformation. However, ΦH was highly unstable, due to the activity of insertion sequences and inversion of the 'L-fragment', which could act as an autonomous plasmid. For this reason, work on ΦH was discontinued in the late 1990s.

## Current Euryarchaeal Viruses and VLPs

The published viruses and VLPs infecting members of the kingdom Euryarchaeota in the readily accessible literature are listed in **Table 1**. This table excludes nine uncharacterized head-and-tail viruses with *c.* 50 nm diameter heads, isolated in 1977 from the Great Salt Lake in Utah, USA, on uncharacterized *Halobacterium* isolates. The remainder of this article focuses on detailing the advances

**Table 1**    Viruses and virus-like particles of the kingdom Euryarchaeota

| Virus | Publication date | Isolating host | Isolated from | Infection pathway | Genome size (kbp) | GC content (%) | Particle size (nm) | Number of proteins; size (kDa) | Lipids |
|---|---|---|---|---|---|---|---|---|---|
| *Order Caudovirales, family Myoviridae* | | | | | | | | | |
| Viruses with an isometric head, contractile tail, and linear, double-stranded DNA genome | | | | | | | | | |
| ΦCh1 | 1997 | *Natrialba magadii* DSM 3394 | *Natrialba magadii* | Lytic, temperate | 58.5[a,b] AF440695 | 61.9 | 70 (head); 130 (tail) | 9; 15–80 | nd[c] |
| ΦH | 1982 | *Halobacterium salinarum* ATCC 29341 | *Halobacterium salinarum* | Temperate | 59[d] | 65 | 64 (head); 170 (tail) | >3; 22–80 | nd |
| HF1 | 1993 | *Haloferax lucentense* NCIMB 13854 | Cheetham, VIC, Australia | Lytic, carrier state | 75.7[b] AY190604 | 55.8 | 58 (head); 94 (tail) | >4; 20–55 | nd |
| HF2 | 1993 | *Halorubrum coriense* ACAM 3911 | Cheetham, VIC, Australia | Lytic, carrier state | 77.7[b] AF222060 | 55.8 | 58 (head); 94 (tail) | >4; 20–55 | nd |
| Hs1 | 1974 | *Halobacterium salinarum* strain 1 | *Halobacterium salinarum* | Lytic, carrier state | nd | nd | 50 (head); 120 (tail) | nd | nd |
| Ja.1 | 1975 | *Halobacterium salinarum* NRC 34001 | The Salt Ponds of Yallahs, Jamaica | Lytic | 230 | nd | 90 (head); 150 (tail) | nd | nd |
| S41 | 1998 | *Halobacterium salinarum* NRC 34001 | Little Salt Pond in Yallahs, Jamaica | Lytic, carrier state | nd | nd | 89 (head); 141 (tail) | nd | nd |
| S50.2 | 1998 | *Halobacterium salinarum* NRC 34001 | Little Salt Pond in Yallahs, Jamaica | Lytic, carrier state | nd | nd | 63 (head); 78 (tail) | nd | nd |
| S4100 | 1998 | *Halobacterium salinarum* NRC 34001 | Little Salt Pond in Yallahs, Jamaica | Lytic, carrier state | nd | nd | 56 (head); 85 (tail) | nd | nd |
| S5100 | 1990 | *Halobacterium salinarum* NRC 34001 | Little Salt Pond in Yallahs, Jamaica | Lytic, carrier state | nd | nd | 65 (head); 76 (tail) | nd | nd |
| *Order Caudovirales, family Siphoviridae* | | | | | | | | | |
| Viruses with an isometric head, noncontractile tail, and linear, double-stranded DNA genome | | | | | | | | | |
| ΦF1 | 1993 | *Methanobacterium thermoformicium* FF1 | Anaerobic sludge-bed reactor | Lytic | 85 | nd | 70 (head); 160 (tail) | nd | nd |
| ΦF3 | 1993 | *Methanobacterium thermoformicium* FF1 | Anaerobic sludge-bed reactor | Lytic | 36 | nd | 55 (head); 230 (tail) | nd | nd |
| ΦN | 1988 | *Halobacterium salinarum* NRL/JW | *Halobacterium salinarum* | nd | 56[e] | 70 | 55 (head); 85 (tail) | >1; 53 | nd |
| ψM1 | 1989 | *Methanothermobacter marburgensis* DSM 2133 | Experimental anaerobic sludge digester | Lytic, possible integration | 26.8[b] AF065411, AF065412 | 46.3 | 55 (head); 210 (tail) | 3; 10–35 | nd |
| ψM2 | 1989 | *Methanothermobacter marburgensis* DSM 2133 | Spontaneous deletion mutant of ψM1 | Lytic, possible integration | 26.1[b] AF065411 | 46.3 | 55 (head); 210 (tail) | 3; 10–35 | nd |
| ψM100 | 2001 | *Methanothermobacter wolfeii* | Defective provirus in host chromosome | Defective provirus | 28.8[b] AF301375 | 45.4 | nd | nd | nd |
| B10 | 1982 | *Halobacterium* sp. B10 | nd | Lytic | nd | nd | nd | nd | nd |

| Virus | Year | Host | Source | Replication | Genome (kbp); accession | %GC | Particle size (nm) | Structural proteins | Sequenced |
|---|---|---|---|---|---|---|---|---|---|
| Hh-1 | 1982 | *Halobacterium salinarum* ATCC 29341 | Fermented anchovy sauce | No lysis during release, carrier state | 37.2 | 67.05 | 60 (head); 100 (tail) | >1; 35 | nd |
| Hh-3 | 1982 | *Halobacterium salinarum* ATCC 29341 | Fermented anchovy sauce | Lytic, carrier state | 29.4 | 62.15 | 75 (head); 50 (tail) | lt; 1; 47 | nd |
| PG | 1986 | *Methanobrevibacter smithii* strain G | Rumen fluid samples | Lytic | 50 | nd | nd | nd | nd |
| PMS1 | 1986 | *Methanobrevibacter smithii* | nd | Lytic | 35 | nd | nd | nd | nd |
| S45 | 1984 | *Halobacterium salinarum* NRC 34001 | The Salt Ponds of Yallahs, Jamaica | No lysis, persistent infection | nd | nd | 40 (head); 70 (tail) | nd | nd |
| VTA | 1999 | *Methanococcus voltae* PS | *Methanococcus voltae* | nd | 4.4 | nd | 40 (head); 61 (tail) | nd | nd |
| **Genus *Salterprovirus*** | | | | | | | | | |
| *Viruses that are spindle-shaped, with a tail and a linear, double-stranded DNA genome, with terminal-bound proteins.* | | | | | | | | | |
| His1 | 1998 | *Haloarcula hispanica* ATCC 36930 | Avalon saltern, VIC, Australia | Lytic, carrier state | 14.9[b] AF191796 | 40 | 74 × 44 (body); 7 (tail) | nd | Possible |
| His2 | 2006 | *Haloarcula hispanica* ATCC 36930 | Pink Lakes, VIC, Australia | Lytic, carrier state | 16.1[b] AF191797 | 40 | 67 × 44 (body); nd (tail) | >4; 21–62 | Possible |
| **Unclassified** | | | | | | | | | |
| *Viruses that are spherical, with a linear, double-stranded DNA genome* | | | | | | | | | |
| SH1 | 2005 | *Haloarcula hispanica* ATCC 36930 | Serpentine Lake, WA, Australia | Lytic, carrier state | 30.9[b] AY950802 | 68.4 | 70 | 15; 4–185 | Yes |
| **Unclassified** | | | | | | | | | |
| *Virus-like particles that are polyhedral* | | | | | | | | | |
| CWP | 1988 | *Pyrococcus woesei* | nd | nd | No nucleic acid | nd | nd | 3 | nd |
| **Unclassified** | | | | | | | | | |
| *Virus-like particles that are oblate, with a circular, double-stranded DNA genome* | | | | | | | | | |
| VLPA3 | 1989 | *Methanococcus voltae* A3 | *Methanococcus voltae* A3 | Temperate | 23 | nd | 52 × 70 | 1 (and 3 minor); 13 | nd |
| **Unclassified** | | | | | | | | | |
| *Virus-like particles that are lemon-shaped, with a tail, and a circular, double-stranded DNA genome* | | | | | | | | | |
| VLP PAV1 | 2003 | '*Pyrococcus abysii*' GE23 | '*Pyrococcus abysii*' | Nonlytic, persistent infection | 17.5[b] | nd | 120 × 80 (body); 15 (tail) | >3; 6–36 | Possible |

[a]Genome completely sequenced.
[b]Also packages host derived RNA. Some genome adenine residues are methylated.
[c]nd, not determined.
[d]Some sequence data available: 405323, 405325, AH004327, S63323, S63933, S63992, S63994, X00805, X80161, X80162, X80163, X80164, X52504.
[e]All genome cytosine residues are methylated.

in research for euryarchaeal viruses and VLPs that have been studied since 2001.

## ψM1, ψM2, and ψM100; Viruses of the Methanogenic Archaea

A monovalent virus of *M. marburgensis*, ψM1 was isolated several times from an anaerobic sludge-bed reactor in 1989. The particles resemble bacteriophages of the family *Siphoviridae*, with a head diameter of *c.* 55 nm and a tail of *c.* 210 nm × 10 nm, composed of individual segments and an enlarged terminal segment (**Figure 1**). The ψM1 virion contains a 26.8 kbp genome and three major structural proteins. The proteins appear to be encoded by two open reading frames (ORFs), designated 13 and 18, whose products are post-translationally modified to produce the three proteins. To form the larger protein, the products of the ORFs are covalently cross-linked. The smaller proteins are then formed by processing of this protein at the N- and C-termini. The product of ORF 13 is similar to proteins found in Gram-positive Bacteria and bacteriophages; for example, it shows 28% identity over 330 amino acids to prophage PBSX protein XkdG in *Bacillus subtilis*.

The linear dsDNA genome of ψM1 is terminally redundant and circularly permuted, and packaged via a headful packing mechanism. Upon passage in laboratory cultures a spontaneous ψM1 deletion mutant designated ψM2, which lacked a 0.7 kbp segment (DR1), was found to become dominant. The 26.1 kbp ψM2 genome (AF065411) (**Figure 2**) and the DR1 ψM1 segment (AF065412) were sequenced. The ψM2 genome has a guanine–cytosine (GC) content of 46.3% and encodes 31 ORFs, seven of which have been assigned putative functions, again similar to those in Gram-positive Bacteria and bacteriophages. This suggests some gene exchange between bacterial and archaeal viruses, or a common ancestor of the bacterial and archaeal viruses. DR1 encodes ORF A, a duplication of ψM2 ORF 27. Although this element affects the stability of ψM1, the insertion and deletion of DR1 does not appear to interrupt any downstream ORFs.

Under laboratory conditions, ψM1 is a lytic virus, with no evidence of lysogen formation. The virus produces a pseudomurein endoisopeptidase, a lytic enzyme that cleaves host pseudomurein, encoded by *peiP* (ORF 28). Unexpectedly, ORF 29 encodes a putative site-specific integrase/recombinase, suggesting that ψM1 and ψM2 are actually temperate. This theory is supported by the absence of a viral DNA polymerase, which is usually found in lytic viruses, and the capacity of ψM1 particles to mediate transduction of resistance and biosynthesis markers, an ability as yet unobserved in other archaeal viruses. In addition, ψM1-resistant cultures of *Methanothermobacter wolfeii* spontaneously lyse and carry a chromosomal prophage, known as ψM100, which is

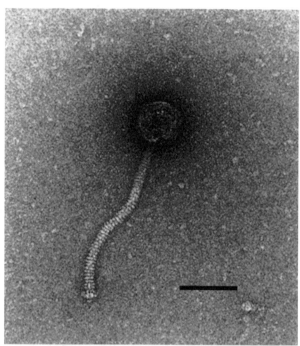

**Figure 1**  Electron micrograph of ψM1, negatively stained with uranyl acetate. Scale = 70 nm. Adapted from *Archives of Microbiology*, 152, 1989, p. 106, Characterization of ψM1, a virulent phage of *Methanobacterium thermoautotrophicum* Marburg, Meile L, Jenal U, Studer D, Jordan M, and Leisinger T, figure 1, © Springer-Verlag 1989, with kind permission from Springer Science and Business Media.

homologous to ψM1 and ψM2. ψM100 appears to be a defective virus, as no VLPs are observed in autolysates but pseudomurein endoisopeptidase PeiW, encoded by ψM100 ORF 28, is present. The 28.8 kbp ψM100 sequence (AF301375) (**Figure 2**) has a GC content of 45.4%. It contains a 2.8 kbp fragment, IRFa, which has a GC content of 33.4% and apparently originates from a source not homologous to ψM1 and ψM2. The remaining 26.0 kbp of the ψM100 genome is 70.8% identical to ψM2. The lytic/temperate relationship between ψM1-like viruses and *M. marburgensis* remains unresolved.

## Viruses of the Extremely Halophilic Archaea

### Head-and-Tail Viruses HF1 and HF2

In 1993, a deliberate search for haloviruses infecting a wider range of haloarchaea resulted in the isolation of HF1 and HF2 from Cheetham Saltworks in Victoria, Australia. Both viruses are lytic, but can enter unstable carrier states in laboratory cultures. They have mutually exclusive host ranges, HF1 infecting a wide range of hosts from the genera *Haloarcula*, *Halobacterium*, and *Haloferax*, while HF2 strictly infects *Halorubrum* species. HF2 is sensitive to chloroform exposure, but HF1 is relatively

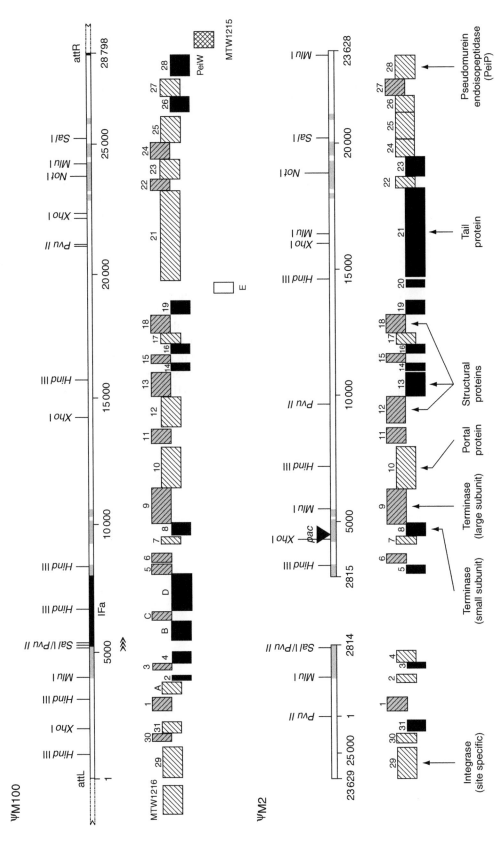

**Figure 2** Schematic representation of ψM100 with its flanking regions and comparison to that of ψM2. The ORFs are represented by numbered boxes and their vertical placement indicates the gene location in one of the six possible reading frames. Homologous ORFs carry the same numbers, and the assigned functions for some ORFs of ψM2 are reported. MTW1215 and MTW1216 represent the two ORFs encoded by the chromosome sequences flanking ψM100. *orfA* to *orfE* are unique to ψM100. The experimentally determined *pac* locus for ψM2 is shown as a solid black triangle. The IFa fragment (black bar) and the DNA regions with at least 200 bp with >98% identity in ψM100 and ψM2 (gray bars) are indicated. Three arrowheads represent three contiguous copies of a direct repeat of 125 nt in the vicinity of the left end of the IFa fragment. Adapted from Luo Y, Pfister P, Leisinger T, and Wasserfallen A (2001) The genome of archaeal prophage ψM100 encodes the lytic enzyme responsible for autolysis of *Methanothermobacter wolfeii*. *Journal of Bacteriology* 183: 5789, with permission from American Society for Microbiology.

insensitive to this solvent. In aspects other than host range and chloroform sensitivity, HF1 and HF2 are very similar. Their particles have identical morphologies, resembling bacteriophages of the family *Myoviridae*, with heads of

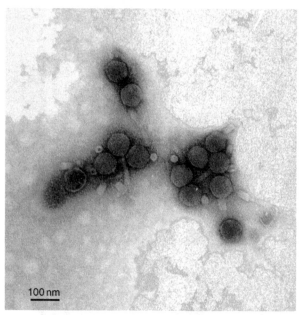

**Figure 3**  Electron micrograph of HF2, negatively stained with uranyl acetate.

*c.* 58 nm in diameter and tails of *c.* 94 nm in length (**Figure 3**). The structural proteins of HF1 and HF2 are very similar, with four major and several minor proteins. They also share similarly sized genomes of linear dsDNA.

The genome of HF2 (AF222060) replicates via concatamer formation. It is 77.7 kbp in length (**Figure 4**), has a GC content of 55.8%, and contains 121 closely spaced ORFs. Approximately 12% of ORFs show similarity to known sequences. The HF2 ORFs are transcribed as operons, with distinct early, middle, and late transcripts. The ORFs are likely to be strategically organized into three groups: (1) genes involved in establishing infection; (2) genes involved in DNA synthesis, modification, and replication; (3) and genes involved in virus assembly and release. There are long intergenic repeats throughout the genome, which appear to be linked to transcription regulation. The genomic arrangement suggests that such viruses mediate genetic exchange across a range of hosts, resulting in mosaic virus genomes (see below).

The HF1 genome (AY190604) is 75.9 kbp in length (**Figure 4**), has a GC content of 55.8%, and encodes 117 ORFs, of which 13% show similarity to known sequences (excluding those of HF2). The first 48 kbp of the HF1 genome is identical to that of HF2, apart from one silent base change, and the remaining sequence is 87% identical. In the latter region, HF2 contains two unique ORFs, two pairs of ORFs that are joined in HF1, and several ORFs

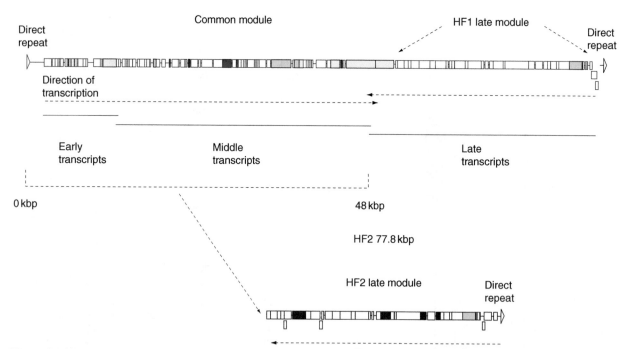

**Figure 4**  Closely related haloviruses HF1 (75.898 kbp) and HF2 (77.670 kbp) have genomes that are identical from 0 to 48 kbp, after which there is significantly lower homology. Direction of transcription is indicated below the genes in the diagram, as is the pattern of gene expression. Genes are drawn to scale. Genes highlighted in red are involved in transcription; dark blue – virion structure; yellow–nucleic acid modification; light blue – replication and repair.

with less than 70% amino acid identity to those in HF1. Divergence in this region of the genome probably explains the wide differences in viral host range and chloroform sensitivities of the two viruses. The path of sequence divergence also indicates that a recent recombination event exchanged the end of one virus for that of a third, unknown but related, virus.

## The Haloalkaliphilic Virus, ΦCh1

Although most extremely halophilic Archaea live at a neutral pH, there is a group that is not only extremely halophilic, but is also alkaliphilic. In 1997, a haloalkaliphilic virus, ΦCh1, was isolated after spontaneous lysis of a culture of the haloalkaliphilic archaeon *Natrialba magadii*. ΦCh1 is monovalent, producing plaques on lawns of ΦCh1-cured *Nab. magadii* cells. The virus is also temperate, with lysogens containing genomic ΦCh1 DNA integrated into the *Nab. magadii* chromosome. Virus integration is potentially mediated by putative site-specific recombinases, Int1 and Int2, encoded by ORFs 35 (*int1*, which has been shown to mediate inversion and excision reactions, resulting in small, circular molecules) and 45 (*int2*).

ΦCh1 particles resemble the family *Myoviridae*, with a head of *c.* 70 nm in diameter and a contractile tail *c.* 130 nm × 20 nm (**Figure 5**). The ΦCh1 virion contains at least nine structural proteins, designated A to I in decreasing size order. Proteins A and H are encoded by ORF 19 and protein E is encoded by ORF 11 (gene *E*). Gene *E* is transcribed late in cell infection and protein E is found to be associated with the host membrane, suggesting a role in DNA packaging or assembly of coat proteins during viral exit.

ΦCh1 virus particles contain both linear dsDNA and host-derived RNA species. Genomic ΦCh1 DNA is modified at adenine residues within various sequences, including 5′-GATC-3′. Although DNA methylation is a common viral mechanism for avoiding host-mediated restriction, it was unexpected in ΦCh1, as *Nab. magadii* does not have methylated DNA. An $N^6$-adenine methyltransferase, encoded by ORF 94 of ΦCh1, is transcribed and expressed late in cell infection. These factors suggest that ΦCh1 may infect other hosts.

The ΦCh1 genome has a circular replicative form and is circularly permuted and terminally redundant, suggesting a headful packing mechanism. The 58.5 kbp genome (AF440695) has a GC content of 61.9% and is predicted to contain 98 ORFs (**Figure 6**). In a similar manner to head-and-tail bacteriophages, the ORFs appear to be organized into three transcriptional units encoding (1) structural and morphogenesis proteins; (2) replication, stabilization, and gene regulation proteins; and (3) proteins of mostly unknown functions. Around half of the ORFs show similarity to sequences in the databases, although most of these are proteins of unknown function. The genome sequence of

ΦCh1 shows strong similarity to the incomplete genome of ΦH, which is surprising given that the two viruses were isolated from distinctly different environments and hosts. This unexpected relationship between supposedly diverse viruses suggests that similar viruses may be widely distributed throughout various hypersaline environments across the planet.

## His1 and His2: Spindle-Shaped Haloviruses of the Genus *Salterprovirus*

From 1974 to 1998, all of the viruses described for the kingdom Euryarchaeota were of head-and-tail morphology. Nevertheless, in waters such as the Dead Sea, the most abundant VLPs observed by direct electron microscopy were spindle shaped. In a study of a Spanish saltern, spindle-shaped VLPs were found to increase in abundance with increasing salinity. In 1998, a spindle-shaped halovirus, His1, was reported. Isolated from the Avalon saltern in Victoria, Australia, on a lawn of *Haloarcula hispanica*, the His1 virion is *c.* 74 nm × 44 nm, with a short 7 nm tail

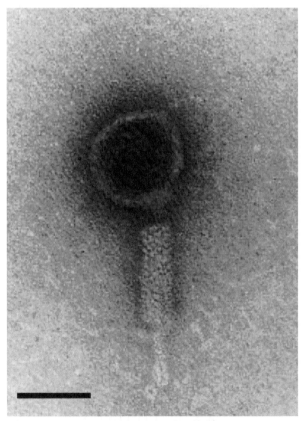

**Figure 5** Electron micrograph of ΦCh1, negatively stained with phosphotungstate. A contracted tail and the anchor structure between head and tail are visible. Scale = 50 nm. Adapted from Witte A, Baranyi U, Klein R, *et al.* (1997) Characterization of *Natronobacterium magadii* phage ΦCh1, a unique archaeal phage containing DNA and RNA. *Molecular Microbiology* 23: 605, with permission from Blackwell Science Ltd.

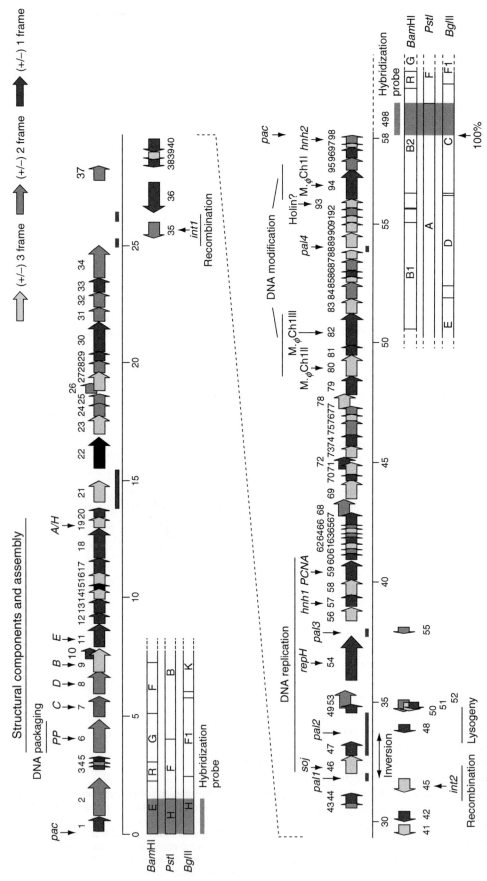

**Figure 6** Linear representation of the 58 498 bp ΦCh1 genome, starting at the *pac* site. ORFs are represented by arrows and numbered. Putative and verified functions of predicted gene products are indicated. The shades of the arrows indicate the frames of the ORFs: light gray, third reading frame; mid-gray, second reading frame; and dark gray, first reading frame for both orientations. A partial restriction map showing the region embedding the *pac* site and the fragments that are created during the cut at *pac* is given beneath the genome map. Both maps are correlated with each other. The binding region for the hybridization probe that was used to map the *pac* site is shaded. Low G+C regions are indicated by black bars, and the segment that is inverted in pΦHL with respect to ΦCh1 is indicated by an arrow. The putative binding sites for site-specific recombinases, *pal1* to *pal4*, are also indicated. Adapted from Klein R, Baranyi U, Rössler N, Greineder B, Scholz H, and Witte A (2002) *Natrialba magadii* virus ΦCh1: First complete nucleotide sequence and functional organization of a virus infecting a haloalkaliphilic archaeon. *Molecular Microbiology* 45: 852, with permission from Blackwell Science Ltd.

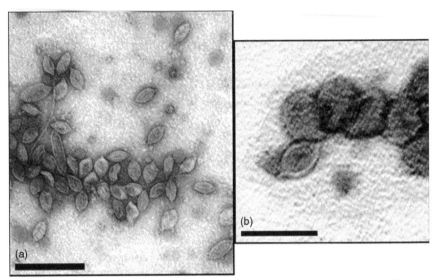

**Figure 7** Electron micrograph of (a) His1 and (b) His2, negatively stained with uranyl acetate. Scale = 200 nm (a); 100 nm (b).

(**Figure 7(a)**). His1 resembles crenarchaeal virus SSV1 and due to the morphological similarities and comparable genome sizes of these two viruses, His1 was initially, and mistakenly, placed in the *Fuselloviridae* family of archaeal viruses (type species, SSV1).

In 2006, a second spindle-shaped virus named His2 was described. It was isolated from the Pink Lakes in Victoria, Australia, and also plaques on *Har. hispanica.* By negative-stain electron microscopy, His2 particles are more flexible than His1 particles, with the virions being *c.* 67 nm × 44 nm, with a short tail (**Figure 7(b)**). The His2 virion contains at least four structural proteins, designated viral protein (VP) 1 (62 kDa) to VP 4 (21 kDa). To date, the ORFs encoding VPs 2 and 3 have not been determined. VP 1 is encoded by ORF 29 and predicted to be exported to the cell surface and glycosylated. ORF 29, and the downstream ORFs 30, 31, and 33, have closely similar sequences in at least four species of extremely halophilic Archaea, although the segments of similarity do not appear to be part of provirus genomes. The functions of these archaeal homologs have not yet been determined.

Although both monovalent haloviruses are virulent, they appear to enter a carrier state and have the capacity to exit cells without causing cell lysis. His1 and His2 are relatively stable in the pH range 3–9; however, His1 is more resistant than His2 to exposure to both increased temperature and lowered ionic environments. Both His1 and His2 are sensitive to chloroform and have low buoyant densities and flexible virus particles. These factors suggest that the virions contain lipids.

The genomes of haloviruses His1 (AF191796) and His2 (AF191797) are linear dsDNA of 14.5 and 16.1 kbp, respectively (**Figure 8**). The genomes have a GC content of *c.* 40%, about 23% lower than *Har. hispanica*, suggesting that the haloviruses are not well equipped to replicate in

*Haloarcula.* Moreover, no tRNA genes have been detected in the genomes of these viruses.

The His1 and His2 genomes each contain 35 ORFs and show almost no sequence similarity to one another or to known sequences. The notable exceptions are the putative DNA polymerases of the two viruses, which are weakly similar to one another at the nucleotide level and show 42% identity at the protein level. The DNA polymerases appear to be members of family B DNA polymerases that use the protein-priming mechanism. The His1 and His2 genomes have inverted terminal repeat (ITR) sequences at each end (105 and 525 nt, respectively), and the 5′ end of each is linked to a terminal protein (TP), which is essential for DNA replication. These characteristics are typical of systems that replicate DNA via protein priming.

At the molecular level, His1 and His2 are distantly related to one another; however, they do not appear to be related to fuselloviruses at all, with distinctly different genome structures, replication strategies, virus–host relationships, and genome sequences. Consequently, haloviruses His1 and His2 have been placed in an independent virus genus, *Salterprovirus.*

## Spherical Halovirus SH1

In addition to the spindle-shaped and head-and-tail VLPs observed in hypersaline waters such as the Dead Sea, isometric particles were also present in high numbers. These could have been classical head-and-tail VLPs, which had lost their tails through the negative-stain treatment, which tends to disrupt halophilic virus particles. However, in 2003, a spherical halovirus named SH1 that resembled these isometric particles was first noted. It was isolated from Serpentine Lake, Rottnest Island, Western Australia, on *Har. hispanica.* The SH1 virion is *c.* 70 nm in diameter and

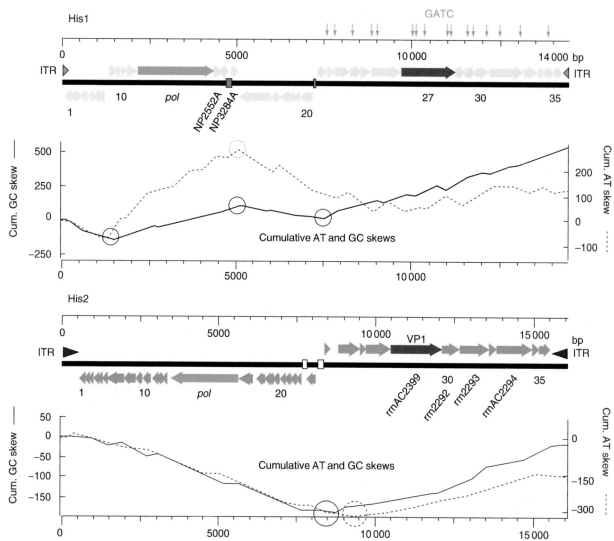

**Figure 8** Diagram of the His1 and His2 genomes. The major features are shown, including the predicted ORFs (yellow and green arrows), putative DNA polymerases (blue arrows), VP1 and its His1 homolog (red arrows), terminal inverted repeat sequences (purple arrowheads), and regions of nucleotide sequence repeats (gray boxes). Scale bars, in bp, are shown above each genome diagram. ORFs are numbered (left to right), and some have been named (pol, DNA polymerase; VP1, major capsid protein) or the accession numbers of closely related sequences given. The template strand for each ORF is indicated by the direction of arrows and their position above or below the black line. The vertical arrows about the His1 genome scale bar show positions of the sequence GATC. Plots of cumulative GC skew (solid black line) and AT skew (dashed blue line) are shown below each genome diagram, with inflection points indicated by circles. Adapted from Bath C, Cukalac T, Porter K, and Dyall-Smith ML (2006) His1 and His2 are distantly related, spindle-shaped haloviruses belonging to the novel virus group, *Salterprovirus*, *Virology* 350: 233, with permission from Elsevier.

displays an outer capsid layer with a compact core particle of *c.* 50 nm in diameter (**Figure 9**). Morphologically, it resembles viruses such as the bacteriophage PRD1, human adenovirus, and archaeal virus STIV, which all share common architecture.

SH1 is virulent, infecting both *Har. hispanica* and an uncharacterized isolate of the genus *Halorubrum*. The virion is stable to exposure to temperatures of 50 °C and in a pH range of 6–9, but is sensitive to exposure to both chloroform and lowered ionic environments. SH1 particles contain a lipid layer and 15 structural proteins, designated VP 1 to VP 15 in decreasing size order. Details

on the locations and possible functions of the SH1 virion proteins are available.

The genome of SH1 (AY950802) is linear dsDNA of 30.9 kbp (**Figure 10**), with a GC content of 68.4%. The viral genome contains 56 ORFs, which show very little sequence similarity to known sequences. It contains 309 bp ITRs. The molecular features of SH1 indicate that it is a member of a novel virus group. Based on the evidence from electron microscopy surveys, haloviruses similar to SH1 are likely to be widespread and dominant members of hypersaline systems.

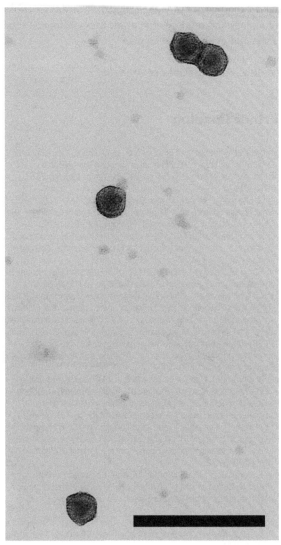

**Figure 9** Electron micrograph of SH1, stained with uranyl acetate. Scale = 200 nm.

## PAV1, A VLP of the Hyperthermophilic Order Thermococcales

No virus has ever been reported to infect the hyperthermophilic Euryarchaeota. However, two major groups of VLPs, rod-shaped particles and spindle-shaped particles, have been observed in enrichment cultures of samples obtained from deep-sea hydrothermal vents. In 2003, such spindle-shaped VLPs were discovered in supernatant of a '*Pyrococcus abysii*' culture and were designated '*P. abysii*' virus 1 (PAV1). PAV1 is continuously released, but does not cause lysis of host cells and cannot be induced to infectivity using ultraviolet or γ irradiation, mitomycin C, or heat or pressure shock. No viral genomes integrated into the host chromosome have been detected.

PAV1 particles are flexible and similar in appearance to both the fuselloviruses and the salterproviruses, being *c.* 120 nm × 80 nm, with a tail of *c.* 15 nm and tail fibers (**Figure 11**). The virion is composed of at least three structural proteins, of *c.* 6, 13, and 36 kDa. PAV1 is sensitive to exposure to chloroform, Triton X-100, proteinase K, and sodium dodecyl sulfate. Combined with its low buoyant density and flexible particles, this suggests that the particles contain lipid.

The genome of PAV1 is circular dsDNA of 17.5 kbp. It contains 24 putative ORFs, which show no similarity to sequences in the databases. A detailed description of the PAV1 genome should be published soon.

## Conclusion

At first glance, it may appear that the virus representatives of the kingdom Euryarchaeota resemble the more thoroughly studied bacterial and eukaryal viruses, or the viruses of the kingdom Crenarchaeota. However, on a

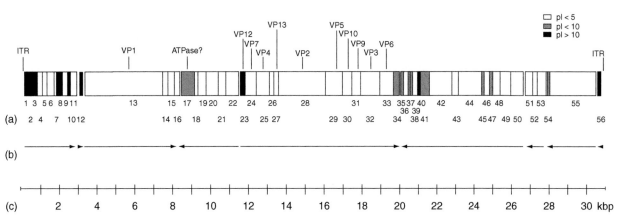

**Figure 10** Genome organization of SH1. (a) Predicted ORFs are numbered 1–56 from left to right and shaded according to the calculated isoelectric point of the predicted gene products. Structural virion components (VP 1 to VP 14) determined by protein chemistry methods are marked. (b) Direction of transcription is depicted by arrows. (c) Scale bar. Adapted from Bamford DH, Ravantti JJ, Rönnholm G, *et al.* (2005) Constituents of SH1, a novel, lipid-containing virus infecting the halophilic euryarchaeon *Haloarcula hispanica*. *Journal of Virology* 79: 9102, with permission from American Society for Microbiology.

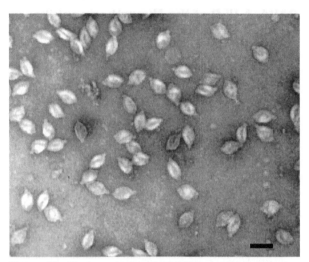

**Figure 11** Electron micrograph of PAV1, negatively stained with 2% uranyl acetate. Scale = 100 nm. Adapted from Geslin C, Le Romancer M, Erauso G, Gaillard M, Perrot G, and Prieur D (2003) PAV1, the first virus-like particle isolated from a hyperthermophilic euryarchaeote, "*Pyrococcus abyssi*". *Journal of Bacteriology* 185: 3890, with permission from American Society for Microbiology.

molecular level, the euryarchaeal viruses are clearly distinct and radically different from any other known viruses. Many of the representatives, such as PAV1 and SH1, show almost no similarity to any sequences in the databases and even the head-and-tail representatives, which appear to resemble the 'classical' bacteriophages in both morphology and genome structure, encode many previously unobserved genes.

Fortunately, it appears that we are now in a good position to culture euryarchaeal viruses. Whether all the dominant morphological forms of euryarchaeal viruses have been isolated is still uncertain; however, the current cultivation techniques appear to have isolated all of the dominant morphological forms of haloviruses (head-and-tail, spindle shaped, and spherical) that have been observed in hypersaline waters. The current representatives suggest that there may be relatively few dominant virus families infecting the kingdom Euryarchaeota, and that these virus families may be widespread. This view may change radically when the metagenomic studies of archaeal environments, such as those performed by the Venter Institute program, begin to bear fruit. In any case, the major goal now is to develop genetic systems to analyze the viruses already isolated, in order to explore and understand their genetic properties, ecological significance, and evolutionary impact.

*See also:* Fuselloviruses of Archaea.

## Further Reading

Bamford DH, Ravantti JJ, Rönnholm G, *et al.* (2005) Constituents of SH1, a novel, lipid-containing virus infecting the halophilic euryarchaeon *Haloarcula hispanica. Journal of Virology* 79: 9097–9107.

Bath C, Cukalac T, Porter K, and Dyall-Smith ML (2006) His1 and His2 are distantly related, spindle-shaped haloviruses belonging to the novel virus group, *Salterprovirus. Virology* 350: 228–239.

Bath C and Dyall-Smith ML (1998) His1, an archaeal virus of the. *Fuselloviridae* family that infects *Haloarcula hispanica. Journal of Virology* 72: 9392–9395.

Dyall-Smith M, Tang S-L, and Bath C (2003) Haloarchaeal viruses: How diverse are they? *Research in Microbiology* 154: 309–313.

Fauquet CM, Mayo MA, Maniloff J, Desselberger U, and Ball LA (eds.) (2005) *Virus Taxonomy: Eighth Report of the International Committee on Taxonomy of Viruses.* San Diego, CA: Elsevier Academic Press.

Geslin C, Le Romancer M, Erauso G, Gaillard M, Perrot G, and Prieur D (2003) PAV1, the first virus-like particle isolated from a hyperthermophilic euryarchaeote, "*Pyrococcus abyssi*". *Journal of Bacteriology* 185: 3888–3894.

Klein R, Baranyi U, Rössler N, Greineder B, Scholz H, and Witte A (2002) *Natrialba magadii* virus ΦCh1: First complete nucleotide sequence and functional organization of a virus infecting a haloalkaliphilic archaeon. *Molecular Microbiology* 45: 851–863.

Luo Y, Pfister P, Leisinger T, and Wasserfallen A (2001) The genome of archaeal prophage ψM100 encodes the lytic enzyme responsible for autolysis of *Methanothermobacter wolfeii. Journal of Bacteriology* 183: 5788–5792.

Meile L, Jenal U, Studer D, Jordan M, and Leisinger T (1989) Characterization of ψM1, a virulent phage of *Methanobacterium thermoautotrophicum* Marburg. *Archives of Microbiology* 152: 105–110.

Pfister P, Wasserfallen A, Stettler R, and Leisinger T (1998) Molecular analysis of. *Methanobacterium* phage ψM2. *Molecular Microbiology* 30: 233–244.

Porter K, Kukkaro P, Bamford JKH, *et al.* (2005) SH1: A novel, spherical halovirus isolated from an Australian hypersaline lake. *Virology* 335: 22–33.

Rössler N, Klein R, Scholz H, and Witte A (2004) Inversion within the haloalkaliphilic virus ΦCh1 DNA results in differential expression of structural proteins. *Molecular Microbiology* 52: 413–426.

Tang S-L, Nuttall S, and Dyall-Smith M (2004) Haloviruses HF1 and HF2: Evidence for a recent and large recombination event. *Journal of Bacteriology* 186: 2810–2817.

Tang S-L, Nuttall S, Ngui K, Fisher C, Lopez P, and Dyall-Smith M (2002) HF2: A double-stranded DNA tailed haloarchaeal virus with a mosaic genome. *Molecular Microbiology* 44: 283–296.

Witte A, Baranyi U, Klein R, *et al.* (1997) Characterization of *Natronobacterium magadii* phage √Ch1, a unique archaeal phage containing DNA and RNA. *Molecular Microbiology* 23: 603–616.

# SUBJECT INDEX

## Notes

Cross-reference terms in italics are general cross-references, or refer to subentry terms within the main entry (the main entry is not repeated to save space). Readers are also advised to refer to the end of each article for additional cross-references - not all of these cross-references have been included in the index cross-references.

The index is arranged in set-out style with a maximum of three levels of heading. Major discussion of a subject is indicated by bold page numbers. Page numbers suffixed by T and F refer to Tables and Figures respectively. *vs.* indicates a comparison.

This index is in letter-by-letter order, whereby hyphens and spaces within index headings are ignored in the alphabetization. Prefixes and terms in parentheses are excluded from the initial alphabetization.

To save space in the index the following abbreviations have been used

CJD - Creutzfeldt–Jakob disease

CMV - cytomegalovirus

EBV - Epstein–Barr virus

HCMV - human cytomegalovirus

HHV - human herpesvirus

HIV - human immunodeficiency virus

HPV - human papillomaviruses

HSV - herpes simplex virus

HTLV - human T-cell leukemia viruses

KSHV - Kaposi's sarcoma-associated herpesvirus

RdRp - RNA-dependent RNA polymerase

RNP - ribonucleoprotein

SARS - severe acute respiratory syndrome

TMEV - Theiler's murine encephalomyelitis virus

For consistency within the index, the term "bacteriophage" has been used rather than the term "bacterial virus."

Printed and bound by CPI Group (UK) Ltd, Croydon, CR0 4YY

03/10/2024

01040316-0015